2007
MOSBY'S
NURSING DRUG
REFERENCE

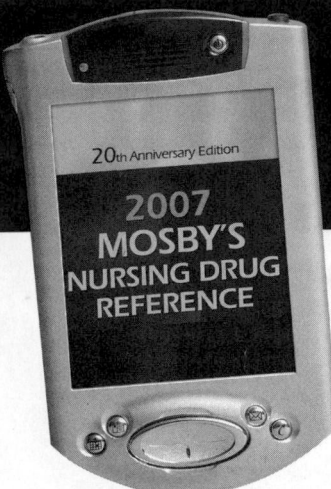 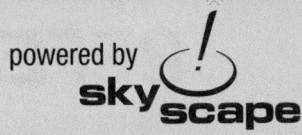
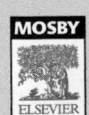

2007
MOSBY'S
NURSING DRUG REFERENCE

Linda Skidmore-Roth, RN, MSN, NP
Consultant
Littleton, Colorado

Formerly, Nursing Faculty
New Mexico State University
Las Cruces, New Mexico
El Paso Community College
El Paso, Texas

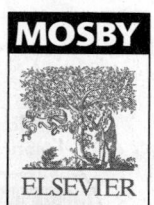

MOSBY

ELSEVIER

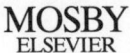

MOSBY
ELSEVIER

11830 Westline Industrial Drive
St. Louis, Missouri 63146

MOSBY'S 2007 NURSING DRUG REFERENCE

ISBN-13: 978-0-323-04590-2
ISBN-10: 0-323-04590-1

NOTICE

Knowledge and best practice in this field are constantly changing. As new research and experience broaden our knowledge, changes in practice, treatment and drug therapy may become necessary or appropriate. Readers are advised to check the most current information provided (i) on procedures featured or (ii) by the manufacturer of each product to be administered, to verify the recommended dose or formula, the method and duration of administration, and contraindications. It is the responsibility of the practitioner, relying on their own experience and knowledge of the patient, to make diagnoses, to determine dosages and the best treatment for each individual patient, and to take all appropriate safety precautions. To the fullest extent of the law, neither the Publisher nor the Author assumes any liability for any injury and/or damage to persons or property arising out of or related to any use of the material contained in this book.

The Publisher

ISBN-13: 978-0-323-04590-2
ISBN-10: 0-323-04590-1

Executive Publisher: Darlene Como
Managing Editor: Tamara Myers
Developmental Editor: Laura M. Selkirk
Publishing Services Manager: Melissa Lastarria
Senior Project Manager: Joy Moore
Design Direction: Mark Oberkrom

Printed in the United States of America.

Last digit is the print number:
9 8 7 6 5 4 3 2 1

Working together to grow
libraries in developing countries

www.elsevier.com | www.bookaid.org | www.sabre.org

ELSEVIER   BOOK AID International   Sabre Foundation

Consultants

Victoria Agyekum, RN, MSN
Department Head
Savannah Technical College
Savannah, Georgia

Timothy L. Brenner, PharmD
Assistant Professor
University of Arizona College of Pharmacy
Tucson, Arizona

Jennifer Chan, PharmD
Clinical Assistance Professor of Pharmacy
   and Pharmacology
University of Texas Health Science Center
San Antonio, Texas

Bruce D. Clayton, BS, PharmD, RPh
Professor of Pharmacy Practice
College of Pharmacy and Health Sciences
Butler University
Indianapolis, Indiana

Daryl D. DePestel, PharmD
Clinical Assistant Professor/Infectious
   Diseases
University of Michigan Health System
Ann Arbor, Michigan

Amanda Gross, RPh
Pharmacist
University Hospital
Denver, Colorado

Dana H. Hamamura, PharmD
Clinical Pharmacist
University of Colorado Hospital
Denver, Colorado

Peter Huynh, PharmD
Diabetes Fellow
Washington State University
Spokane, Washington

Joan Knape, RN, BSEd
I Can Do That Services
St. Louis, Missouri

Amy E. Miller, PharmD
Assistant Professor of Clinical Pharmacy
Philadelphia College of Pharmacy
University of the Sciences in Philadelphia
Philadelphia, Pennsylvania

Teresa L. Moore, PharmD
Camilla, Georgia

Lisa Nagle, CMA
Program Director – Medical Assisting
Augusta Technical College
Augusta, Georgia

Randolph E. Regal, BS, PharmD, RPh
Clinical Assistant Professor
College of Pharmacy
University of Michigan Hospital
Ann Arbor, Michigan

Roberta J. Secrest, PhD, PharmD, RPh
Eli Lilly and Company
Indianapolis, Indiana

Stephen M. Setter, PharmD, CDE,
   CGP, DVM
Assistant Professor of Pharmacotherapy
Washington State University
Elder Services/Visiting Nurses Association
Spokane, Washington

John J. Smith, EdD
Director – Health Sciences
Corinthian Colleges, Inc.
Santa Ana, California

Travis Sonnett, PharmD
Clinical Research Associate/Geriatric Resident
Washington State University
Spokane, Washington

Patricia R. Teasley, MSN, RN,
   APRN, BC
Professor, Nursing Department
Central Texas Collge
Killeen, Texas

Preface

Since the first publication of *Mosby's Nursing Drug Reference* in 1988, more than 100 U.S. and Canadian pharmacists and consultants have reviewed the book's content closely. Today, *Mosby's 2007 Nursing Drug Reference* is more up-to-date than ever—with features that make it easy to find critical information fast!

New facts
This edition features more than 2000 new drug facts, including:
- New drugs and new dosage information
- Newly researched side effects and adverse reactions
- The latest precautions, interactions, and contraindications
- IV therapy updates
- Revised nursing considerations
- Updated patient/family teaching guidelines
- Updates on key new drug research

New features for the twentieth anniversary edition
- A cleaner, easier to use internal design
- A color insert featuring drug mechanisms illustrations and sites of action
- Key clinical drugs added (fluticasone, docetaxel, and desipramine)
- Current immunization schedules for both the United States and Canada
- Appendix A, "Selected new drugs," provides detailed monographs for 13 drugs and a brief monograph for 1 rarely used drug recently approved by the FDA. (See Table of Contents for a complete list.) Included are monographs for exenatide (Byetta), approved for Type 2 diabetes mellitus; pramlintide (Synlin), approved for Type 1 and 2 diabetes mellitus; and abatacept (Orencia), approved for rheumatoid arthritis.
- Appendix B, "Recent FDA drug approvals," lists generic/trade names and uses for six of the most recently approved drugs
- In addition to a drug interactions tool, patient teaching guides and herbal monographs, the companion CD-ROM now offers complete and printable monographs for 28 of the most commonly prescribed drugs in the United States

Organization
This reference is organized into four main sections:
- Drug categories
- Full-color insert of drug mechanisms
- Individual drug monographs (in alphabetical order by generic name)
- Appendixes (identified by the wide dark blue thumb tabs on the edge)

The guiding principle behind this book is to provide fast, easy access to drug information and nursing considerations. Every detail—from the paper, typeface, cover, binding, use of color, and appendixes—has been carefully chosen with the user in mind.

Color Insert

This insert features 14 detailed, four-color illustrations to help enhance the understanding of the mechanisms or sites of action for the following select drugs and drug classes:

- ACE inhibitors
- Adrenocortical steroids
- Antidepressants
- Antidiabetic agents
- Antifungal agents
- Antiinfective agents
- Antiplatelet agents
- Antiretroviral agents
- Benzodiazepines
- Diuretics
- Drugs used to treat GERD
- Narcotic agonist-antagonist analgesics
- Narcotic analgesics
- Sympatholytics

Also included in the color insert is the 2006 Recommended Childhood and Adolescent Immunization Schedule for the United States.

Individual Drug Monographs

This book contains monographs for more than 1300 generic and 4500 trade medications. Common trade names are given for all drugs regularly used in the United States and Canada, with drugs available only in Canada identified by a maple leaf 🍁.

The following information is provided, whenever possible, for safe, effective administration of each drug:

High-alert status: Identifies high-alert drugs with a label and icon.

Pronunciation: Helps the nurse master complex generic names.

R/OTC: Identifies prescription or over-the-counter drugs.

Functional and chemical classifications: Allows the nurse to see similarities and dissimilarities among drugs in the same functional but different chemical classes.

Controlled-substance schedule: Includes schedules for the United States and Canada.

Do not confuse: Presents drug names within each appropriate monograph that might easily be confused.

Action: Describes pharmacologic properties concisely.

Uses: Lists the conditions the drug is used to treat.

Investigational uses: Describes drug uses that may be encountered in practice but are not yet FDA approved.

Dosages and routes: Lists all available and approved dosages and routes for adult, pediatric, and geriatric patients.

Available forms: Includes tablets, capsules, extended-release, injectables (IV, IM, SUBCUT), solutions, creams, ointments, lotions, gels, shampoos, elixirs, suspensions, suppositories, sprays, aerosols, and lozenges.

Side effects: Groups these reactions by alphabetical body system, with common side effects *italicized* and life-threatening reactions in ***bold italic type*** for emphasis.

Contraindications: Lists conditions under which the drug absolutely should not be given, including FDA pregnancy safety categories D or X.

Precautions: Lists conditions that require special consideration when the drug is prescribed, including FDA pregnancy safety categories A, B, and C.

Pharmacokinetics: Outlines metabolism, distribution, and elimination.

Interactions: Includes confirmed drug interactions, followed by the drug or nutrient causing that interaction, when applicable.

Drug/herb: Highlights more than 400 potential interactions between herbal products and prescription or OTC drugs.

Drug/food: Identifies many common drug interactions with foods.

Drug/lab test: Identifies how the drug may affect lab test results.

Nursing considerations: Identifies key nursing considerations for each step of the nursing process: Assess, Administer, Perform/Provide, Evaluate, and Teach Patient/Family. Instructions for giving drugs by various routes (e.g., PO, IM, IV) are included, with route subheadings in bold.

Compatibilities: Lists syringe, Y-site, and additive compatibilities and incompatibilities. If no compatibilities are listed for a drug, the necessary compatibility testing has not been done and that compatibility information is unknown. To ensure safety, assume that the drug may not be mixed with other drugs unless specifically stated.

"Nursing Alert" icon ⚠: Highlights a critical consideration.

Treatment of overdose: Provides drugs and treatment for overdoses where appropriate.

Appendixes

Selected new drugs: Includes comprehensive information on 14 key drugs approved by the FDA during the last 12 months.

Recent FDA drug approvals: Summarizes basic information, such as generic name, trade name and uses, for drugs so recently approved by the FDA that complete information was not yet available when this book went to press.

Ophthalmic, otic, nasal, and topical products: Provides essential information for more than 150 ophthalmic, otic, nasal, and topical products commonly used today, grouped by chemical drug class.

Commonly used antiinfectives in adults and children: Presents at-a-glance adult and pediatric dosage information for common antiinfectives.

Vaccines and toxoids: Features an easy-to-use table with generic and trade names, uses, dosages and routes, and contraindications for 29 key vaccines and toxoids.

Antitoxins and antivenins: Provides names, uses, dosages and contraindications.

Less frequently used antihistamines: Includes names, uses, doses, forms, interactions and contraindications.

Herbal products: Features basic usage information on more than 47 common herbs and natural supplements.

Combination products: Provides details on the forms and uses of more than 700 combination products.

High-alert drugs: Lists the 105 drugs in *Mosby's Nursing Drug Reference* that cause significant harm to patients if administered incorrectly.

Drugs metabolized by known P450s: Convenient table provides a quick metabolization reference.

Look-alike/sound-alike drug names: Includes all current ISMP pairs of generic and trade drug names that are easily confused.

FDA pregnancy categories: Explains the 5 FDA pregnancy categories.

Controlled substance chart: Covers the drug schedules for the United States, with examples.

Abbreviations: Lists abbreviations alphabetically with their meanings.

Weights and equivalents: Provides the conversion for weight and volume among the metric, apothecary, and avoirdupois systems.

High-alert Canadian medications: Lists the drugs that the Institute for Safe Medication Practices Canada considered high-alert because of their potential to cause significant harm to patients.

Canadian controlled substance chart: Covers the drug schedules for Canada, with examples.

Canadian recommended immunization schedules for infants and children: Convenient, up-to-date reference table for Canadian patients.

Bibliography: Lists key resources used in creating and updating *Mosby's 2007 Nursing Drug Reference*.

I am indebted to the nursing and pharmacology consultants who reviewed the manuscript and galley pages and thank them for their criticism and encouragement. I would also like to thank Darlene Como, Tamara Myers, and Laura Selkirk, my editors, whose active encouragement and enthusiasm have made this book better than it might otherwise have been. I am likewise grateful to Joy Moore and Graphic World Inc. for the coordination of the production process and assistance with the development of the new edition.

Linda Skidmore-Roth

Contents

Drug categories, 1

Color Insert

Individual drugs, 69

Bibliography, 1061

Appendixes, 1063

Index, 1191

ALPHA-ADRENERGIC BLOCKERS

Action: cts by binding to α-adrenergic receptors, causing dilation of peripheral blood vessels. Lowers peripheral resistance, resulting in decreased blood pressure.

Uses: Used for pheochromocytoma, prevention of tissue necrosis and sloughing associated with extravasation of IV vasopressors.

Side effects: The most common side effects are hypotension, tachycardia, nasal stuffiness, nausea, vomiting, and diarrhea.

Contraindications: Hypersensitive reactions may occur, and allergies should be identified before these products are given. Patients with myocardial infarction, coronary insufficiency, angina, or other evidence of coronary artery disease should not use these products.

Pharmacokinetics: Onset, peak, and duration vary among products.

Interactions: Vasoconstrictive and hypertensive effects of epINEPHrine are antagonized by α-adrenergic blockers.

Possible nursing diagnoses:
- Tissue perfusion, ineffective *[uses]*
- Injury, risk for *[adverse reactions]*
- Sleep pattern, disturbed *[adverse reactions]*

Nursing Considerations

Assess:
- Electrolytes: K, Na, Cl, CO_2
- Weight daily, I&O
- B/P lying, standing before starting treatment, q4h thereafter
- Nausea, vomiting, diarrhea
- Skin turgor, dryness of mucous membranes for hydration status

Administer:
- Starting with low dose, gradually increasing to prevent side effects
- With food or milk for GI symptoms

Evaluate:
- Therapeutic response: decreased B/P, increased peripheral pulses

Teach patient/family:
- To avoid alcoholic beverages
- To report dizziness, palpitations, fainting
- To change position slowly or fainting may occur
- To take drug exactly as prescribed
- To avoid all OTC products (cough, cold, allergy) unless directed by prescriber

Selected Generic Names

phentolamine

ANESTHETICS— GENERAL/LOCAL

Action: Anesthetics (general) act on the CNS to produce tranquilization and sleep before invasive procedures. Anesthetics (local) inhibit conduction of nerve impulses from sensory nerves.

Uses: General anesthetics are used to premedicate for surgery, induction and maintenance in general anesthesia. For local anesthetics, refer to individual product listing for indications.

Side effects: The most common side effects are dystonia, akathisia, flexion of arms, fine tremors, drowsiness, restlessness, and hypotension. Also common are chills, respiratory depression, and laryngospasm.

Contraindications: Persons with CVA, increased intracranial pressure, severe hypertension, cardiac decompensation should not use these products, since severe adverse reactions can occur.

Precautions: Anesthetics (general) should be used with caution in the elderly, cardiovascular disease (hypotension, bradydysrhythmias), renal disease, hepatic disease, Parkinson's disease, children <2 yr. The precaution for anesthetics (local) is pregnancy.

Pharmacokinetics: Onset, peak, and duration vary widely among products. Most products are metabolized in the liver and excreted in urine.

Interactions: MAOIs, tricyclics, phenothiazines may cause severe hypotension or hypertension when used with local anesthetics. CNS depressants will potentiate general and local anesthetics.

Possible nursing diagnoses:
General:
• Injury, risk for *[adverse reactions]*
• Knowledge, deficient *[teaching]*
Local:
• Acute pain *[uses]*
• Knowledge, deficient *[teaching]*

Nursing Considerations

Assess:
• VS q10min during IV administration, q30min after IM dose

Administer:
• Anticholinergic preoperatively to decrease secretions
• Only with crash cart, resuscitative equipment nearby

Perform/provide:
• Quiet environment for recovery to decrease psychotic symptoms

Evaluate:
• Therapeutic response: maintenance of anesthesia, decreased pain

Selected Generic Names (Injectables Only)

General anesthetics
droperidol
etomidate
fentanyl
fentanyl/droperidol
fentanyl transdermal
midazolam
propofol
thiopental

Local anesthetics
lidocaine
procaine
ropivacaine
tetracaine

ANTACIDS

Action: Antacids are basic compounds that neutralize gastric acidity and decrease the rate of gastric emptying. Products are divided into those containing aluminum, magnesium, calcium, or a combination of these.

Uses: Hyperacidity is decreased by antacids in conditions such as peptic ulcer disease, reflux esophagitis, gastritis, and hiatal hernia.

Side effects: The most common side effect caused by aluminum-containing antacids is constipation, which may lead to fecal impaction and bowel obstruction. Diarrhea occurs often when magnesium products are given. Alkalosis may occur when systemic products are used. Constipation occurs more frequently than laxation with calcium carbonate. The release of CO_2 from carbonate containing antacids causes belching, abdominal distention, and flatulence. Sodium bicarbonate may act as a systemic antacid and produce systemic electrolyte disturbances and alkalosis. Calcium carbonate and sodium bicarbonate may cause rebound hyperacidity and milk-alkali syndrome. Alkaluria may occur when products are used on a long-term basis, particularly in persons with abnormal renal function.

Contraindications: Sensitivity to aluminum or magnesium products may cause hypersensitive reactions. Aluminum products should not be used by persons sensitive to aluminum; magnesium products should not be used by persons sensitive to magnesium. Check for sensitivity before administering.

Precautions: Magnesium products should be given cautiously to patients with renal insufficiency and during pregnancy and lactation. Sodium content of antacids may be significant; use with caution for patients with hypertension or CHF or those on a low-sodium diet.

Pharmacokinetics: Duration is 20-40 min. If ingested 1 hr after meals, acidity is reduced for at least 3 hr.

Interactions: Drugs whose effects may be increased by some antacids: quinidine, amphetamines, pseudoephedrine, levodopa, valproic acid, dicumarol. Drugs whose effects may be decreased by some antacids: cimetidine, corticosteroids, ranitidine, iron salts, phenothiazines, phenytoin, digoxin, tetracyclines, ketoconazole, salicylates, isoniazid.

Possible nursing diagnoses:
- Chronic pain *[uses]*
- Constipation *[adverse reactions]*
- Diarrhea *[adverse reactions]*

Nursing Considerations

Assess:
- Aggravating and alleviating factors of epigastric pain or hyperacidity; identify the location, duration, and characteristics of epigastric pain
- GI symptoms, including constipation, diarrhea, abdominal pain; if severe abdominal pain with fever occurs, these drugs should not be given
- Renal symptoms, including increasing urinary pH, electrolytes

Administer:
- All products with an 8-oz glass of water to ensure absorption in the stomach
- Another antacid if constipation occurs with aluminum products
- Not to take other drugs within 1-2 hr of antacid administration, since antacids may impair absorption of other drugs

Evaluate:
- The therapeutic effectiveness of the drug; absence of epigastric pain and decreased acidity should occur

Selected Generic Names

aluminum hydroxide
bismuth subsalicylate
calcium carbonate
magaldrate
magnesium oxide
sodium bicarbonate

ANTIANGINALS

Action: The antianginals are divided into the nitrates, calcium channel blockers, and β-adrenergic blockers. The nitrates dilate coronary arteries, causing decreased preload, and dilate systemic arteries, causing decreased afterload. Calcium channel blockers dilate coronary arteries, decrease SA/AV node conduction. β-Adrenergic blockers decrease heart rate so that myocardial O_2 use is decreased. Dipyridamole selectively dilates coronary arteries to increase coronary blood flow.

Uses: Antianginals are used in chronic stable angina pectoris, unstable angina, vasospastic angina. Some (i.e., calcium channel blockers and β-blockers) may be used for dysrhythmias and in hypertension.

Side effects: The most common side effects are postural hypotension, headache, flushing, dizziness, nausea, edema, and drowsiness. Also common are rash, dysrhythmias, and fatigue.

Contraindications: Persons with known hypersensitivity, increased intracranial pressure, or cerebral hemorrhage should not use some of these products.

Precautions: Antianginals should be used with caution in postural hypotension, pregnancy, lactation, children, renal disease, and hepatic injury.

Pharmacokinetics: Onset, peak, and duration vary widely among coronary products. Most products are metabolized in the liver and excreted in urine.

Interactions: Please check individual monographs since interactions vary widely among products.

Possible nursing diagnoses:
• Tissue perfusion, ineffective *[uses]*
• Acute pain *[uses]*
• Injury, risk for *[uses]*
• Knowledge, deficient *[teaching]*
• Cardiac output, decreased *[adverse reactions]*

Nursing Considerations
Assess:
• Orthostatic B/P, pulse
• Pain: duration, time started, activity being performed, character
• Tolerance if taken over long period
• Headache, light-headedness, decreased B/P; may indicate a need for decreased dosage

Perform/provide:
• Storage protected from light, moisture; place in cool environment

Evaluate:
• Therapeutic response: decrease, prevention of anginal pain

Teach patient/family:
• To keep tabs in original container
• Not to use OTC products unless directed by prescriber
• To report bradycardia, dizziness, confusion, depression, fever
• To take pulse at home, advise when to notify prescriber
• To avoid alcohol, smoking, sodium intake
• To comply with weight control, dietary adjustments, modified exercise program
• To carry emergency ID to identify drug that you are taking, allergies
• To make position changes slowly to prevent fainting

Selected Generic Names
Nitrates
amyl nitrite
isosorbide
nitroglycerin
β-Adrenergic blockers
atenolol
dipyridamole
metoprolol
nadolol
propranolol
Calcium channel blockers
amlodipine
bepridil
diltiazem
niCARdipine
NIFEdipine
verapamil

ANTICHOLINERGICS

Action: Anticholinergics inhibit the muscarinic actions of acetylcholine at receptor sites in the autonomic nervous system; anticholinergics are also known as antimuscarinic drugs.

Uses: Anticholinergics are used for a variety of conditions: gastrointestinal anticholinergics are used to decrease motility (smooth muscle tone) in the GI, biliary, and urinary tracts and for their ability to decrease gastric secretions (propantheline, glycopyrrolate); decreasing involuntary movements in parkinsonism (benztropine, trihexyphenidyl); bradydysrhythmias (atropine); nausea and vomiting (scopolamine); and as cycloplegic mydriatics (atropine, homatropine, scopolamine, cyclopentolate, tropicamide).

Side effects: The most common side effects are dry mouth, constipation, urinary retention, urinary hesitancy, headache, and dizziness. Also common is paralytic ileus.

Contraindications: Persons with narrow-angle glaucoma, myasthenia gravis, or GI/GU obstruction should not use some of these products.

Precautions: Anticholinergics should be used with caution in patients who are elderly, pregnant, or lactating or in those with prostatic hypertrophy, CHF, or hypertension; use with caution in presence of high environmental temp.

Pharmacokinetics: Onset, peak, and duration vary widely among products. Most products are metabolized in the liver and excreted in urine.

Interactions: Increased anticholinergic effects may occur when used with MAOIs and tricyclic antidepressants and amantadine. Anticholinergics may cause a decreased effect of phenothiazines and levodopa.

Possible nursing diagnoses:
- Cardiac output, decreased *[uses]*
- Constipation *[adverse reactions]*
- Knowledge, deficient *[teaching]*

Nursing Considerations
Assess:
- I&O ratio; retention commonly causes decreased urinary output
- Urinary hesitancy, retention; palpate bladder if retention occurs
- Constipation; increase fluids, bulk, exercise if this occurs
- For tolerance over long-term therapy, dose may need to be increased or changed
- Mental status: affect, mood, CNS depression, worsening of mental symptoms during early therapy

Administer:
- Parenteral dose with patient recumbent to prevent postural hypotension
- With or after meals to prevent GI upset; may give with fluids other than water
- Parenteral dose slowly; keep in bed for at least 1 hr after dose; monitor vital signs
- After checking dose carefully; even slight overdose can lead to toxicity

Perform/provide:
- Storage at room temp
- Hard candy, frequent drinks, sugarless gum to relieve dry mouth

Evaluate:
- Therapeutic response: decreased secretions, absence of nausea and vomiting

Teach patient/family:
- To avoid driving or other hazardous activities; drowsiness may occur
- To avoid OTC medication: cough, cold preparations with alcohol, antihistamines unless directed by prescriber

Selected Generic Names
atropine
benztropine
biperiden
dicyclomine
glycopyrrolate
hyoscyamine
propantheline
scopolamine (transdermal)
solifenacin
trihexyphenidyl

ANTICOAGULANTS

Action: Anticoagulants interfere with blood clotting by preventing clot formation.

Uses: Anticoagulants are used for deep vein thrombosis, pulmonary emboli, myocardial infarction, open-heart surgery, disseminated intravascular clotting syndrome, atrial fibrillation with embolization, transfusion, and dialysis.

Side effects: The most serious adverse reactions are hemorrhage, agranulocytosis, leukopenia, eosinophilia, and thrombocytopenia, depending on the specific product. The most common side effects are diarrhea, rash, and fever.

Contraindications: Persons with hemophilia and related disorders, leukemia with bleeding, peptic ulcer disease, thrombocytopenic purpura, blood dyscrasias, acute nephritis, and subacute bacterial endocarditis should not use these products.

Precautions: Anticoagulants should be used with caution in alcoholism, elderly, and pregnancy.

Pharmacokinetics: Onset, peak, and duration vary widely among products. Most products are metabolized in the liver and excreted in urine.

Interactions: Salicylates, steroids, and nonsteroidal antiinflammatories will potentiate the action of anticoagulants. Anticoagulants may cause serious effects; please check individual monographs.

Possible nursing diagnoses:
- Tissue perfusion, ineffective *[uses]*
- Injury, risk for *[side effects]*
- Knowledge, deficient *[teaching]*

Nursing Considerations

Assess:
- Blood studies (Hct, platelets, occult blood in stools) q3mo
- Partial prothrombin time, which should be 1½-2 × control PPT daily, also APTT, ACT
- B/P, watch for increasing signs of hypertension
- Bleeding gums, petechiae, ecchymosis; black, tarry stools; hematuria
- Fever, skin rash, urticaria
- Needed dosage change q1-2wk

Administer:
- At same time each day to maintain steady blood levels
- Do not massage area or aspirate when giving SUBCUT injection; give in abdomen between pelvic bone, rotate sites; do not pull back on plunger; leave in for 10 sec; apply gentle pressure for 1 min
- Without changing needles
- Avoiding all IM injections that may cause bleeding

Perform/provide:
- Storage in tight container

Evaluate:
- Therapeutic response: decrease of deep vein thrombosis

Teach patient/family:
- To avoid OTC preparations that may cause serious drug interactions unless directed by prescriber
- That drug may be held during active bleeding (menstruation), depending on condition
- To use soft-bristle toothbrush to avoid bleeding gums, avoid contact sports, use electric razor
- To carry emergency ID identifying drug taken
- To report any signs of bleeding: gums, under skin, urine, stools

Selected Generic Names

ardeparin
argatroban
dalteparin
danaparoid
desirudin
enoxaparin
fondaparinux
heparin
lepirudin
tinzaparin
warfarin

ANTICONVULSANTS

Action: Anticonvulsants are divided into the barbiturates (p. 29), benzodiazepines (p. 30), hydantoins, succinimides, and miscellaneous products. Barbiturates and benzodiazepines are discussed in separate sections. Hydantoins act by inhibiting the spread of seizure activity in the motor cortex. Succinimides act by inhibiting spike and wave formation; they also decrease amplitude, frequency, duration, and spread of discharge in seizures.

Uses: Hydantoins are used in generalized tonic-clonic seizures, status epilepticus, and psychomotor seizures. Succinimides are used for absence (petit mal) seizures. Barbiturates are used in generalized tonic-clonic and cortical focal seizures.

Side effects: Bone marrow depression is the most life-threatening adverse reaction associated with hydantoins or succinimides. The most common side effects are GI symptoms. Other common side effects for hydantoins are gingival hyperplasia and CNS effects such as nystagmus, ataxia, slurred speech, and mental confusion.

Contraindications: Hypersensitive reactions may occur, and allergies should be identified before these products are given.

Precautions: Persons with renal or hepatic disease should be watched closely.

Pharmacokinetics: Onset, peak, and duration vary widely among products. Most products are metabolized in the liver and excreted in urine, bile, and feces.

Interactions: Decreased effects of estrogens, oral contraceptives (hydantoins).

Possible nursing diagnoses:
- Injury, risk for *[uses]*
- Noncompliance *[teaching]*
- Sleep pattern, disturbed *[adverse reactions]*

Nursing Considerations

Assess:
- Renal studies, including BUN, creatinine, serum uric acid, urine creatinine clearance before and during therapy
- Blood studies: RBC, Hct, Hgb, reticulocyte counts qwk for 4 wk then qmo
- Hepatic studies: AST, ALT, bilirubin, creatinine
- Mental status, including mood, sensorium, affect, behavorial changes; if mental status changes, notify prescriber
- Eye problems, including need for ophthalmic exam before, during, and after treatment (slit lamp, funduscopy, tonometry)
- Allergic reactions, including red, raised rash; if this occurs, drug should be discontinued
- Blood dyscrasia, including fever, sore throat, bruising, rash, jaundice
- Toxicity, including bone marrow depression, nausea, vomiting, ataxia, diplopia, cardiovascular collapse, Stevens-Johnson syndrome

Administer:
- With food, milk to decrease GI symptoms

Perform/provide:
- Good oral hygiene is important for hydantoins

Evaluate:
- Therapeutic response, including decreased seizure activity; document on patient's chart

Teach patient/family:
- To carry emergency ID stating drugs taken, condition, prescriber's name, phone number
- To avoid driving, other activities that require alertness

Selected Generic Names

Hydantoins
fosphenytoin
phenytoin
Succinimides
ethosuximide
Miscellaneous
acetaZOLAMIDE
carbamazepine

clonazepam
diazepam
felbamate
gabapentin
lamotrigine
magnesium sulfate
paraldehyde
paramethadione

phenacemide
phenobarbital
primidone
tiagabine
topiramate
valproate/valproic acid, divalproex
    sodium
zonisamide

ANTIDEPRESSANTS

Action: Antidepressants are divided into the tricyclics, MAOIs, and miscellaneous antidepressants (SSRIs). The tricyclics work by blocking reuptake of norepinephrine and serotonin into nerve endings and increasing action of norepinephrine and serotonin in nerve cells. MAOIs act by increasing concentrations of endogenous epinephrine, norepinephrine, serotonin, dopamine in storage sites in CNS by inhibition of MAO; increased concentration reduces depression.

Uses: Antidepressants are used for depression and, in some cases, enuresis in children.

Side effects: The most serious adverse reactions are paralytic ileus, acute renal failure, hypertension, and hypertensive crisis, depending on the specific product. Common side effects are dizziness, drowsiness, diarrhea, dry mouth, urinary retention, and orthostatic hypotension.

Contraindications: The contraindications to antidepressants are convulsive disorders, prostatic hypertrophy and severe renal, hepatic, cardiac disease depending on the type of medication.

Precautions: Antidepressants should be used cautiously in suicidal patients, severe depression, schizophrenia, hyperactivity, diabetes mellitus, pregnancy, and the elderly.

Pharmacokinetics: Onset, peak, and duration vary widely among products. Most products are metabolized in the liver and excreted in urine.

Interactions: Please check individual monographs since interactions vary widely among products.

Possible nursing diagnoses:
- Coping, ineffective *[uses]*
- Injury, risk for *[uses/adverse reactions]*
- Knowledge, deficient *[teaching]*

Nursing Considerations

Assess:
- B/P (lying, standing), pulse q4h; if systolic B/P drops 20 mm Hg, hold drug, notify prescriber; take vital signs q4h in patients with cardiovascular disease
- Blood studies: CBC, leukocytes, differential, cardiac enzymes if patient is receiving long-term therapy
- Hepatic studies: AST, ALT, bilirubin, creatinine
- Weight qwk; appetite may increase with drug
- EPS, primarily in elderly: rigidity, dystonia, akathisia
- Mental status: mood, sensorium, affect, suicidal tendencies, increase in psychiatric symptoms: depression, panic
- Urinary retention, constipation; constipation is more likely to occur in children, elderly
- Withdrawal symptoms: headache, nausea, vomiting, muscle pain, weakness; do not usually occur unless drug was discontinued abruptly
- Alcohol consumption; if alcohol is consumed, hold dose until morning

Administer:
- Increased fluids if urinary retention occurs, bulk in diet, if constipation occurs
- With food or milk for GI symptoms

Perform/provide:
- Storage in tight container at room temp; do not freeze
- Assistance with ambulation during beginning therapy, since drowsiness, dizziness occur
- Safety measures including side rails primarily in elderly
- Checking to see PO medication swallowed
- Gum, hard candy, or frequent sips of water for dry mouth

Evaluate:
- Therapeutic response: decreased depression

Teach patient/family:
- That therapeutic effects may take 2-3 wk

- To use caution in driving, other activities requiring alertness because of drowsiness, dizziness, blurred vision
- To avoid alcohol ingestion, other CNS depressants
- Not to discontinue medication quickly after long-term use; may cause nausea, headache, malaise
- To wear sunscreen or wide-brimmed hat, since photosensitivity may occur

Selected Generic Names

Tetracyclics
mirtazapine

Tricyclics
amitriptyline
amoxapine
clomiPRAMINE
desipramine
doxepin
imipramine
nortriptyline
trimipramine

Miscellaneous
buPROPion
duoxetine
trazodone
venlafaxine

MAOIs
phenelzine
tranylcypromine

SSRIs
citalopram
escitalopram
fluoxetine
fluvoxamine
paroxetine
sertraline

ANTIDIABETICS

Action: Antidiabetics are divided into the insulins that decrease blood glucose, phosphate, and potassium and increase blood pyruvate and lactate; and oral antidiabetics that cause functioning β-cells in the pancreas to release insulin, improve the effect of endogenous and exogenous insulin.

Uses: Insulins are used for ketoacidosis and diabetes mellitus types 1 and 2; oral antidiabetics are used for stable adult-onset diabetes mellitus type 2.

Side effects: The most common side effect of insulin and oral antidiabetics is hypoglycemia. Other adverse reactions to oral antidiabetics include blood dyscrasias, hepatotoxicity, and rarely, cholestatic jaundice. Adverse reactions to insulin products include allergic responses and, more rarely, anaphylaxis.

Contraindications: Hypersensitive reactions may occur, and allergies should be identified before these products are given. Oral antidiabetics should not be used in juvenile or brittle diabetes, diabetic ketoacidosis, severe renal disease, or severe hepatic disease.

Precautions: Oral antidiabetics should be used with caution in the elderly, in cardiac disease, pregnancy, lactation, and in the presence of alcohol.

Pharmacokinetics: Onset, peak, and duration vary widely among products. Oral antidiabetics are metabolized in the liver, with metabolites excreted in urine, bile, and feces.

Interactions: Interactions vary widely among products. Check individual monographs for specific information.

Possible nursing diagnoses:
• Imbalanced nutrition: more than body requirements [uses]

Nursing Considerations

Assess:
• Blood, urine glucose levels during treatment to determine diabetes control (oral products)
• Fasting blood glucose, 2 hr PP (60-100 mg/dl normal fasting level) (70-130 mg/dl normal 2-hr level)

• Hypoglycemic reaction that can occur during peak time

Administer:
• Insulin after warming to room temp by rotating in palms to prevent lipodystrophy from injecting cold insulin
• Human insulin to those allergic to beef or pork
• Oral antidiabetic 30 min before meals

Perform/provide:
• Rotation of injection sites when giving insulin; use abdomen, upper back, thighs, upper arm, buttocks; rotate sites within one of these regions; keep a record of sites

Evaluate:
• Therapeutic response, including decrease in polyuria, polydipsia, polyphagia, clear sensorium, absence of dizziness, stable gait

Teach patient/family:
• To avoid alcohol and salicylates except on advice of prescriber
• Symptoms of ketoacidosis: nausea, thirst, polyuria, dry mouth, decreased B/P; dry, flushed skin; acetone breath, drowsiness, Kussmaul respiration
• Symptoms of hypoglycemia: headache, tremors, fatigue, weakness; and that candy or sugar should be carried to treat hypoglycemia
• To test urine for glucose/ketones tid if this drug is replacing insulin
• To continue weight control, dietary restrictions, exercise, hygiene
• Obtain yearly eye exams

Selected Generic Names

chlorproPAMIDE
glipiZIDE
glyBURIDE
insulin aspart
insulin glargine
insulin glulisine
insulin lispro
insulin, regular
insulin, regular concentrated
insulin, zinc suspension (Lente)
insulin, zinc suspension extended (Ultralente)
metformin
miglitol
pioglitazone
repaglinide
rosiglitazone

ANTIDIARRHEALS

Action: Antidiarrheals work by various actions, including direct action on intestinal muscles to decrease GI peristalsis; by inhibiting prostaglandin synthesis responsible for GI hypermotility; by acting on mucosal receptors responsible for peristalsis; or by decreasing water content of stools.

Uses: Antidiarrheals are used for diarrhea of undetermined causes.

Side effects: The most serious adverse reactions of some products are paralytic ileus, toxic megacolon, and angioneurotic edema. The most common side effects are constipation, nausea, dry mouth, and abdominal pain.

Contraindications: Persons with severe ulcerative colitis, pseudomembranous colitis with some products.

Precautions: Antidiarrheals should be used with caution in the elderly, pregnancy, lactation, children, dehydration.

Pharmacokinetics: Onset, peak, and duration vary widely among products. Most products are metabolized in the liver and excreted in urine.

Interactions: Please check individual monographs, since interactions vary widely among products.

Possible nursing diagnoses:
• Diarrhea *[uses]*
• Constipation *[adverse reactions]*
• Fluid volume, deficient *[adverse reactions]*
• Knowledge, deficient *[teaching]*

Nursing Considerations
Assess:
• Electrolytes (K, Na, Cl) if on long-term therapy
• Bowel pattern before; for rebound constipation after termination of medication
• Response after 48 hr; if no response, drug should be discontinued
• Dehydration in children
Administer:
• For 48 hr only
Evaluate:
• Therapeutic response: decreased diarrhea
Teach patient/family:
• To avoid OTC products
• Not to exceed recommended dose

Selected Generic Names
bismuth subsalicylate
kaolin/pectin
loperamide

ANTIDYSRHYTHMICS

Action: Antidysrhythmics are divided into four classes and miscellaneous antidysrhythmics:

• Class I increases the duration of action potential and effective refractory period and reduces disparity in the refractory period between a normal and infarcted myocardium; further subclasses include Ia, Ib, Ic

• Class II decreases the rate of SA node discharge, increases recovery time, slows conduction through the AV node, and decreases heart rate, which decreases O_2 consumption in the myocardium

• Class III increases the duration of action potential and the effective refractory period

• Class IV inhibits calcium ion influx across the cell membrane during cardiac depolarization; decreases SA node discharge, decreases conduction velocity through the AV node

• Miscellaneous antidysrhythmics include those such as adenosine, which slows conduction through the AV node, and digoxin, which decreases conduction velocity and prolongs the effective refractory period in the AV node

Uses: These products are used for PVCs, tachycardia, hypertension, atrial fibrillation, angina pectoris.

Side effects: Side effects and adverse reactions vary widely among products.

Contraindications: Contraindications vary widely among products.

Precautions: Precautions vary widely among products.

Pharmacokinetics: Onset, peak, and duration vary widely among products.

Interactions: Interactions vary widely among products; check individual monographs for specific information.

Possible nursing diagnoses:
• Cardiac output, decreased *[uses]*
• Tissue perfusion, ineffective *[uses]*
• Diarrhea *[adverse reactions]*
• Gas exchange, impaired *[adverse reactions]*

Nursing Considerations

Assess:
• ECG continuously to determine drug effectiveness, PVCs, or other dysrhythmias
• IV infusion rate to avoid causing nausea, vomiting
• For dehydration or hypovolemia
• B/P continuously for hypotension, hypertension
• I&O ratio
• Serum potassium
• Edema in feet and legs daily

Evaluate:
• Therapeutic response, including decrease in B/P in hypertension; decreased B/P, edema, moist crackles in CHF

Teach patient/family:
• To comply with dosage schedule, even if patient is feeling better
• To report bradycardia, dizziness, confusion, depression, fever

Selected Generic Names

Class I
moricizine
Class Ia
disopyramide
procainamide
quinidine
Class Ib
lidocaine
mexiletine
phenytoin
tocainide
Class Ic
flecainide
propafenone
Class II
acebutolol
esmolol
propranolol
sotalol
Class III
amiodarone
ibutilide
Class IV
verapamil
Miscellaneous
adenosine
atropine
digoxin

ANTIFUNGALS (SYSTEMIC)

Action: Antifungals act by increasing cell membrane permeability in susceptible organisms by binding sterols and decreasing potassium, sodium, and nutrients in the cell.

Uses: Antifungals are used for infections of histoplasmosis, blastomycosis, coccidioidomycosis, cryptococcosis, aspergillosis, phycomycosis, candidiasis, sporotrichosis causing severe meningitis, septicemia, and skin infections.

Side effects: The most serious adverse reactions include renal tubular acidosis, permanent renal impairment, anuria, oliguria, hemorrhagic gastroenteritis, acute hepatic failure, and blood dyscrasias. Some common side effects include hypokalemia, nausea, vomiting, anorexia, headache, fever, and chills.

Contraindications: Persons with severe bone depression or hypersensitivity should not use these products.

Precautions: Antifungals should be used with caution in renal disease, pregnancy, and hepatic disease.

Pharmacokinetics: Onset, peak, and duration vary widely among products. Most products are metabolized in the liver and excreted in urine.

Interactions: Please check individual monographs since interactions vary widely among products.

Possible nursing diagnoses:
- Infection, risk for *[uses]*
- Injury, risk for *[adverse reactions]*
- Knowledge, deficient *[teaching]*

Nursing Considerations

Assess:
- VS q15-30min during first infusion; note changes in pulse, B/P
- I&O ratio; watch for decreasing urinary output, change in specific gravity; discontinue drug to prevent permanent damage to renal tubules
- Blood studies: CBC, K, Na, Ca, Mg q2wk
- Weight weekly; if weight increases over 2 lb/wk, edema is present; renal damage should be considered

- For renal toxicity: increasing BUN, if >40 mg/dl or if serum creatinine >3 mg/dl; drug may be discontinued or dosage reduced
- For hepatotoxicity: increasing AST, ALT, alk phosphatase, bilirubin
- For allergic reaction: dermatitis, rash; drug should be discontinued, antihistamines (mild reaction) or epINEPHrine (severe reaction) administered
- For hypokalemia: anorexia, drowsiness, weakness, decreased reflexes, dizziness, increased urinary output, increased thirst, paresthesias
- For ototoxicity: tinnitus (ringing, roaring in ears), vertigo, loss of hearing (rare)

Administer:
- IV using in-line filter (mean pore diameter >1 µm) using distal veins; check for extravasation, necrosis q8h
- Drug only after C&S confirms organism, drug needed to treat condition; make sure drug is used in life-threatening infections

Perform/provide:
- Protection from light during infusion, cover with foil
- Symptomatic treatment as ordered for adverse reactions: aspirin, antihistamines, antiemetics, antispasmodics
- Storage protected from moisture and light; diluted sol is stable for 24 hr

Evaluate:
- Therapeutic response: decreased fever, malaise, rash, negative C&S for infecting organism

Teach patient/family:
- That long-term therapy may be needed to clear infection (2 wk-3 mo depending on type of infection)

Selected Generic Names

amphotericin B
fluconazole
griseofulvin
itraconazole
ketoconazole
nystatin
voriconazole

ANTIHISTAMINES

Action: Antihistamines compete with histamines for H_1-receptor sites. They antagonize in varying degrees most of the pharmacologic effects of histamines.
Uses: Products are used to control the symptoms of allergies, rhinitis, and pruritus.
Side effects: Most products cause drowsiness; however, fexofenadine and loratadine produce little, if any, drowsiness. Other common side effects are headache and thickening of bronchial secretions. Serious blood dyscrasias may occur, but are rare. Urinary retention, GI effects occur with many of these products.
Contraindications: Hypersensitivity to H_1-receptor antagonists occurs rarely. Patients with acute asthma and lower respiratory tract disease should not use these products since thick secretions may result. Other contraindications include narrow-angle glaucoma, bladder neck obstruction, stenosing peptic ulcer, symptomatic prostatic hypertrophy, newborn, lactation.
Precautions: These products must be used cautiously in conjunction with intraocular pressure since they increase intraocular pressure. Caution should also be used in patients with renal and cardiac disease, hypertension, seizure disorders, pregnancy, lactation, and in the elderly.
Pharmacokinetics: Onset varies from 20-60 min, with duration lasting 4-24 hr. In general, pharmacokinetics vary widely among products.
Interactions: Barbiturates, opioids, hypnotics, tricyclic antidepressants, or alcohol can increase CNS depression when taken with antihistamines.
Possible nursing diagnoses:
• Airway clearance, ineffective *[uses]*

Nursing Considerations
Assess:
• I&O ratio; be alert for urinary retention, frequency, dysuria; drug should be discontinued if these occur
• CBC during long-term therapy, since hemolytic anemia, although rare, may occur
• Blood dyscrasias: thrombocytopenia, agranulocytosis (rare)
• Respiratory status, including rate, rhythm, increase in bronchial secretions, wheezing, chest tightness
• Cardiac status, including palpitations, increased pulse, hypotension
Administer:
• With food or milk to decrease GI symptoms; absorption may be decreased slightly
• Whole (sustained release tabs)
Perform/provide:
• Hard candy, gum, frequent rinsing of mouth for dryness
Evaluate:
• Therapeutic response, including absence of allergy symptoms, itching
Teach patient/family:
• To notify prescriber if confusion, sedation, hypotension occur
• To avoid driving, other hazardous activity if drowsiness occurs
• To avoid concurrent use of alcohol, other CNS depressants
• To discontinue a few days before skin testing

Selected Generic Names
brompheniramine
budesonide
cetirizine
chlorpheniramine
cyproheptadine
desloratadine
diphenhydrAMINE
fexofenadine
loratadine
promethazine

ANTIHYPERTENSIVES

Action: Antihypertensives are divided into angiotensin-converting enzyme (ACE) inhibitors, β-adrenergic blockers, calcium channel blockers, centrally acting adrenergics, diuretics, peripherally acting antiadrenergics, and vasodilators. β-Blockers, calcium channel blockers, and diuretics are discussed in separate sections. Angiotensin-converting enzyme inhibitors act by selectively suppressing renin-angiotensin I to angiotensin II; dilation of arterial and venous vessels occurs. Centrally acting adrenergics act by inhibiting the sympathetic vasomotor center in the CNS that reduces impulses in the sympathetic nervous system; blood pressure, pulse rate, and cardiac output decrease. Peripherally acting antiadrenergics inhibit sympathetic vasoconstriction by inhibiting release of norepinephrine and/or depleting norepinephrine stores in adrenergic nerve endings. Vasodilators act on arteriolar smooth muscle by producing direct relaxation or vasodilation; a reduction in blood pressure, with concomitant increases in heart rate and cardiac output, occurs.

Uses: Used for hypertension and some products are used for heart failure not responsive to conventional therapy. Some products are used in hypertensive crisis, angina, and for some cardiac dysrhythmias.

Side effects: The most common side effects are hypotension, bradycardia, tachycardia, headache, nausea, and vomiting. Side effects and adverse reactions may vary widely between classes and specific products.

Contraindications: Hypersensitive reactions may occur, and allergies should be identified before these products are given. Antihypertensives should not be used in patients with heart block or in children.

Precautions: Antihypertensives should be used with caution in the elderly, in dialysis patients, and in the presence of hypovolemia, leukemia, and electrolyte imbalances.

Pharmacokinetics: Onset, peak, and duration vary widely among products. Most products are metabolized in the liver, with metabolites excreted in urine, bile, and feces.

Interactions: Interactions vary widely among products; check individual monographs for specific information.

Possible nursing diagnoses:
• Tissue perfusion, ineffective *[uses]*
• Cardiac output, decreased *[uses]*
• Diarrhea *[adverse reactions]*
• Gas exchange, impaired *[adverse reactions]*

Nursing Considerations

Assess:
• Blood stuies: neutrophil; decreased platelets occur with many of the products
• Renal studies: protein, BUN, creatinine; watch for increased levels that may indicate nephrotic syndrome; obtain baselines in renal and hepatic function studies before beginning treatment
• Edema in feet and legs daily
• Allergic reaction, including rash, fever, pruritus, urticaria: drug should be discontinued if antihistamines fail to help
• Symptoms of CHF: edema, dyspnea, wet crackles, B/P
• Renal symptoms: polyuria, oliguria, frequency

Perform/provide:
• Supine or Trendelenburg position for severe hypotension

Evaluate:
• Therapeutic response, including decrease in B/P in hypotension; decreased B/P, edema, moist crackles in CHF

Teach patient/family:
• To comply with dosage schedule, even if feeling better
• To rise slowly to sitting or standing position to minimize orthostatic hypotension

Selected Generic Names

Aldosterone receptor antagonist
eplerenone

Angiotensin-converting enzyme inhibitors
benazepril
enalapril
fosinopril
quinapril
ramipril
trandolapril

Angiotensin II receptor blockers
candesartan
eprosartan
irbesartan
losartan
olmesartan
telmisartan
valsartan

Centrally acting adrenergics
clonidine
guanfacine
methyldopa

Peripherally acting antiadrenergics
prazosin
reserpine
terazosin

Vasodilators
diazoxide
fenoldopam
hydrALAZINE
minoxidil
nitroprusside

Antiadrenergic combined α-/β-blocker
labetalol

ANTIINFECTIVES

Action: Antiinfectives are divided into several groups, which include but are not limited to penicillins, cephalosporins, aminoglycosides, sulfonamides, tetracyclines, monobactam, erythromycins, and quinolones. These drugs act by inhibiting the growth and replication of susceptible bacterial organisms.

Uses: Used for infections of susceptible organisms. These products are effective against bacterial, rickettsial, and spirochetal infections.

Side effects: The most common side effects are nausea, vomiting, and diarrhea. Adverse reactions include bone marrow depression and anaphylaxis.

Contraindications: Hypersensitivity reactions may occur, and allergies should be identified before these products are given. Cross-sensitivity can occur between products of different classes (penicillins and cephalosporins). Many persons allergic to penicillins are also allergic to cephalosporins.

Precautions: Antiinfectives should be used with caution in persons with renal and hepatic disease.

Pharmacokinetics: Onset, peak, and duration vary widely among products. Most products are metabolized in the liver, and metabolites are excreted in urine, bile, and feces.

Interactions: Interactions vary widely among products; check individual monographs for specific information.

Possible nursing diagnoses:
- Infection, risk for *[uses]*
- Diarrhea *[adverse reactions]*

Nursing Considerations

Assess:
- Nephrotoxicity, including increased BUN, creatinine
- Blood studies: AST, ALT, CBC, Hct, bilirubin; test monthly if patient is on long-term therapy
- Bowel pattern daily; if severe diarrhea occurs, drug should be discontinued
- Urine output; if decreasing, notify prescriber; may indicate nephrotoxicity
- Allergic reaction, including rash, fever, pruritus, urticaria; drug should be discontinued
- Bleeding: ecchymosis, bleeding gums, hematuria, stool guaiac daily
- Overgrowth of infection: perineal itching, fever, malaise, redness, pain, swelling, drainage, rash, diarrhea, change in cough, sputum

Administer:
- For 10-14 days to ensure organism death, prevention of superinfection
- Drug after C&S completed; drug may be taken as soon as C&S is drawn

Evaluate:
- Therapeutic response, including absence of fever, fatigue, malaise, draining wounds

Teach patient/family:
- To comply with dosage schedule, even if feeling better
- To report sore throat, bruising, bleeding, joint pain; may indicate blood dyscrasias (rare)

Selected Generic Names

Aminoglycosides
amikacin
azithromycin
clarithromycin
gentamicin
kanamycin
neomycin
streptomycin
tobramycin

Cephalosporins
cefaclor
cefadroxil
cefamandole
cefazolin
cefdinir
cefditoren
cefepime
cefixime
cefmetazole
cefonicid
cefoperazone
cefotaxime

cefprozil
ceftibuten
cefuroxime
cephalexin
cephapirin
cephradine
Fluoroquinolones
alatrofloxacin/trovafloxacin
ciprofloxacin
enoxacin
gemifloxacin
levofloxacin
lomefloxacin
norfloxacin
ofloxacin
sparfloxacin
Ketolides
telithromycin
Miscellaneous
adefovir dipivoxil
daptomycin
ertapenem
meropenem
peginterferon alfa-2a

Penicillins
amoxicillin/clavulanate
ampicillin/sulbactam
cloxacillin
dicloxacillin
imipenem/cilastatin
mezlocillin
nafcillin
oxacillin
penicillin G benzathine
penicillin G
penicillin G procaine
penicillin V
piperacillin
ticarcillin
ticarcillin/clavulanate
Sulfonamides
sulfasalazine
sulfiSOXAZOLE
Tetracyclines
demeclocycline
doxycycline
minocycline
tetracycline

ANTINEOPLASTICS

Action: Antineoplastics are divided into alkylating agents, antimetabolites, antibiotic agents, hormonal agents, and miscellaneous agents. Alkylating agents act by cross-linking strands of DNA. Antimetabolites act by inhibiting DNA synthesis. Antibiotic agents act by inhibiting RNA synthesis and by delaying or inhibiting mitosis. Hormones alter the effects of androgens, luteinizing hormone, follicle-stimulating hormone, and estrogen by changing the hormonal environment.

Uses: Uses vary widely among products and classes of drugs. They are used to treat leukemia, Hodgkin's disease, lymphomas, and other tumors throughout the body.

Side effects: Most products cause thrombocytopenia, leukopenia, and anemia, and if these reactions occur, the drug may have to be stopped until the problem is corrected. Other side effects include nausea, vomiting, glossitis, and hair loss. Some products also cause hepatotoxicity, nephrotoxicity, and cardiotoxicity.

Contraindications: Hypersensitive reactions may occur, and allergies should be identified before these products are given. Also, persons with severe hepatic and renal disease should not use these products unless the benefits outweigh the risks.

Precautions: Persons with bleeding, severe bone marrow depression, or renal or hepatic disease should be watched closely.

Pharmacokinetics: Onset, peak, and duration vary widely among products. Most products cross the placenta and are excreted in breast milk and in urine.

Interactions: Toxicity may occur when used with other antineoplastics or radiation.

Possible nursing diagnoses:
- Infection, risk for *[adverse reactions]*
- Nutrition: less than body requirements, imbalanced *[adverse reactions]*
- Oral mucous membrane, impaired *[adverse reactions]*

Nursing Considerations

Assess:
- CBC, differential, platelet count weekly; withhold drug if WBC is <4000/mm^3 or platelet count is <75,000/mm^3; notify prescriber of results
- Renal function studies, including BUN, creatinine, serum uric acid, and urine creatinine clearance before and during therapy
- I&O ratio; report fall in urine output of 30 ml/hr
- Monitor temp q4h (may indicate beginning infection)
- Liver function tests before and during therapy (bilirubin, AST, ALT, LDH) as needed or monthly
- Bleeding, including hematuria, guaiac, bruising or petechiae, mucosa, or orifices q8h; obtain prescription for viscous Xylocaine (lidocaine)
- Yellowing of skin, sclera, dark urine, clay-colored stools, itchy skin, abdominal pain, fever, diarrhea
- Edema in feet, joint pain, stomach pain, shaking
- Inflammation of mucosa, breaks in skin

Administer:
- Checking IV site for irritation; phlebitis
- EpINEPHrine for hypersensitivity reaction
- Antibiotics for prophylaxis of infection

Perform/provide:
- Strict asepsis, protective isolation if WBC levels are low
- Comprehensive oral hygiene, using careful technique and soft-bristle brush

Evaluate:
- Therapeutic response, including decreased tumor size

Teach patient/family:
- To report signs of infection, including increased temp, sore throat, malaise
- To report signs of anemia, including fatigue, headache, faintness, shortness of breath, irritability
- To report bleeding and avoid use of razors or commercial mouthwash

Selected Generic Names

Alkylating agents
busulfan
carboplatin
carmustine
chlorambucil
cisplatin
cyclophosphamide
dacarbazine
lomustine
mechlorethamine
melphalan
oxaliplatin
thiotepa
Antimetabolites
capecitabine
cytarabine
etoposide
fludarabine
fluorouracil
mercaptopurine
pemetrexed
thioguanine (6-TG)
Antibiotic agents
bleomycin
dactinomycin
DAUNOrubicin
DOXOrubicin
epirubicin
methotrexate
mitomycin
mitoxantrone
plicamycin
Hormonal agents
aminoglutethimide
estramustine

flutamide
fulvestrant
goserelin
irinotecan
leuprolide
megestrol
mitotane
nilutamide
tamoxifen
testolactone
topotecan
Miscellaneous
altretamine
anastrozole
arsenic trioxide
asparaginase
azacitidine
bortezomib
cetuximab
cladribine
erlotinib
gefitinib
gemcitabine
ibritumomab
interferon alfa-2a
interferon alfa-2b
irinotecan
pentostatin
porfimer
procarbazine
rituximab
vinBLAStine
vinCRIStine
vinorelbine

ANTIPARKINSON AGENTS

Action: Antiparkinson agents are divided into cholinergics and dopamine agonists. Cholinergics work by blocking or competing at central acetylcholine receptors; dopamine agonists work by decarboxylation to dopamine or by activation of dopamine receptors; monoamine oxidase type B inhibitors work by increasing dopamine activity by inhibiting MAO type B activity.

Uses: Antiparkinson agents are used alone or in combination for patients with Parkinson's disease.

Side effects: Side effects and adverse reactions vary widely among products. The most common side effects include involuntary movements, headache, numbness, insomnia, nightmares, nausea, vomiting, dry mouth, and orthostatic hypotension.

Contraindications: Persons with hypersensitivity, narrow-angle glaucoma, and undiagnosed skin lesions should not use these products.

Precautions: Antiparkinson agents should be used with caution in pregnancy, lactation, children, renal, cardiac, and hepatic disease, and affective disorder.

Pharmacokinetics: Onset, peak, and duration vary widely among products. Most products are metabolized in the liver and excreted in urine.

Interactions: Please check individual monographs since interactions vary widely among products.

Possible nursing diagnoses:
- Injury, risk for *[uses]*
- Mobility, physical, impaired *[uses]*
- Knowledge, deficient *[teaching]*

Nursing Considerations

Assess:
- B/P, respiration
- Mental status: affect, mood, behavioral changes, depression, complete suicide assessment

Administer:
- Drug up until NPO before surgery
- Adjust dosage depending on patient response
- With meals; limit protein taken with drug
- Only after MAOIs have been discontinued for 2 wk

Perform/provide:
- Assistance with ambulation, during beginning therapy
- Testing for diabetes mellitus, acromegaly if on long-term therapy

Evaluate:
- Therapeutic response: decrease in akathisia, increased mood

Teach patient/family:
- To change positions slowly to prevent orthostatic hypotension
- To report side effects: twitching, eye spasm; indicate overdose
- To use drug exactly as prescribed; if drug is discontinued abruptly, parkinsonian crisis may occur

Selected Generic Names

amantadine
apomorphine
benztropine
biperiden
bromocriptine
cabergoline
carbidopa-levodopa
levodopa
pramipexole
selegiline
tolcapone
trihexyphenidyl

ANTIPSYCHOTICS

Action: Antipsychotics/neuroleptics are divided into several subgroups: phenothiazines, thioxanthenes, butyrophenones, dibenzoxazepines, dibenzodiazepines, and indolones and other heterocyclic compounds. Although chemically different, these subgroups share many pharmacologic and clinical properties. All antipsychotics work to block postsynaptic dopamine receptors in the brain that are responsible for psychotic behavior, including hallucinations, delusions, and paranoia.

Uses: Antipsychotic behavior is decreased in conditions such as schizophrenia, paranoia, and mania. These agents are also effective for severe anxiety, intractable hiccups, nausea, vomiting, behavioral problems in children, and for relaxation before surgery.

Side effects: The most common side effects include EPS such as pseudoparkinsonism, akathisia, dystonia, and tardive dyskinesia, which may be controlled by use of antiparkinsonian agents. Serious adverse reactions such as hypotension, agranulocytosis, cardiac arrest, and laryngospasm have occurred. Other common side effects include dry mouth and photosensitivity.

Contraindications: Persons with hepatic damage, severe hypertension or coronary disease, cerebral arteriosclerosis, blood dyscrasias, bone marrow depression, parkinsonism, severe depression, narrow-angle glaucoma, children <12 yr, or persons withdrawing from alcohol or barbiturates should not use antipsychotics until these conditions are corrected.

Precautions: Caution must be used when antipsychotics are given to the elderly since metabolism is slowed and adverse reactions can occur rapidly. Hepatic and renal disease may cause poor metabolism and excretion of the drug. Seizure threshold is decreased with these products; increases in the dose of anticonvulsants may be required. Persons with diabetes mellitus, prostatic hypertrophy, chronic respiratory disease, and peptic ulcer disease should be monitored closely.

Pharmacokinetics: Onset, peak, and duration vary widely with different products and routes. Products are metabolized by the liver, are excreted in urine as metabolites, are highly bound to plasma proteins, cross the placenta, and enter breast milk. Half-life can be extended over 3 days.

Interactions: Because other CNS depressants can cause oversedation, these combinations should be used carefully. Anticholinergics may decrease the therapeutic actions of phenothiazines and also cause increased anticholinergic effects.

Possible nursing diagnoses:

- Thought processes, disturbed *[uses]*
- Sensory perception, disturbed *[uses]*

Nursing Considerations

Assess:

- Bilirubin, CBC, hepatic studies qmo, since these drugs are metabolized in the liver and excreted in urine
- I&O ratio: palpate bladder if low urinary output occurs, since urinary retention occurs with many of these products
- Affect, orientation, LOC, reflexes, gait, coordination, sleep pattern disturbances
- Dizziness, faintness, palpitations, tachycardia on rising
- B/P lying and standing; wide fluctuations between lying and standing B/P may require dosage or product change, since orthostatic hypotension is occurring
- EPS, including akathisia, tardive dyskinesia, pseudoparkinsonism

Administer:

- Antiparkinsonian agent if EPS occur
- Liquid concentrates mixed in glass of juice or cola, since taste is unpleasant; avoid contact with skin when preparing liquid concentrate or parenteral medications
- Patient should remain lying down for at least 30 min after IM injections

Perform/provide:
- Supervised ambulation until stabilized on medication; do not involve in strenuous exercise program because fainting is possible; patient should not stand still for long periods
- Increased fluids to prevent constipation
- Sips of water, candy, gum for dry mouth

Evaluate:
- Therapeutic response: decrease in excitement, hallucinations, delusions, paranoia, reorganization of thought patterns, speech

Teach patient/family:
- To rise from sitting or lying position gradually, since fainting may occur
- To avoid hot tubs, hot showers, or tub baths, since hypotension may occur
- To wear a sunscreen or protective clothing to prevent burns
- To take extra precautions during hot weather to stay cool; heat stroke can occur
- To avoid driving, other activities requiring alertness until response to medication is known
- That drowsiness or impaired mental/motor activity is evident the first 2 wk, but tends to decrease over time

Selected Generic Names

Phenothiazines
chlorproMAZINE
fluphenazine
perphenazine
prochlorperazine
thioridazine
thiothixene
trifluoperazine
Butyrophenone
haloperidol
Miscellaneous
aripiprazole
loxapine
olanzapine
quetiapine
risperidone
ziprasidone

ANTITUBERCULARS

Action: Antituberculars act by inhibiting RNA or DNA, or interfering with lipid and protein synthesis, thereby decreasing tubercle bacilli replication.

Uses: Antituberculars are used for pulmonary tuberculosis.

Side effects: They vary widely among products. Most products can cause nausea, vomiting, anorexia, and rash. Serious adverse reactions include renal failure, nephrotoxicity, ototoxicity, and hepatic necrosis.

Contraindications: Persons with severe renal disease or hypersensitivity should not use these products.

Precautions: Antituberculars should be used with caution with pregnancy, lactation, and hepatic disease.

Pharmacokinetics: Onset, peak, and duration vary widely among products. Most products are metabolized in the liver and excreted in urine.

Interactions: Please check individual monographs since interactions vary widely among products.

Possible nursing diagnoses:
• Infection, risk for *[uses]*
• Injury, risk for *[adverse reactions]*
• Knowledge, deficient *[teaching]*
• Noncompliance *[teaching]*

Nursing Considerations

Assess:
• Signs of anemia: Hct, Hgb, fatigue
• Hepatic studies qwk: ALT, AST, bilirubin
• Renal status before, qmo: BUN, creatinine, output, specific gravity, urinalysis
• Hepatic status: decreased appetite, jaundice, dark urine, fatigue

Administer:
• For some of these agents on empty stomach, 1 hr ac (only for isoniazid and rifampin) or 2 hr pc
• Antiemetic if vomiting occurs
• After C&S is completed; qmo to detect resistance

Evaluate:
• Therapeutic response: decreased symptoms of TB, culture negative

Teach patient/family:
• That compliance with dosage schedule, duration is necessary
• That scheduled appointments must be kept; relapse may occur
• To avoid alcohol while taking drug
• To report flulike symptoms: excessive fatigue, anorexia, vomiting, sore throat; unusual bleeding, yellowish discoloration of skin/eyes

Selected Generic Names

ethambutol
isoniazid
pyrazinamide
rifabutin
rifampin
streptomycin

ANTITUSSIVES/EXPECTORANTS

Action: Antitussives act by suppressing the cough reflex by direct action on the cough center in the medulla. Expectorants act by liquefying and reducing the viscosity of thick, tenacious secretions.

Uses: Antitussives/expectorants are used to treat cough occurring in pneumonia, bronchitis, TB, cystic fibrosis, and emphysema; as an adjunct in atelectasis (expectorants); and nonproductive cough (antitussives).

Side effects: The most common side effects are drowsiness, dizziness, and nausea.

Contraindications: Some products are contraindicated in hypothyroidism, pregnancy, and lactation.

Precautions: Some products should be used cautiously in asthmatic, elderly, and debilitated patients.

Pharmacokinetics: Onset, peak, and duration vary widely among products. Some products are metabolized in the liver and excreted in urine.

Interactions: Please check individual monographs since interactions vary widely among products.

Possible nursing diagnoses:
• Breathing pattern, ineffective *[uses]*
• Airway clearance, ineffective *[uses]*
• Knowledge, deficient *[teaching]*

Nursing Considerations

Assess:
• Cough: type, frequency, character (including sputum)

Administer:
• Decreased dose to elderly patients; their metabolism may be slowed

Perform/provide:
• Increased fluids to liquefy secretions
• Humidification of patient's room

Evaluate:
• Therapeutic response: absence of cough

Teach patient/family:
• To avoid driving, other hazardous activities until patient is stabilized on this medication
• To avoid smoking, smoke-filled rooms, perfumes, dust, environmental pollutants, cleaners that increase cough

Selected Generic Names

acetylcysteine
ammonium chloride
benzonatate
codeine
dextromethorphan
guaifenesin
hydrocodone

ANTIVIRALS/ANTIRETROVIRALS

Action: Antivirals act by interfering with DNA synthesis that is needed for viral replication.

Uses: Antivirals are used for mucocutaneous herpes simplex virus, herpes genitalis (HSV_1, HSV_2), advanced HIV infections, herpes simplex virus encephalitis, varicella-zoster encephalomyelitis.

Side effects: Serious adverse reactions are fatal metabolic encephalopathy, blood dyscrasias, and acute renal failure. Common side effects are nausea, vomiting, anorexia, diarrhea, headache, vaginitis, and moniliasis.

Contraindications: Persons with hypersensitivity, or immunosuppressed individuals with herpes zoster should not use these products.

Precautions: Antivirals should be used with caution in renal disease, hepatic disease, lactation, pregnancy, and dehydration.

Pharmacokinetics: Onset, peak, and duration vary widely among products. Most products are metabolized in the liver and excreted in urine.

Interactions: Please check individual monographs since interactions vary widely among products.

Possible nursing diagnoses:
- Infection, risk for *[uses]*
- Injury, risk for *[adverse reactions]*
- Knowledge, deficient *[teaching]*

Nursing Considerations

Assess:
- Signs of infection, anemia
- I&O ratio; report hematuria, oliguria, fatigue, weakness; may indicate nephrotoxicity; check for protein in urine during treatment
- Any patient with compromised renal system, since drug is excreted slowly in poor renal system function; toxicity may occur rapidly
- Hepatic studies: AST, ALT
- Blood studies: WBC, RBC, Hct, Hgb, bleeding time; blood dyscrasias may occur; drug should be discontinued

- Renal studies: urinalysis, protein, BUN, creatinine, CCr
- C&S before drug therapy; drug may be taken as soon as culture is taken; repeat C&S after treatment
- Bowel pattern before, during treatment; if severe abdominal pain with bleeding occurs, drug should be discontinued
- Skin eruptions: rash, urticaria, itching
- Allergies before treatment, reaction of each medication; record allergies on chart in bright red letters

Administer:
- Increased fluids to 3 L/day to decrease crystalluria when given IV

Perform/provide:
- Storage at room temp for up to 12 hr after reconstitution
- Adequate intake of fluids (2 L) to prevent deposit in kidneys

Evaluate:
- Therapeutic response: absence or control of infection

Teach patient/family:
- That drug does not cure infection, just controls symptoms
- To report sore throat, fever, fatigue; could indicate superinfection
- That drug must be taken in equal intervals around the clock to maintain blood levels for duration of therapy
- To notify prescriber of side effects of bruising, bleeding, fatigue, malaise; may indicate blood dyscrasias

Selected Generic Names

abacavir
acyclovir
amantadine
atazanavir
cidofovir
delavirdine
didanosine
emtricitabine
enfuvirtide
famciclovir
fosamprenavir
foscarnet
ganciclovir
indinavir

nelfinavir
nevirapine
rimantadine
ritonavir
saquinavir

stavudine
tenofovir
valganciclovir
zalcitabine
zidovudine

BARBITURATES

Action: Barbiturates act by decreasing impulse transmission to the cerebral cortex.

Uses: All forms of epilepsy can be controlled, since the seizure threshold is increased. Uses also include febrile seizures in children, sedation, insomnia, hyperbilirubinemia, chronic cholestasis with some of these products. Ultra–short-acting barbiturates are used as anesthetics.

Side effects: The most common side effects are drowsiness and nausea. Serious adverse reactions such as Stevens-Johnson syndrome and blood dyscrasias may occur with high doses and long-term treatment.

Contraindications: Hypersensitivity may occur, and allergies should be identified before administering. Barbiturates are identified as pregnancy category D and should not be used in pregnancy. Other contraindications include porphyria and marked impairment of hepatic function.

Precautions: Caution must be used when these products are given to the elderly or debilitated; usually smaller doses are needed since metabolism is slowed. Persons with renal and hepatic disease may show delayed excretion. Barbiturates may produce excitability in children.

Pharmacokinetics: Onset of action can be slow, up to 1 hr, with a peak of 8 hr and a duration of 3-10 hr. These drugs are metabolized by the liver, excreted by the kidneys, cross the placenta, and enter breast milk.

Interactions: Increased CNS depressant effect may occur with alcohol, MAOIs, sedatives, or opioids. These products should be used together cautiously. Oral anticoagulants, corticosteroids, griseofulvin, quinidine, oral contraceptives, and theophylline may show a decreased effect when used with barbiturates.

Possible nursing diagnoses:
- Sleep pattern, disturbed *[uses]*
- Injury, risk for *[adverse reactions]*

Nursing Considerations

Assess:
- Hepatic and renal studies: AST, ALT, bilirubin, creatinine, LDH, phosphatase, BUN if patient is on long-term therapy, since these products are metabolized and excreted by the liver and kidneys
- Blood studies: CBC, hematocrit, hemoglobin, and prothrombin time if patient is on long-term therapy, since these products increase the possibility of bleeding and blood dyscrasias
- Barbiturate toxicity: hypotension, pulmonary constriction; cold, clammy skin; cyanosis of lips, insomnia, nausea, vomiting, hallucinations, delirium, weakness

Evaluate:
- Therapeutic response, including appropriate sedation or seizure control

Teach patient/family:
- That physical dependency may result when used for extended periods (45-90 days, depending on dose)
- To avoid driving, activities that require alertness since drowsiness and dizziness may occur
- To abstain from alcohol or other psychotropic medications unless directed by prescriber
- Not to discontinue medication abruptly after long-term use; withdrawal symptoms will occur

Selected Generic Names

pentobarbital
phenobarbital
secobarbital
thiopental

BENZODIAZEPINES

Action: Benzodiazepines potentiate the effects of γ-aminobutyric acid (GABA), including any other inhibitory transmitters in the CNS, resulting in decreased anxiety.

Uses: Anxiety is relieved in conditions such as phobic disorders. Benzodiazepines are also used for acute alcohol withdrawal to relieve the possibility of delirium tremens, and some products are used for relaxation before surgery.

Side effects: The most common side effects are dizziness, drowsiness, blurred vision, and orthostatic hypotension. Most adverse effects are mediated through the CNS. There is a risk of physical dependence and abuse.

Contraindications: Hypersensitivity, acute narrow-angle glaucoma, children <6 mo, hepatic disease (clonazepam), lactation (diazepam).

Precautions: Caution must be used when these products are given to the elderly or debilitated; usually smaller doses are needed, since metabolism is slowed. Persons with renal and hepatic disease may show delayed excretion. Clonazepam may increase incidence of seizures.

Pharmacokinetics: Onset of action is ½-1 hr, with a peak of 1-2 hr and a duration of 4-6 hr. These drugs are metabolized by the liver, excreted by the kidneys, cross the placenta, and enter breast milk.

Interactions: Increased CNS depressant effect may occur with other CNS depressants. These products should be used together cautiously. Alcohol should not be used; fatal reactions can occur. The serum concentration and toxicity of digoxin may be increased.

Possible nursing diagnoses:
- Anxiety *[uses]*
- Injury, risk for *[adverse reactions]*

Nursing Considerations

Assess:
- B/P (lying, standing), pulse; if systolic B/P drops 20 mm Hg, hold drug, notify prescriber; orthostatic hypotension is severe
- Hepatic and renal studies: AST, ALT, bilirubin, creatinine, LDH, alk phosphatase
- Physical dependency, withdrawal symptoms, including headache, nausea, vomiting, muscle pain, weakness after long-term use

Administer:
- With food or milk for GI symptoms; may give crushed if patient is unable to swallow medication whole

Evaluate:
- Therapeutic response, including relaxation or decreased anxiety

Teach patient/family:
- That drug should not be used for everyday stress or long-term; not to take more than prescribed amount since drug is habit-forming
- To avoid driving and activities that require alertness since drowsiness and dizziness occur
- To abstain from alcohol, other psychotropic medications unless directed by prescriber
- Not to discontinue medication abruptly after long-term use; withdrawal symptoms will occur

Selected Generic Names

alprazolam
chlordiazepoxide
clonazepam
diazepam
flurazepam
lorazepam
midazolam
oxazepam
temazepam
triazolam

BETA-ADRENERGIC BLOCKERS

Action: β-Blockers are divided into selective and nonselective blockers. Nonselective blockers produce a fall in blood pressure without reflex tachycardia or reduction in heart rate through a mixture of β-blocking effects; elevated plasma renins are reduced. Selective β-blockers competitively block stimulation of β_1-receptors in cardiac smooth muscle; these drugs produce chronotropic and inotropic effects.

Uses: β-Blockers are used for hypertension, ventricular dysrhythmias, and prophylaxis of angina pectoris.

Side effects: The most common side effects are orthostatic hypotension, bradycardia, diarrhea, nausea, vomiting. Serious adverse reactions include blood dyscrasias, bronchospasm, and CHF.

Contraindications: Hypersensitive reactions may occur, and allergies should be identified before these products are given. β-Adrenergic blockers should not be used in heart block, CHF, or cardiogenic shock.

Precautions: β-Blockers should be used with caution in the elderly or in renal and thyroid disease, COPD, CAD, diabetes mellitus, pregnancy, or asthma.

Pharmacokinetics: Onset, peak, and duration vary widely among products. Most products are metabolized in the liver, with metabolites excreted in urine, bile, and feces.

Interactions: Interactions vary widely among products; check individual monographs for specific information.

Possible nursing diagnoses:
- Tissue perfusion, ineffective *[uses]*
- Cardiac output, decreased *[uses]*
- Diarrhea *[adverse reactions]*
- Gas exchange, impaired *[adverse reactions]*

Nursing Considerations

Assess:
- Renal studies, including protein, BUN, creatinine; watch for increased levels that may indicate nephrotic syndrome; obtain baselines in renal and hepatic function studies before beginning treatment
- I&O, weight daily
- B/P during beginning treatment and periodically thereafter; pulse q4h, note rate, rhythm, quality
- Apical/radial pulse before administration; notify prescriber of significant changes
- Edema in feet and legs daily

Administer:
- PO ac, bedtime; tablets may be crushed or swallowed whole
- Reduced dosage in renal dysfunction

Evaluate:
- Therapeutic response, including decrease in B/P in hypertension, decreased B/P, edema, moist crackles in CHF

Teach patient/family:
- To comply with dosage schedule, even if feeling better
- To rise slowly to sitting or standing position to minimize orthostatic hypotension
- To report bradycardia, dizziness, confusion, depression, fever
- To take pulse at home; advise when to notify prescriber
- To comply with weight control, dietary adjustment, modified exercise program
- To wear support hose to minimize effects of orthostatic hypotension
- Not to discontinue drug abruptly; taper over 2 wk; may precipitate angina

Selected Generic Names

Selective β_1-receptor blockers
acebutolol
atenolol
esmolol
metoprolol

Combined α_1-, β_1-, and β_2-receptor blocker
labetalol

Nonselective β_1- and β_2-blockers
carteolol
nadolol
pindolol
propranolol
timolol

BRONCHODILATORS

Action: Bronchodilators are divided into anticholinergics, α/β-adrenergic agonists, β-adrenergic agonists, and phosphodiesterase inhibitors. Anticholinergics act by inhibiting interaction of acetylcholine at receptor sites on bronchial smooth muscle; α/β-adrenergic agonists by relaxing bronchial smooth muscle and increasing diameter of nasal passages; β-adrenergic agonists by action on β_2-receptors, which relaxes bronchial smooth muscle; phosphodiesterase inhibitors by blocking phosphodiesterase and increasing cAMP, which mediates smooth muscle relaxation in the respiratory system.

Uses: Bronchodilators are used for bronchial asthma, bronchospasm associated with bronchitis, emphysema, or other obstructive pulmonary diseases, Cheyne-Stokes respirations, prevention of exercise-induced asthma.

Side effects: The most common side effects are tremors, anxiety, nausea, vomiting, and irritation in throat. The most serious adverse reactions include bronchospasm and dyspnea.

Contraindications: Persons with hypersensitivity, narrow-angle glaucoma, tachydysrhythmias, and severe cardiac disease should not use some of these products.

Precautions: Bronchodilators should be used with caution in lactation, pregnancy, hyperthyroidism, hypertension, prostatic hypertrophy, and seizure disorders.

Pharmacokinetics: Onset, peak, and duration vary widely among products. Most products are metabolized in the liver and excreted in urine.

Interactions: Please check individual monographs since interactions vary widely among products.

Possible nursing diagnoses:
- Airway clearance, ineffective *[uses]*
- Activity intolerance *[uses]*
- Injury, risk for *[adverse reactions]*
- Knowledge, deficient *[teaching]*

Nursing Considerations

Assess:
- Respiratory function: vital capacity, forced expiratory volume, ABGs, lung sounds, heart rate and rhythm

Administer:
- After shaking, exhale, place mouthpiece in mouth, inhale slowly, hold breath, remove, exhale slowly
- PO with meals to decrease gastric irritation

Perform/provide:
- Storage in light-resistant container, do not expose to temps over 86° F (30° C)
- Gum, sips of water for dry mouth

Evaluate:
- Therapeutic response: absence of dyspnea, wheezing

Teach patient/family:
- Not to use OTC medications; extra stimulation may occur
- Use of inhaler; review package insert with patient
- To avoid getting aerosol in eyes
- To wash inhaler in warm water daily and dry
- To avoid smoking, smoke-filled rooms, persons with respiratory infections

Selected Generic Names

albuterol
aminophylline
atropine
bitolterol
dyphylline
epHEDrine
epINEPHrine
formoterol
ipratropium
isoproterenol
levalbuterol
metaproterenol
pirbuterol
terbutaline
theophylline
tiotropium

CALCIUM CHANNEL BLOCKERS

Action: These products act by inhibiting calcium ion influx across the cell membrane in cardiac and vascular smooth muscle. This action produces relaxation of coronary vascular smooth muscle, dilates coronary arteries, slows SA/AV node conduction, and dilates peripheral arteries.

Uses: These products are used for chronic stable angina pectoris, vasospastic angina, dysrhythmias, hypertension, and unstable angina.

Side effects: The most common side effects are dysrhythmias and edema. Also common are headache, fatigue, drowsiness, and flushing.

Contraindications: Persons with 2nd- or 3rd-degree heart block, sick sinus syndrome, hypotension of <90 mm Hg systolic, Wolff-Parkinson-White syndrome, or cardiogenic shock should not use these products since worsening of those conditions may occur.

Precautions: CHF may worsen since edema may be increased. Hypotension may worsen since B/P is decreased. Patients with renal and hepatic disease should use these products cautiously since they are metabolized in the liver and excreted by the kidneys.

Pharmacokinetics: Onset, peak, and duration vary widely with route of administration. Drugs are metabolized by the liver and excreted in the urine primarily as metabolites.

Interactions: Increased levels of digoxin and theophylline may occur when used with these products. Increased effects of β-blockers and antihypertensives may occur with calcium channel blockers.

Possible nursing diagnoses:
• Tissue perfusion, ineffective *[uses]*
• Cardiac output, decreased *[adverse reactions]*

Nursing Considerations

Assess:
• Cardiac system, including B/P, pulse, respirations, ECG intervals (PR, QRS, QT)

Administer:
• PO before meals and at bedtime

Evaluate:
• Therapeutic response, including decreased anginal pain, decreased B/P, dysrhythmias

Teach patient/family:
• How to take pulse before taking drug; patient should record or graph pulses to identify changes
• To avoid hazardous activities until stabilized on this drug, since dizziness commonly occurs
• Need for compliance in all areas of medical regimen, including diet, exercise, stress reduction, drug therapy

Selected Generic Names

diltiazem
felodipine
niCARdipine
NIFEdipine
verapamil

CARDIAC GLYCOSIDES

Action: Products act by inhibiting sodium and potassium ATPase and then making more calcium available to activate contracted proteins. Cardiac contractility and cardiac output are increased.

Uses: These products are used for CHF, atrial fibrillation, atrial flutter, atrial tachycardia, and rapid digitalization in these disorders.

Side effects: The most common side effects are cardiac disturbances, headache, hypotension, GI symptoms. Also common are blurred vision and yellow-green halos.

Contraindications: Hypersensitive reactions may occur, and allergies should be identified before these products are given. Also, persons with ventricular tachycardia, ventricular fibrillation, and carotid sinus syndrome should not use these products.

Precautions: Persons with acute MI and those who have or may develop serum potassium, calcium, or magnesium imbalances should use these products cautiously. Also, persons with AV block, severe respiratory disease, hypothyroidism, or renal and hepatic disease and the elderly should exercise caution when these drugs are prescribed.

Pharmacokinetics: Onset, peak, and duration vary widely with the route of administration. Digitoxin is inactivated by the liver, and inactive metabolites are excreted in urine. Digoxin is excreted in urine mainly as the parent drug and metabolites.

Interactions: Toxicity may occur when used with diuretics, succinylcholine, quinidine, and thioamines. Increased blood levels may occur with propantheline bromide, spironolactone, quinidine, verapamil, aminoglycosides (PO), amiodarone, anticholinergics, and quinine. Diuretics may increase toxicity.

Possible nursing diagnoses:
• Tissue perfusion, ineffective *[uses]*
• Cardiac output, decreased *[adverse reactions]*

Nursing Considerations

Assess:
• Cardiac system, including B/P, pulse, respirations, and increased urine output
• Apical pulse for 1 min before giving drug; if pulse <60 bpm, take again in 1 hr; if still <60 bpm, notify prescriber
• Electrolytes, including K, Na, Cl, Mg; renal function studies, including BUN and creatinine; and blood studies, including AST, ALT, bilirubin
• I&O ratio, daily weights
• Monitor therapeutic drug levels

Administer:
• K supplements if ordered for K levels <3 mg/dl

Evaluate:
• Therapeutic response, including decreased weight, edema, pulse, respiration, and increased urine output

Teach patient/family:
• How to take pulse before taking drug; patient should record or graph pulse to identify changes
• To avoid hazardous activities until stabilized on this drug, since dizziness commonly occurs
• Need for compliance in all areas of medical regimen, including diet, exercise, stress reduction, drug therapy

Selected Generic Name

digoxin

CHOLINERGICS

Action: Cholinergics act by preventing destruction of acetylcholine, which increases concentration at sites where acetylcholine is released; this exaggerates the effects of acetylcholine and facilitates transmission of impulses across the myoneural junction. Cholinergics may also act by stimulating receptors for acetylcholine.

Uses: Cholinergics are used for myasthenia gravis, as antagonists of nondepolarizing neuromuscular blockade, postoperative bladder distention and urinary distention, and postoperative ileus.

Side effects: The most serious adverse reactions are respiratory depression, bronchospasm, constriction, laryngospasm, respiratory arrest, convulsions, and paralysis. The most common side effects are nausea, diarrhea, and vomiting.

Contraindications: Persons with obstruction of the intestine or renal system should not use these products.

Precautions: Caution should be used in patients with bradycardia, hypotension, seizure disorders, bronchial asthma, coronary occlusion, hyperthyroidism, lactation, and in children.

Pharmacokinetics: Onset, peak, and duration vary widely among products. Most products are metabolized in the liver and excreted in urine.

Interactions: Please check individual monographs since interactions vary widely among products.

Possible nursing diagnoses:
- Urinary elimination, impaired *[uses]*
- Breathing pattern, ineffective *[uses]*
- Knowledge, deficient *[teaching]*
- Noncompliance *[teaching]*

Nursing Considerations

Assess:
- VS, respiration q8h
- I&O ratio; check for urinary retention or incontinence
- Bradycardia, hypotension, bronchospasm, headache, dizziness, convulsions, respiratory depression; drug should be discontinued if toxicity occurs

Administer:
- Only with atropine sulfate available for cholinergic crisis
- Only after all other cholinergics have been discontinued
- Increased doses if tolerance occurs
- Larger doses after exercise or fatigue
- On empty stomach for better absorption

Perform/provide:
- Storage at room temp

Evaluate:
- Therapeutic response: increased muscle strength, hand grasp, improved muscle gait, absence of labored breathing (if severe)

Teach patient/family:
- That drug is not a cure; it only relieves symptoms (myasthenia gravis)
- To carry emergency ID specifying myasthenia gravis, drugs taken

Selected Generic Names

bethanechol
edrophonium
neostigmine
physostigmine
pyridostigmine

CHOLINERGIC BLOCKERS

Action: Cholinergic blockers inhibit or block acetylcholine at receptor sites in the autonomic nervous system.

Uses: Many products are used to decrease secretions before surgery, to reverse neuromuscular blockade, and to decrease motility of GI, biliary, urinary tracts. Other products are used for parkinsonian symptoms, including dystonia associated with neuroleptic drugs.

Side effects: The most common side effects are dryness of the mouth and constipation, which can be prevented by frequent rinsing of the mouth and by increasing water and bulk in the diet.

Contraindications: Hypersensitivity can occur, and allergies should be identified before administering these products. Persons with GI and GU obstruction should not use these products since constipation and urinary retention may occur. They are also contraindicated in angle-closure glaucoma and myasthenia gravis.

Precautions: Caution must be used when these products are given to the elderly, since metabolism is slowed. Also, persons with tachycardia or prostatic hypertrophy should use these products with caution.

Pharmacokinetics: Onset, peak, and duration vary with route.

Interactions: Increase in anticholinergic effect occurs when used with opioids, barbiturates, antihistamines, MAOIs, phenothiazines, and amantadine.

Possible nursing diagnoses:
- Mobility, physical, impaired *[uses]*
- Chronic pain *[uses]*

Nursing Considerations

Assess:
- I&O ratio; be alert for urinary retention, frequency, dysuria; drug should be discontinued if these occur
- Urinary hesitancy, retention; palpate bladder if retention occurs
- Constipation; increase fluids, bulk, exercise
- For tolerance over long-term therapy, dose may have to be increased or changed
- Mental status: affect, mood, CNS depression, worsening of mental symptoms during early therapy

Administer:
- With food or milk to decrease GI symptoms
- Parenteral dose with patient recumbent to prevent postural hypotension; give parenteral dose slowly, monitoring vital signs

Perform/provide:
- Hard candy, gum, frequent rinsing of mouth for dryness

Evaluate:
- Therapeutic response, including absence of cramps and EPS

Teach patient/family:
- To avoid driving, other hazardous activity if drowsiness occurs
- To avoid concurrent use of cough, cold preparations with alcohol, antihistamines unless directed by prescriber
- To use with caution in hot weather since medication may increase susceptibility to heat stroke

Selected Generic Names

atropine
benztropine
biperiden
glycopyrrolate
scopolamine
trihexyphenidyl

CORTICOSTEROIDS

Action: Corticosteroids are divided into glucocorticoids and mineralocorticoids. Glucocorticoids decrease inflammation by the suppression of migration of polymorphonuclear leukocytes, fibroblasts, increased capillary permeability, and lysosomal stabilization. They also have varied metabolic effects and modify the body's immune responses to many stimuli. Mineralocorticoids act by increasing resorption of sodium by increasing hydrogen and potassium excretion in the distal tubule.

Uses: Glucocorticoids are used to decrease inflammation and for immunosuppression. In addition, some products may be given for allergy, adrenal insufficiency, or cerebral edema. Mineralocorticoids are given for adrenal insufficiency or adrenogenital syndrome.

Side effects: The most common side effects include change in behavior, including insomnia and euphoria; GI irritation, including peptic ulcer; metabolic reactions, including hypokalemia, hyperglycemia, and carbohydrate intolerance; and sodium and fluid retention. Most adverse reactions are dose dependent.

Contraindications: Hypersensitivity may occur and should be identified before administering. Since these products mask infection, they should not be used in systemic fungal infections or amebiasis. Mothers taking pharmacologic doses of corticosteroids should not nurse.

Precautions: Caution must be used when these products are prescribed for diabetic patients since hyperglycemia may occur. Also, patients with glaucoma, seizure disorders, peptic ulcer, impaired renal function, CHF, hypertension, ulcerative colitis, or myasthenia gravis should be monitored closely if corticosteroids are given. Use with caution in children and the elderly and during pregnancy.

Pharmacokinetics: For oral preparations, the onset of action occurs between 1 and 2 hr, and duration can be up to 2 days, with a half-life of 2-4 days. Pharmacokinetics vary widely among products. These products cross the placenta and appear in breast milk.

Interactions: Decreased corticosteroid effect may occur with barbiturates, rifampin, phenytoin; corticosteroid dose may have to be increased. There is a possibility of GI bleeding when used with salicylates, indomethacin. Steroids may reduce salicylate levels. When using with digitalis glycosides, potassium-depleting diuretics, and amphotericin, serum potassium levels should be monitored.

Possible nursing diagnoses:
• Infection, risk for *[adverse reactions]*
• Body image, disturbed *[adverse reactions]*
• Suicide, risk for *[adverse reactions]*

Nursing Considerations

Assess:

• Potassium, blood glucose, urine glucose while on long-term therapy; hypokalemia and hyperglycemia are common

• Weight daily; notify prescriber of weekly gain >5 lb, since these products alter fluid and electrolyte balance

• I&O ratio; be alert for decreasing urinary output and increasing edema

• Plasma cortisol levels during long-term therapy (normal level is 138-635 nmol/L SI units when drawn at 8 AM)

• Infection, including increased temp, WBC, even after withdrawal of medication; drug masks symptoms of infection

• Adrenal insufficiency: nausea, anorexia, fatigue, dizziness, dyspnea, weakness, joint pain

• Potassium depletion, including paresthesias, fatigue, nausea, vomiting, depression, polyuria, dysrhythmias, weakness

• Mental status, including affect, mood, behavioral changes, aggression; if severe personality changes occur, including depression, drug may have to be tapered and then discontinued

Administer:
- With food or milk to decrease GI symptoms
- Take single daily or alternate-day doses in the morning before 9 AM (for replacement therapy)

Evaluate:
- Therapeutic response, including decreased inflammation

Teach patient/family:
- That emergency ID as steroid user should be carried
- Not to discontinue this medication abruptly, or adrenal crisis can result
- Teach patient all aspects of drug use, including cushingoid symptoms
- To take with meals or a snack
- If taking immunosuppressives, avoid exposure to chickenpox or measles

Selected Generic Names

Glucocorticoids
beclomethasone
betamethasone
cortisone
dexamethasone
hydrocortisone
hydrocortisone sodium phosphate
methylPREDNISolone
prednisoLONE
predniSONE
triamcinolone

Mineralocorticoid
fludrocortisone

DIURETICS

Action: Diuretics are divided into subgroups: thiazides and thiazide-like diuretics, loop diuretics, carbonic anhydrase inhibitors, osmotic diuretics, and potassium-sparing diuretics. Each one of these subgroups has its own mechanism of action. Thiazides and thiazide-like diuretics increase excretion of water and sodium by inhibiting resorption in the early distal tubule. Loop diuretics inhibit resorption of sodium and chloride in the thick ascending limb of the loop of Henle. Carbonic anhydrase inhibitors increase sodium excretion by decreasing sodium-hydrogen ion exchange throughout the renal tubule. Carbonic anhydrase inhibitors also decrease secretion of aqueous humor in the eye and thus decrease intraocular pressure. Osmotic diuretics increase the osmotic pressure of glomerular filtrate, thus decreasing net absorption of sodium. The potassium-sparing diuretics interfere with sodium resorption at the distal tubule, thus decreasing potassium excretion.

Uses: B/P is reduced in hypertension; edema is reduced in CHF; intraocular pressure is decreased in glaucoma.

Side effects: Hypokalemia, hyperuricemia, and hyperglycemia occur most frequently with thiazide diuretics. Aplastic anemia, blood dyscrasias, volume depletion, and dehydration may occur when thiazide-like diuretics, loop diuretics, or carbonic anhydrase inhibitors are given. Side effects and adverse reactions vary widely for the miscellaneous products.

Contraindications: Persons with electrolyte imbalances (Na, Cl, K), dehydration, or anuria should not be given these products until the problem is corrected.

Precautions: Caution must be used when diuretics are given to the elderly, since electrolyte disturbances and dehydration can occur rapidly. Hepatic and renal disease may cause poor metabolism and excretion of the drug.

Pharmacokinetics: Onset, peak, and duration vary widely among the different subgroups of these drugs.

Interactions: Cholestyramine and colestipol will decrease the absorption of thiazide diuretics. Concurrent use of thiazides with diazoxide may increase hyperuricemia, hyperglycemia, and antihypertensive effects of thiazides. Ototoxicity may occur when loop diuretics are used with aminoglycosides. Thiazide and loop diuretics may increase therapeutic and toxic effects of lithium.

Possible nursing diagnoses:
- Fluid volume, excess *[uses]*
- Cardiac output, decreased *[adverse reactions]*

Nursing Considerations

Assess:
- Weight, I&O daily to determine fluid loss; check skin turgor for dehydration
- Electrolytes: K, Na, Cl; include BUN, blood glucose, CBC, serum creatinine, blood pH, ABGs, uric acid, Ca; electrolyte imbalances may occur quickly
- B/P lying, standing; postural hypotension may occur since fluid loss occurs first from intravascular spaces
- Signs of metabolic alkalosis, including drowsiness and restlessness
- Signs of hypokalemia with some products, including postural hypotension, malaise, fatigue, tachycardia, leg cramps, weakness

Administer:
- In AM to avoid interference with sleep if using drug as a diuretic
- K replacement if K is less than 3 mg/dl

Evaluate:
- Therapeutic response: improvement in edema of feet, legs, sacral area daily if medication is being used in CHF; improvement in B/P if medication is being used as a diuretic; improvement in intraocular pressure if medication is being used to decrease aqueous humor in the eye

Teach patient/family:
• To take drug early in the day (diuretic) to prevent nocturia

Selected Generic Names

Thiazides
chlorothiazide
hydrochlorothiazide
Thiazide-like
chlorthalidone
indapamide
metolazone

Loop
bumetanide
furosemide
torsemide
Carbonic anhydrase inhibitor
acetaZOLAMIDE
Potassium-sparing
amiloride
spironolactone
triamterene
Osmotics
mannitol
urea

HISTAMINE H₂ ANTAGONISTS

Action: Histamine H_2 antagonists act by inhibiting histamine at the H_2-receptor site in parietal cells, which inhibits gastric acid secretion.

Uses: Histamine H_2 antagonists are used for short-term treatment of duodenal and gastric ulcers and maintenance therapy for duodenal ulcer; gastroesophageal reflux disease.

Side effects: The most serious adverse reactions are agranulocytosis, thrombocytopenia, neutropenia, aplastic anemia, exfoliative dermatitis. The most common side effects are confusion (not with ranitidine), headache, and diarrhea.

Contraindications: Persons with hypersensitivity should not use these products.

Precautions: Caution should be used in pregnancy, lactation, child <16 yr, organic brain syndrome, hepatic disease, renal disease.

Pharmacokinetics: Onset, peak, and duration vary widely among products. Most products are metabolized in the liver and excreted in urine.

Interactions: Antacids interfere with absorption of histamine H_2 antagonists. Check individual monographs for other interactions.

Possible nursing diagnoses:
- Chronic pain *[uses]*
- Injury, risk for *[bleeding]*
- Knowledge, deficient *[teaching]*

Nursing Considerations

Assess:
- Gastric pH (>5 should be maintained)
- I&O ratio, BUN, creatinine

Administer:
- With meals for prolonged drug effect
- Antacids 1 hr before or 1 hr after cimetidine
- IV slowly; bradycardia may occur; give over 30 min

Perform/provide:
- Storage of diluted sol at room temp for up to 48 hr

Evaluate:
- Therapeutic response: decreased pain in abdomen

Teach patient/family:
- That gynecomastia, impotence may occur, but are reversible
- To avoid driving, other hazardous activities until patient is stabilized on this medication
- To avoid black pepper, caffeine, alcohol, harsh spices, extremes in temp of food
- To avoid OTC preparations: aspirin, cough, cold preparations
- That drug must be continued for prescribed time to be effective
- To report bruising, fatigue, malaise; blood dyscrasias may occur

Selected Generic Names

cimetidine
famotidine
ranitidine

IMMUNOSUPPRESSANTS

Action: Immunosuppressants act by inhibiting lymphocytes (T).

Uses: Most products are used for organ transplants to prevent rejection.

Side effects: The most serious adverse reactions are albuminuria, hematuria, proteinuria, renal failure, and hepatotoxicity. The most common side effects are overgrowth of oral *Candida,* gum hyperplasia, tremors, and headache. The most serious adverse reactions for azathioprine are hematologic (leukopenia and thrombocytopenia) and GI (nausea and vomiting). There is a risk of secondary infection.

Contraindications: Products are contraindicated in hypersensitivity.

Precautions: Caution should be used in severe renal disease, severe hepatic disease, and pregnancy.

Pharmacokinetics: Onset, peak, and duration vary widely among products. Most products are metabolized in the liver and excreted in urine.

Interactions: Please check individual monographs since interactions vary widely among products.

Possible nursing diagnoses:
- Infection, risk for *[adverse reactions]*
- Injury, risk for *[uses]*
- Knowledge, deficient *[teaching]*

Nursing Considerations

Assess:
- Renal studies: BUN, creatinine at least qmo during treatment, 3 mo after treatment
- Hepatic studies: alk phosphatase, AST (SGOT), ALT (SGPT), bilirubin
- Drug blood levels during treatment
- Hepatotoxicity: dark urine, jaundice, itching, light-colored stools; drug should be discontinued

Administer:
- For several days before transplant surgery
- With meals for GI upset or drug mixed with chocolate milk
- With oral antifungal for *Candida* infections

Evaluate:
- Therapeutic response: absence of rejection

Teach patient/family:
- To report fever, chills, sore throat, fatigue, since serious infections may occur
- To use contraceptive measures during treatment, for 12 wk after ending therapy

Selected Generic Names

azathioprine
basiliximab
cycloSPORINE
muromonab-CD3
sirolimus
tacrolimus

LAXATIVES

Action: Laxatives are divided into bulk products, lubricants, osmotics, saline laxative stimulants, and stool softeners. Bulk laxatives work by absorbing water and expanding to increase moisture content and bulk in the stool. Lubricants increase water retention in the stool, causing reabsorption of water in the bowel. Stimulants act by increasing peristalsis by direct effect on the intestine. Saline draws water into the intestinal lumen. Osmotics increase distention and promote peristalsis. Stool softeners reduce surface tension of liquids of the bowel.

Uses: Laxatives are used as a preparation for bowel and rectal exam, constipation, and stool softener.

Side effects: The most common side effects are nausea, abdominal cramps, and diarrhea.

Contraindications: Persons with GI obstruction, perforation, gastric retention, toxic colitis, megacolon, abdominal pain, nausea, vomiting, or fecal impaction should not use these products.

Precautions: Caution should be used in rectal bleeding, large hemorrhoids, and anal excoriation.

Pharmacokinetics: Onset, peak, and duration vary among products.

Interactions: Please check individual monographs since interactions vary widely among products.

Possible nursing diagnoses:
- Constipation *[uses]*
- Diarrhea *[adverse reactions]*
- Knowledge, deficient *[teaching]*

Nursing Considerations

Assess:
- Blood, urine electrolytes if drug is used often by patient
- I&O ratio: to identify fluid loss
- Cause of constipation; identify whether fluids, bulk, or exercise is missing from lifestyle
- Cramping, rectal bleeding, nausea, vomiting; if these symptoms occur, drug should be discontinued

Administer:
- Swallow tabs whole; do not break, crush, or chew
- Alone only with water for better absorption; do not take within 1 hr of antacids, milk, or cimetidine

Evaluate:
- Therapeutic response: decrease in constipation

Teach patient/family:
- Not to use laxatives for long-term therapy; bowel tone will be lost
- That normal bowel movements do not always occur daily
- Not to use in presence of abdominal pain, nausea, vomiting
- To notify prescriber of abdominal pain, nausea, vomiting
- To notify prescriber if constipation is unrelieved or if symptoms of electrolyte imbalance: muscle cramps, pain, weakness, dizziness

Selected Generic Names

Bulk laxatives
calcium polycarbophil
methylcellulose
psyllium
Osmotic agents
glycerin
lactulose
Saline laxatives
magnesium salts
sodium biphosphate/phosphate
Stimulants
bisacodyl
cascara sagrada
senna
Stool softener
docusate

NEUROMUSCULAR BLOCKING AGENTS

Action: Neuromuscular blocking agents are divided into depolarizing and nondepolarizing blockers. They act by inhibiting transmission of nerve impulses by binding with cholinergic receptor sites.

Uses: Neuromuscular blocking agents are used to facilitate endotracheal intubation and skeletal muscle relaxation during mechanical ventilation, surgery, or general anesthesia.

Side effects: The most serious adverse reactions are prolonged apnea, bronchospasm, cyanosis, respiratory depression, and malignant hyperthermia. The most common side effects are bradycardia and decreased motility.

Contraindications: Persons who are hypersensitive should not be given this product.

Precautions: Caution should be used in pregnancy, thyroid disease, collagen disease, cardiac disease, lactation, children <2 yr, electrolyte imbalances, dehydration, neuromuscular disease (myasthenia gravis), and respiratory disease.

Pharmacokinetics: Onset, peak, and duration vary widely among products. Most products are metabolized in the liver and excreted in urine.

Interactions: Aminoglycosides potentiate neuromuscular blockade. See individual monographs.

Possible nursing diagnoses:
- Breathing pattern, ineffective *[uses]*
- Injury, risk for *[adverse reactions]*
- Knowledge, deficient *[teaching]*

Nursing Considerations

Assess:
- For electrolyte imbalances (K, Mg); may lead to increased action of this drug

- VS (B/P, pulse, respirations, airway) q15min until fully recovered; rate, depth, pattern of respirations, strength of hand grip
- I&O ratio; check for urinary retention, frequency, hesitancy
- Recovery: decreased paralysis of face, diaphragm, leg, arm, rest of body
- Allergic reactions: rash, fever, respiratory distress, pruritus; drug should be discontinued

Administer:
- Using nerve stimulator by anesthesia provider to determine neuromuscular blockade
- Anticholinesterase to reverse neuromuscular blockade
- IV undiluted over 1-2 min (only by qualified person, usually an anesthesiologist)

Perform/provide:
- Storage in light-resistant container, cool area
- Reassurance if communication is difficult during recovery from neuromuscular blockade

Evaluate:
- Therapeutic response: paralysis of jaw, eyelid, head, neck, rest of body

Selected Generic Names

atracurium
doxacurium
gallamine
mivacurium
pancuronium
pipecuronium
rocuronium
succinylcholine
tubocurarine
vecuronium

NONSTEROIDAL ANTIINFLAMMATORIES

Action: Nonsteroidals decrease prostaglandin synthesis by inhibiting an enzyme needed for biosynthesis.

Uses: Nonsteroidal antiinflammatories are used to treat mild to moderate pain, osteoarthritis, rheumatoid arthritis, and dysmenorrhea.

Side effects: The most serious adverse reactions are nephrotoxicity (dysuria, hematuria, oliguria, azotemia), blood dyscrasias, and cholestatic hepatitis. The most common side effects are nausea, abdominal pain, anorexia, dizziness, and drowsiness.

Contraindications: Persons with hypersensitivity, asthma, severe renal disease, and severe hepatic disease should not use these products.

Precautions: Caution should be used in pregnancy, lactation, children, bleeding disorders, GI disorders, cardiac disorders, hypersensitivity to other antiinflammatory agents, and the elderly.

Pharmacokinetics: Onset, peak, and duration vary widely among products. Most products are metabolized in the liver and excreted in urine.

Interactions: Please check individual monographs since interactions vary widely among products.

Possible nursing diagnoses:
- Pain, chronic *[uses]*
- Mobility, physical, impaired *[uses]*
- Knowledge, deficient *[teaching]*
- Noncompliance *[teaching]*

Nursing Considerations

Assess:
- Renal, hepatic, blood studies: BUN, creatinine, AST, ALT, Hgb, before treatment, periodically thereafter
- Audiometric, ophthalmic examination before, during, and after treatment
- For eye, ear problems: blurred vision, tinnitus; may indicate toxicity

Administer:
- With food to decrease GI symptoms; however, best to take on empty stomach to facilitate absorption

Perform/provide:
- Storage at room temp

Evaluate:
- Therapeutic response: decreased pain, stiffness in joints, decreased swelling in joints, ability to move more easily

Teach patient/family:
- To report blurred vision, ringing, roaring in ears; may indicate toxicity
- To avoid driving, other hazardous activities if dizziness, drowsiness occur, especially elderly
- To report change in urine pattern, increased weight, edema, increased pain in joints, fever, blood in urine; indicate nephrotoxicity
- That therapeutic effects may take up to 1 mo

Selected Generic Names

celecoxib
diclofenac
etodolac
fenoprofen
ibuprofen
indomethacin
ketoprofen
ketorolac
nabumetone
naproxen
piroxicam
sulindac

OPIOID ANALGESICS

Action: Opioid analgesics act by depressing pain impulse transmission at the spinal cord level by interacting with opioid receptors. Products are divided into opiates and nonopiates.

Uses: Most products are used to control moderate to severe pain and are used before and after surgery.

Side effects: GI symptoms, including nausea, vomiting, anorexia, constipation, and cramps are the most common side effects. Other common side effects include light-headedness, dizziness, sedation. Serious adverse reactions such as respiratory depression, respiratory arrest, circulatory depression, and increased intracranial pressure may result but are less common and usually dose dependent.

Contraindications: Hypersensitive reactions occur frequently. Check for sensitivity before administering. These drugs should be used cautiously if opiate addiction is suspected.

Precautions: Caution must be used when these products are given to a person with an addictive personality since the possibility of addiction is so great. Also, they may worsen intracranial pressure. Persons with severe heart disease, hepatic or renal disease, respiratory conditions, or seizure disorders should be monitored closely for worsening condition.

Pharmacokinetics: Onset of action is immediate by IV route and rapid by IM and PO routes. Peak occurs from 1-2 hr, depending on route, with a duration of 2-8 hr. These agents cross the placenta and appear in breast milk.

Interactions: Barbiturates, other opioids, hypnotics, antipsychotics, or alcohol can increase CNS depression when taken with opioids.

Possible nursing diagnoses:
• Acute pain *[uses]*
• Gas exchange, impaired *[adverse reactions]*

Nursing Considerations
Assess:
• I&O ratio; be alert for urinary retention, frequency, dysuria; drug should be discontinued if these occur
• Respiratory dysfunction, including respiratory depression, rate, rhythm, character; notify prescriber if respirations are <12/min
• CNS changes: dizziness, drowsiness, hallucinations, euphoria, LOC, pupil reaction
• Allergic reactions: rash, urticaria
• Need for pain medication; use pain scoring

Administer:
• With antiemetic if nausea or vomiting occurs
• When pain is beginning to return; determine dosage interval by response

Perform/provide:
• Assistance with ambulation; patient should not be ambulating during drug peak

Evaluate:
• Therapeutic response, including decrease in pain

Teach patient/family:
• To report any symptoms of CNS changes, allergic reactions, or shortness of breath
• That physical dependency may result when used for extended periods
• That withdrawal symptoms may occur, including nausea, vomiting, cramps, fever, faintness, anorexia
• To avoid alcohol and other CNS depressants

Selected Generic Names
alfentanil
buprenorphine
butorphanol
codeine
fentanyl
fentanyl transdermal
hydromorphone
meperidine
methadone
morphine
nalbuphine
oxycodone
oxymorphone
pentazocine
propoxyphene
remifentanil

SALICYLATES

Action: Salicylates have analgesic, anti-pyretic, and antiinflammatory effects. The antiinflammatory and analgesic activities may be mediated through the inhibition of prostaglandin synthesis. Antipyretic action results from inhibition of the hypothalamic heat-regulating center.

Uses: The primary uses of salicylates are relief of mild to moderate pain and fever and in inflammatory conditions such as arthritis, thromboembolic disorders, and rheumatic fever.

Side effects: The most common side effects are GI symptoms and rash. Serious blood dyscrasias and hepatotoxicity may result when used for long periods at high doses. Tinnitus or impaired hearing may indicate that blood salicylate levels are reaching or exceeding the upper limit of the therapeutic range.

Contraindications: Hypersensitivity to salicylates is common. Check for sensitivity before administering. Persons with bleeding disorders, GI bleeding, and vit K deficiency should not use these products since salicylates increase prothrombin time. Children should not use these products since salicylates have been associated with Reye's syndrome.

Precautions: Caution is needed when salicylates are given to patients with anemia, hepatic or renal disease, or Hodgkin's disease. Caution should also be exercised in pregnancy and lactation.

Pharmacokinetics: Onset of action occurs in 15-30 min, with a peak of 1-2 hr and a duration up to 6 hr. These drugs are metabolized by the liver and excreted by the kidneys.

Interactions: Increased effects of anticoagulants, insulin, methotrexate, heparin, valproic acid, and oral sulfonylureas may occur when used with salicylates. Aspirin may decrease serum concentrations of nonsteroidal antiinflammatory agents.

Possible nursing diagnoses:
- Acute, chronic pain *[uses]*
- Mobility, physical, impaired *[uses]*
- Activity intolerance *[uses]*
- Sensory/perceptual alterations: auditory *[adverse reactions]*
- Thermoregulation, ineffective *[uses]*

Nursing Considerations

Assess:
- Hepatic and renal studies: AST, ALT, bilirubin, creatinine, LDH, alk phosphatase, BUN if patient is on long-term therapy, since these products are metabolized and excreted by the liver and kidney
- Blood studies: CBC, hematocrit, hemoglobin, and prothrombin time if patient is on long-term therapy, since these products increase the possibility of bleeding and blood dyscrasias
- Hepatotoxicity: dark urine, clay-colored stools; yellowing of skin, sclera; itching, abdominal pain, fever, diarrhea, which may occur with long-term use
- Ototoxicity: tinnitus; ringing, roaring in ears; audiometric testing is needed before and after long-term therapy

Administer:
- With food or milk to decrease gastric irritation; give 30 min before or 1 hr after meals with a full glass of water

Evaluate:
- Therapeutic response, including decreased pain, fever

Teach patient/family:
- That blood glucose levels should be monitored closely if patient is diabetic
- Not to exceed recommended dosage; acute poisoning may result
- That therapeutic response takes 2 wk in arthritis
- To avoid use of alcohol, since GI bleeding may result
- To notify prescriber of ringing in the ears or persistent GI pain
- To take with full glass of water to reduce risk of lodging in esophagus

Selected Generic Names

aspirin
choline salicylate
magnesium salicylate
salsalate

THROMBOLYTICS

Action: Thrombolytics act by activating conversion of plasminogen to plasmin (fibrinolysin): plasmin is able to break down clots (fibrin).

Uses: Thrombolytics are used to treat deep vein thrombosis, pulmonary embolism, arterial thrombosis, arterial embolism, arteriovenous cannula occlusion, lysis of coronary artery thrombi after MI, and acute, evolving transmural MI.

Side effects: Serious adverse reactions include GI, GU, intracranial retroperitoneal bleeding, and anaphylaxis. The most common side effects are decreased Hct, urticaria, headache, and nausea.

Contraindications: Persons with hypersensitivity, active bleeding, intraspinal surgery, neoplasms of the CNS, ulcerative colitis/enteritis, severe hypertension, renal disease, hepatic disease, hypocoagulation, COPD, subacute bacterial endocarditis, rheumatic valvular disease, cerebral embolism/thrombosis/hemorrhage, recent intraarterial diagnostic procedure or surgery (10 days), and recent major surgery should not use these products.

Precautions: Caution should be used in arterial emboli from left side of heart and pregnancy.

Pharmacokinetics: Onset, peak, and duration vary widely among products. Most products are metabolized in the liver and excreted in urine.

Interactions: Please check individual monographs since interactions vary widely among products.

Possible nursing diagnoses:
• Injury, risk for *[uses]*

Nursing Considerations

Assess:
• VS, B/P, pulse, resp, neurologic signs, temp at least q4h; temp >104° F (40° C) indicator of internal bleeding; cardiac rhythm following intracoronary administration; systolic pressure increase of >25 mm Hg should be reported to prescriber
• For neurologic changes that may indicate intracranial bleeding

• Retroperitoneal bleeding: back pain, leg weakness, diminished pulses
• Allergy: fever, rash, itching, chill; mild reaction may be treated with antihistamines
• For bleeding during 1st hr of treatment: hematuria, hematemesis, bleeding from mucous membranes, epistaxis, ecchymosis
• Blood studies (Hct, platelets, PTT, PT, TT, APTT) before starting therapy; PT or APTT must be less than 2× control before starting therapy; or PT q3-4h during treatment

Administer:
• As soon as thrombi identified; not useful for thrombi over 1 wk old
• Cryoprecipitate or fresh, frozen plasma if bleeding occurs
• Loading dose at beginning of therapy; may require increased loading doses
• Heparin after fibrinogen level is over 100 mg/dl; heparin infusion to increase PTT to 1.5-2 × baseline for 3-7 days
• About 10% of patients have high streptococcal antibody titers requiring increased loading doses
• IV therapy using 0.8 μm filter

Perform/provide:
• Storage of reconstituted drug in refrigerator; discard after 24 hr
• Bed rest during entire course of treatment
• Avoidance of venous or arterial puncture, inj, rectal temp
• Treatment of fever with acetaminophen or aspirin
• Pressure for 30 sec to minor bleeding sites; inform prescriber if this does not attain hemostasis; apply pressure dressing

Evaluate:
• Therapeutic response: resolution of thrombosis, embolism

Selected Generic Names

alteplase
anistreplase
drotrecogin alfa
streptokinase
tenecteplase
urokinase

THYROID HORMONES

Action: Acts by increasing metabolic rates, resulting in increased cardiac output, O_2 consumption, body temp, blood volume, growth, development at cellular level, respiratory rate, enzyme system activity.

Uses: Products are used for thyroid replacement.

Side effects: The most common side effects include insomnia, tremors, tachycardia, palpitations, angina, dysrhythmias, weight loss, and changes in appetite. Serious adverse reactions include thyroid storm.

Contraindications: Persons with adrenal insufficiency, myocardial infarction, or thyrotoxicosis should not use these products.

Precautions: The elderly and patients with angina pectoris, hypertension, ischemia, cardiac disease, or diabetes mellitus or insipidus should be watched closely when using these products. Caution should be used in pregnancy (A) and lactation.

Pharmacokinetics: Pharmacokinetics vary widely among products; check specific monographs.

Interactions:

• Impaired absorption of thyroid products may occur when administered with cholestyramine, iron products (separate by 4-5 hr)

• Increased effects of anticoagulants, sympathomimetics, tricyclic antidepressants, catecholamines may occur

• Decreased effects of digitalis, glycosides, insulin, hypoglycemics may occur

• Decreased effects of thyroid products may occur with estrogens

Possible nursing diagnoses:

• Knowledge, deficient *[teaching]*

• Noncompliance *[teaching]*

• Body image, disturbed *[adverse reactions]*

Nursing Considerations

Assess:

• B/P, pulse before each dose

• I&O ratio

• Weight daily in same clothing, using same scale, at same time of day

• PT should be closely monitored and dosage of anticoagulant therapy may need adjustment

• Height, growth rate if given to a child

• T_3, T_4, which are decreased; radioimmunoassay of TSH, which is increased; ratio uptake, which is decreased if patient is on too low a dosage of medication

• Increased nervousness, excitability, irritability; may indicate overdosage, usually after 1-3 wk of treatment

• Cardiac status: angina, palpitation, chest pain, change in VS

Administer:

• At same time each day to maintain drug level

• Only for hormone imbalances, not to be used for obesity, male infertility, menstrual conditions, lethargy

Perform/provide:

• Removal of medication 4 wk before RAIU test

Evaluate:

• Therapeutic response: absence of depression; increased weight loss; diuresis; pulse; appetite; absence of constipation; peripheral edema; cold intolerance; pale, cool, dry skin; brittle nails; alopecia; coarse hair; menorrhagia; night blindness; paresthesias; syncope; stupor; coma; rosy cheeks

Teach patient/family:

• That hair loss will occur in child and is temporary

• To report excitability, irritability, anxiety, chest pain, palpitations, increased pulse, excessive sweating, heat intolerance; indicates overdose

• Not to switch brands unless directed by prescriber

• That hypothyroid child will show almost immediate behavior/personality change

• That treatment drug is not to be taken to reduce weight
• To avoid OTC preparations with iodine; read labels
• To avoid iodine in food, iodinized salt, soybeans, tofu, turnips, some seafood, some bread

Selected Generic Names

levothyroxine (T_4)
liothyronine (T_3)
liotrix
thyroid USP

VASODILATORS

Action: Vasodilators have various modes of action. Please check individual monographs for specific action.

Uses: Vasodilators are used to treat intermittent claudication, arteriosclerosis obliterans, vasospasm and muscular ischemia, ischemic cerebral vascular disease, hypertension, and angina.

Side effects: The most common side effects are headache, nausea, hypotension or hypertension, and ECG changes.

Contraindications: Some drugs are contraindicated in acute MI, paroxysmal tachycardia, and thyrotoxicosis.

Precautions: Caution should be used in uncompensated heart disease or peptic ulcer disease.

Pharmacokinetics: Onset, peak, and duration vary widely among products. Most products are metabolized in the liver and excreted in urine.

Interactions: Please check individual monographs since interactions vary widely among products.

Possible nursing diagnoses:
• Cardiac output, decreased *[uses]*
• Tissue perfusion, ineffective *[uses]*
• Knowledge, deficient *[teaching]*

Nursing Considerations

Assess:
• Bleeding time in individuals with bleeding disorders
• Cardiac status: B/P, pulse, rate, rhythm, character; watch for increasing pulse

Administer:
• With meals to reduce GI symptoms

Perform/provide:
• Storage in tight container at room temp

Evaluate:
• Therapeutic response: ability to walk without pain, increased temp in extremities, increased pulse volume

Teach patient/family:
• That medication is not cure; may need to be taken continuously
• That it is necessary to quit smoking to prevent excessive vasoconstriction
• That improvement may be sudden, but usually occurs gradually over several wk
• To report headache, weakness, increased pulse, as drug may have to be decreased or discontinued
• To avoid hazardous activities until stabilized on medication; dizziness may occur

Selected Generic Names

amyl nitrite
bosentan
dipyridamole
hydrALAZINE
isoxsuprine
midodrine
minoxidil
nesiritide
papaverine

VITAMINS

Action: Action varies widely among products and classes; check specific monographs.

Uses: Vitamins are used to correct and prevent vitamin deficiencies.

Side effects: There are no side effects or adverse reactions with the water-soluble vitamins (C, B). However, fat-soluble vitamins (A, D, E, K) may accumulate in the body and cause adverse reactions (see specific monographs).

Contraindications: Hypersensitive reactions may occur, and allergies should be identified before these products are given.

Pharmacokinetics: Onset, peak, and duration vary widely among products; check individual monographs for specific information.

Possible nursing diagnoses:
• Nutrition: less than body requirements, imbalanced *[uses]*

Nursing Considerations

Administer:
• PO with food for better absorption

Perform/provide:
• Storage in tight, light-resistant container

Evaluate:
• Therapeutic response: no vitamin deficiency

Teach patient/family:
• Not to take more than prescribed amount

Selected Generic Names

Fat-soluble
phytonadione (vitamin K_1)
vitamin A
vitamin D
vitamin E

Water-soluble
ascorbic acid (C)
cyanocobalamin B_{12}
pyridoxine (B_6)
riboflavin (B_2)
thiamine (B_1)

Miscellaneous
multivitamins

MECHANISMS AND SITES OF ACTION

*For Canadian Recommended Immunization Schedule for Infants and Children, see Appendix S

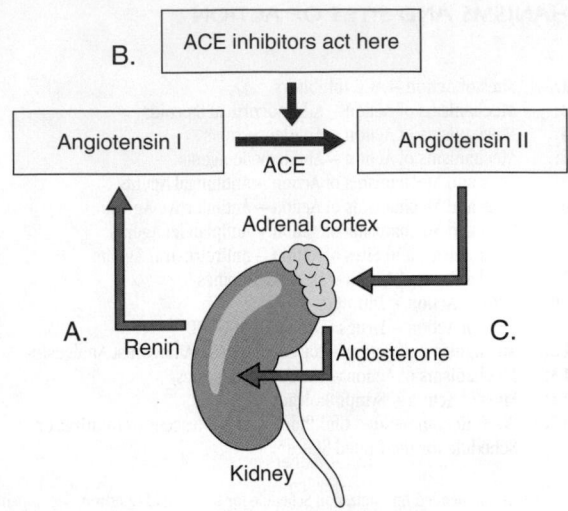

Plate 1:   Sites of Action – ACE Inhibitors

The renin-angiotensin-aldosterone system plays a major role in regulating BP. Any condition that decreases renal blood flow, reduces BP, or stimulates beta$_1$-adrenergic receptors prompts the kidneys to release renin (A). Renin acts on angiotensinogen, which is converted to angiotensin I, a weak vasoconstrictor. Angiotensin-converting enzyme (ACE) converts angiotensin I to angiotensin II, which causes systemic and renal blood vessels to constrict (B). Systemic vasoconstriction increases peripheral vascular resistance, raising the BP. Renal vasoconstriction decreases glomerular filtration, resulting in sodium and water retention and increasing blood volume and BP. In addition, angiotensin II also acts on the adrenal cortex causing it to release aldosterone (C). This makes the kidneys retain additional sodium and water, which further increases the BP.

ACE inhibitors, such as captopril, enalapril, and lisinopril, block the action of ACE. As a result, angiotensin II can't form, which prevents systemic and renal vasoconstriction and the release of aldosterone. (From Prosser S, Worster B, Dewar K: *Applied Pharmacology for Nurses and Other Health Care Professionals*, St. Louis, 2000, Mosby.)

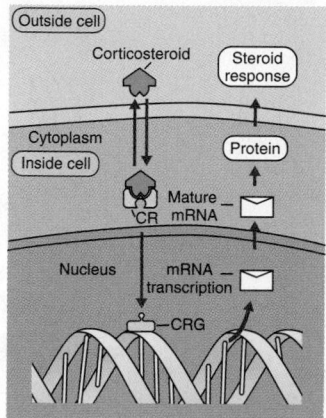

Plate 2: Mechanisms of Action – Adrenocortical Steroids

Adrenocortical steroids (also called corticosteroids) are available in many forms, such as predniSONE, and produce a wide range of effects, such as immunosupression and anti-inflammation. Here's how these drugs work at the cellular level.

Corticosteroids are hormones that are naturally produced by the body (endogenous hormones). Synthetic corticosteroids work much the same as the endogenous hormones. When a corticosteroid enters a cell, it binds to corticosteroid receptors (CRs) in the cell's cytoplasm, forming a complex. The complex moves to the nucleus where it causes the transcription of corticosteroid responsive genes (CRGs) to messenger ribonucleic acid (mRNA), eventually translating to a protein that produces a steroid response in target tissues. (From Taylor: *Mosby's Crash Course Pharmacology*, St. Louis, 1998, Mosby.)

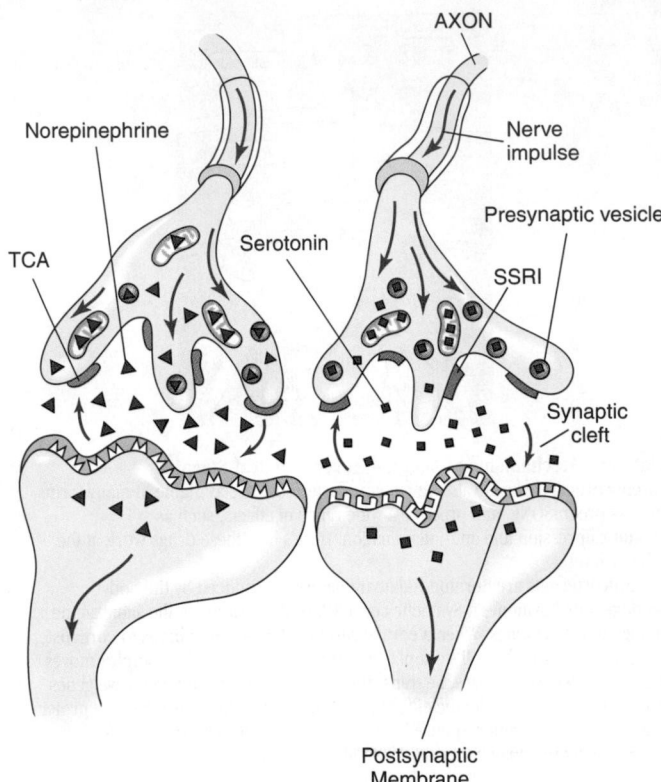

Plate 3:   Mechanisms of Action – Antidepressants

Depression is thought to occur when levels of neurotransmitters, such as norepinephrine and serotonin, are reduced at postsynaptic receptor sites. These neurotransmitters affect a wide array of functions, including mood, obsessions, appetite, and anxiety. Antidepressants work by increasing the availability of these neurotransmitters at postsynaptic membranes and by enhancing and prolonging their effects. As a result, these agents improve mood, reduce anxiety, and minimize obsessions.

Antidepressants typically are classified as tricyclic antidepressants (TCAs), monoamine oxidase inhibitors (not shown), selective serotonin reuptake inhibitors (SSRIs), and atypical antidepressants (not shown). TCAs, such as amitriptyline and desipramine, primarily block norepinephrine reuptake at presynaptic membranes, thereby increasing the norepinephrine concentration at synapses and making more available at postsynaptic receptors (A).

SSRIs, such as fluoxetine and paroxetine, selectively inhibit serotonin uptake at presynaptic membranes. This action leads to increased serotonin availability at postsynaptic receptors (B). (From Gutierrez K: *Pharmacotherapeutics: Clinical Decision Making in Nursing*, Philadelphia, 1999, Saunders.)

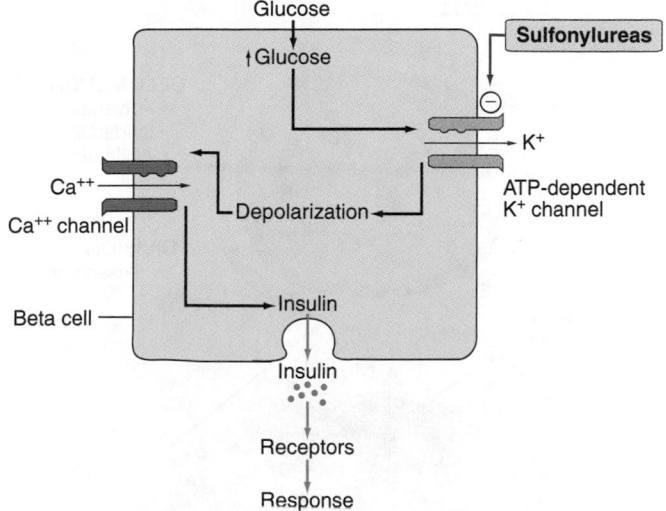

Plate 4:   Mechanisms of Action – Antidiabetic Agents

Diabetes mellitus takes two forms: type 1 diabetes characterized by a complete lack of insulin and type 2 diabetes marked by insufficient insulin secretion, insulin resistance in peripheral tissues, or both. Normally, the beta cells in the pancreatic islets of Langerhans are responsible for secreting insulin. When glucose levels rise in the beta cell, it triggers adenosine triphosphate (ATP)-dependent potassium (K^+) channels in the membranes of beta cells to close. Then the beta cells depolarize and calcium (Ca^{++}) enters the cell through Ca^{++} channel, and insulin is released from the cell. When circulating insulin engages with insulin receptors on cell membranes, it facilitates the movement of glucose into the cell, among other actions.

Type 1 diabetes is treated with the use of exogenous insulin, which mimics natural insulin in the body. Insulin takes many forms with varying degrees of onset, peak and duration, including rapid, regular, intermediate, and long-acting.

Type 2 diabetes is usually treated with oral agents. Sulfonylureas, such as glyburide for example, block ATP-dependent K^+ channels in the cell membranes of beta cells, ultimately resulting in the release of insulin. (From Taylor: *Mosby's Crash Course Pharmacology*, St. Louis, 1998, Mosby.)

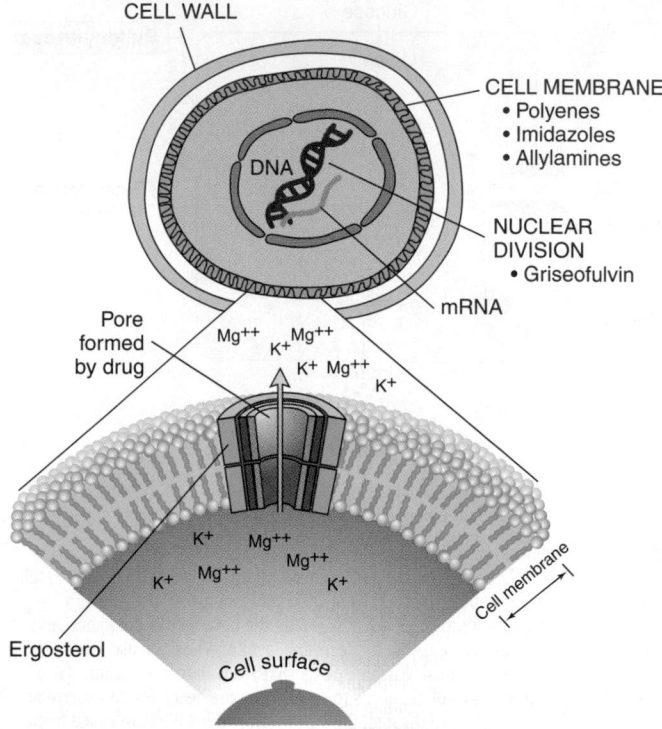

CELL WALL

CELL MEMBRANE
• Polyenes
• Imidazoles
• Allylamines

DNA

NUCLEAR
DIVISION
• Griseofulvin

mRNA

Pore
formed
by drug

Mg^{++} Mg^{++}

K^+ K^+ Mg^{++}

K^+

Ergosterol

K^+ Mg^{++} Mg^{++} K^+

K^+ Mg^{++} Mg^{++} K^+

Cell membrane

Cell surface

Plate 5:   Sites and Mechanisms of Action – Antifungal Agents
Antifungal agents primarily affect fungi at one of two sites: the cell membrane or the
cell nucleus. Most of these agents, such as polyene, imidazole, and allylamine
antifungals, act on the fungal cell membrane. Polyene antifungals, such as
amphotericin B, bind to ergosterol and increase cell membrane permeability.
Imidazole antifungals, such as fluconazole and ketoconazole, interfere with
ergosterol synthesis by inhibiting the cytochrome P_{450} enzyme system, altering the
cell membrane, and inhibiting fungal growth. Allylamine antifungals, such as
terbinafine, inhibit the enzyme squaline epoxidase, which disrupts ergosterol
production—and cell membrane integrity. When cell membrane permeability
increases, cellular components, including potassium (K^+) and magnesium (Mg^{++}),
leak out. Loss of these cellular components leads to cell death.
    Another antifungal agent, griseofulvin directly affects the fungal nucleus,
interfering with mitosis. By binding to structures in the mitotic spindle, it prevents
cells from dividing, which eventually leads to their death. (From Gutierrez K:
Pharmacotherapeutics: Clinical Decision Making in Nursing, Philadelphia, 1999,
Saunders.)

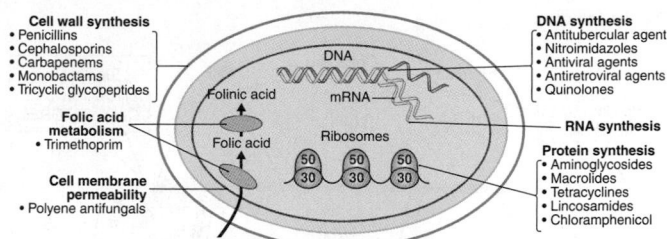

Plate 6:   Sites and Mechanisms of Action – Antiinfective Agents

The goal of anti-infective therapy is to kill or inhibit the growth of microorganisms, such as bacteria, viruses, and fungi. To achieve this goal, anti-infective agents must reach their targets, which usually occurs through absorption and distribution by the circulatory system. When the target is reached, a drug can kill or suppress microorganisms by:

- inhibiting cell wall synthesis or activating enzymes that disrupt the cell wall, which leads to cellular weakening, lysis, and death. Penicillins (ampicillin), cephalosporins (cefazolin), carbapenems (imipenem), monobactams (aztreonam), and tricyclic glycopeptides (vancomycin) act in this way.
- altering cell membrane permeability through direct action on the cell wall, which allows intracellular substances to leak out and destabilizes the cell. Polyene antifungals (amphotericin) work by this mechanism.
- altering protein synthesis by binding to bacterial ribosomes (50/30) or affecting ribosomal function, which leads to cell death or slowed growth respectively. Aminoglycosides (gentamicin), macrolides (erythromycin), tetracyclines (doxycycline), lincosamides (clindamycin), and the miscellaneous antiinfective chloramphenicol act in this way.
- inhibiting DNA or RNA, including messenger RNA (mRNA), by synthesis by binding to nucleic acids or interacting with enzymes required for their synthesis. Antitubercular agents (rifampin), nitroimidazoles (metronidazole), antiviral agents (acyclovir), antiretroviral agents (stavudine), and quinolones (ciprofloxacin) act like this.
- inhibiting the metabolism of folic acid and folinic acid or other cellular components that are essential for bacterial cell growth. The miscellaneous anti-infective trimethoprim employs this mechanism of action. (From Page C, et al: *Integrated Pharmacology*, ed 2, St. Louis, 2002, Mosby.)

Platelet Activation

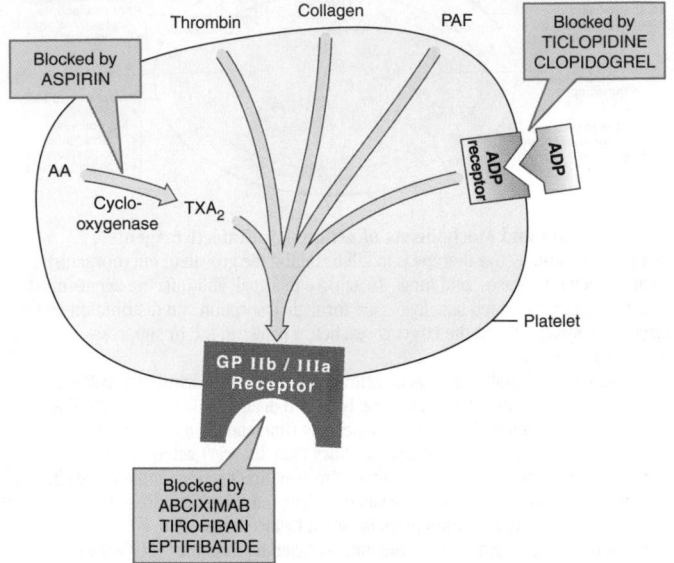

Plate 7:   Sites and Mechanisms of Action – Antiplatelet Agents

Antiplatelet drugs are prescribed to prevent arterial thrombosis because they prevent platelet aggregation. These drugs include aspirin, adenosine diphosphate (ADP) receptor antagonists, or glycoprotein (GP) receptor IIb/IIIa antagonists. The degree of antiplatelet activity exerted by each drug or drug class depends on where the drug acts in the platelet activation pathway.

Aspirin suppresses platelet aggregation and vasoconstriction by inhibiting cylooxygenase, an enzyme that's needed to create thromboxane A_2 (TXA_2) from arachidonic acid (AA). TXA_2 is responsible for platelet activation and vasoconstriction.

ADP receptor antagonists, such as ticlopidine and clopidogrel, block ADP receptors on the surface of platelets, preventing platelet aggregation.

GP receptor IIb/IIIa inhibitors, such as abciximab, tirofiban, and eptifibatide, are powerful antiplatelet agents because they prevent platelet aggregation in the common pathway, whether aggregation is triggered by thromboxane, ADP, or another factor. These drugs block GP IIb/IIIa receptors from the effects of fibrinogen, thrombin, platelet activating factor (PAF), collagen, and other adhesive molecules. (From Lehne RA: *Pharmacology for Nursing Care*, ed 5, St. Louis, 2004, Saunders.)

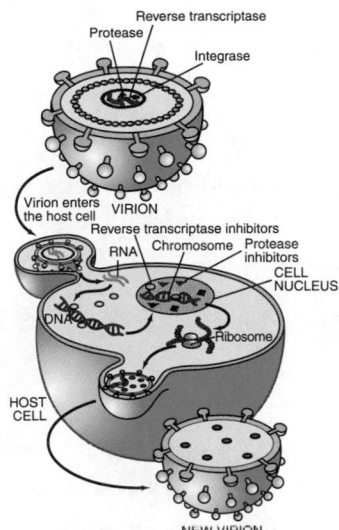

Plate 8: Mechanisms and Sites of Action – Antiretroviral Agents

To understand how antiretroviral agents work, you need to know how viruses reproduce. First, the infectious viral particle or virion (A) enters the host cell. The virion attaches to the cell's surface and then inserts itself into the host cell (B). Once inside, the virion uncoats, and the enzyme reverse transcriptase makes two copies of the viral RNA: one copy is identical; the other is a mirror image. These two copies merge to form double-stranded viral DNA. This newly formed viral DNA enters the host cell's nucleus, where it inserts itself into the host cell's DNA with the help of the enzyme integrase. Then viral DNA reprograms the host cell to produce additional viral RNA, which begins the process of forming new viruses. Specifically, messenger RNA (mRNA) instructs ribosomal RNA (rRNA) to produce a new chain of proteins and enzymes that are used to form new viruses. Protease, another enzyme, cuts the chains of proteins, creating individual proteins. These individual proteins combine with new RNA to create new virions, which bud and are then released from the host cell (C).

Antiretroviral agents target specific enzymes during viral reproduction. Many of them work to inhibit reverse transcriptase. Nucleoside reverse transcriptase inhibitors, such as stavudine, interfere with the action of reverse transcriptase by mimicking naturally occurring nucleosides. Nucleotide reverse transcriptase inhibitors, such as tenofovir, block reverse transcriptase by competing with the natural substrate deoxyadenosine triphosphate and by causing DNA chain termination. Nonnucleoside reverse transcriptase inhibitors, such as delavirdine, work by directly binding to reverse transcriptase. All of these actions block the conversion of single-stranded viral RNA into double-stranded DNA. As a result, no viral DNA is available to insert itself into the host cell's DNA. Protease inhibitors, such as indinavir, bind to and interefere with the action of protease. By blocking protease, the new chain of proteins formed by rRNA can't be cut into individual proteins to make new viruses. (From Gutierrez K: *Pharmacotherapeutics: Clinical Decision Making in Nursing*, Philadelphia, 1999, Saunders.)

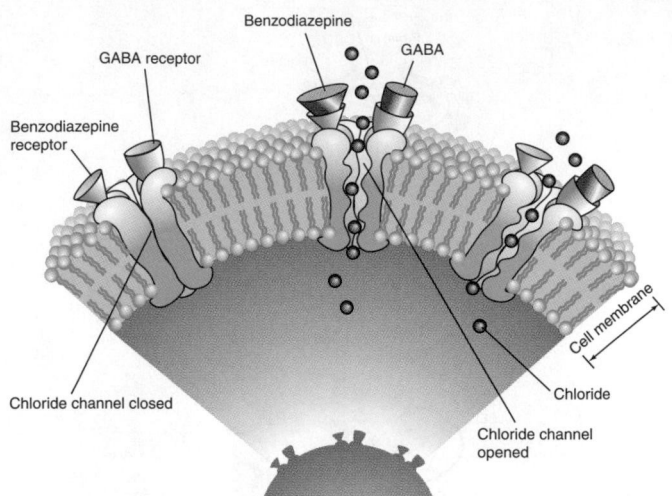

Plate 9:   Mechanisms of Action – Benzodiazepines

Benzodiazepines reduce anxiety by stimulating the action of the inhibitory neurotransmitter, gamma-aminobutyric acid (GABA), in the limbic system. The limbic system plays an important role in the regulation of human behavior. Dysfunction of GABA neurotransmission in the limbic system may be linked to the development of certain anxiety disorders.

The limbic system contains a highly dense area of benzodiazepine receptors that may be linked to the antianxiety effects of benzodiazepines. These benzodiazepine receptors are located on the surface of neuronal cell membranes and are adjacent to GABA receptors. The binding of a benzodiazepine to its receptor enhances the affinity of a GABA receptor for GABA. In the absence of a benzodiazepine, the binding of GABA to its receptor causes the chloride channel in the cell membrane to open, which increases the influx of chloride into the cell. This influx of chloride results in hyperpolarization of the neuronal cell membrane and reduces the neuron's ability to fire, which is why GABA is considered an inhibitory neurotransmitter.

A benzodiazepine acts only in the presence of GABA. When it binds to a benzodiazepine receptor, it prolongs the time that the chloride channel remains open. This results in greater depression of neuronal function and a reduction in anxiety. (From Gutierrez K: *Pharmacotherapeutics: Clinical Decision Making in Nursing*, Philadelphia, 1999, Saunders.)

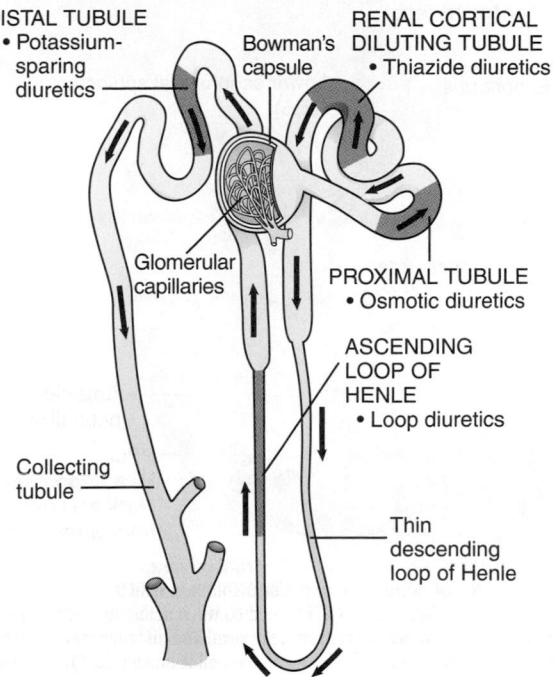

Plate 10: Sites of Action – Diuretics

Diuretics act primarily to increase water and sodium excretion by the kidneys, thereby increasing urine output. In the process, chloride, potassium, and other electrolytes may also be excreted. Most diuretics act by blocking sodium, water, and chloride reabsorption by peritubular capillaries in the nephrons. Water and electrolytes remain in the convoluted tubules to be excreted as urine. The increased water and electrolyte excretion reduces blood volume—and ultimately blood pressure.

Diuretics belong to four major subclasses:

1. Thiazide diuretics, such as hydrochlorothiazide, act in the cortical diluting segment. These drugs block sodium, chloride, and water reabsorption and promote their excretion along with potassium.

2. Loop diuretics, such as furosemide, act primarily in the thick ascending limb of the loop of Henle, blocking sodium, water, and chloride reabsorption. Then these substances are excreted along with potassium.

3. Potassium-sparing diuretics, such as spironolactone, act in the late portion of the distal convoluted tubule and collecting tubule. Here, they inhibit the action of aldosterone, leading to sodium excretion and potassium retention. Although triamterene and amiloride act at the same site they don't affect aldosterone. Instead, these drugs directly block the exchange of sodium and potassium, leading to decreased sodium reabsorption and decreased potassium excretion.

4. Osmotic diuretics, such as mannitol, work in the proximal convoluted tubule. As their name implies, these diuretics increase the osmotic pressure of the glomerular filtrate, inhibiting the passive reabsorption of water, sodium, and chloride. (From Gutierrez K: *Pharmacotherapeutics: Clinical Decision Making in Nursing*, Philadelphia, 1999, Saunders.)

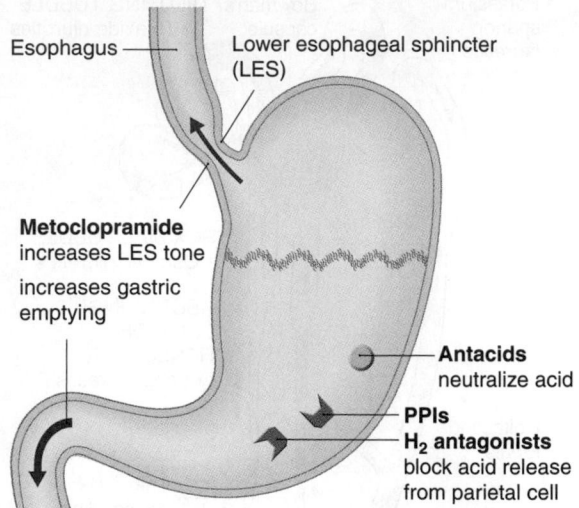

Esophagus

Lower esophageal sphincter (LES)

Metoclopramide
increases LES tone

increases gastric emptying

Antacids
neutralize acid

PPIs
H₂ antagonists
block acid release from parietal cell

Plate 11:   Sites of Action – Drugs Used To Treat GERD

Gastroesophageal reflux disease (GERD) occurs when acidic stomach contents regurgitate into the esophagus, causing heartburn. The disorder may result from a weakness or incompetence of the lower esophageal sphincter (LES). Because the malfunctioning LES makes the reflux leave the esophagus and re-enter the stomach slowly, the esophageal mucosa is exposed to the acid for a long time. Because the enzymatic action of parietal cells in the stomach makes the reflux highly acidic, GERD causes irritation and possible erosion of the esophageal mucosa.

Treatment of GERD can employ drugs from several classes: histamine (H_2) antagonists, proton pump inhibitors (PPIs), the miscellaneous GI agent metoclopramide, and antacids. H_2 antagonists, such as cimetidine, act in parietal cells of the stomach. Normally, H_2-receptor stimulation results in gastric acid secretion. By blocking these receptors, H_2 antagonists decrease the amount and acidity of gastric secretion, including secretion that occurs with fasting, food consumption at night, and stomach distension.

PPIs, such as esomeprazole, also suppress gastric acid secretion. However, they do it by inhibiting the hydrogen-potassium-adenosine triphsophatase enzyme system, which is located on the surface of parietal cells and controls their gastric acid secretion. PPIs block acid secretion that results from fasting or abdominal distension caused by food ingestion.

Metoclopramide increases the tone and motility of the upper GI tract. It works by stimulating the release of acetylcholine from GI nerve endings, which improves LES tone and leads to decreased reflux. The drug also stimulates gastric emptying, which reduces gastric contents.

Antacids, such as aluminum hydroxide, act primarily in the stomach by chemically combining with the hydrogen ions (H^+) in gastric acid and raising the pH of gastric contents. They don't prevent reflux. However, they make the reflux less acidic, so it causes less damage to the esophageal mucosa. (From Page C, et al: *Integrated Pharmacology*, ed 2, St. Louis, 2002, Mosby.)

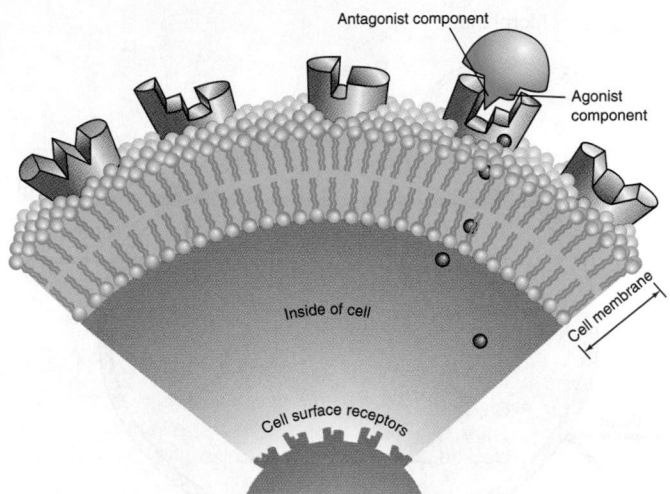

Plate 12: Mechanisms of Action – Narcotic Agonist-Antagonists Analgesics

Cell membranes have different types of opioid receptors, such as mu, kappa, and delta receptors. Opioid agonist-antagonists work by stimulating one type of receptor, while simultaneously blocking another type. As agonists, they work primarily by activating kappa receptors to produce analgesia and such other effects as CNS and respiratory depression, decreased GI motility, and euphoria. As antagonists, they compete with opioids at mu receptors, helping to reverse or block some of the other effects of agonists. (From Gutierrez K: *Pharmacotherapeutics: Clinical Decision Making in Nursing*, Philadelphia, 1999, Saunders.)

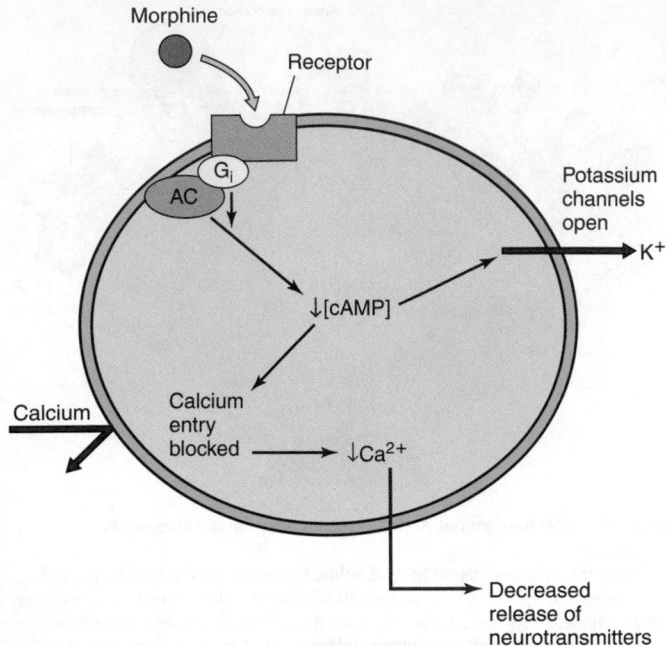

Plate 13:   Mechanisms of Action – Narcotic Analgesics
Narcotic analgesics bind to three types of opioid receptors: mu, kappa, and delta receptors. They produce analgesia primarily by activating mu receptors. However, they also engage with and activate kappa and delta receptors, producing other effects, such as sedation and vasomotor stimulation.

When morphine or another narcotic analgesic binds to opioid receptors, activation occurs. The receptors send signals to the enzyme adenyl cyclase (AC) to slow activity by way of G proteins (G_i). Decreased adenyl cyclase activity causes less cyclic adenosine monophosphate (cAMP) to be produced. A secondary messenger substance, cAMP is important for regulating cell membrane channels. A reduced cAMP level allows fewer potassium ions to leave the cell and blocks calcium ions from entering the cell. This ion imbalance—especially the reduced intracellular calcium level—ultimately decreases the release of neurotransmitters from the cell, thereby blocking or reducing pain impulse transmission. (From Brody TM, Larner J, Minneman KP: *Human Pharmacology: Molecular to Clinical*, ed 3, St. Louis, 1998, Mosby.)

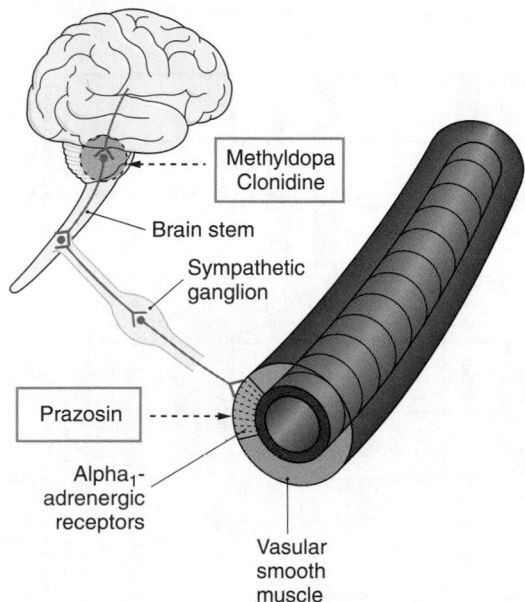

Plate 14:   Sites of Action – Sympatholytics

Sympatholytics inhibit sympathetic nervous system (SNS) activity, which plays a major role in regulating BP. Normally when the SNS is stimulated, nerve impulses travel from the cardiovascular center of the CNS to the sympathetic ganglia. From there, the impulses travel along postganglionic fibers to specific effector organs, such as the heart and blood vessels. SNS stimulation also triggers the release of norepinephrine, which acts primarily at alpha-adrenergic receptors.

Sympatholytics fall into two subclasses: central-acting alpha$_2$ agonists and peripheral-acting alpha$_1$-adrenergic antagonists. Central-acting alpha$_2$ agonists, such as methyldopa and clonidine, stimulate alpha$_2$-adrenergic receptors in the cardiovascular center of the CNS and reduce activity in the vasomotor center of the brain, interfering with sympathetic stimulation of the heart and blood vessels. This causes blood vessel dilation and decreased cardiac output, which leads to reduced BP.

Peripheral-acting alpha$_1$-adrenergic antagonists, such as prazosin, inhibit the stimulation of alpha$_1$-adrenergic receptors by norepinephrine in vascular smooth muscle, interfering with SNS-induced vasoconstriction. As a result, the blood vessels dilate, reducing peripheral vascular resistance and venous return to the heart. These effects, in turn, lead to decreased BP. (From Prosser S, Worster B, Dewar K: *Applied Pharmacology for Nurses and Other Health Care Professionals*, St. Louis, 2000, Mosby.)

Recommended Childhood and Adolescent Immunization Schedule · UNITED STATES · 2006

Vaccine ▼ / Age ▶	Birth	1 month	2 months	4 months	6 months	12 months	15 months	18 months	24 months	4–6 years	11–12 years	13–14 years	15 years	16–18 years
Hepatitis B[1]	HepB	HepB		HepB[1]		HepB					HepB Series			
Diphtheria, Tetanus, Pertussis[2]			DTaP	DTaP	DTaP		DTaP	DTaP		DTaP	Tdap		Tdap	
Haemophilus influenzae type b[3]			Hib	Hib	Hib[3]		Hib							
Inactivated Poliovirus			IPV	IPV	IPV		IPV			IPV				
Measles, Mumps, Rubella[4]						MMR	MMR			MMR	MMR	MMR	MMR	
Varicella[5]						Varicella		Varicella			Varicella	Varicella		
Meningococcal[6]							Vaccines within broken line are for selected populations		MPSV4		MCV4		MCV4 / MCV4	
Pneumococcal[7]			PCV	PCV	PCV	PCV	PCV		PCV	PCV	PPV			
Influenza[8]						Influenza (Yearly)	Influenza (Yearly)				Influenza (Yearly)			
Hepatitis A[9]										HepA Series				

This schedule indicates the recommended ages for routine administration of currently licensed childhood vaccines, as of December 1, 2005, for children through age 18 years. Any dose not administered at the recommended age should be administered at any subsequent visit when indicated and feasible. ▪ Indicates age groups that warrant special effort to administer those vaccines not previously administered. Additional vaccines may be licensed and recommended during the year. Licensed combination vaccines may be used whenever any components of the combination are indicated and other components of the vaccine are not contraindicated and if approved by the Food and Drug Administration for that dose of the series. Providers should consult the respective ACIP statement for detailed recommendations. Clinically significant adverse events that follow immunization should be reported to the Vaccine Adverse Event Reporting System (VAERS). Guidance about how to obtain and complete a VAERS form is available at www.vaers.hhs.gov or by telephone, 800-822-7967.

Range of recommended ages   Catch-up immunization   11–12 year old assessment

Vaccines within broken line are for selected populations

For more information, go to http://www.cdc.gov/nip/recs/child-schedule.htm#printable

abacavir (℞)
(ah-bak′ah-veer)
Ziagen
Func. class.: Antiretroviral
Chem. class.: Nucleoside reverse
transcriptase inhibitor (NRTI)

Action: A synthetic nucleoside analog
with inhibitory action against HIV. Inhibits replication of the virus by incorporating into cellular DNA by viral reverse
transcriptase, thereby terminating the
cellular DNA chain

Uses: In combination with other antiretroviral agents for HIV-1 infection

DOSAGE AND ROUTES

• *Adult:* **PO** 300 mg bid or 600 mg daily
with other antiretrovirals
• *Adolescents and child ≥3 mo:* **PO** 8
mg/kg bid, max 300 mg bid with other
antiretrovirals
Hepatic dose
• *Adult:* **PO** (oral sol) (Child-Pugh 5-6)
200 mg bid
Available forms: Tabs 300 mg; oral
sol 20 mg/ml

SIDE EFFECTS

CNS: Fever, headache, malaise, insomnia, paresthesia
GI: Nausea, vomiting, diarrhea, anorexia, cramps, abdominal pain, increased AST, ALT, **hepatotoxicity**
*HEMA: **Granulocytopenia, anemia, lymphopenia***
INTEG: Rash, urticaria
*META: **Lactic acidosis***
OTHER: Increased CPK, **fatal hypersensitivity reactions**
RESP: Dyspnea

Contraindications: Hypersensitivity,
lactic acidosis

Precautions: Pregnancy (C), granulocyte count <1000/mm^3 or Hgb <9.5 g/dl,
lactation, children, severe renal disease,
impaired hepatic function

PHARMACOKINETICS

50% plasma protein binding, extensively metabolized to inactive metabolites, half-life 1½ hr, excreted in urine,
feces

INTERACTIONS

Possible lactic acidosis: ribavirin
Increase: abacavir levels—alcohol
Decrease: levels of—methadose

NURSING CONSIDERATIONS
Assess:
⚠ For lactic acidosis (elevated lactate
levels, increased LFTs, severe hepatomegaly) with steatosis, discontinue treatment and do not restart
⚠ For fatal hypersensitivity reactions:
fever, rash, nausea, vomiting, fatigue,
cough, dyspnea, diarrhea, abdominal
discomfort; treatment should be discontinued and not restarted
• For blood dyscrasias (anemia,
granulocytopenia): bruising, fatigue,
bleeding, poor healing
• For increased temp, may indicate
beginning infection
• Renal studies: BUN, serum uric acid,
CCr before, during therapy; these may be
elevated throughout treatment
• Hepatic studies before and during
therapy: bilirubin, AST, ALT, amylase, alk
phosphatase, creatine phosphokinase,
creatinine, q mo
• Blood counts q2wk; monitor viral load
and CD4 counts during treatment; watch
for decreasing granulocytes, Hgb; if low,
therapy may have to be discontinued and
restarted after hematologic recovery;
blood transfusions may be required
Administer:
• Give in combination with other antiretrovirals with or without food
• Reduce dose in hepatic disease, use
oral sol
Perform/provide:
• Storage in cool environment; protect
from light; do not freeze, oral sol stored
at room temp

Teach patient/family:
- That drug is not a cure for AIDS but will control symptoms
- To notify prescriber of sore throat, swollen lymph nodes, malaise, fever; other infections may occur; to stop drug if skin rash, fever, cough, shortness of breath, GI symptoms, notify prescriber immediately; advise all health care providers that allergic reaction has occurred with abacavir
- That patient is still infective, may pass AIDS virus on to others
- That follow-up visits must be continued since serious toxicity may occur; blood counts must be done
- To use contraception during treatment
- Give patient Medication Guide and Warning Card, discuss points on guide
- That other drugs may be necessary to prevent other infections
- Do not drink alcohol while taking this drug

---

abarelix (℞)
(a-ba-rel′iks)
Plenaxis
Func. class.: Gonadotropin-releasing hormone antagonist
Chem. class.: Synthetic decapeptide

Action: Inhibitor of pituitary gonadotropin secretion; inhibits LH, FSH, thereby reducing testosterone
Uses: Palliative treatment of prostate cancer

DOSAGE AND ROUTES

- *Adult:* **IM** 100 mg in buttock on day 1, 15, 29 (wk 4), and every 4 wk thereafter
Available forms: Powder for inj 113 mg

SIDE EFFECTS

CNS: Headache, dizziness, fatigue, sleep disturbance
ENDO: Breast enlargement, nipple tenderness
GI: Nausea, constipation, diarrhea
GU: Dysuria, frequency, retention, UTI

INTEG: Pain on inj; local site reactions
MISC: Pain including back pain, hot flashes
*SYST: **Anaphylaxis, systemic allergic reaction,** decreased bone density* (long-term treatment)
Contraindications: Pregnancy (X), hypersensitivity, latex allergy, lactation, children

PHARMACOKINETICS

Excreted in urine, half-life depends on dosage, protein binding 96%-99%

NURSING CONSIDERATIONS

Assess:
- Anaphylaxis: swelling of face, throat, eyes, tongue, chest tightness, difficulty breathing; hypotension, fainting, shock, if these occur, usually occur within ½ hr of administration
- For ALT, AST, GGT, alk phosphatase

Administer:
- Reconstitute 1 vial with provided diluent (50 mg/ml)
- Before reconstituting gently shake vial; hold at 45-degree angle and tap lightly to break caking; withdraw 2.2 ml of 0.9% NaCl inj using 18-gauge, 1½-inch needle and 3-ml syringe enclosed; discard remaining unused diluent
- Keeping vial upright, insert needle all the way in the vial and inject diluent quickly; withdraw needle, removing 2.2 ml of air; shake for several seconds; allow vial to stand for 2 min; tap to remove foam, swirl

Perform/provide:
- Storage between 59°-80° F; use within 1 hr of reconstitution

Evaluate:
- Therapeutic response: reduction in growth of tumor

Teach patient/family:
- To notify prescriber if family members have QTc interval prolongation
- To notify prescriber immediately of chest, throat tightness, flushing, lightheadedness, shortness of breath

---

⚠ Safety alert   *"Tall Man" lettering

⚠ Chances of serious or life-threatening allergic reaction may increase with each inj

abatacept
See Appendix A—Selected New Drugs

Rarely Used ⚠ High Alert

abciximab (℞)
(ab-six'i-mab)
ReoPro
Func. class.: Platelet aggregation inhibitor

Uses: Used with heparin and aspirin to prevent acute cardiac ischemia following percutaneous transluminal coronary angioplasty (PTCA) in patients at high risk for reclosure of affected arteries

DOSAGE AND ROUTES
Percutaneous coronary intervention (PCI)
• *Adult:* **IV BOL** 250 mcg (0.25 mg)/kg 10-60 min prior to PCI, followed by 125 mcg/kg/min **CONT INF** for 12 hr
MI
• *Adult:* **IV BOL** 0.25 mg over 5 min, then 0.125 mcg/kg/min, max 10 mcg/min; **IV INF** for 12 hr unless complications

Contraindications: Hypersensitivity to this drug or murine protein; GI, GU bleeding; CVA within 2 yr, bleeding disorders, intracranial neoplasm, intracranial arteriovenous malformations, intracranial aneurysm, platelet count <100,000/mm³, recent surgery, aneurysm, uncontrolled severe hypertension, vasculitis, coagulopathy

Rarely Used

acamprosate (℞)
(a-kam-proe'sate)
Campral
Func. class.: Antialcoholic agent

Uses: For maintenance of abstinence from alcohol in alcohol dependence

DOSAGE AND ROUTES
• *Adult:* **PO** 666 mg tid
Renal dose
• *Adult:* **PO** 333 mg tid
Contraindications: Hypersensitivity, severe renal disease, CCr <30 ml/hr

acarbose (℞)
(ay-car'bose)
Prandese ✦ Precose
Func. class.: Oral antidiabetic
Chem. class.: α-Glucosidase inhibitor

Do not confuse:
Precose/PreCare
Action: Delays digestion of ingested carbohydrates, results in smaller rise in postprandial blood glucose after meals; does not increase insulin production
Uses: Type 2 diabetes, mellitus, alone or in combination with a sulfonylurea

DOSAGE AND ROUTES
• *Adult:* **PO** 25 mg tid initially, with first bite of meal; maintenance dose may be increased to 50-100 mg tid; dosage adjustment at 4-8 wk intervals
• *Adult <60 kg:* **PO** Not to exceed 50 mg tid
Available forms: Tabs 25, 50, 100 mg

SIDE EFFECTS
GI: Abdominal pain, diarrhea, flatulence, increased serum transaminase level
Contraindications: Hypersensitivity, diabetic ketoacidosis, cirrhosis, inflam-

---

matory bowel disease, colonic ulceration, partial intestinal obstruction, chronic intestinal disease, serum creatinine >2 mg/dl

Precautions: Pregnancy (B), renal disease, lactation, children, hepatic disease

PHARMACOKINETICS

Peak 1 hr, metabolized in GI tract, excreted as intact drug in urine, half-life 2 hr

INTERACTIONS

Increase: hypoglycemia—sulfonylureas, insulin
Decrease: effect, increase hyperglycemia—digestive enzymes, intestinal absorbents, thiazide diuretics, loop diuretics, corticosteroids, estrogen, progestins, oral contraceptives, sympathomimetics, calcium channel blockers, isoniazid, phenothiazines, digoxin
Drug/Herb
Increase: hypoglycemia—alfalfa, aloe, basil, bay, bilberry, bitter melon, black cohosh, buchu, burdock, chromium, coenzyme Q-10, coriander, eyebright (PO), fenugreek, garlic, ginseng *(Panax)*, glucomannan, glucosamine, goat's rue, gymnema, horehound, horse chestnut, jambul, myrrh, myrtle, raspberry, Siberian ginseng
Decrease: hypoglycemia—bee pollen, blue cohosh, broom chromium, elecampane, eucalyptus, gotu kola, senega
Drug/Lab Test
Increase: AST, bilirubin
Decrease: Calcium, vit B_6

NURSING CONSIDERATIONS

Assess:
• Hypoglycemia (weakness, hunger, dizziness, tremors, anxiety, tachycardia, sweating), hyperglycemia; even though drug does not cause hypoglycemia, if patient is on sulfonylureas or insulin, hypoglycemia may be additive; if hypoglycemia occurs, treat with dextrose, or if severe, IV glucose or glucagon.

• 1 hr postprandial for establishing effectiveness, then A1c q3mo
• Monitor AST, ALT q3mo × 1 yr and periodically thereafter; if elevated, dose may need to be reduced or discontinued; obtain A1c periodically
Administer:
PO route
• Tid with first bite of each meal
Perform/provide:
• Storage in tight container in cool environment
Evaluate:
• Therapeutic response: improved signs/symptoms of diabetes mellitus (decreased polyuria, polydipsia, polyphagia; clear sensorium, absence of dizziness, stable gait)
Teach patient/family:
• The symptoms of hypo/hyperglycemia, what to do about each
• That medication must be taken as prescribed; explain consequences of discontinuing medication abruptly; that insulin may need to be used for stress, including trauma, surgery, fever
• To avoid OTC medications, herbal supplements unless approved by health care provider
• That diabetes is lifelong illness; that this drug is not a cure
• To carry emergency ID for emergency purposes
• That diet and exercise regimen must be followed

---

acebutolol (R)
(a-se-byoo'toe- lole)
Monitan ✤ Sectral
Func. class.: Antihypertensive, β_1-blocker, antidysrhythmic (II)

Action: Competitively blocks stimulation of β-adrenergic receptors within vascular smooth muscle; decreases rate of SA node discharge, increases recovery time, slows conduction of AV node resulting in decreased heart rate (negative chronotropic effect), which decreases O_2 consumption in myocardium due to

---

β_1-receptor antagonism; also decreases renin-aldosterone-angiotensin system at high doses, inhibits β_2-receptors in bronchial system (high doses)

Uses: Mild to moderate hypertension, sinus tachycardia, persistent atrial extrasystoles, tachydysrhythmias, management of PVCs

Investigational uses: Prophylaxis of MI, treatment of angina pectoris, tremor, mitral valve prolapse, thyrotoxicosis, idiopathic hypertrophic subaortic stenosis

DOSAGE AND ROUTES

Hypertension
• *Adult:* **PO** 400 mg daily or in 2 divided doses; may be increased to desired response; maintenance 200-1200 mg/daily in 2 divided doses

Ventricular dysrhythmia
• *Adult:* **PO** 200 mg bid, may increase gradually, usual range 600-1200 mg daily; should be tapered over 2 wk before discontinuing
• *Geriatric:* not to exceed 800 mg daily

Renal dose
• *Adult:* **PO** CCr 25-50 ml/min, reduce dose by 50%; if <25 ml/min reduce dose by 75%

Available forms: Caps 200, 400 mg; tabs 100, 200; 400 mg ✤

SIDE EFFECTS

CNS: Insomnia, fatigue, dizziness, mental changes, memory loss, hallucinations, depression, lethargy, drowsiness, strange dreams, catatonia

CV: **Profound hypotension, bradycardia, CHF,** *cold extremities, postural hypotension,* **2nd-/3rd-degree heart block**

EENT: Sore throat; dry, burning eyes

ENDO: Increased hypoglycemic response to insulin

GI: Nausea, diarrhea, vomiting, **mesenteric arterial thrombosis, ischemic colitis,** *flatulence*

GU: Impotence, decreased libido, dysuria, nocturia

HEMA: **Agranulocytosis, thrombocytopenia, purpura**

INTEG: Rash, flushing, pruritus, sweating, alopecia, dry skin

MISC: Facial swelling, weight gain, decreased exercise tolerance

MS: Joint pain, cramping

RESP: **Bronchospasm,** dyspnea, wheezing, cough

Contraindications: Hypersensitivity to β-blockers, cardiogenic shock, heart block (2nd, 3rd degree), sinus bradycardia, CHF, cardiac failure

Precautions: Pregnancy (B), major surgery, lactation, peripheral vascular disease, children, diabetes mellitus, renal disease, thyroid disease, COPD, asthma, well-compensated heart failure, hepatic disease

PHARMACOKINETICS

PO: Onset 1-1½ hr, peak 2-4 hr, duration 10-12 hr, half-life 3-4 hr, metabolized in liver, 30%-40% excreted in urine, protein binding 26%

INTERACTIONS

Attenuated effects: oral sulfonylureas
Peripheral ischemia: ergots

Increase: hypotension, bradycardia—reserpine, hydralazine, methyldopa, prazosin, anticholinergics, cardiac glycosides, diltiazem, verapamil, diuretics, other antihypertensives, calcium channel blockers, cimetidine

Increase: hypoglycemic effect—insulin

Decrease: antihypertensive effects—NSAIDs, calcium, cholestyramine, colestipol

Decrease: bronchodilation—theophyllines, β_2-agonists

Drug/Herb
May increase acebutolol effect—aloe, buckthorn bark/berry, betel palm, butterbur, cola tree, figwort, fumitory, guarana, hawthorn, lily of the valley, motherwort, plantain, rhubarb root, senna leaf/fruits, cascara sagrada bark
Toxicity/death: aconite

Decrease: antihypertensive effect—coenzyme Q10, yohimbe

Drug/Lab Test

Increase: Serum lipoprotein levels, BUN, potassium, triglyceride, uric acid, LDH, AST, ALT, blood glucose, alk phosphatase

Positive: ANA titer

NURSING CONSIDERATIONS

Assess:

• B/P during beginning treatment, periodically thereafter; pulse q4h; note rate, rhythm, quality

• Apical/radial pulse before administration; notify prescriber of any significant changes (pulse <50 bpm); signs of CHF (dyspnea, crackles, weight gain, jugular vein distention)

• Baselines in renal, hepatic studies before therapy begins

• Edema in feet, legs daily: monitor I&O

• Skin turgor, dryness of mucous membranes for hydration status, especially elderly

Administer:

PO route

• Drug ac, at bedtime, tablet may be crushed or swallowed whole; give with food to prevent GI upset

Perform/provide:

• Storage protected from light, moisture; place in cool environment

Evaluate:

• Therapeutic response: decreased B/P after 1-2 wk; decreased dysrhythmias

Teach patient/family:

⚠ Not to discontinue drug abruptly, severe cardiac reactions may occur, taper over 2 wk; do not double dose; if a dose is missed, take as soon as remembered up to 4 hr before next dose

• Drug may mask signs of hypoglycemia or alter blood glucose levels

• Not to use OTC products containing α-adrenergic stimulants (such as nasal decongestants, OTC cold preparations) unless directed by prescriber

• To report low pulse, dizziness, confusion, depression, fever

• To take pulse, B/P at home, advise when to notify prescriber

• To comply with weight control, dietary adjustments, modified exercise program

• To carry emergency ID to identify drug, allergies

• To avoid hazardous activities if dizziness, drowsiness is present

• To report symptoms of CHF: difficult breathing, especially on exertion or when lying down, night cough, swelling of extremities

• To continue with required life-style changes (exercise, diet, weight loss, stress reduction)

Treatment of overdose: Lavage, IV atropine for bradycardia, IV theophylline for bronchospasm, digitalis, O_2, diuretic for cardiac failure, IV glucose for hypoglycemia, IV diazepam (or phenytoin) for seizures

---

acetaminophen (OTC)

(a-seat-a-mee'noe-fen)
Abenol ✤, Acephen, Aceta, Actimol, Aminofen, Apacet, APAP, Apo-Acetaminophen ✤, Arthritis Foundation Pain Reliever Aspirin-Free, Aspirin-Free Anacin, Aspirin-Free Pain Relief, Atasol ✤, Banesin, Children's Feverall, Dapa, Dapacin, Datril, Exdol ✤, FemEtts, Genapap, Genebs, Halenol, Liquiprin, Mapap, Maranox, Meda, Neopap, Oraphen-PD, Panadol, Redutemp, Robigesic ✤, Rounax ✤, Silapap, Tapanol, Tempra, Tylenol

Func. class.: Nonopioid analgesic, antipyretic

Chem. class.: Nonsalicylate, paraaminophenol derivative

Action: May block pain impulses peripherally that occur in response to inhibition of prostaglandin synthesis; does not possess antiinflammatory properties;

antipyretic action results from inhibition of prostaglandins in the CNS (hypothalamic heat-regulating center)

Uses: Mild pain or fever

DOSAGE AND ROUTES

- *Adult and child >12 yr:* **PO/RECT** 325-650 mg q4h prn, max 4 g/day
- *Child:* **PO** 10-15 mg/kg q4h
- *Child 6-12 yr:* **RECT** 325 mg q4-6h, max 2.6 g/day
- *Child 3-6 yr:* **RECT** 125 mg q4-6h, max 720 mg/day
- *Child 1-3 yr:* **RECT** 80 mg q4h
- *Child 3-11 mo:* **RECT** 80 mg q6h

Available forms: Rect supp 80, 120, 125, 325, 600, 650 mg; soft chew tabs 80, 160 mg; caps 500 mg; elix 120, 160, 325 mg/5 ml; liq 160 mg/5 ml, 500 mg/15 ml; sol 100 mg/1 ml, 120 mg/2.5 ml; granules 80 mg/packet, 80 mg/cap; tabs 160, 325, 500, 650 mg

SIDE EFFECTS

CNS: Stimulation, drowsiness

GI: Nausea, vomiting, abdominal pain; ***hepatotoxicity, hepatic seizure (overdose)***

GU: ***Renal failure (high, prolonged doses)***

HEMA: ***Leukopenia, neutropenia, hemolytic anemia (long-term use)***, thrombocytopenia, pancytopenia

INTEG: Rash, urticaria

SYST: Hypersensitivity

TOXICITY: ***Cyanosis, anemia, neutropenia, jaundice, pancytopenia, CNS stimulation, delirium followed by vascular collapse, convulsions, coma, death***

Contraindications: Hypersensitivity, intolerance to tartrazine (yellow dye #5), alcohol, table sugar, saccharin, depending on product

Precautions: Pregnancy (B), anemia, hepatic disease, renal disease, chronic alcoholism, elderly, lactation

PHARMACOKINETICS

Well absorbed PO, rectal absorption varies; 85%-90% metabolized by liver, excreted by kidneys; metabolites may be toxic if overdose occurs; widely distributed, crosses placenta in low concentrations, excreted in breast milk, half-life 1-4 hr

PO: Onset 10-30 min, peak ½-2 hr, duration 3-4 hr

RECT: Onset slow, peak 1-2 hr, duration 3-4 hr

INTERACTIONS

Hypoprothrombinemia—warfarin, long-term use, high doses of acetaminophen

Bone marrow suppression—zidovudine

Renal adverse reactions—NSAIDs, salicylates

Decrease: effect, increase hepatotoxicity—barbiturates, alcohol, carbamazepine, hydantoins, rifampin, rifabutin, isoniazid, diflunisal, sulfinpyrazone

Decrease: absorption—colestipol, cholestyramine

Drug/Lab Test

Interference: Chemstrip G, Dextrostix, Visidex II, 5-HIAA

NURSING CONSIDERATIONS

Assess:

- Hepatic studies: AST, ALT, bilirubin, creatinine prior to therapy if long-term therapy is anticipated; may cause hepatic toxicity at doses >4 g/day with chronic use
- Renal studies: BUN, urine creatinine, occult blood, albumin, if patient is on long-term therapy; presence of blood or albumin indicates nephritis
- Blood studies: CBC, PT if patient is on long-term therapy
- I&O ratio; decreasing output may indicate renal failure (long-term therapy)
- For fever and pain: type of pain, location, intensity, duration
- For chronic poisoning: rapid, weak pulse; dyspnea; cold, clammy

extremities; report immediately to prescriber
- Hepatotoxicity: dark urine; clay-colored stools; yellowing of skin, sclera; itching, abdominal pain; fever; diarrhea if patient is on long-term therapy
- Allergic reactions: rash, urticaria; if these occur, drug may have to be discontinued

Administer:

PO route
- Crushed or whole; chewable tablets may be chewed; give with full glass of water
- With food or milk to decrease gastric symptoms if needed

Perform/provide:
- Storage of suppositories <80° F (27° C)

Evaluate:
- Therapeutic response: absence of pain, fever

Teach patient/family:

⚠ Not to exceed recommended dosage; acute poisoning with liver damage may result

⚠ That acute toxicity includes symptoms of nausea, vomiting, abdominal pain; prescriber should be notified immediately

- To read label on other OTC drugs; many contain acetaminophen and may cause toxicity if taken concurrently
- To recognize signs of chronic overdose: bleeding, bruising, malaise, fever, sore throat
- To notify prescriber of pain or fever lasting over 3 days

Treatment of overdose: Drug level, gastric lavage, activated charcoal; administer oral acetylcysteine to prevent hepatic damage *(see acetylcysteine monograph),* monitor for bleeding

---

*acetaZOLAMIDE (R)
(a-set-a-zole′a- mide)
acetaZOLAMIDE,
Apo-Acetazolamide ✿,
Dazamide, Diamox, Diamox
Sequels
Func. class.: Diuretic, carbonic anhydrase inhibitor, antiglaucoma agent, antiepileptic
Chem. class.: Sulfonamide derivative

Do not confuse:
acetaZOLAMIDE/acetoHEXAMIDE
Diamox/Trimox
Diamox/Dobutrex

Action: Inhibits carbonic anhydrase activity in proximal renal tubules to decrease reabsorption of water, sodium, potassium, bicarbonate; decreases carbonic anhydrase in CNS, increasing seizure threshold; able to decrease aqueous humor in eye, which lowers intraocular pressure

Uses: Open-angle glaucoma, narrow-angle glaucoma (preoperatively, if surgery delayed), epilepsy (petit mal, grand mal, mixed), edema in CHF, drug-induced edema, acute mountain sickness

Investigational uses: Prevention of uric acid/cystine renal stones, decrease CSF production in infants with hydrocephalus

DOSAGE AND ROUTES

Closed-angle glaucoma
- *Adult:* **PO/IM/IV** 250 mg q4h or 250 mg bid, to be used for short-term therapy

Open-angle glaucoma
- *Adult:* **PO/IM/IV** 250 mg-1 g/day in divided doses for amounts over 250 mg or 500 mg SR bid

Edema in CHF
- *Adult:* **IM/IV** 250-375 mg/day in AM
- *Child:* **IM/IV** 5 mg/kg/day in AM

Seizures
- *Adult:* **PO/IM/IV** 4-30 mg/kg/day, in 1-4 divided doses usual range 375-1000 mg/day
- *Child:* **PO/IM/IV** 8-30 mg/kg/day in

---

divided doses tid or qid, or 300-900 mg/m^2/day, not to exceed 1 g/day

Mountain sickness

• *Adult:* **PO** 250 mg q8-12h

Renal stones

• *Adult:* **PO** 250 mg at bedtime

Infants with hydrocephalus

• *Infant:* **IV** 5 mg/kg/dose q6h, may be increased up to 100 mg/kg/day if tolerated

Available forms: Tabs 125, 250 mg; caps sust rel 500 mg; inj 500 mg

SIDE EFFECTS

CNS: Drowsiness, paresthesia, anxiety, depression, headache, dizziness, confusion, stimulation, fatigue, *convulsions,* sedation, nervousness

EENT: Myopia, tinnitus

ENDO: Hyperglycemia

GI: Nausea, vomiting, anorexia, constipation, diarrhea, melena, weight loss, *hepatic insufficiency,* taste alterations

GU: Frequency, polyuria, *uremia,* glucosuria, hematuria, dysuria, crystalluria, renal calculi

HEMA: Aplastic anemia, hemolytic anemia, leukopenia, agranulocytosis, thrombocytopenia, purpura, pancytopenia

INTEG: Rash, pruritus, urticaria, fever, *Stevens-Johnson syndrome,* photosensitivity

META: Hypokalemia, hyperchloremic acidosis

Contraindications: Hypersensitivity to sulfonamides, severe renal disease, severe hepatic disease, electrolyte imbalances (hyponatremia, hypokalemia), hyperchloremic acidosis, Addison's disease, long-term use in narrow-angle glaucoma

Precautions: Pregnancy (C), hypercalciuria, lactation, respiratory acidosis, COPD

PHARMACOKINETICS

PO: Onset 1-1½ hr, peak 2-4 hr, duration 8-12 hr

PO-SUS REL: Onset 2 hr, peak 3-6 hr, duration 18-24 hr

IV: Onset 2 min, peak 15 min, duration 4-5 hr, 65% absorbed if fasting (oral), 75% absorbed if given with food; half-life 2½-5½ hr; excreted unchanged by kidneys (80% within 24 hr), crosses placenta

INTERACTIONS

Toxicity: cycloSPORINE

Increase: action of amphetamines, procainamide, quinidine, anticholinergics

Increase: excretion of lithium

Increase: toxicity—salicylates

Increase: side effects—diflunisal

Decrease: acetaZOLAMIDE effect—methenamine

Decrease: primidone levels

Drug/Lab Test

Decrease: Thyroid iodine uptake

False positive: Urinary protein, 17 hydroxysteroid

NURSING CONSIDERATIONS

Assess:

• Weight daily, I&O daily to determine fluid loss; effect of drug may be decreased if used daily; monitor the elderly for dehydration

• For cross-sensitivity between other sulfonamides and this drug

• B/P lying, standing; postural hypotension may occur

• Electrolytes: K, Na, Cl; also BUN, blood glucose, CBC, serum creatinine, blood pH, ABGs, LFTs; I&O, glucose, patient may need to be on a high-potassium diet

Administer:

• In AM to avoid interference with sleep if using drug as diuretic

• Potassium replacement if potassium level is less than 3.0 mg/dl

PO route

• Do not break, crush, or chew sus rel caps

• With food if nausea occurs; absorption may be decreased slightly

IV route

- After diluting 500 mg in >5 ml sterile H_2O for injection; direct IV—give at 100-500 mg/min; may be diluted further in LR, D_5W, $D_{10}W$, 0.45% NaCl, 0.9% NaCl, or Ringer's sol and infused over 4-8 hr; use within 24 hr of dilution

Additive compatibilities: Cimetidine, ranitidine

Perform/provide:

- Storage in dark, cool area; use reconstituted solution within 24 hr

Evaluate:

- Therapeutic response: improvement in edema of feet, legs, sacral area daily if medication is being used in CHF; or decrease in aqueous humor if medication is being used in glaucoma

Teach patient/family:

- To take exactly as prescribed; if dose is missed, take as soon as remembered; do not double dose
- To notify prescriber if sore throat, unusual bleeding, bruising, paresthesias, tremors, flank pain, or skin rash occurs
- To use sunscreen to prevent photosensitivity; to monitor blood glucose and urine for sugar
- To avoid hazardous activities if drowsiness occurs
- Increase fluids to 2-3 L/day if not contraindicated
- Report nausea, vertigo, rapid weight gain, change in stools

Treatment of overdose: Lavage if taken orally; monitor electrolytes; administer dextrose in saline; monitor hydration, CV, renal status

---

acetylcholine ophthalmic

See Appendix C

---

acetylcysteine (R)

(a-se-teel-sis'tay-een)

Acetadote, Mucomyst ✦, Mucosil, Parvolex ✦

Func. class.: Mucolytic; antidote—acetaminophen

Chem. class.: Amino acid L-cysteine

Action: Decreases viscosity of secretions by breaking disulfide links of mucoproteins; increases hepatic glutathione, which is necessary to inactivate toxic metabolites in acetaminophen overdose

Uses: Acetaminophen toxicity; bronchitis; pneumonia; cystic fibrosis; emphysema; atelectasis; tuberculosis; complications of thoracic, cardiovascular surgery; diagnosis in bronchial lab tests

Investigational uses: Prevention of contrast medium nephrotoxicity

DOSAGE AND ROUTES

Mucolytic

- *Adult and child:* **INSTILL** 1-2 ml (10%-20% sol) q1-4h prn or 3-5 ml (20% sol) or 6-10 ml (10% sol) tid or qid; nebulization (face mask, mouthpiece, tracheostomy) 1-10 ml of a 20% sol, or 2-20 ml of a 10% sol, q2-6h; nebulization (tent, croupette) may require large dose, up to 300 ml/treatment

Acetaminophen toxicity

- *Adult and child:* **PO** 140 mg/kg, then 70 mg/kg q4h × 17 doses to total of 1330 mg/kg; **IV** loading dose 150 mg/kg over 15 min (dilution 150 mg/kg in 200 ml of D_5); maintenance dose 1: 50 mg/kg over 4 hr (dilution 50 mg/kg in 500 ml D_5): maintenance dose 2: 100 mg/kg over 16 hr (dilution 100 mg/kg in 1000 ml D_5)

Available forms: Oral sol 10%, 20%; Inj 20% (200 mg/ml)

SIDE EFFECTS

CNS: Dizziness, drowsiness, headache, fever, chills

CV: Hypotension

EENT: Rhinorrhea, tooth damage

GI: Nausea, stomatitis, constipation, vomiting, anorexia, ***hepatotoxicity***
INTEG: Urticaria, rash, fever, clamminess, pruritus
RESP: ***Bronchospasm,*** burning, ***hemoptysis,*** chest tightness
Contraindications: Hypersensitivity, increased intracranial pressure, status asthmaticus
Precautions: Pregnancy (B), hypothyroidism, Addison's disease, CNS depression, brain tumor, asthma, hepatic disease, renal disease, COPD, psychosis, alcoholism, convulsive disorders, lactation

PHARMACOKINETICS

INH/INSTILL: Onset 1 min, duration 5-10 min, metabolized by liver, excreted in urine, half-life 5.6 hr (adult) 11 hr (newborn)
IV: Protein binding 83%

INTERACTIONS

Do not use with iron, copper, rubber
Do not mix with antibiotics: tetracycline, chlortetracycline, oxytetracycline, erythromycin lactobionate, amphotericin B, sodium ampicillin; iodized oil, chymotrypsin, trypsin, hydrogen peroxide

NURSING CONSIDERATIONS

Assess:
• Cough: type, frequency, character, including sputum
• Rate, rhythm of respirations, increased dyspnea; sputum; discontinue if bronchospasm occurs
• VS, cardiac status including checking for dysrhythmias, increased rate, palpitations
• ABGs for increased CO_2 retention in asthma patients
• Antidotal use: LFTs, PT, BUN, glucose, electrolytes, acetaminophen levels; inform prescriber if dose is vomited or vomiting is persistent
• Nausea, vomiting, rash; notify prescriber if these occur

Administer:
PO route
• Antidotal use: give within 24 hr; give with cola or soft drink to disguise taste; can be given with H_2O through tubes; use within 1 hr
INSTILL route
• By syringe 2-3 doses of 1-2 ml of 20% or 2-4 ml of 10% solution
• Decreased dose to elderly patients; their metabolisms may be slowed
• Only if suction machine is available
• Before meals ½-1 hr for better absorption, to decrease nausea
• 20% solutions diluted with NS or water for injection; may give 10% solution undiluted
• Only after patient clears airway by deep breathing, coughing
IV route
• Dilute with D_5
Incompatibilities: Rubber, metals, stability with other drugs not known
Perform/provide:
• Storage in refrigerator; use within 96 hr of opening
• Assistance with inhaled dose: bronchodilator if bronchospasm occurs
• Mechanical suction if cough insufficient to remove excess bronchial secretions
• Gum, hard candy, frequent rinsing of mouth for dryness of oral cavity
Evaluate:
• Therapeutic response: absence of purulent secretions when coughing; absence of hepatic damage in acetaminophen toxicity
Teach patient/family:
• About mucolytic use
• That unpleasant odor will decrease after repeated use
• That discoloration of solution after bottle is opened does not impair its effectiveness

---

---

activated charcoal (oᴛᴄ)
Actidose-Aqua, CharcoAid,
CharcoAid 2000, Liqui-Char
Func. class.: Antiflatulent; antidote

Action: Binds poisons, toxins, irritants; increases adsorption in GI tract; inactivates toxins and binds until excreted
Uses: Poisoning
Investigational uses: Diarrhea, flatulence

DOSAGE AND ROUTES

Children should not get more than 1 dose of products with sorbitol
Poisoning
• *Adult and child:* **PO** 30-100 g or 1 g/kg, minimum dose 30 g/250 ml of water, may give 20-40 g q6h for 1-2 days in severe poisoning
Available forms: Powder 15, 25 ✹, 30, 40, 120, 125, 240 g/container; oral susp 12.5 g/60 ml, 15 g/72 ml, 15 g/120 ml, 25 g/120 ml, 30 g/120 ml, 50 g/240 ml; Canada 15 g/120 ml, 25 g/125 ml, 50 g/225 ml, 50 g/250 ml
• Tabs/caps should not be used in poisonings

SIDE EFFECTS

GI: Nausea, black stools, vomiting, constipation, diarrhea
Contraindications: Hypersensitivity to this drug, unconsciousness, semiconsciousness, poisoning of cyanide, mineral acids, alkalis, gag reflex, depression, ethanol intoxication
Precautions: Pregnancy (C)

PHARMACOKINETICS

PO: Excreted in feces

INTERACTIONS

Inactivation of: acetylcysteine

NURSING CONSIDERATIONS

Assess:
• Respiration, pulse, B/P to determine charcoal effectiveness if taken for

barbiturate/opiate poisoning, intact gag reflex
Administer:
PO route
• After inducing vomiting unless vomiting contraindicated (i.e., cyanide or alkalis)
• After mixing with water or fruit juice to form thick syrup; do not use dairy products to mix charcoal
• Repeat dose if vomiting occurs soon after dose; give with a laxative to promote elimination
• After spacing at least 1 hr before or after other drugs, or absorption will be decreased
NG route
• Through a nasogastric tube if patient unable to swallow
Perform/provide:
• Container closed tightly to prevent absorption of gases
Evaluate:
• Therapeutic response: LOC alert (poisoning)
Teach patient/family:
• That stools will be black
• How to prevent further poisonings

---

acyclovir (℞)
(ay-sye′kloe-veer)
Avirax ✹, Zovirax
Func. class.: Antiviral
Chem. class.: Acyclic purine nucleoside analog

See Topical Appendix for Topical Product
Action: Interferes with DNA synthesis by conversion to acyclovir triphosphate, causing decreased viral replication, time of lesional healing
Uses: Mucocutaneous herpes simplex virus, herpes genitalis (HSV-1, HSV-2), varicella infections, herpes zoster, herpes simplex encephalitis
Investigational uses: Cytomegalovirus, HSV after transplant, mononucleosis, herpes simplex

---

DOSAGE AND ROUTES

Renal dose
• *Adult and child:* **PO/IV** CCr >50 ml/min 100% dose q8h, CCr 25-50 ml/min 100% dose q12h, CCr 10-25 ml/min 100% dose q24h, CCr 0-10 ml/min 50% of dose q24h

Herpes simplex
• *Adult and child >12 yr:* **IV INF** 5 mg/kg over 1 hr q8h × 5 days
• *Child <12 yr:* **IV INF** 250 mg/m² or 30 mg/kg/day divided q8h over 1 hr × 5 days

Genital herpes
• *Adult:* **PO** 200 mg q4h (5×/day while awake) for 5 days to 6 mo depending on whether initial, recurrent, or chronic; **IV** 5 mg/kg q8h × 5 days

Herpes simplex encephalitis
• *Adult:* **IV** 10 mg/kg over 1 hr q8h × 10 days
• *Child 3 mo-12 yr:* **IV** 20 mg/kg q8h × 10 days
• *Child birth-3 mo:* **IV** 10 mg/kg q8h × 10 days

Herpes zoster
• *Adult:* **PO** 800 mg q4h while awake × 7-10 days; **IV** 5 mg/kg q8h

Varicella-zoster
• *Adult:* **PO** 1000 mg q6h × 5 days or 600-800 mg q4h (5×/day while awake); **IV** 500 mg/m² q8h or 10 mg/kg q8h × 7 days
• *Child:* **PO** 10-20 mg/kg (max 800 mg) qid × 5 days; **IV** 500 mg/m² q8h or 10 mg/kg q8h × 7 days

Mucosal/cutaneous herpes simplex infections in immunosuppressed patients
• *Adult and child >12 yr:* **IV** 5 mg/kg q8h × 7 days
• *Child <12:* **IV** 10 mg/kg q8h × 7 days

Chickenpox
• *Adult and child >40 kg:* **PO** 800 mg qid × 5 days
• *Child 2 yr or older <40 kg:* **PO** 20 mg/kg qid × 5 days
Available forms: Caps 200 mg; inj 500 mg, oral susp, tabs 400, 800 mg

SIDE EFFECTS

CNS: Tremors, confusion, lethargy, hallucinations, ***seizures,*** dizziness, *headache,* encephalopathic changes
EENT: Gingival hyperplasia
GI: Nausea, vomiting, diarrhea, increased ALT, AST, abdominal pain, glossitis, colitis
GU: ***Oliguria, proteinuria, hematuria,*** vaginitis, moniliasis, ***glomerulonephritis, acute renal failure,*** changes in menses, polydipsia
HEMA: ***Thrombotic thrombocytopenia purpura, hemolytic uremic syndrome*** (immunocompromised patients)
INTEG: Rash, urticaria, pruritus, pain or phlebitis at IV site, unusual sweating, alopecia
MS: Joint pain, leg pain, muscle cramps
Contraindications: Hypersensitivity
Precautions: Pregnancy (B), lactation, hepatic disease, renal disease, electrolyte imbalance, dehydration

PHARMACOKINETICS

Distributed widely; crosses placenta, CSF concentrations are 50% plasma
IV: Onset immediate, peak immediate, duration unknown, half-life 20 min-3 hr (terminal); metabolized by liver, excreted by kidneys as unchanged drug (95%)
PO: Absorbed minimally; onset unknown, peak 1½-2 hr, terminal half-life 3½ hr

INTERACTIONS

Synergistic effect: interferon
CNS side effects: zidovudine
Increase: levels, toxicity—probenecid

NURSING CONSIDERATIONS
Assess:
• Signs of infection, anemia
🅐 Any patient with compromised renal system, since drug is excreted slowly in poor renal system function; toxicity may occur rapidly
• Hepatic studies: AST, ALT

- Blood studies: WBC, RBC, Hct, Hgb, bleeding time; blood dyscrasias may occur; drug should be discontinued
- Renal studies: urinalysis, protein, BUN, creatinine, CCr, watch for increasing BUN and serum creatinine or decreased CCr, may indicate nephrotoxicity; I&O ratio; report hematuria, oliguria, fatigue, weakness; may indicate nephrotoxicity; check for protein in urine during treatment
- C&S before drug therapy; drug may be taken as soon as culture is taken; repeat C&S after treatment; determine the presence of other sexually transmitted diseases
- Bowel pattern before, during treatment; if severe abdominal pain with bleeding occurs, drug should be discontinued
- Skin eruptions: rash, urticaria, itching
- Allergies before treatment, reaction of each medication; place allergies on chart in bright red letters

Administer:

PO route
- Do not break, crush, or chew caps
- May give without regard to meals, with 8 oz of water
- Shake suspension before use
- Lower dose in acute or chronic renal failure

IV route
- Increased fluids to 3 L/day to decrease crystalluria
- After reconstituting with 10 ml compatible sol/500 mg of drug, concentration of 50 mg/ml, shake, further dilute in 50-100 ml compatible sol; use within 12 hr; give over at least 1 hr (constant rate) by infusion pump to prevent nephrotoxicity; do not reconstitute with sol containing benzyl alcohol in neonates

Additive compatibilities: Fluconazole

Solution compatibilities: D$_5$W, LR, or NaCl (D$_5$ 0.9% NaCl, 0.9% NaCl) solutions

Y-site compatibilities: Allopurinol, amikacin, ampicillin, amphotericin B, cefamandole, cefazolin, cefonicid, cefoperazone, cefotaxime, cefoxitin, ceftazidime, ceftizoxime, ceftriaxone, cefuroxime, cephapirin, chloramphenicol, cholesteryl sulfate complex, cimetidine, clindamycin, dexamethasone sodium phosphate, dimenhyDRINATE, diphenhydrAMINE, DOXOrubicin, doxycycline, erythromycin, famotidine, filgrastim, fluconazole, gallium, gentamicin, granisetron, heparin, hydrocortisone sodium succinate, hydromorphone, imipenem/cilastatin, lorazepam, magnesium sulfate, melphalan, methylPREDNISolone sodium succinate, metoclopramide, metronidazole, multivitamin, nafcillin, oxacillin, paclitaxel, penicillin G potassium, pentobarbital, perphenazine, piperacillin, potassium chloride, propofol, ranitidine, remifentanil, sodium bicarbonate, tacrolimus, teniposide, theophylline, thiotepa, ticarcillin, tobramycin, trimethoprim-sulfamethoxazole, vancomycin, zidovudine

Perform/provide:
- Storage at room temperature for up to 12 hr after reconstitution; if refrigerated, sol may show a precipitate that clears at room temperature, yellow discoloration does not affect potency
- Adequate intake of fluids (2 L) to prevent deposit in kidneys

Evaluate:
- Therapeutic response: absence of itching, painful lesions; crusting and healed lesions; decreased symptoms of chickenpox

Teach patient/family:
- To take as prescribed; if dose is missed, take as soon as remembered up to 1 hr before next dose; do not double dose; that drug does not cure the condition
- That drug may be taken orally before infection occurs; drug should be taken when itching or pain occurs, usually before eruptions
- That sexual partners need to be told that patient has herpes; they can become infected; condoms must be worn to prevent reinfections

---

⚠ Safety alert   *"Tall Man" lettering

- Not to touch lesions to avoid spreading infection to new sites
- That drug does not cure infection, just controls symptoms and does not prevent infecting others

A To report sore throat, fever, fatigue (may indicate superinfection)
- That drug must be taken in equal intervals around the clock to maintain blood levels for duration of therapy
- To notify prescriber of side effects of bruising, bleeding, fatigue, malaise; may indicate blood dyscrasias
- To seek dental care during treatment to prevent gingival hyperplasia
- That women with genital herpes are more likely to develop cervical cancer; to keep all gynecologic appointments

Treatment of overdose: Discontinue drug, hemodialysis, resuscitate if needed

---

acyclovir topical
See Appendix C

---

adalimumab (℞)
(add-a-lim'yu-mab)
Humira
Func. class.: Antirheumatic agent (disease modifying), immunomodulator
Chem. class.: Recombinant human IgG1 monoclonal antibody, DMARDs

Action: A form of human IgG1 monoclonal antibody specific for human tumor necrosis factor (TNF). Elevated levels of TNF are found in patients with rheumatoid arthritis.

Uses: Reduction in signs and symptoms and inhibiting progression of structural damage in patients with moderate to severe active rheumatoid arthritis in patients ≥18 years of age who have not responded to other disease-modifying agents

DOSAGE AND ROUTES

- *Adult:* SUBCUT 40 mg every other wk
Available form: Inj 40 mg/0.8 ml

SIDE EFFECTS

CNS: Headache
EENT: Sinusitis
GI: Abdominal pain, nausea
INTEG: Rash, *inj site reaction*
MISC: Flulike symptoms, UTI, hypertension, back pain, lupuslike syndrome
RESP: URI

Contraindications: Hypersensitivity, active infections

Precautions: Pregnancy (B), lactation, children, elderly, CNS demyelinating disease, lymphoma, latent TB

PHARMACOKINETICS

Terminal half-life 2 wk

INTERACTIONS

Do not give concurrently with vaccines; immunizations should be brought up to date before treatment

NURSING CONSIDERATIONS

Assess:
- Pain, stiffness, ROM, swelling of joints during treatment
- For inj site pain, swelling; usually occur after 2 inj (4-5 days)

A For infections (fever, flulike symptoms, dyspnea, change in urination, redness/swelling around any wounds), stop treatment if present, some serious infections including sepsis may occur; patients with active infections should not be started on this drug

Administer:
SUBCUT route
- Do not admix with other sol or medications, do not use filter, protect from light
- Other DMARDs should be continued during this therapy

Evaluate:
- Therapeutic response: decreased inflammation, pain in joints, decreased joint destruction

Teach patient/family:
- About self-administration if appropriate: inj should be made in thigh, abdomen, upper arm; rotate sites at least 1 inch from old site, do not inject in areas that are bruised, red, hard

- That if medication is not taken when due, inject next dose as soon as remembered and inject next dose as scheduled
- Not to take any live virus vaccines during treatment

---

adefovir dipivoxil (℞)
(add-ee-foh'veer)
Hepsera
Func. class.: Antiviral
Chem. class.: Adenosine monophosphate analog

Action: Inhibits hepatitis B virus DNA polymerase by competing with natural substrates and by causing DNA termination after its incorporation into viral DNA; causes viral DNA death
Uses: Chronic hepatitis B

DOSAGE AND ROUTES
- *Adult:* **PO** 10 mg daily, optimal duration unknown
Renal dose
- *Adult:* **PO** CCr ≥50 ml/min 10 mg q24h; CCr 20-49 ml/min 10 mg q48h; CCr 10-19 ml/min 10 mg q72h; hemodialysis 10 mg q7 days following dialysis
Available forms: Tabs 10 mg

SIDE EFFECTS
CNS: Headache
GI: Dyspepsia, abdominal pain
Contraindications: Hypersensitivity
Precautions: Pregnancy (C), lactation, child, severe renal disease, impaired hepatic disease, elderly

PHARMACOKINETICS
PO: Rapidly absorbed from GI tract, peak 1¾ hr, excreted by kidneys 45%; terminal half-life 7.48 hr

INTERACTIONS
Granulocytopenia: cetaminophen, aspirin, indomethacin
Increase: serum concentration and possible toxicity—amphotericin B, dapsone, flucytosine, Adriamycin, interferon, vinCRIStine, vinBLAStine, pentamidine, probenecid, experimental nucleoside analogs, benzodiazepines, cimetidine, morphine, sulfonamides, acyclovir, ganciclovir, DOXOrubicin, acetaminophen, indomethacin, fluconazole, phenytoin, trimethoprim

NURSING CONSIDERATIONS
Assess:
- For nephrotoxicity: increasing CCr, BUN
- For HIV before beginning treatment, because HIV resistance may occur in chronic hepatitis B patients
- For lactic acidosis, severe hepatomegaly with stenosis
- Elderly patients more carefully; may develop renal, cardiac symptoms more rapidly
- For exacerbations of hepatitis after discontinuing treatment, monitor LFTs
Administer:
- By mouth without regard to food
Perform/provide:
- Storage in cool environment; protect from light
Evaluate:
- Therapeutic response: decreased symptoms of chronic hepatitis B, improving LFTs
Teach patient/family:
- That optimal duration of treatment is unknown
- To avoid use with other medications unless approved by prescriber
- To notify prescriber of decreased urinary output

⚠ High Alert

adenosine (℞)
(a-den'oh-seen)
Adenocard, Adenoscan
Func. class.: Antidysrhythmic
Chem. class.: Endogenous nucleoside

Do not confuse:
Adenocard/adenosine phosphate
Action: Slows conduction through AV node, can interrupt reentry pathways through AV node, and can restore normal

---

sinus rhythm in patients with supraventricular tachycardia (SVT)

Uses: SVT, as a diagnostic aid to assess myocardial perfusion defects in CAD

DOSAGE AND ROUTES

Antidysrhythmic

• *Adult:* **IV BOL** 6 mg; if conversion to normal sinus rhythm does not occur within 1-2 min, give 12 mg by rapid **IV BOL;** may repeat 12 mg dose again in 1-2 min

• *Infants and children:* 0.05 mg/kg, if not effective, increase dose by 0.05 mg/kg q2min to a max of 0.25 mg/kg or 12 mg

Diagnostic use

• *Adult:* 140 mcg/kg/min × 6 min

Available forms: Inj 3 mg/ml vial, 6 mg/2 ml vial

SIDE EFFECTS

CNS: Lightheadedness, dizziness, arm tingling, numbness, apprehension, blurred vision, headache

CV: Chest pain, pressure, ***atrial tachydysrhythmias,*** sweating, palpitations, hypotension, *facial flushing*

GI: Nausea, metallic taste, throat tightness, groin pressure

RESP: Dyspnea, chest pressure, hyperventilation

Contraindications: Hypersensitivity, 2nd- or 3rd-degree heart block, AV block, sick sinus syndrome, atrial flutter, atrial fibrillation

Precautions: Pregnancy (C), lactation, children, asthma, elderly

PHARMACOKINETICS

Cleared from plasma in <30 sec, half-life 10 sec

INTERACTIONS

Higher degree of heart block: carbamazepine

Possible ventricular fibrillation: digoxin

Smoking: increase tachycardia

Increase: effects of adenosine—dipyridamole

Decrease: activity of adenosine—theophylline or other methylxanthines (caffeine)

Drug/Herb

Increase: toxicity/death—aconite

Increase: adenosine effect—aloe, broom, buckthorn, cascara sagrada, figwort, fumitory, goldenseal, kudzu, licorice, rhubarb, senna

Increase: serotonin effect—horehound

Decrease: adenosine effect—coltsfoot, guarana

NURSING CONSIDERATIONS

Assess:

• I&O ratio, electrolytes (K, Na, Cl)

• Cardiopulmonary status: B/P, pulse, respiration, ECG intervals (PR, QRS, QT); check for transient dysrhythmias (PVCs, PACs, sinus tachycardia, AV block)

• Respiratory status: rate, rhythm, lung fields for crackles, watch for respiratory depression; bilateral crackles may occur in CHF patient; increased respiration, increased pulse, drug should be discontinued

• CNS effects: dizziness, confusion, psychosis, paresthesias, convulsions; drug should be discontinued

Administer:

IV BOLUS route

• Undiluted; give 6 mg or less by rapid inj; if using an IV line, use port near insertion site, flush with NS (50 ml)

CONT INF route

• Give 30 ml vial, undiluted, by peripheral vein

Solution compatibilities: D_5LR, D_5W, LR, 0.9% NaCl

Perform/provide:

• Storage at room temperature; sol should be clear; discard unused drug

Evaluate:

• Therapeutic response: normal sinus rhythm or diagnosis of perfusion defect

Teach patient/family:
• To report facial flushing, dizziness, sweating, palpitations, chest pain
• To rise from sitting or standing slowly to prevent orthostatic hypotension
Treatment of overdose: Defibrillation, vasopressor for hypotension

---

alatrofloxacin (℞)
(ah-lat-troh-floks′ah-sin)
Trovan IV

trovafloxacin (℞)
(tro-vah-floks′ah-sin)
Trovan (oral)
Func. class.: Antiinfective
Chem. class.: Fluoroquinolone

Do not confuse:
Trovan/Tenormin
Action: Interferes with conversion of intermediate DNA fragments into high-molecular-weight DNA in bacteria; DNA gyrase inhibitor
Uses: Nosocomial pneumonia; *Escherichia coli, Proteus aeruginosa, Haemophilus influenzae, Staphylococcus aureus*; community-acquired pneumonia: *Streptococcus pneumoniae, H. influenzae, S. aureus, Klebsiella pneumoniae, Mycoplasma pneumoniae, Moraxella catarrhalis, Legionella pneumophila, Chlamydia pneumoniae;* chronic bronchitis, acute sinusitis, complicated intraabdominal infections, gynecologic/pelvic infections, skin/skin structure infections, UTIs, chronic bacterial prostatitis, urethral gonorrhea in males, PID, cervicitis caused by susceptible organisms

DOSAGE AND ROUTES
Alatrofloxacin—serious infections
• *Adult:* IV 300 mg q24h
Other infections
• *Adult:* IV 200 mg q24h
Perioperative prophylaxis
• *Adult:* IV 200 mg ½-4 hr prior to surgery

Trovafloxacin—gonorrhea
• *Adult:* PO 100 mg as a single dose
Other infections
• *Adult:* PO 100-200 mg q24h
Perioperative prophylaxis
• *Adult:* PO 200 mg ½-4 hr prior to surgery

Available forms: Conc sol for inj 5 mg/ml (200 mg/40 ml, 300 g/60 ml) (alatrofloxacin); tabs 100, 200 mg (trovafloxacin)

SIDE EFFECTS
CNS: Headache, *dizziness,* insomnia, anxiety, psychosis, *seizures*
GI: Nausea, flatulence, vomiting, diarrhea, abdominal pain, *pseudomembranous colitis, hepatotoxicity, fatal hepatitis*
GU: Vaginitis, crystalluria, increased BUN, creatinine
HEMA: Anemia, *thrombocytopenia, leukopenia,* decreased Hgb; Hct, increased platelets
INTEG: Rash, pruritus, photosensitivity
MS: Arthralgia, myalgia
SYST: **Anaphylaxis, Stevens-Johnson syndrome**
Contraindications: Hypersensitivity to quinolones, seizure disorders, cerebral atherosclerosis, photosensitivity
Precautions: Pregnancy (C), lactation, children

PHARMACOKINETICS
Metabolized in liver, excreted in urine unchanged

INTERACTIONS
May increase theophylline level, lead to toxicity
May increase warfarin level
Nephrotoxicity may occur with cyclo-SPORINE
Decrease: absorption of trovafloxacin—IV morphine
Decrease: absorption—antacids with aluminum, magnesium, citric acid buffered with sodium citrate, sucralfate, iron products, IV morphine

---

Drug/Herb

Do not use acidophilus concurrently with antiinfectives

Increase: antiinfective effect—cola tree

NURSING CONSIDERATIONS

Assess:

• For hepatic toxicity, use only for serious or life-threatening infections

• For previous sensitivity reaction to fluoroquinolones

• For signs and symptoms of infection: characteristics of sputum, WBC >10,000, fever; obtain baseline information before and during treatment

• For CNS disorders, since other quinolones can cause CNS stimulation, seizures

• C&S before beginning drug therapy to identify if correct treatment has been initiated

• For allergic reactions and anaphylaxis: rash, urticaria, pruritus, chills, fever, joint pain; may occur a few days after therapy begins; epINEPHrine and resuscitation equipment should be available for anaphylactic reaction

• Bowel pattern daily; if severe diarrhea occurs, drug should be discontinued

• For overgrowth of infection, perineal itching, fever, malaise, redness, pain, swelling, drainage, rash, diarrhea, change in cough, sputum

⚠ Hepatic studies: AST; ALT, alk phosphatase, bilirubin; identify hepatotoxicity, fatal hepatitis

Administer:

• Do not use theophylline with this product, will cause toxicity

• Drug may be taken without regard to meals; separate aluminum, magnesium, iron, or sucralfate by 4 hr; to increase fluid intake to 2 L/day to prevent crystalluria

Intermittent INF route

• Dilute with compatible solution to a concentration of 1-2 mg/ml, run over 1 hr

Solution compatibilities: D_5, ½NaCl, D_5 ½NaCl, D_5/0.2% NaCl

Y-site compatibilities: Amikacin, cycloSPORINE, DOPamine, droperidol, fentanyl, gentamicin, ketorolac, lorazepam, midazolam, nitroglycerin, ondansetron, tobramycin, vancomycin

Evaluate:

• Therapeutic response: absence of signs/symptoms of infection (WBC <10,000/mm³, temp WNL)

Teach patient/family:

• To avoid hazardous activities until response is known

• To contact prescriber if vaginal itching, loose foul-smelling stools, or furry tongue occurs (may indicate superinfection); to report itching, rash, pruritus, urticaria, tendon pain

• To use frequent rinsing of mouth, sugarless candy or gum for dry mouth

• To avoid other medication unless approved by prescriber

• To contact prescriber if taking theophylline

• To take as prescribed, not to double or miss doses

• To notify prescriber of diarrhea with blood or pus, may indicate pseudomembranous colitis

• To prevent sun exposure or use sunscreen to prevent phototoxicity

---

albumin, normal serum 5%/25% (℞)

(al-byoo´min)

Albuminar 5%, Albuminar 25%, Albutein 5%, Albutein 25%, Buminate 5%, Buminate 25%, Plasbumin 5%, Plasbumin 25%

Func. class.: Blood derivative

Chem. class.: Placental human plasma

Action: Exerts oncotic pressure, which expands volume of circulating blood and maintains cardiac output

Uses: Restores plasma volume in burns, hyperbilirubinemia, shock, hypoproteinemia, prevention of cerebral edema, cardiopulmonary bypass procedures, ARDS, nephrotic syndrome

---

DOSAGE AND ROUTES

Burns
• *Adult:* IV dose to maintain plasma albumin at 30-50 g/L, use 5% sol initially, then 25% sol after 24 hr

Shock
• *Adult:* IV 500 ml of 5% sol q30 min, as needed
• *Child:* IV 0.5-1 g/kg/dose

Hypoproteinemia
• *Adult:* IV 1000-2000 ml of 5% sol daily, not to exceed 5-10 ml/min or 25-100 g of 25% sol daily, not to exceed 3 ml/min, titrated to patient response

Hyperbilirubinemia/erythroblastosis fetalis
• *Infant:* IV 1 g of 25% sol/kg before transfusion

Available forms: Inj 50, 250 mg/ml (5%, 25%)

SIDE EFFECTS

CNS: Fever, chills, flushing, headache
CV: Fluid overload, hypotension, erratic pulse, tachycardia
GI: Nausea, vomiting, increased salivation
INTEG: Rash, urticaria
RESP: Altered respirations, ***pulmonary edema***

Contraindications: Hypersensitivity, CHF, severe anemia, renal insufficiency
Precautions: Pregnancy (C), decreased salt intake, decreased cardiac reserve, lack of albumin deficiency, hepatic disease, renal disease

PHARMACOKINETICS

In hyponutrition states, metabolized as protein/energy source

Drug/Lab Test
False increase: Alk phosphatase

NURSING CONSIDERATIONS

Assess:
• Blood studies Hct, Hgb; if serum protein declines, dyspnea, hypoxemia can result
• Decreased B/P, erratic pulse, respiration
• I&O ratio: urinary output may decrease

⚠ CVP, pulmonary wedge pressure will increase if overload occurs
• Allergy: fever, rash, itching, chills, flushing, urticaria, nausea, vomiting, hypotension, requires discontinuation of infusion, use of new lot if therapy reinstituted; premedicate with diphenhydrAMINE
• CVP reading: distended neck veins indicate circulatory overload; shortness of breath, anxiety, insomnia, expiratory crackles, frothy blood-tinged cough, cyanosis indicate pulmonary overload

Administer:
IV route
• Slowly, to prevent fluid overload; dilute with NS for injection or D_5W; 5% may be given undiluted; 25% may be given diluted or undiluted, give over 4 hr, use infusion pump

Solution compatibilities: LR, NaCl, Ringer's, D_5W, $D_{10}W$, $D_{2\frac{1}{2}}W$, dextrose/saline, dextran$_6$ D_5, dextran$_6$ NaCl 0.9%, dextrose/Ringer's, dextrose/LR

Y-site compatibilities: Diltiazem

Perform/provide:
• Adequate hydration before, during administration
• Check type of albumin; some stored at room temperature, some need to be refrigerated

Evaluate:
• Therapeutic response: increased B/P, decreased edema, increased serum albumin levels, increased plasma protein

---

albuterol (℞)
(al-byoo'ter-ole)
AccuNeb, Airet, albuterol, Gen-Salbutamol ✚, Novo-Salmol ✚, Proventil, Salbutamol, Ventodisk, Ventolin
Func. class.: Adrenergic β_2-agonist, sympathomimetic, bronchodilator

Do not confuse:
albuterol/atenolol
Ventolin/Vantin

⚠ Safety alert   *"Tall Man" lettering

Volmax/Flomax
Proventil/Prinivil
Salbutamol/salmeterol

Action: Causes bronchodilation by action on β_2 (pulmonary) receptors by increasing levels of cAMP, which relaxes smooth muscle; produces bronchodilation, CNS, cardiac stimulation, as well as increased diuresis and gastric acid secretion; longer acting than isoproterenol

Uses: Prevention of exercise-induced asthma, acute bronchospasm, bronchitis, emphysema, bronchiectasis, or other reversible airway obstruction

Investigational uses: Hyperkalemia in dialysis patients

DOSAGE AND ROUTES

To prevent exercise-induced bronchospasm
• *Adult:* INH (metered dose inhaler) 2 puffs 15 min before exercising
Other respiratory conditions
• *Adult and child ≥12 yr:* INH (metered dose inhaler) 2 puffs q4h; PO 2-4 mg tid-qid, not to exceed 8 mg; NEB/IPPB 2.5 mg tid-qid
• *Geriatric:* PO 2 mg tid-qid, may increase gradually to 8 mg tid-qid
• *Child 2-12 yr:* INH (metered dose inhaler) 0.1 mg/kg tid (max 2.5 mg tid-qid); NEB/IPPB 0.1-0.15 mg/kg/dose tid-qid or 1.25 mg tid-qid for child 10-15 kg or 2.5 mg tid-qid >15 kg

Available forms: Aerosol 90 mcg/actuation; oral sol 2 mg/5 ml; tabs 2, 4 mg; ext rel 4, 8 mg; INH sol 0.83, 0.5, 1, 2, 5 mg/ml; powder for INH (Ventodisk) 200, 400 mcg; INH cap 200 mcg; 100 mcg/spray, 80 INH/canister, 200 INH/canister

SIDE EFFECTS

CNS: Tremors, anxiety, insomnia, headache, dizziness, stimulation, *restlessness,* hallucinations, flushing, irritability
CV: Palpitations, tachycardia, hypertension, angina, hypotension, dysrhythmias
EENT: Dry nose, irritation of nose and throat

GI: Heartburn, nausea, vomiting
MISC: Flushing, sweating, anorexia, bad taste/smell changes, hypokalemia
MS: Muscle cramps
RESP: Cough, wheezing, dyspnea, ***bronchospasm,*** dry throat

Contraindications: Hypersensitivity to sympathomimetics, tachydysrhythmias, severe cardiac disease, heart block

Precautions: Pregnancy (C), lactation, cardiac disorders, hyperthyroidism, diabetes mellitus, hypertension, prostatic hypertrophy, narrow-angle glaucoma, seizures, exercise-induced bronchospasm (aerosol) in children <12 years, hypoglycemia

PHARMACOKINETICS

Well absorbed PO, extensively metabolized in the liver and tissues, crosses placenta, breast milk, blood-brain barrier
PO: Onset ½ hr, peak 2½ hr, duration 4-6 hr, half-life 2½ hr
PO-ER: Onset ½ hour; peak 2-3 hr; duration 12 hr
INH: Onset 5 min, peak 1-1½ hr, duration 4-6 hr, half-life 4 hr

INTERACTIONS

May inhibit action of albuterol: other β-blockers
Severe hypotension: oxytocics
Toxicity: theophylline
ECG changes/hypokalemia: potassium-losing diuretics
Increase: action of aerosol bronchodilators
Increase: action of albuterol—tricyclics, MAOIs, other adrenergics; do not use together
Drug/Herb
Increase: stimulation—caffeine (cola nut, green/black tea, guarana, yerba maté, coffee, chocolate)

NURSING CONSIDERATIONS
Assess:
• Respiratory function: vital capacity, forced expiratory volume, ABGs; lung

sounds, heart rate and rhythm, B/P, sputum (baseline and peak)
• That patient has not received theophylline therapy before giving dose
• Patient's ability to self-medicate
• For evidence of allergic reactions
• Paradoxical bronchospasm, hold medication, notify prescriber if bronchospasm occurs

Administer:

PO route
• Do not break, crush, or chew ext rel tabs
• With meals to decrease gastric irritation
• Oral solution to children (no alcohol, sugar)

Inhalation route
• In geriatric patients and children, a spacing device is advised
• After shaking metered dose inhaler, exhale, place mouthpiece in mouth, inhale slowly, while depressing inhaler, hold breath, remove, exhale slowly; give INH at least 1 min apart
• NEB/IPPB diluting 5 mg/ml sol/2.5 ml 0.9% NaCl for INH; other sol do not require dilution; for neb O_2 flow or compressed air 6-10 L/min
• Gum, sips of water for dry mouth

Perform/provide:
• Storage in light-resistant container, do not expose to temperatures over 86° F (30° C)

Evaluate:
• Therapeutic response: absence of dyspnea, wheezing after 1 hr, improved airway exchange, improved ABGs

Teach patient/family:
• To use exactly as prescribed; take missed dose when remembered, alter dosing schedule
• Not to use OTC medications; excess stimulation may occur
• Use of inhaler; review package insert with patient; use demonstration, return demonstration
• To avoid getting aerosol in eyes; blurring of vision may result
• To wash inhaler in warm water daily and dry

• To avoid smoking, smoke-filled rooms, persons with respiratory infections
⚠ That paradoxic bronchospasm may occur and to stop drug immediately, call prescriber
• To limit caffeine products such as chocolate, coffee, tea, and colas

Treatment of overdose: Administer a β_1-adrenergic blocker

---

alclometasone topical
See Appendix C

⚠ High Alert

aldesleukin (℞)
(al-dess-loo'ken)
Interleukin-2, IL-2, Proleukin
Func. class.: Miscellaneous antineoplastic
Chem. class.: Interleukin-2, human recombinant (cytokine)

Do not confuse:
aldesleukin/oprelvekin
Proleukin/oprelvekin
Proleukin/Prokine

Action: Enhancement of lymphocyte mitogenesis and stimulation of IL-2–dependent cell lines; enhancement of lymphocyte cytotoxicity; induction of killer cell activity; induction of interferon-γ production; results in activation of cellular immunity, production of cytokines, and inhibition of tumor growth

Uses: Metastatic renal cell carcinoma in adults, phase II for HIV in combination with zidovudine; melanoma (metastatic)

Investigational uses: Kaposi's sarcoma given with zidovudine, metastatic melanoma given with cyclophosphamide, non-Hodgkin's lymphoma given with lymphokine-activated killer cells, AIDS (phase I) given with zidovudine

---

DOSAGE AND ROUTES

• *Adult:* **IV INF** 600,000 international units/kg (0.037 mg/kg) over 15 min q8h × 14 doses; off 9 days, repeat schedule for another 14 doses, for a max of 28 doses/course

Available forms: Powder for inj 22 million international units/vial

SIDE EFFECTS

CNS: Mental status changes, dizziness, sensory dysfunction, syncope, motor dysfunction, *fever, chills,* headache, impaired memory, depression, sleep disturbances, hallucinations, rigors, neuropathy

CV: Hypotension, sinus tachycardia, dysrhythmias, bradycardia, PVCs, PACs, myocardial ischemia, *myocardial infarction, cardiac arrest, capillary leak syndrome, CVA*

EENT: Reversible visual changes

GI: Nausea, vomiting, diarrhea, stomatitis, anorexia, GI bleeding, dyspepsia, constipation, *intestinal perforation/* ileus, jaundice, ascites

GU: Oliguria/anuria, proteinuria, hematuria, dysuria, *renal failure*

HEMA: Anemia, *thrombocytopenia, leukopenia, coagulation disorders, leukocytosis, eosinophilia*

INTEG: Pruritus, *erythema, rash,* dry skin, *exfoliative dermatitis,* purpura, petechiae, urticaria

MS: Arthralgia, myalgia

RESP: Pulmonary congestion, *dyspnea, pulmonary edema, respiratory failure, apnea,* tachypnea, pleural effusion, wheezing

SYST: Infection

Contraindications: Hypersensitivity, abnormal thallium stress test or pulmonary function tests, organ allografts

Precautions: Pregnancy (C), CNS metastases, bacterial infections, renal/hepatic/cardiac/pulmonary disease, lactation, children, anemia, thrombocytopenia

PHARMACOKINETICS

Renal elimination half-life 85 min; onset 4 wk, duration, variable

INTERACTIONS

Potentiate hypotension: antihypertensives
Reduced antitumor effectiveness: glucocorticoids
Unpredictable reactions: psychotropics
Increase: toxicity—aminoglycosides, indomethacin, cytotoxic chemotherapy, methotrexate, asparaginase, DOXOrubicin

Drug/Lab Test
Increase: Bilirubin, BUN, serum creatinine, transaminase, alk phosphatase; hypomagnesemia, acidosis hypocalcemia, hypophosphatemia, hypokalemia, hyperuricemia, hypoalbuminemia, hypoproteinemia, hyponatremia, hyperkalemia, alkalosis (toxic effect of drug)

NURSING CONSIDERATIONS

Assess:
• CBC, differential, platelet count weekly; withhold drug if WBC is <2000/mm^3 or platelet count is <75,000/mm^3; notify prescriber of these results

⚠ Capillary leak syndrome including a drop in mean arterial pressure (2-12 hr after initiating therapy); hypotension and hypoperfusion will occur; if B/P <90 mm Hg, use CVP, ECG, VS

• Renal studies: BUN, serum uric acid, urine CCr, electrolytes before, during therapy; I&O ratio; report fall in urine output to <30 ml/hr

• Monitor temp q4h

• Hepatic studies before, during therapy: bilirubin, AST, ALT, alk phosphatase, LDH as needed or monthly

• ECG; ST-T wave changes, low QRS and T, possible dysrhythmias (sinus tachycardia, PVCs)

⚠ Baselines in pulmonary function; document FEV >2 L or ≥75% prior to therapy; check VS q4h, monitor temp q4h, pulse oximetry, dyspnea, crackles, ABGs; watch for respiratory failure, intubate if necessary

---

• Stress thallium study prior to therapy; document normal ejection fraction, unimpaired wall motion

• Bleeding: hematuria, guaiac, bruising petechiae, mucosa or orifices q8h

• Buccal cavity q8h for dryness, sores, ulceration, white patches, oral pain, bleeding, dysphagia

• Local irritation, pain, burning at inj site

• GI symptoms: frequency of stools, cramping; acidosis, signs of dehydration: rapid respirations, poor skin turgor, decreased urine output, dry skin, restlessness, weakness

Administer:

IV, Intermittent INF routes

• Hydrocortisone, dexamethasone or sodium bicarbonate (1 mEq/1 ml) for extravasation, apply ice compresses

• Antiemetic 30-60 min before giving drug to prevent vomiting

• IV after diluting 22 million international units (1.3 mg)/1.2 ml sterile H_2O for inj at site of vial and swirl, do not shake; dilute dose with 50 ml D_5W and give over 15 min; use plastic bag; do not use an in-line filter, give through Y-tube or 3-way stopcock

• DOPamine 1-5 kg/min before onset of hypotension; decreased dose preserves kidney output

Y-site compatibilities: Amikacin, amphotericin B, calcium gluconate, diphenhydrAMINE, DOPamine, fluconazole, foscarnet, gentamicin, heparin, IV fat emulsion, magnesium sulfate, metoclopramide, morphine, ondansetron, piperacillin, potassium chloride, ranitidine, ticarcillin, tobramycin, TPN #145, trimethoprim-sulfamethoxazole

Perform/provide:

• Liquid diet: carbonated beverage, gelatin (Jell-O) may be added if patient is not nauseated or vomiting

• Rinsing of mouth tid-qid with water, club soda; brushing of teeth bid-tid with soft brush or cotton-tipped applicators for stomatitis; use unwaxed dental floss

• Storage in refrigerator of diluted drug; protect from light, do not freeze; administer within 48 hr; bring to room temperature before infusing; discard unused portion

Evaluate:

• Therapeutic response: decreased tumor size, spread of malignancy

Teach patient/family:

• To use a nonhormonal contraceptive method during therapy

• To report any complaints, side effects to nurse or prescriber

• To avoid foods with citric acid, hot or rough texture

• To avoid alcohol, NSAIDs, salicylates; GI bleeding may occur

• To report any bleeding, white spots, ulcerations in mouth to prescriber; tell patient to examine mouth daily

• To avoid crowds and persons with infections when granulocyte count is low

• Visual problems may occur, but are reversible

Rarely Used

alefacept (℞)

(ah-leh'fa-cept)
Amevive
Func. class.: Immunosuppressive

Uses: Adults with moderate to severe plaque psoriasis

DOSAGE AND ROUTES

• *Adult:* **IV BOL** 7.5 mg qwk or IM 15 mg qwk, for 12 wk

Contraindications: Hypersensitivity

alemtuzumab (℞)

(al-em-tuz'uh-mab)
Campath
Func. class.: Miscellaneous antineoplastic
Chem. class.: Monoclonal antibody

Action: Composed of recombinant DNA-derived humanized monoclonal antibody (campath-1H), binds to CD52 antigen that is present on surface of B and T lymphocytes, causes lysis of leukemic cells

Uses: B-cell chronic lymphocytic leukemia that has been treated with alkylating agents and that has failed fludarabine therapy

Investigational uses: Multiple sclerosis

DOSAGE AND ROUTES

• *Adult:* IV 3 mg over 2 hr daily; when tolerated, increase to 10 mg; when 10 mg tolerated increase to 30 mg daily, maintenance is 30 mg/day 3×/wk on alternate days for 12 wk, titration usually takes 3-7 days, max single dose 30 mg; max weekly dose 90 mg

Available forms: Sol for inj 30 mg/3 ml

SIDE EFFECTS

CNS: Dizziness, insomnia, depression, headache, tremor, somnolence, fatigue
CV: Hypotension, tachycardia, hypertension, edema, chest pain, supraventricular tachycardia
GI: Anorexia, diarrhea, constipation, *nausea, stomatitis, vomiting, abdominal pain, dyspepsia*
*HEMA: **Anemia, neutropenia, thrombocytopenia, pancytopenia,*** purpura, epistaxis
INTEG: Rash, local reaction, pruritus
MISC: Rigors, fever
RESP: Cough, pneumonia, rhinitis, ***bronchospasm,*** dyspnea, pharyngitis
Contraindications: Hypersensitivity, active systemic infection, immunodeficiency
Precautions: Pregnancy (C), lactation, children

PHARMACOKINETICS

Steady state 6 wk

INTERACTIONS

Do not give live virus vaccines
Drug/Lab Test
Interference: Diagnostic tests using antibodies

NURSING CONSIDERATIONS
Assess:
• CBC, platelets qwk or more often if myelosuppression occurs; CD4$^+$ after therapy until recovery of >200 cells/µl; irradiate blood if transfusions are required to prevent graft vs. host disease
• For symptoms of infection; chills, fever, headache, may be masked by drug fever; do not administer drug if infection is present
• CNS reaction: LOC, mental status, dizziness, confusion
• Cardiac status: lung sounds; ECG before and during treatment, especially in those with cardiac disease; monitor B/P hypotensive effect during administration
• Bone marrow depression: bruising, bleeding, blood in stools, urine, sputum, emesis
Administer:
IV route
• Do not give IV push or bolus
• Withdraw amount needed, use 5-µm filter before dilution, check for particulate matter and discoloration; inject into 100 ml sterile 0.9% NaCl or D$_5$W, gently invert to mix; do not add other drugs or infuse in same IV tubing
• Do not shake ampule
• Give diphenhydrAMINE 50 mg and acetaminophen 650 mg ½ hr prior to infusion; give hydrocortisone 200 mg to decrease severe infusion reactions; give TMP-sulfa DS bid 3×/wk and famciclovir 250 mg bid; continue for 2 mo or until CD4+ ≥200 cells/mm^3, whichever is later
Perform/provide:
• Storage of reconstituted sol for ≤8 hr at room temperature, do not freeze; protect from light
Evaluate:
• Therapeutic response: decrease in production of malignant lymphocytes
Teach patient/family:
• To take acetaminophen for fever
• To avoid hazardous tasks, because confusion, dizziness may occur

---

Side effects: *italics* = common; ***bold italics*** = life-threatening

• To report signs of infection: sore throat, fever, diarrhea, vomiting
• To avoid breastfeeding, effects are unknown, do not resume for ≥3 mo after last dose

---

alendronate (R)

(al-en-drone′ate)
Fosamax
Func. class.: Bone-resorption inhibitor
Chem. class.: Bisphosphonate

Do not confuse:
Fosamax/Flomax
Action: Absorbs calcium phosphate crystal in bone and may directly block dissolution of hydroxyapatite crystals of bone; inhibits normal and abnormal bone resorption, mineralization
Uses: Treatment and prevention of osteoporosis in postmenopausal women, treatment of osteoporosis in men, Paget's disease, treatment of corticosteroid-induced osteoporosis in postmenopausal women not receiving estrogen and men who are on continuing corticosteroid treatment with low bone mass

DOSAGE AND ROUTES

Osteoporosis in postmenopausal women
• *Adult and geriatric:* **PO** 10 mg daily or 70 mg qwk
Paget's disease
• *Adult and geriatric:* **PO** 40 mg daily × 6 mo, consider retreatment for relapse
Prevention of osteoporosis
• *Adult:* **PO** 5 mg daily or 35 mg qwk
Corticosteroid-induced osteoporosis in postmenopausal women (not receiving estrogen)
• *Adult:* **PO** 10 mg daily
Corticosteroid-induced osteoporosis in men or premenopausal women
• *Adult:* **PO** 5 mg daily
Available forms: Tabs 5, 10, 35, 40, 70 mg; oral sol 70 mg

SIDE EFFECTS

CNS: Headache
GI: Abdominal pain, anorexia, constipation, nausea, vomiting, esophageal ulceration, acid reflux, dyspepsia
META: Anemia, hypokalemia, hypomagnesemia, hypophosphatemia, hypocalcemia
MS: Bone pain
Contraindications: Hypersensitivity to bisphosphonates, delayed esophageal emptying, inability to sit or stand for 30 min, hypocalcemia
Precautions: Pregnancy (C), children, lactation, CCr <35 ml/min, esophageal disease, ulcers, gastritis

PHARMACOKINETICS

Rapidly cleared from circulation, taken up mainly by bones, eliminated primarily through kidneys

INTERACTIONS

Possible GI reactions: NSAIDs, salicylates
Increase: alendronate effect—ranitidine (IV)
Decrease: absorption—antacids, calcium supplements
Drug/Food
Decrease: absorption when used with caffeine, orange juice

NURSING CONSIDERATIONS

Assess:
• Hormonal status if a woman, prior to treatment
• For osteoporosis: bone density test
• For Paget's disease: increased skull size, bone pain, headache
• Electrolytes; renal function studies; Ca, P, Mg, K
• For hypercalcemia: paresthesia, twitching, laryngospasm, Chvostek's, Trousseau's signs
• Alk phosphatase levels, baseline and periodically, 2 × upper limit of normal is indicative of Paget's disease
Administer:
• For 6 months to be effective in Paget's disease; take with 8 oz of water 30 min

---

...ge, or medication

Continuous anesthesia

Induction
• *Adult:* IV 50-75 mcg/kg

Maintenance
• *Adult:* IV 0.5-3.0 mcg/kg/min: rate should be decreased by 30%-50% after 1 hr maintenance or INF; may be increased to 4 mcg/kg/min or BOL doses of 7 mcg/kg

Induction of anesthesia >45 min
• *Adult:* IV 130-245 mcg/kg, then 0.5-1.5 mcg/kg/min

MAC

Induction
• *Adult:* IV duration ≤½ hr 3-8 mcg/kg

Maintenance
• *Adult:* 3-5 mcg/kg (5-20 min to 1 mcg/kg/min, total dose 3-40 mcg/kg

Contraindications: Child <12 yr, hypersensitivity

---

alfuzosin (R)

[al-fyoo'zoe-sin]
Uroxatral
Func. class.: Antiadrenergics
Chem. class.: Quinazoline

Action: Binds preferentially to α₁-adrenoceptor subtype located mainly in the prostate

Uses: Symptoms of benign prostatic hyperplasia; use not indicated for the treatment of high blood pressure

DOSAGE AND ROUTES
• *Adult:* PO ext rel to g d, 10 mg after same meal each day

Available forms: Tabs...

SIDE ...potenc...e, ...gue
CNS ...ess, fati..., pain,
...administer...
...a, Abdom...n, dyspepsia,
...ea, ...om...
...s 3...m
...potence, ...ral
...; Body pain

Rarely Used

alfentanil (R)

[al-fen'ta-nil]
Alfenta, Rapifen
Func. class.: Opioid analgesic

Controlled Substance Schedule II

Uses: In combination with other drugs in general anesthesia, as a primary anesthetic in general surgery, monitored anesthesia care (MAC)

DOSAGE AND ROUTES

Anesthesia <30 min

Combination
• *Adult:* IV 8-50 mcg/kg, may increase by 3-15 mcg/kg

Anesthetic induction
• *Adult:* IV 3-5 mcg/kg, then 0.5-1.5 mcg/kg/min; total dose is 8-40 mcg/kg

Anesthesia 30-60 min

Induction
• *Adult:* IV 20-50 mcg/kg

Maintenance
• *Adult:* IV 5-15 mcg...
75 mcg/kg total dos...

...response: increased bone
...fractures

.../family:
...right for 30 min after
...t esophageal irritation, if
...d, skip dose, do not double
...d later in day
...le later in day
...an before food, other meds,
...8 oz of water only (no min-
...an before food, other meds,
...e calcium, vit D if instructed by
...e bone density
...rease weight-bearing exercise to
...are provider
...o let health care provider know if
...gnant or if pregnancy is planned or if
...ursing

pper respiratory infection, phar-
as, bronchitis, sinusitis

ontraindications: Hypersensitivity,
moderate to severe hepatic impairment,
not indicated for use in women or children

Precautions: Pregnancy (B), lactation,
coronary artery disease, coronary insufficiency, mild hepatic disease, mild/
moderate/severe renal disease, history of
QT prolongation or coadministration
with meds known to prolong QT interval

PHARMACOKINETICS

PO: Elimination half-life: 10 hr; extensively metabolized in liver by CYP3A4
enzyme; excreted via urine (11%
unchanged); moderately protein binding (82%-90%)

INTERACTIONS

Possible increased effects of alfuzosin:
alcohol
Not to be taken with: prazosin, terazosin,
doxazosin
Not to be taken with: CYP3A4 inhibitors
(ketoconazole, itraconazole, and
ritonavir)

NURSING CONSIDERATIONS

Asses:
• rstatic hyperplasia: change in uri-
na patterns, baseline and throughout
trent
• ith difind LFTsB/P and heart
ate
• B diac ac un dynamic studies
(urin y ras, nal volume)
• &d wei
weigh eder edema, report
Admi
PO ro
• Do no crush,
Perform
• Storage: contai
ronment
Evaluate:
• Therapeut ve: d
symptoms of be p at
sia

⚠ Safety alert

• Not to drive or operate machinery for
4 hr after first dose or after dosage increase

---

alitretinoin (℞)
(a-li-tret'i-noyn)
Panretin
Func. class.: Retinoid, 2nd generation, topical antineoplastic

---

Action: Controls cellular differentiation
and proliferation of neoplastic and
healthy cells by binding to retinoid receptors
Uses: Kaposi's sarcoma cutaneous lesions

DOSAGE AND ROUTES

• *Adult:* **TOP** Apply enough gel to cover
lesions with a generous coating, allow to
dry for 3-5 min, before covering with
clothing, do not apply near mucosal
areas, apply as long as benefit occurs; do
not rub gel into the lesion
Available forms: Gel 0.1%

SIDE EFFECTS

INTEG: Rash, stinging, warmth, redness,
erythema, blistering, crusting, peeling,
contact dermatitis, *pain*
Contraindications: Pregnancy (D),
hypersensitivity to retinoids
Precautions: Lactation, eczema, sunburn, elderly, cutaneous T-cell lymphoma

PHARMACOKINETICS

TOP: Poor systemic absorption

INTERACTIONS

Do not use around DEET (an insect re-
pellant agent)

NURSING CONSIDERATIONS

Assess:
• Area of body involved, what helps or
ravates condition; cysts, dryness,
lesions may worsen at beginning
nt

- Dermal toxicity that may start as erythema, then edema, may need to be discontinued and restarted

Administer:
- Bid initially to lesions, can be increased to tid-qid according to tolerance

Perform/provide:
- Storage at room temperature
- Hand washing after application

Evaluate:
- Therapeutic response: decrease in size and number of lesions

Teach patient/family:
- To avoid application on normal skin, getting cream in eyes, nose, other mucous membranes, not to rub into lesion, do not use occlusive dressing, wait 20 min after bath, shower to apply; wait at least 3 hr after using to shower, bathe, swim
- To avoid sunlight, sunlamps, or use protective clothing, sunscreen
- That treatment may cause warmth, stinging, dryness, peeling will occur
- That drug does not cure condition; only relieves symptoms
- That therapeutic results may be seen in 2-3 wk but may not be optimal until after 6 wk

---

allopurinol (℞)

(al-oh-pure′i-nole)
Alloprim, allopurinol,
Apo-Allopurinol ✦, Lopurin ✦,
Purimol ✦, Zyloprim
Func. class.: Antigout drug
Chem. class.: Xanthene oxidase inhibitor

Do not confuse:
allopurinol/apresoline
Lopurin/Lupron
Action: Inh
oxidase
Use
asso
cal
cut
aci

Side effects: *italics* = common; **bold italics** = life-threatening

---

Investigational uses: Stomatitis (mouthwash)

DOSAGE AND ROUTES

Increased uric acid levels in malignancies
- *Adult:* **IV INF** 200-400 mg/m²/day, max 600 mg/day
- *Child:* **IV INF** 200 mg/m²/day, initially

Gout/hyperuricemia
- *Adult:* **PO** 200-600 mg daily depending on severity, not to exceed 800 mg/day
- *Child 6-10 yr:* 300 mg daily
- *Child <6 yr:* 150 mg daily

Impaired renal function
- *Adult:* **PO** 200 mg daily (CCr is 20 to 30 ml/min); 100 mg daily (CCr <20 ml/min); **IV** CCr 10-20 ml/min 200 mg/day; CCr 3-10 ml/min 100 mg/day; CCr <3 ml/min 100 mg/day at intervals

Recurrent calculi
- *Adult:* **PO** 200-300 mg daily

Uric acid nephropathy prevention
- *Adult and child >10 yr:* **PO** 600-800 mg daily × 2-3 days

Stomatitis
- *Adult:* Mouthwash dose varies, do not swallow

Available forms: Tabs, scored 100, 300 mg; inj 500g/vial

SIDE EFFECTS

CNS: Headache, drowsiness, neuritis, paresthesia, *peripheral neuropathy, cataract, ataxia, malaise*
EENT: Retinopathy, peptic ulcer,
GI: Nausea, hepatitis, thrombocytopenia, aplastic anemia, pancytopenia, eosinophilia
fever, chills, dermatitis, pruritus, erythema, ecchymosis, alopecia myopathy, arthralgia, hepatomegaly, cholestatic jaundice, renal failure, exfoliative dermatitis

Contraindications: Hypersensitivity
Precautions: Pregnancy (C), lactation, renal disease, hepatic disease, children

PHARMACOKINETICS

PO: Peak 2-4 hr; excreted in feces, urine; half-life 2-3 hr, terminal half-life 18-30 hr
IV: Half-life 1 hr

INTERACTIONS

Possible kidney stone formation: ammonium chloride, vit C, potassium/sodium phosphate
Rash: ampicillin, amoxicillin, bacampicillin
Increase: action of oral anticoagulants, chlorpropamide, cyclophosphamide, hydantoin, theophylline, vidarabine, ACE inhibitors, mercaptopurine azathioprine
Increase: allopurinol toxicity—thiazide diuretics
Increase: bone marrow depression—antineoplastics
Decrease: effects of probenecid
Decrease: effects of allopurinol—aluminum salts

NURSING CONSIDERATIONS

Assess:
• Uric acid levels q w k; uric acid levels should be 6 mg/dl o les
• CBC, AST, BUN, creatine before starting treatment, month
• I&O ratio; increase ds to 2 L/day to prevent stone formation
• Nutritional status: discorage organ meat, sardine, salmon, le mes, gravies (aline foods), acoh

Admir
PO route
• With meal
• A few days b symptoms
apy

IV INF route
• Reconstitute 30 tic thersterile water for inj;
conc with 0.9% NaCl
begin inf within 10 hr

Solution incompati
Amikacin, amphotericin
tine, cefotaxime, chlorpro
cimetidine, clindamycin, cy
dacarbazine, DAUNOrubicin

drAMINE, DOXOrubicin, doxycycline, droperidol, floxuridine, gentamicin, haloperidol, hydrOXYzine, idarubicin, imipenem, cilastatin, mechlorethamine, meperidine, metoclopramide, methylPREDNISolone, minocycline, nalbuphine, netilmicin, ondansetron, prochlorperazine, promethazine, sodium bicarbonate, streptozocin, tobramycin, vinorelbine

Evaluate:
• Therapeutic response: decreased pain in joints, decreased stone formation in kidneys

Teach patient/family:
• That tabs may be crushed
• To take as prescribed; if dose is missed, take as soon as remembered; do not double dose
• To increase fluid intake to 2 L/day
• To report skin rash, stomatitis, malaise, fever, aching; drug should be discontinued
• To avoid hazardous activities if drowsiness or dizziness occurs
• To avoid alcohol, caffeine; will increase uric acid levels
• To avoid large doses of vit C; kidney stone formation may occur
• To maintain a diet enhancing urine alkalinity (e.g., dairy products)
• To reduce dairy products, refined sugars, sodium, meat if taking for calcium oxalate stones

almotriptan (℞)
(al-moh-trip'tan)
Axert
Func. class.: Antimigraine agent
Chem. class.: 5-HT$_1$-receptor agonist

: Binds selectively to the vascular receptors, exerts antimigraine vasoconstriction in cranial

t of migraine with

⚠ Safety alert   *"Tall Man" letterin

DOSAGE AND ROUTES

Adult: **PO** may use the 6.25-mg dose initially, but 12.5 mg is more effective; may repeat dose after 2 hr; do not give more than 2 doses/24 hr or 4 treatment cycles within any 30-day period

Hepatic/renal dose
• *Adult:* **PO** 6.25 mg initially, max 12.5 mg

Available forms: Tabs 6.25, 12.5 mg

SIDE EFFECTS

CV: Flushing, palpitations, tachycardia, ***coronary artery vasospasm, MI, ventricular fibrillation, ventricular tachycardia***
EENT: Throat, mouth, nasal discomfort; vision changes
GI: Nausea, xerostomia
INTEG: Sweating
MS: Weakness, neck stiffness, myalgia
NEURO: Tingling, hot sensation, burning, feeling of pressure, tightness, numbness, dizziness, sedation, headache, anxiety, fatigue, cold sensation
RESP: Chest tightness, pressure

Contraindications: Hypersensitivity, cluster headache, hemiplegia, vascular migraine, ischemic heart disease, peripheral vascular syndrome, concurrent use of ergotamine-containing preparations, uncontrolled hypertension, basilar or hemiplegic migraine; concurrent MAO inhibitor therapy or within 2 wk
Precautions: Pregnancy (C), postmenopausal women, men >40 yr, risk factors for CAD, hypercholesterolemia, obesity, diabetes, impaired hepatic or renal function, lactation, children <18 yr, elderly

PHARMACOKINETICS

Onset of pain relief 2 hr, got
duration 3-4'
live

Increase: almotriptan effect—MAOIs, CYP2D6 inhibitors
Increase: plasma concentration of almotriptan—ketoconazole
Drug/Herb
Increase: almotriptan effect—butterbur

NURSING CONSIDERATIONS

Assess:
• B/P; signs/symptoms of coronary vasospasms
• Tingling, hot sensation, burning, feeling of pressure, numbness, flushing
• For stress level, activity, recreation, coping mechanisms
• Neurologic status: LOC, blurring vision, nausea, vomiting, tingling in extremities preceding headache
• Ingestion of tyramine foods (pickled products, beer, wine, aged cheese), food additives, preservatives, colorings, artificial sweeteners, chocolate, caffeine, which may precipitate these types of headaches

Administer:
• Swallow tabs whole; do not break, crush, or chew

Perform/provide:
• Quiet, calm environment with decreased stimulation from noise, bright light, excessive talking

Evaluate:
• Therapeutic response: decrease in severity of migraine

Teach patient/family:
• To report chest pain, drowsiness, dizziness, tingling, flushing, ~~ncy is~~
• To use contrac~~...~~ breastfeed-
drug, not~~...~~diet environment
~~...~~graine attacks ~~...not prevent or reduce~~

alprazolam (R)

(al-pray′zoe-lam)
Apo-Alpraz ✤, Novo-
Alprazol ✤, Nu-Alpraz ✤,
Xanax, Xanax XR
Func. class.: Antianxiety
Chem. class.: Benzodiazepine

Controlled Substance Schedule IV
Do not confuse:
alprazolam/lorazepam
Xanax/Lanoxin
Xanax/Tylox
Xanax/Zantac

Action: Depresses subcortical levels of CNS, including limbic system, reticular formation

Uses: Anxiety, panic disorders, anxiety with depressive symptoms

Investigational uses: Depression, social phobia, premenstrual dysphoric disorders

DOSAGE AND ROUTES

Anxiety disorder
• *Adult:* **PO** 0.25-0.5 mg tid, not to exceed 4 mg/day in divided doses
• *Geriatric:* **PO** 0.125-0.25 mg bid; increase by 0.125 as needed

Panic disorder
• *Adult:* **PO** 0.5 mg tid may increase, max 10 mg/day; ext rel tabs (Xanax XR) give daily in AM 0.5-1 mg initially, mainte-
nⷮce 1-10 mg daily
• *ⷮenstrual dysphoric disorders*
day ⷮ **PO** 0.25 mg bid-qid, starting on
when ⷮ doses, taper over 2-3 days
Social Pⷮses
• *Adult:* **P**ⷮ
Hepatic dosⷮ
• Reduce dose ⷮ
Available forms:ⷮ
mg; oral sol 1 mg/ml;ⷮ
XR) 0.5, 1, 2, 3 mg

SIDE EFFECTS
CNS: *Dizziness, drowsiness,* coⷮ
headache, anxiety, tremors, stimuⷮ

⚠ Safety alert   *"Tall Man" lettering

fatigue, depression, insomnia, hallucinations
*CV: Orthostatic hypotension, **ECG changes, tachycardia,** hypotension*
EENT: Blurred vision, tinnitus, mydriasis
GI: Constipation, dry mouth, nausea, vomiting, anorexia, diarrhea
INTEG: Rash, dermatitis, itching
Contraindications: Pregnancy (D), hypersensitivity to benzodiazepines, narrow-angle glaucoma, psychosis, lactation, addiction
Precautions: Elderly, debilitated, hepatic disease

PHARMACOKINETICS

PO: Onset 30 min, peak 1-2 hr, duration 4-6 hr, therapeutic response 2-3 days; metabolized by liver, excreted by kidneys; crosses placenta, breast milk; half-life 12-15 hr

INTERACTIONS

A substrate of CYP3A4
Increase: alprazolam action—cimetidine, disulfiram, erythromycin, fluoxetine, isoniazid, ketoconazole, metoprolol, propoxyphene, propanolol, valproic acid
Increase: CNS depression—anticonvulsants, alcohol, antihistamines, sedative/hypnotics
Decrease: sedation—xanthines
Decrease: alprazolam action—barbiturates, rifampin
Decrease: action of levodopa
Drug/Herb
Increase: CNS depression—cat's claw, chamomile, cowslip, echinacea, goldenseal, hops, kava, licorice, Queen Anne's lace, skullcap, St. John's wort, valerian, wild cherry
Drug/Food
Increase: drug level; grapefruit juice
Drug/Lab Test
ⷮ AST/ALT, alk phosphatase

ⷮNSIDERATIONS
ⷮsen-

drowsiness, dizziness, especially in elderly

• B/P lying, standing; pulse; if systolic B/P drops 20 mm Hg, hold drug, notify prescriber

• Hepatic, blood studies: AST, ALT, bilirubin, creatinine, LDH, alk phosphatase, CBC; may cause neutropenia, decreased Hct, increased LFTs

• For indications of increasing tolerance and abuse

⚠ Physical dependency, withdrawal symptoms: anxiety, panic attacks, agitation, convulsions, headache, nausea, vomiting, muscle pain, weakness; withdrawal seizures may occur after rapid decrease in dose or abrupt discontinuation; since duration of action is short, considered to be the drug of choice in the elderly

Administer:

PO route

• With food or milk for GI symptoms

• Crushed, mixed with food or fluids if patient is unable to swallow medication whole

• May divide total daily doses into more times/day, if anxiety occurs between doses

Evaluate:

• Therapeutic response: decreased anxiety, restlessness, sleeplessness

Teach patient/family:

• Not to double doses; take exactly as prescribed; if dose is missed, take within 1 hr as scheduled

• That drug may be taken with food

• Not to use for everyday stress or longer than 4 mo unless directed by prescriber; not to take more than prescribed amount; may be habit forming; memory impairment is a sign of long-term use

• To avoid OTC preparations unless approved by prescriber

• To avoid driving, activities that require alertness, since drowsiness may occur

• To avoid alcohol ingestion or other psychotropic medications unless directed by prescriber

• Not to discontinue medication abruptly after long-term use

• To rise slowly or fainting may occur, especially elderly

• That drowsiness may worsen at beginning of treatment

Treatment of overdose: Lavage, VS, supportive care, flumazenil

---

Rarely Used

alprostadil (℞)

(al-pros'ta-dil)

Caverject, Edex, Muse, PGEI, prostaglandin E₁, Prostin VR ✦, Prostin VR Pediatric

Func. class.: Hormone

Uses: To maintain patent ductus arteriosus (temporary treatment), erectile dysfunction

DOSAGE AND ROUTES

Patent ductus arteriosus

• *Infants:* **IV INF** 0.1 mcg/kg/min, until desired response, then reduce to lowest effective amount, 0.4 mcg/kg/min not likely to produce greater beneficial effects

Erectile dysfunction of vasculogenic or mixed etiology, psychogenic

• *Men:* **INTRACAVERNOSAL** 2.5 mcg may increase by 2.5 mcg; may then increase by 5-10 mcg until adequate response occurs; **INTRAURETHRAL:** administer as needed to achieve erection

Contraindications: Hypersensitivity, respiratory distress syndrome (RDS)

⚠ High Alert

alteplase (℞)

(al-ti-plaze')

Activase, Activase rt-PA ✦, Cathflo, Lysatec-rt-PA ✦, tissue plasminogen activator, t-PA

Func. class.: Thrombolytic enzyme

Chem. class.: Tissue plasminogen activator (TPA)

Do not confuse:

alteplace/Altace

Action: Produces fibrin conversion of plasminogen to plasmin; able to bind to fibrin, convert plasminogen in thrombus to plasmin, which leads to local fibrinolysis, limited systemic proteolysis

Uses: Lysis of obstructing thrombi associated with acute MI, ischemic conditions requiring thrombolysis (i.e., PE, DVT, unclotting arteriovenous shunts, acute ischemic CVA)

Investigational uses: Unstable angina, occluded central venous catheters

Dosage and routes:
Myocardial infarction (standard INF)
• *Adult >65 kg:* **IV** a total of 100 mg; 6-10 mg given **IV BOL** over 1-2 min, 60 mg given over 1st hr, 20 mg given over 2nd hr, 20 mg given over 3rd hr; or 1.25 mg/kg given over 3 hr for patients <65 kg
• *Adult <65 kg:* **IV** 0.75 mg over 1st hr, 0.075-0.125 mg/kg given **IV BOL** over 1st 1-2 min; 0.25 mg/kg over 2nd hr, 0.25 mg/kg over 3rd hr to a total dose of 1.25 mg/kg, max 100 mg total

Myocardial infarction (accelerated INF)
• *Adult:* **IV BOL** 15 mg; then 0.75 mg/kg over ½ hr; then 0.5 mg/kg over 1 hr, usually given with heparin

Pulmonary embolism
• *Adult:* **IV** 100 mg over 2 hr, then heparin

Acute ischemic stroke
• *Adult:* **IV** 0.9 mg/kg, max 90 mg; give as **INF** over 1 hr, give 10% of dose **IV BOL** over 1st min

Occluded central venous catheters
• *Adult:* 2 mg/2 ml infused in each port of dual-lumen catheter, dwell time varies widely

Available forms: Powder for inj 50 mg (29 million international units/vial), 100 mg (58 million international units/vial)

SIDE EFFECTS

CV: **Sinus bradycardia, ventricular tachycardia, accelerated idioventricular rhythm, bradycardia**
INTEG: Urticaria, rash

SYST: **GI, GU, intracranial, retroperitoneal bleeding,** *surface bleeding,* **anaphylaxis**

Contraindications: Hypersensitivity, active internal bleeding, recent CVA, severe uncontrolled hypertension, intracranial/intraspinal surgery/trauma, aneurysm, brain tumor

Precautions: Pregnancy (C), lactation, children, elderly, neurologic deficits, mitral stenosis, recent GI, GU bleeding

PHARMACOKINETICS

Cleared by liver, 80% cleared within 10 min of drug termination, onset immediate, peak 45 min, duration 4 hr, half-life 35 min

INTERACTIONS

Increase: bleeding—anticoagulants, salicylates, dipyridamole, other NSAIDs, abciximab, eptifibatide, tirofiban, clopidogrel, ticlopidine, some cephalosporins, plicamycin, valproic acid

Drug/Herb
Increase: risk of bleeding—agrimony, alfalfa, angelica, anise, basil, bay, bilberry, black haw, bogbean, bromelain, buchu, chondroitin, cinchona bark, dong quai, fenugreek, feverfew, garlic, ginger, ginkgo, ginseng, horse chestnut, Irish moss, kelp, kelpware, khella, lovage, lungwort, meadowsweet, mother wort, mugwort, nettle, papaya, parsley (large amts), pau d'arco, pineapple, poplar, prickly ash, safflower, saw palmetto, tonka bean, tumeric, wintergreen, yarrow

Decrease: anticoagulant effect—chamomile, coenzyme Q10, flax, glucomannan, goldenseal, guar gum

Drug/Lab Test
Increase: PT, APTT, TT

NURSING CONSIDERATIONS

Assess:
• VS, B/P, pulse, respirations, neurologic signs, temperature at least q4h; temp >104° F (40° C) indicates internal bleeding; monitor rhythm closely; ven-

tricular dysrhythmias may occur with hyperfusion; monitor heart, breath sounds, neurologic status, peripheral pulses; assess neurologic status, neurologic change may indicate intracranial bleeding

A For bleeding during first hour of treatment and 24 hr after procedure: hematuria, hematemesis, bleeding from mucous membranes, epistaxis, ecchymosis; guaiac all body fluids, stools. Do not use 150 mg or more total dose; intracranial bleeding may occur

A Hypersensitivity: fever, rash, itching, chills, facial swelling, dyspnea, notify prescriber immediately; stop drug, keep resuscitative equipment nearby; mild reaction may be treated with antihistamines

• Blood studies (Hct, platelets, PTT, PT, TT, APTT) before starting therapy; PT or APTT must be less than 2 × control before starting therapy TT or PT q3-4h during treatment

• ECG continuously, cardiac enzymes, radionuclide myocardial scanning/coronary angiography

Administer:

Intermittent IV INF route

• After reconstituting with provided diluent, add appropriate amount of sterile water for inj (no preservatives) 20 mg vial/20 ml or 50 mg vial/50 ml to make 1 mg/ml, mix by slow inversion or dilute with NaCl, D₅W to a concentration of 0.5 mg/ml; 1.5 to <0.5 mg/ml may result in precipitation of drug; use 18G needle; flush line with NaCl after administration, give over 3 hr for MI, 2 hr for pulmonary embolism

• Heparin therapy after thrombolytic therapy is discontinued, TT, ACT, or APTT less than 2 × control (about 3-4 hr)

• Reconstituted IV solution within 8 hr or discard

• Within 6 hr of coronary occlusion for best results

Additive compatibilities: Lidocaine, morphine, nitroglycerin

Y-site compatibilities: Lidocaine, metoprolol, propranolol

Perform/provide:

• Avoidance of invasive procedures, injection, rectal temp

• Pressure for 30 sec to minor bleeding sites; 30 min to sites of atrial puncture, followed by pressure dressing; inform prescriber if this does not attain hemostasis; apply pressure dressing

• Storage of powder at room temperature or refrigerate; protect from excessive light

Evaluate:

• Therapeutic response: lysis of thrombi

Teach patient/family:

• The purpose and expected results of the treatment; to report adverse reactions

---

Rarely Used

altretamine (℞)
(al-tret′a-meen)
Hexalen, hexamethylmelamine, Hexastat ✦
Func. class.: Misc. antineoplastic

Uses: Palliative treatment of recurrent, persistent ovarian cancer following first-line treatment with cisplatin or alkylating agent–based combination

Investigational uses: Lymphoma, lung cancer

DOSAGE AND ROUTES

• *Adult:* **PO** 260 mg/m²/day for 14 or 21 days in a 28-day cycle; give in 4 divided doses after meals and at bedtime

Contraindications: Pregnancy (D), hypersensitivity, severe bone marrow depression, severe neurologic toxicity

---

Side effects: *italics* = common; ***bold italics*** = life-threatening

aluminum hydroxide (otc)

AlternaGEL, Alu-Cap, Alugel ✤, Aluminet, aluminum hydroxide, Alu-Tab, Amphojel, Basal gel, Dialume

Func. class.: Antacid, hypophosphatemic, antiulcer

Chem. class.: Aluminum product, phosphate binder

Action: Neutralizes gastric acidity, binds phosphates in GI tract; these phosphates are excreted

Uses: Antacid, hyperphosphatemia in chronic renal failure; adjunct in gastric, peptic, duodenal ulcers; hyperacidity, reflux esophagitis, heartburn, stress ulcer prevention in critically ill, GERD

Investigational uses: GI bleeding

DOSAGE AND ROUTES

Antacid
• **Adult: SUSP** 5-10 ml 1 hr pc, at bedtime; **PO** 600 mg 1 hr pc, at bedtime, chewed; max 6 times per day

Hyperphosphatemia in renal failure
• **Adult: SUSP** 500 mg-2 g bid-qid

GI bleeding
• **Infant:PO** 2-5 ml/dose q1-2h
• **Child: PO** 5-15 ml/dose q1-2h

Available forms: Caps 475, 500 mg; tabs 300, 500, 600 mg; susp 320 mg/5 ml, 450 mg/5 ml, 600 mg/5 ml, 675 mg/5 ml

SIDE EFFECTS

GI: Constipation, anorexia, **obstruction,** fecal impaction
META: Hypophosphatemia, hypercalciuria

Contraindications: Hypersensitivity to this drug or aluminum products

Precautions: Pregnancy (C), elderly, fluid restriction, decreased GI motility, GI obstruction, dehydration, renal disease, sodium-restricted diets, lactation

PHARMACOKINETICS

PO: Onset 20-40 min, duration 1-3 hr, excreted in feces

INTERACTIONS

Decrease: effectiveness of allopurinol, amprenavir, cephalosporins, ciprofloxacin, corticosteroids, delavirdine, diflunisal, digitalis, gabapentin, gatifloxacin, H_2-antagonists, iron salts, isoniazid, ketoconazole, penicillamine, phenothiazines, phenytoin, quinidine, tetracyclines, thyroid hormones, ticlopidine anticholinergics, warfarin; separate by at least 2 hr

Drug/Herb
Decrease: action of buckthorn, cascara sagrada, castor, Chinese rhubarb

NURSING CONSIDERATIONS

Assess:
• Pain: location, intensity, duration, character
• Phosphate levels, since drug is bound in GI system
• Hypophosphatemia: anorexia, weakness, fatigue, bone pain, hyporeflexia
• Constipation; increase bulk in diet if needed
• Urinary pH, Ca^{++}, electrolytes

Administer:
• 2 tsp (10 ml) will neutralize 20 mEq of acid; 2 tabs will neutralize 16 mEq of acid

PO route
• Give with 8 oz water for hyperphosphatemia, unless contraindicated
• Tablets must be chewed well, then give 8 oz water
• Laxatives or stool softeners if constipation occurs, especially elderly
• After shaking liquid
• With small amount of water or milk

NG route
• By nasogastric tube if patient unable to swallow

Evaluate:
• Therapeutic response: absence of pain, decreased acidity, healed ulcers

---

🅐 Safety alert   *"Tall Man" lettering

Teach patient/family:
• To increase fluids to 2 L/day unless contraindicated; measures to prevent constipation
• To avoid phosphate foods (most dairy products, eggs, fruits, carbonated beverages) during drug therapy for hyperphosphatemia
• Not to use for prolonged periods in patients with low serum phosphate or if on a low-sodium diet
• To add cheese, corn, pasta, plums, prunes, lentils after drug is discontinued
• That stools may appear white or speckled
• To check with prescriber after 2 wk of self-prescribed antacid use
• To separate other medications by 2 hr

---

amantadine (℞)

(a-man'ta-deen)
amantadine HCl, Symadine, Symmetrel
Func. class.: Antiviral, antiparkinsonian agent
Chem. class.: Tricyclic amine

Do not confuse:
amantadine/ranitidine
amantadine/rimantidine
Symmetrel/Synthroid
Action: Prevents uncoating of nucleic acid in viral cell, preventing penetration of virus to host; causes release of dopamine from neurons
Uses: Prophylaxis or treatment of influenza type A, extrapyramidal reactions, parkinsonism, Parkinson's disease
Investigational uses: Neuroleptic malignant syndrome, cocaine dependency, enuresis

DOSAGE AND ROUTES
Influenza type A
• *Adult and child >12 yr:* **PO** 200 mg/day in single dose or divided bid, max 400 mg/day
• *Geriatric:* **PO** No more than 100 mg daily
• *Child 9-12 yr:* **PO** 100 mg bid

• *Child 1-9 yr:* **PO** 5 mg/kg/day divided bid-tid, not to exceed 150 mg/day
Extrapyramidal reaction/parkinsonism
Adult: **PO** 100 mg bid, up to 400 mg/day in EPS; give for 1 wk, then 100 mg as needed up to 400 mg in parkinsonism
MS-associated fatigue (off-label)
• *Adult:* **PO** 200 mg daily or 100 mg bid
Neuroleptic malignant syndrome (off-label)
• *Adult:* **PO** 100 mg bid × 3 wk
Renal dose
• CCr 40-50 ml/min 100 mg/day; CCr 30 ml/min 200 mg 2×/wk; CCr 20 ml/min 100 mg 3×/wk; CCr <10 ml/min 100 mg alternating with 200 mg q7days
Available forms: Caps 100 mg; syr 50 mg/5 ml

SIDE EFFECTS
CNS: Headache, dizziness, drowsiness, fatigue, *anxiety,* psychosis, *depression, hallucinations,* tremors, ***convulsions,*** confusion, *insomnia*
CV: Orthostatic hypotension, ***CHF***
EENT: Blurred vision
GI: Nausea, vomiting, constipation, dry mouth
GU: Frequency, retention
HEMA: ***Leukopenia***
INTEG: Photosensitivity, dermatitis
Contraindications: Hypersensitivity, lactation, child <1 yr, eczematic rash
Precautions: Pregnancy (C), epilepsy, CHF, orthostatic hypotension, psychiatric disorders, hepatic disease, renal disease, peripheral edema, elderly

PHARMACOKINETICS
PO: Onset 48 hr, half-life 24 hr, not metabolized, excreted in urine (90%) unchanged, crosses placenta, excreted in breast milk

INTERACTIONS
Increase: anticholinergic response—atropine, other anticholinergics
Increase: CNS stimulation—CNS stimulants

Side effects: *italics* = common; ***bold italics*** = life-threatening

Decrease: renal excretion of amantadine—triamterene, hydrochlorothiazide

Drug/Herb

Increase: anticholinergic effect—belladonna, henbane

Increase: action/side effects—pheasant's eye, quinine, scopolia root

Decrease: effect—kava

NURSING CONSIDERATIONS

Assess:
• I&O ratio; report frequency, hesitancy
• CHF, confusion, mottling of skin
• Bowel pattern before, during treatment
• Skin eruptions, photosensitivity after administration of drug
• Respiratory status: rate, character, wheezing, tightness in chest
• Allergies before initiation of treatment, reaction of each medication
• Signs of infection

Administer:
• Before exposure to influenza; continue for 10 days after contact
• At least 4 hr before bedtime to prevent insomnia
• After meals for better absorption, to decrease GI symptoms
• In divided doses to prevent CNS disturbances: headache, dizziness, fatigue, drowsiness

Perform/provide:
• Storage in tight, dry container

Evaluate:
• Therapeutic response: absence of fever, malaise, cough, dyspnea in infection; tremors, shuffling gait in Parkinson's disease

Teach patient/family:
• To change body position slowly to prevent orthostatic hypotension
• About aspects of drug therapy: need to report dyspnea, weight gain, dizziness, poor concentration, dysuria, behavioral changes
• To avoid hazardous activities if dizziness, blurred vision occurs
• To take drug exactly as prescribed; parkinsonian crisis may occur if drug is discontinued abruptly; do not double dose; if a dose is missed, do not take within 4 hr of next dose; caps may be opened and mixed with food
• To avoid alcohol

Treatment of overdose: Withdraw drug, maintain airway, administer epINEPHrine, aminophylline, O_2, IV corticosteroids, physostigmine

---

amcinonide topical
See Appendix C

---

amifostine (R)
(a-mi-foss′teen)
Ethyol
Func. class.: Cytoprotective agent for cisplatin

Action: Binds and detoxifies damaging metabolites of cisplatin by converting this drug by alk phosphatase in tissue to an active free thiol compound

Uses: Used to reduce renal toxicity when cisplatin is given repeatedly in ovarian cancer, non–small cell lung cancer; reduces xerostomia (dry mouth) in radiation therapy for head, neck cancer

Investigational uses: To prevent or reduce cisplatin-induced neurotoxicity, cyclophosphamide-induced granulocytopenia; prevent or reduce toxicity of radiation therapy; reduce toxicity of paclitaxel

DOSAGE AND ROUTES

Reduction of renal damage with cisplatin
• *Adult:* **IV** 910 mg/m^2 daily, within ½ hr before chemotherapy, give over 15 min; may reduce dose to 740 mg/m^2 if higher dose is poorly tolerated

Xerostomia
• *Adult:* **IV** 200 mg/m^2 daily over 3 min as an infusion 15-30 min before radiation therapy

---

Available forms: Powder for inj, lyophilized 500 mg/vial

SIDE EFFECTS

CNS: Dizziness, somnolence
CV: Hypotension
EENT: Sneezing
GI: Nausea, vomiting, hiccups
INTEG: Flushing, feeling of warmth
MISC: Hypocalcemia, rash, chills
Contraindications: Hypersensitivity
to mannitol, aminothiol; hypotension,
dehydration, lactation
Precautions: Pregnancy (C), elderly,
CV disease, children

PHARMACOKINETICS

Metabolized to free thiol compound,
half-life 8 min, onset 5-8 min

INTERACTIONS

Increase: hypotension—antihypertensives

NURSING CONSIDERATIONS

Assess:
• For xerostomia: mouth lesions, dry
mouth during therapy
• Fluid status before administration;
administer antiemetic prior to administration to prevent severe nausea and
vomiting; also, dexamethasone 20 mg IV
and a serotonin antagonist such as ondansetron, dolasetron, or granisetron
• Calcium levels before and during treatment, may cause hypocalcemia; calcium
supplements may be given for hypocalcemia
• B/P prior to and q5min during
infusion; antihypertensive should be
discontinued 24 hr prior to infusion if
severe hypotension occurs, give IV 0.9%
NaCl to expand fluid volume, place in
modified Trendelenburg position
Administer:
Intermittent IV INF route
• Intermittent inf after reconstituting
with 9.5 ml of sterile 0.9% NaCl, further
dilute with 0.9% NaCl to a concentration

of 5-40 mg/ml, give over 15 min within
½ hr of chemotherapy
• Supine position during infusion
Y-site compatibilities: Amikacin,
aminophylline, ampicillin, ampicillin/
sulbactam, aztreonam, bleomycin,
bumetanide, buprenorphine, butorphanol, calcium gluconate, carboplatin,
carmustine, cefazolin, cefonicid, cefotaxime, cefotetan, cefoxitin, ceftazidime,
ceftizoxime, ceftriaxone, cefuroxime,
cimetidine, ciprofloxacin, clindamycin,
cyclophosphamide, cytarabine, dacarbazine, dactinomycin, DAUNOrubicin,
dexamethasone, diphenhydrAMINE,
DOBUTamine, DOPamine, DOXOrubicin,
doxycycline, droperidol, enalaprilat,
etoposide, famotidine, floxuridine, fluconazole, fludarabine, fluorouracil,
furosemide, gallium, gentamicin, granisetron, haloperidol, heparin, hydrocortisone, hydromorphone, idarubicin,
ifosfamide, imipenem-cilastatin, leucovorin, lorazepam, magnesium sulfate, mannitol, mechlorethamine, meperidine,
mesna, methotrexate, methylPREDNISolone, metoclopramide, metronidazole,
mezlocillin, mitomycin, mitoxantrone,
morphine, nalbuphine, netilmicin, ondansetron, piperacillin, plicamycin,
potassium chloride, promethazine, ranitidine, sodium bicarbonate, streptozocin, teniposide, thiotepa, ticarcillin,
ticarcillin/clavulanate, tobramycin,
trimethoprim-sulfamethoxazole, trimetrexate, vancomycin, vinBLAStine, vinCRIStine, zidovudine
Additive incompatibilities: Do not
mix with other drugs or solutions
Evaluate:
• Therapeutic response: prevention of
renal toxicity associated with cisplatin
therapy; decreased xerostomia associated with radiation therapy of head, neck
cancer
Teach patient/family:
• The reason for the medication and
expected results
• That side effects may cause severe
nausea, vomiting, decreased B/P, chills,
dizziness, somnolence, hiccups, sneezing

Side effects: *italics* = common; ***bold italics*** = life-threatening

amikacin (R)
(am-i-kay'sin)
amikacin sulfate, Amikin
Func. class.: Antiinfective
Chem. class.: Aminoglycoside

Do not confuse:
Amikin/Amicar

Action: Interferes with protein synthesis in bacterial cell by binding to ribosomal subunit, which causes misreading of genetic code; inaccurate peptide sequence forms in protein chain, causing bacterial death

Uses: Severe systemic infections of CNS, respiratory, GI, urinary tract, bone, skin, soft tissues caused by *Staphylococcus, Pseudomonas aeruginosa, Escherichia coli, Enterobacter, Acinetobacter, Providencia, Citrobacter, Serratia, Proteus, Klebsiella* pneumonia

Investigational uses: *Mycobacterium avium* complex (intrathecal or intraventricular) in combination; aerosolization

DOSAGE AND ROUTES
Severe systemic infections
• *Adult and child:* **IV INF** 15 mg/kg/day in 2-3 divided doses q8-12h in 100-200 ml D5W over 30-60 min, not to exceed 1.5 g; decreased doses are needed in poor renal function as determined by blood levels, renal studies; **IM** 15 mg/kg/day in divided doses q8-12h; daily or extended interval dosing as an alternative dosing regimen
• *Infant:* **IV/IM** 10 mg/kg initially; then 7.5 mg/kg q12h
• *Neonate:* **IV/IM** 10 mg/kg, initially, 7.5 mg/kg q12h
• *Premature neonate:* 10 mg/kg initially, then 7.5 mg/kg q8-12h
Severe urinary tract infections
• *Adult:* **IM** 250 mg q12h
Renal dose
Adult: **IV/IM** 7.5 mg/kg initially, then increased as determined by blood levels, renal function studies

Available forms: Inj 50, 250 mg/ml

SIDE EFFECTS
CNS: Confusion, depression, numbness, tremors, **convulsions,** muscle twitching, **neurotoxicity,** dizziness, vertigo, tinnitus
CV: Hypotension or hypertension, palpitations
EENT: Ototoxicity, deafness, visual disturbances
GI: Nausea, vomiting, anorexia; increased ALT, AST, bilirubin; hepatomegaly, **hepatic necrosis,** splenomegaly
GU: **Oliguria, hematuria, renal damage, azotemia, renal failure, nephrotoxicity**
HEMA: **Agranulocytosis, thrombocytopenia,** leukopenia, eosinophilia, anemia
INTEG: **Rash,** burning, urticaria, dermatitis, alopecia
Contraindications: Pregnancy (D), mild to moderate infections, hypersensitivity to aminoglycosides, sulfites
Precautions: Neonates, mild renal disease, myasthenia gravis, lactation, hearing deficits, Parkinson's disease, elderly

PHARMACOKINETICS
IM: Onset rapid, peak 1-2 hr
IV: Onset immediate, peak 15-30 min; plasma half-life 2-3 hr, prolonged up to 7 hr in infants; not metabolized, excreted unchanged in urine, crosses placental barrier, poor penetration into CSF, removed by hemodialysis

INTERACTIONS
May increase serum trough and peak: indomethacin
Inactivation of amikacin: parenteral penicillins, cephalosporins; do not use together
Mask ototoxicity: dimenhydrinate, ethacrynic acid
Nephrotoxicity: cephalosporins

⚠ Safety alert   *"Tall Man" lettering

Increase: neuromuscular blockade, respiratory depression—anesthetics, nondepolarizing neuromuscular blockers

Drug/Herb
Do not use acidophilus with antiinfectives
Toxicity: lysine (large amounts)

Drug/Lab Test
Increase: BUN, ALT, AST, bilirubin, LDH, alk phosphatase, creatinine
Decrease: Ca, Na, K, Mg

NURSING CONSIDERATIONS

Assess:
• Weight before treatment; calculation of dosage is usually based on ideal body weight but may be calculated on actual body weight
• I&O ratio; urinalysis daily for proteinuria, cells, casts; report sudden change in urine output
• VS during infusion; watch for hypotension, change in pulse
• IV site for thrombophlebitis including pain, redness, swelling q30 min; change site if needed; apply warm compresses to discontinued site
• Serum peak, drawn at 30-60 min after IV infusion or 60 min after IM injection, trough level drawn just before next dose; peak 20-30 mcg/ml, trough 4-8 mcg/ml; adjust dosage per levels
• Urine pH if drug is used for UTI; urine should be kept alkaline
• Renal impairment by securing urine for CCr, BUN, serum creatinine; lower dosage should be given in renal impairment (CCr <80 ml/min); nephrotoxicity may be reversible if drug stopped at first sign
⚠ Deafness by audiometric testing, ringing, roaring in ears, vertigo; assess hearing before, during, after treatment
• Dehydration: high specific gravity, decrease in skin turgor, dry mucous membranes, dark urine
• Overgrowth of infection, including increased temp, malaise, redness, pain, swelling, perineal itching, diarrhea, stomatitis, change in cough, sputum

• C&S before starting treatment to identify organism
• Vestibular dysfunction: nausea, vomiting, dizziness, headache; drug should be discontinued if severe
• Inj sites for redness, swelling, abscesses; use warm compresses at site

Administer:

IM route
• Inj in large muscle mass; rotate inj sites
• Bicarbonate to alkalinize urine if ordered for UTI because drug is most active in alkaline environment

Intermittent IV INF route
• Dilute 500 mg of drug/100-200 ml of IV D$_5$W, D$_5$RL, D$_5$NaCl, or 0.9% NaCl and give over ½-1 hr; flush after administration with D$_5$W or 0.9% NaCl; solution is clear or pale yellow; discard if precipitate or dark color develops
• In evenly spaced doses to maintain blood level

Additive compatibilities: Avoid admixing

Syringe compatibilities: Clindamycin, doxapram

Y-site compatibilities: Acyclovir, amifostine, amiodarone, amsacrine, aztreonam, cefepime, cisatracurium, cyclophosphamide, dexamethasone, diltiazem, enalaprilat, esmolol, filgrastim, fluconazole, fludarabine, foscarnet, furosemide, granisetron, idarubicin, IL-2, labetalol, lorazepam, magnesium sulfate, melphalan, midazolam, morphine, ondansetron, paclitaxel, perphenazine, remifentanil, sargramostim, teniposide, thiotepa, TPN #54, #61, #91, #203, #204, #212, vinorelbine, warfarin, zidovudine

Perform/provide:
• Adequate fluids of 2-3 L/day, unless contraindicated, to prevent irritation of tubules
• Flush of IV line with NS or D$_5$W after infusion
• Supervised ambulation, other safety measures with vestibular dysfunction

---

Evaluate:
• Therapeutic response: absence of fever, draining wounds, negative C&S after treatment

Teach patient/family:
• To report headache, dizziness, symptoms for overgrowth of infection, renal impairment

⚠ To report loss of hearing, ringing, roaring in ears or feeling of fullness in head

• To report hypersensitivity: rash, itching, trouble breathing, facial edema and notify health care provider

Treatment of hypersensitivity:
Hemodialysis, exchange transfusion in the newborn, monitor serum levels of drug, may give ticarcillin or carbenicillin

---

amiloride (R)
(a-mill'oh-ride)
amiloride HCl, Midamor
Func. class.: Potassium-sparing diuretic
Chem. class.: Pyrazine

Do not confuse:
amiloride/amlodipine

Action: Acts primarily on proximal distal tubule by inhibiting reabsorption of sodium, H_2O, and increasing potassium retention

Uses: Edema in CHF in combination with other diuretics, for hypertension, adjunct with other diuretics to maintain potassium

DOSAGE AND ROUTES
• *Adult:* **PO** 5 mg daily, may be increased to 10-20 mg daily if needed
Available forms: Tabs 5 mg

SIDE EFFECTS

CNS: Headache, dizziness, fatigue, weakness, paresthesias, tremor, depression, anxiety
CV: Orthostatic hypotension, dysrhythmias, angina
EENT: Loss of hearing, tinnitus, blurred vision, nasal congestion, increased intraocular pressure

ELECT: **Hyperkalemia**
GI: Nausea, diarrhea, dry mouth, *vomiting, anorexia,* cramps, constipation, abdominal pain, jaundice, bleeding
GU: Polyuria, dysuria, urinary frequency, impotence
HEMA: **Aplastic anemia, neutropenia**
INTEG: Rash, pruritus, alopecia, urticaria
MS: Cramps, joint pain
RESP: Cough, dyspnea, shortness of breath

Contraindications: Anuria, hypersensitivity, hyperkalemia, impaired renal function

Precautions: Pregnancy (B), dehydration, diabetes, acidosis, lactation, elderly

PHARMACOKINETICS
PO: 15%-25% absorbed from GI tract; widely distributed; onset 2 hr, peak 6-10 hr, duration 24 hr; excreted in urine, feces, half-life 6-9 hr

INTERACTIONS
Enhanced action of antihypertensives
Hyperkalemia: other potassium-sparing diuretics, potassium products, ACE inhibitors, salt substitutes
Lithium toxicity: lithium
Decrease: effect of amiloride—NSAIDs
Drug/Herb
Fatal hypokalemia: arginine
Hypokalemia: bearberry, gossypol
Severe photosensitivity: St. John's wort
Increase: effect—cucumber, dandelion, horsetail, licorice, nettle, pumpkin, Queen Anne's lace
Increase: hypotension—khella
Drug/Food
Possible hyperkalemia: foods high in potassium
Drug/Lab Test
Interference: GTT

NURSING CONSIDERATIONS
Assess:
• Weight, I&O daily to determine fluid loss; effect of drug may be decreased if used daily

---

⚠ Safety alert   *"Tall Man" lettering

- B/P lying, standing; postural hypotension may occur
- Electrolytes: K, Na, Cl; glucose (serum), BUN, CBC, serum creatinine, blood pH, ABGs
- Improvement in CVP q8h
- Rashes, temp elevation daily
- Confusion, especially in elderly; take safety precautions if needed

Administer:
- In AM to avoid interference with sleep if using drug as a diuretic; if second daily dose is needed, give in late afternoon
- With food; if nausea occurs, absorption may be decreased slightly

Evaluate:
- Therapeutic response: improvement in edema of feet, legs, sacral area daily if medication is being used in CHF

Teach patient/family:
- To take as prescribed; if dose is missed, take when remembered within 1 hr of next dose
- About adverse reactions: muscle cramps, weakness, nausea, dizziness, blurred vision
- To take with food or milk for GI symptoms
- To take early in day to prevent nocturia
- To avoid potassium-rich foods: oranges, bananas; salt substitutes, dried fruits

Treatment of overdose: Lavage if taken orally, monitor electrolytes, administer sodium bicarbonate for potassium >6.5 mEq/L, monitor hydration, CV, renal status

---

amino acid injection (℞)
(a-mee'noe)
FreAmine, HepatAmine
Func. class.: Nitrogen product

Action: Needed for anabolism to maintain structure, decrease catabolism, promote healing
Uses: Hepatic encephalopathy, cirrhosis, hepatitis, nutritional support in cancer

DOSAGE AND ROUTES
- *Adult:* **IV** 80-120 g/day; 500 ml of amino acids/500 ml D_{50} given over 24 hr
Available forms: Inj; many strengths, types

SIDE EFFECTS
CNS: Dizziness, headache, confusion, **loss of consciousness**
CV: Hypertension, **CHF, pulmonary edema**
ENDO: Hyperglycemia, rebound hypoglycemia, electrolyte imbalances, hyperosmolar syndrome, hyperosmolar hyperglycemic nonketotic syndrome, alkalosis, acidosis, hypophosphatemia, hyperammonemia, dehydration, hypocalcemia
GI: Nausea, vomiting, liver fat deposits, abdominal pain
GU: Glycosuria, osmotic diuresis
INTEG: Chills, flushing, warm feeling, rash, urticaria, extravasation necrosis, phlebitis at inj site
Contraindications: Hypersensitivity, severe electrolyte imbalances, anuria, severe liver damage, maple syrup urine disease, PKU
Precautions: Pregnancy (C), renal disease, lactation, children, diabetes mellitus, CHF

INTERACTIONS
Tetracycline—decrease: protein sparing effects

NURSING CONSIDERATIONS
Assess:
- Electrolytes (K, Na, Ca, Cl, Mg), blood glucose, ammonia, phosphate, ketones
- Renal, hepatic studies: BUN, creatinine, ALT, AST, bilirubin
- Inj site for extravasation: redness along vein, edema at site, necrosis, pain, hard tender area; site should be changed immediately
- Respiratory function q4h: auscultate lung fields bilaterally for crackles, respirations, quality, rate, rhythm

• Temp q4h for increased fever, indicating infection; if infection suspected, infusion is discontinued, tubing and solution cultured

⚠ For impending hepatic coma: asterixis, confusion, uremic fetor, lethargy

• Hyperammonemia: nausea, vomiting, malaise, tremors, anorexia, convulsions

Administer:
CONT IV route

• Up to 40% protein and dextrose (up to 12.5%) via peripheral vein; stronger solutions require central IV administration

• TPN only mixed with dextrose to promote protein synthesis

• Immediately after mixing under strict aseptic technique, use infusion pump, in-line filter (0.22 µm) unless mixed with fat emulsion and dextrose (3 in 1)

⚠ Using careful monitoring technique; do not speed up infusion; pulmonary edema, glucose overload will result

Additive compatibilities: Amikacin, aminophylline, aztreonam, calcium gluconate, cefamandole, cefazolin, cefepime, cefotaxime, cefoxitin, cefsulodin, ceftazidime, ceftriaxone, cefuroxime, cimetidine, clindamycin, cyanocobalamin, cyclophosphamide, cycloSPORINE, cytarabine, DOPamine, epoetin, erythromycin, famotidine, folic acid, fosphenytoin, furosemide, heparin, insulin (regular), isoproterenol, lidocaine, meperidine, metaraminol, methicillin, methotrexate, methyldopate, methylPREDNISolone, metoclopramide, morphine, nafcillin, netilmicin, nizatidine, norepinephrine, ondansetron, oxacillin, penicillin G potassium, penicillin G sodium, phytonadione, polymyxin B, sodium bicarbonate, tacrolimus, tobramycin, vancomycin

Y-site compatibilities: Amikacin, aminophylline, amoxicillin, ampicillin, ascorbic acid inj, atracurium, azlocillin, aztreonam, bumetanide, buprenorphine, calcium gluconate, carboplatin, cefamandole, cefonicid, cefoperazone, cefotaxime, cefotetan, cefoxitin, ceftazidime, ceftizoxime, ceftriaxone, cefuroxime, cephalothin, cephapirin, chloramphenicol, chlorproMAZINE, cimetidine, clindamycin, clonazepam, dexamethasone, diazepam, digoxin, diphenhydrAMINE, DOBUTamine, DOPamine, doxycycline, droperidol, enalaprilat, epINEPHrine, erythromycin, famotidine, fentanyl, flucloxacillin, fluconazole, folic acid, foscarnet, gentamicin, granisetron, haloperidol, heparin, hydrocortisone, hydromorphone, hydrOXYzine, idarubicin, ifosfamide, IL-2, imipenem/cilastatin, insulin (regular), isoproterenol, kanamycin, leucovorin, levorphanol, lidocaine, lorazepam, magnesium sulfate, mannitol, meperidine, mesna, methicillin, metronidazole, mezlocillin, miconazole, morphine, moxalactam, multivitamins, nafcillin, netilmicin, nitroglycerin, nitroprusside, norepinephrine, octreotide, ofloxacin, ondansetron, oxacillin, paclitaxel, penicillin G, penicillin G potassium, pentobarbital, phenobarbital, piperacillin, potassium chloride, prochlorperazine, ranitidine, salbutamol, sargramostim, tacrolimus, thiotepa, ticarcillin, ticarcillin/clavulanate, tobramycin, trimethoprim-sulfamethoxazole, urokinase, vancomycin, vecuronium, zidovudine

Perform/provide:
• Storage depends on type of solution; consult manufacturer
• Changing dressing and IV tubing to prevent infection q24-48h

Evaluate:
• Therapeutic response: weight gain, decrease in jaundice in liver disorders, increased LOC

Teach patient/family:
• The reason for use of TPN
• If chills, sweating are experienced, report at once
• About infusion pump and blood glucose monitoring

**amino acid
solution (R)**
Aminees, Aminosyn, Branch
Amin, FreAmine III,
NeprAmine, Novamine,
ProcalAmine, Ren Amin,
Travasol, Troph Amine
Func. class.: Nitrogen product

Action: Needed for anabolism to maintain structure, decrease catabolism, promote healing
Uses: Nutritional support in cancer, trauma, intestinal obstruction, short bowel syndrome, severe malabsorption

DOSAGE AND ROUTES

• *Adult:* **IV** 1-1.5 g/kg/day titrated to patient's needs
• *Child:* **IV** 2-3 g/kg/day titrated to patient's needs
Available forms: Inj, many types, strengths

SIDE EFFECTS

CNS: Dizziness, headache, confusion, ***loss of consciousness***
CV: Hypertension, ***CHF, pulmonary edema***
ENDO: Hyperglycemia, rebound hypoglycemia, electrolyte imbalances, hyperosmolar syndrome, hyperosmolar hyperglycemic nonketotic syndrome, alkalosis, acidosis, hypophosphatemia, hyperammonemia, dehydration, hypocalcemia
GI: Nausea, vomiting, liver fat deposits, abdominal pain, jaundice
GU: Glycosuria, osmotic diuresis
INTEG: Chills, flushing, warm feeling, rash, urticaria, extravasation necrosis, phlebitis at inj site
Contraindications: Hypersensitivity, severe electrolyte imbalances, anuria, severe liver damage, maple syrup urine disease, PKU
Precautions: Pregnancy (C), renal disease, lactation, children, diabetes mellitus, CHF

NURSING CONSIDERATIONS

Assess:
• Electrolytes (K, Na, Ca, Cl, Mg), blood glucose, ammonia, phosphate
• Renal, hepatic studies: BUN, creatinine, ALT, AST, bilirubin
• Inj site for extravasation: redness along vein, edema at site, necrosis, pain, hard tender area; site should be changed immediately
• Monitor respiratory function q4h: auscultate lung fields bilaterally for crackles, respirations, quality, rate, rhythm
• Monitor temp q4h for increased fever, indicating infection; if infection suspected, discontinue infusion, culture tubing, bottle
• Urine glucose q6h using Tes-Tape, Clinistix, which are not affected by infusion substances; blood glucose is preferred testing method
• Hyperammonemia: nausea, vomiting, malaise, tremors, anorexia, convulsions
Administer:
CONT IV route
• Up to 40% protein and dextrose (up to 12.5%) via peripheral vein; stronger solutions require central IV administration, use infusion pump
• TPN only mixed with dextrose to promote protein synthesis
• Immediately after mixing in pharmacy under strict aseptic technique using laminar flow hood, use infusion pump, in-line filter (0.22 μm) unless mixed with fat emulsion and dextrose (3 in 1)
⚠ Using careful monitoring technique; do not speed up infusion; pulmonary edema, glucose overload will result
Y-site compatibilities: Cefamandole, cefazolin, cefoperazone, cefotaxime, cefoxitin, cephalothin, cephapirin, chloramphenicol, clindamycin, digoxin, DOBUTamine, DOPamine, doxycycline, erythromycin lactobionate, fat emulsion, foscarnet, furosemide, gentamicin, isoproterenol, kanamycin, lidocaine, meperidine, methicillin, mezlocillin, miconazole, morphine, nafcillin, netilmicin,

norepinephrine, oxacillin, penicillin G potassium, piperacillin, sargramostim, ticarcillin, tobramycin, urokinase, vancomycin

Perform/provide:

• Storage depends on type of solution; consult label

• Dressing and IV tubing change q24-48h to prevent infection

Evaluate:

• Therapeutic response: weight gain, decrease in jaundice in liver disorders, increased serum albumin

Teach patient/family:

• The reason for use of TPN

• That any chills, sweating should be reported at once

• About infusion pump and blood glucose monitoring

Rarely Used

aminocaproic acid (℞)

(a-mee-noe-ka-proe'ik)

Amicar, aminocaproic acid, EACA

Func. class.: Hemostatic

Uses: Hemorrhage from hyperfibrinolysis, adjunctive therapy in hemophilia

DOSAGE AND ROUTES

• *Adult:* **PO/IV** 5 g loading dose, then 1-1.25 g q1h

Contraindications: Hypersensitivity, abnormal bleeding, postpartum bleeding, DIC, upper urinary tract bleeding, new burns

---

Rarely Used

aminoglutethimide (℞)

(a-meen-oh-gloo-teth'i-mide)

Cytadren

Func. class.: Antineoplastic, adrenal steroid inhibitor

Chem. class.: Hormone

Uses: Suppression of adrenal function in Cushing's syndrome, adrenal cancer

DOSAGE AND ROUTES

• *Adult:* **PO** 250 mg qid at 6 hr intervals, may increase by 250 mg/day q1-2wk, not to exceed 2 g/day, concurrent hydrocortisone supplementation is recommended

Contraindications: Pregnancy (D), hypersensitivity, hypothyroidism

---

Rarely Used

aminolevulinic acid (℞)

Levulan Kerastick

Func. class.: Photochemotherapy

Uses: Face/scalp nonhyperkeratotic actinic keratoses

DOSAGE AND ROUTES

• *Adult:* **TOP** 1 application of solution and 1 dose of illumination/treatment site × 8 wk

Contraindications: Hypersensitivity to porphyrins

---

aminophylline (theophylline ethylenediamine) (℞)

(am-in-off'i-lin)

Phyllocontin, Truphylline

Func. class.: Bronchodilator, spasmolytic

Chem. class.: Xanthine, ethylenediamide

Action: Exact mechanism unknown, relaxes smooth muscle of respiratory system by blocking phosphodiesterase,

---

which increases cAMP; increased cAMP alters intracellular calcium ion movements; produces bronchodilation, increased pulmonary blood flow, relaxation of respiratory tract

Uses: Bronchial asthma, bronchospasm associated with chronic bronchitis, emphysema, bradycardia

Investigational uses: Apnea in infancy for respiratory/myocardial stimulation

DOSAGE AND ROUTES

• *Adult:* **PO** 6 mg/kg, then 3 mg/kg q6h × 2 doses, then 3 mg/kg q8h maintenance, max 900 mg/day or 13 mg/kg; **PO** in CHF 6 mg/kg, then 2 mg/kg q8h × 2 doses, then 1-2 mg/kg q12h maintenance; **IV** 4.7 mg/kg, then 0.55 mg/kg/hr × 12 hr, then 0.36/kg/hr maintenance; **IV** in CHF 4.7 mg/kg, then 0.39 mg/kg/hr × 12 hr, then 0.08-0.16 mg/kg/hr maintenance

• *Geriatric and in cor pulmonale:* **PO** 6 mg/kg, then 2 mg/kg q6h × 2 doses, then 2 mg/kg q8h maintenance; **IV** 4.7 mg/kg, then 0.47 mg/kg/hr × 12 hr, then 0.24 mg/kg/hr maintenance

• *Child 9-16 yr:* **PO** 6 mg/kg, then 3 mg/kg q4h × 3 doses, then 3 mg/kg q6h maintenance, max 18 mg/kg/day 12-16 yr, or 20 mg/kg/day 9-12 yr; **IV** 4.7 mg/kg, then 0.79 mg/kg/hr × 12 hr, then 0.63 mg/kg/hr maintenance

• *Child 6 mo-9 yr:* **PO** 4 mg/kg q4h × 3 doses, then 4 mg/kg q6h maintenance, max 24 mg/kg/day; **IV** 4.7 mg/kg, then 0.95 mg/kg/hr × 12 hr, then 0.79 mg/kg/hr maintenance

• *Infants 6-52 wk:* Dose (0.2 × age in wk) ÷ 5 × kg = 24 hr dose in mg

• *Neonate—up to 40 wk premature postconception age:* **PO/IV** 1 mg/kg q12h

• *Neonate at birth or 40 wk postconception age:* **PO/IV** over 8 wk postnatal 1-3 mg/kg q6h; 4-8 wk postnatal 1-2 mg/kg q8h; up to 4 wk postnatal 1-2 mg/kg q12h

Hepatic disease

• *Adult:* **PO** 6 mg/kg/ then 2 mg/kg q8h × 2 doses, then 1-2 mg/kg q12h maintenance; **IV** 4.7 mg/kg, then 0.39 mg/kg/hr × 12 hr, then 0.08-0.16 mg/kg/hr maintenance

Available forms: Inj 250 mg/10 ml, 500 mg/20 ml, 100 mg/100 ml in 0.45% NaCl, 200 mg/100 ml in 0.45% NaCl; rect supp 250, 500 mg, oral liq 105 mg/5 ml; tabs 100, 200 mg, tabs con rel 225, 350 mg

SIDE EFFECTS

CNS: Anxiety, restlessness, insomnia, *dizziness, seizures,* headache, lightheadedness, muscle twitching
CV: Palpitations, sinus tachycardia, hypotension, flushing, ***dysrhythmias***
GI: Nausea, vomiting, diarrhea, dyspepsia, anal irritation (suppositories), epigastric pain, reflux
GU: Urinary frequency, SIADH
INTEG: Flushing, urticaria
RESP: Tachypnea, increased respiratory rate

Contraindications: Hypersensitivity to xanthines, tachydysrhythmias, active peptic ulcer disease

Precautions: Pregnancy (C), elderly, CHF, cor pulmonale, hepatic disease, diabetes mellitus, hyperthyroidism, hypertension, seizure disorder, irritation of the rectum or lower colon, children, lactation, alcoholism

PHARMACOKINETICS

Well absorbed PO; extended rel well absorbed slowly, rect supp is erratic, rect sol is absorbed quickly; metabolized by liver (caffeine); excreted in urine; crosses placenta; appears in breast milk; half-life 3-12 hr; half-life increased in geriatric patients, hepatic disease, CHF, smokers, neonates, premature infants
PO: Onset ¼ hr, peak 1-2 hr, duration 6-8 hr
PO-ER: Unknown, peak 4-7 hr, duration 8-12 hr
IV: Onset rapid, duration 6-8 hr
REC: Onset erratic, peak 1-2 hr, duration 6-8 hr

INTERACTIONS

Dose-dependent reversal of: neuromuscular blockade

Dysrhythmias: halothane

May increase or decrease aminophylline levels: carbamazepine, loop diuretics, isoniazid

Increase: action of aminophylline, toxicity—cimetidine, nonselective β-blockers, erythromycin, clarithromycin, oral contraceptives, corticosteroids, interferons, fluoroquinolones, disulfiram, mexiletine, fluvoxamine, high doses of allopurinol, influenza vaccines, interferon, benzodiazepines

Increase: adverse reactions—tetracyclines

Increase: elimination—smoking

Decrease: effects of lithium

Decrease: effect of aminophylline—nicotine products, adrenergics, barbiturates, phenytoin, ketoconazole, rifampin

Drug/Herb

Increase: effects—cola tree, guarana, yerba maté, tea (black, green), horsetail, ginseng, Siberian ginseng

Decrease: effects—St. John's wort

Drug/Food

Increase: effect—xanthines

Increase: elimination by low-carbohydrate, high-protein diet; charcoal-broiled beef

Decrease: elimination by high-carbohydrate and low-protein diet

Drug/Lab Test

Increase: Plasma free fatty acids

NURSING CONSIDERATIONS

Assess:

• Theophylline blood levels (therapeutic level is 10-20 mcg/ml); toxicity may occur with small increase above 20 mcg/ml, especially elderly

• Monitor I&O; diuresis occurs; dehydration may occur in elderly or children

• Whether theophylline was given recently (24 hr)

• Respiratory rate, rhythm, depth; auscultate lung fields bilaterally; notify prescriber of abnormalities

• Allergic reactions: rash, urticaria; if these occur, drug should be discontinued

Administer:

• Avoid IM injection; pain and tissue damage may occur

PO route

• Do not break, crush, or chew enteric-coated or cont rel tabs

• Avoid giving with food

Rectal route

• If patient is unable to take PO; retain rectal dose for ½ hr

• Remain in bed 15-20 min after rect supp is inserted to avoid removal

IV route

• Only clear sol; flush IV line before dose

• May be diluted for IV INF in 100-200 ml in D_5W, $D_{10}W$, $D_{20}W$, 0.9% NaCl, 0.45% NaCl, LR

• Give loading dose over ½ hr; max rate of inf 25 mg/min, use infusion pump; after loading dose give by cont inf

Additive compatibilities: Amobarbital, bretylium, calcium gluconate, chloramphenicol, cibenzoline, cimetidine, dexamethasone, diphenhydrAMINE, DOPamine, erythromycin lactobionate, esmolol, floxacillin, flumazenil, furosemide, heparin, hydrocortisone, lidocaine, mephentermine, meropenem, methyldopate, metronidazole/sodium bicarbonate, nitroglycerin, pentobarbital, phenobarbital, potassium chloride, ranitidine, secobarbital, sodium bicarbonate, terbutaline

Syringe compatibilities: Heparin, metoclopramide, pentobarbital, thiopental

Y-site compatibilities: Allopurinol, amifostine, amphotericin B, amrinone, aztreonam, ceftazidime, cholesteryl sulfate complex, cimetidine, cladribine, DOXOrubicin liposome, enalaprilat, esmolol, famotidine, filgrastim, fluconazole, fludarabine, foscarnet, gallium, granisetron, heparin sodium with hydrocortisone sodium succinate, labetalol, melphalan, meropenem, netilmicin, paclitaxel, pancuronium, piperacillin/tazobactam, potassium chloride, propofol, ranitidine, remifentanil, sargramostim, tacrolimus, teniposide, thiotepa, tolazoline, vecuronium

Perform/provide:
• Storage of diluted solution for 24 hr if refrigerated

Evaluate:
• Therapeutic response: decreased dyspnea, respiratory stimulation in infancy, clear lung fields bilaterally

Teach patient/family:
• To take doses as prescribed, not to skip dose, not to double dose
• To check OTC medications, current prescription medications for ephedrine; will increase CNS stimulation; not to drink alcohol or caffeine products (tea, coffee, chocolate, colas)
• To avoid hazardous activities; dizziness may occur
• If GI upset occurs, to take drug with 8 oz water; avoid food, since absorption may be decreased
⚠ To notify prescriber of toxicity: insomnia, anxiety, nausea, vomiting, rapid pulse, seizures, flushing, headache, diarrhea; notify prescriber immediately
• To notify prescriber of change in smoking habit; a change in dose may be required
• To increase fluids to 2 L/day to decrease secretion viscosity
• To avoid smoking; decreases blood levels and terminal half-life

---

⚠ High Alert

amiodarone (℞)
(a-mee-oh′da-rone)
Cordarone, Pacerone
Func. class.: Antidysrhythmic (class III)
Chem. class.: Iodinated benzofuran derivative

Do not confuse:
amiodarone/amrinone
Cordarone/Inocor
Action: Prolongs duration of action

potential and effective refractory period, noncompetitive α- and β-adrenergic inhibition; increases PR and QT intervals, decreases sinus rate, decreases peripheral vascular resistance
Uses: Severe ventricular tachycardia, supraventricular tachycardia, atrial fibrillation, ventricular fibrillation not controlled by first-line agents, cardiac arrest

DOSAGE AND ROUTES
Ventricular dysrhythmias
• *Adult:* **PO** loading dose 800-1600 mg/day for 1-3 wk; then 600-800 mg/day × 1 mo; maintenance 400 mg/day; **IV** loading dose (first rapid) 150 mg over the first 10 min then slow 360 mg over the next 6 hr; maintenance 540 mg given over the remaining 18 hr, decrease rate of the slow infusion to 0.5 mg/min
• *Child:* **PO** loading dose 10-15 mg/kg/day in 1-2 divided doses for 4-14 days then 5 mg/kg/day (not recommended in children)
• *Child/infants:* **IV/Intraosseous** 5 mg/kg as a bolus (PALS guidelines)
Perfusion tachycardia
• **IV** 5 mg/kg loading dose given over 20-60 min
Supraventricular tachycardia
• *Adult:* **PO** 600-800 mg/day × 7 days or until desired response, then 400 mg/day × 21 days, then 200-400 mg/day maintenance
• *Child:* **PO** 10 mg/kg/day (800 mg/1.72 m²/day) × 10 days or until desired response, then 5 mg/kg/day (400 mg/1.72 m²/day) × 21-28 days, then 2.5 mg/kg/day (200 mg/1.72 m²/day) (not recommended in children)
Available forms: Tabs 200, 400 mg; inj 50 mg/ml

SIDE EFFECTS
CNS: Headache, dizziness, involuntary movement, tremors, peripheral neuropathy, malaise, fatigue, ataxia, paresthesias, insomnia
*CV: Hypotension, bradycardia, **sinus arrest, CHF, dysrhythmias, SA node dysfunction***

EENT: Blurred vision, halos, photophobia, **corneal microdeposits,** dry eyes
ENDO: Hyperthyroidism or hypothyroidism
GI: Nausea, vomiting, diarrhea, abdominal pain, anorexia, constipation, **hepatotoxicity**
INTEG: Rash, photosensitivity, bluegray skin discoloration, alopecia, spontaneous ecchymosis, **toxic epidermal necrolysis**
MISC: Flushing, abnormal taste or smell, edema, abnormal salivation, coagulation abnormalities
MS: Weakness, pain in extremities
RESP: **Pulmonary fibrosis,** pulmonary inflammation, **ARDS; gasping syndrome if used in neonates**
Contraindications: Pregnancy (D), lactation, 2nd-, 3rd-degree AV block, bradycardia, severe sinus node dysfunction, neonates, infants
Precautions: Goiter, Hashimoto's thyroiditis, electrolyte imbalances, CHF, severe hepatic, respiratory disease, children

PHARMACOKINETICS

PO: Onset 1-3 wk, peak 2-10 hr; half-life 15-100 days; metabolized by liver, excreted by kidneys

INTERACTIONS

Bradycardia: β-blockers, calcium channel blockers
Increase: levels of cycloSPORINE, dextromethorphan, digoxin, disopyramide, flecainide, methotrexate, phenytoin, procainamide, quinidine, theophylline
Increase: anticoagulant effects: warfarin
Drug/Herb
Serotonin effect: horehound
Toxicity/death: aconite
May increase amiodarone effect—aloe, broom, buckthorn, cascara sagrada, Chinese rhubarb, figwort, fumitory, goldenseal, kudzu, licorice, rhubarb, senna
Decrease: amiodarone effect—coltsfoot

Drug/Lab Test
Increase: T_4

NURSING CONSIDERATIONS

Assess:
• I&O ratio; electrolytes (K, Na, Cl); hepatic studies: AST, ALT, bilirubin, alk phosphatase
• Chest x-ray, thyroid function tests
• ECG continuously to determine drug effectiveness, measure PR, QRS, QT intervals, check for PVCs, other dysrhythmias, B/P continuously for hypotension, hypertension
• For dehydration or hypovolemia
• For rebound hypertension after 1-2 hr
• For ARDS, pulmonary fibrosis
• CNS symptoms: confusion, psychosis, numbness, depression, involuntary movements; if these occur, drug should be discontinued
• Hypothyroidism: lethargy, dizziness, constipation, enlarged thyroid gland, edema of extremities, cool, pale skin
• Hyperthyroidism: restlessness, tachycardia, eyelid puffiness, weight loss, frequent urination, menstrual irregularities, dyspnea; warm, moist skin
• Ophthalmic exams
⚠ Pulmonary toxicity: dyspnea, fatigue, cough, fever, chest pain; drug should be discontinued
• Cardiac rate, respiration: rate, rhythm, character, chest pain; start with patient hospitalized and monitored up to 1 wk
Administer:
PO route
• Loading dose with food to decrease nausea
Intermittent IV INF route
• 1000 mg/24 hr during loading/maintenance
• Initial loading: Add 3 ml (150 mg) 100 ml D_5W (1.5 mg/ml) give over 10 min
• Loading inf: Add 18 ml (900 mg) 500 ml D_5W (1.8 mg/ml) give over next 6 hr
• Maintenance inf: Give remainder of loading inf 540 mg over 18 hr (0.5 mg/min)

⚠ Safety alert   *"Tall Man" lettering

CONT INF route

• After 24 hr, give 1-6 mg/ml at 0.5 mg/ml, do not exceed 30 mg/min

Additive compatibilities: DOBUTamine, lidocaine, potassium chloride, procainamide, verapamil

Y-site compatibilities: Amikacin, bretylium, clindamycin, DOBUTamine, DOPamine, doxycycline, erythromycin, esmolol, gentamicin, insulin, isoproterenol, labetalol, lidocaine, metaraminol, metronidazole, midazolam, morphine, nitroglycerin, norepinephrine, penicillin G potassium, phentolamine, phenylephrine, potassium chloride, procainamide, tobramycin, vancomycin

Solution compatibility: D_5W, 0.9% NaCl

Evaluate:

• Therapeutic response: decrease in ventricular tachycardia, supraventricular tachycardia or fibrillation

Teach patient/family:

• To take this drug as directed; avoid missed doses

• To use sunscreen or stay out of sun to prevent burns

• To report side effects immediately

• That skin discoloration is usually reversible

• That dark glasses may be needed for photophobia

Treatment of overdose: O_2, artificial ventilation, ECG, administer DOPamine for circulatory depression, administer diazepam or thiopental for convulsions, isoproterenol

---

amitriptyline (℞)

(a-mee-trip′ti-leen)
amitriptyline HCl,
Apo-Amitriptyline ✦, Endep,
Levate ✦, Novotriptyn ✦
Func. class.: Antidepressant—tricyclic
Chem. class.: Tertiary amine

Do not confuse:
amitriptyline/nortriptyline
Elavil/Mellaril/Oruvail/Plavix

Action: Blocks reuptake of norepinephrine, serotonin into nerve endings, increasing action of norepinephrine, serotonin in nerve cells

Uses: Major depression

Investigational uses: Chronic pain management, prevention of cluster/migraine headaches, fibromyalgia

DOSAGE AND ROUTES

Depression

• *Adult:* **PO** 75 mg/day in divided doses, may increase to 150 mg daily, not to exceed 300 mg/day; **IM** 20-30 mg qid, or 80-120 mg at bedtime

• *Geriatric and adolescent:* **PO** 30 mg/day in divided doses, may be increased to 100 mg/day

Cluster/migraine headache

• *Adult:* **PO** 50-150 mg/day

Chronic pain

• *Adult:* **PO** 75-150 mg/day

Fibromyalgia

• *Adult:* **PO** 10-50 mg nightly

Available forms: Tabs 10, 25, 50, 75, 100, 150 mg; inj 10 mg/ml; syr 10 mg/5 ml

SIDE EFFECTS

CNS: Dizziness, drowsiness, confusion, headache, anxiety, tremors, stimulation, weakness, insomnia, nightmares, EPS (elderly), increased psychiatric symptoms, *seizures*

*CV: Orthostatic hypotension, **ECG changes, tachycardia, hypertension,** palpitations, **dysrhythmias***

EENT: Blurred vision, tinnitus, mydriasis, ophthalmoplegia

GI: Constipation, dry mouth, weight gain, nausea, vomiting, ***paralytic ileus,*** increased appetite, cramps, epigastric distress, jaundice, ***hepatitis,*** stomatitis

GU: Urinary retention

*HEMA: **Agranulocytosis, thrombocytopenia, eosinophilia, leukopenia***

INTEG: Rash, urticaria, sweating, pruritus, photosensitivity

Contraindications: Hypersensitivity

---

to tricyclics, recovery phase of myocardial infarction

Precautions: Pregnancy (C), suicidal patients, convulsive disorders, prostatic hypertrophy, schizophrenia, psychosis, severe depression, increased intraocular pressure, narrow-angle glaucoma, urinary retention, cardiac disease, hepatic disease, renal disease, hyperthyroidism, electroshock therapy, elective surgery, child <12 yr, lactation, elderly

PHARMACOKINETICS

PO/IM: Onset 45 min, peak 2-12 hr, therapeutic response 4-10 days; metabolized by liver; excreted in urine, feces; crosses placenta, excreted in breast milk, half-life 10-46 hr

INTERACTIONS

⚠ Hyperpyretic crisis, convulsions, hypertensive episode: MAOIs

Increase: risk of agranulocytosis—antithyroid agents

Increase: amitriptyline levels, toxicity—cimetidine, fluoxetine, phenothiazines, oral contraceptives, antidepressants, carbamazepine, IC antidysrhythmics

Increase: effects of—direct-acting sympathomimetics (epINEPHrine), alcohol, barbiturates, benzodiazepines, CNS depressants, opioids, sedative/hypnotics

Decrease: effects of—guanethidine, clonidine, indirect-acting sympathomimetics (epHEDrine)

Drug/Herb

Serotonin syndrome: SAM-e, St. John's wort

Increase: CNS depression—kava, skullcap, hops, chamomile, lavender, valerian

Increase: anticholinergic effect—belladonna leaf/root, henbane leaf, jimsonweed, scopolia

Increase: action of amitriptyline—scopolia root

Increase: hypertension—yohimbe

Drug/Lab Test

Increase: Serum bilirubin, blood glucose, alk phosphatase

NURSING CONSIDERATIONS

Assess:

• B/P lying, standing; pulse q4h; if systolic B/P drops 20 mm Hg, hold drug, notify prescriber; take vital signs q4h in patients with cardiovascular disease

• Blood studies: CBC, leukocytes, differential, cardiac enzymes if patient is receiving long-term therapy

• Hepatic studies: AST, ALT, bilirubin

• Weight qwk; appetite may increase with drug

• ECG for flattening of T wave, prolongation of QTc interval, bundle branch block, AV block, dysrhythmias in cardiac patients

• EPS primarily in elderly: rigidity, dystonia, akathisia

• Mental status: mood, sensorium, affect, suicidal tendencies; increase in psychiatric symptoms: depression, panic

• Urinary retention, constipation; constipation is most likely to occur in children and elderly

• Withdrawal symptoms: headache, nausea, vomiting, muscle pain, weakness; do not usually occur unless drug was discontinued abruptly

• Alcohol consumption; if alcohol is consumed, hold dose until morning

Administer:

PO route

• Increased fluids, bulk in diet if constipation, urinary retention occur, especially elderly

• With food or milk for GI symptoms

• Crushed if patient is unable to swallow medication whole

• Dosage at bedtime if oversedation occurs during day; may take entire dose at bedtime; elderly may not tolerate once/day dosing

Perform/provide:

• Storage at room temperature; do not freeze

• Assistance with ambulation during beginning therapy, since drowsiness/dizziness occurs

• Gum; hard, sugarless candy; or frequent sips of water for dry mouth

---

Evaluate:
- Therapeutic response: decrease in depression, absence of suicidal thoughts

Teach patient/family:
- To take medication as directed; do not double dose; that therapeutic effects may take 2-3 wk
- To use caution in driving, other activities requiring alertness because of drowsiness, dizziness, blurred vision; to avoid rising quickly from sitting to standing, especially elderly
- To avoid alcohol ingestion, other CNS depressants
- Not to discontinue medication quickly after long-term use: may cause nausea, headache, malaise
- To wear sunscreen or large hat, since photosensitivity occurs
- That contraception is recommended during treatment

Treatment of overdose: ECG monitoring, lavage, administer anticonvulsant, sodium bicarbonate

---

amlodipine (℞)

(am-loe'di-peen)

Norvasc

Func. class.: Antianginal, antihypertensive, calcium channel blocker

Chem. class.: Dihydropyridine

Do not confuse:

amlodipine/amiloride

Norvasc/Navane

Action: Inhibits calcium ion influx across cell membrane during cardiac depolarization; produces relaxation of coronary vascular smooth muscle, peripheral vascular smooth muscle; dilates coronary vascular arteries; increases myocardial oxygen delivery in patients with vasospastic angina

Uses: Chronic stable angina pectoris, hypertension, vasospastic angina (Prinzmetal's angina); may coadminister with other antihypertensives, antianginals

DOSAGE AND ROUTES

Angina
- *Adult:* **PO** 5-10 mg daily

Hypertension
- *Adult:* **PO** 2.5-5 mg daily initially, max 10 mg/day

Hepatic dose/elderly
- *Adult:* **PO** 2.5 mg/day; may increase up to 10 mg/day (antihypertensive); 5 mg/day, may increase up to 10 mg/day (antianginal)

Available forms: Tabs 2.5, 5, 10 mg

SIDE EFFECTS

CNS: Headache, fatigue, dizziness, asthenia, anxiety, depression, insomnia, paresthesia, somnolence

CV: Dysrhythmia, peripheral edema, bradycardia, hypotension, palpitations, syncope, chest pain

GI: Nausea, vomiting, diarrhea, gastric upset, constipation, flatulence, anorexia, gingival hyperplasia, dyspepsia, dysphagia

GU: Nocturia, polyuria, sexual difficulties

INTEG: Rash, pruritus, urticaria, hair loss

OTHER: Flushing, sexual difficulties, muscle cramps, cough, weight gain, tinnitus, epistaxis

Contraindications: Sick sinus syndrome, 2nd- or 3rd-degree heart block, hypersensitivity, severe aortic stenosis, obstructive coronary artery disease

Precautions: Pregnancy (C), CHF, hypotension, hepatic injury, lactation, children, elderly

PHARMACOKINETICS

PO: Onset not determined, peak 6-12 hr, half-life 30-50 hr, increased in geriatric, hepatic disease; metabolized by liver, excreted in urine (90% as metabolites), protein binding >95%

INTERACTIONS

Neurotoxicity: lithium

Increase: hypotension—alcohol, antihypertensives, nitrates

Increase: amlodipine level—diltiazem

Side effects: *italics* = common; ***bold italics*** = life-threatening

Decrease: antihypertensive effect—NSAIDs

Drug/Herb

Increase: effects—barberry, betel palm, burdock, goldenseal, khat, khella, lily of the valley, plantain

Decrease: effect—yohimbe

Drug/Food

May increase hypotensive effect: grapefruit juice

NURSING CONSIDERATIONS

Assess:

• Cardiac status: B/P, pulse, respiration, ECG; some patients have developed severe angina, acute MI after calcium channel blockers if obstructive CAD is severe

• I&O ratio, weight daily; peripheral edema, dyspnea, jugular vein distention, crackles that are signs of CHF

Administer:

PO route

• Once a day, without regard to meals

Evaluate:

• Therapeutic response: decreased anginal pain, decreased B/P, increased exercise tolerance

Teach patient/family:

• To take drug as prescribed, do not double or skip dose

• To avoid hazardous activities until stabilized on drug, dizziness is no longer a problem

• To avoid OTC drugs, grapefruit juice unless directed by prescriber

• To comply in all areas of medical regimen: diet, exercise, stress reduction, drug therapy, smoking cessation

• To notify prescriber of irregular heartbeat, shortness of breath, swelling of feet and hands, severe dizziness, constipation, nausea, hypotension

• To use correct technique in monitoring pulse, to contact prescriber if pulse <50 bpm

• To change positions slowly, to prevent orthostatic hypotension

• To continue with good oral hygiene to prevent gingival disease

• To notify all health care providers of this drug use

Treatment of overdose: Defibrillation, β-agonists, IV calcium inotropic agents, diuretics, atropine for AV block, vasopressor for hypotension

---

amoxapine (℞)

(a-mox′a-peen)

amoxapine, Asendin

Func. class.: Antidepressant

Chem. class.: Dibenzoxazepine derivative—secondary amine

Do not confuse:

amoxapine/amoxicillin/Amoxil

Action: Blocks reuptake of norepinephrine, serotonin into nerve endings, increasing action of norepinephrine, serotonin in nerve cells

Uses: Depression

DOSAGE AND ROUTES

• *Adult:* **PO** 50 mg tid, may increase to 100 mg tid on 3rd day of therapy; not to exceed 300 mg/day unless lower doses have been given for at least 2 wk, may be given daily dose at bedtime, not to exceed 600 mg/day in hospitalized patients

• *Geriatric:* **PO** 25 mg at bedtime, may increase by 25 mg/wk, up to 150 mg/day in divided doses

Available forms: Tabs 25, 50, 100, 150 mg

SIDE EFFECTS

CNS: Dizziness, drowsiness, confusion, headache, anxiety, tremors, stimulation, weakness, insomnia, nightmares, EPS (elderly), increased psychiatric symptoms, paresthesia, ***neuroleptic malignant syndrome,*** impairment of sexual functioning

CV: Orthostatic hypotension, ECG changes, tachycardia, hypertension, palpitations

EENT: Blurred vision, tinnitus, mydriasis, ophthalmoplegia

GI: Dry mouth, weight gain, *constipation,* nausea, vomiting, ***paralytic ileus,*** increased appetite, cramps, epigas-

---

tric distress, jaundice, *hepatitis,*
stomatitis
GU: Urinary retention, *acute renal
failure*
*HEMA: Agranulocytosis, thrombocy-
topenia, eosinophilia, leukopenia*
INTEG: Rash, urticaria, sweating, pruritus,
photosensitivity
META: Increased prolactin levels
Contraindications: Hypersensitivity
to tricyclics, recovery phase of myocardial infarction, convulsive disorders,
prostatic hypertrophy, narrow-angle
glaucoma
Precautions: Pregnancy (C), suicidal
patients, severe depression, increased
intraocular pressure, urinary retention,
cardiac disease, hepatic disease, hyperthyroidism, electroshock therapy, elective surgery, elderly

PHARMACOKINETICS

PO: Steady state 2-7 days; metabolized
by liver, excreted by kidneys, crosses
placenta, half-life 8 hr

INTERACTIONS

⚠ Hyperpyretic crisis, convulsions,
hypertensive episode: MAOIs
Increase: CNS depression—CNS depressants
Increase: amoxapine level—cimetidine,
fluoxetine, fluvoxamine, paroxetine,
sertraline
Increase: hypertensive effect—
clonidine, epinephrine, norepinephrine
Decrease: amoxapine effect—
barbiturates
Drug/Herb
Increase: CNS depression—chamomile,
hops, kava, lavender, skullcap, St. John's
wort, valerian
Increase: anticholinergic effects—
belladonna, corkwood, henbane, jimsonweed
Increase: action of amoxapine—
scopolia root
Drug/Lab Test
Increase: LFTs, blood glucose
Decrease: WBC, blood glucose

NURSING CONSIDERATION

Assess:
• B/P lying, standing; pulse q4h; if systolic B/P drops 20 mm Hg, hold drug,
notify prescriber; take vital signs q4h in
patients with cardiovascular disease
• Blood studies: CBC, leukocytes, differential, cardiac enzymes if patient is receiving long-term therapy
• Blood level: ther 20-100 ng/ml
• Hepatic studies: AST, ALT, bilirubin
• Weight qwk, appetite may increase
with drug
• ECG for flattening of T wave, bundle
branch block, AV block, dysrhythmias in
cardiac patients
• EPS primarily in elderly: rigidity, dystonia, akathisia
• Mental status: mood, sensorium, affect, suicidal tendencies; increase in
psychiatric symptoms: depression, panic;
confusion (elderly)
• Urinary retention, constipation; constipation is more likely to occur in children, elderly
• Withdrawal symptoms: headache,
nausea, vomiting, muscle pain,
weakness; do not usually occur unless
drug is discontinued abruptly
• Alcohol consumption; if alcohol is
consumed, hold dose until morning
Administer:
PO route
• Increased fluids, bulk in diet if constipation, urinary retention occur, especially in elderly
• Crushed if patient is unable to swallow
medication whole, with food or milk for
GI symptoms
• Dosage at bedtime if oversedation
occurs during day; may take entire dose
at bedtime; elderly may not tolerate once/
day dosing
Perform/provide:
• Storage at room temperature; do not
freeze
• Check to see PO medication swallowed
• Gum, hard candy, or frequent sips of
water for dry mouth

Evaluate:

• Therapeutic response: decreased depression, absence of suicidal thoughts

Teach patient/family:

• To take as directed, not to double dose

• That therapeutic effects may take 2-3 wk

• To use caution in driving or other activities requiring alertness because of drowsiness, dizziness, blurred vision

• To avoid alcohol ingestion, other CNS depressants, may potentiate effects

• Not to discontinue medication quickly after long-term use; may cause nausea, headache, malaise

• To wear sunscreen or large hat, since photosensitivity occurs

Treatment of overdose: ECG monitoring, induce emesis, lavage, activated charcoal, administer anticonvulsant

---

amoxicillin (R)

(a-mox-i-sill'in)

amoxicillin, Amoxil, Apo-Amoxi ✿, Novamoxin ✿, Nu-Amoxi ✿, Trimox, Wymox

Func. class.: Antiinfective, antiulcer

Chem. class.: Aminopenicillin

Do not confuse:

amoxicillin/amoxapine/Amoxil

Trimox/Diamox/Tylox

Wymox/Tylox

Action: Interferes with cell wall replication of susceptible organisms; the cell wall, rendered osmotically unstable, swells and bursts from osmotic pressure

Uses: Treatment of skin, respiratory, GI, GU infections; otitis media, gonorrhea. For gram-positive cocci (*Staphylococcus aureus, Streptococcus pyogenes, Streptococcus faecalis, Streptococcus pneumoniae*), gram-negative cocci (*Neisseria gonorrhoeae, Neisseria meningitidis*), gram-positive bacilli (*Corynebacterium diphtheriae, Listeria monocytogenes*), gram-negative bacilli (*Haemophilus influenzae, Escherichia coli, Proteus mirabilis, Salmonella*); prophylaxis of bacterial

endocarditis; in combination with other drugs used for treatment of *Helicobacter pylori*

Investigational uses: Lyme disease

DOSAGE AND ROUTES

Systemic infections

• *Adult:* PO 750 mg-1.5 g daily in divided doses q8h

• *Child:* PO 20-50 mg/kg/day in divided doses q8h

Renal disease

• *Adult:* PO CCr 10-50 ml/min dose q12h; CCr <10 ml/min dose q24h

Gonorrhea/urinary tract infections

• *Adult:* PO 3 g given with 1 g probenecid as a single dose; followed by tetracycline or erythromycin therapy

Chlamydia trachomatis

• *Adult:* PO 500 mg/day × 1 wk

Bacterial endocarditis prophylaxis

• *Child:* PO 50 mg/kg/hr before and 25 mg/kg 6 hr after procedure

Helicobacter pylori

• *Adult:* PO 1000 mg bid, given with lansoprazole 30 mg bid, clarithromycin 500 mg bid × 2 wk or 1000 mg bid given with omeprazole 20 mg bid, clarithromycin 500 mg bid × 2 wk, or 1000 mg tid given with lansoprazole 30 mg tid × 2 wk

Available forms: Caps 250, 500 mg; chew tabs 125, 200, 250, 400 mg; tabs 500, 875 mg; susp pediatric drops 50 mg/ml; susp 125, 200, 250, 400 mg/5 ml

SIDE EFFECTS

CNS: Headache, **seizures**

GI: Nausea, vomiting, diarrhea, increased AST, ALT, abdominal pain, glossitis, colitis, **pseudomembranous colitis**

HEMA: Anemia, increased bleeding time, **bone marrow depression, granulocytopenia**

INTEG: Urticaria, rash

SYST: **Anaphylaxis, respiratory distress, serum sickness**

Contraindications: Hypersensitivity to penicillins

Precautions: Pregnancy (B), lactation,

---

hypersensitivity to cephalosporins, neonates, renal disease

PHARMACOKINETICS

PO: Peak 2 hr, duration 6-8 hr; half-life 1-1⅓ hr, metabolized in liver, excreted in urine, crosses placenta, enters breast milk

INTERACTIONS

Increase: amoxicillin level—probenecid

Increase: anticoagulant action—warfarin

Decrease: effectiveness of oral contraceptives

Drug/Herb

Do not use with acidophilus

Delayed or reduced absorption: khat; separate by 2 hr

Drug/Lab Test

False positive: Urine glucose, urine protein, direct Coombs' test

NURSING CONSIDERATIONS

Assess:

• I&O ratio; report hematuria, oliguria, since penicillin in high doses is nephrotoxic

• Any patient with a compromised renal system, since drug is excreted slowly in poor renal system function; toxicity may occur rapidly

• Hepatic studies: AST, ALT

• Blood studies: WBC, RBC, Hgb and Hct, bleeding time

• Renal studies: urinalysis, protein, blood, BUN, creatinine

• C&S before drug therapy; drug may be given as soon as culture is taken

• Bowel pattern before, during treatment; diarrhea, cramping, blood in stools, report to prescriber; pseudomembranous colitis may occur

• Skin eruptions after administration of penicillin to 1 wk after discontinuing drug

• Respiratory status: rate, character, wheezing, tightness in the chest

• Anaphylaxis: rash, itching, dyspnea, facial/laryngeal edema

Administer:

PO route

• Shake suspension well before each dose, may be used alone or mixed in drinks, use immediately

• Give around the clock, caps may be emptied and mixed with liquids if needed

Perform/provide:

• Adrenaline, suction, tracheostomy set, endotracheal intubation equipment on unit

• Adequate intake of fluids (2 L) during diarrhea episodes

• Scratch test to assess allergy after securing order from prescriber; usually done when penicillin is only drug of choice

• Storage in tight container; after reconstituting, oral suspension refrigerated for 14 days

Evaluate:

• Therapeutic response: absence of infection; prevention of endocarditis, resolution of ulcer symptoms

Teach patient/family:

• That caps may be opened and contents taken with fluids; chewable form is available

• To take as prescribed, not to double dose

• All aspects of drug therapy: need to complete entire course of medication to ensure organism death (10-14 days); culture may be taken after completed course of medication

⚠ To report sore throat, fever, fatigue, diarrhea (may indicate superinfection or agranulocytopenia)

• That drug must be taken in equal intervals around the clock to maintain blood levels; take on empty stomach with a full glass of water

• To wear or carry emergency ID if allergic to penicillins

Treatment of anaphylaxis: Withdraw drug, maintain airway, administer epINEPHrine, aminophylline, O_2, IV corticosteroids

amoxicillin/clavulanate potassium (℞)

(a-mox-i-sill′in)
Augmentin, Augmentin ES-600, Augmentin XR, Clavulin ✦

Func. class.: Broad-spectrum antiinfective

Chem. class.: Aminopenicillin β-lactamase inhibitor

Action: Interferes with cell wall replication of susceptible organisms; the cell wall, rendered osmotically unstable, swells and bursts from osmotic pressure; combination increases spectrum of activity against β-lactamase–resistant organisms

Uses: Sinus infections, pneumonia, otitis media, skin infection, UTI; effective for strains of *Escherichia coli, Proteus mirabilis, Haemophilus influenzae, Streptococcus faecalis, Streptococcus pneumoniae,* and some β-lactamase–producing organisms

DOSAGE AND ROUTES

• *Adult:* **PO** 250-500 mg q8h or 500-875 mg q12h depending on severity of infection

• *Child ≤40 kg:* **PO** 20-40 mg/kg/day in divided doses q8h or 25-45 mg/kg/day in divided doses q12h

Renal disease

• *Adult:* **PO** CCr 10-30 ml/min dose q12h; CCr <10 ml/min dose q24h

Available forms: Tabs 250, 500, 875 mg/125 mg clavulanate; chew tabs 125, 200, 250, 400 mg; powder for oral susp 125, 200, 250, 400 mg/5 ml; (XR) ext rel tabs 1000 mg amoxicillin, 62.5 mg clavulanate; (ES) powder for oral susp 600 mg amoxicillin, 42.9 mg clavulanate

SIDE EFFECTS

CNS: Headache, fever, *seizures*
GI: Nausea, diarrhea, vomiting, increased AST, ALT, abdominal pain, glossi-tis, colitis, black tongue, *pseudomembranous colitis*
GU: Oliguria, proteinuria, hematuria, *vaginitis, moniliasis, glomerulonephritis*
HEMA: Anemia, *bone marrow depression, granulocytopenia, leukopenia, eosinophilia,* thrombocytopenic purpura
INTEG: Rash, urticaria
META: Hyperkalemia, hypokalemia, alkalosis, hypernatremia
SYST: Anaphylaxis, respiratory distress, serum sickness, superinfection

Contraindications: Hypersensitivity to penicillins

Precautions: Pregnancy (B), lactation, hypersensitivity to cephalosporins; neonates, renal disease

PHARMACOKINETICS

PO: Peak 2 hr, duration 6-8 hr; half-life 1-1⅓ hr, metabolized in liver, excreted in urine, crosses placenta, excreted in breast milk, removed by hemodialysis

INTERACTIONS

Increase: amoxicillin levels—probenecid
Increase: anticoagulant effect—warfarin
Decrease: action of—oral contraceptives

Drug/Herb
Delayed/reduced absorption: khat; separate by 2 hr
Do not use acidophilus with antiinfectives

Drug/Lab Test
False positive: Urine glucose, urine protein, direct Coombs' test

NURSING CONSIDERATIONS

Assess:
• I&O ratio; report hematuria, oliguria since penicillin in high doses is nephrotoxic
• Any patient with a compromised renal system since drug is excreted slowly in

poor renal system function; toxicity may occur

- Hepatic studies: AST, ALT
- Blood studies: WBC, RBC, Hgb and Hct, bleeding time
- Renal studies: urinalysis, protein, blood, BUN, creatinine
- C&S before drug therapy; drug may be given as soon as culture is taken
- Bowel pattern before, during treatment; diarrhea, cramping, blood in stools, report to prescriber; pseudomembranous colitis may occur
- Skin eruptions after administration of penicillin to 1 wk after discontinuing drug
- Respiratory status: rate, character, wheezing, tightness in chest
- Anaphylaxis: rash, itching, dyspnea, facial/laryngeal edema

Administer:

PO route

⚠ Only as directed, 2 (250 mg tab) not equivalent to 1 (500 mg tab) due to strength of clavulanate

- Shake suspension well before each dose, may be used alone or mixed in drinks, use immediately
- Give around the clock

Perform/provide:

- Adrenaline, suction, tracheostomy set, endotracheal intubation equipment on unit
- Adequate intake of fluids (2 L) during diarrhea episodes
- Scratch test to assess allergy after securing order from prescriber; usually done when penicillin is only drug of choice
- Storage refrigerated for 10 days

Evaluate:

- Therapeutic response: absence of infection

Teach patient/family:

- To take as prescribed, not to double dose
- All aspects of drug therapy: need to complete entire course of medication to ensure organism death (10-14 days);

culture may be taken after completed course of medication

⚠ To report sore throat, fever, fatigue (may indicate superinfection or agranulocytosis)

- That drug must be taken in equal intervals around the clock to maintain blood levels
- To wear or carry emergency ID if allergic to penicillins
- To notify prescriber of diarrhea, cramping, blood in stools; pseudomembranous colitis may occur
- To use alternative contraceptive measures, if using oral contraceptives

Treatment of hypersensitivity:
Withdraw drug, maintain airway, administer epINEPHrine, aminophylline, O$_2$, IV corticosteroids for anaphylaxis

---

amphotericin B deoxycholate
(am-foe-ter′i-sin)
Fungizone
amphotericin B cholesteryl sulfate
Amphotec
amphotericin B lipid based
Abelcet
amphotericin B liposome
AmBisome
Func. class.: Antifungal
Chem. class.: Amphoteric polyene

Action: Increases cell membrane permeability in susceptible fungi by binding sterols; alters cell membrane, causing leakage of cell components and cell death

Uses: Histoplasmosis, blastomycosis, coccidioidomycosis, cryptococcosis, aspergillosis, zygomycosis, candidiasis, sporotrichosis, cryptococcal meningitis
Investigational uses: Candiduria (bladder irrigation)

DOSAGE AND ROUTES
Deoxycholate
- *Adult:* **IV** Give test dose of 1 mg (not required); then 0.25 mg/kg, increase daily slowly to 0.5 mg/kg, may give 1 mg/kg/day or 1.5 mg/kg/day, alternate-day dosing may be used
- *Child:* **IV** 0.25 mg/kg infused initially, increase by 0.25 mg/kg every other day to max of 1 mg/kg/day
- *Adult/child:* **TOP** apply 2-4 × daily
- *Adult/child:* **PO** 1 ml (100 mg) qid
Amphotec
- *Adult/child:* **IV** 3-4 mg/kg/day, max 7.5 mg/kg/day
Abelcet
- *Adult/child:* **IV** 5 mg/kg/day as a 1 mg/ml inf given 2.5 mg/kg/hr
AmBisome
Fungal infections
- *Adult/child:* **IV** 3-5 mg/kg q24h
Visceral leishmaniasis
- 3-4 mg/kg q24h days 1-5

Available forms: *Amphotericin deoxycholate* inj 50 mg vial; oral susp 100 mg/ml, cream, ointment, lotion 3%; *amphotericin B cholesteryl* powder for inj 50 mg/20 ml, 100 mg/50 ml; *amphotericin B lipid complex* susp for inj 100 mg/20 ml vial; amphotericin B liposome powder for inj 50 mg vial

SIDE EFFECTS

CNS: Headache, fever, chills, peripheral nerve pain, paresthesias, peripheral neuropathy, *convulsions,* dizziness
EENT: Tinnitus, deafness, diplopia, blurred vision
GI: Nausea, vomiting, anorexia, diarrhea, cramps, *hemorrhagic gastro-enteritis, acute liver failure*
GU: Hypokalemia, azotemia, hyposthe-nuria, *renal tubular acidosis,* neph-rocalcinosis, *permanent renal im-pairment, anuria, oliguria*
HEMA: Normochromic, normocytic ane-mia, *thrombocytopenia, agranulo-cytosis, leukopenia, eosinophilia,* hypokalemia, hyponatremia, hypomag-nesemia

INTEG: Burning, irritation, pain, necro-sis at inj site with extravasation, flushing, dermatitis, skin rash (topical route)
MS: Arthralgia, myalgia, generalized pain, weakness, weight loss
Contraindications: Hypersensitivity, severe bone marrow depression
Precautions: Pregnancy (B), renal disease, lactation

PHARMACOKINETICS
IV: Peak 1-2 hr, initial half-life 24 hr, metabolized in liver, excreted in urine (metabolites), breast milk, highly bound to plasma proteins; penetrates poorly CSF, bronchial secretions, aque-ous humor, muscle, bone

INTERACTIONS
Increase: nephrotoxicity—other neph-rotoxic antibiotics (aminoglycosides, cisplatin, vancomycin, cycloSPORINE, polymyxin)
Increase: hypokalemia—corticoste-roids, digitalis, skeletal muscle relaxants, thiazides
Drug/Herb
Do not use acidophilus with antiinfectives
Increase: possibility of nephrotoxicity—gossypol

NURSING CONSIDERATIONS
Assess:
- VS q15-30min during first infusion; note changes in pulse, B/P
- I&O ratio; watch for decreasing uri-nary output, change in specific gravity; discontinue drug to prevent permanent damage to renal tubules
- Blood studies: CBC, K, Na, Ca, Mg q2wk, BUN, creatinine weekly
- Weight weekly; if weight increases over 2 lb/wk, edema is present; renal damage should be considered
- ⚠ For renal toxicity: increasing BUN, serum creatinine; if BUN is >40 mg/dl or if serum creatinine >3 mg/dl, drug may be discontinued or dosage reduced
- ⚠ For hepatotoxicity: increasing AST, ALT, alk phosphatase, bilirubin

• For allergic reaction: dermatitis, rash; drug should be discontinued, antihistamines (mild reaction) or epINEPHrine (severe reaction) administered

• For hypokalemia: anorexia, drowsiness, weakness, decreased reflexes, dizziness, increased urinary output, increased thirst, paresthesias

• For ototoxicity: tinnitus (ringing, roaring in ears) vertigo, loss of hearing (rare)

Administer:

• Do not confuse three different types; these are not interchangeable: conventional amphotericin B, amphotericin B cholesteryl, amphotericin B lipid complex, amphotericin B liposome

IV route

• Drug only after C&S confirms organism, drug needed to treat condition; make sure drug is used in life-threatening infections

Deoxycholate

• After diluting 50 mg/10 ml sterile water (no preservatives) (5 mg per 1 ml), shake, dilute with 500 ml of D_5W to concentration of 0.1 mg/ml

• Test dose of 1 mg/20 ml D_5W; give over 10-30 min

Intermittent IV INF route

• IV using in-line filter (mean pore diameter >1 micron) using distal veins; check for extravasation, necrosis q8h; use an infusion pump; infuse over 2-6 hr; rapid infusion may result in circulation collapse; use central line if possible

Additive compatibilities: Heparin, hydrocortisone, sodium bicarbonate

Syringe compatibilities: Heparin

Y-site compatibilities: Aldesleukin, diltiazem, DOXOrubicin liposome, famotidine, remifentanil, tacrolimus, teniposide, thiotepa, zidovudine

Solution compatibilities: D_5W

Cholesteryl

IV route

• Reconstitute 50 mg vial/10 ml, 100 mg vial/20 ml sterile water for inj (5 mg/5 ml); swirl or shake gently until dissolved, further dilute with D_5W (0.6 mg/ml); wear gloves while preparing

• Test dose 10 ml of final solution (1.6-8.3 mg) over ½ hr, observe for next ½ hr for reactions

• Give 1 mg/kg/hr using infusion pump, do not give rapidly, may increase infusion, if tolerated

Additive compatibilities: Heparin

Liposomal complex

IV route

• Reconstitute with 12 ml sterile water/50 ml vial (4 mg/ml), shake, use 5-micron filter, dilute in D_5W (1-2 mg/ml), give over 2 hr

• Do not admix

Lipid complex

IV route

• Shake vial until dissolved, withdraw dose using 18G needle, replace needle from syringe with drug using 5 micron filter needle (use needle for 4 vials or less), empty contents in IV of D_5W (1 mg/ml), give at 2.5 mg/kg/hr, use infusion pump

• Do not admix

Perform/provide:

• Acetaminophen and diphenhydrAMINE 30 min prior to infusion to reduce fever, chills, headache

• Storage protected from moisture and light; diluted solution is stable for 24 hr at room temperature

Evaluate:

• Therapeutic response: decreased fever, malaise, rash, negative C&S for infecting organism

Teach patient/family:

• That long-term therapy may be needed to clear infection (2 wk-3 mo depending on type of infection)

• To notify prescriber of bleeding, bruising, or soft tissue swelling

---

amphotericin B topical
See Appendix C

---

ampicillin (R)
(am-pi-sill'in)
Ampicin ✦, Apo-Ampi ✦,
Marcillin, NovoAmpicillin ✦,
Nu- Ampi ✦, Omnipen,
Penbriten ✦, Polycillin,
Principen, Totacillin
Func. class.: Broad-spectrum antiinfective
Chem. class.: Aminopenicillin

Do not confuse:
Omnipen/imipenem

Action: Interferes with cell wall replication of susceptible organisms; the cell wall, rendered osmotically unstable, swells, bursts from osmotic pressure

Uses: Effective for gram-positive cocci *(Staphylococcus aureus, Streptococcus pyogenes, Streptococcus faecalis, Streptococcus pneumoniae)*, gram-negative cocci *(Neisseria gonorrhoeae, Neisseria meningitidis)*, gram-negative bacilli *(Haemophilus influenzae, Proteus mirabilis, Salmonella, Shigella, Listeria monocytogenes)*, gram-positive bacilli

Investigational uses: High-risk for infection in patients having C-section

DOSAGE AND ROUTES
Systemic infections
• *Adult and child ≥40 kg (88 lb):* **PO** 1-2 g daily in divided doses q6h; **IV/IM** 2-8 g daily in divided doses q4-6h
• *Child <40 kg:* **PO** 25-100 mg/kg/day in divided doses q6h; **IV/IM** 25-50 mg/kg/day in divided doses q8h
Renal disease
• CCr 10-30 ml/min dose q8-12h; CCr 30-50 ml/min q6-8hr; <10 ml/min dose q12h
Bacterial meningitis
• *Adult:* **IV** 8-14 g/day in divided doses q3-4h
• *Child:* **IV** 100-200 mg/kg/day in divided doses q3-4h
Gonorrhea
• *Adult and child ≥45 kg (99 lb):* **PO**

3.5 g given with 1 g probenecid as a single dose; **IM/IV** 500 mg q6h (≥40 kg); **IM/IV** 50 mg/kg/day in divided doses q6-8h (<40 kg)

Available forms: Powder for inj 125, 250, 500 mg, 1, 2, 10 g; IV inj 500 mg, 1, 2 g; caps 250, 500 mg; powder for oral susp 125, 250, 500 mg/5 ml

SIDE EFFECTS
CNS: Lethargy, hallucinations, anxiety, depression, twitching, ***coma, seizures***
GI: Nausea, vomiting, diarrhea, ***pseudomembranous colitis***
GU: Oliguria, proteinuria, hematuria, *vaginitis, moniliasis, **glomerulonephritis***
HEMA: Anemia, increased bleeding time, ***bone marrow depression, granulocytopenia***
INTEG: Rash, urticaria
MISC: ***Anaphylaxis, serum sickness***

Contraindications: Hypersensitivity to penicillins

Precautions: Pregnancy (B), lactation; hypersensitivity to cephalosporins; neonates, renal disease

PHARMACOKINETICS
PO: Peak 2 hr, duration 6-8 hr
IV: Peak 5 min
IM: Peak 1 hr
Half-life 50-110 min; metabolized in liver; excreted in urine, bile, breast milk; crosses placenta, removed by dialysis

INTERACTIONS
Increase: ampicillin concentrations—probenecid
Increase: ampicillin-induced skin rash—allopurinol
Decrease: effectiveness of oral contraceptives
Drug/Herb
Delayed/reduced absorption—khat; separate by 2 hr
Do not use acidophilus with antiinfectives
Drug/Lab Test
Increase: AST, ALT

Decrease: Conjugated estrone in pregnancy, conjugated estrial
False positive: Urine glucose, urine protein, direct Coombs'

NURSING CONSIDERATIONS
Assess:
• I&O ratio; report hematuria, oliguria, since penicillin in high doses is nephrotoxic
⚠ Any patient with compromised renal system, since drug is excreted slowly in poor renal system function; toxicity may occur
• Hepatic studies: AST, ALT
• Blood studies: WBC, RBC, Hgb and Hct, bleeding time
• Renal studies: urinalysis, protein, blood, BUN, creatinine
• C&S before drug therapy; drug may be taken as soon as culture is taken
• Bowel pattern before, during treatment
• Skin eruptions after administration of penicillin to 1 wk after discontinuing drug
• Respiratory status: rate, character, wheezing, tightness in chest
• Anaphylaxis: rash, itching, dyspnea, facial swelling; stop drug, notify prescriber, have emergency equipment available

Administer:
PO route
• On empty stomach for best absorption (1-2 hr ac or 2-3 hr pc)
• Shake suspension well before each dose

IM route
• Reconstitute by adding 0.9-1.2 ml/125 mg vial; 0.9-1.9 ml/250 mg vial; 1.2-1.8 ml/500 mg vial; 2.4-7.4 ml/1 g vial; 6.8 ml/2 g vial

IV route
• After diluting with sterile H₂O 0.9-1.2 ml/125 mg drug, administer over 3-5 min (up to 500 mg), 10-15 min (>500 mg) by direct IV; may be diluted in 50 ml or more of D₅W, D₅ 0.45% NaCl to a concentration of 30 mg/ml or less; IV sol is stable for 1 hr; give at prescribed rate

Additive compatibilities: Clindamycin, erythromycin, floxacillin, furosemide
Syringe compatibilities: Chloramphenicol, heparin, procaine
Y-site compatibilities: Acyclovir, allopurinol, amifostine, aztreonam, cyclophosphamide, DOXOrubicin liposome, enalaprilat, esmolol, famotidine, filgrastim, fludarabine, foscarnet, granisetron, heparin, insulin (regular), labetalol, magnesium sulfate, melphalan, meperidine, morphine, multivitamins, ofloxacin, perphenazine, phytonadione, potassium chloride, propofol, remifentanil, tacrolimus, teniposide, theophylline, thiotepa, tolazoline, vit B/C

Perform/provide:
• Adrenaline, suction, tracheostomy set, endotracheal intubation equipment on unit
• Adequate intake of fluids (2 L) during diarrhea episodes
• Scratch test to assess allergy after securing order from prescriber; usually done when penicillin is only drug of choice
• Storage in tight container; after reconstituting, oral suspension refrigerated for 2 wk or stored at room temperature for 1 wk

Evaluate:
• Therapeutic response: absence of temp, draining wounds, other symptoms of infections

Teach patient/family:
• That tabs may be crushed; caps may be opened and mixed with water
• To take oral ampicillin on empty stomach with full glass of water
• All aspects of drug therapy: need to complete entire course of medication to ensure organism death (10-14 days); culture may be taken after completed course of medication
⚠ To report sore throat, fever, fatigue, diarrhea (may indicate superinfection); report rash or other signs of allergy
• That drug must be taken in equal intervals around the clock to maintain blood levels

Side effects: *italics* = common; ***bold italics*** = life-threatening

• To wear or carry emergency ID if allergic to penicillins

Treatment of anaphylaxis: Withdraw drug, maintain airway, administer epINEPHrine, aminophylline, O_2, IV corticosteroids

---

ampicillin, sulbactam (R)

Unasyn

Func. class.: Broad-spectrum antiinfective

Chem. class.: Aminopenicillin with β-lactamase inhibitor

Action: Interferes with cell wall replication of susceptible organisms; the cell wall, rendered osmotically unstable, swells, bursts from osmotic pressure; combination extends spectrum of activity by β-lactamase inhibition

Uses: Skin infections, intraabdominal infections, pneumonia *(Staphylococcus aureus, Escherichia coli, Klebsiella, Proteus mirabilis, Bacteroides fragilis, Haemophilus influenzae, Enterobacter, Acinetobacter calcoaceticus)*, intraabdominal infections *(Enterobacter, Klebsiella, Bacteroides, E. coli)*, gynecologic infections *(E. coli, Bacteroides)*, meningitis, septicemia

DOSAGE AND ROUTES

• *Adult/child ≥40 kg:* **IM/IV** 1 g ampicillin, 0.5 g sulbactam to 2 g ampicillin and 1 g sulbactam q6h, not to exceed 4 g/day sulbactam

• *Child ≤40 kg:* **IV** 100-200 mg/kg/day (ampicillin component) divided q6h, max 8 g/day

Renal disease

• *Adult ≥40 kg:* **IM/IV** CCr 15-29 ml/min dose q12h; CCr 5-14 ml/min dose q24h

Available forms: Powder for inj 1.5 g (1 g ampicillin, 0.5 g sulbactam), 3 g (2 g ampicillin, 1 g sulbactam), 10 g (10 g ampicillin, 5 g sulbactam)

SIDE EFFECTS

CNS: Lethargy, hallucinations, anxiety, depression, twitching, ***coma, seizures***

GI: Nausea, vomiting, diarrhea, increased AST, ALT, abdominal pain, glossitis, colitis, ***pseudomembranous colitis***

GU: Oliguria, proteinuria, hematuria, *vaginitis, moniliasis, **glomerulonephritis,*** dysuria

HEMA: Anemia, increased bleeding time, ***bone marrow depression, granulocytopenia***

*MISC: **Anaphylaxis, serum sickness***

Contraindications: Hypersensitivity to penicillins, ampicillin, or sulbactam

Precautions: Pregnancy (B), lactation, hypersensitivity to cephalosporins, neonates, renal disease

PHARMACOKINETICS

IV: Peak 5 min; half-life 50-110 min; little metabolized in liver, 75% to 85% of both drugs excreted in urine, diffuses to breast milk, crosses placenta

INTERACTIONS

Ampicillin-induced skin rash: allopurinol

Increase: ampicillin level—probenecid

Decrease: oral contraceptive effect

Drug/Herb

Delayed/reduced absorption—khat; separate by 2 hr

Do not use acidophilus with antiinfectives

Drug/Lab Test

False positive: Urine glucose, urine protein

NURSING CONSIDERATIONS

Assess:

• Bowel pattern before, during treatment

• Respiratory status: rate, character, wheezing, tightness in chest

• I&O ratio; report hematuria, oliguria, since penicillin in high doses is nephrotoxic

⚠ Any patient with compromised renal system, since drug is excreted slowly in

---

poor renal system function; toxicity may occur rapidly

• Hepatic studies: AST, ALT if on long-term therapy

• Blood studies: WBC, RBC, Hct, Hgb, bleeding time

• Renal studies: urinalysis, protein, blood, BUN, creatinine

• C&S before drug therapy; drug may be given as soon as culture is taken

• Skin eruptions after administration of ampicillin to 1 wk after discontinuing drug

• Allergies before initiation of treatment; reaction of each medication; report allergies

Administer:

IM route

• Reconstitute by adding 3.2 ml sterile water/1.5 g vial; 6.4 ml/3 g vial, give deep in large muscle

IV route

• After diluting 1.5 g/3.2 ml sterile H_2O for inj or 3 g/6.4 ml (250 mg ampicillin/125 mg sulbactam); allow to stand until foaming stops; may give over 15 min as direct IV; dilute further in 50 ml or more of D_5W, NaCl, administer within 1 hr after reconstitution; give as an intermittent inf over 15-30 min

Additive compatibilities: Aztreonam

Y-site compatibilities: Amifostine, aztreonam, cefepime, enalaprilat, famotidine, filgrastim, fluconazole, fludarabine, gallium, granisetron, heparin, insulin (regular), meperidine, morphine, paclitaxel, remifentanil, tacrolimus, teniposide, theophylline, thiotepa

Perform/provide:

• Adrenaline, suction, tracheostomy set, endotracheal intubation equipment on unit for possible anaphylaxis

• Adequate intake of fluids (2 L) during diarrhea episodes

• Scratch test to assess allergy after securing order from prescriber; usually done when penicillin is only drug choice

• Storage in tight container, out of light

Evaluate:

• Therapeutic response: absence of fever, draining wounds, negative C&S

Teach patient/family:

• That oral contraceptives may be reduced and a nonhormonal contraceptive should be taken while on this drug if pregnancy is to be prevented

• To report superinfection: vaginal itching, loose, foul-smelling stools, black furry tongue

⚠ To report immediately pseudomembranous colitis: fever, diarrhea with pus, blood, or mucus; may occur up to 4 wk after treatment

• To wear or carry emergency ID if allergic to penicillin products

Treatment of anaphylaxis: Withdraw drug, maintain airway, administer epINEPHrine, aminophylline, O_2, IV corticosteroids

---

amprenavir (R)

(am-pren'ah-veer)

Agenerase

Func. class.: Antiretroviral

Chem. class.: Protease inhibitor

Action: Inhibits human immunodeficiency virus (HIV-1) protease, which prevents replication, proliferation of the infectious virus

Uses: HIV-1 in combination with other antiretroviral agents

DOSAGE AND ROUTES

Caps and sol are not interchangeable

• *Adult:* **PO** (cap) 1200 mg bid; **SOL** 1400 mg bid

• *Child ≥50 kg:* **PO** (cap) 1200 mg bid; **SOL** 1400 mg bid

• *Child <50 kg:* **PO** Caps: 20 mg/kg bid or 15 mg/kg tid, max 2400 mg/day; **SOL:** 22.5 mg/kg bid or 17 mg/kg tid daily, max 2800 mg/day

Amprenavir/Ritonavir regimen

• *Adult:* **PO** 600 mg amprenavir, 100 mg ritonavir bid or 1200 mg amprenavir, 200 mg ritonavir bid

Hepatic dose

• *Adult:* **PO** (Child-Pugh score 5-8) 450 mg bid (caps), 513 mg bid (sol) in

---

combination; (Child-Pugh score 9-12) 300 mg bid (caps), 342 mg bid (sol) in combination

Available forms: Caps 50 mg; oral sol 15 mg/ml

SIDE EFFECTS

CNS: Paresthesia, headache
ENDO: New-onset diabetes, hyperglycemia, exacerbation of preexisting diabetes mellitus, hypertriglyceridemia
*GI: Diarrhea, abdominal pain, nausea, **hepatotoxicity***
*HEMA: **Acute hemolytic anemia***
INTEG: Rash, **Stevens-Johnson syndrome**

Contraindications: Hypersensitivity; oral sol: renal failure
Precautions: Pregnancy (C), liver renal disease, lactation, children, hemophilia, sulfonamide sensitivity, elderly

PHARMACOKINETICS

Rapidly absorbed, peak 1-2 hr, 90% protein bound, metabolized in liver, excreted unchanged in urine/feces (minimal), half-life 7-10½ hr

INTERACTIONS

Toxicity: alprazolam, atorvastatin, bepridil, carbamazepine, clonazepam, clozapine, dapsone, diazepam, diltiazem, ergots, erythromycin, fentanyl, flurazepam, itraconazole, loratadine, lovastatin, midazolam, niCARdipine, NIFEdipine, pimozide, triazolam, verapamil
⚠ Serious life-threatening interactions: amiodarone, lidocaine, quinidine, tricyclics, warfarin
Increase: amprenavir levels—cimetidine, clarithromycin, erythromycin, indinavir, itraconazole, ketoconazole, ritonavir
Decrease: amprenavir levels—antacids, carbamazepine, didanosine, efavirenz, methadone, nevirapine, phenobarbital, phenytoin, rifamycins
Decrease: effects of—oral contraceptives, methadone

Drug/Herb
Decrease: amprenavir levels—St. John's wort
Drug/Food
Decrease: bioavailability after high-fat meal
Drug/Lab Test
Increase: Glucose, cholesterol, triglycerides

NURSING CONSIDERATIONS

Assess:
⚠ For renal or hepatic failure, pregnancy, or those receiving disulfiram, metronidazole; oral solution contains propylene glycol in greater quantities
• Signs of infection, anemia
• Hepatic studies: ALT, AST
• Bowel pattern before, during treatment; if severe abdominal pain with bleeding occurs, drug should be discontinued; monitor hydration
• Viral load, CD4 count throughout treatment
• Skin eruptions, rash, urticaria, itching
• Allergies before treatment, reaction of each medication; place allergies on chart
Administer:
• Do not interchange caps and oral sol; they are not the same on a mg/mg basis.
• With or without food; avoid high-fat meals
Evaluate:
• Therapeutic response: increasing CD4 counts; decreased viral load, resolution of symptoms of HIV
Teach patient/family:
• To take as prescribed with or without food, avoid high-fat foods; if dose is missed, take as soon as remembered up to 1 hr before next dose; do not double dose, do not share with others
• That drug must be taken in equal intervals around the clock to maintain blood levels for duration of therapy
• To use a nonhormonal method of contraception during treatment, use condoms
• To notify prescriber if diarrhea, nausea, vomiting, rash occurs
• That drug does not cure AIDs or pre-

vent transmission to others, only controls symptoms

Rarely Used

amyl nitrite (R)
(am'il nye'trite)
amyl nitrite, Amyl Nitrite
Aspirols, Amyl Nitrite
Vaporole
Func. class.: Coronary vasodilator

Uses: Acute angina pectoris, cyanide poisoning
Investigational uses: Cardiac murmur diagnosis

DOSAGE AND ROUTES
Angina
• *Adult:* **INH** 0.18-0.3 ml as needed, 1-6 inhalations from 1 cap, may repeat in 3-5 min
Cyanide poisoning
• *Adult:* **INH** 0.3 ml ampule inhaled 15 sec until preparation of sodium nitrite infusion is ready
Contraindications: Pregnancy (X), hypersensitivity to nitrites, severe anemia, increased intracranial pressure, hypertension

anagrelide (R)
(a-na'gre-lide)
Agrylin
Func. class.: Antiplatelet
Chem. class.: Imidazo-quinazolinone

Action: Reduces platelet count and prevents early platelet shape changes in response to aggregating agents thus inhibiting platelet aggregation
Uses: Thrombocythemia, secondary to myeloproliferative disorders, to reduce elevated platelet count

DOSAGE AND ROUTES
Adult: **PO** 0.5 mg qid or 1 mg bid, may be adjusted after 1 wk, max 10 mg/day or 2.5 mg single dose; maintenance: titrate to lowest dose to maintain platelets <600,000
Available forms: Caps 0.5, 1 mg

SIDE EFFECTS
*CNS: Headache, dizziness, **seizures,** paresthesia, **CVA,** fever*
*CV: Postural hypotension, tachycardia, palpitations, **CHF, MI, cardiomyopathy, cardiomegaly, complete heart block, atrial fibrillation,** dysrhythmia, **chest pain***
GI: Diarrhea, abdominal pain, nausea, flatulence, vomiting, anorexia, constipation, pancreatitis
GU: Dysuria
*HEMA: **Anemia, thrombocytopenia, ecchymosis, lymphadenoma***
*INTEG: **Rash,** photosensitivity*
MISC: Edema, pain,
MS: Asthenia, back pain
RESP: Dyspnea
Contraindications: Hypersensitivity, hypotension
Precautions: Pregnancy (C), lactation, child <16 yr, cardiac, renal, hepatic disease

PHARMACOKINETICS
PO: Peak 1 hr, duration >24 hr: metabolized in liver: excreted in feces/urine

INTERACTIONS
Increase: bleeding risk—anticoagulants, aspirin, NSAIDs, abciximab, eptifibatide, tirofiban, thrombolytics, ticlopidine
Decrease: absorption—sucralfate
Drug/Herb
Gastric irritation: arginine
Increase: effect—bogbean, dong quai, feverfew, ginger, ginkgo
Increase: bleeding risk; green tea
Decrease: effect—bilberry, saw palmetto
Drug/Food
Decrease: bioavailability, plasma concentrations

Side effects: *italics* = common; ***bold italics*** = life-threatening

NURSING CONSIDERATIONS

Assess:

• Platelet counts q2day × 1 wk, and qwk thereafter, response should begin after 1-2 wk; Hgb, WBC, LFTs, renal function studies

• B/P, pulse during treatment until stable; take B/P lying, standing; orthostatic hypotension is common

• Cardiac status: chest pain, what aggravates or ameliorates condition

Administer:

• May give with food, monitor closely for dosage adjustment, there is better absorption on empty stomach

Perform/provide:

• Storage at room temperature

Evaluate:

• Therapeutic response: decreased platelet count

Teach patient/family:

• That medication is not a cure: may have to be taken continuously in evenly spaced doses only as directed

• That it is necessary to quit smoking to prevent excessive vasoconstriction

• To avoid hazardous activities until stabilized on medication; dizziness may occur

• To rise slowly from sitting or lying to prevent orthostatic hypotension

• Not to use alcohol or OTC medications unless approved by prescriber; to use sunscreen, protective clothing to prevent burns

• To report cardiac reactions, increased bruising, bleeding

• To use contraception (female, childbearing age), fetal harm may occur

anakinra (℞)

(an-ah-kin′rah)
Kineret
Func. class.: Antirheumatic agent (disease modifying), immunomodulator
Chem. class.: Recombinant form of human interleukin-1 receptor antagonist (IL-1Ra)

Action: A form of human interleukin-1 receptor antagonist (IL-1Ra) produced by DNA technology; blocks activity of IL-1, resulting in decreased cartilage degradation and decreased bone resorption

Uses: Reduction in signs and symptoms of moderate to severe active rheumatoid arthritis in patients ≥18 years of age who have not responded to other disease-modifying agents

DOSAGE AND ROUTES

• *Adult:* **SUBCUT** 100 mg daily
Available form: Inj 100 mg/ml

SIDE EFFECTS

CNS: Headache
EENT: Sinusitis
GI: Abdominal pain, nausea, diarrhea
HEMA: **Neutropenia**
INTEG: Rash, *inj site reaction*
MISC: Flulike symptoms
MS: Worsening of RA, arthralgia
RESP: URI

Contraindications: Hypersensitivity to *Escherichia coli*–derived proteins or this product, sepsis
Precautions: Pregnancy (B), lactation, children, renal impairment, elderly

PHARMACOKINETICS

Terminal half-life 4-6 hr

INTERACTIONS

Do not give concurrently with vaccines, immunizations should be brought up to date before treatment

Increase: risk of severe infection—TNF blocking agents, etanercept

NURSING CONSIDERATIONS
Assess:
• Pain, stiffness, ROM, swelling of joints during treatment
• For inj site pain, swelling; usually occur after 2 inj (4-5 days)
• For infections, stop treatment if present
• Neutrophil counts prior to treatment and monthly × 3 mo and quarterly for up to 1 yr thereafter
Administer:
• Do not use if cloudy or discolored or if particulate is present, protect from light
• Do not admix with other sol or medications, do not use filter
Evaluate:
• Therapeutic response: decreased inflammation, pain in joints
Teach patient/family:
• Not to receive vaccines while taking this drug
• About self-administration if appropriate: inj should be made in thigh, abdomen, upper arm; rotate sites at least 1 inch from old site, give at same time of day
• To notify prescriber if pregnancy is planned or suspected, avoid breastfeeding

anastrozole
(an-a-stroh′zole)
Arimidex
Func. class.: Antineoplastic
Chem. class.: Aromatase inhibitor

Action: Highly selective nonsteroidal aromatase inhibitor that lowers serum estradiol concentrations; many breast cancers have strong estrogen receptors
Uses: Advanced breast carcinoma not responsive to other therapy in estrogen-receptor–positive patients (usually postmenopausal)

DOSAGE AND ROUTES
• *Adult:* **PO** 1 mg daily
Available forms: Tabs 1 mg

SIDE EFFECTS
CNS: Hot flashes, headache, light-headedness, depression, dizziness, confusion, insomnia, anxiety
CV: Chest pain, hypertension, thrombophlebitis, edema
GI: Nausea, vomiting, altered taste leading to anorexia, diarrhea, constipation, abdominal pain, dry mouth
GU: Vaginal bleeding, vaginal dryness, pelvic pain, pruritus vulvae, UTI
HEMA: **Leukopenia**
INTEG: Rash
MS: Bone pain, myalgia, *asthenia*
RESP: Cough, sinusitis, dyspnea
Contraindications: Pregnancy (D), hypersensitivity
Precautions: Lactation, children, elderly, liver disease, renal disease

PHARMACOKINETICS
PO: Peak 4-7 hr, half-life 50 hr, excreted in feces, urine

Drug/Lab Test
Increase: GGT, AST, ALT, alk phosphatase, cholesterol, LDL

NURSING CONSIDERATIONS
Assess:
• For side effects during treatment
Administer:
• Give with food
Perform/provide:
• Storage in light-resistant container at room temperature
Evaluate:
• Therapeutic response: decreased tumor size, spread of malignancy
Teach patient/family:
• To report any complaints, side effects to prescriber
• That vaginal bleeding, pruritus, hot flashes are reversible after discontinuing treatment
• To report vaginal bleeding immediately
• That tumor flare—increase in size of

tumor, increased bone pain—may occur and will subside rapidly; may take analgesics for pain

> ### ⚠ High Alert
>
> **anistreplase** (R̥)
> (ah-nis'tre-place)
> anisoylated plasminogen, APSAC, Eminase
> *Func. class.:* Thrombolytic enzyme
> *Chem. class.:* Plasminogen activator

Action: Promotes thrombolysis by promoting conversion of plasminogen to plasmin

Uses: Acute MI for lysis of coronary artery thrombi

DOSAGE AND ROUTES

• *Adult:* **IV INJ** 30 units over 2-5 min as soon as possible after onset of symptoms
Available forms: Powder, lyophilized 30 units/vial

SIDE EFFECTS

CNS: Headache, fever, sweating, agitation, dizziness, paresthesia, tremor, vertigo, ***intracranial hemorrhage***
CV: Hypotension, ***dysrhythmias,*** conduction disorders
GI: Nausea, vomiting
HEMA: Decreased Hct; ***GI, GU, intracranial, retroperitoneal,*** surface bleeding; ***thrombocytopenia***
INTEG: Rash, urticaria, phlebitis at inj site, itching, flushing
MS: Low back pain, arthralgia
RESP: Altered respirations, dyspnea, ***bronchospasm, lung edema***
SYST: ***Anaphylaxis (rare)***
Contraindications: Hypersensitivity, active internal bleeding, intraspinal or intracranial surgery, neoplasms of CNS, severe, uncontrolled hypertension, cerebral embolism/thrombosis/hemorrhage, hypersensitivity to this drug or streptokinase, recent trauma/history of CVA
Precautions: Pregnancy (C), arterial emboli from left side of heart, ulcerative

colitis/enteritis, renal disease, hepatic disease, hypocoagulation, COPD, subacute bacterial endocarditis, rheumatic valvular disease, intraarterial diagnostic procedure or surgery (10 days), recent major surgery, lactation, elderly

PHARMACOKINETICS

Half-life 105 min

INTERACTIONS

Increase: bleeding potential—aspirin, other NSAIDs, heparin, antiplatelets, abciximab, eptifibatide, tirofiban, clopidogrel, ticlopidine, some cephalosporins, plicamycin, valproic acid, anticoagulants, dipyridamole
Decrease: action of anistreplase—aminocaproic acid, aprotinin, trahexamic acid
Drug/Herb
Increase: risk of bleeding—agrimony, alfalfa, angelica, anise, basil, bay, bilberry, black haw, bogbean, bromelain, buchu, chondroitin, cinchona bark, dong quai, fenugreek, feverfew, garlic, ginger, ginkgo, ginseng, horse chestnut, Irish moss, kelp, kelpware, khella, lovage, lungwort, meadowsweet, motherwort, mugwort, nettle, papaya, parsley (large amts), Pau D'arco, pineapple, poplar, prickly ash, safflower, saw palmetto, tonka bean, tumeric, wintergreen, yarrow
Decrease: anticoagulant effect—chamomile, coenzyme Q10, flax, glucomannan, goldenseal, guar gum
Drug/Lab Test
Increase: PT, APTT, TT
Decrease: Fibrinogen, plasminogen

NURSING CONSIDERATIONS

Assess:
• VS, B/P, pulse, respirations, neurologic signs, temp at least q4h, temp >104° F (40° C) or indicators of internal bleeding, monitor ECG, treat bradycardia, ventricular changes; assess neurologic status, neurologic change may indicate intracranial bleeding; ECG continuously,

cardiac enzymes, radionuclide, myocardial scanning/coronary angiography
• Hypersensitivity: fever, rash, itching, chills, facial swelling dyspnea; notify prescriber immediately, stop drug, keep resuscitative equipment nearby; mild reaction may be treated with antihistamines

⚠ Bleeding during first hr of treatment (hematuria, hematemesis, bleeding from mucous membranes, epistaxis, ecchymosis), continue to monitor for 24 hr after treatment
• Blood studies (Hct, platelets, PTT, PT, TT, APTT) before starting therapy; PT or APTT must be less than 2 × control before starting therapy; TT or PT q3-4h during treatment

Administer:

IV, direct route
• Reconstitute single-dose vial/5 ml sterile water for inj (not bacteriostatic water), and roll (not shake) to enhance reconstitution; give over 2-5 min by direct IV, give within ½ hr of reconstitution or discard, do not add other meds to vial or syringe; give within 6 hr of thrombi identification for best results
• Pressure of 30 sec to minor bleeding sites, 30 min to sites of arterial puncture followed by dressing; inform prescriber if hemostasis not attained; apply pressure dressing
• Use powder within 30 min after reconstitution
• Cryoprecipitate or fresh frozen plasma if bleeding occurs
• Heparin therapy after thrombolytic therapy is discontinued, TT or APTT less than 2 × control (about 3-4 hr)
• About 10% of patients have high streptococcal antibody titers, requiring increased loading doses

Perform/provide:
• Bed rest during entire course of treatment; handle patient as little as possible during therapy
• Storage of powder in refrigerator
• Avoid invasive procedures: inj, rectal temperature
• Treat fever with acetaminophen

Evaluate:
• Therapeutic response: absence of thrombi formation in MI, improved ventricular function

---

⚠ High Alert

antihemophilic factor VIII (AHF) (℞)
(an-tee-hee-moe-fill'ik)
antihemophilic factor, Alphanate, Bioclate, Helixate FS, Hemofil M, Humate-P, Hyate C, Koate-DVI, Kogenate, Kogenate FS, Monoclate-P, Recombinate, ReFacto
Func. class.: Hemostatic
Chem. class.: Factor VIII

Do not confuse:
Kogenate/Kogenate 2
Action: Necessary for clotting; activates factor X in conjunction with activated factor IX; transforms prothrombin to thrombin
Uses: Hemophilia A, patients with acquired circulating factor VIII inhibitors, factor VIII deficiency

DOSAGE AND ROUTES
Massive hemorrhage
• *Adult and child:* **IV** 40-50 units/kg, then 20-25 units/kg q8-12h
Overt bleeding
• *Adult and child:* **IV** 15-25 units/kg, then 8-15 units/kg q8-12h × 4 days
Hemorrhage near vital organs
• *Adult and child:* **IV** 15 units/kg, then 8 units/kg q8h × 2 days, then 4 units/kg q8h × 2 days
Minor hemorrhage
• *Adult and child:* **IV** 8-10 units/kg q24h × 2-3 days or 8 units/kg q12h × 2 days, then q24h × 2 days
Joint bleeding
• *Adult and child:* **IV** 5-10 units/kg q8-12h × 1-2 days
Available forms: Inj 250, 500, 1000,

1500 units/vial (number of units noted on label)

SIDE EFFECTS

CNS: Headache, *lethargy, chills, fever, flushing*

CV: Hypotension, tachycardia

GI: Nausea, vomiting, abdominal cramps, constipation, diarrhea, anorexia, jaundice, *viral hepatitis*

*HEMA: **Thrombosis, hemolysis, risk of hepatitis B, risk of HIV***

INTEG: Rash, flushing, *urticaria,* stinging at inj site

*MISC: **Anaphylaxis,*** blurred vision

*RESP: **Bronchospasm,*** rhinitis, dyspnea, nosebleeds, wheezing

Contraindications: Hypersensitivity; mouse, hamster, bovine, porcine protein, lactation, HIV, viral infection

Precautions: Pregnancy (C), neonates/infants, hepatic disease; blood types A, B, AB; factor VIII inhibitor

PHARMACOKINETICS

IV: Half-life 4 hr, terminal 15 hr

NURSING CONSIDERATIONS

Assess:

- Blood studies (coagulation factors assay by % normal: 5% prevents spontaneous hemorrhage, 30%-50% for surgery, 80%-100% for severe hemorrhage)
- I&O, urine color; notify prescriber if urine becomes orange, red
- Pulse: discontinue infusion if significant increase
- Hct, Coombs' test with blood types A, B, AB
- Test for factor VIII inhibitors before starting treatment, may require concomitant antiinhibitor coagulant complex therapy
- Allergy: fever, rash, itching, jaundice; give diphenhydrAMINE HCl (Benadryl), continue therapy if reaction is mild
- Blood group of patient, donors (if applicable; most factor VIII not from specific blood group donors)

A Bleeding: ankles, knees, elbows, other joints

Administer:

IV route

- To prepare, administer factor VIII concentrates at first sign of danger
- After rotating gently to mix
- Using plastic syringe to reconstitute, and administer; adheres to glass; use another needle as a vent when reconstituting
- After dilution with warm NS, D_5W, LR, give within 3 hr

IV INF route

- Give at ≤2 ml/min if concentration exceeds 34 units/ml or over 3 min if concentration is less than 34 units/ml

Perform/provide:

- Storage in refrigerator; do not freeze; after reconstitution, do not refrigerate; give within 3 hr

Evaluate:

- Therapeutic response: absence of bleeding

Teach patient/family:

- To report any signs of bleeding: gums, under skin, urine, stools, emesis; review methods to prevent bleeding
- To avoid salicylates, NSAIDs (increase bleeding tendencies)
- To advise health professionals of treatment for hemophilia
- The signs of viral hepatitis, AIDS
- That immunization for hepatitis B may be given first
- To report hives, urticaria, chest tightness, hypotension; may be monoclonal antibody-derived factor VIII
- To be checked q2-3mo for HIV screen
- To carry emergency ID describing disease process

A Safety alert   *"Tall Man" lettering

⚠ High Alert

antithrombin III, human (℞)

(an'tee-throm-bin)
ATnativ, Thrombate III
Func. class.: Antithrombin
Chem. class.: Pooled human plasma

Action: Inactivates thrombin and the activated forms of factors IX, X, XI, XII, resulting in inhibition of coagulation
Uses: During surgical or obstetric procedures, or for thromboembolism in patients with known antithrombin III deficiency

DOSAGE AND ROUTES

Dosage is individualized
• Expect a 1.4% rise from baseline for every 1 international unit/kg administered

Units required =

$$\frac{(\text{Desired level} - \text{Baseline}) \times \text{Weight in kg}}{1.4\%}$$

Available forms: 500 international units in 10 ml; 1000 international units in 20 ml

SIDE EFFECTS

CNS: Dizziness, chills, severe lightheadedness
GI: Nausea, cramps, bowel fullness
RESP: Shortness of breath
SYST: **Bleeding,** surface bleeding, **anaphylaxis,** vasodilatory effects
Precautions: Pregnancy (B), lactation, children

PHARMACOKINETICS

Biologic half-life 2-5 days, peak 15-30 min

INTERACTIONS

Do not administer with other drugs in syringe or solutions
Increase: anticoagulant effect—anticoagulants

NURSING CONSIDERATIONS
Assess:
• AT-III levels q12h, maintain at >80% of normal activity until stabilized, then daily before dose
• VS, B/P, pulse, respirations, neurologic signs, temp at least q4h, temp 104° F (40° C) or indicators of internal bleeding, cardiac rhythm
⚠ For child born of parents with hereditary AT-III deficiency, obtain AT-III levels immediately after birth
⚠ For neurologic changes that may indicate intracranial bleeding
⚠ Retroperitoneal bleeding: back pain, leg weakness, diminished pulses
Administer:
• Heparin after fibrinogen level is over 100 mg/dl; heparin infusion to increase PTT to 1.5-2 × baseline for 3-7 days
IV route
• After reconstituting 500 international units/10 ml of NS or D_5W; do not shake; rotate to dissolve; allow to warm to room temperature; use within 3 hr of reconstitution; give 50 international units or less/min; do not exceed 100 international units/min using 0.22 or 0.45 microfilter
Evaluate:
• Therapeutic response: absence of thrombi formation
Teach patient/family:
• About drug use and expected results; to report adverse reactions; bleeding, bruising

antithymocyte
See lymphocyte immune globulin

apomorphine (℞)
(a-poe-mor'feen)
Apokyn
Func. class.: Antiparkinson agent
Chem. class.: Dopamine-receptor agonist, nonergot

Action: Selective agonist for D_2 subfamily receptors (presynaptic/postsynaptic sites); binding at D_3 receptor may contribute to antiparkinson effects
Uses: Parkinsonism: for acute, intermittent treatment of hypomobility (off) episodes in advanced Parkinsonism

DOSAGE AND ROUTES

• *Adult:* **SUBCUT** 0.2 ml (2 mg) titrate upward, max 0.6 ml (6 mg); administer a test dose of 0.2 ml (2 mg) and closely monitor B/P; to be used concomitantly with antiemetic
Renal dose
• Reduce test dose and starting dose to 0.1 ml (1 mg)
Available forms: Inj 10 mg/ml

SIDE EFFECTS

CNS: Agitation, psychosis, hallucination, depression, dizziness, headache, confusion, *sleep attacks,* yawning, dykinesias, drowsiness, somnolence
CV: Orthostatic hypotension, edema, syncope, tachycardia
EENT: Blurred vision, rhinorrhea, sweating
GI: Nausea, vomiting, *anorexia,* constipation, dysphagia, dry mouth
GU: Impotence, urinary frequency
HEMA: Hemolytic anemia, leukopenia, agranulocytosis
Contraindications: Hypersensitivity
Precautions: Pregnancy (C), renal, hepatic, cardiac disease, MI with dysrhythmias, affective disorders, psychosis, preexisting dyskinesias, elderly

PHARMACOKINETICS

Minimally metabolized

INTERACTIONS

Increased effect of: levodopa
⚠ Do not give with 5-HT_3 antagonists: ondansetron, granisetron, dolasetron: profound hypotension may occur
Increase: apomorphine levels— levodopa, cimetidine, ranitidine, diltiazem, triamterene, verapamil, quinidine
Decrease: apomorphine levels— DOPamine antagonists, phenothiazines, metoclopramide, butyrophenones
Drug/Herb
Decrease: effect of apomorphine— chaste tree fruit, kava

NURSING CONSIDERATIONS
Assess:
• B/P supine/standing before dose, and 20, 40, 60 min after dose
• Renal, hepatic, cardiac studies baseline
• Involuntary movements in parkinsonism: akinesia, tremors, staggering gait, muscle rigidity, drooling
• Mental status: affect, mood, behavioral changes, depression; complete suicide assessment
• For risk of QT prolongation, this drug may increase QT prolongation and possibility of prodysrhythmias
Administer:
• Adjust dosage to patient response
⚠ Do not give IV
• Use a test dose of 0.2 ml (2 mg); those who tolerate this dose but achieve no response, give 0.4 ml (4 mg) at the next "off"
• Give antiemetic, usually trimethobenzamide, 300 mg tid PO 3 days before beginning apomorphine and continue for 2 months
Perform/provide:
• Assistance with ambulation during beginning therapy
• Storage at 77° F, excursion permitted to 59°-86° F
Evaluate:
• Therapeutic response: decrease in end of dose wearing off and unpredictable on/off episodes

---

⚠ Safety alert   *"Tall Man" lettering

Teach patient/family:
• To notify prescriber if pregnancy is planned or suspected

apraclonidine ophthalmic
See Appendix C

aprepitant (℞)
(ap-re′pi-tant)
Emend
Func. class.: Antiemetic
Chem. class.: Miscellaneous

Action: A selective antagonist of human substance P/neurokinin 1 (NK$_1$) receptors
Uses: Prevention of nausea, vomiting associated with cancer chemotherapy including high-dose cisplatin, used in combination with other antiemetics

DOSAGE AND ROUTES
• *Adult:* **PO** Day 1 (1 hour prior to chemotherapy) aprepitant 125 mg with 12 mg dexamethasone **PO**, with 32 mg ondansetron IV; day 2 aprepitant 80 mg with 8 mg dexamethasone **PO**; day 3 aprepitant 80 mg with 8 mg dexamethasone **PO**; day 4 only dexamethasone 8 mg **PO**
Available forms: Caps 80, 125 mg

SIDE EFFECTS
CNS: Headache, dizziness, insomnia, anxiety, depression, confusion, peripheral neuropathy
CV: Bradycardia, DVT, hypertension
GI: Diarrhea, constipation, abdominal pain, anorexia, gastritis, increased AST, ALT, *nausea,* vomiting, heartburn
GU: Increased BUN, serum creatine, proteinuria, dysuria
HEMA: Anemia, ***thrombocytopenia, neutropenia***
MISC: Asthenia, fatigue, dehydration, fever, hiccups, tinnitus
Contraindications: Hypersensitivity

Precautions: Pregnancy (B), lactation, children, hepatic disease, elderly

PHARMACOKINETICS
Metabolized in liver by CYP3A4 enzymes to an active metabolite; half-life 10-12 hr; 95% protein bound; not excreted in kidneys

INTERACTIONS
Increase: aprepitant action—CYP3A4 inhibitors (ketoconazole, itraconazole, nefazodone, troleandomycin, clarithromycin, ritonavir, nelfinavir, diltiazem)
Increase: action of—CYP3A4 substrates (pimozide, cisapride, dexamethasone, methylPREDNISolone, midazolam, alprazolam, triazolam, docetaxel, paclitaxel, etoposide, irinotecan, imatinib, ifosfamide, vinorelbine, vinBLAStine, vinCRIStine)
Decrease: aprepitant action—CYP3A4 inducers (rifampin, carbamazepine, phenytoin)
Decrease: action of—CYP2C9 substrates (warfarin, tolbutamide, phenytoin), oral contraceptives
Decrease: action of both drugs—paroxetine

NURSING CONSIDERATIONS
Assess:
• For absence of nausea, vomiting during chemotherapy
Administer:
• PO on 3-day schedule
Perform/provide:
• Storage at room temperature
Evaluate:
• Therapeutic response: absence of nausea, vomiting during cancer chemotherapy
Teach patient/family:
• To report diarrhea, constipation
• To take only as prescribed, take 1st dose 1 hr prior to chemotherapy
• To report all medication to prescriber prior to taking this medication
• Advise to use nonhormonal form of contraception while taking this agent

Side effects: *italics* = common; ***bold italics*** = life-threatening

• Advise those on warfarin to have clotting monitored closely during 2-wk period following administration of aprepitant

---

⚠ High Alert

ardeparin (R̸)
(are-de-pear'in)
Normiflo
Func. class.: Anticoagulant
Chem. class.: Low-molecular- weight heparin

Action: Prevents conversion of fibrinogen to fibrin and prothrombin to thrombin by enhancing inhibitory effects of antithrombin III
Uses: Prevention of deep vein thrombosis after knee replacement surgery

DOSAGE AND ROUTES

• *Adult:* **SUBCUT** 50 anti–factor Xa units/kg q12h beginning the evening of the day of knee replacement surgery or the following AM continued until patient is fully ambulatory or 2 wk, whichever is first
Available forms: Inj 5000, 10,000 anti–factor Xa units/0.5 ml

SIDE EFFECTS

CNS: ***Intracranial bleeding***, fever, dizziness, headache
CV: Chest pain
GI: Nausea, vomiting
HEMA: ***Thrombocytopenia***, anemia
INTEG: Pruritus, superficial wound infection, ecchymosis, rash, inj site reactions
RESP: Dyspnea
SYST: Hypersensitivity, ***hemorrhage***, ***anaphylaxis*** possible
Contraindications: Hypersensitivity to this drug, pork products, heparin, or other anticoagulants; hemophilia, leukemia with bleeding, thrombocytopenic purpura, cerebrovascular hemorrhage, cerebral aneurysm, severe hypertension, other severe cardiac disease

Precautions: Pregnancy (C), elderly, hepatic disease, severe renal disease, blood dyscrasias, subacute bacterial endocarditis, acute nephritis, lactation, child, recent childbirth, peptic ulcer disease, pericarditis, pericardial effusion, recent lumbar puncture, vasculitis, other diseases where bleeding is possible

PHARMACOKINETICS

Unknown

INTERACTIONS

Increase: risk of bleeding—aspiration, oral anticoagulants, platelet inhibitors, NSAIDs
Drug/Herb
May increase risk of bleeding: agrimony, alfalfa, angelica, anise, bilberry, black haw, bogbean, bromelain, buchu, chondroitin, cinchona bark, dong quai, fenugreek, feverfew, garlic, ginger, ginkgo, ginseng, horse chestnut, Irish moss, kelp, kelpware, khella, lovage, lungwort, meadowsweet, mother wort, mugwort, nettle, papaya, parsley, pau d'arco, pineapple, poplar, prickly ash, safflower, saw palmetto, senega, tonka bean, tumeric, wintergreen, yarrow
Decrease: action—chamomile, coenzyme Q10, flax, glucomannan, goldenseal, guar gum

NURSING CONSIDERATIONS

Assess:
• For blood studies (Hct, occult blood in stools, CBC, platelets, urinalysis) during treatment since bleeding can occur
⚠ For bleeding gums, petechiae, ecchymosis, black tarry stools, hematuria, epistaxis, decrease in Hct, B/P; may indicate bleeding, possible hemorrhage; notify prescriber immediately, drug should be discontinued, protamine should be = to dose of drug given; 1 mg protamine = 100 anti–factor Xa units of drug
• For hypersensitivity: fever, skin rash, urticaria; notify prescriber immediately

---

⚠ Safety alert   *"Tall Man" lettering

Administer:
• By SUBCUT only; have patient sit or lie down; SUBCUT inj may be around the navel in a U-shape, upper outer side of thigh or upper outer quadrangle of the buttocks; rotate inj sites
• Changing needles is not recommended
Evaluate:
• Therapeutic response: absence of deep-vein thrombosis
Teach patient/family:
• To avoid OTC preparations that may cause serious drug interactions unless directed by prescriber; may contain aspirin; other anticoagulants, NSAIDs
• To use soft-bristle toothbrush to avoid bleeding gums, avoid contact sports, use electric razor, avoid IM inj
• To report any signs of bleeding: gums, under skin, urine, stools; unusual bruising, hematoma at inj site
Treatment of overdose: Protamine sulfate 1% given IV

> **⚠ High Alert**
>
> **argatroban** (℞)
> (are-ga-troe′ban)
> Argatroban
> *Func. class.:* Anticoagulant
> *Chem. class.:* Thrombin inhibitor

Do not confuse:
argatroban/Aggrastat
Action: Direct inhibitor of thrombin that is derived from ʟ-arginine; it reversibly binds to the thrombin active site
Uses: Thrombosis, prophylaxis or treatment; percutaneous coronary intervention (PCI), anticoagulation prevention/treatment of thrombosis in heparin-induced thrombocytopenia

DOSAGE AND ROUTES
Heparin-induced thrombocytopenia/ thrombosis syndrome (HIT or HITTS)
• *Adult:* **IV:** 2 mcg/kg/min (1 mg/ml) give at 6 ml/hr for 50 kg of weight, at 8 ml/hr for 70 kg of weight, at 11 ml/hr for 90 kg of weight, at 13 ml/hr for 110 kg of weight, at 16 ml/hr for 130 kg of weight
Hepatic dose
• *Adult:* **CONT INF** 0.5 mcg/kg/min, adjust rate based on aPTT
• Heparin-induced thrombocytopenia or heparin-induced thrombocytopenia and thrombosis syndrome
Percutaneous coronary intervention (PCI) in HIT
• *Adult:* **IV INF** 25 mcg/kg/min and a bolus of 350 mcg/kg given over 3-5 min, check ACT 5-10 min after bolus is completed; proceed if ACT >300 sec
Available forms: Inj 100 mg/ml (must dilute 100-fold)

SIDE EFFECTS
CNS: Fever
*CV: **Atrial fibrillation, coronary thrombosis, MI, myocardial ischemia, coronary occlusion, ventricular tachycardia, bradycardia,** chest pain, hypotension*
GI: Nausea, vomiting, abdominal pain, diarrhea, GI bleeding
*GU: **Hematuria,** abnormal kidney function, UTI*
*HEMA: **Hemorrhage, thrombocytopenia***
MISC: Back pain, headache, CV disorder, infection, UTI
RESP: Pneumonia, dyspnea, coughing
*SYST: **Sepsis***
Contraindications: Hypersensitivity, overt major bleeding
Precautions: Pregnancy (B), intracranial bleeding, renal function impairment, lactation, children, hepatic disease

PHARMACOKINETICS
Metabolized in the liver by P450 CYP3A 4/5, distributed to extracellular fluid, 54% plasma protein binding, half-life 39-51 min, excreted in feces

INTERACTIONS
Increase: bleeding risk—antiplatelets, thrombolytics, other anticoagulants

Drug/Herb

Increase: bleeding risk—agrimony, alfalfa, angelica, anise, bilberry, black haw, bogbean, buchu, chondroitin, dong quai, fenugreek, feverfew, garlic, ginger, ginkgo, ginseng, horse chestnut, Irish moss, kelp, kelpware, khella, lovage, lungwort, meadowsweet, mother wort, mugwort, nettle, papaya, parsley, pau d'arco, pineapple, poplar, prickly ash, safflower, saw palmetto, senega, turmeric, wintergreen

Decrease: argatroban effect—chamomile, coenzyme Q10, flax, glucomannan, goldenseal, guar gum

NURSING CONSIDERATIONS

Assess:

• Obtain baseline in aPTT before treatment; do not start treatment if aPTT ratio ≥2.5, then aPTT 4 hr after initiation of treatment and at least daily thereafter, if aPTT above target, stop inf for 2 hr, then restart at 50%, take aPTT in 4 hr; if below target, increase inf rate by 20%, take aPTT in 4 hr, do not exceed inf rate of 0.21 mg/kg/hr without checking for coagulation abnormalities

• aPTT, which should be 1.5-3 × control

⚠ Bleeding gums, petechiae, ecchymosis, black tarry stools, hematuria/epistaxis, B/P, vaginal bleeding and possible hemorrhage

• Fever, skin rash, urticaria

Administer:

• Avoiding all IM inj that may cause bleeding

IV INF route

• Dilute in 0.9% NaCl, D_5, LR to a final conc 1 mg/ml. Dilute each 2.5 ml vial 100-fold by mixing with 250 ml of diluent, mix by repeated inversion of the diluent bag for 1 min; may be slightly hazy

• Dosage adjustment may be made after review of aPTT, not to exceed 10 mcg/kg/min

Evaluate:

• Therapeutic response: absence or decrease of thrombosis

Teach patient/family:

• To use soft-bristle toothbrush to avoid bleeding gums, avoid contact sports, use electric razor, avoid IM inj

• To report any signs of bleeding: gums, under skin, urine, stools

• To notify prescriber if planning to become pregnant or breastfeeding

---

aripiprazole (℞)

(a-rip-ip-pra′zol)

Abilify

Func. class.: Antipsychotic/neuroleptic

Chem. class.: Quinolinone

Action: Exact mechanism unknown; may be mediated through both dopamine type 2 (D_2, D_3) and serotonin type 2 (5-HT$_{1A}$, 5-HT$_{2A}$) antagonism

Uses: Schizophrenia

DOSAGE AND ROUTES

• *Adult:* **PO** 10-15 mg/day; if needed, dosage may be increased to 30 mg daily after 2 wk; maintenance 15 mg/day, periodically reassess

Available forms: Tabs 5, 10, 15, 20, 30 mg

SIDE EFFECTS

*CNS: Drowsiness, insomnia, agitation, anxiety, headache, **seizures, neuroleptic malignant syndrome,** lightheadedness, akathisia, asthenia, tremor*

*CV: Orthostatic hypotension, **tachycardia***

EENT: Blurred vision, rhinitis

GI: Constipation, nausea, vomiting, jaundice, weight gain

INTEG: Rash

RESP: Cough

Contraindications: Hypersensitivity, lactation, seizure disorders

Precautions: Pregnancy (C), children, renal disease, hepatic disease, elderly

---

PHARMACOKINETICS

PO: Absorption 87%, extensively metabolized by liver to a major active metabolite, plasma protein binding >99%, terminal ½ life 75-146 hr, excretion urine 25%, feces 55%; clearance decreased in elderly

INTERACTIONS

Increase: effects of aripiprazole—CYP 3A4 inhibitors (ketoconazole, erythromycin), CYP 2D6 inhibitors (quinidine, fluoxetine, paroxetine); reduce dose of aripiprazole

Increase: sedation—other CNS depressants, alcohol

Increase: EPS—other antipsychotics, lithium

Increase: dose of aripiprazole—CYP 3A4 inducers

Decrease: aripiprazole level—famotidine, valproate

Decrease: effects of aripiprazole—CYP 3A4 inducers (carbamazepine)

Drug/Herb

Increase: EPS—betel palm, kava

Increase: neuroleptic effect—cola tree, hops, nettle, nutmeg

NURSING CONSIDERATIONS

Assess:

• Mental status before initial administration

• Swallowing of PO medication; check for hoarding or giving of medication to other patients

• I&O ratio; palpate bladder if urinary output is low

• Bilirubin, CBC, LFTs qmo

• Affect, orientation, LOC, reflexes, gait, coordination, sleep pattern disturbances

• B/P standing and lying; also pulse, respirations; take q4h during initial treatment; establish baseline before starting treatment; report drops of 30 mm Hg; watch for ECG changes

• Dizziness, faintness, palpitations, tachycardia on rising

• EPS, including akathisia (inability to sit still, no pattern to movements), tardive dyskinesia (bizarre movements of the jaw, mouth, tongue, extremities), pseudoparkinsonism (rigidity, tremors, pill rolling, shuffling gait)

⚠ For neuroleptic malignant syndrome: hyperthermia, increased CPK, altered mental status, muscle rigidity

• Constipation, urinary retention daily; if these occur, increase bulk and water in diet, stool softeners, laxatives may be needed

Administer:

• Reduced dose in elderly

Perform/provide:

• Supervised ambulation until patient is stabilized on medication; do not involve in strenuous exercise program because fainting is possible; patient should not stand still for a long time

• Storage in tight, light-resistant container

Evaluate:

• Therapeutic response: decrease in emotional excitement, hallucinations, delusions, paranoia; reorganization of patterns of thought, speech

Teach patient/family:

• That orthostatic hypotension may occur and to rise from sitting or lying position gradually

• To avoid hot tubs, hot showers, tub baths; hypotension may occur

• To avoid abrupt withdrawal of this drug; EPS may result; drug should be withdrawn slowly

• To avoid OTC preparations (cough, hay fever, cold) unless approved by prescriber, serious drug interactions may occur; avoid use with alcohol, CNS depressants; increased drowsiness may occur

• To avoid hazardous activities if drowsy or dizzy

• Compliance with drug regimen

• To report impaired vision, tremors, muscle twitching, urinary retention

• In hot weather, that heat stroke may occur; take extra precautions to stay cool

• To notify prescriber if pregnant or

intend to become pregnant; not to breast-feed

Treatment of overdose:
• Lavage if orally ingested; provide airway; *do not induce vomiting*

⚠ High Alert

arsenic trioxide (℞)
Trisenox
Func. class.: Antineoplastic—miscellaneous

Action: Not understood, causes morphologic changes and DNA fragmentation
Uses: Acute promyelocytic leukemia patients who are refractory to or have relapsed from retinoid and anthracycline chemotherapy

DOSAGE AND ROUTES

Induction
• *Adult:* IV 0.15 mg/kg/day until bone marrow remission, max 60 doses
Consolidation treatment
Wait 3-6 wk after completion of induction
• *Adult:* IV 0.15 mg/kg/day × 25 doses over a period of up to 5 wk
Available forms: Inj 1 mg/ml

SIDE EFFECTS

CNS: Anxiety, confusion, insomnia, headache, paresthesia, depression, dizziness, tremor, seizures, agitation, coma, weakness
CV: Hypotension, hypertension, prolonged QT interval, other ECG changes, chest pain, *tachycardia,* torsades de pointes
GI: Abdominal pain, constipation, diarrhea, dyspepsia, fecal incontinence, GI hemorrhage, dry mouth, *nausea, vomiting, anorexia*
GU: Vaginal hemorrhage, renal failure, incontinence
HEMA: Leukocytosis, anemia, thrombocytopenia, neutropenia, DIC
META: Increased ALT/AST, hyperkalemia, *hypokalemia,* hypomagnesemia, *hyperglycemia*

MISC: Weight gain or loss, fatigue, severe edema, rigors, herpes simplex/zoster
*RESP: **Pleural effusion,** dyspnea, cough,* epistaxis, hypoxia, sinusitis, wheezing, crackles, tachypnea
Contraindications: Pregnancy (D), hypersensitivity
Precautions: Elderly, lactation, children

PHARMACOKINETICS

Metabolized in the liver, stored in the liver, kidney, heart, lung, hair, nails, excreted in urine

NURSING CONSIDERATIONS

Assess:
⚠ For APL differentiation syndrome: fever, dyspnea, pulmonary infiltrates, pleural or pericardial effusions, weight gain; this condition can be fatal; give high-dose steroids
• For ECG changes: QT interval prolongation, complete AV block; obtain baseline ECG prior to drug therapy; watch drug-drug interactions with other drugs that prolong QT interval
• Electrolytes: K, Ca, Mg, creatine; hematologic, coagulation lab studies twice weekly or more; ECG qwk
Administer:
IV route
• Dilute with 100-250 ml D$_5$ or 0.9% NaCl immediately after withdrawing from ampule, give over 1-2 hr may give over 4 hr if reactions occur
Evaluate:
• Therapeutic response: decrease in malignant cells
Teach patient/family:
• To report planned or suspected pregnancy
• That fertility impairment has not been studied
• Symptoms of APL differentiation syndrome
Treatment of overdose:
• Dimercaprol 3 mg/kg IM q4hr, then 250 mg penicillamine PO, max 4 ×/day (≤1 g/day)

⚠ Safety alert   *"Tall Man" lettering

ascorbic acid (vit C) (OTC, ℞)
(a-skor'bic)
Apo-C ✦, ascorbic acid, Ascorbicap, Cebid, Cecon, Cecore-500, Cemill, Cenolate, Cetane, Cevalin, Cevi-Bid, Ce-Vi-Sol, C-Span, Flavorcee, Mega-C/A Plus, Ortho/CS, Sunkist
Func. class.: Vit C—water-soluble vitamin

Action: Needed for wound healing, collagen synthesis, antioxidant, carbohydrate metabolism

Uses: Vit C deficiency, scurvy, delayed wound and bone healing, chronic disease, urine acidification, before gastrectomy, acidification of urine, dietary supplement

Investigational uses: Common cold prevention

DOSAGE AND ROUTES

• *Child <6 mo:* PO 30 mg/day
Dietary supplementation
• *Adults/child >14 yr:* 50-200 mg daily
• *Child 11-14 yr:* PO 50 mg/day
• *Child 4-10 yr:* PO 45 mg/day
• *Child 1-3 yr:* PO 40 mg/day
• *Child 6 mo-1 yr:* PO 35 mg/day
Scurvy
• *Adult:* PO/SUBCUT/IM/IV 100 mg-500 mg daily × 2 wk, then 50 mg or more daily
• *Child:* PO/SUBCUT/IM/IV 100-300 mg daily × 2 wk, then 35 mg or more daily
Wound healing/chronic disease/fracture(may be given with zinc)
• *Adult:* SUBCUT/IM/IV/PO 200-500 mg daily for 1-2 mo
• *Child:* SUBCUT/IM/IV/PO 100-200 mg added doses for 1-2 mo
Urine acidification
• *Adult:* 4-12 g daily in divided doses
• *Child:* 500 mg q6-8h

Available forms: Tabs 25, 50, 100, 250, 500, 1000, 1500 mg; tabs effervescent 1000 mg; tabs chewable 100, 250, 500 mg; tabs timed release 500, 750, 1000, 1500 mg; caps timed release 500 mg; crys 4 g/tsp; powd 4 g/tsp; liq 35 mg/0.6 ml; sol 100 mg/ml; syr 20 mg/ml, 500 mg/5 ml; inj SUBCUT, IM, IV 100, 250, 500 mg/ml

SIDE EFFECTS

CNS: Headache, insomnia, dizziness, fatigue, flushing
GI: Nausea, vomiting, diarrhea, anorexia, heartburn, cramps
GU: Polyuria, urine acidification, oxalate or urate renal stones, dysuria
HEMA: **Hemolytic anemia in patients with G6PD**
INTEG: Inflammation at inj site
Contraindications: Tartrazine, sulfite sensitivity; G6PD deficiency
Precautions: Pregnancy (C), gout, diabetes, renal calculi (large doses)

PHARMACOKINETICS

PO, INJ: Readily absorbed PO, metabolized in liver, unused amounts excreted in urine (unchanged) and metabolites, crosses placenta, breast milk

INTERACTIONS

None known

Drug/Lab Test
False positive: Negatives in glucose tests
False negative: Occult blood, urine bilirubin, leukocyte determination

NURSING CONSIDERATIONS
Assess:
• I&O ratio
• Ascorbic acid levels throughout treatment if continued deficiency is suspected
• Nutritional status: citrus fruits, vegetables
• Inj sites for inflammation

Side effects: *italics* = common; ***bold italics*** = life-threatening

Administer:

PO route

- Do not break, crush, or chew ext rel tab or caps
- That caps may be opened and contents mixed with jelly

IV, direct route

- Undiluted by direct IV 100 mg over at least 1 min, rapid inf may cause fainting

Intermittent IV INF route

- Diluted with D_5W, D_5NaCl, NS, LR, Ringer's, sodium lactate and given over 15 min

Additive compatibilities: Amikacin, calcium chloride, calcium gluceptate, calcium gluconate, cephalothin, chloramphenicol, chlorproMAZINE, colistimethate, cyanocobalamin, diphenhydrAMINE, heparin, kanamycin, methicillin, methyldopate, penicillin G potassium, polymyxin B, prednisolone, procaine, prochlorperazine, promethazine, verapamil

Syringe compatibilities: Metoclopramide, aminophylline, theophylline

Y-site compatibilities: Warfarin

Evaluate:

- Therapeutic response: absence of anorexia, irritability, pallor, joint pain, hyperkeratosis, petechiae, poor wound healing

Teach patient/family:

- The necessary foods in diet, such as citrus fruits
- That smoking decreases vit C levels, not to exceed prescribed dose; increases will be excreted in urine, except timed release

---

> **⚠ High Alert**
>
> **asparaginase** (℞)
> (a-spare′a-gi-nase)
> Elspar, Kidrolase ✦
> *Func. class.:* Antineoplastic
> *Chem. class.:* Escherichia coli enzyme

Action: Indirectly inhibits protein synthesis in tumor cells; without amino acid, DNA, RNA synthesis is halted; asparagine, protein synthesis is halted; G_1 phase of cell cycle specific; a nonvesicant

Uses: Acute lymphocytic leukemia in combination with other antineoplastics

DOSAGE AND ROUTES

In combination

- *Adult and child:* **IV** 1000 international units/kg/day × 10 days given over 30 min; **IM** 6000 international units/m²/day

Sole induction

- *Adult and child:* **IV** 200 international units/kg/day × 28 days

Desensitization

- *Adult and child:* Test dose adult/child **ID** 2 international units, then double dose q10 min, until total dose is administered or reaction occurs

Available forms: Inj 10,000 international units with mannitol

SIDE EFFECTS

CNS: Neuritis, dizziness, headache, **coma,** depression, fatigue, confusion, hallucinations, lethargy, drowsiness, agitation, Parkinson-like syndrome, **seizures,** chills, fever

CV: Chest pain

ENDO: Hyperglycemia

GI: Nausea, vomiting, anorexia, diarrhea, weight loss, cramps, stomatitis, hepatotoxicity, pancreatitis

GU: Urinary retention, **renal failure,** glycosuria, polyuria, azotemia, uric acid neuropathy, proteinuria

*HEMA: **Thrombocytopenia, leukopenia, myelosuppression, anemia, decreased clotting factors (V, VII, VIII, IX), decreased fibrinogen***

INTEG: Rash, urticaria, perspiration

*RESP: **Fibrosis, pulmonary infiltrate***

*SYST: **Anaphylaxis***

Contraindications: Hypersensitivity, infants, lactation, pancreatitis

Precautions: Pregnancy (C), renal disease, hepatic disease

PHARMACOKINETICS

Half-life 4-9 hr, terminal 1.4-1.8 days

INTERACTIONS

May decrease response to live virus vaccines
Increase: toxicity—vinCRIStine, predniSONE
Decrease: action of—methotrexate
Drug/Lab Test
Increase: Uric acid
Decrease: Thyroid function tests

NURSING CONSIDERATIONS
Assess:
A For signs and symptoms of pancreatitis (nausea, vomiting, severe abdominal pain), anaphylaxis (bronchospasm, dyspnea), cyanosis; more toxic in adults than children
• CBC, differential, platelet count weekly; withhold drug if WBC is <4000 or platelet count is <75,000; notify prescriber of these results
• Pulmonary function tests, chest x-ray studies before, during therapy; chest x-ray film should be obtained q2wk during treatment
• Renal studies: BUN, serum uric acid, ammonia urine CCr, electrolytes before, during therapy
• I&O ratio; report fall in urine output of 30 ml/hr
• Monitor temp q4h; elevated temp may indicate beginning infection
• Hepatic studies before, during therapy (bilirubin, AST, ALT, LDH) as needed or monthly
• RBC, Hct, Hgb, since these may be decreased
• Serum, urine glucose levels
• Bleeding: hematuria, guaiac, bruising or petechiae, mucosa or orifices q8h
A Dyspnea, crackles, nonproductive cough, chest pain, tachypnea, fatigue, increased pulse, pallor, lethargy, swelling around eyes or lips; anaphylaxis may occur; risk of hypersensitivity increases with repeated dose
• Jaundice of skin and sclera, dark

urine, clay-colored stools, itchy skin, abdominal pain, fever, diarrhea
• Local irritation, pain, burning, discoloration at inj site
• Symptoms indicating severe allergic reaction: rash, pruritus, urticaria, purpuric skin lesions, itching, flushing, dyspnea
• Frequency of stools, characteristics: cramping, acidosis; signs of dehydration: rapid respirations, poor skin turgor, decreased urine output, dry skin, restlessness, weakness
Administer:
• May be mutagenic, teratogenic, carcinogenic to the staff, prepare according to policy
• Desensipmay be required before 1st dose, 1 unit may be ordered IV and dose doubled q10min, if no reaction, until amount equals patient's dose for that day; be prepared to treat acute allergic reaction if it occurs
IM route
• Reconstitute with 2 ml NaCl/10,000 units/vial, refrigerate, use within 8 hr; discard sooner if sol becomes cloudy, do not give more than 2 ml IM in one inj site
IV, direct route
• After intradermal skin testing and desensitization, give 0.1 ml (2 international units) intradermally after reconstituting with 5 ml sterile H_2O or 0.9% NaCl for inj; then add 0.1 ml of reconstituted drug to 9.9 ml diluent (20 international units/ml); observe for 1 hr, check for wheal
• Allopurinol to reduce uric acid levels, alkalinization of urine
Intermittent IV INF route
• Using 21G, 23G, 25G needle; administer by slow IV infusion via Y-tube or 3-way stopcock of flowing D_5W or NS infusion over 30 min after diluting 10,000 international units/5 ml of sterile H_2O or 0.9% NaCl (no preservatives) (2000 international units/ml); use of filter may be necessary if fibers are present
Y-site compatibilities: Methotrexate, sodium bicarbonate

Side effects: *italics* = common; **bold italics** = life-threatening

Perform/provide:
• Deep-breathing exercises with patient 3-4 ×/day; place in semi-Fowler's position
• Increase fluid intake to 2-3 L/day to prevent urate deposits, calculi formation
• Brushing of teeth 2-3 ×/day with soft brush or cotton-tipped applicators for stomatitis; use unwaxed dental floss
• Warm compresses at inj site for inflammation

Evaluate:
• Therapeutic response: decreased exacerbations in ALL

Teach patient/family:
• To report any changes in breathing or coughing
• Not to obtain vaccination while taking this drug
• To use contraception, since drug is teratogenic

Treatment of anaphylaxis:
• Administer epINEPHrine, diphenhydrAMINE, IV corticosteroids, O_2

---

aspirin (otc)

(as'pir-in)

acetylsalicylic acid, Acuprin, Apo-ASA ✖, Apo-Asen ✖, Arthrinol ✖, Arthrisin ✖, Artria S.R., A.S.A., Aspergum, Aspirin ✖, Aspir-Low, Aspirtab, Astrin ✖, Bayer Aspirin, Coryphen ✖, Easprin, Ecotrin, 8-Hour Bayer Timed Release, Empirin, Entrophen ✖, Halfprin, Norwich Extra-Strength, Novasen ✖, PMS-ASA ✖, Sloprin, St. Joseph Children's, Supasa ✖, Therapy Bayer, ZORprin

Func. class.: Nonopioid analgesic, nonsteroidal antiinflammatory, antipyretic, antiplatelet

Chem. class.: Salicylate

Action: Blocks pain impulses in CNS, reduces inflammation by inhibition of prostaglandin synthesis; antipyretic action results from vasodilation of peripheral vessels; decreases platelet aggregation

Uses: Mild to moderate pain or fever including rheumatoid arthritis, osteoarthritis, thromboembolic disorders; transient ischemic attacks, rheumatic fever, postmyocardial infarction, prophylaxis of MI, ischemic stroke, angina

Investigational uses: Prevention of cataracts (long-term use), prevention of pregnancy loss in women with clotting disorders

DOSAGE AND ROUTES

Arthritis
• *Adult:* **PO** 2.6-5.2 g/day in divided doses q4-6h
• *Child:* **PO** 90-130 mg/kg/day in divided doses q4-6h

Pain/fever
• *Adult:* **PO/RECT** 325-650 mg q4h prn, not to exceed 4 g/day
• *Child:* **PO/RECT** 40-100 mg/kg/day in divided doses q4-6h prn

Kawasaki disease
• *Child:* **PO** 80-120 mg/kg/day in 4 divided doses, maintenance 3-8 mg/day as a single dose × 8 wk

Acute rheumatic fever
• *Adult:* **PO** 5-6 g/day initially
• *Child:* **PO** 100 mg/kg/day × 2 wk, then 75 mg/kg/day × 4-6 wk

Thromboembolic disorders
• *Adult:* **PO** 325-650 mg/day or bid

Transient ischemic attacks
• *Adult:* **PO** 650 mg bid or 350 mg qid

MI, stroke prophylaxis
• *Adult:* **PO** 81-650 mg/day

Available forms: Tabs 81, 162.5, 325, 500, 650, 975 mg; chewable tabs 80, 81 mg; supp 60, 120, 125, 130, 150, 160, 195, 200, 300, 320, 325, 600, 640, 650 mg, 1.2 g; cream; gum 227 mg; dispersible tabs 325, 500 mg, del rel tabs, enteric coated 80, 165, 300, 325, 500, 600, 650, 975 mg; ext rel tabs 325, 650, 800 mg, del rel caps 325, 500 mg

---

⚠ Safety alert   *"Tall Man" lettering

SIDE EFFECTS

CNS: Stimulation, drowsiness, dizziness, confusion, *seizures,* headache, flushing, hallucinations, *coma*

CV: Rapid pulse, pulmonary edema

EENT: Tinnitus, hearing loss

ENDO: Hypoglycemia, hyponatremia, hypokalemia

GI: Nausea, vomiting, *GI bleeding,* diarrhea, heartburn, anorexia, *hepatitis*

HEMA: *Thrombocytopenia, agranulocytosis, leukopenia, neutropenia, hemolytic anemia,* increased PT, APTT, bleeding time

INTEG: Rash, urticaria, bruising

RESP: Wheezing, hyperpnea

SYST: *Reye's syndrome (children), anaphylaxis, laryngeal edema*

Contraindications: Pregnancy (D) 3rd trimester, hypersensitivity to salicylates, tartrazine (FDC yellow dye #5), GI bleeding, NSAIDs, bleeding disorders, children <12 yr, children with flulike symptoms, lactation, vit K deficiency, peptic ulcer

Precautions: Anemia, hepatic disease, renal disease, Hodgkin's disease, pre/postoperatively, gastritis, asthmatic patients with nasal polyps or aspirin sensitivity

PHARMACOKINETICS

Well absorbed PO; enteric metabolized by liver, inactive metabolites excreted by kidneys, crosses placenta, excreted in breast milk; half-life 15-20 min, up to 30 hr in large dose; rectal products may be erratic

PO: Onset 15-30 min, peak 1-2 hr, duration 4-6 hr

REC: Onset slow, duration 4-6 hr

INTERACTIONS

Gastric ulcer: steroids, antiinflammatories, NSAIDs

Increase: bleeding—alcohol, heparin, plicamycin, cefamandole, thrombolytics, ticlopidine, clopidogrel, tirofiban, eptifibatide

Increase: effects of warfarin, insulin, methotrexate, thrombolytic agents, penicillins, phenytoin, valproic acid, oral hypoglycemics, sulfonamides

Increase: salicylate levels—urinary acidifiers, ammonium chloride, nizatidine

Increase: hypotension—nitroglycerin

Decrease: effects of aspirin—antacids (high doses), urinary alkalizers, corticosteroids

Decrease: antihypertensive effect—ACE inhibitors

Decrease: effects of probenecid, spironolactone, sulfinpyrazone, sulfonylamides, NSAIDs, β-blockers, loop diuretics

Drug/Herb

Gastric irritation: arginine, gossypol

Increase: risk of bleeding—anise, arnica, bilberry, bogbean, chamomile, chondroitin, clove, fenugreek, feverfew, garlic, ginger, ginkgo, ginseng *(Panax),* horse chestnut, Irish moss, kelpware, licorice, pansy

Drug/Food

Foods acidifying urine may increase aspirin level

Drug/Lab Test

Increase: Coagulation studies, LFTs, serum uric acid, amylase, CO_2, urinary protein

Decrease: Serum potassium, PBI, cholesterol

Interference: Urine catecholamines, pregnancy test, urine glucose tests (Clinistix, Tes-Tape)

NURSING CONSIDERATIONS

Assess:

• Pain: character, location, intensity; ROM before and 1 hr after administration

• Fever: temperature before and 1 hr after administration

• Hepatic studies: AST, ALT, bilirubin, creatinine if patient is on long-term therapy

• Renal studies: BUN, urine creatinine; I&O ratio; decreasing output may indicate renal failure (long-term therapy)

• Blood studies: CBC, Hct, Hgb, PT if patient is on long-term therapy
⚠ Hepatotoxicity: dark urine, clay-colored stools, yellowing of skin, sclera, itching, abdominal pain, fever, diarrhea if patient is on long-term therapy
• Allergic reactions: rash, urticaria; if these occur, drug may have to be discontinued; patients with asthma, nasal polyps, allergies: severe allergic reaction may occur
• Ototoxicity: tinnitus, ringing, roaring in ears; audiometric testing needed before, after long-term therapy
• Salicylate level: therapeutic level 150-300 mcg/ml for chronic inflammation
• Visual changes: blurring, halos; corneal, retinal damage
• Edema in feet, ankles, legs
• Drug history; many drug interactions
Administer:
PO route
• Do not break, crush, or chew enteric product
• Crushed or whole; chewable tablets may be chewed
• ½ hr before planned exercise
• With food or milk to decrease gastric symptoms; separate by 2 hr of enteric product
• With 8 oz H₂O and sit upright for ½ hr after dose to facilitate drug passing into the stomach
Evaluate:
• Therapeutic response: decreased pain, inflammation, fever
Teach patient/family:
• To report any symptoms of hepatotoxicity, renal toxicity, visual changes, ototoxicity, allergic reactions, bleeding (long-term therapy)
• To avoid if allergic to tartrazine
• Not to exceed recommended dosage; acute poisoning may result
• To read label on other OTC drugs; many contain aspirin or salicylates
• That the therapeutic response takes 2 wk (arthritis)
• To report tinnitus, confusion, diarrhea, sweating, hyperventilation

• To avoid alcohol ingestion; GI bleeding may occur
• That patients who have allergies, nasal polyps, asthma may develop allergic reactions
• To discard tabs if vinegar-like smell is detected
• That medication is not to be given to children or teens with flulike symptoms or chickenpox; Reye's syndrome may develop
Treatment of overdose: Lavage, activated charcoal, monitor electrolytes, VS

---

atazanavir (℞)
(at-a-za-na′veer)
Reyataz
Func. class.: Antiretroviral
Chem. class.: Protease inhibitor

Action: Inhibits human immunodeficiency virus (HIV-1) protease, which prevents maturation of the infectious virus
Uses: HIV-1 infection in combination with other antiretroviral agents

DOSAGE AND ROUTES
Antiretroviral-naive patients
• *Adult:* **PO** 400 mg daily
Antiretroviral-experienced patients
Adult: **PO** 300 mg daily and ritonavir 100 mg daily
Hepatic dose
• *Adult:* **PO** (Child-Pugh B) 300 mg daily; (Child-Pugh C) do not use
Available forms: Caps 100, 150, 200 mg

SIDE EFFECTS
CNS: Headache, depression, dizziness, insomnia, peripheral neurologic symptoms
GI: Vomiting, *diarrhea, abdominal pain, nausea,* **hepatotoxicity**
INTEG: Rash, **Stevens-Johnson syndrome,** *photosensitivity*
MISC: Fatigue, fever, arthralgia, back pain, cough, lipodystrophy, pain, gynecomastia

---

Contraindications: Hypersensitivity
Precautions: Pregnancy (B), liver disease, lactation, children, elderly

PHARMACOKINETICS

Rapidly absorbed, absorption increased with food, peak 2½ hr, 86% protein bound, extensively metabolized in liver, 27% excreted unchanged in urine/feces (minimal), half life 7 hr

INTERACTIONS

Increase: levels resulting in increased toxicity of immunosuppressants (cyclo-SPORINE, sirolimus, tacrolimus, sildenafil), tricylic antidepressants, warfarin, calcium channel blockers, irinotecan, HMG-CoA reductase inhibitors, antidysrhythmics, midazolam, triazolam, ergots, pimozide
Increase: effects of—oral contraceptives
Increase: hyperbilirubinemia indinavir
Decrease: atazanavir levels—rifampin, antacids, didanosine, efavirenz, proton pump inhibitors, H_2-receptor antagonists
Drug/Herb
Decrease: atazanavir levels—St. John's wort
Drug/Lab Test
Increase: AST, ALT, total bilirubin, amylase, lipase

NURSING CONSIDERATIONS

Assess:
A For hepatic failure
• Signs of infection, anemia
• Hepatic studies: ALT, AST, bilirubin
• Bowel pattern before, during treatment; if severe abdominal pain with bleeding occurs, drug should be discontinued; monitor hydration
• Viral load, CD4 count throughout treatment
• Skin eruptions, rash, urticaria, itching
• Allergies before treatment, reaction of each medication; place allergies on chart
Administer:
• With food

Evaluate:
• Therapeutic response: increasing CD4 counts; decreased viral load, resolution of symptoms of HIV-1 infection
Teach patient/family:
• To take as prescribed with other antiretrovirals as prescribed, if dose is missed, take as soon as remembered up to 1 hr before next dose; do not double dose, do not share with others
• That drug must be taken daily to maintain blood levels for duration of therapy
• May cause photosensitivity, use protective clothing, or stay out of the sun
• To notify prescriber if diarrhea, nausea, vomiting, rash occurs; dizziness, light-headedness, ECG may be altered
• That drug interacts with many drugs and St. John's wort, advise prescriber of all drugs, herbal products used
• That redistribution of body fat may occur, the effect is not known
• That drug does not cure HIV-1 infection or prevent transmission to others, only controls symptoms
• That if taking sildenafil with atazanavir, there may be an increased risk of sildenafil-associated adverse events, including hypotension and prolonged penile erection; notify physician promptly of these symptoms

---

atenolol (Ŗ)
(a-ten'oh-lole)
Apo-Atenol ✤, atenolol ✤, Novo-Atenol ✤, Tenormin
Func. class.: Antihypertensive, antianginal
Chem. class.: β-Blocker, $β_1$-, $β_2$-blocker (high doses)

Do not confuse:
atenolol/albuterol/Altenol
Tenormin/thiamine/Imuran/Trovan
Action: Competitively blocks stimulation of β-adrenergic receptor within vascular smooth muscle; produces negative chronotropic activity, negative inotropic activity (decreases rate of SA node discharge, increases recovery time),

---

slows conduction of AV node, decreases heart rate, decreases O_2 consumption in myocardium; also decreases renin-aldosterone-angiotensin system at high doses, inhibits β_2 receptors in bronchial system at higher doses

Uses: Mild to moderate hypertension, prophylaxis of angina pectoris; suspected or known myocardial infarction (IV use)
Investigational uses: Dysrhythmia, mitral valve prolapse, pheochromocytoma, hypertrophic cardiomyopathy, vascular headaches, thyrotoxicosis, tremors, alcohol withdrawal

DOSAGE AND ROUTES

• *Adult:* **IV** 5 mg, repeat in 10 min if initial dose is well tolerated, then start **PO** dose 10 min after last **IV** dose
• *Adult:* **PO** 25-50 mg daily, increasing q1-2wk to 100 mg daily; may increase to 200 mg daily for angina or up to 100 mg for hypertension
• *Geriatric:* **PO** 25 mg/day initially
Renal disease
• *Adult:* **PO** CCr 15-35 ml/min, max 50 mg/day; CCr <15 ml/min max dose 25 mg/day; hemodialysis 25-50 mg after dialysis
MI
• *Adult:* **IV** 5 mg, then 5 mg over 10 min, then after 10 min, give **PO** dose
Available forms: Tabs 25, 50, 100 mg; inj 500 mcg/ml

SIDE EFFECTS

CNS: Insomnia, fatigue, dizziness, mental changes, memory loss, hallucinations, depression, lethargy, drowsiness, strange dreams, catatonia
*CV: **Profound hypotension, bradycardia, CHF,** cold extremities, postural hypotension, 2nd- or 3rd-degree heart block*
EENT: Sore throat, dry burning eyes, blurred vision, stuffy nose
ENDO: Increased hypoglycemic response to insulin
GI: Nausea, diarrhea, vomiting, ***mesenteric arterial thrombosis, ischemic colitis***

GU: Impotence, decreased libido
*HEMA: **Agranulocytosis, thrombocytopenia, purpura***
INTEG: Rash, fever, alopecia
*RESP: **Bronchospasm,** dyspnea, wheezing, pulmonary edema*
Contraindications: Pregnancy (D), hypersensitivity to β-blockers, cardiogenic shock, 2nd- or 3rd-degree heart block, sinus bradycardia, cardiac failure, Raynaud's disease, pulmonary edema
Precautions: Major surgery, lactation, diabetes mellitus, renal disease, thyroid disease, CHF, COPD, asthma, well-compensated heart failure, dialysis, myasthenia gravis

PHARMACOKINETICS

IV: Onset rapid, peak 5 min, duration unknown
PO: Peak 2-4 hr, onset 1 hr, duration 24 hr; half-life 6-9 hr, excreted unchanged in urine, feces protein binding 5%-15%

INTERACTIONS

Mutual inhibition: sympathomimetics (cough, cold preparations)
Increase: hypotension, bradycardia—reserpine, hydrALAZINE, methyldopa, prazosin, anticholinergics, digoxin, diltiazem, verapamil, cardiac glycosides, antihypertensives
Increase: atenolol absorption—atropine
Drug/Herb
Toxicity/death: aconite
Increase: atenolol effect—betel palm, butterbur, cola tree, figwort, fumitory, guarana, hawthorn, jaborandi tree, lily of the valley, motherwort, plantain
Decrease: atenolol effect—coenzyme Q10, yohimbe
Drug/Lab Test
Increase: Blood glucose, BUN, K, triglycerides, uric acid, ANA titer

NURSING CONSIDERATIONS

Assess:
• I&O, weight daily
• B/P, pulse q4h; note rate, rhythm,

quality; apical/radial pulse before administration; notify prescriber of any significant changes (<50 bpm)

• Baselines in renal, hepatic studies before therapy begins

Administer:

PO route

• Drug ac, at bedtime, tablet may be crushed or swallowed whole

• Reduced dosage in renal dysfunction

IV, direct route

• Undiluted over 5 min

IV INF route

• Diluted in 10-50 ml of D_5W, D_5/NaCl, or NS and give as an infusion at prescribed rate

Y-site compatibilities: Meperidine, meropenem, morphine

Perform/provide:

• Storage protected from light, moisture; place in cool environment

Evaluate:

• Therapeutic response: decreased B/P after 1-2 wk

Teach patient/family:

🛦 Not to discontinue drug abruptly, taper over 2 wk (angina), take at same time each day

• Not to use OTC products unless directed by prescriber

• To report bradycardia, dizziness, confusion, depression, fever

• To take pulse at home; advise when to notify prescriber

• To limit alcohol, smoking, sodium intake

• To comply with weight control, dietary adjustments, modified exercise program

• To carry emergency ID to identify drug, allergies, conditions being treated

• To avoid hazardous activities if dizziness is present

• That drug may mask symptoms of hypoglycemia in diabetic patients

• To use contraception while taking this drug, pregnancy category (D)

Treatment of overdose: Lavage, IV atropine for bradycardia, IV theophylline for bronchospasm, dextrose for hypoglycemia, digitalis, O_2, diuretic for cardiac failure, hemodialysis

atomoxetine (R)

(at-o-mox'eh-teen)
Strattera
Func. class.: Miscellaneous psychotherapeutic
Chem. class.: Selective norepinephrine reuptake inhibitor

Action: A selective norepinephrine reuptake inhibitor. May inhibit the presynaptic norepinephrine transporter.
Uses: Attention deficit hyperactivity disorder

DOSAGE AND ROUTES

• *Child ≤70 kg:* **PO** 0.5 mg/kg, increase after 3 days to a target daily dose of 1.2 mg/kg in AM or evenly divided doses AM, late afternoon; max 1.4 mg/kg/day or 100 mg daily, whichever is less

• *Adult/child >70 kg:* **PO** 40 mg daily, increase after 3 days to a target daily dose of 80 mg in AM or evenly divided doses AM, late afternoon; max 100 mg daily

Hepatic dose

• (Child-Pugh B) reduce dose by 50%

• (Child-Pugh C) reduce dose by 75%

Available forms: Caps 10, 18, 25, 40, 60 mg

SIDE EFFECTS

CNS: Insomnia, dizziness, headache, irritability, crying, mood swings, fatigue
CV: Palpitations, hot flushes
ENDO: Growth retardation
GI: Dyspepsia, nausea, anorexia, dry mouth, weight loss, vomiting, diarrhea, constipation
GU: Urinary hesitancy, retention, dysmenorrhea, erectile disturbance, ejaculation failure, impotence, prostatis, orgasm abnormal
*INTEG: **Exfoliative dermatitis,*** sweating
MISC: Cough, rhinorrhea, dermatitis, ear infection
Contraindications: Hypersensitivity, narrow-angle glaucoma
Precautions: Pregnancy (C), hyperten-

sion, lactation, child <6 yr; hepatic, cardiac, or cerebrovascular disease

PHARMACOKINETICS

PO: Peak 1-2 hr, metabolized by liver, excreted by kidneys, 98% protein binding

INTERACTIONS

Hypertensive crisis: MAOIs or within 14 days of MAOIs, vasopressors
Increase: cardiovascular effects of—albuterol, pressor agents
Increase: effects of atomoxetine: CYP 2D6 inhibitors (amiodarone, cimetidine [weak], clomipramine, delavirdine, gefitinib, imatinib, propafenone, quinidine [potent], ritonavir, citalopram, escitalopram, fluoxetine, sertraline, paroxetine, thioridazine, venlafaxine)

NURSING CONSIDERATIONS

Assess:
• VS, B/P; check patients with cardiac disease more often for increased B/P
• Height, growth rate q3mo in children; growth rate may be decreased
• Mental status: mood, sensorium, affect, stimulation, insomnia, aggressiveness
• Appetite, sleep, speech patterns
• For attention span, decreased hyperactivity in ADHD persons
Administer:
• Gum, hard candy, frequent sips of water for dry mouth
Evaluate:
• Therapeutic response: decreased hyperactivity (ADHD)
Teach patient/family:
• To avoid OTC preparations unless approved by prescriber
• To avoid alcohol ingestion
• To avoid hazardous activities until stabilized on medication
• To get needed rest; patients will feel more tired at end of day

---

atorvastatin (℞)
(a-tore′va-stat-in)
Lipitor
Func. class.: Antilipidemic
Chem. class.: HMG-CoA reductase inhibitor

Action: Inhibits HMG-CoA reductase enzyme, which reduces cholesterol synthesis
Uses: As an adjunct in primary hypercholesterolemia (types Ia, Ib), dysbetalipoproteinemia, elevated triglyceride levels, prevention of CV disease by reduction of heart risk in those with mildly elevated cholesterol

DOSAGE AND ROUTES

• *Adult:* **PO** 10-20 mg daily, usual range 10-80, dosage adjustments may be made in 2-4 wk intervals, max 80 mg/day; patients requiring >45% reduction in LDL may be started at 40 mg daily
Available forms: Tabs 10, 20, 40, 80 mg

SIDE EFFECTS

CNS: Headache, asthenia
EENT: Lens opacities
GI: Abdominal cramps, constipation, diarrhea, flatus, heartburn, dyspepsia, *liver dysfunction,* pancreatitis, nausea, increased serum transaminase
GU: Impotence
INTEG: Rash, pruritus, alopecia
MISC: Hypersensitivity
MS: Arthralgia, myalgia, *rhabdomyolysis*
RESP: Pharyngitis, sinusitis
Contraindications: Pregnancy (X), hypersensitivity, lactation, active liver disease
Precautions: Past hepatic disease, alcoholism, severe acute infections, trauma, severe metabolic disorders, electrolyte imbalance

---

⚠ Safety alert   *"Tall Man" lettering

PHARMACOKINETICS

Metabolized in liver, highly protein bound, excreted primarily in urine, half-life 14 hr; protein binding 98%

INTERACTIONS

Risk of possible rhabdomyolysis: azole antifungals, cycloSPORINE, erythromycin, niacin, gemfibrozil, clofibrate
Increase: serum level of digoxin
Increase: levels of oral contraceptives
Increase: levels of atorvastatin—erythromycin
Increase: effects of warfarin
Decrease: atorvastatin levels—colestipol
Drug/Herb
Increase: effect—glucomannan
Decrease: effect—gotu kola
Drug/Food
Possible toxicity when used with grapefruit juice; food increases blood levels
Drug/Lab Test
Increase: Bilirubin, alk phosphatase
Interference: Thyroid function tests

NURSING CONSIDERATIONS
Assess:
• Diet, obtain diet history including fat, cholesterol in diet
• Cholesterol triglyceride levels periodically during treatment; check lipid panel 6 wk after changing dose
• Hepatic studies q1-2mo during the first 1½ yr of treatment; AST, ALT, LFTs may be increased
• Renal studies in patients with compromised renal system: BUN, I&O ratio, creatinine
⚠ For muscle pain, tenderness, obtain CPK baseline and if these occur, drug may need to be discontinued
Administer:
• Total daily dose any time of day
Perform/provide:
• Storage in cool environment in tight container protected from light
Evaluate:
• Therapeutic response: decrease in cholesterol to desired level after 6 wk

Teach patient/family:
• That blood work and eye exam will be necessary during treatment
• To report blurred vision, severe GI symptoms, headache, muscle pain, weakness
• That previously prescribed regimen will continue: low-cholesterol diet, exercise program, smoking cessation
• Not to take drug if pregnant
• To stay out of the sun, or use sunscreen, protective clothing to prevent photosensitivity (rare)

---

atovaquone (R)
(a-toe'va-kwon)
Mepron
Func. class.: Antiprotozoal
Chem. class.: Aromatic diamide derivative, analog of ubiquinone

---

Do not confuse:
Mepron (U.S.)/Mepron (meprobamate in Australia)
Action: Interferes with DNA/RNA synthesis in protozoa
Uses: *Pneumocystis jiroveci* infections in patients intolerant of trimethoprim-sulfamethoxazole, prophylaxis, *Toxoplasma gondii,* toxoplasmosis
Investigational uses: Babesiosis, malaria treatment/prophylaxis, toxoplasmosis prophylaxis, *plasmodium* sp.

DOSAGE AND ROUTES
Acute, mild, moderate Pneumocystis jiroveci *pneumonia (PCP)*
• *Adult and adolescents 13-16 yr:* **PO** 750 mg with food bid for 21 days
Pneumocystis carinii *pneumonia, prophylaxis*
• *Adult/adolescents:* **PO** 1500 mg daily with meal
Available forms: 750 mg/5 ml, susp

SIDE EFFECTS

CNS: Dizziness, headache, anxiety, insomnia
CV: Hypotension
GI: Nausea, vomiting, diarrhea, an-

orexia, increased AST and ALT, acute pancreatitis, constipation, abdominal pain

HEMA: Anemia, *leukopenia,* neutropenia

INTEG: Pruritus, urticaria, *rash,* oral monilia

META: Hyperkalemia, hypoglycemia, hyponatremia

Contraindications: Hypersensitivity or history of developing life-threatening allergic reactions to any component of the formulation, benzyl alcohol sensitivity

Precautions: Pregnancy (C), blood dyscrasias, hepatic disease, diabetes mellitus, lactation, children, elderly, GI disease, respiratory insufficiency

PHARMACOKINETICS

Excreted unchanged in feces (94%), highly protein bound (99%)

INTERACTIONS

Use caution when administering concurrently with other highly plasma protein-bound drugs with narrow therapeutic indices

Decrease: effect of atovaquone—rifampin, rifabutin

NURSING CONSIDERATIONS

Assess:
• Signs of infection, anemia
• Bowel pattern before, during treatment
• Respiratory status: rate, character, wheezing, dyspnea
• Allergies before treatment, reaction of each medication

Administer:
• With high-fat food because of increased absorption of the drug and higher plasma concentrations

Evaluate:
• Therapeutic response: decreased temp, ability to breathe

Teach patient/family:
• To take with food to increase plasma concentrations

Rarely Used

atracurium (R)
(a-tra-kyoor′ee-um)
Tracrium
Func. class.: Neuromuscular blocker (nondepolarizing)

Uses: Facilitation of endotracheal intubation, skeletal muscle relaxation during mechanical ventilation, surgery, or general anesthesia

DOSAGE AND ROUTES

• *Adult and child >2 yr:* **IV BOL** 0.3-0.5 mg/kg, then 0.08-0.10 mg/kg 20-45 min after first dose if needed for prolonged procedures
• *Child, 1 mo-2 yr:* **IV BOL** 0.3-0.4 mg/kg

Contraindications: Hypersensitivity

⚠ High Alert

atropine (R)
(a′troe-peen)
atropine sulfate, Atro-Pen, Sal-Tropine
Func. class.: Antidysrhythmic, anticholinergic parasympatholytic, antimuscarinic
Chem. class.: Belladonna alkaloid

Do not confuse:
atropine/Akarpine

Action: Blocks acetylcholine at parasympathetic neuroeffector sites; increases cardiac output, heart rate by blocking vagal stimulation in heart; dries secretions by blocking vagus

Uses: Bradycardia <40-50 bpm, bradydysrhythmia, reversal of anticholinesterase agents, insecticide poisoning, blocking cardiac vagal reflexes, decreasing secretions before surgery, antispasmodic with GU, biliary surgery, bronchodilator

---

⚠ Safety alert   *"Tall Man" lettering

DOSAGE AND ROUTES

Bradycardia/bradydysrhythmia
- *Adult:* **IV BOL** 0.5-1 mg given q3-5min, not to exceed 2 mg
- *Child:* **IV BOL** 0.01-0.03 mg/kg up to 0.4 mg or 0.3 mg/m²; may repeat q4-6h; min dose 0.1 mg to avoid paradoxical reaction

Organophosphate poisoning
- *Adult and child:* **IM/IV** 2 mg qh until muscarinic symptoms disappear, may need 6 mg qh; *Atro-pen Adult/child 90 lb, usually >10 yr:* 2 mg; *Child 40-90 lb, usually 4-10 yr:* 1 mg; *Child 15-40 lb, 6 mo-4 yr:* 0.05 mg

Presurgery
- *Adult/child >20 kg:* **SUBCUT/IM/IV** 0.4-0.6 mg before anesthesia
- *Child <20 kg:* **IM/SUBCUT** 0.01 mg/kg up to 0.4 mg ½-1 hr preop

Available forms: Inj 0.05, 0.1, 0.3, 0.4, 0.5, 0.8, 1 mg/ml; tabs 0.4 mg; Atropen 0.5, 1, 2 mg inj prefilled auto-injectors

SIDE EFFECTS

CNS: Headache, dizziness, involuntary movement, confusion, psychosis, anxiety, coma, flushing, drowsiness, insomnia, weakness; delirium (elderly)
CV: Hypotension, paradoxical bradycardia, angina, PVCs, hypertension, *tachycardia*, ectopic ventricular beats
EENT: Blurred vision, photophobia, glaucoma, eye pain, pupil dilation, nasal congestion
GI: Dry mouth, nausea, vomiting, abdominal pain, anorexia, constipation, *paralytic ileus*, abdominal distention, altered taste
GU: Retention, hesitancy, impotence, dysuria
INTEG: Rash, urticaria, contact dermatitis, dry skin, flushing
MISC: Suppression of lactation, decreased sweating
Contraindications: Hypersensitivity to belladonna alkaloids, angle-closure glaucoma, GI obstructions, myasthenia gravis, thyrotoxicosis, ulcerative colitis, prostatic hypertrophy, tachycardia/tachydysrhythmias, asthma, acute hemorrhage, hepatic disease, myocardial ischemia
Precautions: Pregnancy (C), renal disease, lactation, CHF, tachydysrhythmia, hyperthyroidism, COPD, hepatic disease, child <6 yr, hypertension, elderly, intraabdominal infection, Down syndrome, spastic paralysis, gastric ulcer

PHARMACOKINETICS

Well absorbed PO, IM, SUBCUT; half-life 13-40 hr, excreted by kidneys unchanged (70%-90% in 24 hr); metabolized in liver, 40%-50% crosses placenta, excreted in breast milk
IV: Peak 2-4 min, duration 4-6 hr
IM/SUBCUT: Onset 15-50 min; peak 30 min, duration 4-6 hr
PO: Onset ½ hr; peak ½-1 hr; duration 4-6 hr

INTERACTIONS

Mucosal lesions: potassium chloride tab
Increase: anticholinergic effects, tricyclics, amantadine, antiparkinson agents
Decrease: absorption—ketoconazole, levodopa
Decrease: effect of atropine—antacids
Drug/Herb
Forms insoluble complex: black root
Serotonin effect: horehound
Increase: atropine effect—aloe, buckthorn, cascara sagrada, figwort, fumitory, goldenseal, jimsonweed, kudzu, licorice, rhubarb, senna, scopolia
Increase: toxicity/death—aconite
Decrease: effect—coltsfoot

NURSING CONSIDERATIONS

Assess:
- I&O ratio; check for urinary retention, daily output
- ECG for ectopic ventricular beats, PVC, tachycardia, in cardiac patients
- For bowel sounds; check for constipation
- Respiratory status: rate, rhythm, cya-

nosis, wheezing, dyspnea, engorged neck veins
• Increased intraocular pressure: eye pain, nausea, vomiting, blurred vision, increased tearing
• Cardiac rate: rhythm, character, B/P continuously
• Allergic reaction: rash, urticaria

Administer:

PO route
• Increased bulk, water in diet if constipation occurs
• ½ hr ac

IM route
• Atropine flush may occur in children and is not harmful

Atro-Pen
• Use no more than 3 Atro-Pen inj unless under the supervision of trained medical provider
• Use as soon as symptoms appear (tearing, wheezing, muscles fasciculations, excessive oral secretions)

IV route
• Undiluted or diluted with 10 ml sterile H₂O, give at 0.6 mg/min, give through Y-tube or 3-way stopcock; do not add to IV sol; may cause paradoxical bradycardia lasting 2 min

Additive compatibilities: DOBUTamine, furosemide, meropenem, netilmicin, sodium bicarbonate, verapamil

Syringe compatibilities: Benzquinamide, butorphanol, chlorproMAZINE, cimetidine, dimenhyDRINATE, diphenhydrAMINE, droperidol, fentanyl, glycopyrrolate, heparin, hydromorphone, hydrOXYzine, meperidine, metoclopramide, midazolam, milrinone, morphine, nalbuphine, pentazocine, perphenazine, prochlorperazine, promazine, promethazine, propiomazine, ranitidine, scopolamine, sufentanil

Y-site compatibilities: Amrinone, etomidate, famotidine, heparin, hydrocortisone, meropenem, nafcillin, potassium chloride, sufentanil, vit B/C

Perform/provide:
• Sugarless hard candy, gum, frequent rinsing of mouth for dryness

Evaluate:
• Therapeutic response: decreased dysrhythmias, increased heart rate, secretions; GI, GU spasms; bronchodilation

Teach patient/family:
• To report blurred vision, chest pain, allergic reactions, constipation, urinary retention
• Not to perform strenuous activity in high temperatures; heat stroke may result
• To take as prescribed; not to skip doses
• Not to operate machinery if drowsiness occurs
• Not to take OTC products without approval of prescriber

Treatment of overdose: O₂, artificial ventilation, ECG; administer DOPamine for circulatory depression; administer diazepam or thiopental for convulsions; assess need for antidysrhythmics

---

atropine ophthalmic
See Appendix C

Rarely Used

auranofin (℞)
(au-rane′oh-fin)
Ridaura
Func. class.: Antiinflammatory

Do not confuse:
Ridaura/Cardura
Uses: Rheumatoid arthritis; not for first-line therapy
Investigational uses: SLE, psoriatic arthritis, pemphigus

DOSAGE AND ROUTES
• *Adult:* PO 6 mg daily or 3 mg bid; may increase to 9 mg/day after 3 mo
Contraindications: Hypersensitivity to gold, necrotizing enterocolitis, bone marrow aplasia, child <6 yr, lactation, pulmonary fibrosis, exfoliative dermatitis, blood dyscrasias, recent radiation

therapy, renal/hepatic disease, marked hypertension, uncontrolled CHF

Rarely Used

aurothioglucose/gold sodium thiomalate (℞)
(aur-oh-thye-oh-gloo′kose)
Solganal/Aurolate
Func. class.: Antiinflammatory

Uses: Rheumatoid arthritis, psoriatic arthritis

DOSAGE AND ROUTES
• *Adult:* **IM** 10 mg, then 25 mg qwk × 2-3 wk, then 50 mg/wk until total of 1 g is administered, then 25-50 mg q3-4wk if there is improvement without toxicity (aurothioglucose) total of 800 mg-1 g
• *Adult:* **IM** 10 mg, then 25 mg after 1 wk, then 50 mg qwk for total of 14-20 doses, then 50 mg q2wk × 4, then 50 mg q3wk × 4, then 50 mg qmo for maintenance (gold sodium thiomalate)
• *Child 6-12 yr:* **IM** 0.25 mg/kg/wk 1st wk, increase by 0.25 mg/kg/wk up to 0.75-1 mg/kg/wk, max 25 mg/dose; give for 20 wk (aurothioglucose)
• *Child:* **IM** 10 mg 1st wk, then 1 mg/kg, max 50 mg/dose; space doses as per adult dosing schedule if improvement without toxicity (gold sodium thiomalate)
Contraindications: Hypersensitivity to gold, SLE, uncontrolled diabetes mellitus, marked hypertension, recent radiation therapy, CHF, lactation, renal disease, hepatic disease

▲ High Alert

azacitidine (℞)
(a-za-sie-ti′deen)
Vidaza
Func. class.: Antineoplastic hormone
Chem. class.: DNA demethylation agent

Action: Cytotoxic by producing damage to double-strand DNA during DNA synthesis
Uses: Myelodysplastic syndrome (MDS)

DOSAGE AND ROUTES
• *Adult:* **SUBCUT** 75 mg/m^2 daily × 7 days, q4wk, premedicate with antiemetic; dose may be increased to 100 mg/m^2 if no response is seen after 2 treatment cycles, minimum treatment 4 cycles
Available forms: Powdered for inj, lyophilized 100 mg

SIDE EFFECTS
CNS: Anxiety, depression, dizziness, fatigue, headache
CV: Cardiac murmur, hypotension, tachycardia
GI: **Diarrhea,** nausea, vomiting, anorexia, constipation, abdominal pain, distention, tenderness, hemorrhoids, mouth hemorrhage, tongue ulceration, stomatitis, dyspepsia, **hepatotoxicity, hepatic coma**
GU: **Renal failure, renal tubular acidosis,** dysuria, UTI
HEMA: **Leukopenia, anemia, thrombocytopenia, neutropenia,** ecchymosis
INTEG: Irritation at site, rash, sweating, pyrexia
META: Hypokalemia
Contraindications: Pregnancy (D), hypersensitivity to this drug or mannitol, advanced malignant hepatic tumors
Precautions: Lactation, children, elderly, renal and hepatic disease; a man should not father a child while taking this drug

---

Side effects: *italics* = common; ***bold italics*** = life-threatening

PHARMACOKINETICS

Rapidly absorbed, peak ½ hr, metabolized in the liver, half-life 35-49 min, excreted in urine

INTERACTIONS

None known

NURSING CONSIDERATIONS

Assess:

• For CNS symptoms: fever, headache, chills, dizziness

• Hematologic response with patients with baseline WBC $\geq 3 \times 10^9$/L, absolute neutrophil count (ANC) $\geq 1.5 \times 10^9$/L, and platelets $\geq 75 \times 10^9$/L, adjust dose; ANC $<0.5 \times 10^9$/L, platelets $<25 \times 10^9$/L, give 50% dose next course; ANC 0.5-1.5 $\times 10^9$/L, platelets 25-50 $\times 10^9$/L, give 67% next course

• Buccal cavity q8h for dryness, sores, or ulceration, white patches, oral pain, bleeding, dysphagia

• Bone marrow depression: bruising, bleeding, blood in stools, urine, sputum, emesis

Administer:

• Antiemetics and dexamethasone 10 mg at least ½ hr before antineoplastics

IV route

• Reconstitute with 4 ml sterile water for inj (25 mg/ml), inject diluent slowly into vial, invert vial 2-3 times and gently rotate; sol will be cloudy, use immediately; divide doses greater than 4 ml into two syringes; resuspend the contents 2-3 times and gently roll syringe between the palms for 30 sec immediately before administration

• Rotate inj site

Perform/provide:

• Increased fluid intake to 2-3 L/day to prevent dehydration, unless contraindicated

• Rinsing of mouth tid-qid with water, club soda; brushing of teeth bid-tid with soft brush or cotton-tipped applicator for stomatitis; use unwaxed dental floss

• Nutritious diet with iron, vitamin supplement, low fiber, few dairy products

Evaluate:

• Therapeutic response: improvement in blood counts in refractory anemia, or refractory anemia with excess blasts

Teach patient/family:

• To avoid foods with citric acid or hot or rough texture if stomatitis is present; to drink adequate fluids

• To report stomatitis; any bleeding, white spots, ulcerations in mouth; tell patient to examine mouth daily, report symptoms

• To use contraception during therapy

• Not to father a child while receiving this drug

---

azathioprine (℞)

(ay-za-thye'oh-preen)

Imuran

Func. class.: Immunosuppressant

Chem. class.: Purine antagonist

Do not confuse:

Imuran/Imferon/Elmiron/IMDUR/Enduron/Tenormin

Action: Produces immunosuppression by inhibiting purine synthesis in cells

Uses: Renal transplants to prevent graft rejection, refractory rheumatoid arthritis, refractory ITP, glomerulonephritis, nephrotic syndrome, bone marrow transplant

Investigational uses: Myasthenia gravis, chronic ulcerative colitis, Crohn's disease, Behçet's disease

DOSAGE AND ROUTES

Prevention of rejection

• *Adult and child:* **PO, IV** 3-5 mg/kg/day, then maintenance (**PO**) of at least 1-2 mg/kg/day

Refractory rheumatoid arthritis

• *Adult:* **PO** 1/mg/kg/day, may increase dose after 2 mo by 0.5 mg/kg/day, not to exceed 2.5 mg/kg/day

Renal disease

• CCr 10-50 ml/min 75% of dose; CCr <10 ml/min 50% of dose

Available forms: Tabs 50 mg; inj 100 mg

SIDE EFFECTS

GI: Nausea, vomiting, stomatitis, esophagitis, ***pancreatitis, hepatotoxicity, jaundice***

HEMA: ***Leukopenia, thrombocytopenia, anemia, pancytopenia***

INTEG: Rash, alopecia

MISC: ***Serum sickness,*** Raynaud's symptoms

MS: Arthralgia, muscle wasting

Contraindications: Pregnancy (D), hypersensitivity, lactation

Precautions: Severe renal disease, severe hepatic disease, elderly

PHARMACOKINETICS

Metabolized in liver, excreted in urine (active metabolite), crosses placenta

INTERACTIONS

Leukopenia: ACE inhibitors; co-trimoxazole

Do not admix with other drugs

Increase: myelosuppression—cycloSPORINE, antineoplastics

Increase: action of azathioprine—allopurinol

Decrease: immune response—vaccines

Decrease: action of warfarin—warfarin

Drug/Herb

Increase: immunosuppression—astragalus, echinacea, melatonin, safflower

Decrease: immunosuppression—ginseng, maitake, mistletoe, schisandra, St. John's wort, tumeric

Drug/Lab Test

Increase: LFTs

Decrease: Uric acid

Interfere: CBC, diff count

NURSING CONSIDERATIONS

Assess:

• For infection: increased temp, WBC; sputum, urine

• For rheumatoid arthritis, pain, mobility, ROM

• I&O, weight daily, report decreasing urine output; toxicity may occur

• Blood studies: Hgb, WBC, platelets during treatment monthly; if leukocytes are <3000/mm³ or platelets <100,000/mm³, drug should be discontinued

⚠ Hepatotoxicity: dark urine, jaundice, itching, light-colored stools, increased LFTs; drug should be discontinued; hepatic studies: alk phosphatase, AST, ALT, bilirubin

• Arthritis: pain; location, ROM, swelling, before and during treatment

Administer:

• All medications PO if possible, avoiding IM inj, since bleeding may occur

PO route

• With meals to reduce GI upset

IV route

• Prepare in biologic cabinet using gown, gloves, mask

• After diluting 100 mg/10 ml of sterile H₂O for inj; rotate to dissolve; may further dilute with 50 ml or more saline or glucose in saline, give over ½-1 hr

• For several days before transplant surgery

Solution compatibilities: D₅W, NaCl 0.9%, NaCl 0.45%

Evaluate:

• Therapeutic response: absence of graft rejection, immunosuppression in autoimmune disorders

Teach patient/family:

• To take as prescribed, do not miss doses, if dose is missed on daily regimen, skip dose; if on multiple dosing/day, take as soon as remembered

• That therapeutic response may take 3-4 mo in rheumatoid arthritis; to continue with prescribed exercise, rest, other medications

• To report fever, rash, severe diarrhea, chills, sore throat, fatigue, since serious infections may occur

• To use contraceptive measures during treatment, for 16 wk after ending therapy; to avoid vaccinations

• To avoid crowds to reduce risk of infection

• To use soft-bristled toothbrush to prevent bleeding

• That treatment is ongoing to prevent transplant rejection

azelaic acid topical
See Appendix C

azelastine nasal agent
See Appendix C

azelastine ophthalmic
See Appendix C

azithromycin (R)
(ay-zi-thro-my'sin)
Zithromax
Func. class.: Antiinfective
Chem. class.: Macrolide (azalide)

Do not confuse:
azithromycin/erythromycin
Zithromax/Zinacef
Action: Binds to 50S ribosomal subunits of susceptible bacteria and suppresses protein synthesis; much greater spectrum of activity than erythromycin
Uses: Mild to moderate infections of the upper respiratory tract, lower respiratory tract, uncomplicated skin and skin structure infections caused by *Moraxella catarrhalis, Streptococcus pneumoniae, Streptococcus pyogenes, Staphylococcus aureus, Streptococcus agalactiae, Mycoplasma pneumoniae, Haemophilus influenzae, Clostridium, Legionella pneumophila;* nongonococcal urethritis or cervicitis due to *Chlamydia trachomatis;* in children: acute otitis media *(H. influenzae, M. catarrhalis, S. pneumoniae)* **PO;** acute pharyngitis/tonsillitis (group A streptococcal) **PO;** acute skin/soft tissue infections **(PO);** community-acquired pneumonia *(Chlamydia pneumoniae, H. influenzae, M. pneumoniae, S. pneumoniae)* **PO;** pharyngitis/tonsillitis *(S. pyogenes);* prophylaxis of disseminated *Mycobacterium avium* complex (MAC)

Investigational uses: Chlamydial infections, gonococcal infections, prophylaxis after sexual assault, bacterial endocarditis prevention

DOSAGE AND ROUTES
Most infections
• *Adult:* PO 500 mg on day 1, then 250 mg daily on days 2-5 for a total dose of 1.5 g
• *Child 2-15 yr:* PO 10 mg/kg on day 1, then 5 mg/kg × 4 days
Pharyngitis/tonsillitis
• *Adult:* PO 12 mg/kg daily × 5 days
Disseminated MAC infections
• *Adult:* PO 600 mg/day in combination with ethambutol
Community-acquired pneumonia
• *Adult:* PO/IV 500 mg IV q24h × 2 doses, then 500 mg PO q24h × 7-10 days
Pelvic inflammatory disease
• *Adult:* PO/IV 500 mg IV q24h × 2 doses, then 500 mg PO q24h × 7-10 days
Cervicitis, chlamydia, chancroid, nongonococcal urethritis
• *Adult:* PO 1 g single dose
Gonorrhea
• *Adult:* PO 2 g single dose
Endocarditis prophylaxis
• *Adult:* PO 500 mg 1 hr prior to procedure
• *Child:* PO 15 mg/kg 1 hr prior to procedure
Lower respiratory tract infections, acute skin/soft tissue infections, acute pharyngitis/tonsillitis
• *Child, 3-day regimen:* PO 10 mg/kg daily × 3 days
Acute otitis media
• *Child:* PO 30 mg/kg as a single dose or 10 mg/kg daily × 3 days or 10 mg/kg as a single dose on day 1 (max 500 mg/day), then 5 mg/kg on days 2-5 (max 250 mg/day)
Prevention of acute otitis media
Child: PO 10 mg/kg q wk × 6 mo
Available forms: Tabs 250, 600 mg; powder for inj 500 mg; powder for oral susp 1 g/packet susp 100, 200 mg/5 ml

SIDE EFFECTS

CNS: Dizziness, headache, vertigo, somnolence

CV: Palpitations, chest pain

*GI: Nausea, vomiting, diarrhea, **hepatotoxicity**,* abdominal pain, stomatitis, heartburn, dyspepsia, flatulence, melena, ***cholestatic jaundice, pseudomembranous colitis***

GU: Vaginitis, moniliasis, nephritis

INTEG: Rash, urticaria, pruritus, photosensitivity

*SYST: **Angioedema***

Contraindications: Hypersensitivity to azithromycin, erythromycin, or any macrolide

Precautions: Pregnancy (B), lactation; hepatic, renal, cardiac disease; elderly, <6 mo for otitis media, <2 yr for pharyngitis, tonsillitis

PHARMACOKINETICS

PO: Peak 2-4 hr, duration 24 hr; *IV:* peak end of inf, duration 24 hr; half-life 11-57 hr, excreted in bile, feces, urine primarily as unchanged drug

INTERACTIONS

Toxicity: ergotamine

⚠ Dysrhythmias: pimozide; fatal reaction

Increase: effects of oral anticoagulants— digoxin, theophylline, methylPREDNISolone, cycloSPORINE, bromocriptine, disopyramide, triazolam, carbamazepine, phenytoin

Decrease: clearance of triazolam

Decrease: absorption of azithromycin—aluminum, magnesium antacids

Drug/Herb

Do not use acidophilus with antiinfectives

Drug/Lab Test

Increase: CPK, ALT, AST, bilirubin, BUN, creatinine, alk phosphatase

NURSING CONSIDERATIONS

Assess:

• I&O ratio; report hematuria, oliguria in renal disease

• Hepatic studies: AST, ALT; CBC with differential

• Renal studies: urinalysis, protein, blood

• C&S before drug therapy; drug may be taken as soon as culture is taken; C&S may be repeated after treatment

• For superinfection: sore throat, mouth, tongue; fever, fatigue, diarrhea, anogenital pruritus

• Bowel pattern before, during treatment

• Respiratory status: rate, character, wheezing, tightness in chest; discontinue drug if these occur

Administer:

PO route

• Susp 1 hr ac or 2 hr pc. Reconstitute 1 g packet for susp with 60 ml water, mix, rinse glass with more water and have patient drink to consume all medication; packets not for pediatric use

IV route

• Reconstitute 500 mg of drug/4.8 ml sterile water for inj (100 mg/ml); shake, dilute with ≥250 ml 0.9% NaCl, 0.45% NaCl, or LR to 1-2 mg/ml; diluted solution is stable for 24 hr or 7 days if refrigerated

• Give 500 mg or more/hr, never give IM or as a bolus

Perform/provide:

• Storage at room temperature

Evaluate:

• Therapeutic response: C&S negative for infection; decreased signs of infection

Teach patient/family:

⚠ To report sore throat, fever, fatigue, severe diarrhea, anal, genital itching (may indicate superinfection)

• Not to take aluminum/magnesium-containing antacids simultaneously with this drug (PO)

⚠ To notify nurse of diarrhea stools, dark urine, pale stools, yellow discoloration of eyes or skin, severe abdominal pain

• To complete dosage regimen

Treatment of hypersensitivity:

Withdraw drug, maintain airway, administer epINEPHrine, aminophylline, O_2, IV corticosteroids

Rarely Used

aztreonam (R)
(az-tree'oh nam)
Azactam
Func. class.: Miscellaneous antibiotic

Uses: Urinary tract infection; septicemia; skin, muscle, bone infection, lower respiratory tract, intraabdominal infections; and other infections caused by gram-negative organisms

DOSAGE AND ROUTES
Urinary tract infections
• *Adult:* **IV/IM** 500 mg-1 g q8-12h
Systemic infections
• *Adult:* **IV/IM** 1-2 g q8-12h
• *Child:* **IV/IM** 90-120 mg/kg/day divided q6-8h
Severe systemic infections
• *Adult:* **IV/IM** 2 g q6-8h; do not exceed 8 g/day
Continue treatment for 48 hr after negative culture or until patient is asymptomatic
Contraindications: Hypersensitivity to this drug, penicillins, cephalosporins

Rarely Used

bacitracin (R)
(bass-i-tray'sin)
BACI-IM, Baciquent, Bacitin ✦
Func. class.: Antiinfective, misc.

Uses: Staphylococcal pneumonia, empyema

DOSAGE AND ROUTES
• *Infant >2.5 kg:* **IM** 1000 units/kg/day in divided doses q8-12h
• *Infant ≤2.5 kg:* **IM** 900 units/kg/day in divided doses q8-12h
Contraindications: Hypersensitivity, severe renal disease (IM use)

bacitracin topical
See Appendix C

baclofen (R)
(bak'loe-fen)
Lioresal, Lioresal Intrathecal
Func. class.: Skeletal muscle relaxant, central acting
Chem. class.: GABA chlorophenyl derivative

Do not confuse:
Lioresal/Lotensin
Action: Inhibits synaptic responses in CNS by stimulating GABAb receptor subtype, which decreases neurotransmitter function; decreases frequency, severity of muscle spasms
Uses: Spasticity in spinal cord injury, multiple sclerosis
Investigational uses: Pain in trigeminal neuralgia, hiccups

DOSAGE AND ROUTES
• *Adult:* **PO** 5 mg tid × 3 days, then 10 mg tid × 3 days, then 15 mg tid × 3 days, then 20 mg tid × 3 days, then titrated to response, not to exceed 80 mg/day. **IT:** Use implantable intrathecal **INF** pump; use screening trial of 3 separate **BOL** doses if needed 24 hr apart (50 mcg/ml, 75 mcg/1.5 ml, 100 mcg/2 ml). Patients that do not respond to 100 mcg should not be considered for chronic **IT** therapy. Initial: double screening dose that produced result and give over 24 hr: increase by 10%-30% q24h only. Maintenance: 1200-1500 mcg/day;
• *Child >2 yr:* **PO** 10-15 mg/kg/day divided q8h titrate every 3 days by 5-15 mg/day to max 40 mg/day
• *Child ≥8 yr:* as above, max 60 mg/day
• *Child:* **IT** Initial test dose same as

adult; for small children, initial dose of 25 mcg/dose may be used; 25-1200 mcg/day infusion, titrated to response in screening phase

Available forms: Tabs 10, 20 mg; intrathecal inj 10 mg/20 ml (500 mcg/ml), 10 mg/5 ml (2000 mcg/ml); pharmacy can prepare extemperaneous liquid preparations

SIDE EFFECTS

CNS: Dizziness, weakness, fatigue, drowsiness, headache, *disorientation,* insomnia, paresthesias, tremors; ***seizures, life-threatening CNS depression*** (IT)

CV: Hypotension, chest pain, palpitations, edema, ***cardiovascular collapse (IT)***

EENT: Nasal congestion, blurred vision, mydriasis, tinnitus

GI: Nausea, constipation, *vomiting,* increased AST, alk phosphatase, abdominal pain, dry mouth, anorexia

GU: Urinary frequency, hematuria

INTEG: Rash, pruritus

RESP: Dyspnea; respiratory failure (IT)

Contraindications: Hypersensitivity

Precautions: Pregnancy (C), peptic ulcer disease, renal disease, hepatic disease, stroke, seizure disorder, diabetes mellitus, lactation, elderly

PHARMACOKINETICS

PO: Onset 3-4 days, peak 2-3 hr, duration >8 hr, half-life 2½-4 hr, partially metabolized in liver, excreted in urine (unchanged)

INTRATHECAL: CSF levels with plasma levels 100 times oral route; peak 4 hr, duration 4-8 hr

BOLUS: Onset ½-1 hr

CONT INF: Onset 6-8 hr, peak 24-48 hr

INTERACTIONS

Increase: CNS depression—alcohol, tricyclics, opiates, barbiturates, sedatives, hypnotics, MAOIs

Drug/Herb

Increase: CNS depression—chamomile, hops, kava, skullcap, valerian

Drug/Lab Test

Increase: AST, alk phosphatase, blood glucose

NURSING CONSIDERATIONS

Assess:

• B/P, weight, blood glucose, and hepatic function periodically

⚠ For increased seizure activity in seizure disorders; this drug decreases seizure threshold

• I&O ratio; check for urinary frequency

• EEG in epileptic patients; poor seizure control has occurred in patients taking this drug

• Allergic reactions: rash, fever, respiratory distress

• Severe weakness, numbness in extremities

• Tolerance: increased need for medication, more frequent requests for medication, increased pain

• For withdrawal symptoms: CNS depression, dizziness, drowsiness, psychiatric symptoms

Administer:

PO route

• With meals for GI symptoms

IT route

• For screening, dilute to a concentration of 50 mcg/ml with NaCl for inj (preservative-free); give test dose over 1 min; watch for decreasing muscle tone or frequency of spasm; if inadequate, use 2 more test doses q24h; maintenance infusion via implantable pump 500-2000 mg/ml

• Dosage, as individual titration is required

• Do not use IT inj IV, IM, SUBCUT, epidural

Additive compatibilities: Morphine

Perform/provide:

• Storage in tight container at room temperature

• Assistance with ambulation if dizziness or drowsiness occurs

Evaluate:

• Therapeutic response: decreased pain, spasticity

Teach patient/family:
• Not to discontinue medication quickly; hallucinations, spasticity, tachycardia will occur; drug should be tapered off over 1-2 wk
• Not to take with alcohol, other CNS depressants
• To avoid hazardous activities if drowsiness or dizziness occurs; rise slowly to prevent orthostatic hypotension
• To avoid using OTC medication: cough preparations, antihistamines, unless directed by prescriber
• To notify prescriber of nausea, headache, tinnitus, insomnia, confusion, constipation, inadequate, painful urination continues
• May require 1-2 months for full response

Treatment of overdose: Induce emesis of conscious patient, lavage, dialysis, physostigmine to reduce life-threatening CNS side effects

---

balsalazide (℞)
(ball-sal′a-zide)
Colazal
Func. class.: GI antiinflammatory
Chem. class.: Salicylate derivative

Do not confuse:
Colazal/Clozaril
Action: Delivered intact to the colon, bioconverted to 5-ASA
Uses: Active, mild to moderate ulcerative colitis

DOSAGE AND ROUTES
• *Adult:* **PO** 2.25 g tid × 8 wk, may take up to 12 wk
Available forms: Tabs 750 mg

SIDE EFFECTS
CNS: Headache, insomnia, fatigue, fever, dizziness
EENT: Dry eyes, rhinitis, sinusitis, watery eyes, blurred vision
GI: Nausea, vomiting, abdominal pain, diarrhea, rectal bleeding, flatulence, dyspepsia, dry mouth, constipation
MS: Arthralgia, back pain, myalgia
SYST: **Anaphylaxis**
Contraindications: Hypersensitivity to salicylates
Precautions: Pregnancy (B), child <14 yr, lactation; pyloric stenosis

PHARMACOKINETICS
PO: Low and variably absorbed, peak 1½ hr, excreted in urine as metabolites, plasma protein binding 99%

Drug/Lab Test
Increase: AST, ALT, GGT, LDH, bilirubin, alk phosphatase
False positive: Urinary glucose test

NURSING CONSIDERATIONS
Assess:
• Renal studies: BUN, creatinine, urinalysis (long-term therapy)
• Allergic reaction: rash, dermatitis, urticaria, pruritus, dyspnea, bronchospasm

Administer:
• With food in evenly divided doses
• With resuscitative equipment available; severe allergic reactions may occur
• Total daily dose evenly spaced to minimize GI intolerance

Perform/provide:
• Storage in tight, light-resistant container at room temperature

Evaluate:
• Therapeutic response: absence of fever, mucus in stools, resolution of symptoms of ulcerative colitis

Teach patient/family:
• To notify prescriber if symptoms do not improve, if rash, hives, or respiratory problems occur

---

⚠ Safety alert   *"Tall Man" lettering

⚠ High Alert

basiliximab (℞)
(bas-ih-liks'ih-mab)
Simulect
Func. class.: Immunosuppressant
Chem. class.: Murine/human monoclonal antibody (interleukin-2) receptor antagonist

Action: Binds to and blocks the IL-2 receptor, which is selectively expressed on the surface of activated T lymphocytes; impairs the immune system to antigenic challenges

Uses: Acute allograft rejection in renal transplant patients when used with cycloSPORINE and corticosteroids

DOSAGE AND ROUTES

• *Adult:* IV 20 mg × 2 doses; 1st dose within 2 hr before transplant surgery; 2nd dose given 4 days after transplantation

• *Child 2-15 yr:* IV 12 mg/m² × 2 doses; 1st dose within 2 hr before transplant surgery; 2nd dose given 4 days after transplantation

Available forms: Powder for inj 20 mg

SIDE EFFECTS

CNS: Pyrexia, chills, tremors, headache, insomnia, weakness
CV: Chest pain, angina, ***cardiac failure***, hypotension, *hypertension, edema*
GI: Vomiting, nausea, diarrhea, constipation, abdominal pain, ***GI bleeding,*** *gingival hyperplasia, stomatitis*
INTEG: Acne
META: Acidosis, hypercholesterolemia, hyperuricemia, hyperkalemia, hypocalcemia, hypokalemia, hypophosphatemia
MISC: Infection, moniliasis, ***anaphylaxis***
MS: Arthralgia, myalgia
RESP: Dyspnea, wheezing, ***pulmonary edema****, cough*

Contraindications: Hypersensitivity, exposure to viral infections, lactation
Precautions: Pregnancy (B), infections, elderly, children

PHARMACOKINETICS

Peak ½ hr (adults) terminal half-life 7 days (adult), 9½ days (children)

INTERACTIONS

Immunosuppression: other immunosuppressants

Drug/Herb
Increase: immunosuppression—astragalus, echinacea, melatonin, safflower
Decrease: immunosuppression—ginseng, maitake, mistletoe, schisandra, St. John's wort, turmeric

Drug/Lab Test
Increase: Cholesterol, BUN, uric acid, creatinine, K, Ca, blood glucose, Hgb, Hct
Decrease: Hgb, Hct, platelets, magnesium, phosphate

NURSING CONSIDERATIONS

Assess:
• For infection: increased temp, WBC, sputum, urine
• Blood studies: Hgb, WBC, platelets during treatment qmo; if leukocytes are <3000/mm³, drug should be discontinued
• Hepatic studies: alk phosphatase, AST, ALT, bilirubin
• Hepatotoxicity: dark urine, jaundice, itching, light-colored stools; drug should be discontinued
⚠ Anaphylaxis, hypersensitivity: dyspnea, wheezing, rash, pruritus, hypotension, tachycardia; if severe hypersensitivity reactions occur, drug should not be used again

Administer:
• All medications PO if possible; avoid IM inj, since infection may occur
IV route
• After adding 5 ml sterile water for inj, shake gently to dissolve, reconstitute to a vol of 50 ml with 0.9% NaCl or D₅, gently

invert bag, do not shake, give over ½ hr, do not admix

Evaluate:

• Therapeutic response: absence of graft rejection

Teach patient/family:

• To report fever, chills, sore throat, fatigue, since serious infection may occur

• To avoid crowds, persons with known upper respiratory infections

• To use contraception during treatment

---

beclomethasone (R)

(be-kloe-meth'a-sone)
Beclodisk ✢, Becloforte
Inhaler ✢, Beclovent, Beclo-
vent Rotocaps ✢, QVAR, Van-
ceril, Vanceril Double Strength
Func. class.: Corticosteroid, syn-
thetic
Chem. class.: Glucocorticoid

Do not confuse:

Vanceril/Vancenase

Action: Prevents inflammation by suppression of migration of polymorphonuclear leukocytes, fibroblasts, reversal of increased capillary permeability and lysosomal stabilization; does not suppress hypothalamus and pituitary function

Uses: Chronic asthma, rhinitis

DOSAGE AND ROUTES

• *Adult:* INH 2-4 puffs bid-qid, max 20 inhalations/day (42 mcg/actuation); 2 puffs bid, max 10 **INH**/day (84 mcg/actuation)

• *Child: 6-12 yr:* INH 1-2 puffs tid-qid, max 10 **INH**/day (42 mcg/actuations); 2 puffs bid, max 5 **INH**/day (84 mcg/actuations)

Available forms: Aerosol 40, 80, 250 ✢ mcg/actuation; INH cap 100 ✢, 200 ✢ mcg

SIDE EFFECTS

CNS: Headache
EENT: Hoarseness, candidal infections of oral cavity, sore throat

GI: Dry mouth, dyspepsia
*MISC: **Angioedema, adrenal insuffi-
ciency,** facial edema, Churg-Strauss syndrome*
*RESP: **Bronchospasm,** wheezing, cough*

Contraindications: Hypersensitivity, status asthmaticus (primary treatment), nonasthmatic bronchial disease; bacterial, fungal, viral infections of mouth, throat, lungs

Precautions: Pregnancy (C), nasal disease/surgery, lactation, children <12 yr

PHARMACOKINETICS

INH: Onset 10 min, excreted in feces, urine (metabolites), half-life 2.8 hr, crosses placenta, metabolized in lungs, liver (by CYP3A)

NURSING CONSIDERATIONS

Assess:

• For fungal infection in mucous membranes

• Adrenal function periodically for HPA axis suppression during prolonged therapy, monitor growth/development

Administer:

• INH with water to decrease possibility of fungal infections

• Titrated dose, use lowest effective dose

Perform/provide:

• Gum, rinsing of mouth for dry mouth

Evaluate:

• Therapeutic response: decreased dyspnea, wheezing, dry crackles

Teach patient/family:

• To carry or wear ID as steroid user

• To gargle/rinse mouth after each use to prevent oral fungal infections

• That in times of stress, systemic corticosteroids may be needed to prevent adrenal insufficiency; do not discontinue oral drug abruptly, taper slowly

• To notify prescriber if therapeutic response decreases; dosage adjustment may be needed

• Proper administration technique

• To wash inhaler with warm water and dry after each use

⚠ Safety alert   ✢"Tall Man" lettering

• All aspects of drug usage, including cushingoid symptoms
• The symptoms of adrenal insufficiency: nausea, anorexia, fatigue, dizziness, dyspnea, weakness, joint pain, depression

---

beclomethasone nasal agent
See Appendix C

---

benazepril (℞)
(ben-aze'uh-pril)
Lotensin
Func. class.: Antihypertensive
Chem. class.: Angiotensin-converting enzyme (ACE) inhibitor

Do not confuse:
Lotensin/Lioresal
Lotensin/Loniten
Action: Selectively suppresses renin-angiotensin-aldosterone system; inhibits ACE, preventing conversion of angiotensin I to angiotensin II
Uses: Hypertension, alone or in combination with thiazide diuretics

DOSAGE AND ROUTES

• *Adult:* **PO** 10 mg daily initially, then 20-40 mg/day divided bid or daily (without a diuretic); 5 mg **PO** daily (with a diuretic)
• *Geriatric:* **PO** 5-10 mg/day initially
Renal dose
• *Adult:* **PO** CCr <30 ml/min 5 mg **PO** daily, max 40 mg/day
Available forms: Tabs 5, 10, 20, 40 mg

SIDE EFFECTS

CNS: Anxiety, hypertonia, insomnia, paresthesia, headache, dizziness, fatigue
CV: Hypotension, postural hypotension, syncope, palpitations, angina
GI: Nausea, constipation, vomiting, gastritis, melena
GU: Increased BUN, creatinine, de-creased libido, impotence, urinary tract infection
INTEG: Rash, flushing, sweating
META: Hyperkalemia, hyponatremia
MISC: ***Angioedema***
MS: Arthralgia, arthritis, myalgia
RESP: Cough, asthma, bronchitis, dyspnea, sinusitis
Contraindications: Pregnancy (D) 2nd/3rd trimester, hypersensitivity to ACE inhibitors, lactation, children
Precautions: Pregnancy (C) 1st trimester, impaired renal, hepatic function, dialysis patients, hypovolemia, blood dyscrasias, CHF, COPD, asthma, elderly, bilateral renal artery stenosis

PHARMACOKINETICS

PO: Peak ½-1 hr, protein binding 97%, half-life 10-11 hr, metabolized by liver (metabolites), excreted in urine

INTERACTIONS

Increase: hypotension—phenothiazines, nitrates, acute alcohol ingestion, diuretics, other antihypertensives
Increase: hyperkalemia—potassium-sparing diuretics, potassium supplements
Increase: serum levels of lithium, digoxin
Drug/Herb
Increase: toxicity/death—aconite
Increase: antihypertensive effect—barberry, betony, black catechu, black cohosh, bloodroot, broom, burdock, cat's claw, dandelion, goldenseal, Irish moss, Jamaican dogwood, kelp, khella, mistletoe, parsley
Increase or decrease: antihypertensive effect—astragalus, cola tree
Decrease: antihypertensive effect—coltsfoot, guarana, khat, licorice, pineapple, yohimbe
Drug/Lab Test
Increase: AST, ALT, alk phosphatase, bilirubin, uric acid, blood glucose
Positive: ANA titer
False positive: ANA titer

NURSING CONSIDERATIONS
Assess:

• Blood studies: neutrophils, decreased platelets; WBC with diff baseline and q3mo, if neutrophils <1000/mm³ discontinue treatment, recommended in collagen-vascular disease

• B/P at peak/trough level of drug, orthostatic hypotension, syncope when used with diuretic

• Renal studies: protein, BUN, creatinine; increased levels may indicate nephrotic syndrome; monitor urine for protein, increased LFTs, uric acid and glucose may be increased

• Potassium levels, although hyperkalemia rarely occurs

• Allergic reactions: rash, fever, pruritus, urticaria; drug should be discontinued if antihistamines fail to help

• Renal symptoms: polyuria, oliguria, frequency, dysuria

• Edema in feet, legs daily, weight daily in CHF; monitor for cough

Administer:

• Do not discontinue drug abruptly

Perform/provide:

• Storage in tight container at 86° F (30° C) or less

Evaluate:

• Therapeutic response: decrease in B/P

Teach patient/family:

• Not to use OTC products (cough, cold, allergy) unless directed by prescriber; do not use salt substitutes containing potassium without consulting prescriber

• The importance of complying with dosage schedule, even if feeling better

• To notify prescriber of pregnancy, drug will need to be discontinued

• To rise slowly to sitting or standing position to minimize orthostatic hypotension

• To notify prescriber of mouth sores, sore throat, fever, swelling of hands or feet, irregular heartbeat, chest pain

• To report excessive perspiration, dehydration, vomiting, diarrhea; may lead to fall in B/P

• That drug may cause dizziness, fainting, light-headedness; may occur during first few days of therapy

• That drug may cause skin rash or impaired perspiration

• How to take B/P, and normal readings for age group

Treatment of overdose: 0.9% NaCl IV INF, hemodialysis

---

benzocaine topical
See Appendix C

Rarely Used

benzonatate (℞)
(ben-zoe′na-tate)
Tessalon Perles
Func. class.: Antitussive, nonopioid

Uses: Nonproductive cough

DOSAGE AND ROUTES

• *Adult and child:* **PO** 100 mg tid, not to exceed 600 mg/day

Contraindications: Hypersensitivity

Rarely Used

benzoyl peroxide (otc)
(ben′zoe-ill per-ox′ide)
Func. class.: Antiacne medication

Uses: Mild to moderate acne

DOSAGE AND ROUTES

• *Adult and child:* **TOP** apply to affected area daily or bid

Contraindications: Hypersensitivity to benzoic acid derivatives

---

benztropine (℞)

(benz'troe-peen)
Apo-Benztropin ✤,
benztropine mesylate,
Cogentin
Func. class.: Cholinergic blocker,
antiparkinson's agent
Chem. class.: Tertiary amine

Action: Blockade of central acetylcholine receptors

Uses: Parkinson's symptoms, EPS associated with neuroleptic drugs, acute dystonic reactions, hypersalivation

DOSAGE AND ROUTES

Drug-induced EPS
• *Adult:* IM/IV 1-4 mg daily-bid; give **PO** dose as soon as possible; **PO** 1-2 mg bid/tid, increase by 0.5 mg q5-6 days
• *Child:* IM/IV 0.02-0.05 mg/kg/dose 1-2 ×/day
• *Geriatric:* **PO** 0.5 mg daily-bid, increase by 0.5 mg q5-6d
Parkinson's symptoms
• *Adult:* **PO** 1-2 mg/day in 1-2 divided doses, increase 0.5 mg q5-6d titrated to patient response, max 6 mg daily
Acute dystonic reactions
• *Adult:* IM/IV 1-2 mg, may increase to 1-2 mg bid (**PO**)
Available forms: Tabs 0.5, 1, 2 mg; inj 1 mg/ml

SIDE EFFECTS

CNS: Anxiety, restlessness, irritability, delusions, hallucinations, headache, sedation, depression, incoherence, dizziness, memory loss; *confusion,* delirium (elderly)
CV: Palpitations, tachycardia, hypotension, bradycardia
EENT: Blurred vision, photophobia, dilated pupils, difficulty swallowing, dry eyes, mydriasis, increased intraocular tension, angle-closure glaucoma
GI: Dryness of mouth, constipation, nausea, vomiting, abdominal distress, ***paralytic ileus,*** epigastric distress

GU: Hesitancy, retention, dysuria
INTEG: Rash, urticaria, dermatoses
MISC: Increased temperature, flushing, decreased sweating, **hyperthermia, heat stroke,** numbness of fingers
MS: Muscular weakness, cramping
Contraindications: Hypersensitivity, narrow-angle glaucoma, myasthenia gravis, GI/GU obstruction, child <3 yr, peptic ulcer, megacolon, prostate hypertrophy
Precautions: Pregnancy (C), elderly, lactation, tachycardia, renal disease, hepatic disease, drug abuse history, dysrhythmias, hypotension, hypertension, psychiatric patients, children

PHARMACOKINETICS

IM/IV: Onset 15 min, duration 6-10 hr
PO: Onset 1 hr, duration 6-10 hr

INTERACTIONS

Increase: anticholinergic effect—antihistamines, phenothiazines, tricyclics, disopyramide, quinidine
Decrease: absorption—antidiarrheals
Drug/Herb
Increase: benztropine effect—butterbur, jimsonweed
Increase: constipation—black catechu
Decrease: benztropine effect—kava, jaborandi, pill-bearing spurge

NURSING CONSIDERATIONS

Assess:
• I&O ratio; commonly causes decreased urinary output; urinary hesitancy, retention; palpate bladder if retention occurs
• Parkinsonism, EPS: shuffling gait, muscle rigidity, involuntary movements, loss of balance
• Constipation; increase fluids, bulk, exercise if this occurs
• Mental status: affect, mood, CNS depression, worsening of mental symptoms during early therapy
• Use caution in hot weather; drug may

increase susceptibility to stroke by decreasing sweating
• For benztropine "buzz" or "high," patients may imitate EPS

Administer:

PO route
• With or after meals to prevent GI upset; may give with fluids other than water
• At bedtime to avoid daytime drowsiness in patient with parkinsonism

IM route
• Use for dystonic reactions only

IV route
• Undiluted IV (1 mg = 1 ml) give 1 mg/1 min; keep in bed for at least 1 hr after dose

Syringe compatibilities: Metoclopramide

Y-site compatibilities: Fluconazole, tacrolimus

Perform/provide:
• Storage at room temperature
• Hard candy, gum, frequent drinks, to relieve dry mouth

Evaluate:
• Therapeutic response: absence of involuntary movements

Teach patient/family:
• That tabs may be crushed and mixed with food
• Not to discontinue this drug abruptly; to taper off over 1 wk, or withdrawal symptoms may occur (EPS, tremors, insomnia, tachycardia, restlessness)
• To avoid driving, other hazardous activities; drowsiness may occur
• To avoid OTC medication: cough, cold preparations with alcohol, antihistamines unless directed by prescriber
• To change positions slowly to prevent orthostatic hypotension
• To use good oral hygiene, frequent sips of water, sugarless gum for dry mouth

---

bepridil (Ⓡ)
(be′pri-dil)
Vascor
Func. class.: Calcium channel blocker, antianginal

Do not confuse:
bepridil/Prepidil

Action: Inhibits calcium ion influx across cell membrane during cardiac depolarization; produces relaxation of coronary vascular smooth muscle, dilates coronary arteries, decreases SA/AV node conduction, inhibits fast sodium inward current, dilates peripheral arteries

Uses: Chronic stable angina, used alone or in combination with β-blockers, nitrates

DOSAGE AND ROUTES

Angina
• *Adult:* **PO** 200 mg daily, after 10 days may increase dose if needed, max dose 400 mg/day

Available forms: Tabs, film-coated, 200, 300 mg

SIDE EFFECTS

CNS: Headache, fatigue, drowsiness, dizziness, anxiety, depression, weakness, insomnia, confusion, light-headedness, nervousness, asthenia

CV: ***Dysrhythmia***, edema, ***CHF,*** bradycardia, hypotension, palpitations, AV block, ***torsades de pointes***

GI: Nausea, vomiting, diarrhea, gastric upset, constipation, increased hepatic studies

GU: Nocturia, polyuria

HEMA: ***Agranulocytosis***

MISC: ***Stevens-Johnson syndrome***

RESP: Pulmonary infiltrate

Contraindications: Hypersensitivity, sick sinus syndrome, 2nd- or 3rd-degree heart block, Wolff-Parkinson-White syndrome, hypotension less than 90 mm Hg systolic, cardiogenic shock, history of

---

serious ventricular dysrhythmias, uncompensated cardiac insufficiency
Precautions: Pregnancy (C), CHF,
hypotension, hepatic injury, lactation,
children, renal disease, idiopathic hypertropic subaortic stenosis (IHSS), concomitant β-blocker therapy, geriatrics,
recent MI

PHARMACOKINETICS

Onset 1 hr, peak 2-3 hr, duration 24 hr,
99% plasma protein bound, half-life 42
hr; completely metabolized in the liver
and excreted in urine and feces

INTERACTIONS

Increase: prolongation of QT, depres-
sion of AV node—cardiac glycosides,
antidysrhythmics, tricyclics
Increase: bepridil levels—ritonavir,
warfarin
Increase: hypotension—fentanyl
Increase: levels of digoxin
Drug/Herb
Increase: antianginal effect—barberry,
betel palm, burdock, cat's claw, chicory,
goldenseal, khat, khella, lily of valley,
plantain
Decrease: effect—yohimbe
Drug/Food
Increase: hypotensive effects—
grapefruit juice
Drug/Lab Test
Increase: LFTs, aminotransferase, CPK,
LDH

NURSING CONSIDERATIONS
Assess:
• Cardiac status: B/P, pulse, respiration,
ECG intervals (PR, QRS, QT),
dysrhythmias; may increase QT interval,
altered T wave
• I&O ratios, weight daily, monitor for
CHF: weight gain, jugular vein distention,
edema, crackles, dyspnea, restlessness
• For loss of glycemic control in diabe-
tes
• Females >60 yr with hypokalemia and
sinus bradycardia, high risk for drug-
induced torsade de pointes

Administer:
• Do not break, crush, or chew tabs
• Before meals, bedtime; adjust no more
frequently than q10 days; may give with
food/fluids to decrease GI upset
Evaluate:
• Therapeutic response: decreased
anginal pain, increased activity tolerance
Teach patient/family:
• How to take pulse before taking drug;
record or graph should be kept; use
demonstration, return demonstration
• To avoid hazardous activities until
stabilized on drug, dizziness no longer a
problem
• To limit caffeine consumption
• To avoid OTC drugs unless directed by
a prescriber
• The importance of compliance with all
areas of medical regimen: diet, exercise,
stress reduction, drug therapy
• To notify prescriber of swelling, weight
gain, dyspnea, irregular heartbeat, ringing in the ears
• To maintain good oral hygiene to prevent gingival hyperplasia
• Avoid breastfeeding
Treatment of overdose: Defibrillation, atropine for AV block, vasopressor
for hypotension

Rarely Used

beractant (℞)
(ber-ak'tant)
Survanta
Func. class.: Natural lung surfactant

Uses: Prevention and treatment (rescue) of respiratory distress syndrome in
premature infants

DOSAGE AND ROUTES
• **INTRATRACHEAL INSTILL:** 4 doses
can be administered in the 1st 48 hr of
life; give doses no more frequently than
q6h; each dose is 100 mg of phospho-
lipids/kg birth weight (4 ml/kg)

Side effects: *italics* = common; ***bold italics*** = life-threatening

betamethasone (℞)

(bay-ta-meth'a-sone)
Betnelan ✳, Betnesol ✳,
Celestone, Cel-U-Jec,
Selestoject ✳
Func. class.: Corticosteroid, synthetic, long-acting

Action: Decreases inflammation by suppressing migration of polymorphonuclear leukocytes, fibroblasts, reversal of increased capillary permeability and lysosomal stabilization

Uses: Immunosuppression, severe inflammation, prevention of neonatal respiratory distress syndrome (by administration to mother)

DOSAGE AND ROUTES

- *Adult:* **PO** 0.6-7.2 mg daily; **IM/IV** 0.6-7.2 mg daily in joint or soft tissue (sodium phosphate)
- *Child:* **PO** 17.5 mcg/kg/day in 3 divided doses; **IM** 17.5 mcg/kg/day in 3 divided doses every 3rd day or 5.8-8.75 mcg/kg/day as a single dose (adrenal insufficiency)
- *Child:* **PO** 62.5-250 mcg/kg/day in 3 divided doses; **IM** 20.8-125 mcg/kg/day of the base q12-24h (other uses)

Available forms: Betamethasone: tabs 500; 600 mcg, tabs, effervescent 500 mcg ✳, syr 600 mcg/5 ml; ext rel tab 1 mg; sol for inj (phosphate) 3 mg/ml; susp for inj (phosphate/acetate) 6 mg/ml

SIDE EFFECTS

CNS: Depression, flushing, sweating, headache, bruising, mood changes
*CV: Hypertension, **circulatory collapse, thrombophlebitis, embolism,** tachycardia, **necrotizing angiitis, CHF***
EENT: Fungal infections, increased intraocular pressure, blurred vision
*GI: Diarrhea, nausea, abdominal distention, **GI hemorrhage,** increased appetite, **pancreatitis***
*HEMA: **Thrombocytopenia***

INTEG: Acne, poor wound healing, ecchymosis, bruising, petechiae
MS: Fractures, osteoporosis, weakness
Contraindications: Psychosis, hypersensitivity, idiopathic thrombocytopenia, acute glomerulonephritis, amebiasis, fungal infections, nonasthmatic bronchial disease, child <2 yr, AIDS, TB
Precautions: Pregnancy (C), lactation, diabetes mellitus, glaucoma, osteoporosis, seizure disorders, ulcerative colitis, CHF, myasthenia gravis, renal disease, esophagitis, peptic ulcer

PHARMACOKINETICS

PO: Onset 1-2 hr, peak 1 hr, duration 3 days
IM/IV: Onset 10 min, peak 4-8 hr, duration 1-1½ days
Metabolized in liver, excreted in urine as steroids, crosses placenta

INTERACTIONS

GI bleeding: NSAIDs, alcohol, salicylates, indomethacin
Decrease: action of betamethasone—barbiturates, rifampin, phenytoin
Decrease: effects of anticoagulants, antidiabetics, insulin, isoniazid, toxoids, vaccines, salicylates
Drug/Herb
Hypokalemia: aloe, buckthorn, cascara sagrada, Chinese rhubarb, rhubarb, senna
Increase: corticosteroid effects—goldenseal, hawthorn, hops, lemon balm, licorice, lily of the valley, mistletoe, perilla, pheasant's eye, squill
Increase: hypokalemia—buckthorn, cascara sagrada, Chinese rhubarb
Drug/Food
Grapefruit juice should be avoided
Drug/Lab Test
Increase: Cholesterol, sodium, blood glucose, uric acid, calcium, urine glucose
Decrease: Calcium, potassium, T_4, T_3, thyroid ^{131}I uptake test, urine 17-OHCS, 17-KS, PBI
False negative: Skin allergy tests

NURSING CONSIDERATIONS
Assess:
• Potassium, blood glucose, urine glucose while on long-term therapy; hypokalemia and hyperglycemia
• Weight daily; notify prescriber of weekly gain >5 lb
• B/P q4h, pulse; notify prescriber if chest pain occurs
• I&O ratio; be alert for decreasing urinary output and increasing edema
• Plasma cortisol levels during long-term therapy (normal level: 138-635 nmol/L SI units when drawn at 8 AM)
Administer:
PO route
• With food or milk to decrease GI symptoms
IM route
• Inject deeply in large muscle mass, rotate sites, avoid deltoid, use 21G needle
• In one dose in AM to prevent adrenal suppression, avoid SUBCUT administration; may damage tissue
IV route
• Only sodium phosphate product; give >1 min; may be given by IV INF in compatible sol
• After shaking suspension (parenteral)
• Titrated dose; use lowest effective dose
Y-site compatibilities: Heparin, hydrocortisone, potassium chloride, vit B/C
Perform/provide:
• Assistance with ambulation in patient with bone tissue disease to prevent fractures
Evaluate:
• Therapeutic response: ease of respirations, decreased inflammation
• Infection: increased temp, WBC even after withdrawal of medication; drug masks infection symptoms
• Potassium depletion: paresthesias, fatigue, nausea, vomiting, depression, polyuria, dysrhythmias, weakness
• Edema, hypertension, cardiac symptoms
• Mental status: affect, mood, behavioral changes, aggression

Teach patient/family:
• That ID as steroid user should be carried
• To notify prescriber if therapeutic response decreases; dosage adjustment may be needed
⚠ Not to discontinue abruptly; adrenal crisis can result
• To avoid OTC products: salicylates, alcohol in cough products, cold preparations unless directed by prescriber
• All aspects of drug usage including cushingoid symptoms
• The symptoms of adrenal insufficiency: nausea, anorexia, fatigue, dizziness, dyspnea, weakness, joint pain

---

betamethasone topical
See Appendix C

---

betamethasone (augmented) topical
See Appendix C

---

betaxolol ophthalmic
See Appendix C

---

bethanechol (℞)
(be-than'e-kole)
bethanechol chloride, Duvoid, Urebeth, Urecholine
Func. class.: Urinary tract stimulant, cholinergic
Chem. class.: Synthetic choline ester

Action: Stimulates muscarinic Ach receptors directly; mimics effects of parasympathetic nervous system stimulation; stimulates gastric motility, stimulates micturition; increases lower esophageal sphincter pressure
Uses: Urinary retention (postoperative, postpartum), neurogenic atony of bladder with retention
Investigational uses: Ileus

Side effects: *italics* = common; ***bold italics*** = life-threatening

DOSAGE AND ROUTES

• *Adult:* **PO** 25-50 mg bid-qid; **SUBCUT** 5 mg tid-qid prn
• *Child:* **PO** 0.6 mg/kg/day divided in 3-4 doses/day; **SUBCUT** 0.06 mg/kg tid or 0.15 mg/kg qid

Test dose
• *Adult:* **SUBCUT** 2.5 mg repeated 15-30 min intervals × 4 doses to determine effective dose

Gastric atony, ileus (off-label)
Adult: **PO** 10-20 mg tid-qid before meals in incomplete retention; **SUBCUT** 10-20 mg tid-qid if retention is complete

Available forms: Tabs 5, 10, 25, 50 mg; inj 5 mg/ml

SIDE EFFECTS

CNS: Dizziness
CV: Hypotension, bradycardia, orthostatic hypotension, reflex tachycardia, ***cardiac arrest, circulatory collapse***
EENT: Miosis, increased salivation, lacrimation, blurred vision
GI: *Nausea, bloody diarrhea, belching, vomiting, cramps, fecal incontinence*
GU: Urgency
INTEG: Rash, urticaria, flushing, increased sweating
RESP: ***Acute asthma, dyspnea, bronchoconstriction***

Contraindications: Hypersensitivity, severe bradycardia, asthma, severe hypotension, hyperthyroidism, peptic ulcer, parkinsonism, seizure disorders, CAD, COPD, coronary occlusion, mechanical obstruction, peritonitis, recent urinary or GI surgery, GI/GU obstruction
Precautions: Pregnancy (C), hypertension, lactation, child <8 yr

PHARMACOKINETICS

PO: Onset 30-90 min, peak 1 hr, duration 6 hr
SUBCUT: Onset 5-15 min, peak 15-30 min, duration 2 hr, excreted by kidneys

INTERACTIONS

Severe hypotension: ganglionic blockers

Increase: action or toxicity—cholinergic agonists, anticholinesterase agents
Decrease: action of anticholinergics
Drug/Herb
Increase: cholinergic effect—jaborandi tree
Decrease: effects—jimsonweed, scopolia
Drug/Lab Test
Increase: AST, lipase/amylase, bilirubin, BSP

NURSING CONSIDERATIONS

Assess:
• B/P, pulse; observe after parenteral dose for 1 hr
• I&O ratio; check for urinary retention or urge incontinence
• Bradycardia, hypotension, bronchospasm, headache, dizziness, convulsions, respiratory depression; drug should be discontinued if toxicity occurs
Administer:
• To avoid nausea and vomiting, take on an empty stomach
SUBCUT route
⚠ Parenteral dose by SUBCUT route; use of IM, IV may result in cardiac arrest
⚠ Only with atropine sulfate available for cholinergic crisis
• Only after all other cholinergics have been discontinued
• Increased doses if tolerance occurs
Perform/provide:
• Storage at room temperature
• Bedpan/urinal if given for urinary retention
• Use of rectal tube if ordered, to increase passage of gas when used for abdominal distention
Evaluate:
• Therapeutic response: absence of urinary retention, abdominal distention
Teach patient/family:
• To take drug exactly as prescribed; 1 hr ac or 2 hr pc
• To make position changes slowly; orthostatic hypotension may occur
Treatment of overdose: Administer atropine 0.6-1.2 mg IV or IM (adult)

⚠ High Alert

bevacizumab (℞)

(beh-va-kiz'you-mab)
Avastin
Func. class.: Antineoplastic—
miscellaneous
Chem. class.: Monoclonal antibody

Action: DNA-derived monoclonal antibody selectively binds to and inhibits activity of human vascular endothelial growth factor to reduce microvascular growth and inhibition of metastatic disease progression
Uses: Metastatic carcinoma of the colon or rectum in combination with 5-FU IV
Investigational uses: Adjunctive in breast, renal cancer

DOSAGE AND ROUTES

• *Adult:* **IV INF** 5 mg/kg q14d given over 90 min; if well tolerated, the next infusion may be given over 60 min; if 60-min infusions are well tolerated, subsequent infusions may be given over 30 min
Available forms: Inj 25 mg/ml

SIDE EFFECTS

CNS: Asthenia, dizziness
*CV: **Deep vein thrombosis,** hypertension, hypotension, **hypertensive crisis***
GI: Nausea, vomiting, anorexia, diarrhea, constipation, abdominal pain, colitis, stomatitis, **GI hemorrhage**
GU: Proteinuria, urinary frequency/urgency, **nephrotic syndrome**
*HEMA: **Leukopenia, neutropenia, thrombocytopenia***
META: Bilirubinemia, hypokalemia
*MISC: **Exfoliative dermatitis, hemorrhage***
RESP: Dyspnea, upper respiratory tract infection
Contraindications: Hypersensitivity
Precautions: Pregnancy (C), lactation, children, elderly, CHF, blood dyscrasias, cardiovascular disease, hypertension

PHARMACOKINETICS

Half-life 20 days, steady state 100 days

INTERACTIONS

None known

NURSING CONSIDERATIONS
Assess:
• B/P q3-4wk
• For symptoms of infection; may be masked by drug
• CNS reaction: dizziness, confusion
⚠ For GI perforation, serious bleeding, nephrotic syndrome, hypertensive crisis, drug should be discontinued permanently; proteinuria or surgery, drug should be discontinued temporarily
Administer:
• Do not give by IV bolus, or IV push
• Give as IV infusion over 90 min for first dose and 60 min thereafter, if well tolerated
Evaluate:
• Therapeutic response: decrease in size of tumors
Teach patient/family:
• To avoid hazardous tasks, since confusion, dizziness may occur
• To report signs of infection: sore throat, fever, diarrhea, vomiting
• Not to become pregnant while taking this drug or for several months after discontinuing treatment
• Notify prescriber if pregnant or planning a pregnancy

bexarotene (℞)

Targretin
Func. class.: Retinoid, 2nd generation

Action: Selectively binds and activates retinoid X receptors (RXRs) that are partially responsible for cellular proliferation and differentiation. Inhibits some tumor cells
Uses: Cutaneous T-cell lymphoma
Investigational uses: Breast cancer, psoriasis (phase II)

Research note: Bexarotene has been proven effective and safe for refractory advanced-stage cutaneous T-cell lymphoma

DOSAGE AND ROUTES

• *Adult:* **PO** 300 mg/day/m^2, may increase to 400 mg/day with proper monitoring

Available forms: Cap 75 mg

SIDE EFFECTS

CNS: Headache, fatigue, lethargy
GI: Nausea, abdominal pain, diarrhea, **acute pancreatitis**
HEMA: **Leukopenia, neutropenia, anemia**
INTEG: Rash, asthenia, dry skin
SYST: Infection, hypothyroidism

Contraindications: Pregnancy (X), hypersensitivity to retinoids
Precautions: Lactation, sunburn, hepatic disease, renal disease, children

PHARMACOKINETICS

Unknown

INTERACTIONS

Limit intake of vit A ≤15,000 international units/day
Increase: action of antidiabetics
Increase: bexarotene levels—azole antiinfectives
Decrease: bexarotene levels—barbiturates, rifampins, phenytoin
Decrease: action of tamoxifen, oral contraceptives

Drug/Food
Increase: bexarotene levels—grapefruit juice

NURSING CONSIDERATIONS

Assess:
• Area of body involved, what helps or aggravates condition; cysts, dryness, itching
• Cholesterol, HDL, triglycerides may be elevated
• CBC for leukopenia, neutropenia, anemia

Administer:
• With food
Perform/provide:
• Storage at room temperature
Evaluate:
• Therapeutic response: decrease in size and number of lesions
Teach patient/family:
• To watch for hypoglycemia in diabetic patients on insulin
• To limit vit A intake to ≤15,000 international units/day to avoid toxicity
• To avoid sunlight, sunlamps, or use protective clothing, sunscreen
• To avoid pregnancy while taking this drug and ≥1 mo after discontinuing therapy, two forms of birth control recommended

---

bicalutamide (℞)
(bye-kal-u′ta-mide)
Casodex
Func. class.: Antineoplastic hormone
Chem. class.: Nonsteroidal antiandrogen

Action: Binds to cytosol androgen in target tissue, which competitively inhibits the action to androgens
Uses: Prostate cancer in combination with luteinizing hormone–releasing hormone (LHRH) analog

DOSAGE AND ROUTES

• *Adult:* **PO** 50 mg daily with LHRH
Available forms: Tabs 50 mg

SIDE EFFECTS

CNS: Dizziness, paresthesia, insomnia, anxiety, neuropathy, headache
CV: **CHF,** edema, *hot flashes,* hypertension, chest pain,
GI: Diarrhea, constipation, nausea, vomiting, increased hepatic enzymes, anorexia, dry mouth, melena, abdominal pain
GU: Nocturia, hematuria, UTI, impotence, gynecomastia, urinary incontinence,

frequency, dysuria, retention, urgency, breast tenderness, decreased libido
INTEG: Rash, sweating, dry skin, pruritus, alopecia
MISC: Infection, anemia, dyspnea, bone pain, headache, asthenia, *back pain,* flulike symptoms
Contraindications: Pregnancy (X), hypersensitivity
Precautions: Renal, hepatic disease, elderly, lactation

PHARMACOKINETICS

Well absorbed, peak 31½ hr, metabolized by liver, excreted in urine, feces; half-life 5.8 days

INTERACTIONS

Increase: anticoagulation—warfarin
Drug/Lab Test
Increase: AST, ALT, bilirubin, BUN, creatinine
Decrease: Hgb, WBC

NURSING CONSIDERATIONS

Assess:
• For diarrhea, constipation, nausea, vomiting
• For hot flashes, gynecomastia (assure patient that these are common side effects)
• Prostate specific antigen (PSA), LFTs
Administer:
• At same time each day, either AM or PM, with/without food
• With LHRH treatment; start at same time for both drugs
Evaluate:
• Therapeutic response: decreased tumor size, decreased spread of malignancy
Teach patient/family:
• To recognize, report signs of anemia, hepatoxicity, renal toxicity
• That hair may be lost, but is reversible after therapy is completed
• Not to use other products, unless approved by prescriber
• To report severe diarrhea

• To use contraception while taking this drug

---

bimatoprost ophthalmic
See Appendix C

---

biperiden (℞)
(bye-per'i-den)
Akineton
Func. class.: Antiparkinson agent, anticholinergic

Action: Centrally acting competitive anticholinergic
Uses: Parkinson's symptoms, EPS secondary to neuroleptic drug therapy

DOSAGE AND ROUTES

Extrapyramidal symptoms
• *Adult:* **PO** 2 mg daily-tid; **IM/IV** 2 mg q30min, if needed, not to exceed 8 mg/24 hr
• *Child:* **IM** 40 mcg/kg or 1.2 mg/m^2, may repeat q½h
Parkinson's symptoms
• *Adult:* **PO** 2 mg tid-qid; max 16 mg/24 hr
Available forms: Tabs 2 mg; inj 5 mg/ml (lactate)

SIDE EFFECTS

CNS: Confusion, anxiety, restlessness, irritability, delusions, hallucinations, headache, sedation, depression, incoherence, dizziness, euphoria, tremors, memory loss
CV: Palpitations, tachycardia, postural hypotension, bradycardia
EENT: Blurred vision, photophobia, dilated pupils, difficulty swallowing, mydriasis, increased intraocular tension, angle-closure glaucoma
GI: Dryness of mouth, constipation, nausea, vomiting, abdominal distress, ***paralytic ileus***
GU: Hesitancy, retention, dysuria
INTEG: Rash, urticaria, dermatoses

✦ Canada only   Side effects: *italics* = common; ***bold italics*** = life-threatening

MISC: Increased temp, flushing, decreased sweating, hyperthermia, **heat stroke,** numbness of fingers
MS: Weakness, cramping

Contraindications: Hypersensitivity, narrow-angle glaucoma, myasthenia gravis, GI/GU obstruction, megacolon, stenosing peptic ulcers, prostatic hypertrophy

Precautions: Pregnancy (C), elderly, lactation, tachycardia, dysrhythmias, liver or kidney disease, drug abuse, hypotension, cognitive impairment, Alzheimer's disease, hypertension, psychiatric patients, children <8 yr

PHARMACOKINETICS

IM/IV: Onset 15 min, duration 6-10 hr
PO: Onset 1 hr, duration 6-10 hr

INTERACTIONS

Increase: schizophrenic symptoms—haloperidol
Increase: anticholinergic effect—antihistamines, phenothiazines, amantadine, tricyclics, quinidine
Increase: sedation—alcohol
Decrease: biperiden absorption—antacids, antidiarrheals

Drug/Herb
Increase: biperiden effect—butterbur, jimsonweed
Increase: constipation—black catechu
Decrease: biperiden effect—kava, jaborandi tree, pill-bearing spurge

NURSING CONSIDERATIONS

Assess:
• I&O ratio; retention commonly causes decreased urinary output
• Parkinsonism, EPS: shuffling gait, muscle rigidity, involuntary movements
• Patient response if anticholinergics are given
• Urinary hesitancy, retention; palpate bladder if retention occurs
• Constipation; increase fluids, bulk, exercise if this occurs, stool softeners, laxatives may be needed
• For tolerance over long-term therapy;

dose may have to be increased or changed
• Mental status: affect, mood, CNS depression, confusion, dementia, worsening of mental symptoms during early therapy

Administer:
PO route
• With or after meals to prevent GI upset; may give with fluids other than water
• At bedtime to avoid daytime drowsiness in patients with parkinsonism
IM/IV route
• With patient recumbent to prevent postural hypotension, give undiluted 2 mg or less over 1 min or more

Perform/provide:
• Storage at room temperature
• Hard candy, gum, frequent drinks to relieve dry mouth

Evaluate:
• Therapeutic response: absence of involuntary movements

Teach patient/family:
• To use caution in hot weather; drug may increase susceptibility to heat stroke, decreases sweating
• Not to discontinue this drug abruptly; to taper off over 1 wk
• To avoid driving, other hazardous activities; drowsiness may occur
• To avoid OTC medication: cough, cold preparations with alcohol, antihistamines unless directed by prescriber

---

bisacodyl (R, OTC)
(bis-a-koe′dill)
Bisac-Evac, Bisaco-Lax, Bisacolax ♣, Bisco-Lax, Carter's Little Pills, Dacodyl, Deficol, Dulcagen, Dulcolax, Feen-a-mint, Fleet Laxative, Laxit ♣, Modane, Reliable Gentle Laxative, Therelax
Func. class.: Laxative, stimulant
Chem. class.: Diphenylmethane

Action: Acts directly on intestine by increasing motor activity; thought to irritate colonic intramural plexus

---

Uses: Short-term treatment of constipation, bowel or rectal preparation for surgery, examination

DOSAGE AND ROUTES

• *Adult/child ≥12 yr:* **PO** 5-15 mg in PM or AM; may use up to 30 mg for bowel or rectal preparation; **RECT** 10 mg, single dose

• *Child 2-11 yr:* **PO** 5-10 mg as a single dose; **RECT** 10 mg as a single dose

• *Child <2 yr:* **RECT** 5 mg as a single dose, do not use oral route

Available forms: Enteric-coated tabs 5 mg; supp 5, 10 mg; rect sol 10 mg/37 ml; enema 0.33 mg/ml, 10 mg/5 ml; powder for rectal sol/1.5 mg bisacodyl/ 2.5 g tannic acid

SIDE EFFECTS

CNS: Muscle weakness
GI: Nausea, vomiting, anorexia, cramps, diarrhea, rectal burning (suppositories)
META: Protein-losing enteropathy, alkalosis, hypokalemia, ***tetany,*** electrolyte, fluid imbalances

Contraindications: Hypersensitivity, rectal fissures, abdominal pain, nausea, vomiting, appendicitis, acute surgical abdomen, ulcerated hemorrhoids, acute hepatitis, fecal impaction, intestinal/ biliary tract obstruction

Precautions: Pregnancy (C), lactation

PHARMACOKINETICS

PO: Onset 6-10 hr
RECT: Onset 15-60 min
Metabolized by liver; excreted in urine, bile, feces, breast milk

INTERACTIONS

Gastric irritation: antacids, milk, H₂-blockers, gastric acid pump inhibitors
Drug/Herb
Increase: action—flax, lily of the valley, pheasant's eye, senna, squill

NURSING CONSIDERATIONS

Assess:
• Blood, urine electrolytes if drug is used often by patient
• I&O ratio to identify fluid loss
• Cause of constipation; identify whether fluids, bulk, or exercise missing from lifestyle, constipating drugs
• Cramping, rectal bleeding, nausea, vomiting; if these symptoms occur, drug should be discontinued

Administer:
PO route
• Swallow tabs whole; do not break, crush, or chew tabs
• Alone only with water for better absorption; do not take within 1 hr of other drugs or within 1 hr of antacids, milk, or cimetidine
• In AM or PM

Evaluate:
• Therapeutic response: decrease in constipation

Teach patient/family:
• Not to use laxatives for long-term therapy; bowel tone will be lost
• That normal bowel movements do not always occur daily
• Not to use in presence of abdominal pain, nausea, vomiting
• To notify prescriber if constipation is unrelieved or if symptoms of electrolyte imbalance occur: muscle cramps, pain, weakness, dizziness

bismuth subsalicylate (otc)

(bis'muth sub-sal-iss'uh-late)
Bismatrol, Bismatrol Extra Strength, Bismed, Pepto-Bismol, Pepto-Bismol Maximum Strength, Pink Bismuth, PMS-Bismuth Subsalicylate
Func. class.: Antidiarrheal
Chem. class.: Salicylate

Action: Inhibits prostaglandin synthesis responsible for GI hypermotility; stimulates absorption of fluid and electrolytes
Uses: Diarrhea (cause undetermined), prevention of diarrhea when traveling; may be included to treat *Helicobacter pylori*

DOSAGE AND ROUTES

Antidiarrheal
• *Adult:* **PO** 524 mg q½h or 1048 mg q1h, max 4.2 mg/24 hr
• *Child 9-12 yr:* **PO** 262 mg q½-1hr, max 2.1 mg/24 hr
• *Child 6-9 yr:* **PO** 174.6 mg q½-1hr, max 1.4 mg/24 hr
• *Child 3-6 yr:* **PO** 88 mg q½-1hr, max 704 mg/24 hr
Available forms: Tabs 262 mg; chewable tabs 262, 300 mg; susp 262 mg/15 ml, 524 mg/15 ml

SIDE EFFECTS

CNS: Confusion, twitching
EENT: Hearing loss, tinnitus, metallic taste, blue gums, black tongue (chew tabs)
GI: Increased fecal impaction (high doses), dark stools
HEMA: Increased bleeding time
Contraindications: Child <3 yr, history of GI bleeding, renal disease, child with chickenpox, flulike symptoms
Precautions: Pregnancy (C), anticoagulant therapy, immobility, elderly, lactation, gout, diabetes mellitus

PHARMACOKINETICS

PO: Onset 1 hr, peak 2 hr, duration 4 hr

INTERACTIONS

Salicylate toxicity: salicylates
Increase: effects of oral anticoagulants, oral antidiabetics
Decrease: absorption of tetracycline
Drug/Herb
Increase: absorption of bismuth—sarsaparilla
Increase: antidiarrheal effect—nutmeg
Drug/Lab Test
Interference: Radiographic studies of GI system

NURSING CONSIDERATIONS

Assess:
• Electrolytes (K, Na, Cl) if diarrhea is severe or continues long term; assess skin turgor
• Bowel pattern before drug therapy, after treatment
Administer:
PO route
• Increased fluids to rehydrate the patient
• Shake liquid before using
Evaluate:
• Therapeutic response: decreased diarrhea or absence of diarrhea when traveling
Teach patient/family:
• To chew or dissolve in mouth; do not swallow whole; shake liquid before using
• To avoid other salicylates unless directed by prescriber; not to give to children, possibility of Reye's syndrome
• That stools may turn black; tongue may darken; impaction may occur in debilitated patients
• To stop use if symptoms do not improve within 2 days or become worse, or if diarrhea is accompanied by high fever

---

⚠ Safety alert   *"Tall Man" lettering

B

bisoprolol (℞)

(bis-oh'pro-lole)

Zebeta

Func. class.: Antihypertensive

Chem. class.: β_1-Blocker

Do not confuse:

Zebeta/Diabeta/Zetia

Action: Preferentially and competitively blocks stimulation of β_1-adrenergic receptors within cardiac muscle (decreases rate of SA node discharge, increases recovery time), slows conduction of AV node, decreases heart rate, which decreases O_2 consumption in myocardium; decreases renin-aldosterone-angiotensin system; inhibits β_2-receptors in bronchial and vascular smooth muscle at high doses

Uses: Mild to moderate hypertension

Investigational uses: Stable angina pectoris, stable CHF

DOSAGE AND ROUTES

• *Adult:* **PO** 5 mg daily; may increase if necessary to 20 mg daily

Renal/hepatic dose

• *Adult:* **PO** 2.5 mg, titrate upward

Available forms: Tabs 5, 10 mg

SIDE EFFECTS

CNS: Vertigo, headache, insomnia, fatigue, dizziness, mental changes, memory loss, hallucinations, depression, lethargy, drowsiness, strange dreams, catatonia, peripheral neuropathy

*CV: **Ventricular dysrhythmias, profound hypotension, bradycardia, CHF,*** cold extremities, postural hypotension, ***2nd- or 3rd-degree heart block***

EENT: Sore throat; dry, burning eyes

ENDO: Increased hypoglycemic response to insulin

GI: Nausea, diarrhea, vomiting, ***mesenteric arterial thrombosis,*** ischemic colitis, flatulence, gastritis, gastric pain

GU: Impotence, decreased libido

*HEMA: **Agranulocytosis, thrombocytopenia,*** purpura, eosinophilia

INTEG: Rash, flushing, alopecia, pruritus, sweating

MISC: Facial swelling, weight gain, decreased exercise tolerance

MS: Joint pain, arthralgia

*RESP: **Bronchospasm,*** dyspnea, wheezing, cough, nasal stuffiness

Contraindications: Hypersensitivity to β-blockers, cardiogenic shock, heart block (2nd, 3rd degree), sinus bradycardia, CHF, cardiac failure

Precautions: Pregnancy (C), major surgery, lactation, children, diabetes mellitus, renal or hepatic disease, thyroid disease, COPD, asthma, well-compensated heart failure, aortic or mitral valve disease, peripheral vascular disease, myasthenia gravis

PHARMACOKINETICS

PO: Peak 2-4 hr; half-life 9-12 hr, 50% excreted unchanged in urine, protein binding 30%; metabolized in liver to inactive metabolites

INTERACTIONS

Hypotension: reserpine, guanethidine

Myocardial depression: calcium channel blockers

Increase: peripheral ischemia—ergots

Decrease: antihypertensive effect—NSAIDs

Drug/Herb

Toxicity/death: aconite

Increase: β-blocking effect—betel palm, butterbur, cola tree, figwort, fumitory, guarana, hawthorn, lily of the valley, motherwort, plantain

Decrease: β-blocking effect—coenzyme Q10, yohimbe

Drug/Lab Test

Increase: AST, ALT, ANA titer, blood glucose, BUN, uric acid, K, lipoprotein

Interference: Glucose/insulin tolerance tests

NURSING CONSIDERATIONS

Assess:

• B/P during beginning treatment, periodically thereafter; pulse q4h: note rate, rhythm, quality

• Apical/radial pulse before administration; notify prescriber of any significant changes (pulse <50 bpm)

• Baselines in renal, hepatic studies before therapy begins

• I&O, weight daily, watch for CHF: increased weight, jugular vein distention, dyspnea, crackles

• Edema in feet, legs daily

• Skin turgor, dryness of mucous membranes for hydration status, especially elderly

Administer:

• Drug ac, bedtime, tablet may be crushed or swallowed whole, may give without regard to meals

• Reduced dosage in renal and hepatic dysfunction

Perform/provide:

• Storage protected from light, moisture; place in cool environment

Evaluate:

• Therapeutic response: decreased B/P after 1-2 wk

Teach patient/family:

• Not to discontinue drug abruptly, may cause precipitate angina, evaluate noncompliance

• Not to use OTC products containing α-adrenergic stimulants (such as nasal decongestants, OTC cold preparations) unless directed by prescriber

• To report bradycardia, dizziness, confusion, depression, fever, cold extremities

• To take pulse at home; advise when to notify prescriber

• To avoid alcohol, smoking, sodium intake

• To comply with weight control, dietary adjustments, modified exercise program

• To carry emergency ID to identify drug taking, allergies

• To avoid hazardous activities if dizziness is present

⚠ To report symptoms of CHF: difficulty breathing, especially on exertion or when lying down, night cough, swelling of extremities

• That if diabetic, may mask signs of hypoglycemia, or alter blood glucose levels

Treatment of overdose: Lavage, IV atropine for bradycardia, IV theophylline for bronchospasm; digitalis, O_2, diuretic for cardiac failure; hemodialysis, IV glucose for hypoglycemia; IV diazepam (or phenytoin) for seizures

---

Rarely Used

bitolterol (Ŗ)

(bye-tole′ter-ole)
Tornalate
Func. class.: Bronchodilator, adrenergic β$_2$-agonist

Uses: Asthma, bronchospasm

DOSAGE AND ROUTES

Inhaler

• *Adult and child >12 yr:* **INH** 2 puffs, wait 1-3 min before 3rd puff if needed, not to exceed 3 **INH** q6h or 2 **INH** q4h

Nebulization

• *Adult and child >12 yr:* **INH** 0.5 ml (1 mg) tid by intermittent flow or 1.25 mg tid by continuous flow, max 8 mg (intermittent), 14 mg (continuous)

Contraindications: Hypersensitivity to bitolterol products

⚠ High Alert

bivalirudin (Ŗ)

(bye-val-i-rue′din)
Angiomax
Func. class.: Anticoagulant
Chem. class.: Thrombin inhibitor

Action: Direct inhibitor of thrombin that is highly specific

Uses: Unstable angina in patients undergoing percutaneous transluminal coronary angioplasty (PTCA)

B

DOSAGE AND ROUTES
• *Adult:* **IV BOL** 1 mg/kg, then **IV INF** 2.5 mg/kg/hr for 4 hr; another **IV INF** may be used at 0.2 mg/kg/hr for ≤20 hr; this drug is intended to be used with aspirin (325 mg daily) adjusted to body weight

Renal dose
• *Adult:* **IV** GFR 30-59 ml/min give 80% of dose; GFR 10-29 ml/min give 40% of dose; dialysis-dependent patients (not on dialysis) give 10% of dose
Available forms: Inj, lyophilized 250 mg/vial

SIDE EFFECTS
CNS: Headache, insomnia, anxiety, nervousness
CV: Hypo/hypertension, bradycardia
GI: Nausea, vomiting, abdominal pain, dyspepsia
HEMA: **Hemorrhage**
MISC: Pain at inj site, pelvic pain, urinary retention, fever
MS: Back pain
Contraindications: Hypersensitivity, active bleeding
Precautions: Pregnancy (B), renal function impairment, elderly, lactation, children, hepatic disease

PHARMACOKINETICS
Excreted in urine, half-life 25 min

INTERACTIONS
Increase: bleeding risk—anticoagulants, thrombolytics
Drug/Herb
Increase: bleeding risk—agrimony, alfalfa, angelica, anise, bilberry, black haw, bogbean, buchu, chondroitin, dong quai, fenugreek, feverfew, garlic, ginger, ginkgo, ginseng, horse chestnut, Irish moss, kelp, kelpware, khella, lovage, lungwort, meadowsweet, motherwort, mugwort, nettle, papaya, parsley (large amts), pau d'arco, pineapple, poplar, prickly ash, safflower, saw palmetto, senega, tonka bean, turmeric, wintergreen, yarrow

Decrease: anticoagulant effect—chamomile, coenzyme Q10, flax, glucomannan, goldenseal, guar gum

NURSING CONSIDERATIONS
Assess:
⚠ Bleeding: check arterial and venous sites, IM inj sites, catheters; all punctures should be minimized; fall in B/P or Hct that may indicate hemorrhage
• Fever, skin rash, urticaria
Administer:
• Prior to PTCA, give with aspirin, 325 mg
IV, direct route
• Dilute by adding 5 ml of sterile water for inj/250 mg bivalirudin, swirl until dissolved, further dilute in 50 ml of D$_5$W or 0.9% NaCl (5 mg/ml), give by bolus inj 1 mg/kg, then intermittent infusion
Intermittent INF route
• To each 250 mg vial add 5 ml of sterile water for inj, swirl until dissolved, further dilute in 500 ml D$_5$W or 0.9% NaCl (0.5 mg/ml); give inf after bolus dose at a rate of 2.5 mg/kg/hr (4 hr inf); may give an additional infusion at 0.2 mg/kg/hr
Evaluate
• Therapeutic response: anticoagulation in PTCA
Teach patient/family:
• Reason for drug and expected results

⚠ High Alert

bleomycin (℞)
(blee-oh-mye′sin)
Blenoxane
Func. class.: Antineoplastic, antibiotic
Chem. class.: Glycopeptide

Action: Inhibits synthesis of DNA, RNA, protein; derived from *Streptomyces verticillus;* phase specific in the G$_2$ and M phases; a nonvesicant, sclerosing agent
Uses: Cancer of head, neck, penis, cervix, vulva of squamous cell origin, Hodgkin's/non-Hodgkin's disease, lym-

phosarcoma, reticulum cell sarcoma, testicular carcinoma, as a sclerosing agent for malignant pleural effusion

DOSAGE AND ROUTES

• *Adult and child:* SUBCUT/IV/IM 0.25-0.5 units/kg 1-2 times/wk or 10-20 units/m^2, then 1 unit/day or 5 units/wk; may also be given by **CONT INF;** do not exceed total dose, 400 units in lifetime

Malignant pleural effusion

• *Adult:* 60 units diluted in 100 ml of 0.9% NaCl intrapleural inj given through a thoracostomy tube following drainage of excess pleural fluid and complete lung expansion, remove after 4 hr

Available forms: Powder for inj, 15, 30 units/vial

SIDE EFFECTS

CNS: Pain at tumor site, headache, confusion

GI: Nausea, vomiting, anorexia, stomatitis, weight loss, ulceration of mouth, lips

IDIOSYNCRATIC REACTION: Hypotension, confusion, fever, chills, wheezing

INTEG: Rash, hyperkeratosis, nail changes, alopecia, pruritus, acne, striae, peeling, hyperpigmentation

RESP: **Fibrosis, pneumonitis,** wheezing, **pulmonary toxicity**

SYST: **Anaphylaxis,** radiation recall, Raynaud's phenomenon

Contraindications: Pregnancy (D), hypersensitivity, prior idiosyncratic reaction

Precautions: Renal, hepatic, respiratory disease, patients >70 yr old

PHARMACOKINETICS

Half-life 2 hr; when CCr >35 ml/min, half-life is increased in lower clearance; metabolized in liver, 50% excreted in urine (unchanged)

INTERACTIONS

Increase: toxicity—other antineoplastics, radiation therapy, general anesthesia

Decrease: serum phenytoin levels—phenytoin, fosphenytoin

Drug/Lab Test

Increase: Uric acid

NURSING CONSIDERATIONS

Assess:

• IM test dose in lymphoma 1-2 units before 1st 2 doses

• Pulmonary function tests: chest x-ray film before and during therapy; should be obtained q2wk during treatment

• Temp q4h; fever may indicate beginning infection

• Serum creatinine

• Dyspnea, crackles, unproductive cough, chest pain, tachypnea, fatigue, increased pulse, pallor, lethargy

• Effects of alopecia and skin color on body image; discuss feelings about body changes

• Buccal cavity q8h for dryness, sores, ulceration, white patches, oral pain, bleeding, dysphagia

• Local irritation, pain, burning, discoloration at inj site

⚠ Symptoms indicating anaphylaxis: rash, pruritus, urticaria, purpuric skin lesions, itching, flushing, wheezing, hypotension; have emergency equipment available

Administer:

• Antiemetic 30-60 min before giving drug to prevent vomiting, continue antiemetics 6-10 hr after treatment

• Topical or systemic analgesics for pain of stomatitis as ordered; antihistamines and antipyretics for fever and chills

IM/SUBCUT route

• After reconstituting 15 units/1-5 ml sterile H$_2$O, D$_5$W, 0.9% NaCl, or bacteriostatic water for inj, rotate inj sites; do not use products containing benzyl alcohol when giving to neonates

IV, direct route

• After reconstituting 15 units or less/5 ml or more of D$_5$W or 0.9% NaCl; after further diluting with 50-100 ml D$_5$W or 0.9% NaCl, give 15 units or less/10 min through Y-tube or 3-way stopcock

• In lymphoma, two test doses 2-5 units

before initial dose; monitor for anaphylaxis

Intrapleural route

• 60 units/50-100 ml of 0.9% NaCl, administered by MD through thoracotomy tube

Additive compatibilities: Amikacin, cephapirin, dexamethasone, diphenhydrAMINE, fluorouracil, gentamicin, heparin, hydrocortisone, phenytoin, streptomycin, tobramycin, vinBLAStine, vinCRIStine

Solution compatibilities: 0.9% NaCl

Syringe compatibilities: Cisplatin, cyclophosphamide, DOXOrubicin, droperidol, fluorouracil, furosemide, heparin, leucovorin, methotrexate, metoclopramide, mitomycin, vinBLAStine, vinCRIStine

Y-site compatibilities: Allopurinol, amifostine, aztreonam, cefepime, cisplatin, cyclophosphamide, DOXOrubicin, DOXOrubicin liposome, droperidol, filgrastim, fludarabine, fluorouracil, granisetron, heparin, leucovorin, melphalan, methotrexate, metoclopramide, mitomycin, ondansetron, paclitaxel, piperacillin/tazobactam, sargramostim, teniposide, thiotepa, vinBLAStine, vinCRIStine, vinorelbine

Perform/provide:

• Storage for 2 wk after reconstituting if refrigerated or 24 hr at room temperature; discard unused portions

• Deep-breathing exercises with patient tid-qid; place in semi-Fowler's position

• Liquid diet: carbonated beverage; gelatin may be added if patient is not nauseated or vomiting

• Rinsing of mouth tid-qid with water, club soda; brushing of teeth with baking soda bid-tid with soft brush or cotton-tipped applicators for stomatitis; use unwaxed dental floss

• HOB raised to facilitate breathing

Evaluate:

• Therapeutic response: decrease in size of tumor

Teach patient/family:

• To report any complaints, side effects to nurse or prescriber

• To report any changes in breathing, coughing, fever

• That hair may be lost during treatment, and wig or hairpiece may make patient feel better; that new hair may be different in color, texture

• To avoid foods with citric acid, hot or rough texture

• To report any bleeding, white spots, ulcerations in mouth; to examine mouth daily and report symptoms

• To use contraception during treatment

• Not to receive vaccines during treatment

---

bortezomib (℞)
(bor-tez′oh-mib)
Velcade
Func. class.: Antineoplastic—miscellaneous
Chem. class.: Proteasome inhibitor

Action: A reversible inhibitor of chymotrypsin-like activity in mammalian cells. Causes a delay in tumor growth by disrupting normal homeostatic mechanisms.

Uses: Multiple myeloma when at least two other treatments have failed.

Investigational uses: Several solid, hematologic tumors

DOSAGE AND ROUTES

• *Adult:* **IV BOL** 1.3 mg/m^2/dose 2×/wk for 2 weeks (days 1, 4, 8, 11) followed by 10-day rest period (days 12 to 21); max 8 cycles

Neuropathic pain

• Grade 1 with pain or grade 2: Reduce to 1 mg/m^2

• Grade 2 with pain or grade 3: Hold drug until toxicity resolves, then start at 0.7 mg/m^2 qwk

• Grade 4 hematologic toxicities, withhold use

Available forms: Lyophilized powder for inj 3.5 mg

SIDE EFFECTS

CNS: Anxiety, insomnia, dizziness, headache, *peripheral neuropathy,* rigors, paresthesia

CV: Hypotension, edema

GI: Abdominal pain, *constipation, diarrhea,* dyspepsia, nausea, *vomiting,* anorexia

HEMA: Anemia, **neutropenia, thrombocytopenia**

MISC: Dehydration, weight loss, herpes zoster, rash, pruritus, blurred vision

MS: Fatigue, malaise, weakness, arthralgia, bone pain, muscle cramps, myalgia, back pain

RESP: Cough, pneumonia, dyspnea, URI

Contraindications: Pregnancy (D), hypersensitivity to this drug, boron, or mannitol

Precautions: Peripheral neuropathy, elderly, hepatic disease, renal disease, hypotension, lactation, children

PHARMACOKINETICS

Half-life 9-15 hrs, protein binding 83%, metabolized by P450 enzymes (3A4, 2D6, 2C19, 2C9, 1A2)

INTERACTIONS

Oral hypoglycemics: may result in hypo, hyperglycemia

Increase: hypotension—antihypertensives

Increase: peripheral neuropathy—amiodarone, antivirals, isoniazid, nitrofurantoin, statins

Increase: toxicity or decrease efficacy when administered with drugs that induce or inhibit cytochrome P4503A4

NURSING CONSIDERATIONS

Assess:
- Hematologic status: platelets, CBC throughout treatment
- For extravasation at inj site
- B/P, fluid status, peripheral neuropathy symptoms

Administer:
- Reconstitute each vial with 3.5 ml 0.9% NaCl

- Use protective clothing during handling, preparation, avoid contact with skin

Evaluate:
- Therapeutic response: improvement of multiple myeloma symptoms

Teach patient/family:
- To use contraception while on this drug, pregnancy (D), avoid breastfeeding
- To monitor blood glucose levels if diabetic
- To contact prescriber of new or worsening peripheral neuropathy, severe vomiting, diarrhea
- To avoid driving, operating machinery until effect is known
- To avoid using other medications unless approved by prescriber

---

bosentan (℞)

(boh'sen-tan)
Tracleer
Func. class.: Vasodilator
Chem. class.: Endothelin receptor antagonist

Action: Peripheral vasodilation occurs via antagonism of the effect of endothelin on endothelium and vascular smooth muscle

Uses: Pulmonary arterial hypertension with WHO class III, IV symptoms

Investigational uses: Septic shock to improve microcirculatory blood flow

DOSAGE AND ROUTES

- *Adult >40 kg/>12 yr:* **PO** 62.5 mg bid × 4 wk, then 125 mg bid
- *Adult <40 kg/>12 yr:* **PO** 62.5 mg bid

Available forms: Tabs 62.5, 125 mg

SIDE EFFECTS

CNS: Headache, flushing, fatigue

CV: Hypotension, palpitations, edema of lower limbs

GI: Abnormal hepatic function, dyspepsia, **hepatotoxicity**

INTEG: Pruritus

MISC: Anemia

Contraindications: Pregnancy (X), hypersensitivity, CVA, CAD
Precautions: Mitral stenosis, elderly, lactation, hepatic function impairment, children

PHARMACOKINETICS

Is metabolized by CYP2C9, CYP3A4, and possibly CYP2C19, metabolized by the liver, terminal half-life 5 hr, steady state 3-5 days

INTERACTIONS

Do not coadminister cycloSPORINE A and bosentan; bosentan is increased, cycloSPORINE is decreased
Do not coadminister glyBURIDE with bosentan; glyBURIDE is decreased significantly, bosentan also is decreased, hepatic enzymes may be increased
Increase: bosentan level—ketoconazole
Decrease: effects of simvastatin, other statins, hormonal contraceptives, warfarin
Drug/Lab Test
Increase: ALT, AST
Decrease: Hgb, Hct

NURSING CONSIDERATIONS
Assess:
• B/P, pulse during treatment until stable
• Hepatic studies: AST, ALT, bilirubin; hepatic enzymes may increase; if ALT/AST >3 and ≤5 × ULN, confirm lab value, decrease dose or interrupt treatment and monitor AST/ALT q2wk; if >8 × ULN, stop treatment
• Blood studies: Hct, Hgb may be decreased
• Hepatic involvement: vomiting, jaundice; drug should be discontinued
Administer:
• Do not stop drug abruptly, taper
Perform/provide:
• Storage at room temperature
Evaluate:
• Therapeutic response: decrease in pulmonary hypertension
Teach patient/family:
• To report jaundice, dark urine, joint

pain, fatigue, malaise, bruising, easy bleeding; may indicate blood dyscrasias
• To avoid pregnancy; to use nonhormonal form of contraception
• Lab work will be required periodically

brimonidine ophthalmic
See Appendix C

brinzolamide ophthalmic
See Appendix C

bromocriptine (R)
(broe-moe-krip′teen)
Alti-Bromocriptine ✤,
Apo-Bromocriptine ✤,
Parlodel
Func. class.: Dopamine receptor agonist, antiparkinson agent
Chem. class.: Ergot alkaloid derivative

Do not confuse:
Parlodel/pindolol/Provera
Action: Inhibits prolactin release by activating postsynaptic dopamine receptors; activation of striatal dopamine receptors may be reason for improvement in Parkinson's disease
Uses: Parkinson's disease, amenorrhea/galactorrhea caused by hyperprolactinemia, infertility, acromegaly, pituitary adenomas
Investigational uses: Neuroleptic malignant syndrome, alcoholism, premenstrual syndrome, mastalgia, cocaine withdrawal

DOSAGE AND ROUTES
Hyperprolactinemia
• *Adult:* **PO** 1.25-2.5 mg with meals; may increase by 2.5 mg q3-7d, usual 5-7.5 mg

Acromegaly
- *Adult:* **PO** 1.25-2.5 mg × 3 days at bedtime; may increase by 1.25-2.5 mg q3-7d; usual range 20-30 mg/day, max 100 mg/day

Parkinson's disease
- *Adult:* **PO** 1.25 mg bid with meals, may increase q2-4wk by 2.5 mg/day, not to exceed 100 mg daily

Pituitary adenoma
- *Adult:* **PO** 1.25 mg bid-tid, may increase over several weeks

Neuroleptic malignant syndrome (off-label)
- *Adult:* **PO** 5 mg daily, max 20 mg/day

Cocaine withdrawal
- *Adult:* **PO** 0.625 mg qid × 42 days

Alcoholism (off-label)
- *Adult:* **PO** 7.5 mg/day

Mastalgia
- *Adult:* **PO** 2.5-7.5 bid, starting 10-14 days prior to menses; discontinue when menses begin

Available forms: Caps 5 mg; tabs 2.5 mg

SIDE EFFECTS

CNS: *Headache,* depression, restlessness, anxiety, nervousness, confusion, ***convulsions, hallucinations,*** dizziness, fatigue, drowsiness, abnormal involuntary movements, psychosis
CV: Orthostatic hypotension, decreased B/P, palpitation, extrasystole, ***shock,*** dysrhythmias, bradycardia, ***MI***
EENT: Blurred vision, diplopia, burning eyes, nasal congestion
GI: *Nausea, vomiting, anorexia,* cramps, constipation, diarrhea, dry mouth, GI hemorrhage
GU: Frequency, retention, incontinence, diuresis
INTEG: *Rash on face, arms,* alopecia; coolness, pallor of fingers, toes

Contraindications: Hypersensitivity to ergot, severe ischemic disease, severe peripheral vascular disease
Precautions: Pregnancy (B), lactation, hepatic disease, renal disease, children, pituitary tumors

PHARMACOKINETICS

PO: Peak 1-3 hr, duration 4-8 hr, 90%-96% protein bound, half-life 3 hr, metabolized by liver (inactive metabolites), 85%-98% of dose excreted in feces

INTERACTIONS

Disulfiram-like reaction: alcohol
Increase: action of antihypertensives, levodopa
Decrease: action of bromocriptine— phenothiazines, oral contraceptives, progestins, estrogens, haloperidol, loxapine, methyldopa, metoclopramide, MAOIs, reserpine

Drug/Herb
Increase: serotonin effect—horehound
Decrease: bromocriptine effect— chaste tree fruit, kava

Drug/Lab Test
Increase: Growth hormone, AST, ALT, CK, BUN, uric acid, alk phosphatase

NURSING CONSIDERATIONS

Assess:
- B/P; establish baseline, compare with other reading; this drug decreases B/P
- Parkinson's symptoms: pill-rolling, shuffling gait, restlessness, tremors, before and during treatment
- For resolution of symptoms of neuroleptic malignant syndrome: decreased temp, seizures, sweating, pulse
- Change in size of soft tissue volume, in acromegaly

Administer:
- With meal to prevent GI symptoms
- At bedtime so dizziness, orthostatic hypotension do not occur

Perform/provide:
- Storage at room temperature in tight container

Evaluate:
- Therapeutic response (Parkinson's disease): decreased dyskinesia, decreased slow movements, decreased drooling

Teach patient/family:
- That tabs may be crushed and mixed with food

⚠ Safety alert   *"Tall Man" lettering

- To change position slowly to prevent orthostatic hypotension
- To use contraceptives during treatment with this drug; pregnancy may occur; to use methods other than oral contraceptives
- That therapeutic effect for Parkinson's disease may take 2 mo: galactorrhea, amenorrhea
- To avoid hazardous activity if dizziness occurs
- To report symptoms of MI immediately

---

brompheniramine (Ŗ)

(brome-fen-ir'a-meen)
Bidhist, Bromfenac, brompheniramine, BroveX, BroveX CT, Chlorphed, Dehist, Dimetane, Dimetane Extentabs, Dimetapp Allergy Liqui-Gels, Lo Hist 12 Hour, Lodrane 24, Lodrane XR, Nasahist-B, VaZol
Func. class.: Antihistamine
Chem. class.: Alkylamine, H_1-receptor antagonist

Action: Acts on blood vessels, GI, respiratory system by competing with histamine for H_1-receptor site; decreases allergic response by blocking histamine
Uses: Allergy symptoms, rhinitis

DOSAGE AND ROUTES

- *Adult and child >12 yr:* **PO** 4-8 mg bid-qid, not to exceed 36 mg/day; **TIME-REL** 6-12 mg bid-tid, not to exceed 36 mg/day
- *Child 6-12 yr:* **PO** 2 mg bid-qid, not to exceed 12 mg/day; **TIME REL** 6-12 mg daily
- *Child 2-6 yr:* 1 mg bid-qid 6h, max 6 mg/day
- *Child <2 yr:* **PO** 0.5 mg/kg/day in divided doses (qid)
Available forms: Tabs 4 mg; elix 2 mg/5 ml; caps 4 mg; chew tab 12 mg; ext rel tab 6 mg, ext rel cap 12 mg; liquid 8, 12 mg/5 ml

SIDE EFFECTS

CNS: Dizziness, drowsiness, poor coordination, fatigue, anxiety, euphoria, confusion, paresthesia, neuritis
CV: Hypotension, palpitations, tachycardia
EENT: Blurred vision, dilated pupils, tinnitus, nasal stuffiness, dry nose, throat, mouth
GI: Nausea, vomiting, anorexia, constipation, diarrhea
GU: Retention, dysuria, frequency, impotence
*HEMA: **Thrombocytopenia, agranulocytosis, hemolytic anemia (rare)***
INTEG: Photosensitivity
RESP: Increased thick secretions, wheezing, chest tightness
Contraindications: Hypersensitivity to H_1-receptor antagonists, acute asthma attack, lower respiratory tract disease, child <2 yr
Precautions: Pregnancy (C), increased intraocular pressure, renal disease, cardiac disease, hypertension, bronchial asthma, seizure disorder, stenosed peptic ulcers, hyperthyroidism, prostatic hypertrophy, bladder neck obstruction, lactation, angle closure glaucoma

PHARMACOKINETICS

PO: Peak 2-5 hr, duration to 48 hr; metabolized in liver, excreted by kidneys, excreted in breast milk, half-life 12-34 hr

INTERACTIONS

Incompatible with aminophylline, insulins, pentobarbital
Increase: CNS depression—barbiturates, opiates, hypnotics, tricyclics, alcohol
Increase: anticholinergic effect—MAOIs
Drug/Herb
Increase: effect—hops, Jamaican dogwood, kava, khat, senega
Increase: anticholinergic effect—corkwood, henbane leaf
Drug/Lab Test
Interference: Skin allergy tests

NURSING CONSIDERATIONS

Assess:

- Be alert for urinary retention, frequency, dysuria; drug should be discontinued if these occur
- CBC during long-term therapy
- Blood dyscrasias: thrombocytopenia, agranulocytosis (rare) during long-term therapy
- Respiratory status: rate, rhythm, increase in bronchial secretions, wheezing, chest tightness

Administer:

PO route

- Do not break, crush, or chew sustained release forms
- With meals if GI symptoms occur; absorption may slightly decrease

Perform/provide:

- Hard candy, gum, frequent rinsing of mouth for dryness
- Storage in tight container at room temperature

Evaluate:

- Therapeutic response: absence of running or congested nose or rashes

Teach patient/family:

- All aspects of drug use; to notify prescriber if confusion/sedation/hypotension occurs
- To avoid driving, other hazardous activities if drowsiness occurs
- To avoid use of alcohol, other CNS depressants while taking drug

Treatment of overdose: Administer vasopressors, barbiturates (short-acting)

---

budesonide (℞)
(byoo-des'oh-nide)
Entocort EC, Pulmicort,
Rhinocort Aqua
Func. class.: Glucocorticoid
Chem. class.: Nonhalogenated

Action: Prevents inflammation by depression of migration of polymorphonuclear leukocytes, fibroblasts, reversal of increased capillary permeability and lysosomal stabilization; does not suppress hypothalamus and pituitary function

Uses: Rhinitis; prophylaxis for asthma; Crohn's disease

DOSAGE AND ROUTES

Rhinitis (Rhinocort Aqua)

- *Adult/child >6 yr:* **SPRAY/INH** 256 mcg daily (2 sprays in each nostril AM, PM or 4 sprays in each nostril, AM)

Asthma

- *Adult and child ≥6 yr:* **INH** 400-600 mcg/day

Crohn's disease

- *Adult:* **PO** 9 mg daily AM × 8 wk

Available forms: Dry powder for INH 200 mcg/metered dose (Palmicort Turbuhaler); inh susp 0.25 mg/2 ml, 0.5 mg/2 ml; 32 mcg/spray (Rhinocort Aqua); caps 3 mg (Entocort EC)

SIDE EFFECTS

CNS: Headache, insomnia, hypertonia, syncope
EENT: Sinusitis, pharyngitis, rhinitis, oral candidiasis
GI: Dry mouth, dyspepsia, nausea, vomiting, abdominal pain
ENDO: Adrenal insufficiency, growth suppression in children
MISC: Ecchymosis, fever, *hypersensitivity,* flulike symptoms
MS: Back pain, myalgias, fractures
RESP: Nasal irritation, cough, nasal bleeding, *respiratory infections, bronchospasm*

Contraindications: Hypersensitivity, status asthmaticus

Precautions: Pregnancy (C), inhaled form (B); lactation, children, TB, fungal, bacterial, systemic viral infections, ocular herpes simplex, nasal septal ulcers; hepatic disease (caps)

PHARMACOKINETICS

Peak: Respules 4-6 wk, Rhinocort Aqua 2 wk, Turbuhaler 1-2 wk, half-life 2-3.6 hr
Onset: Respules 2-8 days; Rhinocort Aqua 10 hr; Turbuhale 24 hr

---

INTERACTIONS

Avoid using with drugs metabolized by CYP3A4 inhibition

Decrease: budesonide metabolism—ketoconazole, cimetidine

Drug/Herb

Increase: Hypokalemia—aloe, buckthorn, Chinese rhubarb, senna

NURSING CONSIDERATIONS

Assess:

• Respiratory status: rate, rhythm, increase in bronchial secretions, wheezing, chest tightness; provide fluids to 2 L/day to decrease thickness of secretions; check for oral candidiasis

• For bronchospasm, stop treatment and give bronchodilator

• With viral infections, corticosteroid use can mask infections

• For increased intraocular pressure, discontinue use if increase occurs

Administer:

PO route (Crohn's disease)

• Swallow caps whole; do not break, crush, or chew

• May repeat 8-wk course if needed; may taper to 6 mg/day for 2 wk before cessation

INH route (asthma)

• Use scissors to open pouch

• Use Turbuhaler upright to load, prime when using first time, turn grip to the right, then left to click in place; to provide dose turn to right, then to the left, click in place. Place mouthpiece between lips, inhale forcefully, do not exhale through Turbuhaler, rinse after use

Perform/provide:

• Storage at 59°-86° F (15°-30° C); keep away from heat, open flame

Evaluate:

• Therapeutic response: absence of asthma, rhinitis

Teach patient/family:

• To notify prescriber of pharyngitis, nasal bleeding

• Not to exceed recommended dose; adrenal suppression may occur

• To carry emergency ID identifying steroid use

• To read and follow package directions

• To prevent exposure to infections, especially viral

• To avoid taking with grapefruit juice (capsule PO)

• To use good oral hygiene if using nebulizer or inhaler

---

budesonide nasal agent
See Appendix C

---

bumetanide (Ŗ)
(byoo-met'a-nide)
Bumex
Func. class.: Loop diuretic, antihypertensive
Chem. class.: Sulfonamide derivative

Do not confuse:
Bumex/Buprenex/Permax

Action: Acts on ascending loop of Henle by inhibiting reabsorption of chloride, sodium

Uses: Edema in CHF, hepatic disease, renal disease (nephrotic syndrome), pulmonary edema, ascites (nephrotic syndrome), hypertension, anasarca

Investigational uses: May be used alone or as adjunct with antihypertensives such as spironolactone, triamterene

DOSAGE AND ROUTES

• *Adult:* **PO** 0.5-2.0 mg daily; may give 2nd or 3rd dose at 4-5 hr intervals, not to exceed 10 mg/day; may be given on alternate days or intermittently; **IV/IM** 0.5-1.0 mg; may give 2nd or 3rd dose at 2-3 hr intervals, not to exceed 10 mg/day

• *Child:* **PO/IM/IV** 0.02-0.1 mg/kg q12h, max 10 mg/day

Available forms: Tabs 0.5, 1, 2 mg; inj 0.25 mg/ml

SIDE EFFECTS

CNS: Headache, fatigue, weakness, vertigo
CV: **Chest pain,** hypotension, **circulatory collapse,** ECG changes, dehydration
EENT: Loss of hearing, ear pain, tinnitus, blurred vision
ELECT: Hypokalemia, hypochloremic alkalosis, hypomagnesemia, hyperuricemia, hypocalcemia, hyponatremia
ENDO: Hyperglycemia
GI: Nausea, diarrhea, dry mouth, vomiting, anorexia, cramps, upset stomach, abdominal pain, **acute pancreatitis, jaundice**
GU: Polyuria, **renal failure,** glycosuria
HEMA: **Thrombocytopenia**
INTEG: Rash, pruritus, purpura, **Stevens-Johnson syndrome,** sweating, photosensitivity
MS: Muscular cramps, arthritis, stiffness, tenderness
Contraindications: Hypersensitivity to sulfonamides, anuria, hepatic coma, severe electrolyte deficiency
Precautions: Pregnancy (C), dehydration, ascites, severe renal disease, hepatic cirrhosis, lactation

PHARMACOKINETICS

PO: Onset ½-1 hr, peak 1-2 hr, duration 3-6 hr
IM: Onset 40 min, peak 1-2 hr, duration 4-6 hr
IV: Onset 5 min, peak 15-30 min, duration 3-6 hr, excreted by kidneys (50% unchanged), feces (20%), crosses placenta, excreted in breast milk, protein binding >91%; half-life 1-1½ hr, 6-15 hr neonates

INTERACTIONS

Ototoxicity: aminoglycosides
Hypokalemia: potassium-wasting drugs, corticosteroids
Increase: toxicity—lithium, digitalis
Increase: diuresis, electrolyte loss—metolazone
Decrease: diuretic effect—indomethacin, NSAIDs, probenecid
Decrease: antidiabetic effects
Drug/Herb
Severe photosensitivity: St. John's wort
Increase: effect—aloe, cucumber, dandelion, horsetail, pumpkin, Queen Anne's lace
Increase: hypotension—khella
Drug/Lab Test
Increase: Urinary phosphate

NURSING CONSIDERATIONS

Assess:
• For tinnitus, obtain audiometric testing for long-term IV treatment
• Weight, I&O daily to determine fluid loss; if urinary output decreases or azotemia occurs, drug should be discontinued; the safest dosage schedule is on alternate days
• B/P lying, standing; postural hypotension may occur
• Electrolytes: K, Na, Cl; include BUN, blood glucose, CBC, serum creatinine, blood pH, ABGs, uric acid, Ca, Mg
• Blood glucose if patient is diabetic; blood uric acid levels in those with gout
• Improvement in edema of feet, legs, sacral area daily if medication is being used in CHF
• Signs of metabolic alkalosis: drowsiness, restlessness
• Signs of hypokalemia: postural hypotension, malaise, fatigue, tachycardia, leg cramps, weakness
• Rashes, temp elevation daily
• Confusion, especially in elderly; take safety precautions if needed
• For digitalis toxicity in patients taking digitalis products (anorexia, nausea, vomiting, confusion, paresthesia, muscle cramps); lithium toxicity in those taking lithium
Administer:
• In AM to avoid interference with sleep if using drug as a diuretic
• Potassium replacement if potassium is less than 3.0
PO route
• With food if nausea occurs; absorption may be decreased slightly

---

⚠ Safety alert   *"Tall Man" lettering

IV, direct route
• Direct IV undiluted over at least 2 min through Y-tube or 3-way stopcock or heplock
Intermittent IV route
• Dilute in LR, D₅W, 0.9% NaCl (rarely given by this method), give over 12 hr in renal disease
Additive compatibilities: Floxacillin, furosemide
Syringe compatibilities: Doxapram
Y-site compatibilities: Allopurinol, amifostine, aztreonam, cefepime, cisatracurium, cladribine, diltiazem, filgrastim, granisetron, lorazepam, melphalan, meperidine, morphine, piperacillin/tazobactam, propofol, remifentanil, teniposide, thiotepa, vinorelbine
Evaluate:
• Therapeutic response: decreased edema, B/P
Teach patient/family:
• To increase fluid intake to 2-3 L/day unless contraindicated, to take potassium supplement, to rise slowly from lying or sitting position
• To recognize adverse reactions: muscle cramps, weakness, nausea, dizziness
• To take with food or milk for GI symptoms
• To take early in day to prevent nocturia
• To use sunscreen to prevent photosensitivity
Treatment of overdose: Lavage if taken orally; monitor electrolytes; administer dextrose in saline; monitor hydration, CV, renal status

---

buprenorphine (℞)
(byoo-pre-nor'feen)
Buprenex
Func. class.: Opioid analgesic, partial agonist
Chem. class.: Thebaine derivative

Controlled Substance Schedule V
Do not confuse:
Buprenex/Bumex
Action: Depresses pain impulse trans-

mission at the spinal cord level by interacting with opioid receptors
Uses: Moderate to severe pain

DOSAGE AND ROUTES
• *Adult:* **IM/IV** 0.3 mg q6h prn, reduce dosage in elderly, may repeat after ½ hr; **EPIDURAL** 60-180 mcg over 48 hr
• *Child 2-12 yr:* **IM/IV** 2-6 mcg/kg q4-6h
• *Geriatric:* **PO** 0.15 mg q6h prn
Available forms: Inj 0.3 mg/ml (1 ml vials)

SIDE EFFECTS
*CNS: Drowsiness, dizziness, confusion, headache, sedation, euphoria, **increased intracranial pressure**,* amnesia
CV: Palpitations, bradycardia, change in B/P, tachycardia
EENT: Tinnitus, blurred vision, *miosis,* diplopia
GI: Nausea, vomiting, anorexia, constipation, cramps, dry mouth
GU: Increased urinary output, dysuria, urinary retention
INTEG: Rash, urticaria, bruising, flushing, diaphoresis, pruritus
*RESP: **Respiratory depression,*** dyspnea, hypo/hyperventilation
Contraindications: Hypersensitivity
Precautions: Pregnancy (C), addictive personality, lactation, increased intracranial pressure, MI (acute), severe heart disease, respiratory depression, hepatic disease, renal disease, hypothyroidism, Addison's disease, addiction (opioid)

PHARMACOKINETICS
IM: Onset 10-30 min, peak ½ hr, duration 3-4 hr
IV: Onset 1 min, peak 5 min, duration 2-5 hr
Metabolized by liver; excreted by kidneys/feces; crosses placenta; excreted in breast milk; half-life 2½-3½ hr; 96% bound to plasma proteins

INTERACTIONS

Increase: effect with other CNS depressants—alcohol, opioids, sedative/hypnotics, antipsychotics, skeletal muscle relaxants, MAOIs

Drug/Herb

Increase: CNS depression—Jamaican dogwood, kava, lavender, mistletoe, nettle, pokeweed, poppy, senega, valerian

Increase: anticholinergic effect—corkwood

NURSING CONSIDERATIONS

Assess:

• I&O ratio; check for decreasing output; may indicate urinary retention
• CNS changes, dizziness, drowsiness, hallucinations, euphoria, LOC, pupil reaction; withdrawal in opioid-dependent persons; if dependence occurs, within 2 wk of discontinuing drug withdrawal symptoms will occur
• Allergic reactions: rash, urticaria
• Respiratory dysfunction: respiratory depression, character, rate, rhythm; notify prescriber if respirations are <12/min
• Need for pain medication, tolerance; location, intensity, severity

Administer:

IM route

• In deep muscle mass

IV, direct route

• Undiluted over 3-5 min (0.3 mg over 2 min), titrate to patient response
• With antiemetic if nausea, vomiting occur
• When pain is beginning to return; determine dosage interval by patient response

Additive compatibilities: Atropine, bupivacaine, diphenhydrAMINE, droperidol, glycopyrrolate, haloperidol, hydrOXYzine, promethazine, scopolamine

Syringe compatibilities: Midazolam

Y-site compatibilities: Allopurinol, amifostine, aztreonam, cefepime, cisatracurium, cladribine, filgrastim, granisetron, melphalan, piperacillin/tazobactam, propofol, remifentanil, teniposide, thiotepa, vinorelbine

Perform/provide:

• Assistance with ambulation if needed

Evaluate:

• Therapeutic response: decrease in pain, absence of grimacing

Teach patient/family:

• To report any symptoms of CNS changes, allergic reactions
• That tolerance may result when used for extended periods
• To avoid hazardous activities

---

*__buPROPion__ (R)

(byoo-proe′pee-on)

buPROPion, Wellbutrin, Wellbutrin SR, Zyban

Func. class.: Misc. antidepressant, smoking deterrent

Chem. class.: Aminoketone

Do not confuse:

buPROPion/busPIRone

Zyban/Diovan/Zagam

Action: Inhibits reuptake of dopamine, serotonin, norepinephrine

Uses: Depression (Wellbutrin), smoking cessation (Zyban)

DOSAGE AND ROUTES

Depression

• *Adult:* **PO** 100 mg bid initially, then increase after 3 days to 100 mg tid if needed; may increase after 1 mo to 150 mg tid; **SR** 150 mg bid, initially 150 mg AM, increase to 300 mg/day if initial dose is tolerated

• *Geriatric:* **PO** 50-100 mg/day, may increase by 50-100 mg q3-4 day

Smoking cessation

• *Adult:* **PO** 150 mg bid, begin with 150 mg daily × 3 days, then 300 mg/day; continue for 7-12 wk; not to exceed 300 mg/day

Available forms: Tabs 75, 100 mg; tabs, sust rel (SR), 100, 150, 200 mg (Zyban), ext rel tab (XL) 150, 300 mg

---

SIDE EFFECTS

CNS: Headache, agitation, dizziness, akinesia, bradykinesia, confusion, **seizures,** delusions, *insomnia, sedation, tremors*

CV: Dysrhythmias, hypertension, palpitations, *tachycardia,* hypotension, **complete AV block**

EENT: Blurred vision, auditory disturbance

GI: Nausea, vomiting, anorexia, diarrhea, *dry mouth,* increased appetite, *constipation*

GU: Impotence, urinary frequency, retention, *menstrual irregularities*

INTEG: Rash, pruritus, *sweating*

MISC: Weight loss or gain

Contraindications: Hypersensitivity, eating disorders, seizure disorders

Precautions: Pregnancy (B), renal disease, hepatic disease, recent MI, cranial trauma, lactation, children <18 yr, elderly, seizure disorder

PHARMACOKINETICS

Onset 2-4 wk, half-life 14 hr; metabolized by liver, steady state 1½-5 wk

INTERACTIONS

⚠ Increase: adverse reactions, seizures—levodopa, MAOIs, phenothiazines, antidepressants, benzodiazepines, alcohol, theophylline, systemic steroids

Increase: buPROPion toxicity—ritonavir

Increase: buPROPion level—cimetidine

Decrease: buPROPion effect—carbamazepine, cimetidine, phenobarbital, phenytoin or other drugs (CYP450)

Drug/Herb

Increase: CNS depression—hops, kava, lavender

Increase: anticholinergic effect—belladonna, corkwood; jimsonweed

NURSING CONSIDERATIONS

Assess:

• For increased risk of seizures; if patient has excessively used CNS depressants and OTC stimulants, dosage of buPROPion should not be exceeded

• For smoking cessation after 7-12 wk; if progress has not been made, drug should be discontinued

• Mental status: mood, sensorium, affect, suicidal tendencies, increase in psychiatric symptoms

Administer:

PO route

• Do not break, crush, or chew sust rel tab

• Increased fluids, bulk in diet if constipation occurs

• With food or milk for GI symptoms

• Sugarless gum, hard candy, or frequent sips of water for dry mouth

Perform/provide:

• Assistance with ambulation during beginning therapy, since sedation occurs

• Safety measures, primarily in elderly

Evaluate:

• Therapeutic response: decreased depression, ability to function in daily activities, ability to sleep throughout the night, smoking cessation

Teach patient/family:

• That therapeutic effects may take 2-4 wk; not to increase dose without prescriber's approval; that treatment for smoking cessation lasts 7-12 wk

• To use caution in driving, other activities requiring alertness; sedation, blurred vision may occur

• To avoid alcohol ingestion, other CNS depressants, alcohol may increase risk of seizures

• Not to use with nicotine patches unless directed by prescriber, may increase B/P

• To notify prescriber immediately if retention occurs

• That risk of seizures is increased when dose is exceeded, or if patient has seizure disorder

• To notify prescriber if pregnancy is suspected or planned

Treatment of overdose: ECG monitoring; induce emesis, lavage, activated charcoal; administer anticonvulsant

busPIRone (Ŗ)

(byoo-spye'rone)
BuSpar
Func. class.: Antianxiety, sedative
Chem. class.: Azaspirodecanedione

Do not confuse:
busPIRone/buPROPion

Action: Acts by inhibiting the action of serotonin (5-HT); has shown little potential for abuse, a good choice in substance abuse

Uses: Management and short-term relief of generalized anxiety disorders

DOSAGE AND ROUTES

• **Adult: PO** 5 mg tid; may increase by 5 mg/day q2-3d, not to exceed 60 mg/day
Available forms: Tabs 5, 7.5, 10, 15, 30 mg

SIDE EFFECTS

CNS: Dizziness, headache, depression, stimulation, insomnia, nervousness, light-headedness, numbness, paresthesia, incoordination, nightmares, *tremors,* excitement, involuntary movements, confusion, akathisia

CV: Tachycardia, palpitations, hypotension, hypertension, *CVA, CHF, MI*

EENT: Sore throat, tinnitus, blurred vision, nasal congestion; red, itching eyes; change in taste, smell

GI: Nausea, dry mouth, diarrhea, constipation, flatulence, increased appetite, rectal bleeding

GU: Frequency, hesitancy, menstrual irregularity, change in libido

INTEG: Rash, edema, pruritus, alopecia, dry skin

MISC: Sweating, fatigue, weight gain, fever

MS: Pain, weakness, muscle cramps, spasms

RESP: Hyperventilation, chest congestion, shortness of breath

Contraindications: Hypersensitivity, child <18 yr

Precautions: Pregnancy (B), lactation, elderly, impaired hepatic, renal function

PHARMACOKINETICS

Half-life 2-3 hr rapidly absorbed, metabolized by liver, excreted in feces

INTERACTIONS

Drugs induced by CYP3A4 (rifampin, phenytoin, phenobarbital, carbamazepine, dexamethasone): decrease busPIRone action

Drug metabolized by CYP450, 3A4 (erythromycin, itraconazole, nefazodone, ketoconazole, ritonavir): increase busPIRone

Increase: B/P—MAOIs; do not use together

Increase: CNS depression—psychotropic drugs, alcohol (avoid use)

Decrease: busPIRone effects—rifampin

Drug/Herb

Increase: CNS depression—cowslip, kava, Queen Anne's lace, valerian

Drug/Food

Increase: peak concentration of busPIRone—grapefruit juice

NURSING CONSIDERATIONS

Assess:

• B/P (lying, standing), pulse; if systolic B/P drops 20 mm Hg, hold drug, notify prescriber

• CNS reactions, since some reactions may be unpredictable

• Mental status: mood, sensorium, affect, sleeping pattern, drowsiness, dizziness

Administer:

• With food or milk for GI symptoms

• Crushed if patient unable to swallow medication whole

• Sugarless gum, hard candy, frequent sips of water for dry mouth

Perform/provide:

• Assistance with ambulation during beginning therapy; drowsiness, dizziness occur

• Safety measures if drowsiness occurs

• Check to see PO medication swallowed

⚠ Safety alert   *"Tall Man" lettering

Evaluate:
• Therapeutic response: decreased anxiety, restlessness, sleeplessness
Teach patient/family:
• That drug may be taken with food
• To avoid OTC preparations unless approved by prescriber
• To avoid activities requiring alertness, since drowsiness may occur
• To avoid alcohol ingestion, other psychotropic medications, unless directed by prescriber
• Not to discontinue medication abruptly after long-term use; if dose is missed, do not double
• To rise slowly because fainting may occur, especially elderly
• That drowsiness may worsen at beginning of treatment
• That 1-2 wk of therapy may be required before therapeutic effects occur
Treatment of overdose: Gastric lavage, VS, supportive care

⚠ High Alert

busulfan (℞)
(byoo-sul'fan)
Busulfex, Myleran
Func. class.: Antineoplastic alkylating agent
Chem. class.: Nitrosourea

Do not confuse:
Myleran/Leukeran
Action: Changes essential cellular ions to covalent bonding with resultant alkylation; this interferes with normal biologic function of DNA; activity is not phase specific; action is due to myelosuppression
Uses: Chronic myelocytic leukemia

DOSAGE AND ROUTES
Chronic myelocytic (granulocytic) leukemia
• *Adult:* **PO** 4-8 mg/day initially until WBC levels fall to 15,000/mm^3, then drug is stopped until WBC levels raise over 50,000/mm^3, then 1-3 mg/day

• *Child:* **PO** 0.06-0.12 mg/kg or 1.8-4.6 mg/m^2 day; dose is titrated to maintain WBC levels at 20,000/mm^3, but never <10,000/mm^3
Allogenic hemopoietic stem cell transplantation in chronic myelogenous leukemia
• *Adult:* **IV** 0.8 mg/kg q6hr × 4 days (total 16 doses); give cyclophosphamide **IV** 60 mg/kg over 1 hr daily for 2 days, starting after 16th dose of busulfan
Available forms: Tabs 2 mg; inj 6 mg/ml

SIDE EFFECTS
PO route
CV: Hypotension, thrombosis, chest pain, tachycardia, atrial fibrillation, heart block, pericardial effusion, ***cardiac tamponade*** (high dose with cyclophosphamide)
GI: Anorexia, constipation, diarrhea, dry mouth, nausea, vomiting
*RESP: **Alveolar hemorrhage,*** atelectasis, cough, hemoptysis, hypoxia, pleural effusion, pneumonia, sinusitis, ***pulmonary fibrosis***
IV route
*CNS: **Cerebral hemorrhage, coma, seizures,** anxiety, depression, dizziness, headache,* encephalopathy, *weakness,* mental changes
EENT: Pharyngitis, epistaxis, cataracts
GI: Nausea, vomiting, diarrhea, weight loss
GU: Impotence, sterility, amenorrhea, gynecomastia, ***renal toxicity,*** hyperuremia, adrenal insufficiency–like syndrome
*HEMA: **Thrombocytopenia, leukopenia, pancytopenia, severe bone marrow depression***
INTEG: Dermatitis, hyperpigmentation, alopecia
*OTHER: **Chromosomal aberrations***
*RESP: **Irreversible pulmonary fibrosis,*** pneumonitis
Contraindications: Pregnancy (D) 3rd trimester, radiation, chemotherapy,

---

Side effects: *italics* = common; ***bold italics*** = life-threatening

lactation, blastic phase of chronic myelocytic leukemia, hypersensitivity
Precautions: Childbearing-age women
and men, leukopenia, thrombocytopenia,
anemia, hepatotoxicity, renal toxicity

PHARMACOKINETICS

Well absorbed orally; excreted in
urine; crosses placenta; excreted in
breast milk, half-life 2.5 hr

INTERACTIONS

Hepatotoxicity: thioguanine
Cardiac tamponade: cyclophosphamide
Increase: toxicity—other antineoplas-
tics, radiation
Increase: risk of bleeding—antico-
agulants, aspirin
Increase: antibody response—live virus
vaccines
Decrease: busulfan level—phenytoin
Decrease: busulfan clearance—
acetaminophen, itraconazole
Drug/Lab Test
False positive: breast, bladder, cervix,
lung cytology tests

NURSING CONSIDERATIONS
Assess:

• CBC, differential, platelet count
weekly; withhold drug if WBC is
<15,000/mm^3 or platelet count is
<150,000/mm^3; notify prescriber of
results; institute thrombocytopenia precautions
• Bone marrow status prior to
chemotherapy; seizure history
• Pulmonary function tests, chest x-ray
films before, during therapy; chest film
should be obtained q2wk during
treatment; pulmonary fibrosis may occur
up to 10 yr after treatment with busulfan
• Renal studies: BUN, serum uric acid,
urine CCr before, during therapy; monitor ALT, alk phosphatase, bilirubin, uric
acid before and during treatment
• I&O ratio; report fall in urine output
<30 ml/hr
• Monitor for cold, fever, sore throat
(may indicate beginning infection)

• Bleeding: hematuria, guaiac, bruising
or petechiae, mucosa or orifices q8h, no
rectal temps
• Dyspnea, crackles, nonproductive
cough, chest pain, tachypnea
• Inflammation of mucosa, breaks in
skin; use viscous xylocaine for oral pain
Administer:
PO route
• Give at same time daily, on empty
stomach
IV route
• Prepared in biologic cabinet, using
gloves, gown, mask; dilute with 10 times
volume of drug with D$_5$W or 0.9% NaCl,
(0.5 mg/ml). When withdrawing drug,
use needle with 5-micron filter provided,
remove amount needed, remove filter
and inject drug into diluent; always add
drug to diluent, not vice versa; stable for
8 hr room temperature (using D$_5$W) or
12 hr refrigerated
• Give antiemetics before IV route, on
schedule
• In those with history of seizures give
phenytoin prior to IV route, to prevent
seizures (using 0.9% NaCl) give by central venous catheter over 2 hr q6h × 4
days, use infusion pump, do not admix
Perform/provide:
• Comprehensive oral hygiene
• Strict medical asepsis, protective isolation if WBC levels are low
• Increase fluid intake to 2-3 L/day to
prevent urate deposits, calculi formation
• Store in tight container
Evaluate:
• Therapeutic response: decreased
exacerbations of chronic myelocytic
leukemia
Teach patient/family:
• About protective isolation precautions
• To avoid use of products containing
aspirin or ibuprofen, razors, commercial
mouthwash
• To report signs of anemia (fatigue,
headache, irritability, faintness, shortness
of breath)
• To report symptoms of bleeding (he-
maturia, tarry stools)
• That impotence or amenorrhea can

occur, are reversible after discontinuing treatment
• To report any changes in breathing or coughing even several years after treatment

butenafine topical
See Appendix C

butoconazole vaginal antifungal
See Appendix C

butorphanol (℞)
(byoo-tor'fa-nole)
Stadol, Stadol NS
Func. class.: Opioid analgesic
Chem. class.: Opioid antagonist, partial agonist

Controlled Substance Schedule IV
Do not confuse:
Stadol/Haldol/sotalol
Action: Depresses pain impulse transmission at the spinal cord level by interacting with opioid receptors
Uses: Moderate to severe pain
Investigational uses: Migraine headache, pain

DOSAGE AND ROUTES
• *Adult:* **IM** 1-4 mg q3-4h prn; **IV** 0.5-2 mg q3-4h prn; **INTRANASAL,** 1 spray in one nostril q3-4h; may give another dose 1-1½ hr later; repeat if needed q3-4h
• *Geriatric:* **IV** ½ adult dose at 2× the interval; **INTRANASAL,** may repeat q1-2h
Severe pain
• *Adult:* **INTRANASAL,** 1 spray in each nostril q3-4h
Renal disease
• CCr 10-50 ml/min 75% dose; CCr <10 ml/min 50% dose
Available forms: Inj 1, 2 mg/ml; nasal spray 10 mg/ml

SIDE EFFECTS
CNS: Drowsiness, dizziness, confusion, headache, sedation, euphoria, weakness, hallucinations
CV: Palpitations, bradycardia, hypotension
EENT: Tinnitus, blurred vision, miosis, diplopia, nasal congestion
GI: Nausea, vomiting, anorexia, constipation, cramps
GU: Increased urinary output, dysuria, urinary retention
INTEG: Rash, urticaria, bruising, flushing, diaphoresis, pruritus
RESP: **Respiratory depression,** pulmonary hypertension
Contraindications: Hypersensitivity to this drug or preservative, addiction (opioid), CHF, myocardial infarction
Precautions: pregnancy (C), addictive personality, lactation, increased intracranial pressure, respiratory depression, hepatic disease, renal disease, child <18 yr

PHARMACOKINETICS
IM: Onset 10-30 min, peak ½ hr, duration 3-4 hr
IV: Onset 1 min, peak 5 min, duration 2-4 hr
INTRANASAL: Onset within 15 min, peak 1-2 hr, duration 4-5 hr
Metabolized by liver; excreted by kidneys; crosses placenta; excreted in breast milk; half-life 2½-3½ hr

INTERACTIONS
⚠ Severe, fatal reactions: MAOIs
Increase: CNS effects—alcohol, opioids, sedative/hypnotics, antipsychotics, skeletal muscle relaxants
Drug/Herb
Increase: anticholinergic effect—corkwood
Increase: CNS depression—chamomile, Jamaican dogwood, kava, lavender, mistletoe, nettle, pokewood, poppy, senega, skullcap, valerian

NURSING CONSIDERATIONS
Assess:
- For decreasing output; may indicate urinary retention

🛆 For withdrawal symptoms in opioid-dependent patients: pulmonary embolus, vascular occlusion, abscesses, ulcerations
- CNS changes: dizziness, drowsiness, hallucinations, euphoria, LOC, pupil reaction
- Allergic reactions: rash, urticaria
- Respiratory dysfunction: respiratory depression, character, rate, rhythm; notify prescriber if respirations are <10/min
- Need for pain medication, physical dependence

Administer:
- With antiemetic if nausea, vomiting occur
- When pain is beginning to return; determine dosage interval by patient response

IM route
- Deeply in large muscle mass

IV route
- Undiluted at a rate of <2 mg/>3-5 min, titrate to patient response

Syringe compatibilities: Atropine, chlorproMAZINE, cimetidine, diphenhydrAMINE, droperidol, fentanyl, hydrOXYzine, meperidine, methotrimeprazine, metoclopramide, midazolam, morphine, pentazocine, perphenazine, prochlorperazine, promethazine, scopolamine, thiethylperazine

Y-site compatibilities: Allopurinol, amifostine, aztreonam, cefepime, cisatracurium, cladribine, DOXOrubicin liposome, enalaprilat, esmolol, filgrastim, fludarabine, granisetron, labetalol, melphalan, paclitaxel, piperacillin/tazobactam, propofol, remifentanil, sargramostim, tenoposide, thiotepa, vinorelbine

Perform/provide:
- Storage in light-resistant container at room temperature
- Assistance with ambulation

- Safety measures: night-light, call bell within easy reach, especially elderly

Evaluate:
- Therapeutic response: decrease in pain

Teach patient/family:
- To report any symptoms of CNS changes, allergic reactions
- That physical dependency may result when used for extended periods
- That withdrawal symptoms may occur: nausea, vomiting, cramps, fever, faintness, anorexia

Treatment of overdose: Naloxone HCl (Narcan) 0.2-0.8 mg IV, O_2, IV fluids, vasopressors

---

calcifediol (℞)
(kal-si-fe-dye′ole)
Calderol
Func. class.: Vit D analog, 25-hydroxyvitamin D_3, fat soluble vitamin
Chem. class.: Sterol

Action: Increases intestinal absorption of calcium, increases renal tubular absorption of phosphate; increases mobilization of calcium from bones, bone resorption

Uses: Metabolic bone disease with chronic renal failure, osteopenia, osteomalacia, hypocalcemia

DOSAGE AND ROUTES
- *Adult:* **PO** 300-350 mcg qwk divided into daily or every other day doses; may increase q4wk or 20-100 mcg/day or 20-200 mcg/day every other day
- *Supplement (elderly):* **PO** 20 mcg daily

Available forms: Caps 20, 50 mcg

SIDE EFFECTS
CNS: Drowsiness, headache, vertigo, fever, lethargy
CV: Dysrhythmias
EENT: Tinnitus, conjunctivitis, photophobia, rhinorrhea
GI: Nausea, diarrhea, vomiting, jaundice,

---

anorexia, dry mouth, constipation, cramps, metallic taste, thirst
GU: Polyuria, hypercalciuria, hyperphosphatemia, hematuria
MS: Myalgia, arthralgia, decreased bone development, weakness
Contraindications: Hypersensitivity, hyperphosphatemia, hypercalcemia, vit D toxicity
Precautions: Pregnancy (C), renal calculi, lactation, CV disease, elderly

PHARMACOKINETICS

Absorbed by the small intestine; stored in liver and fat deposits, activated in kidneys, excreted in bile and feces; peak 4 hr, duration 15-20 days; half-life 12-22 days

INTERACTIONS

Hypercalcemia: thiazide diuretics, calcium supplements
Cardiac dysrhythmias: cardiac glycosides
Hypermagnesemia: magnesium antacids
Toxicity: other vit D products
Increase: metabolism of vit D—phenytoin
Decrease: absorption of calcifediol—cholestyramine, colestipol, mineral oil, fat-soluble vitamins
Decrease: effect of this drug—corticosteroids
Drug/Food
Dairy products, other high-calcium foods may cause hypercalcemia
Drug/Lab Test
False increase: Cholesterol
Interfere: Alk phosphatase, electrolytes

NURSING CONSIDERATIONS
Assess:
• BUN, urinary calcium, AST, ALT, cholesterol, creatinine, uric acid, chloride, magnesium, electrolytes, urine pH, phosphate; may increase; calcium should be kept at 9-10 mg/dl, vit D 50-135 international units/dl, phosphate 70 mg/dl, alk phosphatase may be decreased

• For increased blood level, since toxic reactions may occur rapidly
• For dry mouth, metallic taste, polyuria, bone pain, muscle weakness, headache, fatigue, tinnitus, change in LOC, irregular pulse, dysrhythmias, increased respirations, anorexia, nausea, vomiting, cramps, diarrhea, constipation; may indicate hypercalcemia
• Renal status: decreased urinary output (oliguria, anuria), edema in extremities, weight gain 5 lb, periorbital edema
• Nutritional status, diet for sources of vit D (milk, some seafood), calcium (dairy products, dark green vegetables), phosphates (dairy products)
Administer:
• Do not break, crush, or chew caps
• May be taken without regard to food
• May be increased q4wk depending on blood level
Perform/provide:
• Storage in tight, light-resistant container at room temperature
• Restriction of sodium, potassium if required; ensure adequate calcium intake
• Restriction of fluids if required for chronic renal failure
Evaluate:
• Therapeutic response: calcium levels 9-10 mg/dl, decreasing symptoms of bone disease
Teach patient/family:
• The symptoms of hypercalcemia (renal stones, nausea, vomiting, anorexia, lethargy, thirst, bone or flank pain)
• About foods rich in calcium
• To advise prescriber of all other medications, supplements taken

calcitonin (human) (R)
(kal-sih-toh'nin)
Cibacalcin
calcitonin (salmon) (R)
Calcimir, Miacalcin, Miacalcin
Nasal Spray, Osteocalcin,
Salmonine
Func. class.: Parathyroid agents
(calcium regulator)
Chem. class.: Polypeptide hormone

Action: Decreases bone resorption,
blood calcium levels; increases deposits
of calcium in bones; opposes parathyroid
hormone
Uses: Paget's disease, postmenopausal
osteoporosis, hypercalcemia

DOSAGE AND ROUTES
Human
Paget's disease
• *Adult:* **SUBCUT** 0.5 mg/day initially;
may require 0.5 mg bid × 6 mo, then
decrease until symptoms reappear
Salmon
Postmenopausal osteoporosis
• *Adult:* **SUBCUT/IM** 100 international
units/day; **NASAL** 200 international units
(1 spray) daily alternating nostrils daily,
activate pump before 1st dose
Paget's disease
• *Adult:* **SUBCUT/IM** 100 international
units daily, maintenance 50-100 international units daily or every other day
Hypercalcemia
• Adult: **SUBCUT/IM** 4 international
units/kg q12h, increase to 8 international
units/kg q6h if response is unsatisfactory
Available forms: *Human:* **INJ (SUB-
CUT)** 500 mg vial; *salmon:* **INJ** 100
international units, 200 international
units/ml, **NASAL** spray 200 international
units/actuation

SIDE EFFECTS
CNS: Headache, tetany, chills, weakness,
dizziness, fever
CV: Chest pressure
EENT: Nasal congestion, eye pain

GI: Nausea, diarrhea, vomiting, anorexia,
abdominal pain, salty taste, epigastric
pain
GU: Diuresis, nocturia, urine sediment,
frequency
INTEG: Rash, flushing, pruritus of ear-
lobes, edema of feet, reaction at inj site
MS: Swelling, tingling of hands
RESP: Dyspnea
SYST: **Anaphylaxis**
Contraindications: Hypersensitivity
Precautions: Pregnancy (C), renal
disease, children, lactation, osteogenic
sarcoma, pernicious anemia

PHARMACOKINETICS
IM/SUBCUT: Onset 15 min, peak 4
hr, duration 8-24 hr; metabolized by
kidneys, excreted as inactive metabolites via kidneys

NURSING CONSIDERATIONS
Assess:
• GI symptoms, polyuria, flushing, head
swelling, tingling, headache; may indicate hypercalcemia
• Nutritional status; diet for sources of
vit D (milk, some seafood), calcium
(dairy products, dark green vegetables),
phosphates
• BUN, creatinine, uric acid, chloride,
electrolytes, urine pH, urinary calcium,
magnesium, phosphate, urinalysis (calcium should be kept at 9-10 mg/dl, vit D
50-135 international units/dl), alk phosphatase baseline, q3-6mo, monitor urine
hydroproline in Paget's disease
• Increased drug level, since toxic reactions occur rapidly; have parenteral
calcium on hand if calcium level drops
too low; check for tetany (irritability,
paresthesia, nervousness, muscle twitching, seizures, tetanic spasms)
• Urine for sediment
Administer:
SUBCUT route (Human)
• By SUBCUT route only; rotate inj sites;
use within 6 hr of reconstitution; give at
bedtime to minimize nausea, vomiting

IM route (Salmon)
• After test dose of 10 international units/ml, 0.1 ml intradermally; watch 15 min; give only with epINEPHrine and emergency meds available
• IM inj slowly in deep muscle mass; rotate sites

Perform/provide:
• Storage at <77° F (25° C); protect from light

Evaluate:
• Therapeutic response: calcium levels 9-10 mg/dl, decreasing symptoms of Paget's disease

Teach patient/family:
• The method of inj if patient will be responsible for self-medication
• To report difficulty swallowing or any change in side effects to prescriber immediately

Nasal
• To use alternating nostrils for nasal spray

---

calcitriol (R)
(kal-sih-try′ole)
Calcijex, Rocaltrol (1,25-dihydroxycholecalciferol), vitamin D₃
Func. class.: Parathyroid agent (calcium regulator)
Chem. class.: Vit D hormone

Do not confuse:
calcitriol/Calciferol

Action: Increases intestinal absorption of calcium, provides calcium for bones, increases renal tubular resorption of phosphate

Uses: Hypocalcemia in chronic renal disease, hyperparathyroidism pseudohypoparathyroidism

DOSAGE AND ROUTES

Hypocalcemia
• *Adult:* IV 0.5 mcg tid, initially; may increase by 0.25-0.5 mcg/dose q2-4wk; 0.5-3 mcg tid maintenance

Predialysis
• *Adult:* PO 0.25 mcg/day, max 0.5 mcg/day
• *Child:* PO 0.25 mcg/day, max 0.5 mcg/day
• *Child <3 yr:* PO 10-15 mcg/kg/day

Hypocalcemia during chronic dialysis
• *Adult:* PO 0.5-3 mcg/day
• *Child:* PO 0.25-2 mcg/day

Renal osteodystrophy
• *Adult:* PO 0.25 mcg every other day-3 mcg/day
• *Child:* PO 0.014-0.041 mcg/kg/day

Hypoparathyroidism
• *Adult:* PO 0.25-2.7 mcg/day
• *Child:* PO 0.04-0.08 mcg/kg/day

Available forms: Caps 0.25, 0.5 mcg; inj 1 mcg, 2 mcg/ml

SIDE EFFECTS

CNS: Drowsiness, headache, vertigo, fever, lethargy
CV: Palpitations
EENT: Blurred vision, photophobia
GI: Nausea, diarrhea, vomiting, jaundice, anorexia, dry mouth, constipation, cramps, metallic taste
GU: Polyuria, hypercalciuria, hyperphosphatemia, hematuria, thirst
MS: Myalgia, arthralgia, decreased bone development, weakness

Contraindications: Hypersensitivity, hyperphosphatemia, hypercalcemia, vit D toxicity
Precautions: Pregnancy (C), renal calculi, lactation, CV disease

PHARMACOKINETICS

PO: Absorbed readily from GI tract, peak 10-12 hr, duration 3-5 days, half-life 3-6 hr; undergoes hepatic recycling, excreted in bile

INTERACTIONS

Hypercalcemia: thiazide diuretics, calcium supplements
Cardiac dysrhythmias: cardiac glycosides, verapamil
Hypermagnesemia: magnesium antacids
Toxicity: other vit D products

Side effects: *italics* = common; ***bold italics*** = life-threatening

Increase: metabolism of vit D—phenytoin
Decrease: absorption of calcitriol—cholestyramine, mineral oil, fat-soluble vitamins

Drug/Food
Large amounts of high-calcium foods may cause hypercalcemia

Drug/Lab Test
False increase: Cholesterol
Interfere: Alk phosphatase, electrolytes

NURSING CONSIDERATIONS

Assess:
• BUN, urinary calcium, AST, ALT, cholesterol, creatinine, albumin, uric acid, chloride, magnesium, electrolytes, urine pH, phosphate; may increase calcium, should be kept at 9-10 mg/dl, vit D 50-135 international units/dl, phosphate 70 mg/dl
• Alk phosphatase; may be decreased
• For increased drug level, since toxic reactions may occur rapidly
• For dry mouth, metallic taste, polyuria, bone pain, muscle weakness, headache, fatigue, change in LOC, dysrhythmias, increased respirations, anorexia, nausea, vomiting, cramps, diarrhea, constipation; may indicate hypercalcemia
• Renal status: decreased urinary output (oliguria, anuria), edema in extremities, weight gain 5-7 lb, periorbital edema
• Nutritional status, diet for sources of vit D (milk, some seafood); calcium (dairy products, dark green vegetables), phosphates (dairy products) must be avoided

Administer:
PO route
• Do not break, crush, or chew caps
• Give without regard to meals
IV route
• Give by direct IV over 1 min
Perform/provide:
• Storage protected from light, heat, moisture
• Restriction of sodium, potassium if required
• Restriction of fluids if required for chronic renal failure
Evaluate:
• Therapeutic response: calcium 9-10

mg/dl, decreasing symptoms of hypocalcemia, hypoparathyroidism

Teach patient/family:
• The symptoms of hypercalcemia (renal stones, nausea, vomiting, anorexia, lethargy, thirst, bone or flank pain)
• About foods rich in calcium
• To avoid products with sodium: cured meats, dairy products, cold cuts, olives, beets, pickles, soups, meat tenderizers in chronic renal failure
• To avoid products with potassium: oranges, bananas, dried fruit, peas, dark green leafy vegetables, milk, melons, beans in chronic renal failure
• To avoid OTC products containing calcium, potassium, or sodium in chronic renal failure
• To avoid all preparations containing vit D
• To monitor weight weekly

---

calcium carbonate
(po-otc, iv-℞)
Alka-Mints, Amitone, Apo-Cal ✖, BioCal, Calcarb, Calci-Chew, Calci-Mix, Calcilac, Calcite ✖, Calglycine ✖, Cal-Plus, Calsan ✖, Caltrate 600, Caltrate Jr., Chooz, Dicarbosil, Equilet, Gencalc, Liquid-Cal, Liquid-Cal-600, Maalox Antacid Caplets, Mallamint, Mylanta Lozenges ✖, Nephro-Calci, Nu-Cal ✖, Os-Cal 500, Oysco 500, Oystercal 500, Oyst-Cal 500, Rolaids Calcium Rich, Titralac, Tums, Tums E-X Extra Strength

calcium acetate (otc)
(kal′see-um ass′e-tate)
Calphron, PhosLo
Func. class.: Antacid, calcium supplement
Chem. class.: Calcium product

Action: Neutralizes gastric acidity
Uses: Antacid, calcium supplement; not

suitable for chronic therapy, hyperphosphatemia, hypertension in pregnancy, osteoporosis, prevention, treatment of hypocalcemia, hyperparathyroidism

DOSAGE AND ROUTES

Antacid
• *Adult:* **PO** 0.5-1.5 g or 2 pieces of gum 1 hr pc and at bedtime

Prevention of hypocalcemia, depletion, osteoporosis
• *Adult:* **PO** 1-2 g daily

Hyperphosphatemia
• *Adult:* **PO** 1 g or more in divided doses

Hypertension in pregnancy
• *Adult:* **PO** 500 mg tid during 3rd trimester

Available forms: Chewable tabs 350, 420, 450, 500, 750, 1000, 1250 mg; tabs 500, 600, 650, 1000, 1250 mg; gum 300, 450, 500 mg; susp 1250 mg/5 ml; lozenges 600 mg; caps 1250 mg; powder 6.5 g/packet; calcium acetate: tabs 250 mg (65 mg Ca), 667 mg (169 mg Ca), 668 mg (169 mg Ca), 1 g (250 mg Ca); caps 500 mg (125 mg Ca)

SIDE EFFECTS

GI: Constipation, anorexia, nausea, vomiting, flatulence, diarrhea, rebound hyperacidity, eructation
Contraindications: Hypersensitivity, hypercalcemia, hyperparathyroidism, bone tumors
Precautions: Pregnancy (C), elderly, fluid restriction, decreased GI motility, GI obstruction, dehydration, renal disease, lactation

PHARMACOKINETICS

⅓ of dose absorbed by small intestine, onset 20 min, duration 20-180 min, excreted in feces and urine, crosses placenta

INTERACTIONS

Increase: plasma levels of quinidine, amphetamines
Decrease: levels of salicylates, calcium

channel blockers, ketoconazole, tetracyclines, iron salts, quinolone antibiotics
Drug/Herb
Increase: action/side effects—lily of the valley, pheasant's eye, shark cartilage, squill
Drug/Lab Test
False increase: Chloride
False positive: Benzodiazepines
False decrease: Magnesium, oxylate, lipase

NURSING CONSIDERATIONS

Assess:
• Calcium (serum, urine), calcium should be 8.5-10.5 mg/dl, urine calcium should be 150 mg/day, monitor weekly
⚠ Milk-alkali syndrome: nausea, vomiting, disorientation, headache
• Constipation; increase bulk in the diet if needed
• Hypercalcemia: headache, nausea, vomiting, confusion

Administer:
PO route
• As antacid 1 hr pc and at bedtime
• As supplement 1½ hr pc and at bedtime
• Only with regular tablets or capsules; do not give with enteric-coated tablets
• Laxatives or stool softeners if constipation occurs

Evaluate:
• Therapeutic response: absence of pain, decreased acidity

Teach patient/family:
• To increase fluids to 2 L unless contraindicated, to add bulk to diet for constipation, notify prescriber of constipation
• Not to switch antacids unless directed by prescriber, not to use as antacid for >2 wk without approval by prescriber
• That therapeutic dose recommendations are figured as elemental calcium

calcium chloride
calcium gluceptate
calcium gluconate
calcium lactate (℞)
Func. class.: Electrolyte replacement—calcium product

Action: Cation needed for maintenance of nervous, muscular, skeletal function, enzyme reactions, normal cardiac contractility, coagulation of blood; affects secretory activity of endocrine, exocrine glands

Uses: Prevention and treatment of hypocalcemia, hypermagnesemia, hypoparathyroidism, neonatal tetany, cardiac toxicity caused by hyperkalemia, lead colic, hyperphosphatemia, vit D deficiency, osteoporosis prophylaxis, calcium antagonist toxicity (calcium channel blocker toxicity)

DOSAGE AND ROUTES
Calcium gluceptate
• *Adult:* **IV** 5-20 ml; **IM** 2-5 ml
Calcium chloride
• *Adult:* **IV** 500 mg-1 g q1-3d as indicated by serum calcium levels, give at <1 ml/min; **IV** 200-800 mg injected in ventricle of heart
• *Child:* **IV** 25 mg/kg over several min
Calcium gluconate
• *Adult:* **PO** 0.5-2 g bid-qid; **IV** 0.5-2 g at 0.5 ml/min (10% solution); max **IV** dose 3 g
• *Child:* **PO/IV** 500 mg/kg/day in divided doses
Calcium lactate
• *Adult:* **PO** 325 mg-1.3 g tid with meals
• *Child:* **PO** 500 mg/kg/day in divided doses
Available forms: Many; check product listings

SIDE EFFECTS
CV: Shortened QT, heart block, hypotension, bradycardia, *dysrhythmias; cardiac arrest (IV)*
GI: Vomiting, nausea, constipation

HYPERCALCEMIA: Drowsiness, lethargy, muscle weakness, headache, constipation, *coma,* anorexia, nausea, vomiting, polyuria, thirst
INTEG: Pain, burning at IV site, severe venous thrombosis, necrosis, extravasation

Contraindications: Hypercalcemia, digitalis toxicity, ventricular fibrillation, renal calculi
Precautions: Pregnancy (C), lactation, children, renal disease, respiratory disease, cor pulmonale, digitalized patient, respiratory failure

PHARMACOKINETICS
Crosses placenta, enters breast milk, excreted via urine and feces; half-life unknown
PO: Onset, peak, duration unknown; absorption (PO) from GI tract
IV: Onset immediate, duration ½-2 hr

INTERACTIONS
Milk-alkali syndrome: antacids
Increase: dysrhythmias—digitalis glycosides
Increase: toxicity—verapamil
Increase: hypercalcemia—thiazide diuretics
Decrease: absorption of—fluoroquinolones, tetracyclines, iron salts, phenytoin, when calcium is taken PO
Decrease: effects of—atenolol, verapamil
Drug/Herb
Increase: action/side effects—lily of the valley, pheasant's eye, shark cartilage, squill
Drug/Lab Test
Increase: 11-OHCS
Decrease: 17-OHCS
False decrease: Magnesium

NURSING CONSIDERATIONS
Assess:
• ECG for decreased QT and T wave inversion: hypercalcemia, drug should

be reduced or discontinued, consider cardiac monitoring
• Calcium levels during treatment (8.5-11.5 g/dl is normal level)
• Cardiac status: rate, rhythm, CVP (PWP, PAWP if being monitored directly)

Administer:

PO route
• With or following meals to enhance absorption

IM route
• IM inj may cause severe burning, necrosis, tissue sloughing; warm sol to body temp before administering (only gluconate/gluceptate)

IV route
• Undiluted or diluted with equal amounts of NS to a 5% sol for inj, give 0.5-1 ml/min
• Through small-bore needle into large vein; if extravasation occurs, necrosis will result (IV)
• Remain recumbent ½ hr after IV dose

Calcium chloride
Additive compatibilities: Amikacin, amphotericin B, ampicillin, ascorbic acid, bretylium, ceftriaxone, cephapirin, chloramphenicol, DOPamine, hydrocortisone, isoproterenol, lidocaine, methicillin, norepinephrine, penicillin G potassium, penicillin G sodium, pentobarbital, phenobarbital, verapamil, vit B/C
Syringe compatibilities: Milrinone
Y-site compatibilities: Amrinone, DOBUTamine, epINEPHrine, esmolol, morphine, paclitaxel

Calcium gluceptate
Additive compatibilities: Ascorbic acid inj, isoproterenol, lidocaine, norepinephrine, phytonadione, sodium bicarbonate

Calcium gluconate
Additive compatibilities: Amikacin, aminophylline, ascorbic acid injection, bretylium, cephapirin, chloramphenicol, cisatracurium, corticotropin, dimenhyDRINATE, DOXOrubicin liposome, erythromycin, furosemide, heparin, hydrocortisone, lidocaine, magnesium sulfate, methicillin, norepinephrine, penicillin G

potassium, penicillin G sodium, phenobarbital, potassium chloride, remifentanil, tobramycin, vancomycin, verapamil, vit B/C
Syringe compatibilities: Aldesleukin, allopurinol, amifostine, aztreonam, cefazolin, cefepime, ciprofloxacin, cladribine, DOBUTamine, enalaprilat, epINEPHrine, famotidine, filgrastim, granisetron, heparin/hydrocortisone, labetalol, melphalan, midazolam, netilmicin, piperacillin/tazobactam, potassium chloride, prochlorperazine, propofol, sargramostim, tacrolimus, teniposide, thiotepa, tolazoline, vinorelbine, vit B/C

Perform/provide:
• Seizure precautions: padded side rails, decreased stimuli (noise, light); place airway suction equipment, padded mouth gag if Ca levels are low
• Store at room temperature

Evaluate:
• Therapeutic response: decreased twitching, paresthesias, muscle spasms, absence of tremors, convulsions, dysrhythmias, dyspnea, laryngospasm, negative Chvostek's sign, negative Trousseau's sign

Teach patient/family:
• To add foods high in vit D
• To add calcium-rich foods to diet: dairy products, shellfish, dark green leafy vegetables; decrease oxalate-rich and zinc-rich foods: nuts, legumes, chocolate, spinach, soy
• To prevent injuries, avoid immobilization

---

calcium polycarbophil (otc)
(pol-ee-kar'boe-fil)
Equalactin, Fiberall, FiberCon, Fiber-Lax, Mitrolan
Func. class.: Laxative
Chem. class.: Bulk-forming

Action: Attracts water, expands in intestine to increase peristalsis; also absorbs excess water in stool; decreases diarrhea

Uses: Constipation, irritable bowel syndrome (diarrhea), acute, nonspecific diarrhea

DOSAGE AND ROUTES
• *Adult:* **PO** 1 g daily-qid prn, not to exceed 6 g/24 hr
• *Child 6-12 yr:* **PO** 500 mg bid prn, not to exceed 3 g/24 hr
• *Child 3-6 yr:* **PO** 500 mg bid prn, not to exceed 1.5 g/24 hr
Available forms: Chew tabs 500, 1000 mg; tabs 500 mg

SIDE EFFECTS
GI: **Obstruction,** abdominal distention, flatus, laxative dependence
Contraindications: Hypersensitivity, GI obstruction
Precautions: Pregnancy (C), lactation

PHARMACOKINETICS
PO: Onset 12-24 min, peak 1-3 days

INTERACTIONS
Drug/Herb
Increase: action/side effects—flax, lily of the valley, pheasant's eye, senna, squill

NURSING CONSIDERATIONS
Assess:
• Cause of constipation; identify whether fluids, bulk, or exercise is missing from lifestyle, constipating drugs
• Cramping, rectal bleeding, nausea, vomiting; if these symptoms occur, drug should be discontinued
Administer:
• Alone for better absorption; do not take within 1-2 hr of other drugs
• In morning or evening
Evaluate:
• Therapeutic response: decreased constipation
Teach patient/family:
• Not to use laxatives for long-term therapy; laxative dependence will result
• That normal bowel movements do not always occur daily
• Not to use in presence of abdominal pain, nausea, vomiting
• To notify prescriber if constipation is unrelieved or if symptoms of electrolyte imbalance occur: muscle cramps, pain, weakness, dizziness
• To chew thoroughly (chew tab) and follow with 6-8 oz water

Rarely Used
calfactant (R)
(cal-fak'tant)
Infasurf
Func. class.: Natural lung surfactant extract

Uses: Prevention and treatment (rescue) of respiratory distress syndrome in premature infants

DOSAGE AND ROUTES
• *Newborn:* **INTRATRACHEAL INSTILL:** 3 ml/kg of birth wt, given as 2 doses of 1.5 ml/kg, repeat doses of 3 ml/kg of birth wt until up to 3 doses 12 hr apart have been given

candesartan (R)
(can-deh-sar'tan)
Atacand
Func. class.: Antihypertensive
Chem. class.: Angiotensin II receptor (type AT_1)

Action: Blocks the vasoconstrictor and aldosterone-secreting effects of angiotensin II; selectively blocks the binding of angiotensin II to the AT_1 receptor found in tissues
Uses: Hypertension, alone or in combination

DOSAGE AND ROUTES
• *Adult:* **PO,** single agent 16 mg daily initially in patients who are not volume depleted, range 8-32 mg/day; with diuretic, or volume depletion 2-32 mg/day as single dose or divided bid

Renal disease
• *Adult*: **PO** Give lowest possible dose
Available forms: Tabs 4, 8, 16, 32 mg

SIDE EFFECTS

CNS: Dizziness, fatigue, headache
CV: Chest pain, peripheral edema
EENT: Sinusitis, rhinitis, pharyngitis
GI: Diarrhea, nausea, abdominal pain,
vomiting
*GU: **Renal failure***
MS: Arthralgia, pain
RESP: Cough, upper respiratory infection
*SYST: **Angioedema***

Contraindications: Pregnancy (D)
2nd/3rd trimesters, hypersensitivity
Precautions: Pregnancy (C) 1st trimester, hypersensitivity to ACE inhibitors,
lactation, children, elderly

PHARMACOKINETICS

Extensively metabolized, excreted in
urine and feces

INTERACTIONS

Toxicity/death: aconite

Drug/Herb
Increase or decrease: effect—
astragalus, cola tree
Increase: effect—barberry, betony,
black catechu, black cohosh, bloodroot,
broom, burdock, cats claw, dandelion,
goldenseal, Irish moss, Jamaican dogwood, kelp, khella, mistletoe, parsley,
Queen Anne's lace, rue
Decrease: effect—coltsfoot, guarana,
khat, licorice

NURSING CONSIDERATIONS

Assess:
• For angioedema: facial swelling, difficulty breathing (rare)
• For pregnancy, this drug can cause
fetal death when given in pregnancy
• Response and adverse reactions especially in renal disease
• B/P, pulse q4h; note rate, rhythm,
quality; electrolytes: K, Na, Cl; baselines
in renal, hepatic studies before therapy
begins
Administer:
• Without regard to meals
Evaluate:
• Therapeutic response: decreased B/P
Teach patient/family:
• To comply with dosage schedule, even
if feeling better
• To notify prescriber of mouth sores,
fever, swelling of hands or feet, irregular
heartbeat, chest pain
• That excessive perspiration, dehydration, vomiting, diarrhea may lead to fall
in blood pressure; to consult prescriber
if these occur
• That drug may cause dizziness,
fainting; light-headedness may occur
• To rise slowly to sitting or standing
position to minimize orthostatic hypotension
• To notify prescriber immediately if
pregnant; not to use during lactation
• To avoid all OTC medications, unless
approved by prescriber; to inform all
health care providers of medication use
• To use proper technique for obtaining
B/P and acceptable parameters

---

capecitabine (℞)

(cap-eh-sit′ah-bean)
Xeloda
Func. class.: Antineoplastic, antimetabolite
Chem. class.: Fluoropyrimidine
carbamate

Do not confuse:
Xeloda/Xenical
Action: Competes with physiologic
substrate of DNA synthesis, thus interfering with cell replication in the S phase of
cell cycle (before mitosis), also interferes with RNA and protein synthesis;
drug is converted to 5-FU
Uses: Monotherapy for paclitaxel, anthracycline resistant, metastatic breast,
colorectal cancer when 5-FU monotherapy is preferred; treatment of colorectal cancer patients who have under-

gone complete resection of their primary tumor

DOSAGE AND ROUTES

• *Adult:* **PO** 2500 mg/m²/day in 2 divided doses q12h at end of meal × 2 wk, then 1 wk rest period; given in 3 wk cycles; may be combined with docetaxel, when capecitabine dose is lowered; follow the NCIC (National Cancer Institute of Canada) common toxicity criteria

Available forms: Tabs 150, 500 mg

SIDE EFFECTS

CNS: Dizziness, headache, *paresthesia, fatigue,* insomnia

*GI: Nausea, vomiting, anorexia, diarrhea, stomatitis, abdominal pain, constipation, dyspepsia, **intestinal obstruction***

HEMA: **Neutropenia, lymphopenia, thrombocytopenia,** anemia

INTEG: Hand and foot syndrome, dermatitis, nail disorder

OTHER: Hyperbilirubinemia, eye irritation, edema, myalgia, limb pain, *pyrexia,* dehydration

Contraindications: Pregnancy (D), hypersensitivity to 5-FU, infants, severe renal impairment (CCr <30 ml/min)

Precautions: Renal disease, hepatic disease, lactation, children, elderly

PHARMACOKINETICS

Readily absorbed, peak 1½ hr; food decreases absorption; extensively metabolized in the liver; elimination half-life 45 min

INTERACTIONS

Increase: toxicity—leucovorin

Increase: capecitabine levels—antacids (aluminum, magnesium)

Increase: risk of bleeding—warfarin

Increase: phenytoin level—phenytoin

NURSING CONSIDERATIONS

Assess:

• CBC (RBC, Hct, Hgb), differential, platelet count weekly; withhold drug if

WBC is <4000/mm³, platelet count is <75,000/mm³, or RBC, Hct, Hgb low; notify prescriber of these results

• Renal studies: BUN, serum uric acid, urine CCr, electrolytes before and during therapy

• Monitor temp q4h; fever may indicate beginning infection; no rectal temps

• Hepatic studies before and during therapy: bilirubin, ALT, AST, alk phosphatase, as needed or monthly

• Bleeding: hematuria, heme-positive stools, bruising or petechiae, mucosa or orifices q8h

• Dyspnea, crackles, unproductive cough, chest pain, tachypnea, fatigue, increased pulse, pallor, lethargy; personality changes, with high doses

• For hand and foot syndrome: paresthesia, tingling, painful/painless swelling, blistering, erythema with severe pain of hands or feet

• For toxicity: severe diarrhea, nausea, vomiting, stomatitis

• Buccal cavity q8h for dryness, sores or ulceration, white patches, oral pain, bleeding, dysphagia

• GI symptoms: frequency of stools, cramping, if severe diarrhea occurs, fluid and electrolytes may need to be given

Administer:

• With water within ½ hour of breakfast and dinner

Perform/provide:

• Rinsing of mouth tid-qid with water, club soda; brushing of teeth bid-tid with soft brush or cotton-tipped applicators for stomatitis; use unwaxed dental floss

Evaluate:

• Therapeutic response: decreased tumor size, spread of malignancy

Teach patient/family:

• To avoid foods with citric acid, hot or rough texture if stomatitis is present

• To avoid pregnancy while on this drug; to avoid using while lactating

• Not to double dose, if dose is missed

⚠ To immediately report severe diarrhea, vomiting, stomatitis, fever over 100° F (37.8° C), hand and foot syndrome, anorexia

• To report signs of infection: increased temp, sore throat, flulike symptoms
• To report signs of anemia: fatigue, headache, faintness, shortness of breath, irritability
• To report bleeding; to avoid use of razors, commercial mouthwash

---

captopril (℞)
(kap'toe-pril)
Capoten, Novo-Captoril ✦
Func. class.: Antihypertensive
Chem. class.: Angiotensin-converting enzyme inhibitor (ACE)

Do not confuse:
captopril/Capitrol/carvedilol
Action: Selectively suppresses renin-angiotensin-aldosterone system; inhibits ACE; preventing conversion of angiotensin I to angiotensin II
Uses: Hypertension, CHF, left ventricular dysfunction after MI, diabetic nephropathy

DOSAGE AND ROUTES
Malignant hypertension
• *Adult:* **PO** 25 mg increasing q2h until desired response, not to exceed 450 mg/day
Hypertension
• *Adult:* **PO** initial dose: 25 mg bid-tid; may increase to 50 mg bid-tid at 1-2 wk intervals; usual range: 25-150 mg bid-tid; max 450 mg
• *Child:* **PO** 0.3-0.5 mg/kg/dose, titrate up to 6 mg/kg/day in 2-4 divided doses
• *Neonate:* **PO** 10 mcg (0.01 mg)/kg bid-tid, may increase as needed
CHF
• *Adult:* **PO** 12.5 mg bid-tid; may increase to 50 mg bid-tid; after 14 days, may increase to 150 mg tid if needed
LVD after MI
• *Adult:* **PO** 50 mg tid, may begin treatment 3 days after MI; give 6.25 mg as a single dose, then 12.5 mg tid, increase to 25 mg tid for several days, then to 50 mg tid

Diabetic nephropathy
• *Adult:* **PO** 25 mg tid
Renal dose
• Adult: **PO** 6.25-12.5 mg bid-tid
• *Child:* **PO** 150 mcg (0.15)/kg tid
Available forms: Tabs 12.5, 25, 50, 100 mg

SIDE EFFECTS
CNS: Fever, chills
CV: Hypotension, postural hypotension, *tachycardia,* angina
GI: Loss of taste, increased LFTs
GU: Impotence, dysuria, nocturia, proteinuria, ***nephrotic syndrome, acute reversible renal failure,*** polyuria, oliguria, urinary frequency
*HEMA: **Neutropenia, agranulocytosis, pancytopenia, thrombocytopenia,*** anemia
INTEG: Rash
*MISC: **Angioedema,*** hyperkalemia
*RESP: **Bronchospasm,** dyspnea, cough*
Contraindications: Pregnancy (D) 2nd/3rd trimesters, hypersensitivity, lactation, heart block, children, potassium-sparing diuretics, bilateral renal artery stenosis
Precautions: Pregnancy (C) 1st trimester, dialysis patients, hypovolemia, leukemia, scleroderma, SLE, blood dyscrasias, CHF, diabetes mellitus, renal disease, thyroid disease, COPD, asthma

PHARMACOKINETICS
PO: Peak 1 hr; duration 6-12 hr; half-life <2 hr, increased in renal disease; metabolized by liver (metabolites), excreted in urine; crosses placenta; excreted in breast milk, small amounts

INTERACTIONS
Possible toxicity: lithium, digoxin
Hypoglycemia: insulin, oral antidiabetics
Do not use with potassium-sparing diuretics, sympathomimetics, potassium supplements
Increase: hypotension—diuretics, other

Side effects: *italics* = common; ***bold italics*** = life-threatening

antihypertensives, phenothiazines, nitrates, acute alcohol ingestion
Decrease: captopril effect—antacids, NSAIDs

Drug/Herb
Increase: toxicity/death—aconite
Increase: antihypertensive effect—barberry, betony, black catechu, black cohosh, bloodroot, broom, burdock, cat's claw, dandelion, goldenseal, Irish moss, Jamaican dogwood, kelp, khella, mistletoe, parsley
Increase or decrease: antihypertensive effect—astragalus, cola tree
Decrease: antihypertensive effect—coltsfoot, guarana, khat, licorice

Drug/Lab Test
Increase: AST, ALT, alk phosphatase, bilirubin, uric acid, glucose
False positive: Urine acetone, ANA titer

NURSING CONSIDERATIONS
Assess:
• Blood studies: decreased platelets; WBC with diff baseline and periodically q3mo, if neutrophils <1000/mm³, discontinue treatment (recommended with collagen-vascular or renal disease)
• B/P, pulse rates baseline, frequently
• Renal studies: protein, BUN, creatinine; watch for raised levels that may indicate nephrotic syndrome
• Baselines in renal, hepatic studies before therapy begins and periodically, increased LFTs, uric acid and glucose may be increased
• Edema in feet, legs daily, weight daily in CHF
• Allergic reaction: rash, fever, pruritus, urticaria; discontinue drug if antihistamines fail to help
• Symptoms of CHF: edema, dyspnea, wet crackles, B/P

Administer:
• 1 hr ac or 2 hr pc
• May crush tab and dissolve in water, give within ½ hr, make sure tab is completely dissolved

Perform/provide:
• Storage in tight container at 86° F (30° C) or less

Evaluate:
• Therapeutic response: decrease in B/P in hypertension, edema, moist crackles (CHF)

Teach patient/family:
• That tabs may be crushed and mixed with food; to take 1 hr before meals or 2 hr pc; not to discontinue drug abruptly
• Not to use OTC products (cough, cold, or allergy) unless directed by prescriber
• To avoid sunlight or wear sunscreen if in sunlight; photosensitivity may occur
• To comply with dosage schedule, even if feeling better
• To rise slowly to sitting or standing position to minimize orthostatic hypotension
• To notify prescriber of mouth sores, sore throat, fever, swelling of hands or feet, irregular heartbeat, chest pain, signs of angioedema
• That excessive perspiration, dehydration, vomiting; diarrhea may lead to fall in B/P; consult prescriber if these occur
• That dizziness, fainting, lightheadedness may occur during first few days of therapy
• That skin rash or impaired perspiration may occur
• How to take B/P and when to notify prescriber
• To report if pregnancy is suspected or planned

Treatment of overdose: 0.9% NaCl IV/INF; hemodialysis

---

carbachol ophthalmic
See Appendix C

---

carbamazepine (R)

(kar-ba-maz′e-peen)

Apo-Carbamazepine ✤, Atretol, Carbatrol, Epitol, Equetro, Novo-Carbamaz ✤, Tegretol, Tegretol CR ✤, Tegretol-XR

Func. class.: Anticonvulsant

Chem. class.: Iminostilbene derivative

Do not confuse:

Tegretol/Toradol

Action: Exact mechanism unknown; appears to decrease polysynaptic responses and block posttetanic potentiation

Uses: Tonic-clonic, complex-partial, mixed seizures; trigeminal neuralgia, bipolar disorder

Investigational uses: Diabetes insipidus, neurogenic pain, schizophrenia, psychotic behavior with dementia, rectal administration, diabetic neuropathy, restless leg syndrome

DOSAGE AND ROUTES

Seizures

• *Adult and child >12 yr:* **PO** 200 mg bid, may be increased by 200 mg/day in divided doses q6-8h; maintenance 800-1200 mg/day maximum 1600 mg/day (adult); max child 12-15 yr 1000 mg/day; max child >15 yr 1200 mg/day; adjustment is needed to minimum dose to control seizures; **EXT REL** give bid; rectal administration of oral susp 200 mg/10 ml or 6 mg/kg as a single dose

• *Child 6-12 yr:* **PO** tabs 100 mg bid or susp 50 mg qid; may increase by <100 mg qwk; max 1000 mg/day **EXT REL** tabs daily-bid

• *Child <6 yr:* **PO** 10-20 mg/kg/day in 2-3 divided doses, may increase qwk

Trigeminal neuralgia

• *Adult:* **PO** 100 mg bid with meals; may increase 100 mg q12h until pain subsides, not to exceed 1200 mg/day; maintenance is 200-400 mg bid

Bipolar disorder

• *Adult:* **PO** (Equetro only) 200 mg bid, may adjust dose by 200 mg daily to desired response, max 1600 mg/day

Available forms: Tabs, chewable 100, 200 mg; tabs 200 mg; ext rel tabs (XR) 100, 200, 400 mg; oral susp 100 mg/5 ml; ext rel caps (Carbatrol) 200, 300 mg

SIDE EFFECTS

CNS: Drowsiness, dizziness, unsteadiness, confusion, fatigue, ***paralysis,*** headache, hallucinations, ***worsening of seizures,*** speech disturbance

CV: ***Hypertension, CHF, dysrhythmias, AV block,*** hypotension, aggravation of cardiac artery disease

EENT: Tinnitus, dry mouth, blurred vision, diplopia, nystagmus, conjunctivitis

ENDO: SIADH (elderly)

GI: Nausea, constipation, diarrhea, anorexia, vomiting, abdominal pain, stomatitis, glossitis, increased hepatic enzymes, ***hepatitis***

GU: Frequency, retention, albuminuria, glycosuria, impotence, increased BUN, ***renal failure***

HEMA: ***Thrombocytopenia, leukopenia, agranulocytosis, leukocytosis, aplastic anemia, eosinophilia,*** increased PT

INTEG: Rash, ***Stevens-Johnson syndrome,*** urticaria, photosensitivity

RESP: Pulmonary hypersensitivity (fever, dyspnea, pneumonitis)

Contraindications: Pregnancy (D), hypersensitivity to carbamazepine or tricyclics, bone marrow depression, concomitant use of MAOIs

Precautions: Glaucoma, hepatic disease, renal disease, cardiac disease, psychosis, lactation, child <6 yr

PHARMACOKINETICS

PO: Onset slow, peak 4-8 hr; metabolized by liver; excreted in urine, feces; crosses placenta, blood-brain barrier; excreted in breast milk; half-life 14-16 hr, protein binding 76%

✤ Canada only   Side effects: *italics* = common; ***bold italics*** = life-threatening

INTERACTIONS

CNS toxicity: lithium

⚠ Fatal reaction: MAOIs

Increase: carbamazepine levels—cimetidine, clarithromycin, danazol, diltiazem, erythromycin, fluoxetine, fluvoxamine, isoniazid, propoxyphene, valproic acid, verapamil

Increase: effects of desmopressin, lithium, lypressin, vasopressin

Decrease: effects of benzodiazepines, doxycycline, felbamate, haloperidol, oral contraceptives, phenobarbital, phenytoin, primidone, theophylline, thyroid hormones, warfarin

Decrease: carbamazepine levels—cisplatin, DOXOrubicin, felbamate, rifampin, phenobarbital, phenytoin, primidone, theophylline

Drug/Herb

Decrease: carbamazepine metabolism, increased levels—quinine, ginkgo

Decrease: anticonvulsant effect—ginseng, santonica

Drug/Food

Increase: peak concentration of carbamazepine—grapefruit juice

NURSING CONSIDERATIONS

Assess:

• For seizures: character, location, duration, intensity, frequency, presence of aura

• For trigeminal neuralgia: facial pain including location, duration, intensity, character, activity that stimulates pain

• Renal studies: urinalysis, BUN, urine creatinine q3mo

⚠ Blood studies: RBC, Hct, Hgb, reticulocyte counts qwk for 4 wk then q3-6 months, if on long-term therapy; if myelosuppression occurs, drug should be discontinued

• Hepatic studies: ALT, AST, bilirubin

• Drug levels during initial treatment or when changing dose; should remain at 4-12 mcg/ml; anorexia may indicate increased blood levels

• Mental status: mood, sensorium, affect, behavioral changes; if mental status changes, notify prescriber

• Eye problems: need for ophthalmic examinations before, during, after treatment (slit lamp, funduscopy, tonometry)

• Allergic reaction: purpura, red, raised rash; if these occur, drug should be discontinued

⚠ Blood dyscrasias: fever, sore throat, bruising, rash, jaundice

⚠ Toxicity: bone marrow depression, nausea, vomiting, ataxia, diplopia, cardiovascular collapse, Stevens-Johnson syndrome

Administer:

PO route

• Do not break, crush, or chew ext rel tab; patient should chew chewable tab, not swallow it whole, ext rel cap may be opened and the beads sprinkled over food

• With food, milk to decrease GI symptoms

• Shake oral susp before use

• Mix an equal amount of water, D_5W, 0.9% NaCl when giving by NG tube, flush tube with 100 ml of above sol

Perform/provide:

• Storage at room temperature

• Hard candy, gum, frequent rinsing for dry mouth

Evaluate:

• Therapeutic response: decreased seizure activity, document on patient's chart

Teach patient/family:

• To carry emergency ID stating patient's name, drugs taken, condition, prescriber's name, phone number

• To avoid driving, other activities that require alertness usually the first 3 days of treatment

• Not to discontinue medication quickly after long-term use

• To report immediately chills, rash, light-colored stools, dark urine, yellowing of skin and eyes, abdominal pain, sore throat, mouth ulcers, bruising, blurred vision, dizziness

• That urine may turn pink to brown

Treatment of overdose: Lavage, VS

---

carbidopa-levodopa
(℞)
(kar-bi-doe'pa) (lee-voe-doe'pa)
Atamet, carbidopa/levodopa, Sinemet, Sinemet CR
Func. class.: Antiparkinson agent
Chem. class.: Catecholamine

Action: Decarboxylation of levodopa to periphery is inhibited by carbidopa; more levodopa is made available for transport to brain and conversion to dopamine in the brain

Uses: Parkinson's disease, parkinsonism resulting from carbon monoxide, chronic manganese intoxication, cerebral arteriosclerosis

Investigational uses: Restless leg syndrome

DOSAGE AND ROUTES

Beginning therapy for those not taking levodopa
• *Adult:* **PO** 25 mg carbidopa/100 mg levodopa tid-qid, may increase daily or every other day to desired response; **EXT REL** tabs carbidopa 5 mg/levodopa 200 mg bid

For those not taking levodopa ER
• 50 mg carbidopa/200 mg levodopa bid

For those taking levodopa ER
• Begin treatment with 10% more levodopa/day given q4-8h, may increase or decrease dose q3d

For those taking levodopa <1.5 g/day
• *Adult:* **PO** 25 mg carbidopa/100 mg levodopa tid-qid, may increase daily to desired response

For those taking levodopa >1.5 g/day
• *Adult:* **PO** 25 mg carbidopa/250 mg levodopa tid-qid, may increase daily to desired response

Restless leg syndrome (RLS) (off-label)
• *Adult:* **PO** carbidopa 25 mg/levodopa 100 mg

Available forms: Tabs 10/100, 25/100, 25 mg carbidopa/250 mg levodopa; ext rel tab: 25 mg/100 mg, 50 mg/200 mg carbidopa/levodopa (Sinemet CR)

SIDE EFFECTS

CNS: Involuntary choreiform movements, hand tremors, fatigue, headache, anxiety, twitching, numbness, weakness, confusion, agitation, insomnia, nightmares, psychosis, hallucination, hypomania, severe depression, dizziness

CV: Orthostatic hypotension, tachycardia, hypertension, palpitation

EENT: Blurred vision, diplopia, dilated pupils

GI: Nausea, vomiting, anorexia, abdominal distress, dry mouth, flatulence, dysphagia, bitter taste, diarrhea, constipation

HEMA: **Hemolytic anemia, leukopenia, agranulocytosis**

INTEG: Rash, sweating, alopecia

MISC: Urinary retention, incontinence, weight change, dark urine

Contraindications: Hypersensitivity, narrow-angle glaucoma, malignant melanoma, history of malignant melanoma or undiagnosed skin lesions resembling melanoma

Precautions: Pregnancy (C), renal disease, wide-angle glaucoma, cardiac disease, hepatic disease, respiratory disease, MI with dysrhythmias, convulsions, peptic ulcer, lactation

PHARMACOKINETICS

PO: Peak 1-3 hr, excreted in urine (metabolites)

INTERACTIONS

Hypertensive crisis: MAOIs
Increase: effects of levodopa—antacids, metoclopramide
Decrease: effects of levodopa—anticholinergics, hydantoins, papaverine, pyridoxine, benzodiazepines
Decrease: absorption of levodopa—protein

Side effects: *italics* = common; ***bold italics*** = life-threatening

Drug/Herb

Increase: Parkinson symptoms—kava, octacosanol

Decrease: action, increased EPS—Indian snakeroot

Drug/Food

Increased pyridoxine will decrease levodopa effect

Drug/Lab Test

Increase: BUN, AST, ALT, bilirubin, alk phosphatase, LDH

Decrease: VMA, BUN, creatinine

False positive: Urine ketones (dipstick), Coombs' test

False negative: Urine glucose

False increase: Uric acid, urine protein

NURSING CONSIDERATIONS

Assess:

• For Parkinson's symptoms: tremors, pill rolling, drooling, akinesia, rigidity before and during treatment

• B/P, respiration; orthostatic B/P

• Mental status: affect, mood, behavioral changes, depression, complete suicide assessment

• Muscle twitching, blepharospasm that may indicate toxicity

• Renal, hepatic, hematopoietic tests, also for diabetes, acromegaly if on long-term therapy

Administer:

PO route

• Do not crush or chew ext rel tabs; they may be broken in half

• Drug until NPO before surgery

• Adjust dosage to response

• With meals if GI symptoms occur; limit protein taken with drug

• Only after MAOIs have been discontinued for 2 wk; if previously on levodopa, discontinue for at least 8 hr before change to carbidopa-levodopa

Evaluate:

• Therapeutic response: decrease in akathisia, tremor, rigidity, improved mood

Teach patient/family:

• To change positions slowly to prevent orthostatic hypotension

• To report side effects: twitching, eye spasms; indicate overdose

• To use drug exactly as prescribed; if discontinued abruptly, parkinsonian crisis may occur

• That urine, sweat may darken

• To use physical activities to maintain mobility, lessen spasms

• That improvement may not occur for 2-4 mo

⚠ High Alert

carboplatin (℞)

(kar-boe-pla′-tin)

Paraplatin, Paraplatin-AQ ✦

Func. class.: Antineoplastic alkylating agent

Chem. class.: Platinum coordination compound

Do not confuse:

carboplatin/cisplatin

Paraplatin/Platinol

Action: Produces interstrand DNA cross-links and, to a lesser extent, DNA-protein cross-links; activity is not cell cycle phase specific

Uses: Initial treatment of advanced ovarian cancer in combination with other agents; palliative treatment of ovarian carcinoma recurrent after treatment with other antineoplastic agents

Investigational uses: Endometrial, non–small cell lung, head/neck cancer; refractory/relapsed acute leukemia, recurrent benign tumor in children

DOSAGE AND ROUTES

(single agent):

• *Adult:* **IV INF** initially 300 mg/m^2 given with cyclophosphamide, q4-6wk; refractory tumors 360 mg/m^2 single dose, may repeat q4wk, as needed, do not repeat until neutrophils >2000/mm^3 and platelets >100,000/mm^3

Renal dose

• CCr 41-59 ml/min 250 mg/m^2, CCr 16-40 ml/min 200 mg/m^2, do not use in CCr <15 ml/min

---

Available forms: Inj 50, 150, 450, 600 mg/vial

SIDE EFFECTS

*CNS: **Seizures, central neurotoxicity, peripheral neuropathy,** dizziness, confusion*

CV: Cardiac abnormalities

EENT: Tinnitus, hearing loss, *vestibular toxicity,* visual changes

GI: Severe nausea, vomiting, diarrhea, weight loss, mucositis, anorexia, constipation, taste change

*HEMA: **Thrombocytopenia, leukopenia, pancytopenia, neutropenia, anemia,*** bleeding

INTEG: Alopecia, dermatitis, rash, erythema, pruritus, urticaria

META: Hypomagnesemia, hypocalcemia, hypokalemia, hyponatremia, hyperuremia

*SYST: **Anaphylaxis***

Contraindications: Pregnancy (D), hypersensitivity to this drug, platinum products, mannitol; severe bone marrow depression, significant bleeding, aluminum products used to prepare or administer carboplatin

Precautions: Radiation therapy within 1 mo, chemotherapy within 1 mo, lactation, hepatic disease

PHARMACOKINETICS

Initial half-life 1-2 hr, postdistribution half-life 2½-6 hr, not bound to plasma proteins, excreted by the kidneys

INTERACTIONS

Increase: nephrotoxicity or ototoxicity—aminoglycosides, amphotericin B

Increase: risk of bleeding—aspirin, NSAIDs

Increase: toxicity—radiation, bone marrow suppressants

Increase: myelosuppression—myelosuppressives

Drug/Lab Test

Increase: AST, BUN, alk phosphatase, bilirubin, creatinine

NURSING CONSIDERATIONS

Assess:

• CBC, differential, platelet count weekly; withhold drug if neutrophil count is <2000/mm^3 or platelet count is <100,000/mm^3; notify prescriber of results

• Renal studies: BUN, creatinine, serum uric acid, urine CCr before and during therapy; I&O ratio; report fall in urine output to <30 ml/hr

• Monitor temp q4h (may indicate beginning of infection)

• Hepatic studies tests before and during therapy (bilirubin, AST, ALT, LDH) as needed or monthly; jaundice of skin, sclera, dark urine, clay-colored stools, itchy skin, abdominal pain, fever, diarrhea

⚠ For anaphylaxis: hypotension, rash, pruritus, wheezing, tachycardia; notify prescriber after discontinuing drug, resuscitation equipment should be available

• Bleeding; hematuria, stool guaiac, bruising or petechiae, mucosa or orifices q8h

• Dyspnea, crackles, unproductive cough, chest pain, tachypnea

• Effects of alopecia on body image; discuss feelings about body changes

Administer:

• Antiemetic 30-60 min before giving drug and prn for vomiting

IV route

• After diluting 10 mg/ml of sterile water for inj, D₅W, NS (10 mg/ml); then further dilute with the same sol 1-4 mg/ml; give over 15 min or more (intermittent INF)

• IV INF over 5-6 hr; do not use needles or IV administration sets containing aluminum; may cause precipitate or loss of potency

Additive compatibilities: Cisplatin, etoposide, floxuridine, ifosfamide, ifosfamide/etoposide, paclitaxel

Solution compatibilities: D₅/0.2% NaCl, D₅/0.45% NaCl, D₅/0.9% NaCl, 0.9% NaCl, D₅W, sterile water for inj

Y-site compatibilities: Allopurinol, amifostine, aztreonam, cefepime, cladribine, DOXOrubicin liposome, filgrastim, fludarabine, granisetron, melphalan, ondansetron, paclitaxel, piperacillin/tazobactam, propofol, sargramostim, teniposide, thiotepa, vinorelbine

Perform/provide:
• Storage protected from light at room temperature; reconstituted sol stable for 8 hr at room temperature

Evaluate:
• Therapeutic response: decreasing size of tumor, spread of malignancy

Teach patient/family:
• To report ringing/roaring in the ears, numbness, tingling in face, extremities, weight gain
• That impotence or amenorrhea can occur; reversible after treatment is discontinued, to notify prescriber if pregnancy is suspected or planned; contraception should be used if patient is fertile
• Not to breastfeed during treatment
• To avoid OTC drugs with aspirin, NSAIDs, alcohol or receiving vaccinations during treatment
⚠ To notify prescriber immediately of fever, fatigue, sore throat, and bleeding, bruising, chills, back pain, blood in stools, dyspnea
• That hair may be lost during treatment; a wig or hairpiece may make patient feel better; new hair may be different in color, texture
• To avoid crowds, persons with known infections; avoid use of razors, stiff-bristle toothbrush

---

carboprost (℞)
(kar'boe-prost)
Hemabate, Prostin/15M ✦
Func. class.: Oxytocic, abortifacient
Chem. class.: Prostaglandin

Action: Stimulates uterine contractions, causing complete abortion in approximately 16 hr
Uses: Abortion at 13-20 wk gestation, postpartum hemorrhage caused by uterine atony not controlled by other methods

DOSAGE AND ROUTES

To induce abortion
• *Adult:* **IM** 250 mcg, then 250 mcg q1½-3½hr, may increase to 500 mcg if no response, not to exceed 12 mg total dose

Postpartum hemorrhage
• *Adult:* **IM** 250 mcg, repeat at 15-90 min intervals; max total dosage 2 mg
Available forms: Inj 250 mcg/ml

SIDE EFFECTS

CNS: Fever, chills, headache
GI: Nausea, vomiting, diarrhea
Contraindications: Hypersensitivity, severe hepatic disease, severe renal disease, PID, respiratory disease, cardiac disease
Precautions: Pregnancy (C), asthma, anemia, jaundice, diabetes mellitus, convulsive disorders, past uterine surgery

PHARMACOKINETICS

Onset 15 min, peak 2 hr; metabolized in lungs, liver; excreted in urine (metabolites)

INTERACTIONS

Increase: action—other oxytocics

NURSING CONSIDERATIONS

Assess:
• B/P, pulse; watch for change that may indicate hemorrhage
• Respiratory rate, rhythm, depth; notify prescriber of abnormalities
• For length, duration of contraction; notify prescriber of contractions lasting over 1 min or absence of contractions
• For incomplete abortion, pregnancy must be terminated by another method; drug is teratogenic

Administer:
• In deep muscle mass; rotate inj sites if additional doses are given

---

⚠ Safety alert   *"Tall Man" lettering

Evaluate:
• Therapeutic response: expulsion of fetus, control of bleeding
Teach patient/family:
• To report increased blood loss, abdominal cramps, increased temp, foul-smelling lochia

---

carisoprodol (R)

(kar-eye-soe-proe′dole)
carisoprodol, Soma, Vanadom
Func. class.: Skeletal muscle relaxant, central acting
Chem. class.: Meprobamate congener

Do not confuse:
Soma/Soma Compound
Action: Depresses CNS by blocking interneuronal activity in descending reticular formation, spinal cord, producing sedation
Uses: Relieving pain, stiffness in musculoskeletal disorders

DOSAGE AND ROUTES

• *Adult and child >12 yr:* **PO** 350 mg tid and at bedtime
• *Child 6-12 yr:* **PO** 6.25 mg/kg qid
Available forms: Tabs 350 mg

SIDE EFFECTS

CNS: Dizziness, weakness, drowsiness, headache, tremor, depression, insomnia, ataxia, irritability
CV: Postural hypotension, tachycardia
EENT: Diplopia, temporary loss of vision
GI: Nausea, vomiting, hiccups, epigastric discomfort
HEMA: Eosinophilia
INTEG: Rash, pruritus, fever, facial flushing, ***erythema multiforme***
RESP: Asthmatic attacks
SYST: ***Angioedema, anaphylaxis***
Contraindications: Hypersensitivity, child <12 yr, intermittent porphyria
Precautions: Pregnancy (C), renal disease, hepatic disease, addictive personality, elderly, lactation

PHARMACOKINETICS

PO: Onset ½ hr, peak 4 hr, duration 4-6 hr; metabolized by liver; excreted in urine; crosses placenta; excreted in breast milk (large amounts); half-life 8 hr

INTERACTIONS

Increase: CNS depression—alcohol, tricyclics, opioids, barbiturates, sedatives, hypnotics
Drug/Herb
Increase: CNS depression—chamomile, kava, skullcap, valerian
Drug/Lab Test
Increase: AST, alk phosphatase blood glucose

NURSING CONSIDERATIONS

Assess:
• Pain, stiffness, mobility, activities of daily living baseline and throughout treatment
• ECG in seizure patients; poor seizure control has occurred with patients taking this drug
• Idiosyncratic reaction (weakness, dizziness, blurred vision, confusion, euphoria), anaphylaxis within a few min or hr of 1st to 4th dose
• Allergic reactions: rash, fever, respiratory distress
• CNS depression: dizziness, drowsiness, psychiatric symptoms
Administer:
• With meals for GI symptoms
Perform/provide:
• Storage in tight container at room temperature
• Assistance with ambulation if dizziness, drowsiness occurs, especially elderly
Evaluate:
• Therapeutic response: decreased pain, spasticity
Teach patient/family:
• Not to take with alcohol, other CNS depressants
• To avoid hazardous activities if drowsiness, dizziness occur

---

Side effects: *italics* = common; ***bold italics*** = life-threatening

• To avoid using OTC medication: cough preparations, antihistamines, unless directed by prescriber

Treatment of overdose: Induce emesis of conscious patient, lavage, dialysis

---

⚠ High Alert

carmustine (℞)

(kar-mus'teen)

BiCNU, BCNU, Gliadel

Func. class.: Antineoplastic alkylating agent

Chem. class.: Nitrosourea

Action: Alkylates DNA, RNA; is able to inhibit enzymes that allow synthesis of amino acids in proteins; activity is not cell cycle phase specific

Uses: Brain tumors such as glioblastoma, medulloblastoma, brain stem glioma, astrocytoma, ependymoma, metastatic brain tumors; multiple myeloma (with predniSONE), non-Hodgkin's, Hodgkin's disease, other lymphomas; GI, breast, bronchogenic, renal carcinomas, other lymphomas; wafer, as adjunct to surgery/radiation in newly diagnosed high-grade malignant glioma patients; in recurrent glioblastoma multiforme patients as an adjunct to surgery

Investigational uses: Primary cutaneous T cell lymphoma, malignant melanoma

DOSAGE AND ROUTES

• *Adult:* IV 75-100 mg/m^2 over 1-2 hr × 2 days or 150-200 mg/m^2 × 1 dose q6-8wk or 40 mg/m^2/day × 5 days q6wk; if WBC is 3000-3999/mm^3 give 50% of dose; if WBC is 2000-2999/mm^3 and platelets are 25,000-75,000/mm^3 give 25% of dose; withhold dose if WBC is <2000/mm^3 and platelets are <25,000/mm^3

• *Adult:* **INTRACAVITARY** wafer: 8 inserted into resection cavity

Available forms: Powder for inj 100 mg; wafer 7.7 mg (intracavitary)

SIDE EFFECTS

*GI: Nausea, vomiting, anorexia, stomatitis, **hepatotoxicity***

*GU: Azotemia, **renal failure***

*HEMA: **Thrombocytopenia, leukopenia, myelosuppression, anemia***

INTEG: Pain, burning, hyperpigmentation at inj site

*RESP: **Fibrosis, pulmonary infiltrate***

Contraindications: Pregnancy (D), hypersensitivity, leukopenia, thrombocytopenia

Precautions: Lactation

PHARMACOKINETICS

Degraded within 15 min; crosses blood-brain barrier; 70% excreted in urine within 96 hr; 10% excreted as CO_2; fate of 20% is unknown

INTERACTIONS

Risk of bleeding: aspirin, anticoagulants

Myelosuppression: myelosuppressive agents

Increase: toxicity: other antineoplastics, radiation, cimetidine

Increase: adverse reactions, decreased antibody reaction—live vaccines

Decrease: effects of digoxin, phenytoin

NURSING CONSIDERATIONS

Assess:

• CBC, differential, platelet count weekly; withhold drug if WBC is <4000 or platelet count is <100,000; notify prescriber of results

• Hepatic studies: AST, ALT, bilirubin

• Pulmonary function tests, chest x-ray films before, during therapy; chest film should be obtained q2wk during treatment; monitor for dyspnea, cough, pulmonary fibrosis; infiltrate occurs after high doses or several low-dose courses

• Renal studies: BUN, serum uric acid, urine CCr before, during therapy; I&O ratio; report fall in urine output of 30 ml/hr

---

• Monitor for cold, cough, fever (may indicate beginning infection)
• Bleeding: hematuria, guaiac, bruising, petechiae, mucosa, orifices q8h

Administer:
• Blood transfusions or RBC colony-stimulating factors to combat anemia
• Antiemetic 30-60 min before giving drug to prevent vomiting
• All medications PO, if possible, avoid IM inj if platelets are <100,000/mm^3

Wafer route
• If wafers are broken in several pieces, they should not be used
• Foil pouches may be kept at room temperature for 6 hr if unopened

IV route
• Prepare in biologic cabinet wearing gown, gloves, mask; avoid contact with skin, can cause burning and staining the skin brown
• After diluting 100 mg drug/3 ml ethyl alcohol (provided); then further dilute 27 ml sterile H_2O for inj; then dilute with 100-500 ml 0.9% NaCl or D_5W, give over 1 hr or more, reduce rate if discomfort is felt; use only glass containers, protect from light
• Flush IV line after carmustine with 10 ml 0.9% NaCl to prevent irritation at site

Y-site compatibilities: Amifostine, aztreonam, cefepime, filgrastim, fludarabine, granisetron, melphalan, ondansetron, piperacillin/tazobactam, sargramostim, teniposide, thiotepa, vinorelbine

Perform/provide:
• Storage of reconstituted sol in refrigerator for 24 hr, or room temperature for 8 hr, protect from light
• Rinsing of mouth tid-qid with water or club soda; use of sponge brush for stomatitis
• Warm compresses at inj site for inflammation; reduce flow rate if patient complains of burning at infusion site

Evaluate:
• Therapeutic response: decreasing size of tumor, spread of malignancy

Teach patient/family:
• To report any changes in breathing or coughing, avoid smoking
• To avoid foods with citric acid, hot or rough texture if stomatitis is present; to report any bleeding, white spots, ulceration in mouth to prescriber; tell patient to examine mouth daily
• To avoid use of aspirin, ibuprofen, razors, commercial mouthwash
• To report signs of anemia (fatigue, irritability, shortness of breath, faintness); to report signs of infection (sore throat, fever); pulmonary toxicity can occur up to 15 yr after treatment
• To use contraception during treatment
• Not to receive vaccinations during treatment

---

carteolol (℞)
(kar-tee′oh-lole)
Cartrol
Func. class.: Antihypertensive, antianginal
Chem. class.: Nonselective β-blocker
See ophthalmics, Appendix C

Do not confuse:
carteolol/carvedilol

Action: Produces fall in B/P without reflex tachycardia or significant reduction in heart rate through mixture of α-blocking, β-blocking effects and intrinsic sympathomimetic activity; elevated plasma renins are reduced

Uses: Mild to moderate hypertension, ophthalmic, intraocular, open-angle glaucoma

DOSAGE AND ROUTES
• *Adult:* **PO** 2.5 mg daily initially, may gradually increase to desired response, max 10 mg/day

Renal dose
• *Adult:* **PO** CCr >60 ml/min give dose q24h; CCr 20-60 ml/min give dose q48h; CCr <20 ml/min give dose q72h

Available forms: Tabs 2.5, 5 mg

SIDE EFFECTS

CNS: Dizziness, mental changes, drowsiness, fatigue, headache, catatonia, depression, anxiety, nightmares, paresthesia, lethargy, insomnia, decreased concentration

CV: Orthostatic hypotension, ***bradycardia, CHF, chest pain, ventricular dysrhythmias, AV block, peripheral vascular insufficiency,*** palpitations

EENT: Tinnitus, visual changes, sore throat, double vision, dry, burning eyes

GI: Nausea, vomiting, diarrhea, dry mouth, flatulence, constipation, anorexia

GU: Impotence, dysuria, ejaculatory failure, urinary retention

HEMA: ***Agranulocytosis, thrombocytopenic purpura (rare)***

INTEG: Rash, alopecia, urticaria, pruritus, fever

MS: Joint pain, arthralgia, muscle cramps, pain

OTHER: Facial swelling, decreased exercise tolerance, weight change, Raynaud's disease, lupuslike syndrome

RESP: ***Bronchospasm,*** dyspnea, wheezing, nasal stuffiness, pharyngitis

Contraindications: Hypersensitivity to β-blockers, cardiogenic shock, heart block (2nd or 3rd degree), sinus bradycardia, bronchial asthma

Precautions: Pregnancy (C), major surgery, lactation, CHF, diabetes mellitus, renal disease, thyroid disease, COPD, well-compensated heart failure, nonallergic bronchospasm

PHARMACOKINETICS

PO: Onset 1-2 hr, peak 2-4 hr, duration 8-12 hr, half-life 6-8 hr; metabolized by liver (metabolites inactive); excreted in urine, bile; crosses placenta; excreted in breast milk

INTERACTIONS

Increase: myocardial depression—phenytoin (IV), verapamil

Increase: hypertension—MAOIs, amphetamines

Increase: hypotension—other antihypertensives, clonidine, nitrates, general anesthetics, alcohol (large amts)

Increase: hypoglycemic effect—insulin, oral antidiabetics

Decrease: antihypertensive effect—NSAIDs

Decrease: bronchodilating effects of theophylline, β-agonists

Decrease: CV effect—DOPamine, DOBUTamine

Decrease: carteolol effect—thyroid agents

Drug/Herb

Increase: effect—betel palm, butterbur, cola tree, figwort, fumitory, guarana, hawthorn, jaborandi tree, lily of the valley, motherwort, plantain

Decrease: effect—coenzyme Q10, yohimbe

Drug/Lab Test

Increase: ANA titer, blood glucose, BUN, uric acid, potassium, lipoprotein, triglyceride

NURSING CONSIDERATIONS

Assess:

• I&O, weight daily
• Edema in feet, legs daily, jugular vein distention, dyspnea, crackles
• B/P, pulse q4h; note rate, rhythm, quality; apical/radial pulse before administration; notify prescriber of any significant changes
• Baselines in renal, hepatic studies before therapy begins
• Skin turgor, dryness of mucous membranes for hydration status
• Blood glucose in those taking insulin/oral antidiabetics

Administer:

• Drug ac, at bedtime; tablet may be crushed or swallowed whole

Perform/provide:

• Storage in dry area at room temperature; do not freeze

Evaluate:

• Therapeutic response: decreased B/P after 1-2 wk

Teach patient/family:

• Not to discontinue drug abruptly; taper

over 2 wk or may precipitate hypertension, dysrhythmias, myocardial ischemia
• Not to use OTC products containing α-adrenergic stimulants (nasal decongestants, OTC cold preparations) unless directed by prescriber
• To report bradycardia, dizziness, confusion, depression, fever
• To take pulse, B/P at home, advise when to notify prescriber
• To avoid alcohol, smoking, sodium intake
• To comply with weight control, dietary adjustments, modified exercise program
• To carry emergency ID to identify drug being taken, allergies
• To avoid hazardous activities if dizziness is present
• To report symptoms of CHF: difficulty breathing, especially on exertion or when lying down, night cough, swelling of extremities
• To take medication at bedtime to minimize orthostatic hypotension

Treatment of overdose: Lavage, IV atropine for bradycardia, IV theophylline for bronchospasm, digitalis, O_2, diuretic for cardiac failure; administer vasopressor (norepinephrine) for hypotension, isoproterenol for heart block

---

carteolol ophthalmic
See Appendix C

---

carvedilol (℞)
(kar-ved′i-lole)
Coreg
Func. class.: Antihypertensive, α/β-adrenergic blocker

Do not confuse:
carvedilol/captopril/carteolol
Action: A mixture of nonselective α/β-adrenergic blocking activity; decreases cardiac output, exercise-induced tachycardia, reflex orthostatic tachycardia; causes vasodilation, reduction in peripheral vascular resistance

Uses: Essential hypertension alone or in combination with other antihypertensives, CHF, LV dysfunction following MI
Investigational uses: Angina pectoris, idiopathic cardiomyopathy

DOSAGE AND ROUTES
Essential hypertension
• *Adult:* **PO** 6.25 mg bid × 7-14 days; if tolerated well, then increase to 12.5 mg bid × 7-14 days; if tolerated well, may be increased (if needed) to 25 mg bid; not to exceed 50 mg daily
Congestive heart failure
• *Adult:* **PO** 3.125 mg bid × 2 wk; if tolerated well, give 6.25 mg bid × 2 wk, then double q2wk to max dose, 25 mg bid <85 kg or 50 mg bid >85 kg
Angina pectoris
• *Adult:* **PO** 25-50 mg bid
Idiopathic cardiomyopathy
• *Adult:* **PO** 6.25-25 mg bid
Available forms: Tabs 3.125, 6.25, 12.5, 25 mg

SIDE EFFECTS
CNS: Dizziness, fatigue, weakness, somnolence, insomnia, ataxia, hyperesthesia, paresthesia, vertigo, depression
*CV: **Bradycardia,** postural hypotension,* dependent edema, peripheral edema, ***AV block,*** extrasystoles, hypertension, hypotension, palpitations, peripheral ischemia, ***CHF, pulmonary edema***
GI: Diarrhea, abdominal pain, increased alk phosphatase, ALT/AST
GU: Decreased libido, *impotence*
MISC: Fatigue, injury, back pain, UTI, viral infection, hypertriglyceridemia, ***thrombocytopenia,*** *hyperglycemia*
RESP: Rhinitis, pharyngitis, dyspnea
Contraindications: Hypersensitivity, bronchial asthma, class IV decompensated cardiac failure, 2nd- or 3rd-degree heart block, cardiogenic shock, severe bradycardia, pulmonary edema
Precautions: Pregnancy (C), cardiac failure, hepatic injury, peripheral vascular disease, anesthesia, major surgery, diabetes mellitus, thyrotoxicosis, elderly,

lactation, children, emphysema, chronic bronchitis, renal disease

PHARMACOKINETICS

Readily and extensively absorbed PO, >98% protein binding, extensively metabolized by liver, excreted through bile into feces, terminal half-life 7-10 hr with increases in elderly, hepatic disease

INTERACTIONS

Conduction disturbances: calcium channel blockers

Bradycardia, hypotension: MAOIs, reserpine

Increase: hypoglycemia—antidiabetic agents

Increase: concentrations of digoxin

Increase: toxicity of carvedilol—cimetidine, other antihypertensives, nitrates, acute alcohol ingestion

Decrease: heart rate, B/P—clonidine

Decrease: carvedilol levels—rifampin, NSAIDs, thyroid medications

Drug/Herb

Increase: toxicity/death—aconite

Increase: antihypertensive effect—barberry, betony, black catechu, black cohosh, bloodroot, broom, burdock, cat's claw, dandelion, goldenseal, Irish moss, Jamaican dogwood, kelp, khella, mistletoe, parsley

Increase or decrease: antihypertensive effect—astragalus, cola tree

Decrease: antihypertensive effect—coltsfoot, guarana, khat, licorice

NURSING CONSIDERATIONS

Assess:

⚠ Renal studies, including protein, BUN, creatinine; watch for increased levels that may indicate nephrotic syndrome; obtain baselines in renal, hepatic studies before beginning treatment; I&O, weight daily

• Hepatic studies, jaundice; if LFTs are elevated, drug should be discontinued

• B/P during beginning treatment, periodically thereafter; pulse q4h, note rate, rhythm, quality; apical/radial pulse before administration; notify prescriber of significant changes

• Edema in feet, legs daily, fluid overload: dyspnea, weight gain, jugular vein distention, fatigue, crackles

Administer:

• Pulse: if <50 bpm, hold drug, call prescriber

• Drug ac, bedtime; tablets may be crushed or swallowed whole

• Reduced dosage in renal dysfunction; may give with food

Evaluate:

• Therapeutic response: decreased B/P in hypertension

Teach patient/family:

• To comply with dosage schedule, even if feeling better, that improvement may take several weeks

• To rise slowly to sitting or standing position to minimize orthostatic hypotension

• To report bradycardia, dizziness, confusion, depression, fever, weight gain, SOB, cold extremities, rash, sore throat, bleeding, or bruising

• To take pulse, B/P at home; advise when to notify prescriber

⚠ Not to discontinue drug abruptly, taper over 1-2 wk

• To avoid hazardous activities until stabilized on medication; dizziness may occur

• To avoid all OTC medications unless approved by prescriber

• To carry emergency ID with drug name, prescriber at all times

• To inform all health care providers of drugs, supplements taken

**cascara sagrada/
cascara sagrada
aromatic fluid extract/
cascara sagrada fluid
extract** (otc)
(kas-kar´a)
Func. class.: Laxative
Chem. class.: Anthraquinone

Action: Direct chemical irritation in colon; increases propulsion of stool
Uses: Constipation; bowel or rectal preparation for surgery or examination

DOSAGE AND ROUTES

• *Adult:* **PO** 325 mg at bedtime; **FLUID** 1 ml daily; **AROMATIC FLUID** 5 ml daily
• *Child 2-12 yr:* **PO/FLUID/ AROMATIC FLUID** ½ adult dose
• *Child <2 yr:* **PO/FLUID/AROMATIC FLUID** ¼ adult dose
Available forms: Tabs 325 mg; fluid extract 1 g/ml; aromatic fluid extract 1 g/ml

SIDE EFFECTS

GI: Nausea, vomiting, anorexia, cramps, diarrhea
META: Hypocalcemia, enteropathy, alkalosis, hypokalemia, ***tetany***
Contraindications: Hypersensitivity, GI bleeding, obstruction, CHF, lactation, abdominal pain, nausea/vomiting, appendicitis, acute surgical abdomen, alcoholics (aromatic form)
Precautions: Pregnancy (C)

PHARMACOKINETICS

PO: Peak 6-12 hr; metabolized by liver; excreted in urine, feces, breast milk

INTERACTIONS

Decrease: absorption of—antibiotics, digitalis, nitrofurantoin, salicylates, tetracyclines, oral anticoagulants
Drug/Herb
Increase: action/side effects—flax, lily of the valley, pheasant's eye, senna, squill

NURSING CONSIDERATIONS
Assess:
• Monitor blood, urine electrolytes if drug is used often by patient; check I&O ratio to identify fluid loss
• Cause of constipation; identify whether fluids, bulk, or exercise missing from lifestyle, constipating drugs
• Cramping, rectal bleeding, nausea, vomiting; if these symptoms occur, drug should be discontinued
Administer:
PO route
• Swallow tabs whole; do not break, crush, or chew
• Alone for better absorption; do not take within 1 hr of other drugs or within 1 hr of antacids, milk
• In morning or evening (oral dose)
Evaluate:
• Therapeutic response: decrease in constipation
Teach patient/family:
• Not to use laxatives for long-term therapy; bowel tone will be lost
• That normal bowel movements do not always occur daily
• Not to use in presence of abdominal pain, nausea, vomiting
• To notify prescriber if constipation unrelieved or of symptoms of electrolyte imbalance: muscle cramps, pain, weakness, dizziness

---

cefaclor
See cephalosporins—2nd generation
cefadroxil
cefamandole
cefazolin
See cephalosporins—1st generation
cefdinir
See cephalosporins—3rd generation
cefditoren
See cephalosporins—3rd generation
cefepime
cefixime
See cephalosporins—3rd generation
cefmetazole
See cephalosporins—2nd generation
cefoperazone
cefotaxime
See cephalosporins—3rd generation
cefotetan
cefoxitin
See cephalosporins—2nd generation
cefpodoxime
See cephalosporins—3rd generation
cefprozil
See cephalosporins—2nd generation
ceftazidime
ceftibuten
ceftizoxime
ceftriaxone
See cephalosporins—3rd generation
cefuroxime
See cephalosporins—2nd generation

⚠ High Alert

celecoxib (℞)
(sel-eh-cox′ib)
Celebrex
Func. class.: Nonsteroidal antiin-
flammatory, antirheumatic
Chem. class.: COX-2 inhibitor

Do not confuse:
Celebrex/ Celexa/Cerebra/Cerebyx
Action: Inhibits prostaglandin synthesis
by selectively inhibiting cyclooxygenase

2(COX-2), an enzyme needed for biosynthesis
Uses: Acute, chronic rheumatoid arthritis, osteoarthritis, familial adenomatous
polyposis (FAP), acute pain, primary
dysmenorrhea, ankylosing spondylitis
Investigational uses: Colorectal
polyps

DOSAGE AND ROUTES
**Do not exceed recommended dose,
deaths have occurred**
Acute pain/primary dysmenorrhea
• *Adult:* **PO** 400 mg initially, then 200
mg if needed on first day, then 200 mg
bid prn on subsequent days
Osteoarthritis
• *Adult:* **PO** 200 mg/day as a single dose
or 100 mg bid
Rheumatoid arthritis
• *Adult:* **PO** 100-200 mg bid
Ankylosing spondylitis
Adult: **PO** 200 mg daily or in divided
dose (bid)
*Familial adenomatous polyposis
(FAP)*
• *Adult:* **PO** 400 mg bid
Colorectal polyps
• *Adult:* **PO** 400 mg bid × 6 mo
*Hepatic disease (Child-Pugh class
II)*
• *Adult:* **PO** reduce dose by 50%
Available forms: Caps 100, 200 mg

SIDE EFFECTS
*CNS: Fatigue, anxiety, depression, ner-
vousness, paresthesia, dizziness, insomnia*
*CV: **Stroke, MI, tachycardia, CHF,***
angina, palpitations, dysrhythmias, hypertension, fluid retention
EENT: Tinnitus, hearing loss, blurred
vision, glaucoma, cataract, conjunctivitis,
eye pain
GI: Nausea, anorexia, vomiting, constipation, dry mouth, diverticulitis, gastritis,
gastroenteritis, hemorrhoids, hiatal hernia, stomatitis, ***GI bleeding***
*GU: **Nephrotoxicity:** dysuria, **hematuria, oliguria, azotemia,** cystitis,
UTI*

⚠ Safety alert   *"Tall Man" lettering

HEMA: ***Blood dyscrasias,*** epistaxis, bruising, anemia
INTEG: **Serious sometimes fatal Stevens-Johnson syndrome, toxic epidermal necrolysis,** purpura, rash, pruritus, sweating, erythema, petechiae, photosensitivity, alopecia
RESP: Pharyngitis, shortness of breath, pneumonia, coughing

Contraindications: Pregnancy (D) 3rd trimester, hypersensitivity to aspirin, iodides, other NSAIDs, sulfonamides, asthma triad, asthma

Precautions: Pregnancy (C) 1st/2nd trimesters, lactation, bleeding, GI, cardiac, renal, hepatic, disorders, hypersensitivity to other antiinflammatory agents, glucocorticoids, anticoagulants, geriatrics, hypertension, severe dehydration, children <18 yr

PHARMACOKINETICS

Well absorbed, crosses placenta, bound to plasma proteins, metabolized in liver, excreted by kidneys, peak 3 hr

INTERACTIONS

Increase: effect of anticoagulants
Increase: adverse reactions—glucocorticoids, NSAIDs, aspirin
Increase: toxicity—lithium, antineoplastics
Increase: celecoxib blood level—fluconazole
Decrease: effect of aspirin, ACE inhibitors, thiazide diuretics, furosemide

Drug/Herb
Severe photosensitivity: St. John's wort
Increase: celecoxib effect—bearberry, bilberry
Increase: gastric irritation—arginine, gossypol
Increase: bleeding risk—bogbean, saw palmetto, turmeric

NURSING CONSIDERATIONS
Assess:
• For pain of rheumatoid arthritis, osteoarthritis; check ROM, inflammation of joints, characteristics of pain

• FAP clients for decreasing number of polyps
• Blood counts during therapy; watch for decreasing platelets; if low, therapy may need to be discontinued, restarted after hematologic recovery
⚠ For blood dyscrasias (thrombocytopenia): bruising, fatigue, bleeding, poor healing

Administer:
• With a full glass of water to enhance absorption
• Do not break, crush, chew, or dissolve caps
• With food or milk to decrease gastric symptoms, do not increase dose

Evaluate:
• Therapeutic response: decreased pain, inflammation in arthritic conditions; decreased number of polyps

Teach patient/family:
⚠ **Do not exceed recommended dose, notify prescriber immediately of chest pain, skin eruptions, stop drug**
• To check with prescriber to determine when drug should be discontinued prior to surgery
• That drug must be continued for prescribed time to be effective; to avoid other NSAIDs, aspirin, sulfonamides
• To notify prescriber if pregnancy is planned or suspected
⚠ To notify prescriber of GI symptoms: black, tarry stools; cramping or rash; edema of extremities, weight gain
⚠ To report bleeding, bruising, fatigue, malaise since blood dyscrasias do occur

cephalexin
See cephalosporins—1st generation

CEPHALOSPORINS—1ST GENERATION

cefadroxil (℞)
(sef-a-drox'ill)
cefadroxil, Duricef

cefazolin (℞)
(sef-a'zoe-lin)
Ancef, cefazolin

cephalexin (℞)
(sef-a-lex'in)
Apo-Cephalex ✦, Biocef, cephalexin, Keflex, Keftab, Novo-Lexin ✦, Nu-Cephalex ✦

cephapirin (℞)
(sef-a-pye'rin)
Cefadyl, cephapirin

cephradine (℞)
(sef'ra-deen)
cephradine, Velosef
Func. class.: Antiinfective
Chem. class.: Cephalosporin (1st generation)

Do not confuse:
cephalexin/cefaclor
cephapirin/cephradine
Action: Inhibits bacterial cell wall synthesis, rendering cell wall osmotically unstable, leading to cell death by binding to cell wall membrane
Uses:
cefadroxil: Gram-negative bacilli: *Escherichia coli, Proteus mirabilis, Klebsiella* (UTI only); gram-positive organisms: *Streptococcus pneumoniae, Streptococcus pyogenes, Staphylococcus aureus;* upper, lower respiratory tract, urinary tract, skin infections, otitis media; tonsillitis; and UTIs
cefazolin: Gram-negative bacilli: *Haemophilus influenzae, Escherichia coli, Proteus mirabilis, Klebsiella;* gram-positive organisms: *Staphylococcus aureus;* upper, lower respiratory tract, urinary tract, skin infections, bone, joint, biliary, genital infections, endocarditis, surgical prophylaxis, septicemia

cephalexin: Gram-negative bacilli: *Haemophilus influenzae, Escherichia coli, Proteus mirabilis, Klebsiella;* gram-positive organisms: *Streptococcus pneumoniae, Streptococcus pyogenes, Staphylococcus aureus;* upper, lower respiratory tract, urinary tract, skin, bone infections, otitis media
cephapirin: Gram-negative bacilli: *Haemophilus influenzae, Escherichia coli, Proteus mirabilis, Klebsiella;* gram-positive organisms: *Streptococcus pneumoniae, Streptococcus viridans, Staphylococcus aureus;* lower respiratory tract, skin infections, endocarditis, bacterial peritonitis
cephradine: Gram-negative bacilli: *Haemophilus influenzae, Escherichia coli, Proteus mirabilis, Klebsiella;* gram-positive organisms: *Streptococcus pneumoniae, Streptococcus pyogenes, Staphylococcus aureus;* serious respiratory tract, skin infections, UTIs, otitis media

DOSAGE AND ROUTES
cefadroxil
• *Adult:* **PO** 1-2 g daily or q12h in divided doses, give a loading dose of 1 g initially
• *Child:* **PO** 30 mg/kg/day in divided doses bid
Renal dose: CCr 25-50 ml/min 500 mg q12h; CCr 10-24 ml/min 500 mg q24h; CCr <10 ml/min 500 mg q36h
Available forms: Caps 500 mg; tabs 1 g; oral susp 125, 250, 500 mg/5 ml
cefazolin
Life-threatening infections
• *Adult:* **IM/IV** 1-2 g q6h
• *Child >1 mo:* **IM/IV** 100 mg/kg in 3-4 divided doses
Mild/moderate infections
• *Adult:* **IM/IV** 250 mg-1 g q8h
• *Child >1 mo:* **IM/IV** 25-50 mg/kg in 3-4 equal doses
Renal dose: CCr 35-54 ml/min: 250-1000 mg q12h; CCr 10-34 ml/min: 50%

of dose q12h; CCr <10 ml/min: 50% of dose q18-24h

Available forms: Inj 250, 500 mg, 1, 5, 10, 20 g; infusion 500 mg, 1 g/50 ml vial

cephalexin

Moderate infections

- *Adult:* **PO** 250-500 mg q6h
- *Child:* **PO** 25-50 mg/kg/day in 4 equal doses

Moderate skin infections

- *Adult:* **PO** 500 mg q12h

Endocarditis prophylaxis

- 2 g 1 hr before procedure

Severe infections

- *Adult:* **PO** 500 mg-1 g q6h
- *Child:* **PO** 50-100 mg/kg/day in 4 equal doses

Renal dose: CCr <40 ml/min give q8-12h; CCr 5-10 ml/min give q12h; CCr <5 ml/min give q24h

Available forms: Caps 250, 500 mg; tabs 250, 500 mg, 1 g; oral susp 125, 250 mg/5ml

cephapirin

- *Adult:* **IM/IV** 500 mg-1 g q4-6h
- *Child:* **IM/IV** 40-80 mg/kg/day in divided doses q6h or 10-20 mg/kg q6h

Renal dose: CCr <10 ml/min give q12h

Available forms: Powder for inj 500 mg, 1, 2, 20 g; IV only 1, 2, 4 g

cephradine

- *Adult:* **PO** 250 mg-1 g q6-12h
- *Child >1 yr:* **PO** 6-12 mg/kg q6h

Renal dose: CCr >20 ml/min 500 mg q6h; CCr 5-20 ml/min 250 mg q6h

Available forms: Caps 250, 500 mg; oral susp 125, 250 mg/5ml

SIDE EFFECTS

CNS: Headache, dizziness, weakness, paresthesia, fever, chills, *seizures* (high doses)

GI: Nausea, vomiting, *diarrhea, anorexia,* pain, glossitis, bleeding; increased AST, ALT, bilirubin, LDH, alk phosphatase; abdominal pain, ***pseudomembranous colitis***

GU: Proteinuria, vaginitis, pruritus, candidiasis, increased BUN, ***nephrotoxicity, renal failure***

HEMA: ***Leukopenia, thrombocytopenia, agranulocytosis,*** anemia, ***neutropenia, lymphocytosis, eosinophilia, pancytopenia, hemolytic anemia***

INTEG: Rash, urticaria, dermatitis

RESP: Dyspnea

SYST: ***Anaphylaxis, serum sickness,*** superinfection

Contraindications: Hypersensitivity to cephalosporins, infants <1 mo

Precautions: Pregnancy (B), hypersensitivity to penicillins, lactation, renal disease

PHARMACOKINETICS

cefadroxil: Peak 1-1½ hr, duration 12-24 hr, half-life 1-2 hr; 20% bound by plasma proteins; crosses placenta; excreted in breast milk

cefazolin

IM: Peak ½-2 hr, duration 6-12 hr, half-life 1½-2¼ hr

IV: Peak 10 min, duration 6-12 hr; eliminated unchanged in urine; 70%-86% protein bound

cephalexin: Peak 1 hr, duration 6-12 hr, half-life 30-72 min; 5%-15% bound by plasma proteins; 90%-100% eliminated unchanged in urine; crosses placenta; excreted in breast milk

cephapirin

IV: Peak 5 min, duration 4-6 hr

IM: Peak 30 min, duration 4-6 hr

Half-life 21-47 min; 44%-50% bound by plasma proteins; 40%-70% eliminated unchanged in urine; crosses placenta; excreted in breast milk; metabolized in liver

cephradine: Peak 1-2 hr, duration 6-12 hr, half-life 0.75-1.5 hr; 20% bound by plasma proteins; 80%-90% eliminated unchanged in urine; crosses placenta; excreted in breast milk

INTERACTIONS

Increase: toxicity—aminoglycosides, loop diuretics, probenecid

Drug/Herb

Do not use acidophilus with antiinfectives

Drug/Lab Test

Increase: AST, ALT, alk phosphatase, LDH, BUN, creatinine, bilirubin

False positive: Urinary protein, direct Coombs' test, urine glucose

Interference: Cross-matching

NURSING CONSIDERATIONS

Assess:

• Sensitivity to penicillin and other cephalosporins

⚠ Nephrotoxicity: increased BUN, creatinine

• I&O daily

• Blood studies: AST, ALT, CBC, Hct, bilirubin, LDH, alk phosphatase, Coombs' test monthly if patient is on long-term therapy

• Electrolytes: K, Na, Cl monthly if patient is on long-term therapy

• Bowel pattern daily; if severe diarrhea occurs, drug should be discontinued; may indicate pseudomembranous colitis

• Urine output: if decreasing, notify prescriber; may indicate nephrotoxicity

⚠ Anaphylaxis: rash, urticaria, pruritus, chills, fever, joint pain; angioedema; may occur few days after therapy begins; discontinue drug, notify prescriber immediately, keep emergency equipment nearby

• Bleeding: ecchymosis, bleeding gums, hematuria, stool guaiac daily

⚠ Overgrowth of infection: perineal itching, fever, malaise, redness, pain, swelling, drainage, rash, diarrhea, change in cough, sputum

Administer:

cefadroxil

• For 10-14 days to ensure organism death, prevent superinfection

• With food if needed for GI symptoms

• Shake susp, refrigerate, discard after 2 wk

• After C&S completed

cefazolin

• IV; check for irritation, extravasation often; dilute in 10 ml sterile H_2O for inj and run over 3-5 min; may be further diluted with 50-100 ml of NS, D_5W sol and run over ½-1 hr by Y-tube or 3-way stopcock

• For 10-14 days to ensure organism death, prevent superinfection

• After C&S completed

Additive compatibilities: Aztreonam, clindamycin, famotidine, fluconazole, metronidazole, verapamil

Syringe compatibilities: Heparin, vit B

Y-site compatibilities: Acyclovir, allopurinol, amifostine, atracurium, aztreonam, calcium gluconate, cyclophosphamide, diltiazem, DOXOrubicin liposome, enalaprilat, esmolol, famotidine, filgrastim, fluconazole, fludarabine, foscarnet, heparin, hydromorphone, insulin (regular), labetalol, lidocaine, magnesium sulfate, melphalan, meperidine, midazolam, morphine, multivitamins, ondansetron, perphenazine, pancuronium, remifentanil, sargramostim, tacrolimus, teniposide, theophylline, thiotepa, vecuronium, vit B/C, warfarin

cephalexin

• Shake susp, refrigerate, discard after 2 wk

• For 10-14 days to ensure organism death, prevent superinfection

• With food if needed for GI symptoms

• After C&S

cephapirin

• IV after diluting 1 g or less/10 ml or more NS, D_5W, or bacteriostatic H_2O for inj; give 1 g or less/5 min or more; may be further diluted in 50-100 ml of D_5W, NS; run over 15 min; discontinue primary IV during administration; may also be given by continuous infusion, store refrigerated 96 hr, room temperature 24 hr

• For 10-14 days to ensure organism death, prevent superinfection

• After C&S

Additive compatibilities: Bleomycin, calcium chloride, calcium gluconate, chloramphenicol, diphenhydrA-

MINE, ergonovine, heparin, hydrocortisone, metaraminol, oxacillin, penicillin G potassium, pentobarbital, phenobarbital, phytonadione, potassium chloride, sodium bicarbonate, succinylcholine, verapamil, vit B, warfarin

Y-site compatibilities: Acyclovir, cyclophosphamide, famotidine, heparin, hydrocortisone, hydromorphone, magnesium sulfate, meperidine, morphine, multivitamins, perphenazine, potassium chloride, vit B/C

cephradine

• Shake suspension well before each dose
• For 10-14 days to ensure organism death, prevent superinfection
• With food if needed for GI symptoms
• After C&S

Evaluate:

• Therapeutic response: decreased symptoms of infection, negative C&S

Teach patient/family:

• Not to drink alcohol or use meds with alcohol: reaction may occur
• To use yogurt or buttermilk to maintain intestinal flora, decrease diarrhea
• To take all medication prescribed for length of time ordered
⚠ To report sore throat, bruising, bleeding, joint pain (may indicate blood dyscrasias [rare]); diarrhea with mucus, blood, may indicate pseudomembranous colitis

Treatment of anaphylaxis: EpINEPHrine, antihistamines; resuscitate if needed

CEPHALOSPORINS— 2ND GENERATION

cefaclor (℞)
(sef'a-klor)
Ceclor, Ceclor CD, Raniclor

cefamandole (℞)
(sef-a-man'dole)
Mandol

cefmetazole (℞)
(sef-met'a-zole)
Zefazone

cefotetan (℞)
(sef'oh-tee-tan)
Cefotan

cefoxitin (℞)
(se-fox'i-tin)
Mefoxin

cefprozil (℞)
(sef-proe'zill)
Cefzil

cefuroxime (℞)
(sef-yoor-ox'eem)
Ceftin, cefuroxime, Zinacef

loracarbef (℞)
(lor-a-kar'beff)
Lorabid

Func. class.: Antiinfective
Chem. class.: Cephalosporin (2nd generation)

Do not confuse:
cefaclor/cephalexin
Cefotan/ Ceftin
cefprozil/Cefazolin
cefprozil/cefuroxime
Cefzil/Ceftin

Action: Inhibits bacterial cell wall synthesis, rendering cell wall osmotically unstable, leading to cell death by binding to cell wall membrane

Uses:

cefaclor: Gram-negative bacilli: *Haemophilus influenzae, Escherichia coli, Proteus mirabilis, Klebsiella;* grampositive organisms: *Streptococcus pneu-*

moniae, Streptococcus pyogenes, Staphylococcus aureus; respiratory tract, urinary tract, skin, bone, joint infections, otitis media

cefamandole: Gram-negative bacilli: *Haemophilus influenzae, Escherichia coli, Proteus mirabilis, Klebsiella;* gram-positive organisms: *Streptococcus pneumoniae, Streptococcus pyogenes, Staphylococcus aureus;* upper, lower respiratory tract, urinary tract, skin infections, peritonitis, septicemia, surgical prophylaxis

cefmetazole: Gram-negative bacilli: *Haemophilus influenzae, Escherichia coli, Proteus, Klebsiella, Bacteroides fragilis;* gram-positive organisms: *Streptococcus pneumoniae, Streptococcus pyogenes, Staphylococcus aureus;* anaerobes, including *Clostridium;* infections of lower respiratory tract, urinary tract, skin, bone, intraabdominal infections

cefotetan: Gram-negative organisms: *Haemophilus influenzae, Escherichia coli, Enterobacter aerogenes, Proteus mirabilis, Klebsiella, Citrobacter, Enterobacter, Salmonella, Shigella, Acinetobacter, Bacteroides fragilis, Neisseria, Serratia;* gram-positive organisms: *Streptococcus pneumoniae, Streptococcus pyogenes, Staphylococcus aureus;* upper, lower, serious respiratory tract, urinary tract, skin, bone, joint, gynecologic, gonococcal, intraabdominal infections

cefoxitin: Gram-negative bacilli: *Haemophilus influenzae, Escherichia coli, Proteus, Klebsiella, Bacteroides fragilis, Neisseria gonorrhoeae;* gram-positive organisms: *Streptococcus pneumoniae, Streptococcus pyogenes, Staphylococcus aureus;* anaerobes including *Clostridium,* lower respiratory tract, urinary tract, skin, bone, gynecologic, gonococcal infections, septicemia, peritonitis

cefprozil: Pharyngitis/tonsillitis, otitis media, secondary bacterial infection of acute bronchitis, and acute bacterial exacerbation of chronic bronchitis and uncomplicated skin and skin structure infections; acute sinusitis

cefuroxime: Gram-negative bacilli: *Haemophilus influenzae, Escherichia coli, Neisseria, Proteus mirabilis, Klebsiella;* gram-positive organisms: *Streptococcus pneumoniae, Streptococcus pyogenes, Staphylococcus aureus;* serious lower respiratory tract, urinary tract, skin, bone, joint, gonococcal infections, septicemia, meningitis

loracarbef: Gram-negative bacilli: *Haemophilus influenzae, Escherichia coli, Proteus mirabilis, Klebsiella;* gram-positive organisms: *Streptococcus pneumoniae, Streptococcus pyogenes, Staphylococcus aureus;* upper and lower respiratory tract, urinary tract, skin infections, otitis media, pharyngitis, tonsillitis

DOSAGE AND ROUTES

cefaclor
• *Adult:* **PO** 250-500 mg q8h, not to exceed 4 g/day or 375-500 mg (ext rel) q12h × 7-10 days
• *Child >1 mo:* **PO** 20-40 mg/kg daily in divided doses q8h, or total daily dose may be divided and given q12h, not to exceed 1 g/day

Acute bacterial exacerbations of chronic bronchitis or acute bronchitis
• *Adult:* 500 mg/12 hr × 1 wk (ext rel)

Pharyngitis/tonsillitis
• *Adult:* 375 mg/12 hr × 10 days (ext rel)

Available forms: Caps 250, 500 mg; oral susp 125, 187, 250, 375 mg/5 ml; tabs, ext rel (CD) 375, 500 mg; chew tabs (Raniclor) 125, 187, 250, 375 mg

cefamandole
• *Adult:* **IM/IV** 500 mg-1 g q4-8h; may give up to 2 g q4h for severe infections
• *Child >1 mo:* **IM/IV** 8.3-16.7 mg/kg q4h, not to exceed adult dose
• Dosage reduction indicated in renal impairment (CCr <50 ml/min)
Available forms: Inj 1, 2, 10 g

cefmetazole
- *Adult:* **IV** 2 g divided q6-12h × 5-14 days

Renal dose: CCr <50 ml/min 1-2 g q12h; CCr 10-29 ml/min 1-2 g q24h; CCr <10 ml/min 1-2 g q48h

Available forms: Powder for inj 1, 2 g/vial

cefotetan
- *Adult:* **IV/IM** 1-2 g q12h × 5-10 days

Renal dose: CCr 10-30 ml/min give q24h; CCr <10 ml/min give q48h

Perioperative prophylaxis
- *Adult:* **IV** 1-2 g ½-1 hr before surgery

Available forms: Inj 1, 2, 10 g

cefoxitin
- *Adult:* **IM/IV** 1-2 g q6-8h

Renal dose: CCr <50 ml/min give q8-12h; CCr 10-29 ml/min give q24h; CCr <10 ml/min give q24-48h

Uncomplicated gonorrhea: 2 g IM as single dose with 1 g **PO** probenecid at same time

Severe infections
- *Adult:* **IM/IV** 2 g q4h
- *Child ≥3 mo:* **IM/IV** 80-160 mg/kg/day divided q4-6h; max 12 g/day

Available forms: Powder for inj 1, 2, 10 g

cefprozil
Renal dose: CCr <30 ml/min 50% of dose

Upper respiratory infections
- *Adult:* **PO** 500 mg q24h × 10 days

Otitis media
- *Child 6 mo-12 yr:* **PO** 15 mg/kg q12h × 10 days

Lower respiratory infections
- *Adult:* **PO** 500 mg q12h × 10 days

Skin/skin structure infections
- *Adult:* **PO** 250-500 mg q12h × 10 days

Available forms: Tabs 250, 500 mg; susp 125, 250 mg/5 ml

cefuroxime
- *Adult and child:* **PO** 250 mg q12h; may increase to 500 mg q12h in serious infections
- *Adult:* **IM/IV** 750 mg-1.5 g q8h for 5-10 days

Urinary tract infections
- *Adult:* **PO** 125 mg q12h; may increase to 250 mg q12h if needed

Otitis media
- *Child <2 yr:* **PO** 125 mg bid
- *Child >2 yr:* **PO** 250 mg bid

Surgical prophylaxis
- *Adult:* **IV** 1.5 g ½-1 hr preop

Severe infections
- *Adult:* **IM/IV** 1.5 g q6h; may give up to 3 g q8h for bacterial meningitis
- *Child >3 mo:* **IM/IV** 50-100 mg/day; may give up to 200-240 mg/kg/day **IV** in divided doses for bacterial meningitis (not recommended)
- Dosage reduction indicated in severe renal impairment (CCr <20 ml/min)

Uncomplicated gonorrhea
- *Adult:* 1.5 g **IM** as single dose with oral probenecid in 2 separate sites

Available forms: Tabs 125, 250, 500 mg; inj 150, 750 mg, 1.5, 7.5 g; inj 750 mg; 1.5 g powder; susp 125, 250 mg/5 ml

loracarbef
- *Adult and child >13 yr:* **PO** 200-400 mg q12h
- *Child <12 yr:* **PO** 15-30 mg/kg/day in 2 divided doses q12h

Renal dose: CCr 10-49 ml/min 50% of dose; CCr <10 ml/min q3-5 days

Available forms: Caps 200, 400 mg; 100, 200 mg/5 ml oral susp

SIDE EFFECTS

CNS: Dizziness, headache, fatigue, paresthesia, fever, chills, confusion

GI: *Diarrhea*, nausea, vomiting, anorexia, dysgeusia, glossitis, bleeding; increased AST, ALT, bilirubin, LDH, alk phosphatase; abdominal pain, loose stools, flatulence, heartburn, stomach cramps, colitis, jaundice, *pseudomembranous colitis*

GU: Vaginitis, pruritus, candidiasis, increased BUN, *nephrotoxicity, renal failure,* pyuria, dysuria, reversible interstitial nephritis

HEMA: *Leukopenia, thrombocytopenia, agranulocytosis,* anemia, *neutropenia, lymphocytosis, eosin-*

ophilia, pancytopenia, hemolytic anemia, leukocytosis, granulocytopenia
INTEG: Rash, urticaria, dermatitis, *Stevens-Johnson syndrome*
RESP: Dyspnea
SYST: Anaphylaxis, *serum sickness,* superinfection
Contraindications: Hypersensitivity to cephalosporins or related antibiotics, seizures
Precautions: Pregnancy (B), lactation, children, renal disease

PHARMACOKINETICS
cefaclor
PO: Peak ½-1 hr, ext rel peak 1½-2½ hr, half-life 36-54 min; 25% bound by plasma proteins; 60%-85% eliminated unchanged in urine in 8 hr; crosses placenta; excreted in breast milk (low concentrations)
cefamandole
Peak 1-1½ hr, half-life ½-1 hr; 60%-75% bound by plasma proteins; crosses placenta; excreted in breast milk; poor penetration into CSF
cefmetazole
IM: Peak 30-45 min; 68% bound by plasma proteins, excreted by kidneys; half-life 1-3 hr
cefotetan
IV/IM: Peak 1½-3 hr; half-life 3-5 hr, 70%-90% bound by plasma proteins, 50%-80% eliminated unchanged in urine, crosses placenta, excreted in breast milk
cefoxitin
IV: Peak 3 min
IM: Peak 15-60 min
Half-life 1 hr, 55%-75% bound by plasma proteins, 90%-100% eliminated unchanged in urine; crosses placenta, blood-brain barrier; eliminated in breast milk, not metabolized
cefprozil
PO: Peak 6-10 hr; plasma protein binding 99%; elimination half-life 25 hr; extensively metabolized to an active metabolite

cefuroxime: 65% excreted unchanged in urine, half-life 1-2 hr in normal renal function
loracarbef
PO: Peak 1 hr, half-life 1 hr; excreted in urine as unchanged drug

INTERACTIONS
Disulfiram-like reaction: alcohol
Increase: effect/toxicity—aminoglycosides, furosemide, probenecid
Increase: bleeding risk (cefamandole, cefmetazole, cefotetan)—anticoagulants, thrombolytics, NSAIDs, antiplatelets, plicamycin, valproic acid
Drug/Herb
Do not use acidophilus with antiinfectives
Increase: bleeding risk (cefamandole, cefmetazole, cefotetan)—angelica, anise, arnica, bogbean, boldo, celery, chamomile, clove, fenugreek, feverfew, garlic, ginger, ginkgo, ginseng *(Panax),* horse chestnut, horseradish, licorice, meadowsweet, prickly ash, onion, papain, passion flower, poplar, red clover, turmeric, willow
Drug/Lab Test
False increase: Creatinine (serum urine), urinary 17-KS
False positive: Urinary protein, direct Coombs' test, urine glucose testing (Clinitest)
Interference: Cross-matching

NURSING CONSIDERATIONS
Assess:
⚠ Nephrotoxicity: increased BUN, creatinine
- I&O ratio
- Blood studies: AST, ALT, CBC, Hct, bilirubin, LDH, alk phosphatase, Coombs' test qmo if patient is on long-term therapy
- Electrolytes: K, Na, Cl qmo if patient is on long-term therapy
- Bowel pattern daily; if severe diarrhea occurs, drug should be discontinued; may indicate pseudomembranous colitis
- Urine output; if decreasing, notify prescriber (may indicate nephrotoxicity)

⚠ Anaphylaxis: rash, flushing, urticaria, pruritus, dyspnea, discontinue drug, notify prescriber, have emergency equipment available
• Bleeding: ecchymosis, bleeding gums, hematuria, stool guaiac daily
⚠ Overgrowth of infection: perineal itching, fever, malaise, redness, pain, swelling, drainage, rash, diarrhea, change in cough, sputum

Administer:
• Do not break, crush, or chew ext rel tabs or caps
• On an empty stomach 1 hr before or 2 hr after a meal

cefaclor
• Shake susp, refrigerate, discard after 2 wk
• For 10-14 days to ensure organism death, prevent superinfection
• With food if needed for GI symptoms
• After C&S completed

cefamandole
• IV; check often for irritation, extravasation; dilute 1 g or less of drug/10 ml or more NS or sterile H_2O for inj; run over 3-5 min; may be further diluted with 100 ml of compatible sol and run over 15-30 min via Y-tube or 3-way stopcock; may also be diluted in 1 L compatible sol, run over prescribed rate
• For 10-14 days to ensure organism death, prevent superinfection
• After C&S completed

Additive compatibilities: Clindamycin, floxacillin, furosemide, metronidazole, verapamil
Syringe compatibilities: Heparin
Y-site compatibilities: Acyclovir, cyclophosphamide, hydromorphone, magnesium sulfate, meperidine, morphine, perphenazine

cefmetazole
• For 10-14 days to ensure organism death, prevent superinfection
• After C&S completed

Solution compatibilities: D_5W, 0.9% NaCl
Additive compatibilities: Clindamycin, famotidine, KCl
• IV after diluting 3.7 or 10 ml sterile

H_2O for inj, 2 g/7 or 15 ml, shake, let stand until clear, run over 3-5 min; may be further diluted in 50-100 ml of D_5W, NS, LR to 1-20 mg/ml and run over ½-1 hr by Y-tube or 3-way stopcock

cefotetan
• IV direct after diluting 1 g/10 ml sterile H_2O for inj and give over 3-5 min; may be diluted further with 50-100 ml of NS or D_5W, shake; run over ½-1 hr by Y-tube or 3-way stopcock; discontinue primary inf during administration
• May be stored 96 hr refrigerated or 24 hr room temperature

Y-site compatibilities: Allopurinol, amifostine, aztreonam, diltiazem, famotidine, filgrastim, fluconazole, fludarabine, heparin, insulin (regular), melphalan, meperidine, morphine, paclitaxel, remifentanil, sargramostim, tacrolimus, teniposide, theophylline, thiotepa

cefoxitin
• IV after diluting 1 g or less/10 ml or more D_5W, NS and give over 3-5 min; may be diluted further with 50-100 ml of normal saline or D_5W; run over ½-1 hr by Y-tube or 3-way stopcock; discontinue primary inf during administration; by cont inf at prescribed rate; may store 96 hr refrigerated or 24 hr room temperature
• For 10-14 days to ensure organism death, prevent superinfection
• After C&S completed

Additive compatibilities: Amikacin, cimetidine, clindamycin, gentamicin, kanamycin, multivitamins, sodium bicarbonate, tobramycin, verapamil, vit B/C
Syringe compatibilities: Heparin, insulin
Y-site compatibilities: Acyclovir, amifostine, amphotericin B cholesteryl sulfate complex, aztreonam, cyclophosphamide, diltiazem, DOXOrubicin liposome, famotidine, fluconazole, foscarnet, hydromorphone, magnesium sulfate, meperidine, morphine, ondansetron, perphenazine, remifentanil, teniposide, thiotepa

cefprozil
- For 10-14 days to ensure organism death, prevent superinfection
- After C&S
- Refrigerate/shake susp prior to use

cefuroxime
- For 10-14 days to ensure organism death, prevent superinfection
- With food if needed for GI symptoms
- After C&S

Additive compatibilities: Clindamycin, floxacillin, furosemide, metronidazole, netilmicin

Y-site compatibilities: Acyclovir, allopurinol, amifostine, atracurium, aztreonam, cyclophosphamide, diltiazem, famotidine, fludarabine, foscarnet, hydromorphone, melphalan, meperidine, morphine, ondansetron, pancuronium, perphenazine, remifentanil, sargramostim, tacrolimus, teniposide, thiotepa, vecuronium

loracarbef
- Oral susp should be shaken before giving; store for 2 wk at room temperature, discard after 2 wk
- 1 hr before or 2 hr after a meal
- After C&S is completed
- For 7 days to ensure organism death, prevent superinfection

Evaluate:
- Therapeutic response: negative C&S

Teach patient/family:
- If diabetic, to use blood glucose testing
- Not to drink alcohol or take meds with alcohol or reaction may occur
- To complete full course of drug therapy, to report persistent diarrhea
- To use yogurt or buttermilk to maintain intestinal flora, decrease diarrhea
- To notify prescriber if breastfeeding or of any side effects

⚠ To report sore throat, bruising, bleeding, joint pain (may indicate blood dyscrasias [rare]); diarrhea with mucus, blood, may indicate pseudomembranous colitis

Treatment of anaphylaxis: EpI-NEPHrine, antihistamines; resuscitate if needed

---

CEPHALOSPORINS—3RD GENERATION

cefdinir (℞)
(sef′dih-ner)
Omnicef

cefditoren pivoxil (℞)
(sef-dit′oh-ren pih-vox′il)
Spectracef

cefepime (℞)
(sef′e-peem)
Maxipime

cefixime (℞)
(sef-icks′ime)
Suprax

cefoperazone (℞)
(sef-oh-per′a-zone)
Cefobid

cefotaxime (℞)
(sef-oh-taks′eem)
Claforan

cefpodoxime (℞)
(sef-poe-docks′eem)
Vantin

ceftazidime (℞)
(sef′tay-zi-deem)
Ceptaz, Fortaz, Tazicef, Tazidime

ceftibuten (℞)
(sef-ti-byoo′tin)
Cedax

ceftizoxime (℞)
(sef-ti-zox′eem)
Cefizox

ceftriaxone (℞)
(sef-try-ax′one)
Rocephin
Func. class.: Broad-spectrum antibiotic
Chem. class.: Cephalosporin (3rd generation)

Do not confuse:
Vantin/Ventolin
ceftazidime/ceftizoxime

⚠ Safety alert *"Tall Man" lettering

Action: Inhibits bacterial cell wall synthesis, rendering cell wall osmotically unstable, leading to cell death

Uses:

cefdinir: Gram-negative bacilli: *Haemophilus influenzae, Haemophilus parainfluenzae, Moraxella catarrhalis;* gram-positive organisms: *Streptococcus pneumoniae, Streptococcus pyogenes, Staphylococcus aureus,* acute exacerbations of chronic bronchitis

cefditoren pivoxil: Acute bacterial exacerbation of chronic bronchitis caused by *Haemophilus influenzae, Haemophilus parainfluenzae, Streptococcus pneumoniae, Moraxella catarrhalis;* pharyngitis/tonsillitis caused by *Streptococcus pyogenes;* uncomplicated skin and skin structure infections caused by *Staphylococcus aureus, Streptococcus pyogenes*

cefepime: Gram-negative bacilli: *Escherichia coli, Proteus, Klebsiella;* gram-positive organisms: *Streptococcus pneumoniae, Streptococcus pyogenes, Staphylococcus aureus;* lower respiratory tract, urinary tract, skin, bone infections

cefixime: Uncomplicated UTI *(Escherichia coli, Proteus mirabilis),* pharyngitis and tonsillitis *(Streptococcus pyogenes),* otitis media *(Haemophilus influenzae), Moraxella catarrhalis,* acute bronchitis, and acute exacerbations of chronic bronchitis *(Streptococcus pneumoniae, H. influenzae)*

cefoperazone: Gram-negative bacilli: *Haemophilus influenzae, Escherichia coli, Proteus mirabilis, Klebsiella, Enterobacter, Serratia, Citrobacter, Providencia, Proteus aeruginosa;* lower respiratory tract, urinary tract, skin, bone infections, bacterial septicemia, peritonitis, PID

cefotaxime: Gram-negative organisms: *Haemophilus influenzae, Haemophilus parainfluenzae, Escherichia coli, Enterococcus faecalis, Neisseria gonorrhoeae, Neisseria meningitidis, Proteus mirabilis, Klebsiella, Citrobacter, Serratia, Salmonella, Shigella Pseudomonas;* gram-positive organisms: *Streptococcus pneumoniae, Streptococcus pyogenes, Staphylococcus aureus;* serious lower respiratory tract, urinary tract, skin, bone, gonococcal infections; bacteremia, septicemia, meningitis, skin, skin structure infections, CNS infections; perioperative prophylaxis

cefpodoxime: Gram-negative bacilli: *Neisseria gonorrhoeae, Haemophilus influenzae, Escherichia coli, Proteus mirabilis, Klebsiella;* gram-positive organisms: *Streptococcus pneumoniae, Streptococcus pyogenes, Staphylococcus aureus;* upper and lower respiratory tract, urinary tract, skin infections; otitis media, sexually transmitted diseases

ceftazidime: Gram-negative organisms: *Haemophilus influenzae, Escherichia coli, Enterobacter aerogenes, Pseudomonas aeruginosa, Proteus mirabilis, Klebsiella, Citrobacter, Enterobacter, Salmonella, Shigella, Acinetobacter, Bacteroides fragilis, Neisseria, Serratia;* gram-positive organisms: *Streptococcus pneumoniae, Streptococcus pyogenes, Staphylococcus aureus;* serious upper/lower respiratory tract, urinary tract, skin, gynecologic, bone, joint, intraabdominal infections; septicemia, meningitis

ceftibuten: Pharyngitis/tonsillitis, otitis media, secondary bacterial infection of acute bronchitis

ceftizoxime: Gram-negative bacilli: *Haemophilus influenzae, Escherichia coli, Enterobacter aerogenes, Proteus mirabilis, Klebsiella, Enterobacter;* gram-positive organisms: *Streptococcus pneumoniae, Streptococcus pyogenes, Staphylococcus aureus;* serious lower respiratory tract, urinary tract, skin, intraabdominal infections, septicemia, meningitis, bone and joint infections, PID caused by *Neisseria gonorrhoeae*

ceftriaxone: Gram-negative bacilli: *Haemophilus influenzae, Escherichia* *coli, Enterobacter aerogenes, Proteus mirabilis, Klebsiella, Citrobacter, Enterobacter, Salmonella, Shigella, Acinetobacter, Bacteroides fragilis, Neisseria, Serratia;* gram-positive organisms: *Streptococcus pneumoniae, Streptococcus pyogenes, Staphylococcus aureus;* serious lower respiratory tract, urinary tract, skin, gonococcal, intraabdominal infections, septicemia, meningitis, bone, joint infections

DOSAGE AND ROUTES

cefdinir
Uncomplicated skin and skin structure infections/community-acquired pneumonia
• *Adult and child ≥13 yr:* **PO** 300 mg q12h × 10 days
• *Child 6 mo-12 yr:* **PO** 7 mg/kg q12h or 14 mg/kg q24h × 10 days, max 60 mg daily

Acute exacerbations of chronic bronchitis/acute maxillary sinusitis
• *Adult and child ≥13 yr:* **PO** 300 mg q12h or 600 mg q24h × 10 days or 300 mg bid × 5 days in some infections

Pharyngitis/tonsillitis
• *Adult and child ≥13 yr:* **PO** 300 mg q12h or 600 mg q24h × 10 days
• *Child 6 mo-12 yr:* **PO** 7 mg/kg q12h × 5-10 days or 14 mg/kg q24h × 10 days

Renal dose
• CCr <30 ml/min 300 mg daily (adult); 7 mg/kg daily (child)

Available forms: Caps 300 mg; susp: 125 mg/5 ml

cefditoren pivoxil
• *Adult:* **PO** 200-400 mg bid

Renal dose
• *Adult:* **PO** CCr 30-50 ml/min, max 200 mg bid; CCr <30 ml/min; max 200 mg daily

Available form: Tabs 200 mg

cefepime
Urinary tract infections (mild to moderate)
• *Adult:* **IV/IM** 0.5-1 g q12h × 7-10 days

Urinary tract infections (severe)
• *Adult:* **IV** 2 g q12h × 10 days

Pneumonia (moderate to severe)
• *Adult:* **IV** 1-2 g q12h × 10 days
• Dosage reduction indicated in renal impairment (CCr <50 ml/min)

Uncomplicated gonorrhea
• **IM** 2 g as a single dose with 1 g **PO** probenecid at the same time

Available forms: Powder for inj 500 mg, 1, 2 g

cefixime
• *Adult:* **PO** 400 mg daily as a single dose or 200 mg q12h
• *Child >50 kg or >12 yr:* **PO** use adult dosage
• *Child <50 kg or <12 yr:* **PO** 8 mg/kg/day as a single dose or 4 mg/kg q12h

Renal dose: CCr 21-60 ml/min give 75% of dose; CCr <20 ml/min give 50% of dose

Available forms: Tabs 200, 400 mg; powder for oral susp 100 mg/5 ml

cefoperazone
Hepatic dose: give 50% of dose
Mild/Moderate infections
• *Adult:* **IM/IV** 1-2 g q12h

Severe infections
• *Adult:* **IM/IV** 6-12 g/day divided in 2-4 equal doses

Available forms: Inj 1, 2 g

cefotaxime
• *Adult:* **IM/IV** 1-2 g q12h as a single dose
• *Child 1 mo-12 yr:* **IM/IV** 50-180 mg/kg/day divided q6h

Severe infections
• *Adult:* **IM/IV** 2 g q4h, not to exceed 12 g/day
• *Child 1 mo-12 yr:* **IM/IV** 50-180 mg/kg/day in 4-6 divided doses

Uncomplicated gonorrhea
• *Adult:* **IM** 1 g
• Dosage reduction indicated for severe renal impairment (CCr <30 ml/min)

Available forms: Powder for inj 500 mg, 1, 2, 10 g; inj 1,2 g premixed frozen

cefpodoxime
• *Adult >13 yr: Pneumonia:* 200 mg q12h for 14 days; *uncomplicated gonorrhea:* 200 mg single dose; *skin*

and skin structure: 400 mg q12h for 7-14 days; *pharyngitis and tonsillitis:* 100 mg q12h for 10 days; *uncomplicated UTI:* 100 mg q12h for 7 days; dosing interval increased in presence of severe renal impairment

• *Child 5 mo-12 yr: acute otitis media:* 5 mg/kg q12h for 10 days; *pharyngitis/tonsillitis:* 5 mg/kg q12h (max 100 mg/dose or 200 mg/day) × 5-10 days

Available forms: Tabs 100, 200 mg/granules for susp 50, 100 mg/5 ml

ceftazidime
• *Adult:* **IV/IM** 1-2 g q8-12h × 5-10 days
• *Child:* **IV** 30-50 mg/kg q8h not to exceed 6 g/day
• *Neonate:* **IV** 30-50 mg/kg q12h
Renal dose: CCr <50 ml/min give q12h; CCr 10-30 ml/min give q24h; CCr <10 ml/min give q48h

Available forms: Inj 250,500 mg, 1, 2, 6 g

ceftibuten
• *Adult:* **PO** 400 mg daily × 10 days
• *Child 6 mo-12 yr:* **PO** 9 mg/kg daily × 10 days
Renal dose: CCr <50 ml/min give 200 mg q24h; CCr 5-20 ml/min give 100 mg q24h

Available forms: Caps 400 mg; susp 90, 180 mg/5 ml

ceftizoxime
• *Adult:* **IM/IV** 1-2 g q8-12h, may give up to 4 g q8h in life-threatening infections
• *Child >6 mo:* **IM/IV** 50 mg/kg q6-8h
Renal dose: CCr <80 ml/min give 500-1500 mg q8h; CCr 10-49 ml/min give 250-1000 mg q12h

PID
• *Adult:* **IV** 2 g q8h, may increase to 4 g q8h in severe infections
Available forms: Powder for inj 500 mg, 1, 2, 10 g; premixed 1 g, 2 g/50 ml

ceftriaxone
• *Adult:* **IM/IV** 1-2 g daily, max 2 g q12h
• *Child:* **IM/IV** 50-75 mg/kg/day in equal doses q12h
Uncomplicated gonorrhea
• *Adult:* 250 mg **IM** as single dose
• Reduce dosage in severe renal impairment (CCr <10 ml/min)

Meningitis
• *Adult and child:* **IM/IV** 100 mg/kg/day in equal doses q12h, max 4 g/day
Surgical prophylaxis
• *Adult:* **IV** 1 g ½-2 hr preop
Available forms: Inj 250, 500 mg, 1, 2, 10 g

SIDE EFFECTS

CNS: Headache, dizziness, weakness, paresthesia, fever, chills, ***seizures***
GI: Nausea, vomiting, diarrhea, anorexia, *pain, glossitis, **bleeding;*** increased AST, ALT, bilirubin, LDH, alk phosphatase; abdominal pain, ***pseudomembranous colitis***
GU: **Proteinuria,** vaginitis, pruritus, candidiasis, increased BUN, ***nephrotoxicity, renal failure***
HEMA: ***Leukopenia, thrombocytopenia, agranulocytosis,*** anemia, ***neutropenia, lymphocytosis, eosinophilia, pancytopenia, hemolytic anemia***
INTEG: Rash, urticaria, dermatitis
RESP: Dyspnea
SYST: ***Anaphylaxis, serum sickness***
Contraindications: Hypersensitivity to cephalosporins, infants <1 mo
Precautions: Pregnancy (B), hypersensitivity to penicillins, lactation, renal disease, children

PHARMACOKINETICS

cefdinir
Unchanged in urine; crosses placenta, blood-brain barrier; eliminated in breast milk; not metabolized
cefditoren pivoxil
Absorption well absorbed after it is broken down (prodrug); distribution widely; half-life 100 min; onset rapid, peak 0.5-3 hr, duration 12 hr
cefepime
Peak 79 min, half-life 2 hr, 20% bound by plasma proteins, 90% excreted

---

Side effects: *italics* = common; ***bold italics*** = life-threatening

unchanged in urine; crosses placenta, blood-brain barrier; excreted in breast milk; not metabolized

cefixime
PO: Peak 1-2 hr, half-life 3-4 hr, 65% bound by plasma proteins, 50% eliminated unchanged in urine; crosses placenta; excreted in breast milk

cefoperazone
IV: Onset 5 min, peak 5-20 min, duration 6-8 hr
IM: Peak 1-2 hr, duration 6-8 hr
Half-life 2 hr; 70%-75% is eliminated unchanged in bile; 20%-30% unchanged in urine; excreted in breast milk (small amounts)

cefotaxime
IV: Onset 5 min
IM: Onset 30 min
Half-life 1 hr; 35%-65% is bound by plasma proteins; 40%-65% is eliminated unchanged in urine in 24 hr; 25% metabolized to active metabolites; excreted in breast milk (small amounts)

cefpodoxime
Half-life 2-3 hr; 25% bound by plasma proteins; 30% eliminated unchanged in urine in 8 hr; crosses placenta; excreted in breast milk

ceftazidime
IV/IM: Peak 1 hr, half-life ½-1 hr, 90% bound by plasma proteins, 80% eliminated unchanged in urine, crosses placenta, excreted in breast milk

ceftibuten
PO: Peak 6-10 hr; plasma protein binding 99%; elimination half-life 25 hr; extensively metabolized to an active metabolite

ceftizoxime
IV: Onset 5 min
IM: Peak 1 hr
Half-life 5-8 hr; 90% bound by plasma proteins; 36%-60% eliminated unchanged in urine; crosses placenta; excreted in breast milk

ceftriaxone
IV: Onset 5 min
IM: Peak 1 hr
Half-life 5-8 hr, 90% bound by plasma proteins; 35%-60% eliminated unchanged in urine; crosses placenta; excreted in breast milk

INTERACTIONS
Increase: bleeding—anticoagulants, thrombolytics, plicamycin, valproic acid, NSAIDs
Increase: toxicity—aminoglycosides, furosemide, probenecid
Decrease: absorption of cefdinir—iron

Drug/Herb
Do not use acidophilus with antiinfectives
Increase: bleeding risk (cefoperazone): angelica, anise, arnica, bogbean, boldo, celery, chamomile, clove, fenugreek, feverfew, garlic, ginger, gingko, ginseng *(Panax)*, horse chestnut, horseradish, licorice, meadowsweet, prickly ash, onion, papain, passion flower, poplar, red clover, turmeric, willow

Drug/Lab Test
Increase: ALT, AST, alk phosphatase, LDH, bilirubin, BUN, creatinine
False increase: creatinine (serum urine), urinary 17-KS
False positive: Urinary protein, direct Coombs' test, urine glucose
Interference: Cross-matching

NURSING CONSIDERATIONS
Assess:
• Sensitivity to penicillin, other cephalosporins
⚠ Nephrotoxicity: increased BUN, creatinine; urine output: if decreasing, notify prescriber; may indicate nephrotoxicity
• Blood studies: AST, ALT, CBC, Hct, bilirubin, LDH, alk phosphatase, Coombs' test monthly if patient is on long-term therapy
• Electrolytes: K, Na, Cl monthly if patient is on long-term therapy
• Bowel pattern daily; if severe diarrhea

⚠ Safety alert   *"Tall Man" lettering

occurs, drug should be discontinued; may indicate pseudomembranous colitis
• IV site for extravasation, phlebitis
⚠ Anaphylaxis: rash, urticaria, pruritus, chills, fever, joint pain, angioedema; may occur few days after therapy begins
• Bleeding: ecchymosis, bleeding gums, hematuria, stool guaiac
⚠ Overgrowth of infection: perineal itching, fever, malaise, redness, pain, swelling, drainage, rash, diarrhea, change in cough, sputum

Administer:
• Change IV site q> 2 days

cefdinir
• Oral susp after adding 39 ml water to the 60 ml bottle; 65 ml water to the 120 ml bottle; discard unused portion after 10 days
• After C&S completed

cefditoren pivoxil
• For 10 days to ensure organism death, prevent superinfection
• With food if needed for GI symptoms
• After C&S completed

cefepime
• IV after diluting in 50-100 ml or more D_5, NS and give over 30 min
• For 7-10 days to ensure organism death, prevent superinfection
Solution compatibilities: 0.9% NaCl, D_5, D_5W, 0.5%, 10% lidocaine, bacteriostatic water for inj with parabens/benzyl alcohol
Y-site compatibilities: Doxorubicin liposome

cefixime
• For 10-14 days to ensure organism death, prevent superinfection

cefoperazone
• IV after diluting 1 g/ml sterile H_2O for inj, or 0.9% NaCl; shake, give over 3-5 min; each g may be further diluted with 20-40 ml D_5W, NS given over 30 min or as a cont inf over 6-24 hr to a concentration no greater than 25 mg/ml
• IM for concentration >250 mg/ml, dilute in sterile water, then lidocaine, inject deeply
• For 10-14 days to ensure organism death, prevent superinfection

Additive compatibilities: Cimetidine, clindamycin, furosemide
Syringe compatibilities: Heparin
Y-site compatibilities: Acyclovir, allopurinol, aztreonam, cyclophosphamide, enalaprilat, esmolol, famotidine, foscarnet, fludarabine, hydromorphone, magnesium sulfate, melphalan, morphine, teniposide, thiotepa

cefotaxime
• IV after diluting 1 g/10 ml D_5W, NS, sterile H_2O for inj and give over 3-5 min by Y-tube or 3-way stopcock; may be diluted further with 50-100 ml of normal saline or D_5W; run over ½-1 hr; discontinue primary inf during administration; or may be diluted in larger vol of sol and given as a cont inf over 6-24 hr
• For 10-14 days to ensure organism death, prevent superinfection
• Thaw frozen container at room temperature or refrigeration; do not force thaw by immersion or microwave; visually inspect container for leaks
Additive compatibilities: Clindamycin, metronidazole, verapamil
Syringe compatibilities: Heparin, ofloxacin
Y-site compatibilities: Acyclovir, amifostine, aztreonam, cyclophosphamide, diltiazem, famotidine, fludarabine, hydromorphone, lorazepam, magnesium sulfate, melphalan, meperidine, midazolam, morphine, ondansetron, perphenazine, sargramostim, teniposide, thiotepa, tolazoline, vinorelbine

cefpodoxime
• For 10-14 days to ensure organism death, prevent superinfection
• With food to enhance absorption
Y-site compatibilities: Famotidine, fluconazole, fludarabine, insulin (regular), meperidine, morphine, sargramostim

ceftazidime
• IV after diluting 1 g/10 ml sterile H_2O for inj, shake, invert needle, push plunger, insert needle through stopper and keep in sol, expel bubbles and give over 3-5 min; may be diluted further with

50-100 ml of normal saline or D_5W; run over ½-1 hr, give through Y-tube or 3-way stopcock, discontinue primary inf during administration; store for 96 hr refrigerated, 24 hr room temperature
• For 5-10 days to ensure organism death, prevent superinfection
Syringe compatibilities: Hydromorphone
Additive compatibilities: Ciprofloxacin, clindamycin, fluconazole, metronidazole, ofloxacin
Y-site compatibilities: Acyclovir, allopurinol, amifostine, aztreonam, ciprofloxacin, diltiazem, enalaprilat, esmolol, famotidine, filgrastim, fludarabine, foscarnet, granisetron, heparin, hydromorphone, labetalol, meperidine, melphalan, morphine, ondansetron, paclitaxel, ranitidine, remifentanil, tacrolimus, teniposide, theophylline, thiotepa, vinorelbine, zidovudine

ceftibuten
• For 10 days to ensure organism death, prevent superinfection

ceftizoxime
• IV after diluting 1 g/10 ml sterile water, shake and give over 3-5 min; may be diluted further with 50-100 ml NS or D_5W give through Y-tube or 3-way stopcock; run over ½-1 hr
• For 10-14 days to ensure organism death, prevent superinfection
Additive compatibilities: Clindamycin
Y-site compatibilities: Acyclovir, allopurinol, amphotericin B cholesteryl sulfate complex, aztreonam, DOXOrubicin liposome, enalaprilat, esmolol, famotidine, fludarabine, foscarnet, hydromorphone, labetalol, melphalan, meperidine, morphine, ondansetron, remifentanil, sargramostim, teniposide, vinorelbine

ceftriaxone
• For 10-14 days to ensure organism death, prevent superinfection
• IV after diluting 250 mg/2.4 ml D_5W, H_2O for inj, 0.9% NaCl; may be further diluted with 50-100 ml NS, D_5W, $D_{10}W$, shake; run over ½-1 hr
Additive compatibilities: Amino

acids or sodium bicarbonate, metronidazole
Y-site compatibilities: Acyclovir, allopurinol, aztreonam, cisatracurium, diltiazem, DOXOrubicin liposome, fludarabine, foscarnet, heparin, melphalan, meperidine, methotrexate, morphine, paclitaxel, remifentanil, sargramostim, tacrolimus, teniposide, theophylline, vinorelbine, warfarin, zidovudine
Evaluate:
• Therapeutic response: decreased symptoms of infection; negative C&S
Teach patient/family:
• If diabetic, to check blood glucose
🅐 To report sore throat, bruising, bleeding, joint pain; may indicate blood dyscrasias (rare); diarrhea with mucus, blood, may indicate pseudomembranous colitis
• To report persistent diarrhea
• Cefditoren can be taken with oral contraceptives
Treatment of anaphylaxis: EpINEPHrine, antihistamines; resuscitate if needed

---

cephapirin
cephradine
See cephalosporins—
1st generation

---

cetirizine (R)
(se-teer'i-zeen)
Zyrtec
Func. class.: Antihistamine (2nd generation, peripherally selective)
Chem. class.: Piperazine, H_1-histamine antagonist

Do not confuse:
Zyrtec/Xanax/Zantac
Action: Acts on blood vessels, GI, respiratory system by competing with histamine for H_1-receptor site; decreases allergic response by blocking pharmacologic effects of histamine; minimal anticholinergic action

---

Uses: Rhinitis, allergy symptoms, chronic idiopathic urticaria

DOSAGE AND ROUTES
• *Adult and child ≥6 yr:* **PO** 5-10 mg daily
• *Child 2-5 yr:* **PO** 2.5 mg daily, may increase to 5 mg daily or 2.5 mg bid
• *Child 1-2 yr:* **PO** 2.5 mg daily, may increase to 2.5 mg q12h
• *Child 6-11 mo:* **PO** 2.5 mg daily
• *Geriatric:* **PO** 5 mg daily, may increase to 10 mg/day
Renal dose
• CCr 11-31 ml/min 5 mg daily
Hemodialysis
• *Adult:* **PO** 5 mg daily
Hepatic dose
• *Adult:* **PO** 5 mg daily
Available forms: Tabs 5, 10 mg; syr 5 mg/5 ml

SIDE EFFECTS
CNS: Headache, stimulation, *drowsiness,* sedation, *fatigue,* confusion, blurred vision, tinnitus, restlessness, tremors, paradoxical excitation in children or elderly
GI: Dry mouth, increase LFTs
INTEG: Rash, eczema, photosensitivity, urticaria
RESP: Thickening of bronchial secretions, dry nose, throat
Contraindications: Hypersensitivity to this drug or hydrOXYzine, newborn or premature infants, lactation, severe hepatic disease
Precautions: Pregnancy (B), elderly, children, respiratory disease, narrow-angle glaucoma, prostatic hypertrophy, bladder neck obstruction, asthma

PHARMACOKINETICS
Absorption rapid; onset ½ hr; peak 1-2 hr; duration 24 hr; protein binding 93%; half-life decreased in children; increased in hepatic renal disease

INTERACTIONS
Increase: CNS depression—alcohol, other CNS depressants
Increase: anticholinergic/sedative effect—MAOIs
Drug/Herb
Increase: effect—hops, Jamaican dogwood, kava, senega, valerian
Increase: anticholinergic effect—corkwood
Drug/Food
Food prolongs absorption by 1.7 hr
Drug/Lab Test
False negative: Skin allergy tests

NURSING CONSIDERATIONS
Assess:
• Allergy symptoms: pruritus, urticaria, watering eyes, baseline and during treatment
• Respiratory status: rate, rhythm, increase in bronchial secretions, wheezing, chest tightness
Administer:
• Without regard to meals
Perform/provide:
• Hard candy, gum, frequent rinsing of mouth for dryness
• Storage in tight, light-resistant container
Evaluate:
• Therapeutic response: absence of running or congested nose or rashes
Teach patient/family:
• All aspects of drug use; to notify prescriber if confusion, sedation, hypotension occur
• To avoid driving, other hazardous activity if drowsiness occurs
• To avoid alcohol, other CNS depressants
• That drug is not recommended during lactation
• To avoid exposure to sunlight; burns may occur
• To use sugarless gum, candy, frequent sips of water to minimize dry mouth
Treatment of overdose: Administer diazepam, vasopressors, barbiturates (short-acting)

cetrorelix (℞)

(set-roe-ree′lix)
Cetrotide
Func. class.: Gonadotropin-releasing hormone antagonist
Chem. class.: Synthetic decapeptide

Action: Inhibitor of pituitary gonadotropin secretion; initially increases LH and FSH, induces a rapid suppression of gonadotropin secretion
Uses: For inhibition of premature LH surges in women undergoing controlled ovarian hyperstimulation

DOSAGE AND ROUTES

Single-dose regimen
• *Adult:* **SUBCUT** 3 mg when serum estradiol level is at appropriate stimulation response, usually on stimulation day 7; if hCG has not been given within 4 days after inj of 3 mg cetrorelix, give 0.25 mg daily until day of hCG administration
Multiple-dose regimen
• *Adult:* **SUBCUT** 0.25 mg is given on stimulation day 5 (either morning or evening) or 6 (morning) and continued daily until day hCG is given
Available forms: Inj 0.25, 3 mg

SIDE EFFECTS

CNS: Headache
ENDO: Ovarian hyperstimulation syndrome, abdominal pain (gyn)
GI: Nausea, vomiting, diarrhea
INTEG: Pain on inj; local site reactions
SYST: **Fetal death**
Contraindications: Pregnancy (X), hypersensitivity, latex allergy, lactation

PHARMACOKINETICS

Excreted in feces/urine, half-life depends on dosage, metabolized to metabolites, protein binding 86%

NURSING CONSIDERATIONS

Assess:
• For suspected pregnancy, drug should not be used
• For latex allergy, drug should not be used
• For ALT, AST, GGT, alk phosphatase
Administer:
• **SUBCUT** using abdomen, around navel or upper thigh, swab inj area with disinfectant, clean a 2 in circle and allow to dry, pinch up area between thumb and finger, insert needle 45-90 degrees to surface; if positioned correctly, no blood will be drawn back into syringe, reposition needle without removing it
• Do not administer if patient is pregnant
Perform/provide:
• Protection from light
Evaluate:
• Therapeutic response: pregnancy
Teach patient/family:
• To report abdominal pain, vaginal bleeding, nausea, vomiting, diarrhea, shortness of breath, peripheral edema
• To teach self-administration technique if needed

cetuximab (℞)

(se-tux′i-mab)
Erbitux
Func. class.: Antineoplastic—miscellaneous, monoclonal antibody
Chem. class.: Epidermal growth factor receptor inhibitor

Action: Not fully understood; binds to epidermal growth factor receptors (EGFRs); inhibits phosphorylation and activation of receptor-associated kinase, resulting in inhibition of cell growth
Uses: Alone or in combination with irinotecan for EGFRs expressing metastatic colorectal carcinoma

DOSAGE AND ROUTES

• *Adult:* **IV INF** 400 mg/m² loading dose given over 120 min, max infusion rate 5 ml/min; weekly maintenance dose (all other infusions) is 250 mg/m² given over 60 min, max infusion rate 5 ml/min; premedicate with an H_1 antagonist (diphenhydrAMINE 50 mg IV); dosage adjustments are made for infusion reactions or dermatologic toxicity

Available forms: Inj 50 ml, single use vial with 100 mg of cetuximab (2 mg/ml)

SIDE EFFECTS

CNS: Headache, insomnia, depression
GI: Nausea, diarrhea, vomiting, anorexia, mouth ulceration, dehydration, constipation, abdominal pain
HEMA: **Leukopenia, anemia**
INTEG: Rash, pruritus, acne, dry skin, **toxic epidermal necrolysis, angioedema,** *blepharitis, cheilitis, cellulitis, cysts, alopecia, skin/nail disorder*
MISC: Conjunctivitis, asthma, malaise, fever, **renal failure**
MS: Back pain
RESP: **Interstitial lung disease,** *cough, dyspnea,* **pulmonary embolus,** *peripheral edema*
SYST: **Anaphylaxis, sepsis, infection**
Contraindications: Hypersensitivity to this drug or murine proteins
Precautions: Pregnancy (C), renal/hepatic disease, ocular, pulmonary disorders, lactation, children, elderly

PHARMACOKINETICS

Half-life 114 hr, steady state by 3rd weekly infusion, peak 168-235 g/ml, trough 41-85 g/ml

INTERACTIONS

None known

NURSING CONSIDERATIONS

Assess:

⚠ Pulmonary changes: lung sounds, cough, dyspnea; interstitial lung disease may occur, may be fatal; discontinue therapy if confirmed

⚠ Toxic epidermal necrosis, angioedema, anaphylaxis

• GI symptoms: frequency of stools, dehydration, abdominal pain, stomatitis

Administer:

IV INF route

• By IV infusion only, do not give by IV push or bolus

• Do not shake or dilute

• Infusion pump: draw up volume of a vial using appropriate syringe/needle (a vented spike or other appropriate transfer device); fill Erbitux into sterile evacuated container/bag, repeat until calculated volume has been put into the container; use a new needle for each vial; give through in-line filter (low protein binding 0.22-micrometer); affix infusion line and prime before starting infusion, max rate 5 ml/min; flush line at end of infusion with 0.9% NaCl

• Syringe pump: Draw up volume of a vial using appropriate syringe/needle (a vented spike); place syringe into syringe driver of a syringe pump and set rate; use an in-line filter 0.22-micrometer (low protein binding); connect infusion line and start infusion after priming; repeat until calculated volume has been given

• Use a new needle and filter for each vial, max 5 ml/min rate; use 0.9% NaCl to flush line after infusion

• Do not piggyback to patient infusion line

• Observe patient for adverse reactions for 1 hr after infusion

• Infusion reactions: if mild (grade 1 or 2) reduce all doses by 50%; if severe (grade 3 or 4) permanently discontinue

Perform/provide:

• Storage refrigerated 36°-46° F, discard unused portions

Evaluate:

• Therapeutic response: Decrease growth, spread of EGFR expressing metastatic colorectal carcinoma

Teach patient/family:

• To report adverse reactions immediately: shortness of breath, severe abdominal pain, skin eruptions

• Reason for treatment, expected results

• Use contraception during treatment, pregnancy (C)

• To wear sunscreen and hats to limit sun exposure; sun exposure can exacerbate any skin reactions

chloral hydrate (℞)
(klor-al hye'drate)
Aquachloral, chloral hydrate,
Novo-Chlorhydrate ✦, PMS-
chloral hydrate ✦
Func. class.: Sedative/hypnotic
Chem. class.: Chloral derivative

**Controlled Substance Schedule
IV (USA), Schedule F (Canada)**
Action: Reduction product trichloro-
ethanol produces mild cerebral depression, which causes sleep
Uses: Sedation, short-term treatment of
insomnia

DOSAGE AND ROUTES
Sedation
• *Adult:* **PO/RECT** 250 mg tid pc
• *Child:* **PO** 25-50 mg/kg tid, not to
exceed 500 mg tid
Insomnia
• *Adult:* **PO/RECT** 500 mg-1 g ½ hr
before bedtime
• *Child:* **PO/RECT** 50-75 mg/kg (one
dose)
Procedure sedation
• *Child:* **PO/RECT** 25-50 mg/kg, not to
exceed 100 mg/kg or 2 g
Renal disease
• CCr <50 ml/min avoid use
Available forms: Caps 250, 500, 650
mg; syr 250, 500 mg/5 ml; supp 325, 500
mg

SIDE EFFECTS

CNS: **Drowsiness,** dizziness, stimulation,
nightmares, ataxia, hangover (rare),
light-headedness, headache, paranoia
CV: Hypotension, **dysrhythmias**
GI: Nausea, vomiting, flatulence, diarrhea, unpleasant taste, **gastric necrosis**
HEMA: **Eosinophilia, leukopenia**
INTEG: Rash, urticaria, **angioedema,**
fever, purpura, eczema
RESP: **Depression**
Contraindications: Hypersensitivity
to this drug or triclofos, severe renal

disease, severe hepatic disease, GI disorders (oral forms), gastritis
Precautions: Pregnancy (C), severe
cardiac disease, depression, suicidal
individuals, asthma, intermittent porphyria, lactation, elderly

PHARMACOKINETICS

PO: Onset 30 min-1 hr, duration 4-8
hr
RECT: Onset slow, duration 4-8 hr;
metabolized by liver; excreted by
kidneys (inactive metabolite) and
feces; crosses placenta; excreted in
breast milk; metabolite is highly protein bound

INTERACTIONS

Increase: action—oral anticoagulants,
furosemide
Increase: action of both drugs—
alcohol, CNS depressants
Decrease: effects of—phenytoin
Drug/Herb
Increase: sedative effect—catnip, cham-
omile, clary, cowslip, hops, kava, laven-
der, mistletoe, nettle, pokeweed, poppy,
Queen Anne's lace, senega, skullcap,
valerian
Increase: hypotension—black cohosh
Drug/Lab Test
Interference: Urine catecholamines,
urinary 17-OHCS

NURSING CONSIDERATIONS
Assess:
• Mental status: mood, sensorium, af-
fect, memory (long-, short-term)
• Physical dependency: more frequent
requests for medication, tremors, anxi-
ety, pinpoint pupils
• Respiratory dysfunction: respiratory
depression, character, rate, rhythm; hold
drug if respirations <10/min or if pupils
dilated (rare)
• History of substance abuse, cardiac
disease, gastritis
Administer:
• Do not break, crush, or chew caps
• On empty stomach with full glass of

water or juice for best absorption and to decrease corrosion
• After meals to decrease GI symptoms if using for sedation
• ½-1 hr before bedtime for sleeplessness

Perform/provide:
• Assistance with ambulation after receiving dose, especially elderly
• Safety measure: night-light, call bell within easy reach
• Check to see PO medication swallowed
• Check dose of syrup carefully, fatal overdoses have occurred
• Storage in dark container, suppositories in refrigerator

Evaluate:
• Therapeutic response: ability to sleep at night, decreased amount of early morning awakening if taking drug for insomnia

Teach patient/family:
• To avoid driving, other activities requiring alertness
• To avoid alcohol ingestion, CNS depressants; serious CNS depression may result
• Not to discontinue medication quickly after long-term use; drug should be tapered over 1-2 wk, delirium may occur
• That effects may take 2 nights for benefits to be noticed
• Alternative measures to improve sleep (reading, exercise several hours before bedtime, warm bath, warm milk, TV, self-hypnosis, deep breathing)
• Avoid breastfeeding

Treatment of overdose: Lavage, activated charcoal; monitor electrolytes, vital signs

---

chlorambucil (℞)
(klor-am′byoo-sil)
Leukeran
Func. class.: Antineoplastic alkylating agent
Chem. class.: Nitrogen mustard

Do not confuse:
Leukeran/leucovorin
Leukeran/Leukine

Action: Alkylates DNA, RNA; inhibits enzymes that allow synthesis of amino acids in proteins; activity is not cell cycle phase specific

Uses: Chronic lymphocytic leukemia, non-Hodgkin's/Hodgkin's disease, other lymphomas, nephrotic syndrome, choriocarcinoma

Investigational uses: Macroglobulinemia ovarian, testicular carcinoma, non-Hodgkin's lymphoma

DOSAGE AND ROUTES

• *Adult:* **PO** 0.1-0.2 mg/kg/day for 3-6 wk initially, then 4-10 mg/day maintenance
• *Geriatric:* **PO** initially ≤2-4 mg/day
• *Child:* **PO** 0.1-0.2 mg/kg/day (4.5 mg/m^2/day) in divided doses or 4.5 mg/m^2/day as 1 dose or in divided doses × 3-6 wk

Macroglobulinemia (off-label)
• *Adult:* **PO** 2-10 mg daily × 9 days, or 8 mg/m^2 daily with predniSONE × 10 days, repeat q6-8wk as needed

Nephrotic syndrome
• *Child:* **PO** 0.1-0.2 mg/kg daily with predniSONE × 8-12 wk

Intractable idiopathic uveitis, Behçet's syndrome
• *Adult:* **PO** 6-12 mg or 0.1-0.2 mg/kg × 1 yr or more

Available forms: Tabs 2 mg

SIDE EFFECTS

*CNS: **Seizures,** tremors, confusion, agitation, ataxia*
*GI: Nausea, vomiting, diarrhea, weight loss, **hepatoxicity,** jaundice*
GU: Hyperuremia
*HEMA: **Thrombocytopenia, leukopenia, pancytopenia** (prolonged use), **permanent bone marrow depression***
INTEG: Alopecia (rare), dermatitis, rash, ***Stevens-Johnson syndrome***
*RESP: **Fibrosis, pneumonitis***

Contraindications: Pregnancy (D), radiation therapy within 1 mo, chemotherapy within 1 mo, thrombocytopenia, recent smallpox vaccination, lactation

C

Precautions: *Pneumococcus* vaccination, children

PHARMACOKINETICS

Well absorbed orally; metabolized in liver; excreted in urine; half-life 2 hr

INTERACTIONS

Increase: toxicity—other antineoplastics, radiation
Increase: risk of bleeding—anticoagulants, salicylates

NURSING CONSIDERATIONS

Assess:
• Bleeding: hematuria, guaiac, bruising or petechiae, mucosa or orifices q8h
• Jaundice of skin, sclera, dark urine, clay-colored stools, itchy skin, abdominal pain, fever, diarrhea
• Dyspnea, crackles, unproductive cough, chest pain, tachypnea
• Effects of alopecia on body image; discuss feelings about body changes (rare)
• CBC, differential, platelet count weekly; withhold drug if WBC is <2000 or granulocyte count is <1000/mm^3; notify prescriber of results
• Pulmonary function tests, chest x-ray films before, during therapy; chest film should be obtained q2wk during treatment
• Renal studies: BUN, serum uric acid, urine CCr before, during therapy; I&O ratio; report urine output of <30 ml/hr
• Monitor temp q4h (may indicate beginning infection)
• Hepatic studies before, during therapy (bilirubin, AST, ALT, LDH) as needed or monthly

Administer:
• All drugs PO if possible, avoid IM inj when platelets <100,000/mm^3
• Allopurinol to maintain uric acid levels, alkalinization of urine; increase fluid intake to 2-3 L/day to prevent urate deposits, calculi formation

Perform/provide:
• Storage in tight container, amber glass, store in refrigerator

Evaluate:
• Therapeutic response: decreased size of tumor, spread of malignancy

Teach patient/family:
• To report signs of infection: increased temperature, sore throat, persistent cough, flulike symptoms
• To report signs of anemia: fatigue, headache, faintness, shortness of breath, irritability, seizures, jaundice
• To report bleeding; avoid use of razors, commercial mouthwash
• To avoid use of aspirin products, ibuprofen
• To avoid vaccinations during treatment
• To use contraception during and several months after completion of therapy, may cause irreversible gonadal suppression
• To report any changes in breathing or coughing
• To drink 2-3 L of fluid daily unless contraindicated

chloramphenicol (℞)
(klor-am-fen'i-kole)
chloramphenicol,
Chloromycetin,
Pentamycetin ✦
Func. class.: Antiinfective—miscellaneous
Chem. class.: Dichloroacetic acid derivative

Action: Binds to 50S ribosomal subunit, which interferes with or inhibits protein synthesis
Uses: Infections caused by *Haemophilus influenzae, Salmonella typhi, Rickettsia, Neisseria,* mycoplasma; not to be used if less toxic drugs can be used

DOSAGE AND ROUTES
• *Adult and child:* **PO/IV** 50-75 mg/kg/day in divided doses q6h, 100 mg/kg/day (for meningitis only) max 4 g/day

• *Premature infants and neonates:*
IV/PO 25 mg/kg/day in divided doses
q12-24h
Available forms: Inj 1 g; caps 250 mg

SIDE EFFECTS

CNS: Headache, *depression,* confusion,
peripheral neuritis
CV: **Gray syndrome in newborns:
failure to feed, pallor, cyanosis,
abdominal distention, irregular
respiration, vasomotor collapse**
EENT: Optic neuritis, blindness
GI: *Nausea, vomiting, diarrhea,* abdominal pain, xerostomia, glossitis, colitis, pruritus ani
HEMA: **Anemia, thrombocytopenia,
aplastic anemia, granulocytopenia, leukopenia** (rare)
INTEG: Itching, urticaria, contact dermatitis, rash
Contraindications: Hypersensitivity,
severe renal disease, severe hepatic disease, minor infections
Precautions: Pregnancy (C), hepatic
disease, renal disease, infants, children,
bone marrow depression (drug-
induced), lactation

PHARMACOKINETICS

PO/IV: Peak 1-2 hr, duration 8 hr,
half-life 1½-4 hr; conjugated in liver;
excreted in urine (up to 15% as free
drug, up to 80% in neonates), excreted
in breast milk, feces; crosses placenta

INTERACTIONS

Increase: action of barbiturates, anticoagulants, hydantoins, iron products,
antidiabetics
Decrease: action of vit B_{12}, folic acid,
penicillins, rifampin
Drug/Herb
Do not use acidophilus with antiinfectives

NURSING CONSIDERATIONS

Assess:
• Signs of infection, anemia
A Any patient with compromised renal
system; drug is excreted slowly in poor

renal system function; toxicity may occur
rapidly
• Hepatic studies: AST, ALT
• Blood studies: WBC, RBC, Hct, Hgb,
platelets, serum iron, reticulocytes; drug
should be discontinued if bone marrow
is depressed
• Renal studies: urinalysis, protein,
blood, BUN, creatinine
• C&S before drug therapy; may be given
as soon as culture is taken
• Drug level in impaired hepatic, renal
systems; peak 15-20 mg/ml 3 hr after
dose, trough 5-10 mg/ml prior to next
dose
• Bowel pattern before, during treatment
• Skin eruptions, itching, dermatitis
after administration
• Allergies before treatment, reaction of
each medication
A Neonates for beginning Gray
syndrome: cyanosis, abdominal distention, irregular respiration, failure to feed;
drug should be discontinued immediately
Administer:
• Drug must be taken in equal intervals
around clock to maintain blood levels
• IM route not recommended
PO route
• Do not break, crush, or chew caps
• Oral form on empty stomach with full
glass of water
IV route
• After diluting 1 g/10 ml of sterile H_2O
for inj or D_5W (10% sol); give >1 min;
may be further diluted in 50-100 ml of
D_5W; give through Y-tube, 3-way stopcock, or additive inf set; run over ½-1 hr
Additive compatibilities: Amikacin,
aminophylline, ascorbic acid, calcium
chloride or gluconate, cephalothin,
cephapirin, colistimethate, corticotropin,
cyanocobalamin, dimenhyDRINATE,
DOPamine, epHEDrine, heparin, hydrocortisone, kanamycin, lidocaine, magnesium sulfate, metaraminol, methicillin,
methyldopa, methylPREDNISolone,
metronidazole, nafcillin, oxacillin, oxytocin, penicillin G potassium, penicillin G

Side effects: *italics* = common; **bold italics** = life-threatening

sodium, pentobarbital, phenylephrine, phytonadione, plasma protein fraction, potassium chloride, promazine, ranitidine, sodium bicarbonate, thiopental, verapamil, vit B/C

Syringe compatibilities: Ampicillin, cloxacillin, heparin, methicillin, penicillin G sodium

Y-site compatibilities: Acyclovir, cyclophosphamide, enalaprilat, esmolol, foscarnet, hydromorphone, labetalol, magnesium sulfate, meperidine, morphine, perphenazine, tacrolimus

Perform/provide:

• Storage of capsules in tight container at room temperature, reconstituted sol at room temperature 30 days

Evaluate:

• Therapeutic response: decreased symptoms of infection

Teach patient/family:

• All aspects of drug therapy: the need to complete entire course to ensure organism death (10-14 days); culture may be taken after complete course of medication

• To report sore throat, fever, fatigue, unusual bleeding, bruising; could indicate bone marrow depression (may occur weeks or months after termination of drug)

Treatment of hypersensitivity:

• Withdraw drug, maintain airway, administer epINEPHrine, aminophylline, O_2, IV corticosteroids

---

chloramphenicol ophthalmic
See Appendix C

---

chloramphenicol otic
See Appendix C

---

chlordiazepoxide (℞)
(klor-dye-az-e-pox′ide)
Apo-Chlordiazepoxide ✦, chlordiazepoxide HCl ✦, Librium, Novo-Poxide ✦
Func. class.: Antianxiety
Chem. class.: Benzodiazepine

Controlled Substance Schedule IV

Do not confuse:
Librium/Librax

Action: Potentiates the actions of GABA, especially in the limbic system, reticular formation

Uses: Short-term management of anxiety, acute alcohol withdrawal, preoperatively for relaxation

DOSAGE AND ROUTES

Mild anxiety

• *Adult:* **PO** 5-10 mg tid-qid

• *Geriatric:* **PO** 5 mg bid-qid initially, increase as needed

• *Child >6 yr:* **PO** 5 mg bid-qid, not to exceed 10 mg bid-tid

Severe anxiety

• *Adult:* **PO** 20-25 mg tid-qid; **IM/IV** 50-100 mg initially, then 25-50 mg tid or 25-50 mg initially in geriatrics

Preoperatively

• *Adult:* **PO** 5-10 mg tid-qid on day before surgery; **IM** 50-100 mg 1 hr before surgery

Alcohol withdrawal

• *Adult:* **PO/IM/IV** 50-100 mg, not to exceed 300 mg/day

Available forms: Caps 5, 10, 25 mg; inj 100 mg ampule

SIDE EFFECTS

CNS: Dizziness, drowsiness, confusion, headache, anxiety, tremors, stimulation, fatigue, depression, insomnia, hallucinations

CV: Orthostatic hypotension, ECG changes, tachycardia, hypotension

EENT: Blurred vision, tinnitus, mydriasis

GI: Constipation, dry mouth, nausea, vomiting, anorexia, diarrhea

---

INTEG: Rash, dermatitis, itching

Contraindications: Pregnancy (D), hypersensitivity to benzodiazepines, narrow-angle glaucoma, psychosis, lactation, child <6 yr

Precautions: Elderly, debilitated, hepatic disease, renal disease

PHARMACOKINETICS

PO: Onset 30 min, peak within 2 hr, duration 4-6 hr; metabolized by liver, excreted by kidneys; crosses placenta, excreted in breast milk; half-life 5-30 hr (increased in elderly)

INTERACTIONS

Increase: CNS depression—CNS depressants, alcohol

Increase: chlordiazepoxide—cimetidine, disulfiram, fluoxetine, isoniazid, ketoconazole, metoprolol, oral contraceptives, propranolol, valproic acid

Decrease: action of levodopa

Decrease: action of chlordiazepoxide—barbiturates, rifamycins

Drug/Herb

Decrease: effect—cowslip, kava, Queen Anne's lace, valerian

Drug/Lab Test

False increase: 17-OHCS

False positive: Pregnancy test (some methods)

NURSING CONSIDERATIONS

Assess:

• B/P (lying, standing), pulse; if systolic B/P drops 20 mm Hg, hold drug, notify prescriber

• Blood studies: CBC during long-term therapy; blood dyscrasias have occurred rarely

• Hepatic studies: AST, ALT, bilirubin, creatinine, LDH, alk phosphatase during long-term therapy

• I&O; may indicate renal dysfunction

• For ataxia, oversedation in elderly, debilitated patients

• Mental status: mood, sensorium, affect, sleeping pattern, drowsiness, dizziness

• Physical dependency, withdrawal symptoms: headache, nausea, vomiting, muscle pain, weakness after long-term use

• Suicidal tendencies, paradoxic reactions such as excitement, stimulation, acute rage

• For pregnancy; drug should be avoided during pregnancy

Administer:

PO route

• With food or milk for GI symptoms

• Crushed if patient is unable to swallow medication whole

IM route

• Add 2 ml diluent to powder, rotate until clear, use immediately

• Preferred route is IM

IV route

• 5 ml NS/100 mg powder; agitate ampule gently; give through Y-tube or 3-way stopcock; give 100 mg or less ≥1 min; do not use IM diluent for IV use

• Keep powder from light; refrigerate, mix when ready to use

Solution compatibilities: D$_5$W, 0.9% NaCl

Y-site compatibilities: Heparin, hydrocortisone, potassium chloride, vit B/C

Perform/provide:

• Assistance with ambulation during beginning therapy, since drowsiness/dizziness occurs

• Check to see PO medication has been swallowed if patient is depressed, suicidal

• Sugarless gum, hard candy, frequent sips of water for dry mouth

Evaluate:

• Therapeutic response: decreased anxiety, restlessness, sleeplessness

Teach patient/family:

• That drug may be taken with food

• Not to use drug for everyday stress or use longer than 4 mo, unless directed by prescriber

• Not to take more than prescribed amount; may be habit forming

• To avoid OTC preparations unless approved by prescriber

- To avoid driving, activities that require alertness; drowsiness may occur
- To avoid alcohol ingestion, other psychotropic medications, unless directed by prescriber
- Not to discontinue medication abruptly after long-term use; may precipitate seizures
- To rise slowly or fainting may occur, especially elderly
- That drowsiness may be worse at beginning of treatment
- To notify prescriber if pregnancy is suspected or planned

Treatment of overdose: Lavage, VS, supportive care, give flumazenil

chloroquine (℞)
(klor´oh-kwin)
Aralen HCl, Aralen Phosphate, chloroquine phosphate
Func. class.: Antimalarial
Chem. class.: Synthetic 4-aminoquinoline derivative

Action: Inhibits parasite replications, transcription of DNA to RNA by forming complexes with DNA of parasite

Uses: Malaria of *Plasmodium vivax, P. malariae, P. ovale, P. falciparum* (some strains), amebiasis

DOSAGE AND ROUTES

Malaria suppression
- *Adult and child:* **PO** 5 mg base/kg/wk on same day of week, not to exceed 300 mg base; treatment should begin 1-2 wk before exposure and for 8 wk after; if treatment begins after exposure, 600 mg base for adult and 10 mg base/kg for children in 2 divided doses 6 hr apart

Extraintestinal amebiasis
- *Adult:* **IM** 160-200 mg base daily × 10-12 days or **PO** (HCl) 600 mg base daily × 2 days, then 300 mg base daily × 2-3 wk (phosphate)
- *Child:* **IM/PO** 10 mg/kg daily (HCl) × 2-3 wk, not to exceed 300 mg/day

Available forms: Tabs 250 mg (150 mg base), 500 mg (300 mg base) phosphate; inj 50 mg (40 mg base)/ml HCl

SIDE EFFECTS

CNS: Headache, stimulation, fatigue, *convulsion,* psychosis
CV: Hypotension, *heart block, asystole with syncope,* ECG changes
EENT: Blurred vision, corneal changes, retinal changes, difficulty focusing, tinnitus, vertigo, deafness, photophobia, corneal edema
GI: Nausea, vomiting, anorexia, diarrhea, cramps
HEMA: Thrombocytopenia, agranulocytosis, hemolytic anemia, leukopenia
INTEG: Pruritus, pigmentary changes, skin eruptions, lichen planus–like eruptions, eczema, *exfoliative dermatitis*
Contraindications: Hypersensitivity, retinal field changes
Precautions: Pregnancy (C), children, blood dyscrasias, severe GI disease, neurologic disease, alcoholism, hepatic disease, G6PD deficiency, psoriasis, eczema, lactation

PHARMACOKINETICS
Metabolized in liver; excreted in urine, feces, breast milk; crosses placenta
PO: Peak 1-3 hr, half-life 3-5 days
IM: Peak 30 min

INTERACTIONS
Reduced oral clearance and metabolism of chloroquine: cimetidine
Decrease: action of chloroquine—magnesium, aluminum compounds, kaolin

NURSING CONSIDERATIONS
Assess:
- Ophthalmic test if long-term treatment or dosage >150 mg/day
- Hepatic studies qwk: AST, ALT, bilirubin
- Blood studies: CBC, since blood dyscrasias occur

• ECG during therapy; watch for depression of T waves, widening of QRS complex

• Allergic reactions: pruritus, rash, urticaria

• Blood dyscrasias: malaise, fever, bruising, bleeding (rare)

• For ototoxicity (tinnitus, vertigo, change in hearing); audiometric testing should be done before, after treatment

⚠ For toxicity: blurring vision; difficulty focusing; headache; dizziness; decreased knee, ankle reflexes, seizures, CV collapse; drug should be discontinued immediately

Administer:

• IM after aspirating to avoid inj blood system, which may cause hypotension, asystole, heart block; rotate inj sites

PO route

• Before or after meals at same time each day to maintain drug level

Additive compatibilities: Promethazine

Perform/provide:

• Storage in tight, light-resistant container at room temperature; keep injection in cool environment

Evaluate:

• Therapeutic response: decreased symptoms of infection

Teach patient/family:

• To take with meals or immediately after meals

• To use sunglasses in bright sunlight to decrease photophobia

• That urine may turn rust or brown color

• To report hearing, visual problems, fever, fatigue, bruising, bleeding, which may indicate blood dyscrasias

Treatment of overdose: Induce vomiting, gastric lavage, administer barbiturate (ultrashort-acting), vasopressor; tracheostomy may be necessary

---

chlorothiazide (Ŗ)
(klor-oh-thye′a-zide)
Diuril
Func. class.: Diuretic
Chem. class.: Thiazide; sulfonamide derivative

C

Do not confuse:
chlorothiazide/chlorproMAZINE/
chlorthalidone/chlorproPAMIDE
Action: Acts on distal tubule and thick ascending limb of the loop of Henle by increasing excretion of water, sodium, chloride, potassium, magnesium
Uses: Edema, hypertension, diuresis

DOSAGE AND ROUTES

Edema, hypertension
• *Adult:* **PO/IV** 500 mg-2 g daily may divide bid
Diuresis
• *Adult:* **IV** 250 mg q6-12h
• *Child >6 mo:* **PO** 10-20 mg/kg/day may divide bid
• *Child <6 mo:* **PO** up to 40 mg/kg/day in 2 doses
Available forms: Tabs 250, 500 mg; inj 500 mg; oral susp 250 mg/5 ml

SIDE EFFECTS

CNS: Paresthesia, anxiety, depression, headache, *dizziness, fatigue, weakness,* insomnia
CV: Irregular pulse, orthostatic hypotension, palpitations, volume depletion
EENT: Blurred vision
ELECT: Hypokalemia, hypercalcemia, hyponatremia, hypochloremia, hypophosphatemia, hypomagnesemia
GI: Nausea, vomiting, anorexia, constipation, diarrhea, cramps, pancreatitis, GI irritation, ***hepatitis***
GU: Urinary frequency, polyuria, ***uremia,*** glucosuria, hematuria
*HEMA: **Aplastic anemia, hemolytic anemia, leukopenia, agranulocy-***

---

tosis, thrombocytopenia, neutropenia
INTEG: Rash, urticaria, purpura, photosensitivity, fever, alopecia
META: Hyperglycemia, *hyperuricemia,* increased creatinine, BUN
Contraindications: Hypersensitivity to thiazides or sulfonamides, hepatic coma, anuria, renal decompensation, lactation
Precautions: Pregnancy (B), hypokalemia, renal disease, hepatic disease, gout, COPD, SLE, diabetes mellitus, elderly, hyperlipidemia

PHARMACOKINETICS

Not well absorbed PO
PO: Onset 2 hr, peak 4 hr, duration 6-12 hr; crosses placenta, excreted in breast milk, excreted unchanged by kidneys; half-life 2 hr

INTERACTIONS

Hypokalemia: ticarcillin, glucocorticoids, amphotericin, mezlocillin, piperacillin
Increase: toxicity—lithium, nondepolarizing skeletal muscle relaxants, digitalis, allopurinol
Increase: hypotension—other antihypertensives, alcohol, nitrates
Decrease: absorption of thiazides—cholestyramine, colestipol
Decrease: diuretic action—NSAIDs
Drug/Herb
Hypokalemia: chronic use aloe, buckthorn, cascara sagrada, Chinese rhubarb, gossypol, licorice, nettle, senna
Severe photosensitivity: St. John's wort
Increase: diuretic effect—aloe, cucumber, dandelion, horsetail, pumpkin, Queen Anne's lace
Drug/Lab Test
Increase: BSP retention, Ca, amylase, parathyroid test
Decrease: PBI, PSP
False negative: Phentolamine and tyramine tests
Interference: Urine steroid tests

NURSING CONSIDERATIONS
Assess:
• Weight, I&O daily to determine fluid loss; effect of drug may be decreased if used daily
• Rate, depth, rhythm of respirations; effect of exertion
• B/P lying, standing; postural hypotension may occur, especially in elderly
• Electrolytes: K, Na, Cl; include BUN, blood glucose, CBC, serum creatinine, blood pH, ABGs, uric acid, Ca, Mg
• Glucose in urine if patient is diabetic
• Signs of metabolic alkalosis: drowsiness, restlessness
• Rashes, temp elevation daily
• Confusion, especially in elderly; take safety precautions if needed
Administer:
• In AM to avoid interference with sleep if using drug as a diuretic
• Potassium replacement if potassium < 3 mg/dl
• With food if nausea occurs; absorption may be decreased slightly; dehydration may occur; tablets may be crushed
• After shaking suspension
IV route
• After diluting 0.5 g/18 ml or more of sterile water for inj; may be diluted further with 0.9% NaCl, D_5W, check for extravasation; give over 5 min (0.5 g/5 min)
Additive compatibilities: Cimetidine, lidocaine, nafcillin, ranitidine, sodium bicarbonate
Evaluate:
• Therapeutic response: improvement in edema of feet, legs, sacral area daily if medication is being used for CHF; decreased B/P; increased urinary output
Teach patient/family:
• To rise slowly from lying or sitting position; orthostatic hypotension may occur
• To notify prescriber of muscle weakness, cramps, nausea, dizziness
• That drug may be taken with food or milk; to take at same time each day; not to double dose

⚠ Safety alert   *"Tall Man" lettering

- That blood glucose may be increased in diabetics
- To take early in day to avoid nocturia
- To use sunscreen; use protective clothing to prevent photosensitivity
- To weigh weekly and notify prescriber of change of >3 lb
- To eat diet high in potassium if recommended by prescriber; teach high-potassium foods
- Not to take OTC medications without consulting prescriber

Treatment of overdose: Lavage if taken orally; monitor electrolytes; administer dextrose in saline; monitor hydration, CV, renal status

---

chlorpheniramine
(OTC, ℞)

(klor-fen-ir′a-meen)
Aller-Chlor, Chlo-Amine, Chlorate, chlorpheniramine maleate, Chlor-Trimeton, Chlor-Tripolon ✦, Gen-Allerate, Novo-Pheniram ✦, Pedia Care Allergy Formula, Phenetron, Teldrin

Func. class.: Antihistamine (1st generation, nonselective)
Chem. class.: Alkylamine, H_1-receptor antagonist

Do not confuse:
Teldrin/Tedral

Action: Acts on blood vessels, GI system, respiratory system, by competing with histamine for H_1-receptor site; decreases allergic response by blocking histamine

Uses: Allergy symptoms, rhinitis

DOSAGE AND ROUTES

- *Adult and child ≥12 yr:* **PO** 2-4 mg tid-qid, not to exceed 24 mg/day; **TIME-REL** 8-12 mg bid-tid, not to exceed 24 mg/day; **IM/IV/SUBCUT** 5-40 mg/day, max 40 mg/day
- *Child 6-12 yr:* **PO** 2 mg q4-6h, not to exceed 12 mg/day; **SUS REL** 8 mg bed-time or daily, **SUS REL** not recommended for child <6 yr; **SUBCUT** 87.5 mcg/kg or 2.5 mg/m² q6h
- *Child 2-5 yr:* **PO** 1 mg q4-6h, not to exceed 4 mg/day

Available forms: Tabs, chewable 2 mg; tabs 4, 8, 12 mg; tabs, time-rel 8, 12 mg; caps, time-rel 8, 12 mg; syr 1 mg/5 ml, 2 mg/5 ml, 2.5 mg/5 ml; inj 10, 100 mg/ml

SIDE EFFECTS

CNS: Dizziness, drowsiness, poor coordination, fatigue, anxiety, euphoria, confusion, paresthesia, neuritis
EENT: Blurred vision, dilated pupils, tinnitus, nasal stuffiness, dry nose, throat, mouth
GI: Nausea, anorexia, diarrhea
GU: Retention, dysuria, urinary frequency
*HEMA: **Thrombocytopenia, agranulocytosis, hemolytic anemia***
INTEG: Photosensitivity
RESP: Increased thick secretions, wheezing, chest tightness

Contraindications: Hypersensitivity to H_1-receptor antagonists, acute asthma attack, lower respiratory tract disease, stenosed peptic ulcers, bladder neck obstruction, angle-closure glaucoma, newborns/neonates
Precautions: Pregnancy (B), increased intraocular pressure, renal disease, cardiac disease, hypertension, bronchial asthma, seizure disorder, hyperthyroidism, prostatic hypertrophy, lactation, elderly

PHARMACOKINETICS

PO: Onset ½ hr, duration 4-12 hr
PO-ER: Duration 8-24 hr
SUBCUT/IM/IV: duration 4-12 hr; detoxified in liver; excreted by kidneys (metabolites/free drug); half-life 12-15 hr

INTERACTIONS

Increase: CNS depression—barbiturates, opiates, hypnotics, tricyclics, alcohol

---

Side effects: *italics* = common; ***bold italics*** = life-threatening

Increase: effect of chlorpheniramine—MAOIs

Increase: anticholinergic action—atropine, phenothiazines, quinidine, haloperidol

Drug/Herb

Increase: effect—hops, Jamaican dogwood, kava, khat, senega

Increase: anticholinergic effect—corkwood, henbane leaf

Drug/Lab Test

False negative: Skin allergy tests

NURSING CONSIDERATIONS

Assess:

• Be alert for urinary retention, frequency, dysuria; drug should be discontinued

• Respiratory status: rate, rhythm, increase in bronchial secretions, wheezing, chest tightness

Administer:

• Avoid concurrent use with other CNS depressants

PO route

• Do not break, crush, or chew sustained-release forms

• With meals for GI symptoms; absorption may slightly decrease

IV route

• Undiluted at ≥10 mg/1 min

• Use only 10 mg/ml form for IV use

Perform/provide:

• Hard candy, gum, frequent rinsing of mouth for dryness

• Storage in tight container at room temperature

Evaluate:

• Therapeutic response: absence of running, congested nose, rashes

Teach patient/family:

• All aspects of drug use; to notify prescriber of confusion/sedation/hypotension, difficulty voiding

• To avoid driving, other hazardous activity if drowsiness occurs, especially elderly

• To avoid concurrent use of alcohol

Treatment of overdose: Administer diazepam, vasopressors, barbiturates (short-acting)

---

*chlorproMAZINE (℞)

(klor-proe′ma-zeen)
Chlorpromanyl ✦,
chlorproMAZINE HCl,
Largactil ✦, Novo-
Chlorpromazine ✦,
Thorazine, Thor-Prom
Func. class.: Antipsychotic/neuro-leptic/antiemetic
Chem. class.: Phenothiazine-aliphatic

Do not confuse:

chlorproMAZINE/chlorproPAMIDE
chlorproMAZINE/prochlorperazine

Action: Depresses cerebral cortex, hypothalamus, limbic system, which control activity aggression; blocks neurotransmission produced by dopamine at synapse; exhibits a strong α-adrenergic, anticholinergic blocking action; mechanism for antipsychotic effects is unclear

Uses: Psychotic disorders, mania, schizophrenia, anxiety, intractable hiccups in adults, nausea, vomiting; preoperatively for relaxation; acute intermittent porphyria, behavioral problems in children, nonpsychotic, demented patients, Tourette's syndrome

Investigational uses: Vascular headache

DOSAGE AND ROUTES

Psychosis

• *Adult:* **PO** 10-50 mg q1-4h initially, then increase up to 2 g/day if necessary; **IM** 10-50 mg q1-4h, usual dose 300-800 mg/day

• *Geriatric:* 10-25 mg daily-bid, increase by 10-25 mg/day q4-7 days, max 800 mg/day

• *Child >6 mo:* **PO** 0.5 mg/kg q4-6h; **IM** 0.5 mg/kg q6-8h; **RECT** 1 mg/kg q6-8h

Nausea and vomiting

• *Adult:* **PO** 10-25 mg q4-6h prn; **IM** 25-50 mg q3h prn; **RECT** 50-100 mg

---

q6-8h prn, not to exceed 400 mg/day; **IV** 25-50 mg daily-qid
• *Child ≥6 mo:* **PO** 0.55 mg/kg q4-6h; **IM** q6-8h; **RECT** 1.1 mg/kg q6-8h; max **IM** ≤5 yr or ≤22.7 kg, 40 mg; max **IM** 5-10 yr or 22.7-45.5 kg, 75 mg

Intractable hiccups
• *Adult:* **PO** 25-50 mg tid-qid; **IM** 25-50 mg (only if PO dose does not work); **IV** 25-50 mg in 500-1000 ml **NS** (only for severe hiccups)

Available forms: Tabs 10, 25, 50, 100, 200 mg; sus-rel caps 30, 75, 150, 200, 300 mg; syr 10, 25, 100 mg/5 ml; conc 30, 40, 100 mg/ml; supp 25, 100 mg; inj 25 mg/ml

SIDE EFFECTS

CNS: EPS: pseudoparkinsonism, akathisia, dystonia, tardive dyskinesia, seizures, *headache,* **neuroleptic malignant syndrome,** dizziness
CV: Orthostatic hypotension, hypertension, **cardiac arrest,** ECG changes, **tachycardia**
EENT: Blurred vision, glaucoma, dry eyes
GI: Dry mouth, nausea, vomiting, anorexia, constipation, diarrhea, jaundice, weight gain
GU: Urinary retention, enuresis, impotence, amenorrhea, gynecomastia, breast engorgement
HEMA: Anemia, **leukopenia, leukocytosis, agranulocytosis**
INTEG: Rash, photosensitivity, dermatitis
RESP: **Laryngospasm,** dyspnea, **respiratory depression**

Contraindications: Hypersensitivity, circulatory collapse, liver damage, cerebral arteriosclerosis, coronary disease, severe hyper/hypotension, blood dyscrasias, coma, child <6 mo, brain damage, bone marrow depression, alcohol/ barbiturate withdrawal, narrow-angle glaucoma

Precautions: Pregnancy (C), lactation, seizure disorders, hypertension, hepatic disease, cardiac disease, elderly, prostatic enlargement

PHARMACOKINETICS

PO: Absorption variable, widely distributed; onset erratic 30-60 min, duration 4-6 hr
PO-ER: Onset 30-60 min, peak unknown, duration 10-12 hr
REC: Onset erratic, duration 3 hr
IM: Well absorbed; peak 15-20 min, duration 4-8 hr
IV: Onset 5 min, peak 10 min, duration unknown
Metabolized by liver, excreted in urine (metabolites), crosses placenta, enters breast milk; 95% bound to plasma proteins; elimination half-life 10-30 hr

INTERACTIONS

Lowered seizure threshold: anticonvulsants
Oversedation: other CNS depressants, alcohol, barbiturate anesthetics, antihistamines, sedatives/hypnotics, antidepressants
Toxicity: epINEPHrine
Agranulocystosis: antithyroid agents
Increase: effects of both drugs—β-adrenergic blockers, alcohol
Increase: anticholinergic effects—anticholinergics, antidepressants, antiparkinsonian agents
Increase: valproic acid level
Decrease: absorption—aluminum hydroxide, magnesium hydroxide antacids
Decrease: antiparkinson activity—levodopa, bromocriptine
Decrease: serum chlorproMAZINE—lithium, barbiturates
Decrease: anticoagulant effect—warfarin
Drug/Herb
Increase: action—cola tree, hops, nettle, nutmeg
Increase: anticholinergic effect—henbane leaf
Increase: EPS—betel palm, kava
Drug/Lab Test
Increase: Hepatic studies, cardiac enzymes, cholesterol, blood glucose, pro-

lactin, bilirubin, PBI, cholinesterase,[131]I, alk phosphatase, leukocytes, granulocytes, platelets

Decrease: Hormones (blood and urine)

False positive: Pregnancy tests, PKU

False negative: Urinary steroids, 17-OHCS

NURSING CONSIDERATIONS

Assess:

• Mental status: orientation, mood, behavior, presence and type of hallucinations before initial administration and monthly

• Any potentially reversible causes of behavior problems in the elderly before and during therapy

• Swallowing of PO medication; check for hoarding or giving of medication to other patients

• I&O ratio; palpate bladder if low urinary output occurs, especially in elderly

• Bilirubin, CBC, LFTs, ocular exam; agranulocytosis may occur, monthly

• Urinalysis recommended before, during prolonged therapy

• Affect, orientation, LOC, reflexes, gait, coordination, sleep pattern disturbances

• B/P sitting, standing, lying; take pulse and respirations q4h during initial treatment; establish baseline before starting treatment; report drops of 30 mm Hg; obtain baseline ECG, Q-wave and T-wave changes

• Dizziness, faintness, palpitations, tachycardia on rising

⚠ For neuroleptic malignant syndrome: hyperpyrexia, muscle rigidity, increased CPK, altered mental status, for acute dystonia (check chewing, swallowing, eyes, pill rolling)

• EPS including akathisia (inability to sit still, no pattern to movements), tardive dyskinesia (bizarre movements of the jaw, mouth, tongue, extremities), pseudoparkinsonism (rigidity, tremors, pill rolling, shuffling gait)

• Skin turgor daily

• Constipation, urinary retention daily; increase bulk, H_2O in diet

Administer:

• IM, inject in deep muscle mass, do not give SUBCUT

• Rectal after placing in refrigerator for ½ hr if too soft to insert

• Antiparkinsonian agent for EPS if ordered

PO route

• Do not break, crush, or chew time-rel caps

• With full glass of water, milk; or with food to decrease GI upset

• Drug in liquid form mixed in glass of juice or cola if hoarding is suspected

• Periodically attempt dosage reduction in behavioral problems

• Avoid use with CNS depressants

IV route

• After diluting 1 mg/1 ml with NS, give 1 mg or less/2 min or more; may be further diluted in 500-1000 ml of NS

Additive compatibilities: Ascorbic acid, ethacrynate, netilmicin, theophylline, vit B/C

Syringe compatibilities: Atropine, benztropine, butorphanol, diphenhydrAMINE, doxapram, droperidol, fentanyl, glycopyrrolate, hydromorphone, hydrOXYzine, meperidine, metoclopramide, midazolam, morphine, pentazocine, perphenazine, prochlorperazine, promazine, promethazine, scopolamine

Y-site compatibilities: Amsacrine, cisatracurium, cisplatin, cladribine, cyclophosphamide, cytarabine, DOXOrubicin, DOXOrubicin liposome, famotidine, filgrastim, fluconazole, granisetron, heparin, hydrocortisone, ondansetron, potassium chloride, propofol, teniposide, thiotepa, vinorelbine, vit B/C

Perform/provide:

• Supervised ambulation until stabilized on medication; do not involve in strenuous exercise program because fainting is possible; patient should not stand still for long periods

• Increased fluids and roughage to prevent constipation

• Candy, gum, sips of water for dry mouth

- Storage in tight, light-resistant container, oral sol in amber bottle

Evaluate:

- Therapeutic response: decrease in emotional excitement, hallucinations, delusions, paranoia, reorganization of patterns of thought, speech, increase in target behaviors

Teach patient/family:

- To use good oral hygiene; frequent rinsing of mouth, sugarless gum, candy, ice chips for dry mouth
- To avoid hazardous activities until drug response is determined
- That orthostatic hypotension occurs often and to rise gradually from sitting or lying position
- To remain lying down for at least 30 min after IM inj
- To avoid hot tubs, hot showers, tub baths, since hypotension may occur; that in hot weather, heat stroke may occur; take extra precautions to stay cool
- To avoid abrupt withdrawal of this drug or EPS may result; drug should be withdrawn slowly
- To avoid OTC preparations (cough, hay fever, cold) unless approved by prescriber, since serious drug interactions may occur; avoid use with alcohol, increased drowsiness may occur
- To use a sunscreen and sunglasses to prevent burns
- To take antacids 2 hr before or after this drug
- To report sore throat, malaise, fever, bleeding, mouth sores; CBC should be drawn and drug discontinued
- Contraceptive measures
- That urine may turn pink or reddish-brown

Treatment of overdose: Lavage if orally ingested; provide airway; *do not induce vomiting or use epINEPHrine*

Rarely Used

*chlorproPAMIDE (R)

(klor-proe'pa-mide)
Chloronase ✤,
ChlorproPAMIDE, Diabinese,
Novopropamide ✤
Functional class.: Antidiabetic
Uses: Type 2, non–insulin-dependent diabetes mellitus

Uses: Type 2 diabetes mellitus

DOSAGE AND ROUTES

- *Adult:* **PO** 100-250 mg daily, initially, then 100-500 mg maintenance according to response; not to exceed 750 mg/day

Contraindications: Pregnancy (D), hypersensitivity to sulfonylureas, juvenile or brittle diabetes, lactation, renal failure

chlorthalidone (R)

(klor-thal'i-done)
Apo-Chlorthalidone ✤,
chlorthalidone, Hygroton,
Thalitone, Uridon ✤
Func. class.: Diuretic
Chem. class.: Thiazide-like phthalimidine derivative

Do not confuse:
Uridon/Vicodin
Hygroton/Regroton

Action: Acts on distal tubule and thick ascending limb of the loop of Henle by increasing excretion of water, sodium, chloride, potassium, magnesium, bicarbonate, possible arteriolar dilation

Uses: Edema, hypertension, diuresis, edema in CHF, nephrotic syndrome

DOSAGE AND ROUTES

- *Adult:* **PO** 25-200 mg/day or 100 mg every other day
- *Geriatric:* **PO** 12.5 mg daily, initially
- *Child:* **PO** 2 mg/kg or 60 mg/m^2 3 ×/wk

Available forms: Tabs 25, 50, 100 mg

SIDE EFFECTS

CNS: Paresthesia, headache, *dizziness, fatigue, weakness*

CV: Irregular pulse, orthostatic hypotension, palpitations, volume depletion

EENT: Blurred vision

ELECT: Hypokalemia, hypomagnesemia, hypercalcemia, hyponatremia, hypochloremia

GI: Nausea, vomiting, anorexia, constipation, diarrhea, cramps, pancreatitis, GI irritation, *hepatitis*

GU: Urinary frequency, polyuria, *uremia,* glucosuria, impotence

HEMA: Aplastic anemia, hemolytic anemia, leukopenia, agranulocytosis, thrombocytopenia, neutropenia

INTEG: Rash, urticaria, purpura, photosensitivity, fever

META: Hyperglycemia, hyperuremia, increased creatinine, BUN, gout

Contraindications: Hypersensitivity to thiazides or sulfonamides, anuria, renal decompensation, lactation

Precautions: Pregnancy (B), hypokalemia, renal disease, hepatic disease, gout, diabetes mellitus, elderly, hyperlipidemia

PHARMACOKINETICS

PO: Onset 2 hr, peak 6 hr, duration 24-72 hr; excreted unchanged by kidneys; crosses placenta; enters breast milk; half-life 40 hr

INTERACTIONS

Hyperglycemia, hypotension: diazoxide

Hypokalemia: glucocorticoids, amphotericin B

Increase: toxicity of lithium, nondepolarizing skeletal muscle relaxants, allopurinol

Increase: hypotensive effect—alcohol

Decrease: absorption of thiazides—cholestyramine, colestipol

Drug/Herb

Potassium deficiency: chronic use of buckthorn, cascara sagrada, Chinese rhubarb, gossypol, licorice, nettle, senna

Severe photosensitivity—St. John's Wort

Increase: hypotension—cucumber, dandelion, khella, horsetail, pumpkin, Queen Anne's lace

Drug/Lab Test

Increase: BSP retention, calcium, cholesterol, triglycerides, amylase

Decrease: PBI, PSP, parathyroid test

NURSING CONSIDERATIONS

Assess:

• Weight, I&O daily to determine fluid loss; effect of drug may be decreased if used daily

• Rate, depth, rhythm of respiration, effect of exertion, B/P lying, standing; postural hypotension may occur

• Electrolytes: K, Mg, Na, Cl; include BUN, blood glucose, CBC, serum creatinine, serum creatinine, blood pH, ABGs, uric acid, Ca

• Blood glucose levels if patient is diabetic

• Signs of metabolic alkalosis: drowsiness, restlessness

• Signs of hypokalemia: postural hypotension, malaise, fatigue, tachycardia, leg cramps, weakness

• Rashes, temp elevation daily

• Confusion, especially in elderly; take safety precautions if needed

Administer:

• In AM to avoid interference with sleep if using drug as a diuretic

• Potassium replacement if potassium less than 3 mg/dl

• With food if nausea occurs; absorption may be decreased slightly

Evaluate:

• Therapeutic response: improvement in edema of feet, legs, sacral area daily if medication used in CHF

Teach patient/family:

• To rise slowly from lying or sitting position

• To notify prescriber of muscle weakness, cramps, nausea, dizziness

• That drug may be taken with food or milk

• To maintain adequate potassium intake

⚠ Safety alert   *"Tall Man" lettering

• That blood glucose may be increased in diabetics
• To use sunscreen to protect against photosensitivity
• To take early in day to avoid nocturia
Treatment of overdose: Lavage if taken orally, monitor electrolytes, administer dextrose in NS, monitor hydration, CV, renal status

---

chlorzoxazone (℞)

(klor-zox′a-zone)
EZE-DS, chlorzoxazone, Paraflex, Parafon Forte DSC, Relaxazone, Remular, Remular-S, Strifon Forte DSC
Func. class.: Skeletal muscle relaxant, central acting
Chem. class.: Benzoxazole derivative

Do not confuse:
Parafon Forte DSC/Fam-Pren Forte
Action: Inhibits multisynaptic reflex arcs causing skeletal muscle relaxation
Uses: Relieving pain, spasm in musculoskeletal conditions

DOSAGE AND ROUTES

• *Adult:* **PO** 250-750 mg tid-qid
• *Child:* **PO** 20 mg/kg/day in divided doses bid-tid
Available forms: Tabs 250, 500 mg

SIDE EFFECTS

CNS: Dizziness, drowsiness, headache, insomnia, stimulation, malaise
GI: Nausea, vomiting, anorexia, diarrhea, constipation, *GI bleeding, hepatotoxicity*
GU: Urine discoloration
HEMA: Granulocytopenia, anemia
INTEG: Rash, pruritus, petechiae, ecchymoses, *angioedema*
SYST: Anaphylaxis, angioedema
Contraindications: Hypersensitivity, impaired hepatic function
Precautions: Pregnancy (unknown), lactation, hepatic disease, elderly

PHARMACOKINETICS

PO: Onset 1 hr, peak 1-2 hr, duration 3-4 hr, half-life 1 hr; metabolized in liver; excreted in urine (metabolites)

INTERACTIONS

Increase: CNS depression—alcohol, tricyclics, opiates, barbiturates, sedatives, hypnotics
Drug/Herb
May increase CNS depression—kava

NURSING CONSIDERATIONS

Assess:
• Blood studies: CBC, WBC, differential for blood dyscrasias if on long-term therapy
• Allergic reactions: rash, fever, respiratory distress
• CNS depression: dizziness, drowsiness, psychiatric symptoms
Administer:
• With meals for GI symptoms
Perform/provide:
• Storage in tight container at room temperature
Evaluate:
• Therapeutic response: decreased pain, spasticity
Teach patient/family:
• Not to discontinue abruptly; insomnia, nausea, headache, spasticity, tachycardia will occur; drug should be tapered over 1-2 wk
• To notify prescriber if fever, rash, anorexia, RUQ pain, dark urine, or jaundice occur
• Not to take with alcohol, other CNS depressants; take with food
• To avoid hazardous activities if drowsiness, dizziness occurs
• To avoid using OTC medication: cough preparations, antihistamines, unless directed by prescriber
• That urine may be orange or purple
Treatment of overdose: Gastric lavage or induce emesis, then administer activated charcoal; use other supportive treatment as necessary; monitor cardiac function

---

Side effects: *italics* = common; ***bold italics*** = life-threatening

cholestyramine (℞)

(koe-less-tir'a-meen)
LoCHOLEST, LoCHOLEST
Light, Prevalite, Questran,
Questran Light
Func. class.: Antilipemic
Chem. class.: Bile acid sequestrant

Action: Absorbs, combines with bile acids to form insoluble complex that is excreted through feces; loss of bile acids lowers cholesterol levels

Uses: Primary hypercholesterolemia, pruritus associated with biliary obstruction

Investigational uses: Diarrhea caused by excess bile acid

DOSAGE AND ROUTES

• *Adult:* PO 4 g daily or bid, max 24 g/day
• *Child:* PO 240 mg/kg/day in 3 divided doses with food or drink, max 8 g/day
Available forms: Powder for susp 4 g cholestyramine/packet or scoop

SIDE EFFECTS

CNS: Headache, dizziness, drowsiness, vertigo, tinnitus, anxiety
GI: Constipation, abdominal pain, nausea, fecal impaction, hemorrhoids, flatulence, vomiting, steatorrhea, peptic ulcer
*HEMA: **Bleeding,*** increased PT
INTEG: Rash, irritation of perianal area, tongue, skin
META: Decreased vit A, D, K, red cell folate content; ***hyperchloremic acidosis***
MS: Muscle, joint pain
Contraindications: Hypersensitivity, biliary obstruction
Precautions: Pregnancy (C), lactation, children

PHARMACOKINETICS

PO: Excreted in feces, LDL lowered in 4-7 days, serum cholesterol lowered in 1 mo

INTERACTIONS

Decrease: absorption of—warfarin, thiazides, cardiac glycosides; propranolol, corticosteroids, iron, thyroid hormones, fat-soluble vitamins, clindamycin, penicillin G, tetracyclines, clofibrate, gemfibrozil, glipiZIDE, phenytoin, vit A, D, E, K

Drug/Herb
Increase: effect—glucomannan
Decrease: gotu kola
Drug/Lab Test
Increase: AST, ALT, alk phosphatase
Decrease: Sodium, potassium
Interfere: cholecystography

NURSING CONSIDERATIONS

Assess:
• Cardiac glycoside level, if both drugs are being administered
• For signs of vit A, D, K deficiency
• Fasting LDL, HDL, total cholesterol, triglyceride levels, electrolytes if on extended therapy
• Bowel pattern daily; increase bulk, H_2O in diet for constipation
Administer:
• Drug daily or bid; give all other medications 1 hr before cholestyramine or 4-6 hr after cholestyramine to avoid poor absorption
• Drug mixed with applesauce or stirred into beverage (2-6 oz), let stand for 2 min; do not take dry, avoid inhaling powder
• Supplemental doses of vit A, D, K, if levels are low
Evaluate:
• Therapeutic response: decreased cholesterol level (hyperlipidemia); diarrhea, pruritus (excess bile acids)
Teach patient/family:
⚠ The symptoms of hypoprothrombinemia: bleeding mucous membranes, dark tarry stools, hematuria, petechiae; report immediately
• The importance of compliance
• That risk factors should be decreased: high-fat diet, smoking, alcohol consumption, absence of exercise

- That GI side effects will resolve with continued use

---

choline salicylate (R)
(koe′leen sa-liss′ih-late)
Arthropan
choline/magnesium salicylates
CMT, Tricosal, Trilisate
Func. class.: Nonopioid analgesic
Chem. class.: Salicylate

Action: Blocks pain impulses in CNS that occur in response to inhibition of prostaglandin synthesis; antipyretic action results from inhibition of hypothalamic heat-regulating center to produce vasodilation to allow heat dissipation
Uses: Mild to moderate pain or fever including arthritis, juvenile rheumatoid arthritis

DOSAGE AND ROUTES
Choline salicylate
- *Adult and child >12 yr:* **PO** 870-1740 mg qid; max 6×/day
Pain/fever
- *Adult:* **PO** 435-870 mg q3-4h prn
Choline/magnesium salicylates
- *Adult:* **PO** 2-3 g salicylate/day divided bid-tid
- *Child >37 kg:* **PO** 2.2 g of salicylate/day divided bid
- *Child <37 kg:* **PO** 50 mg of salicylate/kg/day divided bid
Available forms: Choline salicylate liq 870 mg/5 ml; choline/magnesium salicylate tabs 500, 750, 1000 mg; liq 500 mg/5 ml

SIDE EFFECTS
CNS: Stimulation, drowsiness, dizziness, confusion, ***convulsion,*** headache, flushing, hallucinations, ***coma***
CV: Rapid pulse, pulmonary edema
EENT: Tinnitus, hearing loss
ENDO: Hypoglycemia, hyponatremia, hypokalemia
GI: Nausea, vomiting, GI bleeding, *diarrhea, heartburn,* anorexia, ***hepatitis, hepatotoxicity***
HEMA: ***Thrombocytopenia, agranulocytosis, leukopenia, neutropenia, hemolytic anemia,*** increased PT
INTEG: *Rash,* urticaria, bruising, sweating
RESP: Wheezing, hyperpnea, hyperventilation
Contraindications: Hypersensitivity to salicylates, GI bleeding, bleeding disorders, children <3 yr, vit K deficiency, children with flulike symptoms
Precautions: Pregnancy (C), anemia, hepatic disease, renal disease, Hodgkin's disease, lactation

PHARMACOKINETICS
Absorbed via GI tract, onset 15-30 min; metabolized by liver; crosses placenta; excreted in breast milk, by kidneys, half-life 2-3 hr, large doses 15-30 hr

INTERACTIONS
Gastric ulcer: steroids, antiinflammatories, NSAIDs
Increase: bleeding—alcohol, aspirin, heparin, plicamycin
Increase: effects of warfarin, insulin, methotrexate, thrombolytic agents, penicillins, phenytoin, valproic acid, oral hypoglycemics, sulfonamides
Increase: salicylate levels—urinary acidifiers, ammonium chloride, nizatidine
Decrease: effects of aspirin—antacids (high doses), steroids, urinary alkalizers, corticosteroids
Decrease: effects of probenecid, spironolactone, sulfinpyrazone, sulfonylamides, NSAIDs, β-blockers
Drug/Herb
Increase: bleeding risk—bilberry, bogbean, chondroitin, horse chestnut, Irish moss, kelpware, pansy
Drug/Lab Test
Increase: Coagulation studies, LFTs, serum uric acid, amylase, CO_2, urinary protein
Decrease: Serum K, PBI, cholesterol
Interference: Urine catecholamines, pregnancy test

NURSING CONSIDERATIONS
Assess:
- Pain: location, intensity, character baseline and 1-2 hr after dose
- Hepatic studies: AST, ALT, bilirubin, creatinine (long-term therapy)
- Renal studies: BUN, urine creatinine (long-term therapy)
- Blood studies: CBC, Hct, Hgb, PT (long-term therapy)
- I&O ratio; decreasing output may indicate renal failure (long-term therapy)

⚠ Hepatotoxicity: dark urine; clay-colored stools; yellowing of skin, sclera; itching; abdominal pain; fever; diarrhea (long-term therapy)
- Allergic reactions: rash, urticaria; drug may have to be discontinued
- Renal dysfunction: decreased urine output
- Ototoxicity: tinnitus, ringing, roaring in ears; audiometric testing needed before, after long-term therapy
- Visual changes: blurring, halos, corneal, retinal damage
- Edema in feet, ankles, legs
- Drug history; many interactions

Administer:
- Mixed with fruit juice, carbonated beverage, water

Evaluate:
- Therapeutic response: decreased pain, fever, stiffness of joints

Teach patient/family:
- To report any symptoms of hepatotoxicity, renal toxicity, visual changes, ototoxicity, allergic reactions, bleeding (long-term therapy)
- Not to exceed recommended dosage; acute poisoning may result
- To read label on other OTC drugs; many contain aspirin
- That therapeutic response takes 2 wk (arthritis)
- To avoid alcohol ingestion; GI bleeding may occur
- That if anticoagulants are given with this drug, this drug should be decreased 2 wk before surgery

Treatment of overdose: Lavage, activated charcoal, monitor electrolytes, VS

---

ciclopirox topical
See Appendix C

---

cidofovir (R)
(si-doh-foh'veer)
Vistide
Func. class.: Antiviral
Chem. class.: Nucleotide analog

Action: Suppresses cytomegalovirus (CMV) replication by selective inhibition of viral DNA synthesis
Uses: CMV retinitis in patients with HIV, used with probenecid

DOSAGE AND ROUTES
- Dilute in 100 ml 0.9% saline sol before administration; probenecid must be given **PO** 2 g 3 hr prior to the cidofovir infusion and 1 g at 2 and 8 hr after ending the cidofovir infusion; give 1 L of 0.9% saline sol **IV** with each **INF** of cidofovir, give saline **INF** over 1-2 hr period immediately prior to cidofovir; patient should be given a 2nd L if the patient can tolerate the fluid load (2nd L given at time of cidofovir or immediately afterward and should be given over a 1-3 hr period)

Renal dose
- CCr <50 ml/min reduce dose

Induction
- *Adult:* **IV INF** initially, 5 mg/kg given over 1 hr at a constant rate qwk × 2 consecutive wk; then **IV INF** 5 mg/kg given over 1 hr q2wk

Available forms: Inj 75 mg/ml

SIDE EFFECTS
CNS: Fever, chills, **coma,** confusion, abnormal thought, *dizziness,* bizarre dreams, *headache,* psychosis, tremors, somnolence, paresthesia, *amnesia, anxiety, insomnia,* **seizures**

⚠ Safety alert   *"Tall Man" lettering

CV: Dysrhythmias, hypertension/hypotension

EENT: Retinal detachment in CMV retinitis

GI: Abnormal LFTs, *nausea, vomiting, anorexia, diarrhea,* abdominal pain, **hemorrhage**

GU: **Hematuria,** increased creatinine, BUN, **nephrotoxicity**

HEMA: **Granulocytopenia, thrombocytopenia, irreversible neutropenia, anemia, eosinophilia**

INTEG: Rash, alopecia, pruritus, acne, urticaria, pain at inj site, phlebitis

RESP: Dyspnea

Contraindications: Hypersensitivity to this drug or probenecid, sulfa drugs

Precautions: Pregnancy (C), preexisting cytopenias, renal function impairment, lactation, children <6 mo, elderly, platelet count <25,000/mm³

PHARMACOKINETICS

Unknown

INTERACTIONS

Nephrotoxicity: amphotericin B, foscarnet, aminoglycosides, pentamidine IV, NSAIDs, wait 7 days after use to begin cidofovir

NURSING CONSIDERATIONS

Assess:

• Culture before treatment is initiated; cultures of blood, urine, and throat may all be taken; CMV is not confirmed by this method; the diagnosis is made by an ophthalmic exam

• Renal, hepatic, increased hemopoietic studies and BUN; serum creatinine, AST, ALT, creatinine, CCr, A-G ratio, baseline and drip treatment, blood counts should be done q2wk; watch for decreasing granulocytes, Hgb; if low, therapy may have to be discontinued and restarted after hematologic recovery; blood transfusions may be required

• For GI symptoms: severe nausea, vomiting, diarrhea; severe symptoms may necessitate discontinuing drug

• Electrolytes and minerals: calcium,

phosphorus, magnesium, sodium, potassium; watch closely for tetany during first administration

• For symptoms of blood dyscrasias (anemia, granulocytopenia); bruising, fatigue, bleeding, poor healing

• Allergic reactions: flushing, rash, urticaria, pruritus

• For leukopenia, neutropenia, thrombocytopenia: WBCs, platelets q2d during 2×/day dosing and qwk thereafter; check for leukopenias, with daily WBC count in patients with prior leukopenia, with other nucleoside analogs, or for whom leukopenia counts are <1000 cells/mm³ at start of treatment

• Monitor serum creatinine or CCr at least q2wk; give only to those with creatinine levels ≤1.5 mg/dl, CCr >55 ml/min, urine protein <100 mg/dl

Administer:

• Mix under strict aseptic conditions using gloves, gown, and mask, and using precautions for antineoplastic

• After diluting in 100 ml 0.9% NaCl

• Slowly; do not give by bolus IV, SUBCUT inj

• Use diluted sol within 12 hr, do not refrigerate or freeze; do not use sol with particulate matter or discoloration

• Refrigerate up to 24 hr, allow to warm to room temperature before using

Evaluate:

• Therapeutic response: decreased symptoms of CMV

Teach patient/family:

• To notify prescriber if sore throat, swollen lymph nodes, malaise, fever occur; may indicate other infections

• To report perioral tingling, numbness in extremities, and paresthesias

• That serious drug interactions may occur if OTC products are ingested; check first with prescriber

• That drug is not a cure, but will control symptoms

• That regular ophthalmic exams must be continued

• That major toxicities may necessitate discontinuing drug

• To use contraception during treatment

and that infertility may occur; men should use barrier contraception for 90 days after treatment
Treatment of overdose: Discontinue drug; use hemodialysis, and increase hydration

---

cilostazol (℞)
(sih-los'tah-zol)
Pletal
Func. class.: Platelet aggregation inhibitor
Chem. class.: Quinolinone derivative

Do not confuse:
Pletal/Plendil
Action: Reversibly inhibits cellular phosphodiesterase; inhibits platelet aggregation induced by thrombin, ADP, collagen, arachidonic acid, epINEPHrine, stress
Uses: Intermittent claudication

DOSAGE AND ROUTES
• *Adult:* **PO** 100 mg bid taken ≥30 min ac or 2 hr pc breakfast and dinner or 50 mg bid if using drugs that inhibit CYP3A4 and CYP2C19; 12 wk of treatment may be needed for beneficial effect
Available forms: Tabs 50, 100 mg

SIDE EFFECTS
CNS: Dizziness, headache
CV: Palpitations, tachycardia, nodal dysrhythmia, postural hypotension
EENT: Blindness, diplopia, ear pain, tinnitus, retinal hemorrhage
GI: Nausea, vomiting, *diarrhea,* GI discomfort, colitis, cholelithiasis, ulcer, esophagitis, gastritis, anorexia, *flatulence, dyspepsia*
GU: Cystitis, frequency, vaginitis, ***vaginal hemorrhage,*** hematuria
HEMA: **Bleeding (epistaxis, hematuria, retinal hemorrhage, GI bleeding), thrombocytopenia,** anemia, polycythemia
INTEG: Rash, urticaria, dry skin
MISC: Back pain, headache, infection, *myalgia, peripheral edema,* chills, fever, malaise, diabetes mellitus
RESP: Cough, pharyngitis, rhinitis, asthma, pneumonia
Contraindications: Hypersensitivity, CHF, acute MI
Precautions: Pregnancy (C), past liver disease, renal disease, elderly, lactation, children, increased bleeding risk, low platelet count, platelet dysfunction, active bleeding

PHARMACOKINETICS
95%-98% protein binding, metabolism-hepatic extensively by CYPP450 enzymes, excreted urine (74%), feces (20%), half-life 11-13 hr

INTERACTIONS
Increase: bleeding tendencies—anticoagulants, NSAIDs, thrombolytics, abciximab, eptifibatide, tirofiban, ticlopidine
Increase: cilostazol levels—diltiazem, erythromycin, verapamil, protease inhibitors, omeprazole; exercise caution when coadministering with fluvoxamine, fluoxetine, ketoconazole, itraconazole, voriconazole, fluconazole and reduce dose to 50 mg bid
Drug/Herb
Increase: bleeding risk—agrimony, alfalfa, angelica, anise, bilberry, black haw, bogbean, buchu, chondroitin, dong quai, fenugreek, feverfew, garlic, ginger, ginkgo, ginseng, green tea, horse chestnut, Irish moss, kelp, kelpware, khella, lovage, lungwort, meadowsweet, motherwort, mugwort, nettle, papaya, parsley (large amt), pau d'arco, pineapple, poplar, prickly ash, safflower, saw palmetto, senega, tonka bean, turmeric, wintergreen, yarrow
Decrease: action—chamomile, coenzyme Q10, flax, glucomannan, goldenseal
Drug/Food
Do not use with grapefruit juice

NURSING CONSIDERATIONS

Assess:

• For underlying CV disease since CV risk is great; for CV lesions with repeated oral administration

• For congestive heart failure

• Blood studies: CBC q2 wk, Hct, Hgb, PT

Administer:

• Give bid 1 hr ac or 2 hr pc; do not give with grapefruit juice

Evaluate:

• Therapeutic response: improved walking distance and duration, decreased pain

Teach patient/family:

• To report any unusual bleeding

• To report side effects such as diarrhea, skin rashes, subcutaneous bleeding

• That effects may take 2-4 wk, treatment of up to 12 wk may be required for necessary effect

• About potential risk for patients with CHF

• To take 1 hr ac or 2 hr pc

• That reading the patient package insert is necessary

---

cimetidine (otc, ℞)

(sye-met′i-deen)
Apo-Cimetidine ✤, cimetidine, Novo-Cimetidine ✤, Peptol ✤, Tagamet, Tagamet HB
Func. class.: H$_2$-histamine receptor antagonist
Chem. class.: Imidazole derivative

Action: Inhibits histamine at H$_2$-receptor site in the gastric parietal cells, which inhibits gastric acid secretion

Uses: Short-term treatment of duodenal and gastric ulcers and maintenance; management of GERD and Zollinger-Ellison syndrome

Investigational uses: Prevention of aspiration pneumonitis, stress ulcers, upper GI bleeding, herpes infection, hirsutism, cutaneous/nongenital warts, weight loss

DOSAGE AND ROUTES

Treatment of active ulcers

• *Adult:* PO 300 mg qid with meals, at bedtime × 8 wk or 400 mg bid, 800 mg at bedtime; after 8 wk give bedtime dose only; **IV BOL** 300 mg/20 ml 0.9% NaCl over 1-2 min q6h; **IV INF** 300 mg/50 ml D$_5$W over 15-20 min; **IM** 300 mg q6h, not to exceed 2400 mg/day

• *Child:* PO 20-40 mg/kg/day; **IM/IV** 5-10 mg/kg q6-8h

Prophylaxis of duodenal ulcer

• *Adult and child >16 yr:* 400 mg at bedtime

GERD

• *Adult:* PO 800-1600 mg/day in divided doses

Hypersecretory conditions (Zollinger-Ellison syndrome)

• *Adult:* **PO/IM/IV** 300-600 mg q6h; may increase to 12 g/day if needed

Upper GI bleeding prophylaxis

• *Adult:* **IV** 50 mg/hr; lowered in renal disease

Aspiration pneumonitis prophylaxis

• *Adult:* **IM/IV** 300 mg **IM** 1 hr before anesthesia, then 300 mg **IV** q4h until patient is alert, max 2400 mg/day

Hirsutism

• *Adult:* PO 300 mg qid × 5 days or 1600 mg daily up to 6 mo

Warts

• *Adult:* PO 400-800 mg tid × 12 wk or 30-40 mg/kg/day given tid × 3 mo

Weight loss

• *Adult:* PO 200-400 mg tid × 8-12 wk

Renal disease

• CCr 20-40 ml/min 300 mg q8h; CCr <20 ml/min 300 mg q12h

Available forms: Tabs 100, 200, 300, 400, 800 mg; liq 200, 300 mg/5 ml; inj 300 mg/2 ml, 300 mg/50 ml 0.9% NaCl

SIDE EFFECTS

CNS: Confusion, headache, depression, dizziness, anxiety, weakness, psychosis, tremors, **convulsions**

CV: Bradycardia, tachycardia, ***dysrhythmias***

GI: Diarrhea, abdominal cramps, ***paralytic ileus, jaundice***
GU: Gynecomastia, galactorrhea, impotence, increase in BUN, creatinine
*HEMA: **Agranulocytosis, thrombocytopenia, neutropenia, aplastic anemia, increase in PT***
INTEG: Urticaria, rash, alopecia, sweating, flushing, ***exfoliative dermatitis***
Contraindications: Hypersensitivity
Precautions: Pregnancy (B), lactation, child <16 yr, organic brain syndrome, hepatic disease, renal disease, elderly

PHARMACOKINETICS
Well absorbed (PO, IM)
IM/IV: Onset 10 min, peak ½ hr, duration 4-5 hr
PO: Peak 1-1½ hr, half-life 1½-2 hr; 30%-40% metabolized by liver, excreted in urine unchanged, crosses placenta, enters breast milk

INTERACTIONS
Increase: toxicity due to CYP450 pathway—benzodiazepines, β-blockers, calcium channel blockers, carbamazepine, chloroquine, lidocaine, metronidazole, moricizine, phenytoin, quinidine, quinine, sulfonylureas, theophylline, tricyclics, valproic acid, warfarin
Decrease: absorption of cimetidine—antacids, sucralfate
Decrease: absorption—ketoconazole
Drug/Lab Test
Increase: Alk phosphatase, AST, creatinine, prolactin
False positive: Gastroccult, hemoccult
False negative: TB skin tests

NURSING CONSIDERATIONS
Assess:
• Gastric pH (5 or more should be maintained), also epigastric pain and duration, intensity; aggravating, ameliorating factors
• I&O ratio, BUN, creatinine, CBC with differential periodically
Administer:
• With meals for prolonged drug effect;

antacids 1 hr before or 1 hr after cimetidine
IV route
• After diluting 300 mg/20 ml of 0.9% NaCl for inj; give ≥5 min; may be diluted 300 mg/50 ml of D₅W; run over 15-20 min; or total daily dose (900 mg) diluted in 100-1000 ml D₅W given over 24 hr
Additive compatibilities: AcetaZOLAMIDE, amikacin, aminophylline, atracurium, cefoperazone, cefoxitin, chlorothiazide, clindamycin, colistimethate, dexamethasone, digoxin, epINEPHrine, erythromycin, ethacrynate, floxacillin, flumazenil, furosemide, gentamicin, insulin (regular), isoproterenol, lidocaine, lincomycin, meropenem, metaraminol, methylPREDNISolone, norepinephrine, nitroprusside, penicillin G potassium, phytonadione, polymyxin B, potassium chloride, protamine, quinidine, tacrolimus, vancomycin, verapamil, vit B/C
Syringe compatibilities: Atropine, butorphanol, cephalothin, diazepam, diphenhydrAMINE, doxapram, droperidol, fentanyl, glycopyrrolate, heparin, hydromorphone, hydrOXYzine, lorazepam, meperidine, midazolam, morphine, nafcillin, nalbuphine, penicillin G sodium, pentazocine, perphenazine, prochlorperazine, promazine, promethazine, scopolamine
Y-site compatibilities: Acyclovir, amifostine, aminophylline, amrinone, atracurium, aztreonam, cisatracurium, cisplatin, cladribine, cyclophosphamide, cytarabine, diltiazem, DOXOrubicin, DOXOrubicin liposome, enalaprilat, esmolol, filgrastim, fluconazole, fludarabine, foscarnet, gallium, granisetron, haloperidol, heparin, hetastarch, idarubicin, labetalol, melphalan, meropenem, methotrexate, midazolam, ondansetron, paclitaxel, pancuronium, piperacillin/tazobactam, propofol, remifentanil, sargramostim, tacrolimus, teniposide, theophylline, thiotepa, tolazoline, vecuronium, vinorelbine, zidovudine

Perform/provide:

• Storage of diluted sol at room temperature up to 48 hr

Evaluate:

• Therapeutic response: decreased pain in abdomen; healing of ulcers, absence of gastroesophageal reflux, gastric pH 5

Teach patient/family:

• That gynecomastia, impotence may occur, are reversible

• To avoid driving, other hazardous activities until patient is stabilized on this medication; drowsiness or dizziness may occur

• To avoid black pepper, caffeine, alcohol, harsh spices, extremes in temperature of food

• To avoid OTC preparations: aspirin, cough, cold preparations; condition may worsen

• That smoking decreases the effectiveness of the drug

• That drug must be taken exactly as prescribed and continued for prescribed time to be effective; doses not to be doubled

• To report bruising, fatigue, malaise; blood dyscrasias may occur

• To report to prescriber diarrhea, black tarry stools, sore throat, rash

---

cinacalcet (℞)

(sin-a-kal′set)

Sensipar

Func. class.: Calcium receptor agonist

Chem. class.: Polypeptide hormone

Action: Directly lowers PTH levels by increasing sensitivity of calcium sensing receptors to extracellular calcium

Uses: Hypercalcemia in parathyroid carcinoma, secondary hyperparathyroidism in chronic kidney disease on dialysis

DOSAGE AND ROUTES

Parathyroid carcinoma

• *Adult:* **PO** 30 mg bid, titrate q2-4wk, with sequential doses of 30 mg bid, 60 mg bid, 90 mg bid, 90 mg tid-qid to normalize calcium levels

Secondary hyperparathyroidism

• *Adult:* **PO** 30 mg daily, titrate no more frequently than 2-4 wk with sequential doses of 30, 60, 90, 120, 180 mg daily

Available forms: Tab 30, 60, 90 mg

SIDE EFFECTS

CNS: Dizziness

CV: Hypertension

GI: Nausea, diarrhea, vomiting, anorexia

MISC: Access infection, noncardiac chest pain, asthenia

MS: Myalgia

Contraindications: Hypersensitivity

Precautions: Pregnancy (C), children, lactation, seizure disorders, hepatic disease

PHARMACOKINETICS

93%-97% bound to plasma; proteins metabolized by CYP3A4, 2D6, 1A2; half life 30-40 hr; renal excretion of metabolites (80% renal, 15% feces)

INTERACTIONS

Drugs metabolized by CYP3A4 (ketoconazole, erythromycin, itraconazole), CYP2D6 (flecainide, vinBLAStine, thioridazine, tricyclics): adjustments may be necessary

Drug/Food

Increase: action by high-fat meal

NURSING CONSIDERATIONS

Assess:

• Hypocalcemia: cramping, seizures, tetany, myalgia, paresthesia

• Calcium, phosphorous within 1 wk and iPTH 1-4 wk after initiation or dosage adjustment when maintenance is established; measure calcium, phosphorus monthly; iPTH q1-3mo, target range 150-300 pg/ml for iPTH level

• If calcium <8.4 mg/dl, do not start therapy

Administer:

• Swallow tabs whole; do not break, crush, or chew

• Can be used alone or in combination with vit D sterols and/or phosphate binders

Secondary hyperthyroidism

• Titrate q2-4wk to target iPTH consistent with National Kidney Foundation–Kidney Disease Outcomes Quality Initiative (NKF-K/DOQI) for chronic kidney disease patient on dialysis of 150-300 pg/ml; if iPTH drops below 150-300 pg/ml, reduce dose of cinacalcet and/or vit D sterols or discontinue treatment

Perform/provide:

• Storage at <77° F (25° C)

Evaluate:

• Therapeutic response: calcium levels 9-10 mg/dl, decreasing symptoms of hypercalcemia

Teach patient/family:

• Take with food or shortly after a meal
• Report immediately: cramping, seizures, muscle pain, tingling, tetany

---

ciprofloxacin (℞)

(sip-ro-floks′a-sin)
Cipro, Cipro IV, Cipro XR
Func. class.: Broad-spectrum antiinfective
Chem. class.: Fluoroquinolone

Do not confuse:
ciprofloxacin/cephalexin

Action: Interferes with conversion of intermediate DNA fragments into high-molecular-weight DNA in bacteria; DNA gyrase inhibitor

Uses: Infection caused by susceptible *Escherichia coli, Enterobacter cloacae, Proteus mirabilis, Klebsiella pneumoniae, Proteus vulgaris, Citrobacter freundii, Serratia marcescens, Pseudomonas aeruginosa, Staphylococcus aureus, Staphylococcus epidermidis, Enterobacter, Campylobacter jejuni, Salmonella;* chronic bacterial prostatitis, acute sinusitis, postexposure inhalation anthrax, infectious diarrhea, typhoid fever, complicated intraabdominal infections, nosocomial pneumonia, urinary tract infections

DOSAGE AND ROUTES

Uncomplicated urinary tract infections

• *Adult:* **PO** 100-250 mg q12h × 3 days or 500 mg × q24h × 3 days

Complicated/severe urinary tract infections

• *Adult:* **PO** 500 mg q12h or 1000 mg q24h × 7-14 days; **IV** 400 mg q12h

Pyelonephritis, acute uncomplicated

• *Adult:* **PO** 1000 mg × R q24h × 7-14 days

Respiratory, bone, skin, joint infections

• *Adult:* **PO** 500-750 mg q12h; **IV** 400 mg q12h

Nosocomial pneumonia

• *Adult:* **IV** 400 mg q8h × 10-14 days

Intraabdominal infections, complicated

• *Adult:* **PO** 500 mg q12h × 7-14 days, **IV** 400 mg q12h × 7-14 days

Acute sinusitis, mild/moderate

• *Adult:* **PO** 500 mg q12h × 10 days; **IV** 400 mg q12h × 10 days

Inhalational anthrax (postexposure)

• *Adult:* **PO** 500 mg q12h × 60 days; **IV** 400 mg q12h × 60 days
• *Child:* **PO** 15 mg/kg/dose, max 500 mg/dose; **IV** max 400 mg/dose × 60 days

Infectious diarrhea

• *Adult:* **PO** 500 mg q12h × 5-7 days

Chronic bacterial prostatis

• *Adult:* **PO** 500 mg q12h × 28 days; **IV** 400 mg q12h × 28 days

Renal disease

• CCr 30-50 ml/min **PO** 250-500 mg q12h; CCr 5-29 ml/min **PO** 250-500 mg q18h; **IV** 200-400 mg q18-24h

Available forms: Tabs 100, 250, 500, 750 mg; tabs, ext rel 500, 1000 mg (XR); inj 200 mg/20 ml, 400 mg/40 ml, 200 mg/100 ml D$_5$, 400 mg/200 ml D$_5$; oral susp 250, 500 mg/5 ml

SIDE EFFECTS

CNS: Headache, dizziness, fatigue, insomnia, depression, *restlessness,* **seizures,** confusion

GI: Nausea, diarrhea, increased ALT,

AST, dry mouth, flatulence, heartburn, *vomiting*, oral candidiasis, dysphagia, **pseudomembranous colitis**
INTEG: *Rash*, pruritus, urticaria, photosensitivity, flushing, fever, chills
MISC: **Anaphylaxis, Stevens-Johnson syndrome**
MS: Tremor, arthralgia, tendon rupture
Contraindications: Hypersensitivity to quinolones
Precautions: Pregnancy (C), lactation, children, renal disease, epilepsy

PHARMACOKINETICS

PO: Peak 1 hr, half-life 3-4 hr; excreted in urine as active drug, metabolites

INTERACTIONS

Nephrotoxicity: cycloSPORINE
Increase: ciprofloxacin levels— probenecid; monitor for toxicity
Increase: levels of—theophylline, warfarin, monitor blood levels
Decrease: ciproflaxin absorption— antacids containing magnesium, aluminum; zinc, iron, sucralfate, enteral feedings, calcium
Drug/Herb
Do not use acidophilus with antiinfectives
Possible toxicity: yerba maté
Decrease: effect—fennel
Drug/Food
Increase: effect of—caffeine
Decrease: absorption—dairy products, food
Drug/Lab Test
Increase: AST, ALT, BUN, creatinine, LDH, bilirubin, alk phosphatase, glucose, proteinuria, albuminuria
Decrease: WBC, glucose

NURSING CONSIDERATIONS

Assess:
• CNS symptoms: headache, dizziness, fatigue, insomnia, depression
• Renal, hepatic studies: BUN, creatinine, AST, ALT
• I&O ratio, urine pH <5.5 is ideal

⚠ Anaphylaxis: fever, flushing, rash, urticaria, pruritus, dyspnea
Administer:
• Not to use theophylline with this product, will cause toxicity
PO route
• 2 hr before or 2 hr after antacids, zinc, iron, calcium
IV route
• Over 1 hr as an INF, comes in premixed plastic INF container or diluted 20 or 40 ml vial to a final conc of 0.5-2 mg/ml of NS or D_5W; give through Y-tube or 3-way stopcock
• After clean-catch urine for C&S
Additive compatibilities: Amikacin, aztreonam, ceftazidime, cycloSPORINE, gentamicin, metronidazole, netilmicin, piperacillin, potassium acetate, potassium chloride, potassium phosphates, prednisoLONE, promethazine, propofol, ranitidine, Ringer's, sodium chloride, tobramycin, vit B/C
Y-site compatibilities: Amifostine, amino acids, aztreonam, calcium gluconate, ceftazidime, cisatracurium, digoxin, diltiazem, diphenhydrAMINE, DOBUTamine, DOPamine, DOXOrubicin liposome, gallium, gentamicin, granisetron, hydrOXYzine, lidocaine, lorazepam, metoclopramide, midazolam, midodrine, piperacillin, potassium acetate, potassium chloride, potassium phosphates, prednisoLONE, promethazine, propofol, ranitidine, remifentanil, Ringer's, sodium chloride, tacrolimus, teniposide, thiotepa, tobramycin, verapamil
Perform/provide:
• Limited intake of alkaline foods, drugs: milk, dairy products, alkaline antacids, sodium bicarbonate
• That fluids must be increased to 3 L/day to avoid crystallization in kidneys
Evaluate:
• Therapeutic response: decreased pain, frequency, urgency, C&S; absence of infection
Teach patient/family:
• Not to take any products containing magnesium or calcium (such as antac-

ids), iron, or aluminum with this drug or within 2 hr of drug

• That photosensitivity may occur; patient should avoid sunlight or use sunscreen to prevent burns

• If dizziness occurs, to ambulate, perform activities with assistance

• To complete full course of drug therapy, not to double or miss doses

• To contact prescriber if adverse reaction occurs or if inflammation or pain in tendon occurs

• To use frequent rinsing of mouth, sugarless candy or gum for dry mouth

• To contact prescriber if taking theophylline

ciprofloxacin ophthalmic
See Appendix C

⚠ High Alert

cisplatin (℞)
(sis'pla-tin)
Platinol ✿, Platinol-AQ
Func. class.: Antineoplastic alkylating agent
Chem. class.: Inorganic heavy metal

Do not confuse:
cisplatin/carboplatin
Platinol/Paraplatin
Action: Alkylates DNA, RNA; inhibits enzymes that allow synthesis of amino acids in proteins; activity is not cell cycle phase specific
Uses: Advanced bladder cancer, adjunctive in metastatic testicular cancer, osteosarcoma, soft tissue sarcomas, adjunctive in metastatic ovarian cancer, head, neck cancer, esophagus, prostate, lung and cervical cancer, lymphoma

DOSAGE AND ROUTES
Dosage protocols may vary
Metastatic testicular cancer
• *Adult:* IV 20 mg/m² daily × 5 days,

repeat q3wk for 3 cycles or more, depending on response
Advanced bladder cancer
• *Adult:* IV 50-70 mg/m² q3-4wk
Metastatic ovarian cancer
• *Adult:* IV 100 mg/m² q4wk or 75-100 mg/m² q3wk with cyclophosphamide; mix with 2 L NaCl and 37.5 g mannitol over 6 hr
Available forms: Inj 0.5 ✿, 1 mg/ml; powder for inj 10, 50 mg vials

SIDE EFFECTS

CNS: **Seizures,** peripheral neuropathy
CV: Cardiac abnormalities
EENT: **Tinnitus, hearing loss, vestibular toxicity,** blurred vision, altered color perception
GI: **Severe nausea, vomiting, diarrhea, weight loss**
GU: **Renal tubular damage,** renal insufficiency, impotence, sterility, amenorrhea, gynecomastia, hyperuremia
HEMA: **Thrombocytopenia, leukopenia, pancytopenia**
INTEG: **Alopecia,** dermatitis
META: Hypomagnesemia, hypocalcemia, hypokalemia, hypophosphatemia
RESP: **Fibrosis**
SYST: **Anaphylaxis**
Contraindications: Pregnancy (D), radiation therapy or chemotherapy within 1 mo, thrombocytopenia, recent smallpox vaccination, aluminum products used to prepare or administer cisplatin
Precautions: Pneumococcus vaccination, lactation

PHARMACOKINETICS

Absorption complete, metabolized in liver, excreted in urine; half-life 30-100 hr, accumulates in body tissues for several months, enters breast milk

INTERACTIONS

Risk of bleeding: aspirin, NSAIDs, alcohol
Ototoxicity: bumetanide, ethacrynic acid, furosemide

⚠ Safety alert   *"Tall Man" lettering

Increase: myelosuppression—myelosuppressive agents, radiation
Increase: nephrotoxicity—aminoglycosides, loop diuretics
Decrease: effects of phenytoin
Decrease: antibody response—live virus vaccines

Drug/Lab Test
Increase: Uric acid, BUN, creatinine
Decrease: CCr, calcium, phosphate, potassium, magnesium
Positive: Coombs' test

NURSING CONSIDERATIONS
Assess:
For bone marrow depression
• CBC, differential, platelet count weekly; withhold drug if WBC is <4000 or platelet count is <100,000; notify prescriber of results
• Renal studies: BUN, creatinine, serum uric acid, urine CCr before, electrolytes during therapy; dose should not be given if BUN <25 mg/dl; creatinine <1.5 mg/dl; I&O ratio; report fall in urine output of <30 ml/hr
• For anaphylaxis: wheezing, tachycardia, facial swelling, fainting; discontinue drug and report to prescriber; resuscitation equipment should be nearby
• Monitor temp q4h (may indicate beginning infection)
• Hepatic studies before, during therapy (bilirubin, AST, ALT, LDH) as needed or monthly
• Bleeding: hematuria, guaiac, bruising or petechiae, mucosa or orifices q8h; obtain prescription for viscous lidocaine (Xylocaine)
• Effects of alopecia on body image; discuss feelings about body changes
• Jaundice of skin, sclera; dark urine; clay-colored stools; itchy skin; abdominal pain; fever; diarrhea
• Edema in feet, joint pain, stomach pain, shaking

Administer:
IV route
• Do not use aluminum equipment during any preparation or administration, will form precipitate; do not refrigerate unopened powder or solution, protect from sunlight
• Prepare in biologic cabinet using gown, gloves, mask, do not allow drug to come in contact with skin, use soap and water if contact occurs
• For intermittent inf, dilute 10 mg/10 ml or 50 mg/50 ml sterile H_2O for inj; withdraw prescribed dose, dilute ½ dose with 1000 ml D_5 0.2 NaCl or D_5 0.45 NaCl with 37.5 g mannitol; IV INF is given over 3-4 hr; use a 0.45-µm filter; total dose 2 L over 6-8 hr; check site for irritation, phlebitis
• For continuous inf give over 24 hr × 5 days
• Hydrate patient with 0.9% NaCl over 8-12 hr before treatment
• EpINEPHrine, antihistamines, corticosteroids for hypersensitivity reaction
• Antiemetic 30-60 min before giving drug and prn
• Allopurinol to maintain uric acid levels, alkalinization of urine
• Diuretic (furosemide 40 mg IV) or mannitol after infusion

Additive compatibilities: Carboplatin, cyclophosphamide with etoposide, etoposide, etoposide with floxuridine, floxuridine, floxuridine with leucovorin, hydrOXYzine, ifosfamide, ifosfamide with etoposide, leucovorin, magnesium sulfate, mannitol, ondansetron

Solution compatibilities: D_5/0.225% NaCl, D_5/0.45% NaCl, D_5/0.9% NaCl, D_5/0.45% NaCl with mannitol 1.875%, D_5/0.33% NaCl with KCl 20 mEq and mannitol 1.875%, 0.9% NaCl, 0.45% NaCl, 0.3% NaCl, 0.225% NaCl

Syringe compatibilities: Bleomycin, cyclophosphamide, doxapram, DOXOrubicin, droperidol, fluorouracil, furosemide, heparin, leucovorin, methotrexate, metoclopramide, mitomycin, vinBLAStine, vinCRIStine

Y-site compatibilities: Allopurinol, aztreonam, bleomycin, chlorproMAZINE, cimetidine, cladribine, cyclophosphamide, dexamethasone, diphenhydrAMINE, DOXOrubicin, DOXOrubicin liposome, droperidol, famotidine, filgrastim, fludarabine, fluorouracil, furosemide, ganciclovir, granisetron, heparin, hydromorphone, leucovorin, lorazepam, melphalan, methotrexate, methylPREDNISolone, metoclopramide, mitomycin, morphine, ondansetron, paclitaxel, prochlorperazine, promethazine, propofol, ranitidine, sargramostim, teniposide, vinBLAStine, vinCRIStine, vinorelbine

Perform/provide:

• Comprehensive oral hygiene

• All medications PO, if possible, avoid IM inj when platelets <100,000/mm³

• Increase fluid intake to 2-3 L/day to prevent urate deposits, calculi formation; promote elimination of drug

Evaluate:

• Therapeutic response: decreased tumor size, spread of malignancy

Teach patient/family:

• To report signs of infection: increased temp, sore throat, flulike symptoms

• To report signs of anemia: fatigue, headache, faintness, shortness of breath, irritability

• To report bleeding, bruising, petechiae: avoid use of razors, commercial mouthwash

• To avoid aspirin, ibuprofen, NSAIDs, alcohol; may cause GI bleeding

• To report any complaints or side effects to nurse or prescriber

• That impotence or amenorrhea can occur; reversible after discontinuing treatment

• To report any changes in breathing, coughing

• That hair may be lost during treatment; a wig or hairpiece may make patient feel better; new hair may be different in color, texture

• To report numbness, tingling in face or extremities, poor hearing or joint pain, swelling

• Not to receive vaccinations during treatment

• To use contraception during treatment and 4 mo after; this drug may cause infertility

---

citalopram (R̶)
(sigh-tal'oh-pram)
Celexa
Func. class.: Antidepressant
Chem. class.: Selective serotonin reuptake inhibitor (SSRI)

Do not confuse:
Celexa/Celebrex/Cerebyx/Cerebra

Action: Inhibits CNS neuron uptake of serotonin but not of norepinephrine; weak inhibitor of CYP450 enzyme system, making it more appealing than other drugs

Uses: Major depressive disorder

Investigational uses: Fibromyalgia, premenstrual disorders, panic disorder, social phobia, impulsive aggression in children, obsessive-compulsive disorder in adolescents, treatment of psychotic symptoms in nondepressed demented patients

DOSAGE AND ROUTES

Depression

• *Adult:* **PO** 20 mg daily AM or PM, may increase if needed to 40 mg/day after 1 wk; maintenance: after 6-8 wk of initial treatment, continue for 24 wk (32 wk total), reevaluate long-term usefulness (max 60 mg/day)

Fibromyalgia

• *Adult:* **PO** 20 mg daily × 4 wk; increase dose to 40 mg daily × 4 wk

Hepatic dose/elderly

• *Adult:* **PO** 20 mg/day, may increase to 40 mg/day if no response

Panic disorder

• *Adult:* **PO** 20-30 mg/day

Premenstrual dysphoria, social phobia, impulsive aggression in children

• *Adult:* **PO** 20-40 mg/day, used intermittently in premenstrual dysphoria

Available forms: Tabs 10, 20, 40 mg; oral sol 2 mg (as base)/ml

SIDE EFFECTS

CNS: Headache, nervousness, insomnia, drowsiness, anxiety, tremor, dizziness,

---

*fatigue, sedation, poor concentration, abnormal dreams, agitation, **convulsions,*** apathy, euphoria, hallucinations, delusions, psychosis, ***suicidal attempts***

CV: Hot flashes, palpitations, angina pectoris, ***hemorrhage,*** hypertension, tachycardia, 1st-degree AV block, bradycardia, *MI,* thrombophlebitis

EENT: Visual changes, ear/eye pain, photophobia, tinnitus

GI: Nausea, diarrhea, dry mouth, anorexia, dyspepsia, constipation, cramps, vomiting, taste changes, flatulence, decreased appetite

GU: Dysmenorrhea, decreased libido, urinary frequency, UTI, amenorrhea, cystitis, impotence, urine retention

INTEG: Sweating, rash, pruritus, acne, alopecia, urticaria

MS: Pain, arthritis, twitching

RESP: Infection, pharyngitis, nasal congestion, sinus headache, sinusitis, cough, dyspnea, bronchitis, asthma, hyperventilation, pneumonia

SYST: Asthenia, viral infection, fever, allergy, chills

Contraindications: Hypersensitivity

Precautions: Pregnancy (C), lactation, children, elderly

PHARMACOKINETICS

PO: Metabolized in liver; excreted in urine; steady state 28-35 days; peak 2-4 hr; half-life 35 hr

INTERACTIONS

⚠ Fatal reactions: do not use with MAOIs

Increase: effect of tricyclics, use cautiously

Increase: CNS effects—CNS depressants

Increase: citalopram levels—macrolides, azole antifungals

Increase: plasma levels of β-blockers

Increase: serotonergic effects—lithium

Decrease: citalopram levels—carbamazepine

Drug/Herb

Serotonin syndrome: St. John's wort, SAM-e; fatal reaction may occur; do not use concurrently

Increase: CNS stimulation—yohimbe

Drug/Lab Test

Increase: Serum bilirubin, blood glucose, alk phosphatase

Decrease: VMA, 5-HIAA

False increase: Urinary catecholamines

NURSING CONSIDERATIONS

Assess:

• Mental status: mood, sensorium, affect, suicidal tendencies, increase in psychiatric symptoms, depression, panic

• B/P (lying/standing), pulse q4h; if systolic B/P drops 20 mm Hg, hold drug, notify prescriber; take vital signs q4h in patients with cardiovascular disease

• Weight qwk; appetite may decrease or increase with drug

• ECG for flattening of T wave, bundle branch, AV block, dysrhythmias in cardiac patients

• Alcohol consumption; if alcohol is consumed, hold dose until AM

Administer:

• With food or milk for GI symptoms

• Crushed if patient is unable to swallow medication whole

• Dosages at bedtime if oversedation occurs during the day; may take entire dose at bedtime

Perform/provide:

• Storage at room temperature; do not freeze

• Assistance with ambulation during therapy, since drowsiness, dizziness occur

• Safety measures primarily in elderly

• Check to see if PO medication swallowed

• Sugarless gum, hard candy, frequent sips of water for dry mouth

Evaluate:

• Therapeutic response: decreased depression

Teach patient/family:

• That therapeutic effect may take 2-3 wk

- To use caution in driving, other activities requiring alertness because of drowsiness, dizziness, blurred vision
- To avoid alcohol ingestion, other CNS depressants
- To notify prescriber if pregnant or plan to become pregnant or breastfeed

---

Rarely Used

cladribine (CdA) (℞)
(kla′dri-been)
Leustatin
Func. class.: Antineoplastic antiinfective

Uses: Treatment of active hairy cell leukemia; may be useful in chronic lymphocytic leukemia, non-Hodgkin's lymphomas, acute, chronic myeloid leukemia, autoimmune hemolytic anemia

DOSAGE AND ROUTES
- *Adult:* **IV** 0.09 mg/kg diluted with 0.9% NaCl qs to 100 ml; pass through 0.22 μm microfilter, given for cont inf × 5-7 days

Contraindications: Hypersensitivity, lactation

---

clarithromycin (℞)
(klare-ith′row-my-sin)
Biaxin, Biaxin XL
Func. class.: Antiinfective
Chem. class.: Macrolide

Action: Binds to 50S ribosomal subunits of susceptible bacteria and suppresses protein synthesis
Uses: Mild to moderate infections of the upper respiratory tract, lower respiratory tract, uncomplicated skin and skin structure infections caused by *Streptococcus pneumoniae, Mycoplasma pneumoniae, Legionella pneumophila, Moraxella catarrhalis, Neisseria gonorrhoeae, Corynebacterium diphtheriae, Listeria monocytogenes, Haemophilus influenzae, Streptococcus pyogenes,* *Staphylococcus aureus, Mycobacterium avium (MAC)* complex infection in AIDS patients, *Mycobacterium avium intracellulare, Helicobacter pylori* in combination with omeprazole

DOSAGE AND ROUTES
Acute exacerbation of chronic bronchitis
- *Adult:* **PO** 250-500 mg q12h × 7-14 days or 1000 mg daily × 7 days (XL) bid-tid
Pharyngitis/tonsillitis
- *Adult:* **PO** 250 mg q12h × 10 days
Renal dose
- *Adult:* **PO** CCr <30 ml/min 250 mg daily × bid, may use an initial dose of 500 mg
- *Child:* **PO** CCr <30 ml/min reduce dose by 50%
Community-acquired pneumonia
- *Adult:* **PO** 250 mg q12h × 7-14 days or 1000 mg daily × 7 days (XL)
Endocarditis prophylaxis
- *Adult:* **PO** 500 mg 1 hr before procedure
MAC prophylaxis/treatment
- *Adult:* **PO** 500 mg bid, will require an additional antiinfective for active infection
H. pylori *infection*
- *Adult:* **PO** 500 mg daily plus omeprazole 2 × 20 mg q ᴀᴍ (days 1-14), then omeprazole 20 mg q ᴀᴍ (days 15-28)
Acute maxillary sinusitis
- *Adult:* **PO** 500 mg q12h × 14 days
Most infections
- *Child:* **PO** 7.5 mg/kg q12h × 10 days, max 500 mg/dose for MAC

Available forms: Tabs 250, 500 mg; oral susp 125 mg/5 ml, 250 mg/5 ml; ext rel tab 500 mg (XL)

SIDE EFFECTS

*CV: **Ventricular dysrhythmias***
*GI: Nausea, vomiting, diarrhea, **hepatotoxicity**, abdominal pain,* stomatitis, heartburn, anorexia, *abnormal taste, **pseudomembranous colitis***
GU: Vaginitis, moniliasis
HEMA: Leukopenia, thrombocytopenia, increased INR

INTEG: Rash, urticaria, pruritus, ***Stevens-Johnson syndrome***
MISC: Headache

Contraindications: Hypersensitivity to this drug or macrolide antibiotics
Precautions: Pregnancy (C), lactation, hepatic disease, renal disease, elderly

PHARMACOKINETICS

Peak 2 hr, duration 12 hr, half-life 4-6 hr; metabolized by liver; excreted in bile, feces

INTERACTIONS

Dysrhythmias: cisapride, pimozide
Increase: levels, *increase* toxicity—alprazolam, buspirone, Carbamazepine, cycloSPORINE, digoxin, disopyramide, ergots, felodipine, fluconazole, omeprazole, tacrolimus, theophylline
Increase: oral anticoagulants effect—digoxin, theophylline, carbamazepine
Increase: levels of HMG-CoA reductase inhibitors
Increase: action, risk of toxicity—all drugs metabolized by CYP3A enzyme system
Increase or decrease action: zidovudine
Decrease: levels—rifampin, rifabutin
Drug/Herb
Do not use acidophilus with antiinfectives
Drug/Lab Test
Increase: 17-OHCS/17-KS, AST, ALT, BUN, creatinine, LDH, total bilirubin
Decrease: Folate assay, WBC

NURSING CONSIDERATIONS

Assess:
• For infection: wound characteristics, urine, stool, sputum, WBC, temp
• For ulcers: abdominal pain, bleeding in stools, emesis
• Renal, hepatic studies; report hematuria, oliguria
• C&S before drug therapy; drug may be given as soon as culture is taken; C&S may be repeated after treatment
• Bowel pattern before, during treatment
• Skin eruptions, itching
• Respiratory status: rate, character,

wheezing, tightness in chest; discontinue drug
• Allergies before treatment, reaction of each medication
Administer:
• Do not break, crush, or chew tabs
• Adequate intake of fluids (2 L) during diarrhea episodes
• q12h to maintain serum level
Perform/provide:
• Storage at room temperature
Evaluate:
• Therapeutic response: C&S negative for infection
Teach patient/family:
• To take with full glass H_2O; may give with food to decrease GI symptoms
A To report sore throat, fever, fatigue; may indicate superinfection
A To notify nurse of diarrhea, dark urine, pale stools, yellow discoloration of eyes or skin, severe abdominal pain
• To take at evenly spaced intervals; complete dosage regimen
• To notify prescriber if pregnancy is suspected or planned
Treatment of hypersensitivity:
Withdraw drug, maintain airway, administer epINEPHrine, aminophylline, O_2, IV corticosteroids

---

clindamycin HCl (℞)
(klin-da-my'sin)
Cleocin HCl
clindamycin palmitate (℞)
Cleocin Pediatric, Dalacin C Palmitate
clindamycin phosphate (℞)
Cleocin Phosphate, Dalacin C, Dalacin C Phosphate
Func. class.: Miscellaneous antiinfective
Chem. class.: Lincomycin derivative

Action: Binds to 50S subunit of bacterial ribosomes, suppresses protein synthesis
Uses: Infections caused by staphylo-

cocci, streptococci, *Rickettsia, Fuso-bacterium, Actinomyces, Peptococcus, Bacteroides, Pneumocystis jiroveci*

DOSAGE AND ROUTES

• *Adult:* **PO** 150-450 mg q6h, max 1.8 g/day; **IM/IV** 1.2-1.8 g/day in 2-4 divided doses, not to exceed 4800 mg/day

• *Child >1 mo:* **PO** 8-25 mg/kg/day in divided doses q6-8h; **IM/IV** 20-40 mg/kg/day in divided doses q6-8h (3-4 equal doses)

• *Child <1 mo:* 15-20 mg/kg/day divided q6-8h

PID

• *Adult:* **IV** 600 mg qid plus gentamicin or 900 mg q8h

Bacterial endocarditis prophylaxis

• *Adult:* 600 mg 1 hr prior to procedure

Available forms: Phosphate: inj 150, 300, 600 mg base/4 ml; 900 mg base/ml; inj INF in D₅ 300 mg, 600 mg, 900 mg; HCl: caps 75, 150, 300 mg; palmitate: oral sol 75 mg/ml

SIDE EFFECTS

GI: Nausea, vomiting, abdominal pain, diarrhea, **pseudomembranous colitis,** anorexia, weight loss, increased AST, ALT, bilirubin, alk phosphatase; jaundice
GU: Vaginitis, urinary frequency
HEMA: **Leukopenia, eosinophilia, agranulocytosis, thrombocytopenia, polyarthritis**
INTEG: Rash, urticaria, pruritus, erythema, pain, abscess at inj site

Contraindications: Hypersensitivity to this drug or lincomycin, tartrazine dye; ulcerative colitis/enteritis

Precautions: Pregnancy (B), renal disease, liver disease, GI disease, elderly, lactation, tartrazine sensitivity

PHARMACOKINETICS

PO: Peak 45 min, duration 6 hr
IM: Peak 3 hr, duration 8-12 hr; half-life 2½ hr; metabolized in liver; excreted in urine, bile, feces as inactive metabolites; crosses placenta; excreted in breast milk

INTERACTIONS

May block clindamycin effect: erythromycin
Increase: neuromuscular blockade—neuromuscular blockers
Decrease: absorption—kaolin
Drug/Herb
Do not use acidophilus with antiinfectives
Drug/Lab Test
Increase: Alk phosphatase, bilirubin, CPK, AST, ALT

NURSING CONSIDERATIONS
Assess:
• Hepatic studies: AST, ALT if on long-term therapy
• Blood studies: WBC, RBC, Hct, Hgb, platelets, serum iron, reticulocytes; drug should be discontinued if bone marrow depression occurs
• C&S before drug therapy; drug may be given as soon as culture is taken
• B/P, pulse in patient receiving drug parenterally
• Bowel pattern before, during treatment; if severe diarrhea occurs, drug should be discontinued; may indicate pseudomembranous colitis
• Skin eruptions, itching, dermatitis after administration
• Respiratory status: rate, character, wheezing, tightness in chest
• Allergies before treatment, reaction of each medication
Administer:
• That drug must be taken in equal intervals around clock to maintain blood levels
PO route
• Do not break, crush, or chew caps
• Orally with at least 8 oz H₂O
IM route
• IM deep inj; rotate sites
IV route
• By infusion only; do not administer bolus dose; dilute 300 mg or less/50 ml or more of D₅W, NS; may be further diluted in greater amounts of D₅W, NS and given as a cont inf in acute PID; give first dose 10 mg/min over ½ hr, then 0.75

---

mg/min; increased rates may be used to keep serum blood levels higher; run >10 min; no more than 1200 mg in a single 1-hr inf

Additive compatibilities: Amikacin, ampicillin, aztreonam, cefamandole, cefazolin, cefepime, cefonicid, cefoperazone, cefotaxime, cefoxitin, ceftazidime, ceftizoxime, cefuroxime, cephalothin, cimetidine, fluconazole, heparin, hydrocortisone, kanamycin, methylPREDNISolone, metoclopramide, metronidazole, netilmicin, ofloxacin, penicillin G, piperacillin, potassium chloride, sodium bicarbonate, tobramycin, verapamil, vit B/C

Syringe compatibilities: Amikacin, aztreonam, gentamicin, heparin

Y-site compatibilities: Amifostine, amiodarone, amphotericin B cholesteryl, amsacrine, aztreonam, cefpirome, cisatracurium, cyclophosphamide, diltiazem, DOXOrubicin liposome, enalaprilat, esmolol, fludarabine, foscarnet, granisetron, heparin, hydromorphone, labetalol, magnesium sulfate, melphalan, meperidine, midazolam, morphine, multivitamins, ondansetron, perphenazine, piperacillin/tazobactam, propofol, remifentanil, sargramostim, tacrolimus, teniposide, theophylline, thiotepa, vinorelbine, vit B/C, zidovudine

Perform/provide:
• Storage at room temperature (caps) up to 2 wk (reconstituted)
• EpINEPHrine, suction, tracheostomy set, endotracheal intubation equipment on unit
• Adequate intake of fluids (2 L) during diarrhea episodes

Evaluate:
• Therapeutic response: decreased temp, negative C&S

Teach patient/family:
• To take oral drug with full glass H_2O; antiperistaltic drugs may worsen diarrhea
• All aspects of drug therapy: need to complete entire course of medication to ensure organism death (10-14 days);

culture may be taken after medication course completed

⚠ To report sore throat, fever, fatigue; may indicate superinfection
• To take with food to reduce GI symptoms
• To notify nurse or prescriber of diarrhea

Treatment of hypersensitivity:
• Withdraw drug; maintain airway; administer epINEPHrine, aminophylline, O_2, IV corticosteroids

---

clioquinol topical
See Appendix C

---

clobetasol topical
See Appendix C

---

clocortolone topical
See Appendix C

Rarely Used

clofazimine (℞)
(kloe-fa′zi-meen)
Lamprene
Func. class.: Leprostatic

Uses: Lepromatous leprosy, dapsone-resistant leprosy, lepromatous leprosy complicated by erythema nodosum leprosum

DOSAGE AND ROUTES
Erythema nodosum leprosum
• *Adult:* **PO:** 100-200 mg daily × 3 mo, then taper dosage to 100 mg when disease is controlled; do not exceed 200 mg/day
Dapsone-resistant leprosy
• *Adult:* **PO:** 100 mg/day in combination with at least one other antileprosy drug × 3 yr, then 100 mg daily clofazimine (only)

Contraindications: Hypersensitivity to this drug

---

*clomiPHENE (R)

(kloe′mi-feen)
Clomid, clomiphene citrate, Milophene, Serophene
Func. class.: Ovulation stimulant
Chem. class.: Nonsteroidal antiestrogenic

Do not confuse:
clomiPHENE/clomiPRAMINE
Action: Increases LH, FSH release from the pituitary, which increases maturation of ovarian follicle, ovulation, development of corpus luteum
Uses: Female infertility (ovulatory failure)

DOSAGE AND ROUTES

• *Adult:* **PO** 50-100 mg daily × 5 days or 50-100 mg daily beginning on day 5 of cycle; may be repeated until conception occurs or 3 cycles of therapy have been completed
Available forms: Tabs 50 mg

SIDE EFFECTS

CNS: Headache, depression, restlessness, anxiety, nervousness, fatigue, insomnia, dizziness, flushing
CV: Vasomotor flushing, phlebitis, ***deep-vein thrombosis***
EENT: Blurred vision, diplopia, photophobia
GI: Nausea, vomiting, constipation, abdominal pain, bloating
GU: Polyuria, urinary frequency, birth defects, spontaneous abortions, multiple ovulation, breast pain, oliguria, abnormal uterine bleeding
INTEG: Rash, dermatitis, urticaria, alopecia
Contraindications: Pregnancy (X), hypersensitivity, hepatic disease, undiagnosed uterine bleeding, uncontrolled thyroid or adrenal dysfunction, intracranial lesion, ovarian cysts

Precautions: Hypertension, depression, convulsions, diabetes mellitus

PHARMACOKINETICS

Metabolized in liver, excreted in feces

Drug/Lab Test
Increase: FSH/LH, BSP, thyroxine, TBG

NURSING CONSIDERATIONS

Administer:
• After discontinuing estrogen therapy
• At same time daily to maintain drug level
Evaluate:
• Therapeutic response: fertility
Teach patient/family:
• That multiple births are common
• To notify prescriber immediately if low abdominal pain occurs; may indicate ovarian cyst, cyst rupture
• To notify prescriber of photophobia, blurred vision, diplopia, abnormal bleeding, hot flashes, nausea, vomiting, headache
• That if dose is missed, to double it next time; if more than one dose is missed, to call prescriber
• That response usually occurs 4-10 days after last day of treatment
• The method for taking, recording basal body temp to determine whether ovulation has occurred
• If ovulation can be determined (there is a slight decrease in temp, then a sharp increase for ovulation), to attempt coitus 3 days before and every other day until after ovulation
• If pregnancy is suspected, to notify prescriber immediately

---

*clomiPRAMINE (R)

(kloe-mip′ra-meen)
Anafranil
Func. class.: Antidepressant, tricyclic
Chem. class.: Tertiary amine

Do not confuse:
clomiPRAMINE/clomiPHENE/desipramine/Norpramin

⚠ Safety alert   *"Tall Man" lettering

Action: Potentiates serotonin and norepinephrine; also increases dopamine metabolism; moderate anticholinergic effect

Uses: Obsessive-compulsive disorder, depression, dysphoria, phobias, anxiety, agoraphobia

DOSAGE AND ROUTES

Obsessive-compulsive disorder
• *Adult:* **PO** 25 mg at bedtime and increase gradually over 4 wk to 75-250 mg/day in divided doses
• *Child 10-18 yr:* **PO** 25-50 mg/day gradually increased; or 3 mg/kg/day, whichever is smaller, not to exceed 200 mg/day

Depression
• *Adult:* **PO** 50-150 mg/day in a single or divided dose

Anxiety/agoraphobia
• *Adult:* **PO** 25-75 mg/day

Available forms: Caps 25, 50, 75 mg

SIDE EFFECTS

*CNS: Dizziness, tremors, mania, **seizures,** aggressiveness, EPS, drowsiness, headache*
*CV: Hypotension, tachycardia, **cardiac arrest***
EENT: Blurred vision
ENDO: Galactorrhea, hyperprolactinemia
GI: Constipation, dry mouth, nausea, dyspepsia, weight gain
GU: Delayed ejaculation, anorgasmia, urinary retention, decreased libido
*HEMA: **Agranulocytosis, neutropenia, pancytopenia***
INTEG: Diaphoresis, photosensitivity
META: Hyponatremia

Contraindications: Hypersensitivity, immediate post-MI
Precautions: Pregnancy (C), seizures, suicidal patients, elderly, lactation, cardiac disease

PHARMACOKINETICS

Onset ≥2 wk, peak 2-6 hr; extensively bound to tissue and plasma proteins; demethylated in liver; active metabolites excreted in urine; half-life: 19-37 hr; steady state 1-2 wk

INTERACTIONS

Hypertensive crisis, convulsions, hypertensive episode: MAOIs
Increase: clomiPRAMINE levels—cimetidine, fluoxetine, fluvoxamine, sertraline; do not use together
Increase: hypertensive effect—clonidine, epINEPHrine, norepinephrine
Increase: CNS depression—alcohol, CNS depressants
Decrease: clomiPRAMINE levels—barbiturates, carbamazepine, phenytoin

Drug/Herb
Serotonin syndrome: SAM-e, St. John's wort; do not use concurrently
Increase: CNS depression—hops, kava, lavender
Increase: anticholinergic effect—belladonna, corkwood, henbane, jimsonweed
Increase: clomiPRAMINE action—scopolia root

Drug/Lab Test
Increase: Prolactin, TBG
Decrease: Serum thyroid hormone

NURSING CONSIDERATIONS

Assess:
• B/P (lying, standing), pulse q4h; if systolic B/P drops 20 mm Hg, withhold drug, notify prescriber; take vital signs q4h in patients with cardiovascular disease
• ECG for flattening of T wave, QTc prolongation, bundle branch block, AV block, dysrhythmias in cardiac patients
• Blood studies: CBC, leukocytes, differential, cardiac enzymes if patient is receiving long-term therapy
• Hepatic studies: AST, ALT, bilirubin
• Mental status: mood, sensorium, affect, suicidal tendencies; increase in psychiatric symptoms: depression, panic, frequency of obsessive-compulsive behaviors

- Urinary retention, constipation; constipation more likely in children
- Withdrawal symptoms: headache, nausea, vomiting, muscle pain, weakness; not usual unless drug discontinued abruptly
- Alcohol consumption; if alcohol consumed, withhold dose until AM

Administer:

- Do not break, crush, or chew caps
- Increased fluids, bulk in diet for constipation, especially elderly
- With food or milk for GI symptoms

Perform/provide:

- Storage in tight container at room temperature; do not freeze
- Assistance with ambulation during beginning therapy, since drowsiness/dizziness occurs
- Safety measures, primarily in elderly
- Checking to see PO medication swallowed
- Gum, hard candy, or frequent sips of water for dry mouth

Evaluate:

- Therapeutic response: decreased anxiety, depression

Teach patient/family:

- That the effects may take 2-3 wk
- To use caution in driving, other activities requiring alertness because of drowsiness, dizziness, blurred vision
- To avoid alcohol ingestion, other CNS depressants
- Not to discontinue medication quickly after long-term use; may cause nausea, headache, malaise
- To wear sunscreen, protective clothing to prevent photosensitivity
- To notify prescriber if pregnancy is planned or suspected

Treatment of overdose: ECG monitoring; induce emesis; lavage, activated charcoal; anticonvulsant

---

clonazepam (℞)
(kloe-na′zi-pam)
Klonopin, Rivotril ✦,
Syn-Clonazepam ✦
Func. class.: Anticonvulsant
Chem. class.: Benzodiazepine derivative

Controlled Substance Schedule IV
Do not confuse:
clonazepam/lorazepam/clorazepate
Klonopin/clonidine

Action: Inhibits spike, wave formation in absence seizures (petit mal), decreases amplitude, frequency, duration, spread of discharge in minor motor seizures

Uses: Absence, atypical absence, akinetic, myoclonic seizures, Lennox-Gastaut syndrome

Investigational uses: Parkinsonian dysarthrosis, acute manic episodes, adjunction schizophrenia, neuralgias, multifocal tic disorders, restless leg syndrome, rectal administration

DOSAGE AND ROUTES

- *Adult:* **PO** not to exceed 1.5 mg/day in 3 divided doses; may be increased 0.5-1 mg q3d until desired response, not to exceed 20 mg/day; rectal 0.02 mg/kg
- *Geriatric:* **PO** 0.25 daily-bid initially, increase by 0.25 daily q7-14d as needed
- *Child <10 yr or <30 kg:* **PO** 0.01-0.03 mg/kg/day in divided doses q8h, not to exceed 0.05 mg/kg/day; may be increased 0.25-0.5 mg q3d until desired response, not to exceed 0.1-0.2 mg/kg/day; rectal 0.05-0.1 mg/kg

Available forms: Tabs 0.5, 1, 2 mg; oral susp; IV sol

SIDE EFFECTS

CNS: Drowsiness, dizziness, confusion, behavioral changes, tremors, insomnia, headache, ***suicidal tendencies,*** slurred speech
CV: Palpitations, bradycardia, tachycardia

EENT: Increased salivation, nystagmus, diplopia, abnormal eye movements
GI: Nausea, constipation, polyphagia, anorexia, xerostomia, diarrhea, gastritis, sore gums
GU: Dysuria, enuresis, nocturia, retention, libido changes
*HEMA: **Thrombocytopenia, leukocytosis, eosinophilia***
INTEG: Rash, alopecia, hirsutism
*RESP: **Respiratory depression,*** dyspnea, congestion

Contraindications: Hypersensitivity to benzodiazepines, acute narrow-angle glaucoma, psychosis, severe liver disease
Precautions: Pregnancy (C), open-angle glaucoma, chronic respiratory disease, lactation, renal, hepatic disease, elderly

PHARMACOKINETICS

PO: Peak 1-2 hr; metabolized by liver; excreted in urine; half-life 18-50 hr, duration 6-12 hr

INTERACTIONS

Increase: CNS depression—alcohol, barbiturates, opiates, antidepressants, other anticonvulsants, general anesthetics, hypnotics, sedatives
Decrease: clonazepam effect—carbamazepine, phenobarbital, phenytoin

Drug/Herb
Increase: CNS depression—kava
Increase: clonazepam effect—ginkgo
Decrease: clonazepam effect—ginseng, santonica

Drug/Lab Test
Increase: AST, alk phosphatase

NURSING CONSIDERATIONS

Assess:
• Renal studies: urinalysis, BUN, urine creatinine
• Blood studies: RBC, Hct, Hgb, reticulocyte counts qwk for 4 wk, then qmo
• Hepatic studies: ALT, AST, bilirubin, creatinine

• Drug levels during initial treatment (therapeutic 20-80 ng/ml)
• Signs of physical withdrawal if medication suddenly discontinued
• Mental status: mood, sensorium, affect, oversedation, behavioral changes; if mental status changes, notify prescriber
• Eye problems: need for ophthalmic exam before, during, after treatment (slit lamp, funduscopy, tonometry)
• Allergic reaction: red, raised rash; drug should be discontinued
⚠ Blood dyscrasias: fever, sore throat, bruising, rash, jaundice
• Toxicity: bone marrow depression, nausea, vomiting, ataxia, diplopia, cardiovascular collapse

Administer:
• With food, milk for GI symptoms
• Avoid use with CNS depressants

Oral suspension
• May use rectally (1 mg/ml of clonazepam with 1 ml of water); use plastic tube (volume 2.2-3.3 ml)

IV solution
• May use rectally 1-ml syringe inserted 3 cm into rectum

Perform/provide:
• Storage at room temperature
• Assistance with ambulation during early part of treatment; dizziness occurs, especially elderly

Evaluate:
• Therapeutic response: decreased seizure activity, document on patient's chart

Teach patient/family:
• To carry emergency ID bracelet stating name, drugs taken, condition, prescriber's name, phone number
• To avoid driving, other activities that require alertness
• To avoid alcohol ingestion; increased sedation may occur
• Not to discontinue medication quickly after long-term use; taper off over several wk

Treatment of overdose: Lavage, activated charcoal, monitor electrolytes, VS, administer vasopressors

---

clonidine (℞)

(klon′i-deen)

Catapres, Catapres-TTS, clonidine HCl, Dixarit ♣, Duraclon

Func. class.: Antihypertensive, centrally acting analgesic

Chem. class.: Central α-adrenergic agonist

Do not confuse:

clonidine/Klonopin/clonazepam
Catapres/Cataflam/Catarase

Action: Inhibits sympathetic vasomotor center in CNS, which reduces impulses in sympathetic nervous system; blood pressure, pulse rate, cardiac output decrease, prevents pain signal transmission in CNS by α-adrenergic receptor stimulation of the spinal cord

Uses: Mild to moderate hypertension, used alone or in combination; severe pain in cancer patients

Investigational uses: Opioid withdrawal, prevention of vascular headaches, treatment of menopausal symptoms, dysmenorrhea, attention deficit hyperactivity disorder

DOSAGE AND ROUTES

Hypertension

• *Adult:* **PO/TD** 0.1 mg bid, then increase by 0.1-0.2 mg/day at weekly intervals, until desired response; range 0.2-0.6 mg/day in divided doses

• *Geriatric:* **PO** 0.1 mg at bedtime, may increase gradually

• *Child:* 5-10 mcg/kg/day in divided doses q8-12h, max 0.9 mg/day

Opioid withdrawal (unlabeled use)

• *Adult:* **PO** 0.3-1.2 mg/day; may decrease by 50% × 3 days then decrease by 0.1-0.2 mg/day or discontinue

Severe pain

• Adult: **CONT EPIDURAL INF** 30 mcg/hr

• *Child:* **CONT EPIDURAL INF** 0.5 mcg/kg/hr, then titrate to response

ADHD (unlabeled use)

• *Child:* 5 mcg/kg/day in 3-4 divided doses × 8 wk

Menopausal symptoms (unlabeled use)

• *Adult:* **TD** 0.1 mg patch q1wk; **PO** 0.05-0.4 mg daily

Available forms: Tabs 0.025 ♣, 0.1, 0.2, 0.3 mg; TRANS 2.5, 5, 7.5 mg delivering 0.1, 0.2, 0.3 mg/24 hr, respectively; inj 100, 500 mcg/ml

SIDE EFFECTS

CNS: Drowsiness, sedation, headache, fatigue, nightmares, insomnia, mental changes, anxiety, depression, hallucinations, delirium

CV: Orthostatic hypotension, palpitations, **CHF,** ECG abnormalities

EENT: Taste change, parotid pain

ENDO: Hyperglycemia

GI: Nausea, vomiting, malaise, constipation, *dry mouth*

GU: Impotence, dysuria, nocturia, gynecomastia

INTEG: Rash, alopecia, facial pallor, pruritus, hives, edema, burning papules, excoriation (transdermal patches)

MISC: Withdrawal symptoms

MS: Muscle, joint pain; leg cramps

Contraindications: Hypersensitivity; (epidural) bleeding disorders, anticoagulants

Precautions: Pregnancy (C), MI (recent), diabetes mellitus, chronic renal failure, Raynaud's disease, thyroid disease, depression, COPD, child <12 yr (transdermal), asthma, lactation, elderly, noncompliant patients

PHARMACOKINETICS

Absorbed well

PO: Onset ½ to 1 hr, peak 2-4 hr, duration 8-12 hr; half-life 12-21 hr

TD: Onset 3 days, duration 1 wk; metabolized by liver (metabolites), excreted in urine (30% unchanged, inactive metabolites), feces; crosses blood-brain barrier, excreted in breast milk

---

A Safety alert　　*"Tall Man" lettering

INTERACTIONS

AV block: verapamil

Life-threatening elevations of B/P: tricyclics, β-blockers

Increase: CNS depression—opiates, sedatives, hypnotics, anesthetics, alcohol

Increase: hypotensive effects— diuretics, other antihypertensive nitrates

Decrease: hypotensive effects— tricyclics, MAOIs, appetite suppressants, amphetamines, prazosin

Decrease: effect of levodopa

Drug/Herb

Toxicity/death: aconite

Increase: antihypertensive effect— barberry, betony, black catechu, black cohosh, bloodroot, broom, burdock, cat's claw, dandelion, goldenseal, Irish moss, Jamaican dogwood, kelp, khella, mistletoe, parsley, Queen Anne's lace, rue

Decrease: antihypertensive effect— astragalus, capsicum peppers, cola tree, coltsfoot, khat, guarana, licorice

Drug/Lab Test

Increase: Blood glucose

Decrease: VMA, urinary catecholamines, aldosterone

NURSING CONSIDERATIONS

Assess:

• Blood studies: neutrophils, decreased platelets

• Renal studies: protein, BUN, creatinine; increased levels may indicate nephrotic syndrome

• Baselines in renal, hepatic studies before therapy begins; potassium levels, although hyperkalemia rare

• B/P, pulse if used for hypertension, report significant changes

• For opiate withdrawal including fever, diarrhea, nausea, vomiting, cramps, insomnia, shivering, dilated pupils

• Pain: location, intensity, character; alleviating, aggravating factors, baseline and frequently

• Edema in feet, legs daily; monitor I&O; check for falling output

• Allergic reaction: rash, fever, pruritus, urticaria; drug should be discontinued if antihistamines fail to help

• Allergic reaction from patches: rash, urticaria, angioedema; should not continue to use

• Symptoms of CHF: edema, dyspnea, wet crackles, B/P

• Renal symptoms: polyuria, oliguria, frequency

Administer:

• PO: give last dose at bedtime

• Transdermal patch qwk; apply to site without hair; best absorption over chest or upper arm; rotate sites with each application; clean site before application; apply firmly, especially around edges

Perform/provide:

• Storage of patches in cool environment, tablets in tight container

Evaluate:

• Therapeutic response: decrease in B/P in hypertension, decrease in withdrawal symptoms (opioid), decrease in pain

Teach patient/family:

• To avoid hazardous activities, since drug may cause drowsiness

• To notify all health care providers of medication use

• Not to discontinue drug abruptly or withdrawal symptoms may occur: anxiety, increased B/P, headache, insomnia, increased pulse, tremors, nausea, sweating

• Not to use OTC (cough, cold, or allergy) products unless directed by prescriber

• To comply with dosage schedule even if feeling better

• To rise slowly to sitting or standing position to minimize orthostatic hypotension, especially elderly

• To notify prescriber of mouth sores, sore throat, fever, swelling of hands, feet, irregular heartbeat, chest pain, signs of angioedema

• About excessive perspiration, dehydration, vomiting; diarrhea may lead to fall in blood pressure; consult prescriber if these occur

• That drug may cause dizziness, fainting; light-headedness may occur during first few days of therapy

---

Side effects: *italics* = common; ***bold italics*** = life-threatening

• That drug may cause dry mouth; use hard candy, saliva product, or frequent rinsing of mouth

• That compliance is necessary; not to skip or stop drug unless directed by prescriber

• That drug may cause skin rash or impaired perspiration

• To use patch; patch comes in two parts: drug patch and overlay to keep patch in place, do not trim or cut patch

• That response may take 2-3 days if drug is given transdermally; instruct on administration of patch, if switching from tabs to patch, taper tabs to avoid withdrawal

Treatment of overdose: Supportive treatment; administer tolazoline, atropine, DOPamine prn

---

clopidogrel (℞)
(klo-pid′oh-grel)
Plavix
Func. class.: Platelet aggregation inhibitor
Chem. class.: Thienopyridine derivative

Do not confuse:
Plavix/Paxil/Elavil

Action: Inhibits first and second phases of ADP-induced effects in platelet aggregation

Uses: Reducing the risk of stroke, MI, peripheral arterial disease in high-risk patients, acute coronary syndrome, transient ischemic attack (TIA)

DOSAGE AND ROUTES
Recent MI, stroke, peripheral arterial disease
• *Adult:* PO 75 mg daily with or without food

Acute coronary syndrome
• *Adult:* PO loading dose 300 mg then 75 mg daily
Available forms: Tabs 75 mg

SIDE EFFECTS
CNS: Headache, dizziness, depression, syncope, hypesthesia, neuralgia
CV: Edema, hypertension
GI: Nausea, vomiting, diarrhea, GI discomfort, ***GI bleeding***
HEMA: Epistaxis, purpura, ***bleeding, neutropenia***
INTEG: Rash, pruritus
MISC: UTI, hypercholesterolemia, chest pain, fatigue, ***intracranial hemorrhage***
MS: Arthralgia, back pain
RESP: Upper respiratory tract infection, dyspnea, rhinitis, bronchitis, cough
Contraindications: Hypersensitivity, active bleeding
Precautions: Pregnancy (B), past hepatic disease, lactation, children, increased bleeding risk, neutropenia, agranulocytosis, renal disease

PHARMACOKINETICS
Rapidly absorbed, peak 1-3 hr, metabolized by liver, excreted in urine, feces, half-life 8 hr, plasma protein binding 95%, effect on platelets after 3-7 days

INTERACTIONS
Increase: bleeding risk—anticoagulants, aspirin, NSAIDs, abciximab, eptifibatide, tirofiban, thrombolytics, ticlopidine
Increase: action of—some NSAIDs, phenytoin, TOLBUTamide, tamoxifen, torsemide, fluvastatin, warfarin
Drug/Herb
Increase: clopidogrel effect—bogbean, dong quai, feverfew, garlic, ginger, ginkgo, green tea
Increase: gastric irritation—arginine
Decrease: clopidogrel effect—bilberry, saw palmetto

NURSING CONSIDERATIONS
Assess:
• For symptoms of stroke, MI during treatment
• Hepatic studies: AST, ALT, bilirubin, creatinine (long-term therapy)

- Blood studies: CBC, Hct, Hgb, PT, cholesterol (long-term therapy)

Administer:
- With food to decrease gastric symptoms

Evaluate:
- Therapeutic response: absence of stroke, MI

Teach patient/family:
- That blood work will be necessary during treatment
- To report any unusual bruising, bleeding to prescriber, that it may take longer to stop bleeding
- To take with food or just after eating to minimize GI discomfort
- To report diarrhea, skin rashes, subcutaneous bleeding, chills, fever, sore throat
- To tell all health care providers that clopidogrel is used; may be held 3-7 days before surgery

---

clorazepate (℞)

(klor-az′e-pate)
Apo-Clorazepate ✦, clorazepate, Novo-Clopate ✦, Tranxene-SD, Tranxene-SD Half Strength, Tranxene T-tab
Func. class.: Antianxiety, anticonvulsant, sedative/hypnotic
Chem. class.: Benzodiazepine

Controlled Substance Schedule IV
Do not confuse:
clorazepate/clonazepam

Action: Potentiates the actions of GABA, especially in limbic system, reticular formation

Uses: Anxiety, acute alcohol withdrawal, adjunct in seizure disorders

DOSAGE AND ROUTES

Anxiety
- *Adult:* PO 15-60 mg/day or 7.5-15 mg 2-4×/day; **EXT REL** 11.25-22.5 mg at bedtime, do not use **EXT REL** to iniate therapy
- *Geriatric:* PO 7.5 mg daily-bid

Alcohol withdrawal
- *Adult:* PO 30 mg then 30-60 mg in divided doses; day 2, 45-90 mg in divided doses; day 3, 22.5-45 mg in divided doses; day 4, 15-30 mg in divided doses; then gradually reduce daily dose to 7.5-15 mg

Seizure disorders
- *Adult and child >12 yr:* **PO** 7.5 mg tid; may increase by 7.5 mg/wk or less, not to exceed 90 mg/day
- *Child 9-12 yr:* **PO** 3.75-7.5 mg bid; may increase by 3.75 mg/wk or less, not to exceed 60 mg/day

Available forms: Tabs 3.75, 7.5, 15 mg; tab ext rel (Tranxene-SD Half Strength) 11.25 mg; (Tranxene-SD) 22.5 mg

SIDE EFFECTS

CNS: Dizziness, drowsiness, confusion, headache, anxiety, tremors, stimulation, fatigue, depression, insomnia, hallucinations, lethargy
*CV: Orthostatic hypotension, **ECG changes, tachycardia,*** hypotension, chest pain
EENT: Blurred vision, tinnitus, mydriasis
GI: Constipation, dry mouth, nausea, vomiting, anorexia, diarrhea
INTEG: Rash, dermatitis, itching

Contraindications: Pregnancy (D), hypersensitivity to benzodiazepines, narrow-angle glaucoma, psychosis, lactation, child <9 yr
Precautions: Elderly, debilitated, hepatic disease, renal disease

PHARMACOKINETICS

PO: Onset 1 hr, peak 1-2 hr, duration up to 24 hr; metabolized by liver, excreted by kidneys; crosses placenta, breast milk; half-life 30-100 hr

INTERACTIONS

Increase: clorazepate effects—CNS depressants, alcohol, valproic acid, antidepressants, MAOIs, cimetidine, oral contraceptives, disulfiram, fluoxetine, isoniazid, ketoconazole, propoxyphene, some β-blockers

---

Decrease: clorazepate action—
rifampin, barbiturates
Drug/Herb
Increase: CNS depression—catnip,
chamomile, clary, cowslip, kava, mistle-
toe, nettle, pokeweed, poppy, Queen
Anne's lace, senega, valerian
Increase: hypotension—black cohosh
Drug/Lab Test
Increase: AST, ALT
Decrease: Hct

NURSING CONSIDERATIONS
Assess:
• B/P (lying, standing), pulse; if systolic
B/P drops 20 mm Hg, hold drug, notify
prescriber
• Blood studies: CBC during long-term
therapy; blood dyscrasias have occurred
rarely
• Hepatic studies: AST, ALT, bilirubin,
creatinine, LDH, alk phosphatase
• I&O; may indicate renal dysfunction
• Mental status: mood, sensorium, af-
fect, sleeping pattern, drowsiness,
dizziness; for delirium, tremors, halluci-
nation in alcohol withdrawal
• Physical dependency, withdrawal symp-
toms: headache, nausea, vomiting, muscle
pain, weakness after long-term use
• Suicidal tendencies, anxiety level
• Seizures: location, duration, intensity
Administer:
• Do not break, crush, or chew caps
• With food, milk for GI symptoms
• Crushed if patient cannot swallow
whole (tab only)
• Do not break ext rel
Perform/provide:
• Assistance with ambulation during
beginning therapy because of
drowsiness/dizziness, especially elderly
• Safety measures, including side rails
• Check to see PO medication has been
swallowed
• Sugarless gum, hard candy, frequent
sips of water for dry mouth
Evaluate:
• Therapeutic response: decreased
anxiety, restlessness, insomnia

Teach patient/family:
• That drug may be taken with food
• That drug is not to be used for everyday stress or used longer than 4 mo unless directed by prescriber; not to take
more than prescribed amount; may be
habit forming
• To avoid OTC preparations unless
approved by prescriber
• To avoid driving, activities that require
alertness; drowsiness may occur, especially in elderly
• To avoid alcohol ingestion, other psychotropic medications, unless directed
by prescriber
• Not to discontinue medication abruptly
after long-term use; restlessness, insomnia, irritability may occur
• To rise slowly because fainting may
occur
• That drowsiness may worsen at beginning of treatment
Treatment of overdose: Lavage, VS,
supportive care, flumazenil

clotrimazole topical
See Appendix C

**clotrimazole vaginal
antifungal**
See Appendix C

cloxacillin (℞)
(klox-a-sill′in)
Apo-Cloxi ✦, cloxacillin,
Cloxapen, Novo-Cloxin ✦,
Nu-Clox ✦, Orbenin ✦
Func. class.: Broad-spectrum antiin-
fective
Chem. class.: Penicillinase-resistant
penicillin

Action: Interferes with cell wall replication of susceptible organisms; the cell

wall, rendered osmotically unstable, swells, bursts from osmotic pressure, resists the penicillinase action that inactivates penicillin

Uses: Gram-positive cocci *(Staphylococcus aureus, Streptococcus pyogenes, Streptococcus pneumoniae)*, penicillinase-producing staphylococci

DOSAGE AND ROUTES

• *Adult:* **PO** 1-4 g/day in divided doses q6h
• *Child:* **PO** 50-100 mg/kg in divided doses q6h, max 4 g/day
Available forms: Caps 250, 500 mg; oral sol 125 mg/5 ml

SIDE EFFECTS

CNS: Lethargy, hallucinations, anxiety, depression, twitching, ***coma, seizures***
GI: *Nausea, vomiting, diarrhea,* increased AST, ALT, abdominal pain, glossitis, colitis, ***pseudomembranous colitis***
GU: **Oliguria, proteinuria,** hematuria, *vaginitis, moniliasis,* ***glomerulonephritis***
HEMA: Anemia, increased bleeding time, ***bone marrow depression, granulocytopenia***
SYST: ***Anaphylaxis, serum sickness***
Contraindications: Hypersensitivity to penicillins; neonates, severe renal, hepatic disease
Precautions: Pregnancy (B), lactation, hypersensitivity to cephalosporins

PHARMACOKINETICS

PO: Peak 1 hr, duration 6 hr; half-life 30-60 min; metabolized in liver; excreted in urine, bile, breast milk; crosses placenta, poor penetration in CSF

INTERACTIONS

Increase: cloxacillin concentrations—probenecid
Increase: action of anticoagulants

Drug/Herb
Do not use acidophilus with antiinfectives
Decrease: absorption—khat
Drug/Food
Citric juices/food decrease absorption of cloxacillin
Drug/Lab Test
Decrease: Uric acid
False positive: Urine glucose, urine protein

NURSING CONSIDERATIONS
Assess:

⚠ Anaphylaxis: pruritus, rash, dyspnea, laryngeal edema; have emergency equipment available; skin eruptions after administration of penicillin to 1 wk after discontinuing drug
• For infection: temp, draining wounds, WBC, sputum, urine, stool before and during treatment
• I&O ratio; report hematuria, oliguria, since penicillin in high doses is nephrotoxic
⚠ Any patient with compromised renal system, since drug is excreted slowly in poor renal system function; toxicity may occur rapidly
• Hepatic studies: AST, ALT
• Blood studies: WBC, RBC, Hgb, Hct, bleeding time
• Renal studies: urinalysis, protein, blood
• C&S before drug therapy; drug may be taken as soon as culture is taken
• Bowel pattern before, during treatment, report diarrhea
Administer:
• Do not break, crush, or chew caps
• After C&S completed
• Shake suspension well before each dose
Perform/provide:
• Adrenaline, suction, tracheostomy set, endotracheal intubation equipment on unit
• Adequate intake of fluids (2 L) during diarrhea episodes
• Scratch test to assess allergy after securing order from prescriber; usually

done when penicillin is only drug of choice

• Storage in tight container; after reconstituting, store in refrigerator for 2 wk, room temperature 3 days

Evaluate:

• Therapeutic response: absence of fever, draining wounds

Teach patient/family:

• All aspects of drug therapy, including need to complete entire course of medication to ensure organism death (10-14 days); culture may be taken after course of medication completed

• To report sore throat, fever, fatigue (may indicate superinfection)

• To wear or carry emergency ID if allergic to penicillins

• To notify prescriber of diarrhea, fever

• To take on an empty stomach with a full glass of water

Treatment of overdose: Withdraw drug; maintain airway; administer epINEPHrine, aminophylline, O$_2$, IV corticosteroids for anaphylaxis

---

clozapine (℞)

(kloz'a-peen)
clozapine, Clozaril
Func. class.: Antipsychotic
Chem. class.: Tricyclic dibenzodiazepine derivative

Do not confuse:
Clozaril/Clinoril/Colazal

Action: Interferes with dopamine receptor binding with lack of extrapyramidal symptoms; also acts as an adrenergic, cholinergic, histaminergic, serotonergic antagonist

Uses: Management of psychotic symptoms in schizophrenic patients for whom other antipsychotics have failed, recurrent suicidal behavior

DOSAGE AND ROUTES

• *Adult:* **PO** 12.5 mg daily or bid; may increase by 25-50 mg/day; normal range 300-450 mg/day after 2 wk; do not increase dose more than 2 × per wk; max

900 mg/day; use lowest dose to control symptoms

Available forms: Tabs 12.5, 25, 100 mg

SIDE EFFECTS

CNS: **Neuroleptic malignant syndrome,** *sedation, salivation, dizziness, headache, tremors, sleep problems, akinesia, fever,* **seizures,** *sweating, akathisia, confusion, fatigue, insomnia,* depression, slurred speech, anxiety, *agitation*

CV: Tachycardia, hypotension, hypertension, chest pain, ECG changes, orthostatic hypotension

EENT: Blurred vision

GI: Drooling or excessive salivation, constipation, nausea, abdominal discomfort, vomiting, diarrhea, anorexia, *weight gain, dry mouth,* heartburn, *dyspepsia, gastroesophageal reflux*

GU: Urinary abnormalities, incontinence, ejaculation dysfunction, frequency, urgency, retention, dysuria

HEMA: **Leukopenia, agranulocytosis, eosinophilia**

MS: Weakness; pain in back, neck, legs; spasm, *rigidity*

OTHER: Diaphoresis

RESP: Dyspnea, nasal congestion

Contraindications: Hypersensitivity, myeloproliferative disorders, severe granulocytopenia (WBC <3500 before therapy), severe CNS depression, coma, uncontrolled epilepsy

Precautions: Pregnancy (B); lactation; children <16; hepatic, renal, cardiac disease; seizures; prostatic enlargement; elderly, narrow-angle glaucoma

PHARMACOKINETICS

Bioavailability 27%-47%, steady state 2.5 hr; 97% protein bound; completely metabolized by liver enzymes involved in metabolism CYP1A2, 2D6, 3A4; excreted in urine (50%) and feces (30%) (metabolites); half-life 8-12 hr

---

⚠ Safety alert   *"Tall Man" lettering

INTERACTIONS

Increase: CNS depression—CNS depressants, psychoactives, alcohol

Increase: clozapine level—citalopram, fluoxetine, CYP1A2 inhibitors (fluvoxanine), sertraline, CYP3A4 inhibitors (ketoconazole, erythromycin), caffeine, ritonavir, risperidone

Increase: plasma concentration—warfarin, digoxin, other highly protein-bound drugs

Increase: hypotension, respiratory, cardiac arrest, collapse—benzodiazepines

Decrease: clozapine level—CYP1A2 inducers (carbamazepine, omeprazole, rifampin); phenobarbital

Drug/Herb

Increase: CNS depression—kava, St. John's wort

Increase: EPS—betel palm, kava

Increase: clozapine action—cola tree, hops, nettle, nutmeg

Drug/Lab Test

Increase: LFTs, cardiac enzymes, cholesterol, blood glucose, bilirubin, PBI, cholinesterase, ^{131}I

False positive: Pregnancy tests, PKU

False negative: Urinary steroids, 17-OHCS

NURSING CONSIDERATIONS

Assess:

• I&O ratio; obtain baseline before treatment begins; palpate bladder if low urinary output occurs

• Bilirubin, CBC, LFTs monthly; discontinue treatment if WBC <3000/mm³ or ANC <1500/mm³ test qwk; may resume when normal; if WBC <2000/mm³ or ANC <1000/mm³ discontinue

• Urinalysis is recommended before, during prolonged therapy

• Affect, orientation, LOC, reflexes, gait, coordination, sleep pattern disturbances

• B/P standing and lying; take pulse and respirations q4h during initial treatment; establish baseline before starting treatment; report drops of 30 mm Hg

• Dizziness, faintness, palpitations, tachycardia on rising

• EPS including akathisia (inability to sit still, no pattern to movements), tardive dyskinesia (bizarre movements of the jaw, mouth, tongue, extremities), pseudoparkinsonism (rigidity, tremors, pill rolling, shuffling gait)

• For neuroleptic malignant syndrome: tachycardia, seizures, fever, dyspnea, diaphoresis, increased or decreased B/P, notify prescriber immediately

• Skin turgor daily

• Constipation, urinary retention daily; if these occur, increase bulk, water in diet, especially elderly, stool softeners, laxatives may be needed

• If diabetic, check blood glucose levels

Administer:

• Check for swallowing of PO medication; monitor for hoarding or giving of medication to other patients

Perform/provide:

• Supervised ambulation until stabilized on medication; do not involve in strenuous exercise program because fainting is possible; patient should not stand still for long periods

• Storage in tight, light-resistant container

Evaluate:

• Therapeutic response: decrease in emotional excitement, hallucinations, delusions, paranoia, reorganization of patterns of thought, speech

Teach patient/family:

• About symptoms of agranulocytosis and need for blood tests qwk for 6 mo, then q2wk; report flulike symptoms

• That orthostatic hypotension often occurs, and to rise gradually from sitting or lying position; to avoid hot tubs, hot showers, tub baths; hypotension may occur

• To avoid abrupt withdrawal of this drug because EPS may result; drug should be withdrawn over 1-2 wk

• To avoid OTC preparations (cough, hay fever, cold) unless approved by prescriber, since serious drug interactions may occur; avoid use with alcohol or CNS depressants, increased drowsiness may occur

• About compliance with drug regimen

• About EPS and necessity for meticulous oral hygiene, since oral candidiasis may occur

• To report sore throat, malaise, fever, bleeding, mouth sores; if these occur, CBC should be drawn and drug discontinued

• That heat stroke may occur in hot weather; take extra precautions to stay cool

• To avoid driving, other hazardous activities; seizures may occur

• To notify prescriber if pregnant or if pregnancy is intended, not to breastfeed

Treatment of overdose: Lavage, activated charcoal; provide an airway; do not induce vomiting

---

⚠ High Alert

coagulation factor VIIa, recombinant (℞)

NovoSeven

Func. class.: Antihemophilic

Action: Promotes hemostasis by activating the intrinsic pathway of coagulation

Uses: Bleeding in hemophilia A or B, with inhibitors to factor VIII or IX

Investigational uses: Coumarin toxicity, factor VII deficiency

DOSAGE AND ROUTES

• *Adult:* **IV BOL** 90 mcg/kg q2h until hemostasis occurs, or until therapy is deemed to be inadequate; posthemostatic doses q3-6h may be required

Available forms: Lyophilized powder, 1.2 mg/vial (1200 mcg/vial), 4.8 mg/vial (4800 mcg/vial) recombinant human coagulation factor VIIa (rFVIIa)

SIDE EFFECTS

CNS: Fever, headache

INTEG: Pain, redness at inj site, pruritus, purpura, rash

SYST: **Hemorrhage NOS, hemarthro-**sis, fibrinogen plasma decreased, hypertension, bradycardia, **DIC, coagulation disorder, thrombosis**

Contraindications: Hypersensitivity to this product or mouse, hamster, or bovine products

Precautions: Pregnancy (C), lactation, children

PHARMACOKINETICS

Half-life 2.3 hr

INTERACTIONS

Do not use with activated prothrombin complex concentrates or prothrombin complex concentrate

NURSING CONSIDERATIONS

Assess:

• VS, B/P, pulse, respirations, neurologic signs, temp at least q4h, temp 104° F (40° C) or indicators of internal bleeding, cardiac rhythm

• PT, aPTT, plasma FVII clotting

• For thrombosis, dose should be reduced or stopped

Administer:

IV route

• Bring to room temperature; for 1.2 mg vial/2.2 ml sterile water for inj; 4.8 mg vial/8.5 ml sterile water for inj

• Remove caps from stop, cleanse stopper with alcohol, allow to dry, draw back plunger of sterile syringe and allow air into syringe, insert needle of syringe into sterile water for inj, inject the air and withdraw amount required, insert syringe needle with diluent into drug vial, aim to side so liquid runs down vial wall, gently swirl until dissolved, use within 3 hr, give by bol over 3-5 min

• Do not admix, keep refrigerated until ready to use, avoid sunlight

Evaluate:

• Therapeutic response: hemostasis

---

codeine (℞)

(koe'deen)

Paveral ✦

Func. class.: Opiate analgesic, antitussive

Chem. class.: Opiate, phenanthrene derivative

Controlled Substance Schedule II, III, IV, V (depends on route)
Do not confuse:
codeine/Lodine/Iodine/Cardene

Action: Depresses pain impulse transmission at the spinal cord level by interacting with opioid receptors, decreases cough reflex, GI motility

Uses: Moderate to severe pain, nonproductive cough

Investigational uses: Diarrhea

DOSAGE AND ROUTES

Pain
• *Adult:* **PO** 15-60 mg q4h prn; **IM/SUBCUT** 15-60 mg q4h prn
• *Child:* **PO** 3 mg/kg/day in divided doses q4h prn

Cough
• *Adult:* **PO** 10-20 mg q4-6h, not to exceed 120 mg/day
• *Child:* **PO** 1-1.5 mg/kg/day in 4 divided doses, not to exceed 60 mg/day

Diarrhea
• *Adult:* **PO** 30 mg; may repeat qid prn

Renal disease
• CCr 10-50 ml/min 75% of dose; CCr <10 ml/min 50% of dose

Available forms: Inj 30, 60 mg/ml; tabs 15, 30, 60 mg; oral sol 10 mg/5 ml, 15 mg/5 ml

SIDE EFFECTS

CNS: Drowsiness, sedation, dizziness, agitation, dependency, lethargy, restlessness, euphoria, ***seizures***

CV: Bradycardia, palpitations, orthostatic hypotension, tachycardia, ***circulatory collapse***

GI: Nausea, vomiting, anorexia, constipation

GU: Urinary retention

INTEG: Flushing, rash, urticaria, pruritus

*RESP: **Respiratory depression, respiratory paralysis***

*SYST: **Anaphylaxis***

Contraindications: Hypersensitivity to opiates, respiratory depression, increased intracranial pressure, seizure disorders, severe respiratory disorders

Precautions: Pregnancy (C), elderly, cardiac dysrhythmias, lactation, prostatic hypertrophy

PHARMACOKINETICS

Bioavailability 60%-90%, onset 10-30 min, peak ½-1 hr, duration 4-6 hr; metabolized by liver; excreted by kidneys, in breast milk; crosses placenta; half-life 3 hr

INTERACTIONS

Increase: CNS depression—alcohol, opiates, sedative/hypnotics, antipsychotics, skeletal muscle relaxants
Increase: toxicity—MAOIs, use cautiously

Drug/Herb
Increase: CNS depression—Jamaican dogwood, kava, lavender, mistletoe, nettle, pokeweed, poppy, senega, valerian
Increase: anticholinergic effect—corkwood

Drug/Lab Test
Increase: Lipase, amylase

NURSING CONSIDERATIONS

Assess:
• I&O ratio; check for decreasing output; may indicate urinary retention, especially elderly
• GI function: nausea, vomiting, constipation
• By using pain-scoring method
• For productive cough
• Cough: type, duration, ability to raise secretion
• CNS changes, dizziness, drowsiness, hallucinations, euphoria, LOC, pupil reaction
• Allergic reactions: rash, urticaria

• Respiratory dysfunction: respiratory depression, character, rate, rhythm; notify prescriber if respirations are <10/min, shallow
• Need for pain medication, tolerance
Administer:
IV route
• Give slowly by direct inj
• With antiemetic for nausea, vomiting
• When pain is beginning to return; determine dosage interval by patient response
Syringe compatibilities: Glycopyrrolate, hydrOXYzine
Y-site compatibilities: Cefmetazole
Perform/provide:
• Storage in light-resistant container at room temperature
• Assistance with ambulation if needed
• Safety measures: top side rails, night-light, call bell
Evaluate:
• Therapeutic response: decrease in pain, absence of grimacing, decreased cough; decreased diarrhea
Teach patient/family:
• To report any symptoms of CNS changes, allergic reactions
• That physical dependency may result after extended periods
• To change position slowly; orthostatic hypotension may occur
• To avoid hazardous activities if drowsiness, dizziness occurs
• To avoid alcohol, other CNS depressants unless directed by prescriber

---

colchicine (Ŗ)
(kol'chi-seen)
Func. class.: Antigout agent
Chem. class.: Colchicum autumnale alkaloid

Action: Inhibits microtubule formation of lactic acid in leukocytes, which decreases phagocytosis and inflammation in joints
Uses: Gout, gouty arthritis (prevention, treatment); to arrest progression of neurologic disability in multiple sclerosis

Investigational uses: Hepatic cirrhosis, Mediterranean fever, pericarditis, amyloidosis, Behçet's syndrome, biliary cirrhosis, dermatitis herpetiformis, idiopathic thrombocytopenic purpura, Paget's disease, pseudogout, pulmonary fibrosis

DOSAGE AND ROUTES
Gout prevention
• *Adult:* **PO** 0.6-1.8 mg daily depending on severity; **IV** 0.5-1 mg 1-2 × day
Gout treatment
• *Adult:* **PO** 0.6-1.2 mg, then 0.5-1.2 mg q1h, until pain decreases or side effects occur; **IV** 2 mg, then 0.5 mg q6h until response, max 4 mg total
Available forms: Tabs 0.6 mg; inj 0.5 mg/ml

SIDE EFFECTS
GI: Nausea, vomiting, anorexia, malaise, metallic taste, cramps, peptic ulcer, diarrhea
GU: Hematuria, ***oliguria, renal damage***
*HEMA: **Agranulocytosis, thrombocytopenia, aplastic anemia, pancytopenia***
INTEG: Chills, dermatitis, pruritus, purpura, erythema
MISC: Myopathy, alopecia, reversible azoospermia, peripheral neuritis
Contraindications: Pregnancy (D) IV, hypersensitivity; serious GI, renal, hepatic, cardiac disorders
Precautions: Pregnancy (C) PO, blood dyscrasias, hepatic disease, elderly, lactation, children

PHARMACOKINETICS
PO: Peak ½-2 hr, half-life 20 min; deacetylates in liver; excreted in feces (metabolites/active drug)

INTERACTIONS
Toxicity: cycloSPORINE, clarithromycin, erythromycin
Increase: GI effects—NSAIDs, ethanol
Increase: bone marrow depression—

---

radiation, bone marrow depressants, cycloSPORINE
Decrease: action of vit B_{12}, may cause reversible malabsorption
Drug/Lab Test
Increase: Alk phosphatase, AST
False positive: Urine, RBC, Hgb
Interference: Urinary 17-hydroxycortico-steroids

NURSING CONSIDERATIONS
Assess:
• I&O ratio; observe for decrease in urinary output
• CBC, platelets, reticulocytes before, during therapy (q3mo), may cause aplastic anemia, agranulocytosis, decreased platelets
• For toxicity: weakness, abdominal pain, nausea, vomiting, diarrhea; drug should be discontinued
Administer:
PO route
• With food for GI symptoms
IV route
• Do not give IM or SUBCUT
• Do not dilute in D_5W, or change in IV line that contains D_5W
• Give over 2-5 min
• Wait ≥1 wk after giving a full course of IV colchicine before giving subsequent doses
Evaluate:
• Therapeutic response: decreased stone formation on x-ray, decreased pain in kidney region, absence of hematuria, decreased pain in joints
Teach patient/family:
• To avoid alcohol, OTC preparations that contain alcohol
• To report any pain, redness, or hard area, usually in legs; rash, sore throat, fever, bleeding, bruising, weakness, numbness, tingling
• The importance of complying with medical regimen (diet, weight loss, drug therapy); the possibility of bone marrow depression occurring
Treatment of overdose: D/C medication, may need opioids to treat diarrhea

coleseveLAM (R)
(coal-see-vel'am)
Welchol
Func. class.: Antilipemic
Chem. class.: Bile acid sequestrant

Action: Absorbs, combines with bile acids to form insoluble complex that is excreted through feces; loss of bile acids lowers cholesterol levels
Uses: Elevated LDL cholesterol, alone or in combination with HMG-CoA reductase inhibitor

DOSAGE AND ROUTES
• *Adult:* **PO** Monotherapy: 3 625-mg tabs bid with meals or 6 tabs daily with a meal; may increase to 7 tabs if needed
• Combination therapy: 3 tabs bid with meals or 6 tabs daily with a meal given with an HMG-CoA reductase inhibitor
Available forms: Tabs 625 mg

SIDE EFFECTS
CNS: Headache, dizziness, drowsiness, vertigo, tinnitus
GI: Constipation, abdominal pain, nausea, fecal impaction, hemorrhoids, flatulence, vomiting, steatorrhea, peptic ulcer
HEMA: Decreased red cell folate content; *bleeding,* increased PT
INTEG: Rash, irritation of perianal area, tongue, skin
META: Decreased vit A, D, K; *hyperchloremic acidosis*
MS: Muscle, joint pain
Contraindications: Hypersensitivity, biliary obstruction
Precautions: Pregnancy (C), lactation, children

PHARMACOKINETICS
PO: Excreted in feces, LDL decreased in 4-7 days

INTERACTIONS
Decrease: absorption of—gemfibrozil, glipiZIDE, phenytoin, propranolol, warfarin, thiazides, digitalis, penicillin G,

tetracyclines, corticosteroids, iron, thyroid, clindamycin, fat-soluble vitamins

Drug/Herb
Increase: effect—glucomannan
Decrease: antilipidemic effect—gotu kola

Drug/Lab Test
Increase: LFTs, Cl, PO$_4$

NURSING CONSIDERATIONS

Assess:
- Cardiac glycoside level, if both drugs are being administered
- For signs of vit A, D, K deficiency
- Fasting LDL, HDL, total cholesterol, triglyceride levels, electrolytes if on extended therapy
- Bowel pattern daily; increase bulk, H$_2$O in diet for constipation

Administer:
- Drug daily or bid with meals; give all other medications 1 hr before colesevelam or 4 hr after colesevelam to avoid poor absorption take with liquid
- Supplemental doses of vit A, D, K, if levels are low

Evaluate:
- Therapeutic response: decreased cholesterol level (hyperlipidemia); diarrhea, pruritus (excess bile acids)

Teach patient/family:
⚠ The symptoms of hypoprothrombinemia: bleeding mucous membranes, dark tarry stools, hematuria, petechiae; report immediately
- The importance of compliance; toxicity may result if doses missed
- That risk factors should be decreased: high-fat diet, smoking, alcohol consumption, absence of exercise
- Not to discontinue suddenly

---

colestipol (℞)
(koe-les'ti-pole)
Colestid
Func. class.: Antilipemic
Chem. class.: Bile acid sequestrant

Action: Absorbs, combines with bile acids to form insoluble complex excreted through feces; loss of bile acids lowers cholesterol levels

Uses: Primary hypercholesterolemia, xanthomas

Investigational uses: Digitalis toxicity

DOSAGE AND ROUTES

- *Adult:* **PO** tabs 2 g daily-bid, may increase q1mo, max 16 g/day; granules: 5 g daily-bid, may increase q1mo, max 30 g/day

Available forms: Granules 300 g, 450, 500 g bottles; 5 g colestipol/7.5 g powder; tabs 1 g

SIDE EFFECTS

GI: Constipation, abdominal pain, nausea, fecal impaction, hemorrhoids, flatulence, vomiting, steatorrhea, peptic ulcer
HEMA: **Bleeding, increased PT**
INTEG: Rash, irritation of perianal area, tongue, skin
META: Decreased vit A, D, K, red folate content; **hyperchloremic acidosis**
Contraindications: Hypersensitivity, biliary obstruction
Precautions: Pregnancy (B), lactation, children, bleeding disorders

PHARMACOKINETICS

PO: Onset 24-48 hr, peak/duration 30 days, excreted in feces

INTERACTIONS

Decrease: action of—thiazides, digitalis, warfarin, penicillin G, gemfibrozil, glipiZIDE, propranolol, phenytoin, TOLBUTamide, tetracycline, corticosteroids, iron, thyroid agents, clindamycin, fat-soluble vitamins

Drug/Herb
Increase: lipidemic effect—glucomannan
Decrease: lipidemic effect—gotu kola

Drug/Lab Test
Increase: AST, ALT, alk phosphatase, chloride, PO$_4$
Decrease: Na, K, Ca

⚠ Safety alert   *"Tall Man" lettering

NURSING CONSIDERATIONS

Assess:
- Cardiac glycoside levels, if both drugs are being administered
- For signs of vit A, D, K deficiency
- Serum cholesterol, triglyceride levels, electrolytes (extended therapy)
- Bowel pattern daily; increase bulk, water in diet if constipation develops

Administer:
- Swallow tabs whole; do not break, crush, or chew; take tabs one at a time
- Drug daily or bid; give all other medications 1 hr before colestipol or 4 hr after colestipol to avoid poor absorption
- Drug mixed in applesauce or stirred into beverage (2-6 oz); do not take dry; let stand for 2 min
- Supplemental doses of vit A, D, K if levels are low

Evaluate:
- Therapeutic response: decreased triglycerides

Teach patient/family:
⚠ The symptoms of hypoprothrombinemia: bleeding mucous membranes; dark, tarry stools; hematuria, petechiae; report immediately
- That compliance is needed; not to miss or double doses
- That risk factors should be decreased: high-fat diet, smoking, alcohol consumption, absence of exercise

---

contraceptives, oral (℞)

Func. class.: Hormone
Chem. class.: Estrogen, progestin combinations

Action: Prevents ovulation by suppressing FSH, LH; *monophasic:* estrogen/progestin (fixed dose) used during a 21-day cycle; ovulation is inhibited by suppression of FSH and LH; thickness of cervical mucus and endometrial lining prevents pregnancy; *biphasic:* ovulation is inhibited by suppression of FSH and LH; alteration of cervical mucus, endo-metrial lining prevents pregnancy; *triphasic:* ovulation is inhibited by suppression of FSH and LH; change of cervical mucus, endometrial lining prevents pregnancy; variable doses of estrogen/progestin combinations may be similar to natural hormonal fluctuations; *progestin-only pill and implant:* change of cervical mucus and endometrial lining prevents pregnancy; ovulation may be suppressed

Uses: To prevent pregnancy, endometriosis, hypermenorrhea

DOSAGE AND ROUTES
- *Adult:* **PO** 1 daily starting on day 5 of menstrual cycle; day 1 is 1st day of period
21 tablet packs
- *Adult:* **PO** 1 daily starting on day 7 of menstrual cycle; day 1 is 1st day of period, then on 20 or 21 days, off 7 days
28 tablet packs
- *Adult:* **PO** 1 daily continuously
Biphasic
- *Adult:* **PO** 1 daily × 10 days, then next color 1 daily × 11 days
Triphasic
- *Adult:* **PO** 1 daily; check package insert
Implant
- *Adult:* Subdermal 6 cap implanted during 1st wk of menses
Endometriosis
- *Adult:* **PO** 1 daily × 20 days from day 5 to 24 of cycle

Available forms: Check specific brand

SIDE EFFECTS
CNS: Depression, fatigue, dizziness, nervousness, anxiety, headache
CV: Increased B/P, ***cerebral hemorrhage, thrombosis, pulmonary embolism,*** fluid retention, edema
EENT: Optic neuritis, retinal thrombosis, cataracts
ENDO: Decreased glucose tolerance, increased TBG, PBI, T_4, T_3
GI: Nausea, vomiting, cramps, diarrhea, bloating, constipation, change in appetite, ***cholestatic jaundice***
GU: Breakthrough bleeding, amenorrhea,

spotting, dysmenorrhea, galactorrhea, endocervical hyperplasia, vaginitis, cystitis-like syndrome, breast change
HEMA: Increased fibrinogen, clotting factor
INTEG: Chloasma, melasma, acne, rash, urticaria, erythema, pruritus, hirsutism, alopecia, photosensitivity
Contraindications: Pregnancy (X), lactation, reproductive cancer, thrombophlebitis, MI, hepatic tumors, hepatic disease, CAD, women 40 and over, CVA
Precautions: Depression, hypertension, renal disease, seizure disorders, lupus erythematosus, rheumatic disease, migraine headache, amenorrhea, irregular menses, breast cancer (fibrocystic), gallbladder disease, diabetes mellitus, heavy smoking, acute mononucleosis, sickle cell disease

PHARMACOKINETICS

Excreted in breast milk

INTERACTIONS

Decrease: oral contraceptives effectiveness—anticonvulsants, rifampin, analgesics, antibiotics, antihistamines, griseofulvin
Decrease: oral anticoagulants action
Drug/Herb
Altered action: alfalfa, black cohosh, chaste tree
Decrease: oral contraceptives effect—saw palmetto, St. John's wort
Drug/Food
Increase: peak level—grapefruit juice
Drug/Lab Test
Increase: PT; clotting factors VII, VIII, IX, X; TBG, PBI, T_4, platelet aggregability, BSP, triglycerides, bilirubin, AST, ALT
Decrease: T_3, antithrombin III, folate, metyrapone test, GTT, 17-OHCS

NURSING CONSIDERATIONS
Assess:
• Glucose, thyroid function, LFTs
• Reproductive changes: change in breasts, tumors, positive Pap smear; drug should be discontinued

Administer:
• PO with food for GI symptoms; give at same time each day
• Subdermal implant of 6 caps effective for 5 yr; then should be removed
• IM inj deep in large muscle mass after shaking suspension; ensure patient not pregnant if inj are 2 wk or more apart
Evaluate:
• Therapeutic response: absence of pregnancy, endometriosis, hypermenorrhea
Teach patient/family:
• About detection of clots using Homan's sign
• To use sunscreen or avoid sunlight; photosensitivity can occur
• To take at same time each day to ensure equal drug level
• To report GI symptoms that occur after 4 mo
• To use another birth control method during 1st week of oral contraceptive use
• To take another tablet as soon as possible if one is missed
• That after drug is discontinued, pregnancy may not occur for several months
• To report abdominal pain, change in vision, shortness of breath, change in menstrual flow, spotting, breakthrough bleeding, breast lumps, swelling, headache, severe leg pain
• That continuing medical care is needed: Pap smear and gynecologic examinations q6mo
• To notify health care providers and dentists of oral contraceptive

---

Rarely Used

corticotropin (ACTH) (℞)
(kor-ti-koe-troe'pin)
H.P. Acthar Gel
Func. class.: Pituitary hormone

Uses: Testing adrenocortical function, treatment of adrenal insufficiency caused by administration of corticosteroids

---

(long term), multiple sclerosis, infantile spasms

DOSAGE AND ROUTES

Acute exacerbations of multiple sclerosis
• *Adult:* **IM** 80-120 units/day × 14-21 days

Infantile spasms
• *Infant:* **IM GEL** 20 units/day × 2 wks, increase if needed

Contraindications: Hypersensitivity, scleroderma, osteoporosis, CHF, peptic ulcer disease, hypertension, systemic fungal infections, smallpox vaccination, recent surgery, ocular herpes simplex, primary adrenocortical insufficiency/hyperfunction

---

cortisone (℞)
(kor'ti-sone)
Cortone ✦, Cortone Acetate
Func. class.: Corticosteroid, synthetic
Chem. class.: Glucocorticoid, short-acting

Action: Decreases inflammation by suppression of migration of polymorphonuclear leukocytes, fibroblasts, reversal of increased capillary permeability and lysosomal stabilization
Uses: Inflammation, severe allergy, adrenal insufficiency, collagen disorders; respiratory, dermatologic, rheumatic disorders

DOSAGE AND ROUTES
• *Adult:* **PO/IM** 25-300 mg daily or q2d, titrated to response
• *Child:* **PO** 0.7-10 mg/kg/day; **IM** 0.2-5 mg/kg/day
Available forms: Tabs 5, 10, 25 mg; inj 50 mg/ml

SIDE EFFECTS
CNS: Depression, flushing, sweating, headache, mood changes
CV: Hypertension, ***circulatory collapse, thrombophlebitis, embo-lism,*** tachycardia, ***necrotizing angiitis, CHF,*** edema
EENT: Fungal infections, increased intra-ocular pressure, blurred vision
GI: Diarrhea, nausea, abdominal distention, ***GI hemorrhage,*** increased appetite, ***pancreatitis***
HEMA: ***Thrombocytopenia***
INTEG: Acne, poor wound healing, ecchymosis, bruising, petechiae
META: Sodium, fluid retention, potassium loss
MS: Fractures, osteoporosis, weakness, loss of muscle mass
Contraindications: Pregnancy (D), psychosis, hypersensitivity, idiopathic thrombocytopenia, acute glomerulonephritis, amebiasis, fungal infections, nonasthmatic bronchial disease, child <2 yr, AIDS, TB
Precautions: Lactation, diabetes mellitus, glaucoma, osteoporosis, seizure disorders, ulcerative colitis, CHF, myasthenia gravis, renal disease, esophagitis, peptic ulcer, hepatic disease

PHARMACOKINETICS
Half-life 8-12 hrs
PO: Peak 2 hr, duration 1½ days
IM: Peak 20-48 hr, duration 10 days

INTERACTIONS
Increase: action of cortisone—salicylates, estrogens, indomethacin, oral contraceptives, ketoconazole, macrolide antiinfectives
Increase: side effects—alcohol, salicylates, indomethacin, potassium-wasting diuretics
Increase: GI symptoms—salicylates, indomethacin, NSAIDs
Decrease: effects of anticoagulants, antidiabetics, toxoids, vaccines, salicylates
Decrease: cortisone action—barbiturates, rifampin, phenytoin, theophylline, acetyl-cholinesterases

---

Drug/Herb

Potassium deficiency: aloe, buckthorn, cascara sagrada, Chinese rhubarb, rhubarb, senna

Increase: steroid effect—aloe, licorice, perilla

Drug/Lab Test

Increase: Cholesterol, Na, blood glucose, uric acid, Ca, urine glucose

Decrease: Ca, K, T_4, T_3, thyroid ^{131}I uptake test, urine 17-OHCS, 17-KS, PBI

False negative: Skin allergy tests

NURSING CONSIDERATIONS

Assess:

• Potassium, blood, urine glucose while on long-term therapy; hypokalemia and hyperglycemia

• Weight daily; notify prescriber of weekly gain >5 lb

• B/P q4h, pulse; notify prescriber if chest pain occurs

• I&O ratio; be alert for decreasing urinary output and increasing edema

• Plasma cortisol levels during long-term therapy (normal level: 138-635 nmol/L SI units if drawn at 8 AM)

• Infection: fever, WBC even after withdrawal of medication; drug masks infection

• Potassium depletion: paresthesias, fatigue, nausea, vomiting, depression, polyuria, dysrhythmias, weakness

• Edema, hypertension, cardiac symptoms

• Mental status: affect, mood, behavioral changes, aggression

Administer:

• After shaking suspension (parenteral)

• Titrated dose; use lowest effective dose

• IM inj deeply in large mass; rotate sites; avoid deltoid; use a 21G needle

• In one dose in AM to prevent adrenal suppression; avoid SUBCUT administration; tissue may be damaged; never administer by IV route

• With food or milk to decrease GI symptoms

Perform/provide:

• Assistance with ambulation in patient with bone tissue disease to prevent fractures

Evaluate:

• Therapeutic response: ease of respirations, decreased inflammation

Teach patient/family:

• That medical ID as steroid user should be carried at all times

• To notify prescriber if therapeutic response decreases; dosage adjustment may be needed

⚠ Not to discontinue abruptly or adrenal crisis can result

• To avoid OTC products: salicylates, alcohol in cough products, cold preparations unless directed by prescriber

• All aspects of drug usage, including cushingoid symptoms

• The symptoms of adrenal insufficiency: nausea, anorexia, fatigue, dizziness, dyspnea, weakness, joint pain

• Avoid exposure to chickenpox and measles

• To take PO dose in AM with food or fluid (milk)

Rarely Used

cosyntropin (℞)
(koe-sin-troe′pin)
Cortrosyn, Synacthen ✲,
Tetracosactrin
Func. class.: Pituitary hormone

Uses: Testing adrenocortical function

DOSAGE AND ROUTES

• *Adult and child >2 yr:* **IM/IV** 0.25-1 mg between blood sampling

• *Child <2 yr:* **IM/IV** 0.125 mg

Contraindications: Hypersensitivity

cromolyn (otc, R)
(kroe'moe-lin)
Gastrocrom Intal, Nasalcrom,
Rynacrom ✤
Func. class.: Antiasthmatic
Chem. class.: Mast cell stabilizer

Do not confuse:
Nasalcrom/Nasalide

Action: Stabilizes the membrane of the sensitized mast cell, preventing release of chemical mediators after an antigen-IgE interaction

Uses: Severe perennial bronchial asthma, prevention of exercise-induced bronchospasm, acute bronchospasm induced by environmental pollutants, mastocytosis

Investigational uses: Allergic rhinitis, chronic urticarial angioedema

DOSAGE AND ROUTES

Allergic rhinitis
• *Adult and child >2 yr:* **NASAL SOL** 1 spray in each nostril tid-qid, max 6 doses/day

To prevent exercise-induced bronchospasm
• *Adult and child >5 yr:* **INH** 2 metered sprays inhaled ≤1 hr prior to exercise

Bronchial asthma
• *Adult and child >5 yr:* **INH** 2 metered sprays using inhaler qid; **NEB** 20 mg qid by nebulization

Systemic mastocytosis
• *Adult and child >12 yr:* **PO** 200 mg qid ½ hr ac and at bedtime
• *Child 2-12 yr:* **PO** 100 mg qid ½ ac and at bedtime

Available forms: Nasal sol 5.2 mg/metered spray (40 mg/ml); neb sol 20 mg/2 ml; aerosol 800 mcg/actuation; oral conc 100 mg/5 ml

SIDE EFFECTS

CNS: Headache, dizziness, neuritis
EENT: Throat irritation, cough, nasal congestion, burning eyes, nasal stinging, sneezing

GI: Nausea, vomiting, anorexia, dry mouth, bitter taste
GU: Urinary frequency, dysuria
INTEG: Rash, urticaria, angioedema
MS: Joint pain/swelling

Oral conc
CNS: Dizziness, headache, paresthesia, migraine, seizures, psychosis, anxiety, depression, hallucinations, insomnia
CV: Tachycardia, PVCs, palpitations
GI: Diarrhea, nausea, abdominal pain, constipation, dyspepsia, stomatitis, vomiting
HEMA: Polycythemia, neutropenia, pancytopenia
INTEG: Pruritus, rash, flushing, photosensitivity

Contraindications: Hypersensitivity to this drug or lactose, status asthmaticus, acute asthma

Precautions: Pregnancy (B), lactation, renal disease, hepatic disease, safety not established; child <5 yr (aerosol); <2 yr (nebulizer); <2 yr (nasal sol); oral <2 yr

PHARMACOKINETICS

Excreted unchanged in feces; half-life 80 min

NURSING CONSIDERATIONS

Assess:
• Eosinophil count during treatment
• Respiratory status: rate, rhythm, characteristics, cough, wheezing, dyspnea

Administer:
• For oral conc: break open ampule, squeeze contents in glass of water, stir, drink

Perform/provide:
• Gargle, sip of water to decrease irritation in throat

Evaluate:
• Therapeutic response: decrease in asthmatic symptoms; congested, runny nose

Teach patient/family:
Nasal sol
• Blow nose, hold pump between fingers, if first use spray in air until fine mist occurs, insert nozzle in nostril, spray and

Side effects: *italics* = common; ***bold italics*** = life-threatening

breathe in through nose, repeat in other nostril

Aerosol (not for Acute Asthma)

• Take cover off mouthpiece, shake gently, breathe out slowly, place mouthpiece in mouth, close mouth around it, tilt head back, breathe in as the inhaler is depressed, remove, hold breath, then breathe out slowly

Inhalation

• Do not swallow sol

• Empty ampule into power driven nebulizer as directed. Do not combine different meds.

Oral

• To take ½ hr before meals and at bedtime

Rarely Used

crotamiton (℞)
(kroe-tam'i-ton)
Func. class.: Scabicide

Uses: Scabies, pruritus

DOSAGE AND ROUTES

Scabies

• *Adult and child:* **CREAM** wash area with soap, water; remove visible crusts, apply cream, apply another coat in 24 hr, remove with soap, water in 48 hr

Pruritus

• Massage into affected area, repeat as necessary

Contraindications: Hypersensitivity, skin inflammation, abrasions, breaks in skin, mucous membranes

cyanocobalamin
(vit B$_{12}$) (otc, ℞)
(sye-an-oh-koe-bal'a-min)
Alphamin, Anacobin ✸,
Bedoz ✸, Cobex, Cobolin-M,
Crystamine, Crysti-1000,
Cyanabin ✸, Cyanoject,
Cyomin, Ener-B, Hydrobexan,
Hydro Cobex, Hydro-
Crysti-12

hydroxocobalamin
Hydroxycobal, LA-12,
Nascobal, Neuroforte-R,
Rubesol-1000, Rubramin PC,
Shovite, Vibal LA, Vibral,
Vitamin B$_{12}$
Func. class.: Vit B$_{12}$, water-soluble vitamin

Action: Needed for adequate nerve functioning, protein and carbohydrate metabolism, normal growth, RBC development, cell reproduction

Uses: Vit B$_{12}$ deficiency, pernicious anemia, vit B$_{12}$ malabsorption syndrome, Schilling test, increased requirements with pregnancy, thyrotoxicosis, hemolytic anemia, hemorrhage, renal and hepatic disease

DOSAGE AND ROUTES

Cyanocobalamin

• *Adult:* **PO** up to 1000 mcg/day
SUBCUT/IM 30-100 mcg/day × 1 wk, then 100-200 mcg/mo

Schilling test

• *Adult and child:* **IM** 1000 mcg in 1 dose

• Child: **PO** up to 1000 mcg/day
SUBCUT/IM 30-50 mcg/day × 2 wk, then 100 mcg/mo; **NASAL** 500 mcg qwk

Hydroxocobalamin

• *Adult:* **SUBCUT/IM** 30-50 mcg/day × 5-10 days, then 100-200 mcg/mo

• *Child:* **SUBCUT/IM** 30-50 mcg/day × 5-10 days, then 100 mcg/mo

Available forms: Cyanocobalamin: tabs 25, 50, 100, 250, 500, 1000, 5000 mcg; EXT REL tabs: 100, 200, 500, 1000

---

mcg; lozenges: 100, 250, 500 mcg; nasal jel 500 mcg/spray; inj 100, 1000 mcg/ml; hydroxocobalamin: inj 1000 mcg/ml

SIDE EFFECTS

CNS: Flushing, optic nerve atrophy
CV: **CHF,** peripheral vascular thrombosis, ***pulmonary edema***
GI: Diarrhea
INTEG: Itching, rash, pain at inj site
META: Hypokalemia
SYST: **Anaphylactic shock**
Contraindications: Hypersensitivity, optic nerve atrophy
Precautions: Pregnancy (A), lactation, children

PHARMACOKINETICS

Gastric intrinsic factor must be present for absorption to occur; stored in liver, kidneys, stomach; 50%-90% excreted in urine; crosses placenta, excreted in breast milk

INTERACTIONS

Increase: absorption—predniSONE
Decrease: absorption—aminoglycosides, anticonvulsants, colchicine, chloramphenicol, aminosalicylic acid, potassium preparations, cimetidine
Drug/Herb
Decrease: vit B$_{12}$ absorption—goldenseal
Drug/Lab Test
False positive: Intrinsic factor

NURSING CONSIDERATIONS

Assess:
• For vit B$_{12}$ deficiency: red, beefy tongue, psychosis, pallor, neuropathy
• GI function: diarrhea, constipation
• Potassium levels during beginning treatment in megaloblastic anemia; q6mo in pernicious anemia; folic acid, plasma vit B$_{12}$ (after 1 wk), reticulocyte counts
• Nutritional status: egg yolks, fish, organ meats, dairy products, clams, oysters: good sources of vit B$_{12}$

• For pulmonary edema, worsening of CHF in cardiac patients
Administer:
PO route
• With fruit juice to disguise taste; immediately after mixing
• With meals if possible for better absorption
Nasal route
• Avoid use within 1 hr of hot fluids/food
IM route
• By IM inj for pernicious anemia for life unless contraindicated
IV route
• IV route not recommended but may be admixed in TPN solution
Additive compatibilities: Ascorbic acid, chloramphenicol, metaraminol, vit B/C
Solution compatibilities: Dextrose/Ringer's or lactated Ringer's combinations, dextrose/saline combinations, D$_5$W, D$_{10}$W, 0.45% NaCl, Ringer's or lactated Ringer's sol
Y-site compatibilities: Heparin, hydrocortisone, potassium chloride, vit B/C
Perform/provide:
• Protection from light and heat
Evaluate:
• Therapeutic response: decreased anorexia, dyspnea on exertion, palpitations, paresthesias, psychosis, visual disturbances
Teach patient/family:
• That treatment must continue for life for pernicious anemia
• To eat well-balanced diet
• To avoid contact with persons with infection; infections common
Treatment of overdose: Discontinue drug

cyclobenzaprine (℞)

(sye-kloe-ben′za-preen)
cyclobenzaprine HCl,
cycloflex, Flexeril
Func. class.: Skeletal muscle relaxant, central acting
Chem. class.: Tricyclic amine salt

Do not confuse:

cyclobenzaprine/cyproheptadine
Action: Reduction of tonic muscle activity at the brain stem; may be related to antidepressant effects
Uses: Adjunct for relief of muscle spasm and pain in musculoskeletal conditions

DOSAGE AND ROUTES

Muscloskeletal disorders
• *Adult:* **PO** 10 mg tid × 1 wk, not to exceed 60 mg/day × 3 wk
Fibromyalgia
• *Adult:* **PO** 5-40 mg at bedtime
Available forms: Tabs 10 mg

SIDE EFFECTS

CNS: Dizziness, weakness, drowsiness, headache, tremor, depression, insomnia, confusion, paresthesia
CV: Postural hypotension, tachycardia, *dysrhythmias*
EENT: Diplopia, temporary loss of vision
GI: Nausea, vomiting, hiccups, dry mouth, constipation
GU: Urinary retention, frequency, change in libido
INTEG: Rash, pruritus, fever, facial flushing, sweating
Contraindications: Acute recovery phase of myocardial infarction, dysrhythmias, heart block, CHF, hypersensitivity, child <12 yr, intermittent porphyria, thyroid disease
Precautions: Pregnancy (B), renal disease, hepatic disease, addictive personality, lactation, elderly

PHARMACOKINETICS

PO: Onset 1 hr, peak 3-8 hr, duration 12-24 hr, half-life 1-3 days; metabolized by liver; excreted in urine; crosses placenta; excreted in breast milk

INTERACTIONS

Do not use within 14 days of MAOI, tramadol
Increase: CNS depression—alcohol, tricyclics, opiates, barbiturates, sedatives, hypnotics
Drug/Herb
Increase: CNS depression—kava

NURSING CONSIDERATIONS

Assess:
• For pain: location, duration, mobility, stiffness, baseline and periodically
• Blood studies: CBC, WBC, differential for blood dyscrasias
• Hepatic studies: AST, ALT, alk phosphatase; hepatitis may occur
• ECG in epileptic patients; poor seizure control has occurred
• Allergic reactions: rash, fever, respiratory distress
• Severe weakness, numbness in extremities
• Psychologic dependency: increased need for medication, more frequent requests for medication, increased pain
• CNS depression: dizziness, drowsiness, psychiatric symptoms
Administer:
• Without regard to meals
Perform/provide:
• Storage in tight container at room temperature
• Assistance with ambulation if dizziness, drowsiness occur, especially elderly
Evaluate:
• Therapeutic response: decreased pain, spasticity; muscle spasms of acute, painful musculoskeletal conditions generally short term; long-term therapy seldom warranted
Teach patient/family:
• Not to discontinue medication abruptly; insomnia, nausea, headache, spasticity, tachycardia will occur; drug should be tapered off over 1-2 wk

• Not to take with alcohol, other CNS depressants
• To avoid hazardous activities if drowsiness/dizziness occurs
• To avoid using OTC medication: cough preparations, antihistamines, unless directed by prescriber
• To use gum, frequent sips of water for dry mouth

Treatment of overdose: Empty stomach with emesis, gastric lavage, then administer activated charcoal; use anti-convulsants if indicated; monitor cardiac function

---

cyclopentolate ophthalmic
See Appendix C

⚠ High Alert

cyclophosphamide (℞)
(sye-kloe-foss'fa-mide)
Cytoxan, Neosar, Procytox ✦
Func. class.: Antineoplastic alkylating agent
Chem. class.: Nitrogen mustard

Do not confuse:
cyclophosphamide/cycloSPORINE
Cytoxan/Cytosar/Cytotec/Centoxin/ cytarabine
Action: Alkylates DNA is responsible for cross-linking DNA strands; activity is not cell cycle phase specific
Uses: Hodgkin's disease; lymphomas; leukemia; cancer of female reproductive tract, breast; lung, prostate; multiple myeloma; neuroblastoma; retinoblastoma; Ewing's sarcoma

DOSAGE AND ROUTES
• *Adult:* **PO** initially 1-5 mg/kg over 2-5 days, maintenance is 1-5 mg/kg; **IV** initially 40-50 mg/kg in divided doses over 2-5 days, maintenance 10-15 mg/kg q7-10d, or 3-5 mg/kg q3d

• *Child:* **PO/IV** 2-8 mg/kg or 60-250 mg/m² in divided doses for 6 or more days; maintenance 10-15 mg/kg q7-10d or 30 mg/kg q3-4wk; dose should be reduced by half when bone marrow depression occurs
Available forms: Inj 100, 200, 500 mg, 1, 2 g; tabs 25, 50 mg

SIDE EFFECTS
CNS: Headache, dizziness
CV: **Cardiotoxicity** (high doses)
ENDO: Syndrome of inappropriate antidiuretic hormone (SIADH), gonadal suppression
GI: Nausea, vomiting, diarrhea, weight loss, colitis, **hepatotoxicity**
GU: Hemorrhagic cystitis, hematuria, neoplasms, amenorrhea, azoospermia, sterility, ovarian fibrosis
HEMA: Thrombocytopenia, leukopenia, pancytopenia; myelosuppression
INTEG: Alopecia, dermatitis
META: Hyperuricemia
MISC: Secondary neoplasms, **anaphylaxis**
RESP: Fibrosis
Contraindications: Pregnancy (D), lactation, severely depressed bone marrow function, hypersensitivity
Precautions: Radiation therapy

PHARMACOKINETICS
Metabolized by liver; excreted in urine; half-life 4-6½ hr; 50% bound to plasma proteins

INTERACTIONS
Potentiation of neuromuscular blockade: succinylcholine
Increase: cyclophosphamide toxicity— barbiturates
Increase: action of warfarin
Increase: bone marrow depression— allopurinol, thiazides
Increase: hypoglycemia—insulin
Decrease: digoxin levels—digoxin
Decrease: cyclophosphamide effect— chloramphenicol, corticosteroids

---

✦ Canada only   Side effects: *italics* = common; ***bold italics*** = life-threatening

Decrease: antibody response—live virus vaccines

Drug/Lab Test
Increase: Uric acid
Decrease: Pseudocholinesterase
False positive: Pap smear
False negative: PPD, mumps, trichophytin, *Candida*

NURSING CONSIDERATIONS
Assess:
• For hemorrhagic cystitis; renal studies: BUN, serum uric acid, urine CCr before, during therapy; I&O ratio; report fall in urine output <30 ml/hr
• CBC, differential, platelet count baseline, weekly; withhold drug if WBC is <2500 or platelet count is <75,000; notify prescriber of results
• Pulmonary function tests, chest x-ray films before, during therapy; chest film should be obtained q2wk during treatment
• Monitor temp q4h (elevated temp may indicate beginning infection)
• Hepatic studies before, during therapy (bilirubin, AST, ALT, LDH) as needed or monthly
• Bleeding: hematuria, guaiac, bruising or petechiae, mucosa or orifices q8h
• Dyspnea, crackles, unproductive cough, chest pain, tachypnea
• Effects of alopecia on body image, discuss feelings about body changes
• Jaundice of skin, sclera; dark urine; clay-colored stools; itchy skin; abdominal pain; fever; diarrhea
• Buccal cavity q8h for dryness, sores or ulceration, white patches, oral pain, bleeding, dysphagia; obtain prescription for viscous lidocaine (Xylocaine)
⚠ Symptoms indicating severe allergic reaction: rash, pruritus, urticaria, purpuric skin lesions, itching, flushing

Administer:
• In AM so drug can be eliminated before bedtime
• Fluids IV or PO before chemotherapy to hydrate patient
• Antacid before oral agent, give after evening meal, before bedtime

• Antiemetic 30-60 min before giving drug and prn
• Allopurinol or sodium bicarbonate to maintain uric acid levels, alkalinization of urine

IV route
• IV after diluting 100 mg/5 ml of sterile H_2O or bacteriostatic H_2O; shake; let stand until clear; may be further diluted in up to 250 ml D_5 or NS; give 100 mg or less/min through 3-way stopcock of glucose or saline inf
• Using 21, 23, 25G needle; check site for irritation, phlebitis
Additive compatibilities: Cisplatin with etoposide, fluorouracil, hydrOXYzine, methotrexate, methotrexate/fluorouracil, mitoxantrone, ondansetron
Solution compatibilities: Amino acids 4.25%/D_{25}, D_5/0.9% NaCl, D_5W, 0.9% NaCl
Syringe compatibilities: Bleomycin, cisplatin, doxapram, DOXOrubicin, droperidol, fluorouracil, furosemide, heparin, leucovorin, methotrexate, metoclopramide, mitomycin, vinBLAStine, vinCRIStine
Y-site compatibilities: Allopurinol, amifostine, amikacin, ampicillin, azlocillin, aztreonam, bleomycin, cefamandole, cefazolin, cefepime, cefoperazone, cefotaxime, cefoxitin, cefuroxime, cephalothin, cephapirin, chloramphenicol, chlorproMAZINE, cimetidine, cisplatin, cladribine, clindamycin, dexamethasone, diphenhydrAMINE, DOXOrubicin, DOXOrubicin liposome, doxycycline, droperidol, erythromycin, famotidine, filgrastim, fludarabine, fluorouracil, furosemide, gallium, ganciclovir, gentamicin, granisetron, heparin, hydromorphone, idarubicin, kanamycin, leucovorin, lorazepam, melphalan, methotrexate, methylPREDNISolone, metoclopramide, metronidazole, mezlocillin, minocycline, mitomycin, morphine, moxalactam, nafcillin, ondansetron, oxacillin, paclitaxel, penicillin G potassium, piperacillin, piperacillin/tazobactam, prochlorperazine, promethazine, propofol, ranitidine, sargramostim, sodium bicarbonate,

teniposide, thiotepa, ticarcillin, ticarcillin-clavulanate, tobramycin, trimethoprim-sulfamethoxazole, vancomycin, vinBLAStine, vinCRIStine, vinorelbine

Perform/provide:
• Storage in tight container at room temperature
• Strict medical asepsis, protective isolation if WBC levels are low
• Increase fluid intake to 2-3 L/day to prevent urate deposits, calculi formation, reduce incidence of hemorrhagic cystitis
• Diet low in purines: organ meats (kidney, liver), dried beans, peas to maintain alkaline urine
• Rinsing of mouth tid-qid with water, club soda; brushing of teeth bid-tid with soft brush or cotton-tipped applicators for stomatitis; use unwaxed dental floss
• Warm compresses at inj site for inflammation

Evaluate:
• Therapeutic response: decreased tumor size, spread of malignancy

Teach patient/family:
• About protective isolation
• That amenorrhea can occur; reversible after stopping treatment
• To report any changes in breathing or coughing
• That hair may be lost during treatment; a wig or hairpiece may make patient feel better; new hair may be different in color, texture
• To avoid foods with citric acid, hot or rough texture
• To report any bleeding, white spots, ulcerations in mouth to prescriber; tell patient to examine mouth daily
• To report signs of infection: increased temperature, sore throat, flulike symptoms
• To report signs of anemia: fatigue, headache, faintness, shortness of breath, irritability
• To report bleeding (bruising, hematuria, petechiae): avoid use of razors, commercial mouthwash

• To avoid use of aspirin products, ibuprofen
• To avoid vaccinations during therapy

⁕cycloSPORINE (℞)
(sye′kloe-spor-een)
Gengraf, Neoral, Sandimmune, SangCya
Func. class.: Immunosuppressant
Chem. class.: Fungus-derived peptide

Do not confuse:
cycloSPORINE/CycloSERINE
cycloSPORINE/cyclophosphamide
Action: Produces immunosuppression by inhibiting lymphocytes (T)
Uses: Organ transplants (liver, kidney, heart) to prevent rejection, rheumatoid arthritis, psoriasis
Investigational uses: Recalcitrant ulcerative colitis

DOSAGE AND ROUTES
Prevention of transplant rejection
• *Adult and child:* **PO** 15 mg/kg several hr before surgery, daily for 2 wk, reduce dosage by 2.5 mg/kg/wk to 5-10 mg/kg/day; **IV** 5-6 mg/kg several hr before surgery, daily, switch to PO form as soon as possible
Rheumatoid arthritis (Neoral/Gengraf)
• *Adult:* **PO** 2.5 mg/kg/day divided bid, may increase 0.5-0.75 mg/kg/day after 8-12 wk, max 4 mg/kg/day
Psoriasis (Neoral/Gengraf)
• *Adult:* **PO** 2.5 mg/kg/day divided bid, × 4 wk, then increase by 0.5 mg/kg/day q2wk, max 4 mg/kg/day
Available forms: Oral sol 100 mg/ml; soft gel cap 25, 100 mg; inj 50 mg/ml

SIDE EFFECTS
CNS: Tremors, *headache,* **seizures**
GI: Nausea, vomiting, diarrhea, *oral Candida, gum hyperplasia,* **hepatotoxicity,** pancreatitis
GU: **Albuminuria, hematuria, proteinuria, renal failure**

INTEG: Rash, acne, *hirsutism*
META: Hyperkalemia, hypomagnesemia, hyperlipidemia, hyperuricemia
MISC: Infection
Contraindications: Hypersensitivity to polyxyethylated castor oil (inj only), psoriasis or rheumatoid arthritis in renal disease (Neoral/Gengraf); uncontrolled, malignant hypertension; Gengraf/Neoral used with PUVA/UVB, methotrexate, coal tar, radiation in psoriasis, lactation
Precautions: Pregnancy (C), severe renal disease, severe hepatic disease, elderly

PHARMACOKINETICS

Peak 4 hr, highly protein bound, half-life (biphasic) 1.2 hr, 25 hr; metabolized in liver; excreted in feces; crosses placenta; excreted in breast milk

INTERACTIONS

Increase: action, toxicity of cycloSPORINE—allopurinol, amiodarone, amphotericin B, androgens, azole antifungals, beta blockers, bromocriptine, calcium channel blockers, carvedilol, cimetidine, colchicine, corticosteroids, fluoroquinolones, foscarnet, imipenem-cilastatin, macrolides, metoclopramide, oral contraceptives, NSAIDs, melphalan, SSRIs
Increase: effects of—digoxin, etoposide, HMG-CoA reductase inhibitors, methotrexate, potassium-sparing diuretics, sirolimus, tacrolimus
Decrease: cycloSPORINE action—anticonvulsants, nafcillin, orlistat, phenobarbital, phenytoin, probucol, rifamycins, sulfamethoxazole-trimethoprim, terbinafine, ticlopidine
Decrease: antibody reaction—live virus vaccines
Drug/Herb
Increase: immunosuppressant effect—safflower
Decrease: immunosuppressant effect—ginseng, maitake, mistletoe, schisandra, St. John's wort, turmeric

Drug/Food
Slowed metabolism of drug: grapefruit juice, food

NURSING CONSIDERATIONS

Assess:
• Renal studies: BUN, creatinine at least monthly during treatment, 3 mo after treatment
• Drug blood level during treatment
• Hepatic studies: alk phosphatase, AST, ALT, bilirubin; hepatotoxicity: dark urine, jaundice, itching, light-colored stools; drug should be discontinued
• Serum lipids, magnesium, potassium, cycloSPORINE blood concentrations
⚠ For nephrotoxicity: 6 wk postop, acute tubular necrosis, CyA trough level >200 ng/ml, gradual rise in creatinine (0.15 mg/dl/day), creatinine plateau <25% above baseline, intracapsular pressure <40 mm Hg
Administer:
PO route
• Do not break, crush, or chew caps
• Use pipette provided to draw up oral sol; may mix with milk or juice, wipe pipette, do not wash
• For several days before transplant surgery
• With corticosteroids
• With meals for GI upset or in chocolate milk, milk, or orange juice
• With oral antifungal for *Candida* infections
Rheumatoid arthritis
• Give Neoral or Gengraf 2.5 mg/kg/day divided bid, may use with salicylates, NSAIDs, PO corticosteroids
Neoral/Gengraf
• Always give the daily dose in 2 divided doses on consistent schedule
Sandimmune PO
• Give initial dose 4-12 hr prior to transplantation as a single dose of 15 mg/kg, continue the single daily dose for 1-2 wk, then taper 5%/wk to a maintenance dose 5-10 mg/kg/day
IV route
• After diluting each 50 mg/20-100 ml of 0.9% NaCl or D$_5$W; run over 2-6 hr, may

give as a continuous inf over 24 hr; use an infusion pump, glass inf bottles only

Sandimmune, Parenteral

• Give ⅓ of PO dose, initial dose 4-12 hr prior to transplantation as a single IV dose 5-6 mg/kg/day, continue the single daily dose until PO can be used

Additive compatibilities: Ciprofloxacin

Solution compatibilities: D_5W, NaCl 0.9%

Y-site compatibilities: Cefmetazole, propofol, sargramostim

Evaluate:

• Therapeutic response: absence of rejection

Teach patient/family:

• To report fever, chills, sore throat, fatigue, since serious infections may occur; tremors; bleeding gums, increased B/P

• To use contraceptive measures during treatment, for 12 wk after ending therapy

---

cyproheptadine (℞)

(si-proe-hep′ta-deen)

cyproheptadine HCl,

Periactin,

PMS-Cyproheptadine ✤

Func. class.: Antihistamine, H_1-receptor antagonist

Chem. class.: Piperidine

Do not confuse:

cyproheptadine/cyclobenzaprine

Action: Acts on blood vessels, GI, respiratory system by competing with histamine for H_1-receptor site; decreases allergic response by blocking histamine

Uses: Allergy symptoms, rhinitis, pruritus, cold, urticaria

Investigational uses: Appetite stimulant, management of vascular headache, nightmares, posttraumatic stress disorder

DOSAGE AND ROUTES

• *Adult:* **PO** 4 mg tid-qid, not to exceed 0.5 mg/kg/day

• *Child 6-14 yr:* **PO** 4 mg bid-tid, not to exceed 16 mg/day

• *Child 2-5 yr:* **PO** 2 mg bid-tid, not to exceed 12 mg/day

Nightmares, posttraumatic stress disorder

• *Adult:* **PO** 4-12 mg nightly, max 32 mg

Available forms: Tabs 4 mg; syr 2 mg/5 ml

SIDE EFFECTS

CNS: Dizziness, drowsiness, poor coordination, fatigue, anxiety, euphoria, confusion, paresthesia, neuritis

CV: Hypotension, palpitations, tachycardia

EENT: Blurred vision, dilated pupils; tinnitus; nasal stuffiness; dry nose, throat, mouth

GI: Constipation, dry mouth, nausea, vomiting, anorexia, diarrhea, weight gain, increased appctite

GU: Retention, dysuria, urinary frequency

*HEMA: **Hemolytic anemia, leukopenia, thrombocytosis, agranulocytosis***

INTEG: Rash, urticaria, photosensitivity

RESP: Increased thick secretions, wheezing, chest tightness

*SYST: **Anaphylactic shock***

Contraindications: Hypersensitivity to H_1-receptor antagonist, acute asthma attack, lower respiratory tract disease

Precautions: Pregnancy (B), increased intraocular pressure, renal disease, cardiac disease, hypertension, bronchial asthma, seizure disorder, stenosed peptic ulcers, hyperthyroidism, prostatic hypertrophy, bladder neck obstruction, lactation, elderly

PHARMACOKINETICS

PO: Duration 4-6 hr; metabolized in liver; excreted by kidneys; excreted in breast milk

INTERACTIONS

Increase: CNS depression—barbiturates, opiates, hypnotics, tricyclics, alcohol

Increase: anticholinergic effect—
MAOIs
Drug/Herb
Increase: CNS depression—hops,
Jamaican dogwood, kava, khat, senega
Increase: anticholinergic effect—
corkwood, henbane
Drug/Lab Test
False negative: Skin allergy tests

NURSING CONSIDERATIONS

Assess:
• I&O ratio; be alert for urinary reten-
tion, frequency, dysuria; drug should be
discontinued
• CBC during long-term therapy
• Respiratory status: rate, rhythm, in-
crease in bronchial secretions, wheezing,
chest tightness
• Cardiac status: palpitations, increased
pulse, hypotension
Administer:
• With meals for GI symptoms; absorp-
tion may slightly decrease
Perform/provide:
• Hard candy, gum, frequent rinsing of
mouth for dryness
• Storage in airtight container at room
temperature
Evaluate:
• Therapeutic response: absence of
running or congested nose, rashes
Teach patient/family:
• All aspects of drug use; to notify prescriber of confusion, sedation, hypotension
• To avoid driving, other hazardous
activity if drowsiness occurs, especially
elderly
• To avoid concurrent use of alcohol,
other CNS depressants
Treatment of overdose: Ipecac
syrup or lavage, diazepam, vasopressors,
barbiturates (short-acting)

⚠ High Alert

cytarabine (R)
(sye-tare′a-been)
Ara-C, Cytosar ✿, Cytosar-U,
cytosine arabinoside
Func. class.: Antineoplastic, antimetabolite
Chem. class.: Pyrimidine nucleoside

Do not confuse:
Cytosar/Cytoxan/Cytovene
Action: Competes with physiologic
substrate of DNA synthesis, thus interfering with cell replication in the S phase of
the cell cycle (before mitosis)
Uses: Acute myelocytic leukemia, acute
nonlymphocytic leukemia, chronic myelocytic leukemia, lymphomatous meningitis (IT), and in combination for non-
Hodgkin's lymphomas in children

DOSAGE AND ROUTES

Acute nonlymphocytic/lymphocytic
• *Adult:* **IV INF** 200 mg/m^2/day × 5
days q2wk as single agent or 2-6 mg/kg/
day (100-200 mg/m^2/day) as a single
dose or 2-3 divided doses for 5-10 days
until remission, used in combination;
maintenance 70-200 mg/m^2/day for 2-5
days qmo; **SUBCUT/IM** maintenance 1
mg/kg q1-2×/wk
*Refractory acute leukemia/refrac-
tory non-Hodgkin's lymphoma*
• *Adult:* **IV** 3 g/m^2 over 1-3 hr q12h ×
4-12 doses, repeat at 2-3 wk intervals, or
when patient recovers from toxicities
Meningeal leukemia
• *Adult/Child:* **INTRATHECALLY** 5-75
mg/m^2 variable daily × 4 days to q2-7
days
Available forms: Powder for inj 100,
500 mg, 1, 2 g; sus rel, (DepoCyt) liposomal for intrathecal use 10 mg/ml

SIDE EFFECTS

CNS: Neuritis, dizziness, headache, cerebellar syndrome, personality changes,

ataxia, mechanical dysphasia, *coma; chemical arachnoiditis* (IT)

CV: Chest pain, *cardiopathy*

CYTARABINE SYNDROME: Fever, myalgia, bone pain, chest pain, *rash,* conjunctivitis, malaise (6-12 hr after administration)

EENT: Sore throat, conjunctivitis

GI: Nausea, vomiting, anorexia, diarrhea, stomatitis, *hepatotoxicity,* abdominal pain, hematemesis, *GI hemorrhage*

GU: Urinary retention, *renal failure, hyperuricemia*

HEMA: Thrombophlebitis, bleeding, thrombocytopenia, leukopenia, myelosuppression, anemia

INTEG: Rash, fever, freckling, cellulitis

META: Hyperuricemia

RESP: Pneumonia, dyspnea, *pulmonary edema* (high doses)

SYST: Anaphylaxis

Contraindications: Pregnancy (D), hypersensitivity, infants

Precautions: Renal disease, hepatic disease, lactation

PHARMACOKINETICS

INTRATHECAL: Half-life 100-236 hr; metabolized in liver; excreted in urine (primarily inactive metabolite); crosses blood-brain barrier, placenta

IV/SUBCUT: Distribution half-life 10 min, elimination half-life 1-3 hr

INTERACTIONS

Increase: toxicity, bone marrow depression—radiation or other antineoplastics

Decrease: effects of oral digoxin

NURSING CONSIDERATIONS

Assess:

• CBC (RBC, Hct, Hgb), differential, platelet count weekly; withhold drug if WBC is <1000/mm^3, platelet count is <50,000/mm^3, or RBC, Hct, Hgb low; notify prescriber of these results

• Renal studies: BUN, serum uric acid, urine CCr, electrolytes before and during therapy

• I&O ratio; report fall in urine output to <30 ml/hr

• Monitor temp q4h; fever may indicate beginning infection; no rectal temps

• Hepatic studies before and during therapy: bilirubin, ALT, AST, alk phosphatase, as needed or monthly; check for jaundice of skin, sclera; dark urine; clay-colored stools; pruritus; abdominal pain; fever; diarrhea

• Blood uric acid during therapy

A For anaphylaxis: rash, pruritus, facial swelling, dyspnea; resuscitation equipment should be nearby

A Chemical arachnoiditis (IT): headache, nausea, vomiting, fever; neck rigidity pain, meningism; CSF pleocytosis; may be decreased by dexamethasone

• Cytarabine syndrome 6-12 hr after inf: fever, myalgia, bone pain, chest pain, rash, conjunctivitis, malaise; corticosteroids may be ordered

• Bleeding: hematuria, heme-positive stools, bruising or petechiae, mucosa or orifices q8h

A Dyspnea, crackles, unproductive cough, chest pain, tachypnea, fatigue, increased pulse, pallor, lethargy; personality changes, with high doses; pulmonary edema may be fatal (rare)

• Buccal cavity q8h for dryness, sores or ulceration, white patches, oral pain, bleeding, dysphagia

• Local irritation, pain, burning, discoloration at inj site

• GI symptoms: frequency of stools, cramping, antispasmodic may be used

• Acidosis, signs of dehydration: rapid respirations, poor skin turgor, decreased urine output, dry skin, restlessness, weakness

Administer:

• Antiemetic 30-60 min before giving drug and prn

• Allopurinol to maintain uric acid levels and alkalinization of the urine

• Topical or systemic analgesics for pain

IT route
- Use preservative-free NS, add 5 ml/100 mg vial or 10 ml/500 mg vial; use immediately, discard unused drug
- Use dexamethasone with IT administration

IV route
- After diluting 100 mg/5 ml of sterile H_2O for inj; given by direct IV over 1-3 min through free-flowing tubing (IV); may be further diluted in 50-100 ml NS or D_5W, given over 30 min to 24 hr depending on dose; also may be given by continuous inf

Additive compatibilities: Corticotropin, DAUNOrubicin with etoposide, etoposide, hydrOXYzine, lincomycin, mitoxantrone, ondansetron, potassium chloride, prednisoLONE, sodium bicarbonate, vinCRIStine

Solution compatibilities: Amino acids, D_5/LR, D_5/0.2% NaCl, D_5/0.9% NaCl, D_{10}/0.9% NaCl, D_5W, invert sugar 10% in electrolyte #1, Ringer's LR, 0.9% NaCl, sodium lactate ⅙ mol/L, TPN #57

Syringe compatibilities: Metoclopramide

Y-site compatibilities: Amifostine, amsacrine, aztreonam, cefepime, chlorproMAZINE, cimetidine, cladribine, dexamethasone, diphenhydrAMINE, DOXOrubicin liposome, droperidol, famitodine, filgrastim, fludarabine, gentamicin, granisetron, heparin, hydrocortisone, hydromorphone, idarubicin, lorazepam, melphalan, methotrexate, methylPREDNISolone, metoclopramide, morphine, ondansetron, paclitaxel, piperacillin/tazobactam, prochlorperazine, promethazine, propofol, ranitidine, sargramostim, sodium bicarbonate, teniposide, thiotepa, vinorelbine

Perform/provide:
- Strict medical asepsis and protective isolation if WBC levels are low
- Increase fluid intake to 2-3 L/day to prevent urate deposits and calculi formation, unless contraindicated
- Diet low in purines: absence of organ meats (kidney, liver), dried beans, peas to prevent increased urate deposits

- Rinsing of mouth tid-qid with water, club soda; brushing of teeth bid-tid with soft brush or cotton-tipped applicators for stomatitis; use unwaxed dental floss

Evaluate:
- Therapeutic response: decreased tumor size, spread of malignancy

Teach patient/family:
- To report any coughing, chest pain, changes in breathing; may indicate beginning pneumonia, pulmonary edema
- To avoid foods with citric acid, hot or rough texture if stomatitis is present, use sponge brush and rinse with water after each meal; to report stomatitis: any bleeding, white spots, ulcerations in mouth; tell patient to examine mouth daily, report any symptoms
- To report signs of infection: increased temp, sore throat, flulike symptoms; avoid crowds, persons with infections
- To report signs of anemia: fatigue, headache, faintness, shortness of breath, irritability
- To report bleeding; avoid use of razors, commercial mouthwash, salicylates, NSAIDs
- To use thrombocytopenia precautions
- To take fluids to 3 L/day to prevent renal damage
- To use contraception during treatment and 4 mo thereafter
- To avoid receiving vaccines during treatment
- That fever, headache, nausea, vomiting are likely to occur

⚠ High Alert

dacarbazine (℞)
(da-kar'ba-zeen)
dacarbazine, DTIC ✦, DTIC-Dome
Func. class.: Antineoplastic alkylating agent
Chem. class.: Cytotoxic triazine

Action: Alkylates DNA, RNA; inhibits DNA, RNA synthesis; also responsible for breakage, cross-linking DNA strands; activity is not cell cycle phase specific

---

Uses: Hodgkin's disease, sarcomas, neuroblastoma, metastatic malignant melanoma

Investigational uses: Malignant pheochromocytoma in combination with cyclophosphamide and vinCRIStine, metastatic soft tissue sarcoma in combination with other agents, Kaposi sarcoma alone or in combination

DOSAGE AND ROUTES

Metastatic malignant melanoma
• *Adult:* IV 2-4.5 mg/kg daily × 10 days or 250 mg/m² daily × 5 days; repeat q3wk depending on response
Hodgkin's disease
• *Adult:* IV 150 mg/m² daily × 5 days with other agents, repeat q4wk; or 375 mg/m² on day 1 when given in combination, repeat q15d
Available forms: Inj 100, 200 mg

SIDE EFFECTS

CNS: Facial paresthesia, flushing, fever, malaise; confusion, headache, *seizures*, blurred vision (high doses)
*GI: Nausea, anorexia, vomiting, **hepatotoxicity*** (rare)
*HEMA: **Thrombocytopenia, leukopenia,** anemia*
INTEG: Alopecia, dermatitis, pain at inj site, photosensitivity; severe sun reactions (high doses)
MISC: Flulike symptoms, malaise, fever, myalgia
*SYST: **Anaphylaxis***
Contraindications: Lactation
Precautions: Pregnancy (C) 1st trimester, radiation therapy

PHARMACOKINETICS

Metabolized by liver; excreted in urine; half-life 35 min, terminal 5 hr, 5% protein bound

INTERACTIONS

Toxicity, bone marrow suppression: bone marrow suppressants, radiation, other antineoplastics
Bleeding: salicylates, anticoagulants

Increase: adverse reaction decrease antibody reaction—live virus vaccines
Increase: nephrotoxicity—aminoglycosides
Increase: ototoxicity—loop diuretics
Decrease: dacarbazine effect—phenytoin, phenobarbital

D

NURSING CONSIDERATIONS

Assess:
⚠ CBC, differential, platelet count weekly; withhold drug if WBC <4000 or platelet count <75,000; notify prescriber of results
• Monitor temp q4h (may indicate beginning infection)
• Hepatic studies before, during therapy (bilirubin, AST, ALT, LDH) as needed or monthly
• Bleeding: hematuria, guaiac, bruising or petechiae, mucosa or orifices q8h
• Effects of alopecia on body image, discuss feelings about body changes
• Jaundice of skin, sclera; dark urine; clay-colored stools; itchy skin; abdominal pain; fever; diarrhea
• Inflammation of mucosa, breaks in skin
⚠ Hypersensitivity reactions, anaphylaxis, discontinue drug, administer meds for anaphylaxis

Administer:
• Antiemetic 30-60 min before giving drug to prevent vomiting, nausea, vomiting may subside after several doses
• Antibiotics for prophylaxis of infection
IV route
• After diluting 100 mg/9.9 ml of sterile H₂O for inj (10 mg/ml), give by direct IV over 1 min through Y-tube or 3-way stopcock; may be further diluted in 50-250 ml D₅W or NS for inj, given as an inf over ½ hr
• Watch for extravasation; give Na thiosulfate 10% 4 ml plus sterile H₂O 5 ml, 3-5 ml SUBCUT if needed
Additive compatibilities: Bleomycin, carmustine, cyclophosphamide, cytarabine, dactinomycin, DOXOrubicin, fluorouracil, mercaptopurine, methotrexate, ondansetron, vinBLAStine

Additive incompatibilities: Hydrocortisone sodium succinate, cysteine

Y-site compatibilities: Amifostine, aztreonam, filgrastim, fludarabine, granisetron, melphalan, ondansetron, paclitaxel, sargramostim, teniposide, thiotepa, vinorelbine

Perform/provide:

• Storage in light-resistant container, dry area

• Strict medical asepsis, protective isolation if WBC levels are low

• Increase fluid intake to 2-3 L/day to prevent urate deposits, calculi formation

• Warm compresses at infusion site for inflammation

Evaluate:

• Therapeutic response: decreased tumor size, spread of malignancy

Teach patient/family:

• That patient should avoid prolonged exposure to sun, wear sunscreen

• That hair may be lost during treatment; a wig or hairpiece may make the patient feel better; new hair may be different in color, texture

• To report signs of infection: fever, sore throat, flulike symptoms

• To report signs of anemia: fatigue, headache, faintness, shortness of breath, irritability

• To report bleeding; avoid use of razors, commercial mouthwash

• To avoid use of aspirin products or ibuprofen

• To use contraceptives during and for several months after therapy

---

⚠ High Alert

daclizumab (℞)

(dah-kliz'uh-mab)

Zenapax

Func. class.: Immunosuppressant

Chem. class.: Humanized IgG1 monoclonal antibody

Action: Binds to the IL-2 (interleukin-2) receptor antagonist

Uses: Acute allograft rejection in renal transplant patients

DOSAGE AND ROUTES

• *Adult:* **IV** 1 mg/kg as part of a regimen that includes cycloSPORINE and corticosteroids, mix calculated vol with 50 ml of 0.9% NaCl and give via peripheral/central vein over 15 min

Available forms: Inj 25 mg/ml

SIDE EFFECTS

CNS: Chills, tremors, dizziness, insomnia, headache, prickly sensation

CV: Hypertension, **tachycardia, thrombosis,** bleeding

GI: Vomiting, nausea, diarrhea, constipation, abdominal pain, pyrosis

GU: Oliguria, dysuria, **renal tubular necrosis,** renal damage, **hydronephrosis**

INTEG: Acne, impaired wound healing

MISC: Edema, peripheral edema

RESP: Dyspnea, wheezing, **pulmonary edema,** coughing, atelectasis, congestion, hypoxia

Contraindications: Hypersensitivity

Precautions: Pregnancy (C), child 11 mo, lactation, elderly

INTERACTIONS

Drug/Herb

Increase: immunosuppressant effect—safflower

Decrease: immunosuppressant effect—ginseng, maitake, mistletoe, schisandra, St. John's wort, turmeric

NURSING CONSIDERATIONS

Assess:

• Blood studies: Hgb, WBC, platelets during treatment qmo; if leukocytes are <3000/mm^3, drug should be discontinued

• Hepatic studies: alk phosphatase, AST, ALT, bilirubin

⚠ Hepatotoxicity: dark urine, jaundice, itching, light-colored stools; drug should be discontinued

⚠ For anaphylaxis, have corticosteroids, epINEPHrine available

---

Administer:

• All other medications PO if possible

• Avoid IM inj, since infection may occur

• Protect undiluted sol from direct light; should be used with drugs for immunosuppression

Solution compatibilities: 0.9% NaCl

Perform/provide:

• Decreased fluid intake during treatment

Evaluate:

• Therapeutic response: absence of graft rejection

Teach patient/family:

• To report fever, chills, sore throat, fatigue, since serious infection may occur; rash, hives, difficulty breathing, since allergic reactions may occur; nausea, constipation, diarrhea, stomach pain, headache, fast heartbeat, swelling, tremors, chest pain, urinary tract bleeding, fever, cough, pain, redness at site

• To use contraception (women) before, during, and for 4 mo after treatment

• To avoid vaccinations during treatment

• To avoid hazardous activities, dizziness, blurred vision may occur

---

> **⚠ High Alert**

dactinomycin (℞)

(dak-ti-noe-mye′sin)

Cosmegen

Func. class.: Antineoplastic, antibiotic

Action: Inhibits DNA, RNA, protein synthesis; derived from *Streptomyces parvullus;* replication is decreased by binding to DNA, which causes strand splitting; cell cycle nonspecific; a vesicant

Uses: Sarcomas, melanomas, trophoblastic tumors in women, testicular cancer, Wilms' tumor, rhabdomyosarcoma

DOSAGE AND ROUTES

• *Adult:* IV 500 mcg/m²/day × 5 days; stop drug for 2-4 wk; then repeat cycle

• *Child:* IV 15 mcg/kg/day × 5 days, not to exceed 500 mcg/day; stop drug until

bone marrow recovery, then repeat cycle

Available forms: Inj 0.5 mg/vial

SIDE EFFECTS

CNS: Malaise, fatigue, lethargy, fever

EENT: Chelitis, dysphagia, esophagitis

*GI: Nausea, vomiting, anorexia, stomatitis, **hepatotoxicity,*** abdominal pain, diarrhea

HEMA: **Thrombocytopenia, leukopenia, aplastic anemia**

INTEG: Rash, alopecia, pain at injection site, folliculitis, acne, desquamation, *extravasation*

MS: Myalgia

Contraindications: Hypersensitivity, herpes infection, child <6 mo

Precautions: Renal disease, hepatic disease, pregnancy (C), lactation, bone marrow depression

PHARMACOKINETICS

Half-life 36 hr; IV onset 2-5 min; concentrates in kidneys, liver, spleen; does not cross blood-brain barrier; excreted in feces and urine

INTERACTIONS

Increase: toxicity—other antineoplastics, radiation

Drug/Lab Test

Increase: Uric acid

NURSING CONSIDERATIONS

Assess:

• CBC, differential, platelet count weekly; withhold drug if WBC is <4000/mm³ or platelet count is <75,000/mm³; notify prescriber

• Renal studies: BUN, serum uric acid, urine CCr, electrolytes before, during therapy

• I&O ratio; report fall in urine output to <30 ml/hr

• Monitor temp q4h; fever may indicate beginning infection

• Hepatic studies before, during therapy: bilirubin, AST, ALT, alk phosphatase, as needed or monthly; check for jaundice of

---

skin, sclera; dark urine; clay-colored stools; itchy skin; abdominal pain; fever; diarrhea
• Bleeding: hematuria, guaiac stools, bruising, petechiae, mucosa or orifices q8h
• Food preferences; list likes, dislikes
• Effects of alopecia on body image; discuss feelings about body changes
• Inflammation of mucosa, breaks in skin
• Buccal cavity q8h for dryness, sores, ulceration, white patches, oral pain, bleeding, dysphagia
⚠ Symptoms indicating severe allergic reaction: rash, pruritus, urticaria, purpuric skin lesions, itching, flushing
• GI symptoms: frequency of stools, cramping, nausea, vomiting, anorexia
• Acidosis, signs of dehydration: rapid respirations, poor skin turgor, decreased urine output, dry skin, restlessness, weakness, sunken eyeball in children

Administer:
• Antiemetic 30-60 min before giving drug to prevent vomiting
• Increase fluids to 3 L/day

IV route
• After diluting 0.5 mg/1.1 ml of sterile H_2O for inj without preservative; use 2.2 ml (0.25 mg/ml), give by direct IV at 0.5 mg or less/min through Y-tube or 3-way stopcock if inf in progress; may be further diluted if required in 50 ml D_5W or NS for infusion; run over 10-15 min; change needles between reconstitution and direct IV administration
• Hydrocortisone, sodium thiosulfate to infiltration area, and ice compress after stopping infusion

Y-site compatibilities: Allopurinol, amifostine, aztreonam, cefepime, fludarabine, granisetron, melphalan, ondansetron, sargramostim, teniposide, thiotepa, vinorelbine

Perform/provide:
• Strict hand-washing technique, gloves and protective covering
• Liquid diet: carbonated beverages; gelatin may be added if patient is not nauseated or vomiting
• Rinsing of mouth tid-qid with water, club soda; brushing of teeth bid-qid with soft brush or cotton-tipped applicators for stomatitis; use unwaxed dental floss to prevent injury
• Storage in cool, dark environment; do not expose to bright light or freeze
• Fluid increase to 3 L/day

Evaluate:
• Therapeutic response: decreased tumor size, spread of malignancy

Teach patient/family:
• That contraception is needed during treatment and for 4-6 mo after discontinuing therapy
• To avoid vaccinations without order by prescriber
• That hair may be lost during treatment after 1-2 wk and that wig or hairpiece may make patient feel better; that new hair may be different in color, texture
• To avoid foods with citric acid, hot or rough texture when stomatitis is present
• To report any bleeding, white spots, ulcerations in mouth to prescriber; tell patient to examine mouth daily
• To avoid crowds, persons with known infection when granulocyte count is low

---

⚠ High Alert

dalteparin (℞)
(dahl′ta-pear-in)
Fragmin
Func. class.: Anticoagulant
Chem. class.: Low molecular weight heparin

Action: Prevents conversion of fibrinogen to fibrin and prothrombin to thrombin by enhancing inhibitory effects of antithrombin III
Uses: Unstable angina/non–Q-wave MI; prevention of deep vein thrombosis in abdominal surgery, hip replacement or those with restricted mobility during acute illness
Investigational uses: Systemic anticoagulation in venous/arterial thromboembolic complications

---

DOSAGE AND ROUTES

Hip replacement surgery/DVT prophylaxis
• *Adult:* SUBCUT 2500 international units 2 hr prior to surgery and 2nd dose in the evening the day of surgery, then 5000 international units SUBCUT 1st postop day and daily 5-10 days

Unstable angina/non–Q-wave MI
• *Adult:* SUBCUT 120 international units/kg, max 10,000 international units q12h with concurrent aspirin, continue until stable

Systemic anticoagulation
• *Adult:* SUBCUT 200 international units/kg daily or 100 international units/kg bid

DVT, prophylaxis for abdominal surgery
• *Adult:* SUBCUT 2500 international units daily, 1-2 hr prior to abdominal surgery and repeat daily × 5-10 days; in high-risk patients 5000 international units may be used

Available forms: Prefilled syringes, 2500, 5000 international units/0.2 ml; 10,000 international units multidose vials; 7500 international units/0.3 ml, 10,000, 25,000 international units/ml

SIDE EFFECTS

CNS: **Intracranial bleeding**
HEMA: **Thrombocytopenia**
INTEG: Pruritus, superficial wound infection
SYST: Hypersensitivity, **hemorrhage, anaphylaxis** possible

Contraindications: Hypersensitivity to this drug, heparin, or pork products, benzyl alcohol; hemophilia, leukemia with bleeding, thrombocytopenic purpura, cerebrovascular hemorrhage, cerebral aneurysm, severe hypertension, other severe cardiac disease, those undergoing regional anesthesia for unstable angina, non–Q-wave MI
Precautions: Pregnancy (B), elderly, hepatic disease, severe renal disease, blood dyscrasias, subacute bacterial endocarditis, acute nephritis, lactation, children, recent childbirth, peptic ulcer disease, pericarditis, pericardial effusion, recent lumbar puncture, vasculitis, other diseases where bleeding is possible

PHARMACOKINETICS

87% absorbed, excreted by kidneys, elimination half-life 3-5 hr, peak 4 hr, onset and duration unknown

INTERACTIONS

Increase: risk of bleeding—aspirin, oral anticoagulants, platelet inhibitors, NSAIDs, thrombolytics

Drug/Herb
Increase: bleeding risk—agrimony, alfalfa, angelica, anise, bilberry, black haw, bogbean, bromelain, buchu, chondroitin, cinchona bark, dong quai, fenugreek, feverfew, garlic, ginger, ginkgo, ginseng, horse chestnut, Irish moss, kelp, kelpware, khella, lovage, lungwort, meadowsweet, motherwort, mugwort, nettle, papaya, parsley (large amts), pau d'arco, pineapple, poplar, prickly ash, safflower, saw palmetto, senega, tonka bean, turmeric, wintergreen, yarrow
Decrease: anticoagulant action—chamomile, coenzyme , flax, glucomannan, goldenseal, guar gum

NURSING CONSIDERATIONS

Assess:
• For blood studies (Hct, CBC, platelets, occult blood in stools) during treatment since bleeding can occur
⚠ For bleeding gums, petechiae, ecchymosis, black tarry stools, hematuria, epistaxis, decrease in Hct, B/P; may indicate bleeding, possible hemorrhage; notify prescriber immediately, drug should be discontinued
⚠ For neurologic impairment frequently in those when neuraxial anesthesia has been used, spinal/epidural hematomas can occur, with paralysis
• For hypersensitivity: fever, skin rash, urticaria; notify prescriber immediately
• For needed dosage change q1-2wk;

dose may need to be decreased if bleeding occurs

Administer:

• Cannot be used interchangeably (unit for unit) with unfractionated heparin or LMWHs

• Do not give IM or IV drug route; approved is SUBCUT only; do not mix with other inj or sol

• Have patient sit or lie down; SUBCUT inj may be 2 in from umbilicus in a U-shape, upper outer side of thigh, around navel, or upper outer quadrangle of the buttocks; rotate inj sites

• Changing needles is not recommended; change inj site daily; use at same time of day

Evaluate:

• Therapeutic response: absence of deep-vein thrombosis

Teach patient/family:

• To avoid OTC preparations that contain aspirin; other anticoagulants, serious drug interaction may occur unless approved by prescriber

• To use soft-bristle toothbrush to avoid bleeding gums, avoid contact sports, use electric razor, avoid IM inj

• To report any signs of bleeding: gums, under skin, urine, stools; unusual bruising

Treatment of overdose: Protamine sulfate 1% given IV; 1 mg protamine/100 anti-Xa international units of dalteparin given

---

⚠ High Alert

danaparoid (℞)

(dan-a-pair′oid)

Orgaran

Func. class.: Anticoagulant, antithrombotic

Chem. class.: Glycosaminoglycan

Action: Prevents conversion of fibrinogen to fibrin and prothrombin to thrombin by enhancing inhibitory effects of antithrombin III

Uses: Prevention of vein thrombosis in hemodialysis, stroke, elective surgery for malignancy or total hip replacement, hip fracture surgery

DOSAGE AND ROUTES

Prevention of venous thrombosis

• *Adult:* **SUBCUT** 750 anti–factor-Xa units bid × 7-10 days, begin 1-4 hr presurgery and restart 2 hr after surgery; use lower dose in renal failure

Hemodialysis

• *Adult:* **SUBCUT** 2400-4800 anti-Xa units given predialysis

Available forms: Inj 750 anti-Xa units/0.6 ml

SIDE EFFECTS

CNS: Insomnia, headache

CV: Peripheral edema

GI: Nausea, vomiting, constipation

HEMA: **Thrombocytopenia**

INTEG: Rash, pruritus, inj site pain

MS: Asthenia

SYST: Hypersensitivity, **hemorrhage**

Contraindications: Hypersensitivity to this drug, sulfites, pork; hemophilia, leukemia with bleeding, thrombocytopenia, purpura, cerebrovascular hemorrhage, cerebral aneurysm, other severe cardiac disease

Precautions: Pregnancy (B), hypersensitivity to heparin, severe hypertension, elderly, severe renal disease, blood dyscrasias, subacute bacterial endocarditis, acute nephritis, lactation, children, recent childbirth, peptic ulcer disease, pericarditis, pericardial effusion, recent lumbar puncture, vasculitis, other diseases where bleeding is possible

PHARMACOKINETICS

100% absorbed, excreted by kidneys, half-life 24 hr, peak 4 hr

INTERACTIONS

Increase: bleeding risk—aspirin, oral anticoagulants, platelet inhibitors, NSAIDs, penicillin, dextran

Drug/Herb

Increase: bleeding risk—agrimony,

⚠ Safety alert   *"Tall Man" lettering

alfalfa, angelica, anise, bilberry, black haw, bogbean, bromelain, buchu, chondroitin, cinchona bark, dong quai, fenugreek, feverfew, garlic, ginger, ginkgo, ginseng, horse chestnut, Irish moss, kelp, kelpware, khella, lovage, lungwort, meadowsweet, motherwort, mugwort, nettle, papaya, parsley (large amts), pau d'arco, pineapple, poplar, prickly ash, safflower, saw palmetto, senega, tonka bean, turmeric, wintergreen, yarrow
Decrease: anticoagulant action—chamomile, coenzyme Q10, flax, glucomannan, goldenseal, guar gum

NURSING CONSIDERATIONS
Assess:
• For blood studies (Hct, CBC, occult blood in stools) during treatment since bleeding can occur; aPTT, ACT, anti–factor-Xa test, platelets
• For bleeding gums, petechiae, ecchymosis, black tarry stools, hematuria, epistaxis, decrease in Hct, B/P; may indicate bleeding, possible hemorrhage; notify prescriber immediately, drug should be discontinued
• For hypersensitivity: fever, skin, rash, urticaria; notify prescriber immediately
• For needed dosage change q1-2wk; dose may need to be decreased if bleeding occurs
Administer:
• Cannot be used interchangeably (unit for unit) with heparin, LMWHs, or heparinoids
• By SUBCUT only, have patient sit or lie down; SUBCUT inj may be around the navel in a U-shape, upper outer side of thigh or upper outer quadrangle of the buttocks; rotate inj sites
• Changing needles is not recommended
Evaluate:
• Therapeutic response: absence of deep-vein thrombosis
Teach patient/family:
• To avoid OTC preparations that may cause serious drug interactions unless directed by prescriber; may contain aspirin, other anticoagulants
• To use soft-bristle toothbrush to avoid

bleeding gums, avoid contact sports, use electric razor, avoid IM inj
• To report any signs of bleeding: gums, under skin, urine, stools; unusual bruising
Treatment of overdose: Discontinue drug, protamine sulfate 1% given IV; 1 mg protamine/100 anti–factors-Xa international units of danaparoid given

danazol (℞)
(da′na-zole)
Cyclomen ✦, danazol, Danocrine
Func. class.: Androgen, anabolic steroid
Chem. class.: α-Ethinyl testosterone derivative

Do not confuse:
danazol/Dantrium
Action: Atrophy of endometrial tissue; decreases FSH, LH, which are controlled by pituitary; this leads to amenorrhea/anovulation
Uses: Endometriosis, prevention of hereditary angioedema, fibrocystic breast disease

DOSAGE AND ROUTES
Endometriosis
• *Adult:* **PO** 100-500 mg bid uninterrupted for 3-9 mo
Fibrocystic breast disease
• *Adult:* **PO** 100-400 mg daily in 2 divided doses × 2-6 mo
Hereditary angioedema prevention
• *Adult:* **PO** 200 mg bid-tid until desired response, then decrease dose to 100 mg at 1-3 mo intervals
Available forms: Caps 50, 100, 200 mg

SIDE EFFECTS
CNS: Dizziness, headache, fatigue, tremors, paresthesias, flushing, sweating, anxiety, *lability,* insomnia
CV: Increased B/P
EENT: Conjunctival edema, nasal congestion, voice weakness

ENDO: Abnormal GTT
GI: Nausea, vomiting, constipation, *weight gain, **cholestatic jaundice***
GU: Hematuria, *amenorrhea,* atrophic vaginitis, decreased libido, *decreased breast size,* clitoral hypertrophy, testicular atrophy
INTEG: Rash, *acneiform lesions,* oily hair, skin, flushing, sweating, acne vulgaris, alopecia, *hirsutism,* pruritus
MS: Cramps, spasms, joint swelling
Contraindications: Pregnancy (X), severe renal, severe cardiac, severe hepatic disease, hypersensitivity, genital bleeding (abnormal), children, lactation
Precautions: Migraine, lactation headaches, seizure disorders

INTERACTIONS

Nephrotoxicity: cycloSPORINE
Increase: action—anticoagulants, oral antidiabetics, insulin, corticosteroids
Drug/Lab Test
Increase: Cholesterol
Decrease: Cholesterol, T_4, T_3, thyroid ^{131}I uptake test, 17-KS, PBI
Interference: GTT

NURSING CONSIDERATIONS

Assess:
• For pain before and after treatment in endometriosis, fibrocystic breast disease; tenderness, nodules in fibrocystic breast disease
• Potassium, blood, urine glucose while on long-term therapy; LFTs, periodically, semen volume, sperm count, motility in hereditary angioedema
• Weight daily; notify prescriber if weekly weight gain is >5 lb; drug should be decreased or discontinued
• I&O ratio; be alert for decreasing urinary output, increasing edema
• Edema, hypertension, cardiac symptoms, jaundice
• Mental status: affect, mood, behavioral changes, aggression, sleep disorders, depression, anxiety, lability
• Signs of virilization: deepening of voice, decreased libido, facial hair that may not be reversible

• Hypercalcemia: GI symptoms, polydipsia, polyuria, increased calcium levels above 11 mg/dl, loss of muscle tone
Administer:
• Do not break, crush, or chew caps
• Start treatment during menstruation in endometriosis, fibrocystic breast disease
• With food or milk to decrease GI symptoms (i.e., nausea, vomiting, anorexia, dyspepsia)
Perform/provide:
• Storage in airtight container at room temperature; do not freeze
Evaluate:
• Therapeutic response: decreased pain in endometriosis; decreased size, pain in fibrocystic breast disease
Teach patient/family:
• To notify prescriber if therapeutic response decreases
• Not to discontinue medication abruptly; to taper over several wk
• To report menstrual irregularities; that amenorrhea usually occurs but menstruation resumes 2-3 mo after termination of therapy without medical intervention
• About routine breast self-exam and to report any increase in nodule size
• That drug should induce anovulation; reversible within 60-90 days after drug is discontinued and treatment will need to be resumed
• That endometriosis tends to recur after drug is discontinued
• To use nonhormonal contraception
• That virilization may occur, to notify prescriber
• To use sunscreen or stay out of the sun to prevent burns

dantrolene (℞)
(dan'troe-leen)
Dantrium
Func. class.: Skeletal muscle relaxant, direct acting
Chem. class.: Hydantoin

Do not confuse:
Dantrium/danazol
Action: Interferes with intracellular

---

release of calcium from the sarcoplasmic reticulum necessary to initiate contraction; slows catabolism in malignant hyperthermia

Uses: Spasticity in multiple sclerosis, stroke, spinal cord injury, cerebral palsy, malignant hyperthermia

DOSAGE AND ROUTES

Spasticity
• *Adult:* **PO** 25 mg/day; may increase by 25-100 mg bid-qid, not to exceed 400 mg/day × 1 wk
• *Child:* **PO** 1 mg/kg/day given in divided doses bid; dosage may increase gradually, not to exceed 400 mg daily

Prevention of malignant hyperthermia
• *Adult and child:* **PO** 4-8 mg/kg/day in 3-4 divided doses × 1-2 days prior to procedures, give last dose 4 hr preop; **IV** 2.5 mg/kg prior to anesthesia

Malignant hyperthermia
• *Adult and child:* **IV** 1 mg/kg, may repeat to total dose of 10 mg/kg; **PO** 4-8 mg/kg/day in 4 divided doses × 3 days to prevent further hyperthermia; post-crisis follow-up 4-8 mg/kg/day for 1-3 days

Available forms: Caps 25, 50, 100 mg; powder for inj 20 mg/vial

SIDE EFFECTS

CNS: Dizziness, weakness, fatigue, drowsiness, headache, disorientation, insomnia, paresthesias, tremors, ***seizures***

CV: Hypotension, chest pain, palpitations

EENT: Nasal congestion, blurred vision, mydriasis

GI: **Hepatic injury**, *nausea,* constipation, vomiting, increased AST, alk phosphatase, abdominal pain, dry mouth, anorexia, hepatitis, dyspepsia

GU: Urinary frequency, nocturia, impotence, crystalluria

HEMA: **Eosinophilia**

INTEG: Rash, pruritus, photosensitivity

RESP: Pleural effusion

Contraindications: Hypersensitivity, compromised pulmonary function, active hepatic disease, impaired myocardial function

Precautions: Pregnancy (C), peptic ulcer disease, renal disease, hepatic disease, stroke, seizure disorder, diabetes mellitus, lactation, elderly

PHARMACOKINETICS

Oral absorption poor
PO: Peak 5 hr; highly protein bound; half-life 8 hr; metabolized in liver; excreted in urine (metabolites)

INTERACTIONS

Dysrhythmias: verapamil
Hepatotoxicity: estrogens, other hepatotoxics
Considered incompatible in sol or syringe; compatibility unknown
Increase: CNS depression—alcohol, tricyclics, opiates, barbiturates, sedatives, hypnotics, antihistamines

NURSING CONSIDERATIONS

Assess:
• For increased seizure activity, ECG in epilepsy patient; poor seizure control has occurred
• I&O ratio; check for urinary retention, frequency, hesitancy, especially elderly
• Hepatic function by frequent determination of AST, ALT, bilirubin, alk phosphatase, GGTP; renal function studies, BUN, creatinine, CBC
• Allergic reactions: rash, fever, respiratory distress
• Severe weakness, numbness in extremities; prescriber should be notified and drug discontinued
• Tolerance: increased need for medication, more frequent requests for medication, increased pain
• CNS depression: dizziness, drowsiness, insomnia, psychiatric symptoms
⚠ Signs of hepatotoxicity: jaundice, yellow sclera, pain in abdomen, nausea, fever; prescriber should be notified, drug should be discontinued

Administer:
• Avoid use with other CNS depressants

Side effects: *italics* = common; ***bold italics*** = life-threatening

PO route

• Do not break, crush, or chew caps
• Caps may be opened, mixed with juice and swallowed
• With meals for GI symptoms

IV route

• IV after diluting 20 mg/60 ml sterile H_2O for inj without bacteriostatic agent (333 mcg/ml); shake until clear; give by rapid IV push through Y-tube or 3-way stopcock; follow by prescribed doses immediately; may also give by intermittent inf over 1 hr prior to anesthesia

Perform/provide:

• Storage in tight container at room temperature; protect diluted sol from light, use reconstituted solution within 6 hr
• Gum, frequent sips of water for dry mouth
• Assistance with ambulation if dizziness/drowsiness occurs

Evaluate:

• Therapeutic response: decreased pain, spasticity

Teach patient/family:

• Not to discontinue medication quickly; hallucinations, spasticity, tachycardia will occur; drug should be tapered off over 1-2 wk; notify prescriber of abdominal pain, jaundiced sclera, clay-colored stools, change in color of urine
• Not to take with alcohol
• That if improvement does not occur within 6 wk, prescriber may discontinue
• To avoid hazardous activities if drowsiness, dizziness occurs
• To avoid using OTC medication: cough preparations, antihistamines, unless directed by prescriber
• To use sunscreen or stay out of the sun to prevent burns

Treatment of overdose: Induce emesis of conscious patient; lavage, dialysis

---

dapiprazole ophthalmic
See Appendix C

Rarely Used

dapsone (DDS) (℞)
(dap′sone)
Avlosulfon ♣, Dapsone
Func. class.: Leprostatic

Uses: Hansen's disease, PCP (*Pneumocystis jiroveci* pneumonia), malaria, dermatitis herpetiformis

DOSAGE AND ROUTES

Hansen's disease
• *Adult:* **PO** 100 mg daily with rifampin 600 mg daily × 6 mo, then dapsone alone for 3-10 yr
• *Child:* **PO** 1-2 mg/kg/day

PCP
• *Adult:* **PO** 50-100 mg/day usually given with trimethoprim 20 mg/kg/day in 4 divided doses for 3 wk
• *Child:* **PO** 2 mg/kg/day

Contraindications: Hypersensitivity to sulfones, severe anemia

---

daptomycin (℞)
(dap′toe-mye-sin)
Cubicin
Func. class.: Antiinfective, misc
Chem. class.: Lipopeptides

Action: A new class of antiinfective. It binds to the bacterial membrane and results in a rapid depolarization of the membrane potential, thus leading to inhibition of DNA, RNA, and protein synthesis.

Uses: Complicated skin, skin structure infections caused by *Staphylococcus aureus* including methicillin-resistant strains, *Streptococcus pyogenes, Streptococcus agalactiae, Streptococcus dysgalactiae, Enterococcus faecalis* (vancomycin-susceptible strains only).

DOSAGE AND ROUTES

• *Adult:* **IV INF** 4 mg/kg over ½ hr diluted in 0.9% NaCl, give q24h × 7-14 days

---

Renal dose

• *Adult:* **IV INF** CCr ≥30 ml/min 4 mg/kg q24h; CCr <30 ml/min, hemodialysis, CAPD 4 mg/kg q48h

Available forms: Lyophilized powder for inj 250, 500 mg

SIDE EFFECTS

CNS: Headache, insomnia, dizziness

CV: Hypotension, hypertension, increase CPK

GI: Nausea, constipation, diarrhea, vomiting, dyspepsia, ***pseudomembraneous colitis***

GU: Nephrotoxicity: increase BUN, creatinine, albumin

INTEG: Rash, pruritus

MISC: Fungal infections, UTI, anemia

MS: Muscle pain or weakness, arthralgia, pain

Contraindications: Hypersensitivity

Precautions: Renal disease, pregnancy (B), children, lactation, elderly

PHARMACOKINETICS

Site of metabolism unknown, protein binding 92%

INTERACTIONS

Myopathy: HMG-CoA reductase inhibitors

NURSING CONSIDERATIONS

Assess:

• I&O ratio: report hematuria, oliguria; nephrotoxicity may occur

⚠ Any patient with compromised renal system, toxicity may occur; BUN, creatinine

• Blood studies: CBC

• C&S, drug may be given as soon as culture is taken

• B/P during administration; hypo-, hypertension may occur

• Signs of infection

• Respiratory status: rate, character, wheezing

• Allergies before treatment, reaction of each medication

Administer:

• After reconstitution with 5 ml 0.9% NaCl (250 mg/5 ml) or 10 ml 0.9% NaCl (500 mg/10 ml), further dilution is needed with 0.9 NaCl, infuse over ½ hr.

Solution compatibilities: 0.9% NaCl, LR

Evaluate:

• Therapeutic response: Negative culture

Teach patient/family:

• Allergies before treatment, reaction of each medication

• All aspects of drug therapy

• To report sore throat, fever, fatigue, could indicate superinfection

---

darbepoetin alfa (℞)
(dar′bee-poh′eh-tin al′fah)
Aranesp
Func. class.: Hematopoietic agent
Chem. class.: Recombinant human erythropoietin

Action: Stimulates erythropoiesis by the same mechanism as endogenous erythropoietin; in response to hypoxia, erythropoietin is produced in the kidney and released into the bloodstream, where it interacts with progenitor stem cells to increase red cell production

Uses: Anemia associated with chronic renal failure, in patients on and not on dialysis and anemia in nonmyeloid malignancies receiving coadministered chemotherapy

DOSAGE AND ROUTES

Correction of anemia

• *Adult:* **SUBCUT/IV** 0.45 mcg/kg as a single inj, titrate not to exceed a target Hgb of 12 g/dl

Epoetin alfa to darbepoetin conversion

• *Adult:* **SUBCUT/IV** estimate starting dose based on weekly epoetin alfa dose; because of longer serum half-life, darbepoetin must be administered less frequently than epoetin alfa; if epoetin was given 2-3×/wk, give darbepoetin 1×/wk;

if epoetin was given 1×/wk, give darbepoetin 1× q2wk; do not increase doses more often than 1×/mo

Available forms: Sol for inj 25, 40, 60, 100, 150, 200, 300, 500 mcg/ml

SIDE EFFECTS

CNS: **Seizures**, sweating, headache, dizziness, **stroke**

*CV: Hypertension, hypotension, **cardiac arrest**, angina pectoris, **thrombosis, CHF, acute MI, dysrhythmias,** chest pain, transient ischemic attacks*

GI: Diarrhea, vomiting, nausea, abdominal pain, constipation

*MISC: Infection, fatigue, fever, **death**, fluid overload, **vascular access hemorrhage***

MS: Bone pain, myalgia, limb pain, back pain

RESP: URI, dyspnea, cough, bronchitis

SYST: Allergic reactions, **anaphylaxis**

Contraindications: Hypersensitivity to mammalian cell–derived products or human albumin, uncontrolled hypertension, red cell aplasia

Precautions: Pregnancy (C), seizure disorder, porphyria, hypertension, lactation, children, sickle cell disease; vit B$_{12}$, folate deficiency

PHARMACOKINETICS

IV: Onset of increased reticulocyte count 1-6 wk; distributed to vascular space; absorption slow and rate-limiting; terminal half-life 49 hr; peak concentration at 34 hr; increased Hgb levels not generally observed until 2-6 wk after treatment initiated

INTERACTIONS

⚠ Do not use epoetin alfa with this drug

Increase: darbepoetin alfa effect—androgens

NURSING CONSIDERATIONS

Assess:

⚠ Serious allergic reactions: rash, urticaria; if anaphylaxis occurs, stop drug, administer emergency treatment (rare)

• Renal studies: urinalysis, protein, blood, BUN, creatinine

• Blood studies: ferritin, transferrin qmo; transferrin sat ≥20%, ferritin ≥100 ng/ml; Hgb 2×/wk until stabilized in target range (30%-33%), then at regular intervals; those with endogenous erythropoietin levels of <500 units/L respond to this agent; iron stores should be corrected before beginning therapy

• B/P; check for rising B/P as Hgb rises, antihypertensives may be needed

• CV status: hypertension may occur rapidly leading to hypertensive encephalopathy

• I&O; report drop in output to <50 ml/hr

• For seizures if Hgb is increased within 2 wk by 4 pts

• CNS symptoms: sweating, pain in long bones

• Dialysis patients: thrill, bruit of shunts, monitor for circulation impairment

Administer:

IV/SUBCUT route

• Without shaking; check for discoloration, particulate matter, do not use if present; do not dilute, do not mix with other drugs or solutions, discard unused portion, do not pool unused portions

Evaluate:

• Therapeutic response: increase in reticulocyte count, Hgb/Hct; increased appetite, enhanced sense of well-being

Teach patient/family:

• To avoid driving or hazardous activity during beginning of treatment

• To monitor B/P, Hgb

• To take iron supplements, vit B$_{12}$, folic acid as directed

• To report side effects to prescriber, to comply with treatment regimen

• Home administration procedures, if appropriate

⚠ High Alert

*DAUNOrubicin (℞)
(daw-noe-roo'bi-sin)
Cerubidine

*DAUNOrubicin
citrate liposome
DaunoXome

Func. class.: Antineoplastic, antiinfective
Chem. class.: Anthracycline glycoside

Do not confuse:
DAUNOrubicin/DOXOrubicin
Action: Inhibits DNA synthesis, primarily; derived from *Streptomyces coerulorubidus;* replication is decreased by binding to DNA, which causes strand splitting; cell cycle specific (S phase); a vesicant
Uses: Myelogenous, monocytic leukemia, acute nonlymphocytic leukemia, Ewing's sarcoma, rhabdomyosarcoma; DAUNOrubicin citrate liposome: advanced Kaposi's sarcoma in HIV

DOSAGE AND ROUTES
Use decreased dose for those >60 yr of age
DAUNOrubicin
Single agent
• *Adult:* **IV** 60 mg/m^2/day × 3-5 days q4wk
In combination
• *Adult:* **IV** 45 mg/m^2/day × 3 days, then 2 days of subsequent courses in combination
• *Child:* **IV** 25-60 mg/m^2 depending on cycle
DAUNOrubicin citrate liposome
• *Adult:* **IV** 40 mg/m^2 q2wk
Renal dose
• *Adult:* **IV** serum CCr >3 mg/dl reduce dose by 50%
Hepatic dose
• *Adult:* **IV** serum bilirubin 1.2-3 mg/dl reduce dose by 25%; bilirubin >3 mg/dl reduce dose by 50%

Available forms: Inj 20 mg powder/vial, sol for inj 5 mg/ml (DaunoXome); liposome: dispersion for inj 2 mg/ml

SIDE EFFECTS
DAUNOrubicin
CNS: Fever, chills
CV: ***Dysrhythmias, CHF, pericarditis, myocarditis,*** peripheral edema
*GI: Nausea, vomiting, anorexia, mucositis, **hepatotoxicity***
GU: Impotence, sterility, amenorrhea, gynecomastia, hyperuricemia
HEMA: ***Thrombocytopenia, leukopenia, anemia***
*INTEG: Rash, **extravasation,** dermatitis,* reversible alopecia, cellulitis, thrombophlebitis at inj site
SYST: ***Anaphylaxis***
DAUNOrubicin citrate liposome
CNS: Fatigue, headache, depression, insomnia, dizziness, *malaise, neuropathy*
CV: Chest pain, edema
GI: Abdominal pain, stomatitis, *nausea, vomiting, diarrhea,* constipation
INTEG: Alopecia, pruritus, sweating
MISC: Allergic reactions, chest pain, fever, edema, flulike symptoms
MS: Rigors, arthralgia, back pain
RESP: Cough, dyspnea, rhinitis, sinusitis

Contraindications: Pregnancy (D), hypersensitivity, lactation, systemic infections, cardiac disease
Precautions: Renal, hepatic disease; gout; bone marrow depression

PHARMACOKINETICS
Half-life 18½ hr, liposome 55½ hr; metabolized by liver; crosses placenta; excreted in breast milk, urine, bile

INTERACTIONS
Increase: bleeding risk—NSAIDs, salicylates
Increase: toxicity—other antineoplastics, radiation, cyclophosphamide
Decrease: antibody reaction—live virus vaccines

Drug/Lab Test
Increase: Uric acid

NURSING CONSIDERATIONS
Assess:
⚠ CBC, differential, platelet count weekly, leukocyte nadir within 2 wk after administration, recovery within 3 wk; do not administer if absolute granulocyte count is <750/mm^3 (liposome)
• Blood, urine uric acid levels baseline and during therapy
• Renal studies: BUN, urine CCr, electrolytes baseline, before each dose
• I&O ratio; report fall in urine output to <30 ml/hr
• Monitor temp q4h; fever may indicate beginning infection
• Hepatic studies baseline, before each dose: bilirubin, AST, ALT, alk phosphatase; check for jaundice of skin, sclera; dark urine; clay-colored stools; itchy skin; abdominal pain; fever; diarrhea
• Chest x-ray, echocardiography, radionuclide angiography, ECG; watch for ST-T wave changes, low QRS and T, possible dysrhythmias (sinus tachycardia, heart block, PVCs); watch for CHF (jugular vein distention, weight gain, edema, crackles), may occur after 2-6 mo of treatment
• Bleeding: hematuria, guaiac stools, bruising or petechiae, mucosa or orifices q8h
• Effects of alopecia on body image; discuss feelings about body changes
• Buccal cavity q8h for dryness, sores or ulceration, white patches, oral pain, bleeding, dysphagia
• Local irritation, pain, burning at inj site
• GI symptoms: frequency of stools, cramping
• Acidosis, signs of dehydration: rapid respirations, poor skin turgor, decreased urine output, dry skin, restlessness, weakness
Administer:
• Antiemetic 30-60 min before giving

drug and 6-10 hr after treatment to prevent vomiting
• Allopurinol or sodium bicarbonate to reduce uric acid levels, alkalinization of urine
IV route (Cerubidine)
• After diluting 20 mg/4 ml sterile H_2O for inj (5 mg/ml), rotate, further dilute in 10-15 ml 0.9% NaCl; give over 3-5 min by direct IV through Y-tube or 3-way stopcock of inf of D_5 or 0.9% NaCl; or dilute in 50 ml 0.9% NaCl and give over 10-15 min; or dilute in 100 ml and give over 30 min
• Hydrocortisone for extravasation; apply ice compress after stopping infusion
Additive compatibilities: Cytarabine/etoposide, hydrocortisone; not recommended for admixing
Solution compatibilities: $D_{3.3}$/0.3% NaCl, D_5W, Normosol R, Ringer's, 0.9% NaCl
Y-site compatibilities: Amifostine, filgrastim, granisetron, melphalan, methotrexate, ondansetron, sodium bicarbonate, teniposide, thiotepa, vinorelbine
IV route (DaunoXome)
• Dilute with D_5W to (1 mg/ml) give over 60 min, do not use in-line filter, reconstituted sol may be stored ≤6 hr refrigerated; do not admix
Perform/provide:
• Increased fluid intake to 2-3 L/day to prevent urate and calculi formation
• Diet low in purines: absence of organ meats (kidney, liver), dried beans, peas to reduce uric acid level
• Rinsing of mouth tid-qid with water, club soda; brushing of teeth bid-qid with soft brush or cotton-tipped applicators for stomatitis; use unwaxed dental floss
Evaluate:
• Therapeutic response: decreased tumor size, spread of malignancy
Teach patient/family:
• To report signs of infection, bleeding, bruising, shortness of breath, swelling, change in heart rate
• That hair may be lost during treatment and wig or hairpiece may make patient

feel better; tell patient that new hair may be different in color, texture

• To avoid pregnancy while on this drug, and 4 mo thereafter

• To avoid foods with citric acid, hot or rough texture

• To report any bleeding, white spots, ulcerations in mouth; tell patient to examine mouth daily

• That urine and other body fluids may be red-orange for 48 hr

• To avoid vaccines while taking this drug

• To avoid crowds, those with known infections

• To avoid alcohol, aspirin, NSAIDs

Rarely Used

deferoxamine (℞)
(de-fer-ox′a-meen)
Desferal
Func. class.: Heavy metal antagonist

Do not confuse:
deferoxamine/cefuroxime
Uses: Acute, chronic iron intoxication, hemochromatosis, hemosiderosis

DOSAGE AND ROUTES

Acute iron toxicity

• *Adult and child:* **IM/IV** 1 g, then 500 mg q4h × 2 doses, then 500 mg q4-12h × 2 doses, not to exceed 15 mg/kg/hr or 6 g/24 hr

Chronic iron toxicity

• *Adult and child:* **IM** 500 mg-1 g/day plus **IV INF** 2 g given by separate line with each blood transfusion, not to exceed 15 mg/kg/hr or 6 g/24 hr; **SUBCUT** 1-2 g over 8-24 hr by SUBCUT inf pump

Contraindications: Hypersensitivity, anuria, severe renal disease, child <3 yr

delavirdine (℞)
(de-la-veer′deen)
Rescriptor
Func. class.: Antiretroviral
Chem. class.: Nonnucleoside reverse transcriptase inhibitor (NNRTI)

D

Action: Binds directly to reverse transcriptase and blocks RNA, DNA, causing a disruption of the enzyme's site
Uses: HIV-1 in combination with other antiretrovirals

DOSAGE AND ROUTES

• *Adult and child ≥16 yr:* 400 mg tid
Available forms: Tabs 100, 200 mg

SIDE EFFECTS

CNS: Headache, fatigue
GI: Diarrhea, abdominal pain, nausea, anorexia, vomiting, dyspepsia, ***hepatotoxicity***
GU: ***Nephrotoxicity***
HEMA: ***Neutropenia, leukopenia, thrombocytopenia, anemia, granulocytopenia***
INTEG: Rash, pruritus
MS: Pain, myalgia
SYST: ***Stevens-Johnson syndrome***
Contraindications: Hypersensitivity to this drug or atevirdine
Precautions: Pregnancy (C), liver disease, lactation, children, renal disease, myleosuppression

PHARMOCOKINETICS:

98% protein bound, half-life 2-11 hr, peak 1 hr, duration 8 hr, extensively metabolized, excreted in urine/feces

INTERACTIONS

⚠ Serious life-threatening adverse reaction—amphetamines, ergots, benzodiazepines, calcium channel blockers, sedative/hypnotics, antidysrhythmics, sildenafil, pimozide, cisapride
Increase: levels of alprazolam, clarithromycin, dapsone, ergots, felodipine, midazolam, nifedipine, indinavir,

amprenavir, saquinavir, lovastatin, simvastatin, atorvastatin

Increase: delavirdine levels—fluoxetine, ketoconazole

Increase: levels of both drugs—quinidine, warfarin, clarithromycin

Decrease: delavirdine levels—antacids, anticonvulsants, rifamycins, protease inhibitors, didanosine

Decrease: action of oral contraceptives

NURSING CONSIDERATIONS
Assess:

• For signs of infection, anemia
• Hepatic studies: ALT, AST; renal studies
• C&S before drug therapy; drug may be taken as soon as culture is taken; repeat C&S after treatment; determine the presence of other sexually transmitted disease
• Bowel pattern before, during treatment; if severe abdominal pain with bleeding occurs, drug should be discontinued; monitor hydration
• For skin eruptions; rash, urticaria, itching
• For allergies before treatment, reaction to each medication; place allergies on chart
• Plasma delavirdine concentrations (trough 10 micromolar)
• CBC, blood chemistry, plasma HIV RNA, absolute CD4+/CD8+/cell counts/%, serum β-2 microglobulin, serum ICD+24 antigen levels
• For signs of delavirdine toxicity: severe nausea/vomiting, maculopapular rash

Administer:

• Dispersion by adding 4 tab/3-4 oz water, let stand, stir, swallow, rinse glass, swallow; use only 100 mg tabs for dispersion
• Do not give within 1 hr of antacids or didanosine

Evaluate:

• Therapeutic response: increased CD4 cell count, decreased viral load, improvement in symptoms of HIV

Teach patient/family:

• To take as prescribed; if dose is missed, take as soon as remembered up to 1 hr before next dose; do not double dose
• That tabs may be dissolved in ½ cup of water, stir, when dissolved, drink right away, rinse cup with water, and drink that to get all medication
• To make sure health care provider knows of all the medications being taken
• That if severe rash, mouth sores, swelling, aching muscles/joints, or eye redness occur, stop taking and notify health care provider
• Not to breastfeed if taking this drug

demecarium ophthalmic
See Appendix C

Rarely Used

demeclocycline (R)
(dem-e-kloe-sye′kleen)
Declomycin
Func. class.: Antiinfective

Uses: Uncommon gram-positive/gram-negative bacteria, protozoa, *Rickettsia, Mycoplasma, Haemophilus ducreyi, Yersinia pestis, Campylobacter fetus, Chlamydia trachomatis,* psittacosis, granuloma inguinale

DOSAGE AND ROUTES

• *Adult:* **PO** 150 mg q6h or 300 mg q12h
• *Child >8 yr:* **PO** 6-12 mg/kg/day in divided doses q6-12h

Gonorrhea

• *Adult:* **PO** 600 mg, then 300 mg q12h × 4 days, total 3 g

Contraindications: Pregnancy (D), hypersensitivity to tetracyclines, children <8 yr

denileukin diftitox (℞)
(den-ih-loo'kin dif'tih-tox)
Ontak
Func. class.: Antineoplastic—
miscellaneous

Action: A recombinant DNA-derived cytotoxic protein that interacts with high affinity IL-2 receptors on the cell surface and inhibits cellular protein synthesis
Uses: Cutaneous T-cell lymphoma that expresses CD25 component of the IL-2 receptor

DOSAGE AND ROUTES

• *Adult:* IV 9-18 mcg/kg/day given for 5 days q21 days, infused over ≥15 min
Available forms: Sol for inj, frozen 150 mcg/ml

SIDE EFFECTS

CNS: Dizziness, paresthesia, nervousness, confusion, insomnia
CV: Hypotension, vasodilation, tachycardia, thrombosis, hypertension, dysrhythmias
GI: Nausea, anorexia, vomiting, diarrhea, constipation, dyspepsia, dysphagia
GU: Hematuria, albuminuria, pyuria, creatinine increase
*HEMA: **Thrombocytopenia, leukopenia,** anemia*
INTEG: Rash, pruritus, sweating
META: Hypoalbuminemia, edema, hypocalcemia, weight decrease, dehydration, hypokalemia
MISC: Fever, chills, asthenia, infection, pain, headache, chest pain, flulike symptoms
MS: Myalgia, arthralgia
RESP: Dyspnea, cough, pharyngitis, rhinitis
Contraindications: Hypersensitivity to denileukin, diphtheria toxin, IL-2
Precautions: Pregnancy (C), radiation therapy, lactation, elderly, children

PHARMACOKINETICS

Concentrates in liver/kidneys; metabolized by proteolytic degradation

INTERACTIONS

Increase: bone marrow depression—radiation, other antineoplastics
Decrease: antibody reaction—live vaccines

NURSING CONSIDERATIONS
Assess:
• CBC, differential, platelet count weekly; withhold drug if WBC <4000/mm^3 or platelet count <75,000/mm^3; notify prescriber of results
• Monitor temp q4h (may indicate beginning infection)
• Hepatic studies before, during therapy (bilirubin, AST, ALT, LDH) as needed or monthly
• Bleeding: hematuria, guaiac, bruising or petechiae, mucosa or orifices q8h
• Jaundice of skin, sclera; dark urine; clay-colored stools; itchy skin; abdominal pain; fever; diarrhea
• For vascular leak syndrome after 2 wk of treatment, hypotension, edema, hypoalbuminemia; monitor weight, B/P, serum albumin, edema
• Obtain CD25 expression on skin biopsy samples
Administer:
• Antiemetic 30-60 min before giving drug to prevent vomiting
• Antibiotics for prophylaxis of infection
IV route
• Do not shake vigorously
• Prepare and hold sol in plastic syringes or soft plastic IV bags only, no glass containers
• Draw calculated dose from vial, inject into empty IV infusion bag, for each 1 ml of drug removed from vial, no more than 9 ml of sterile saline without preservative should be added to IV bag; infuse over ≥15 min; do not give by bolus; do not admix with other drugs; do not use a filter

D

- Use within 6 hr, discard unused portions

Perform/provide:
- Storage in light-resistant container, dry area
- Warm compresses at infusion site for inflammation

Evaluate:
- Therapeutic response: decreased tumor size, spread of malignancy

Teach patient/family:
- To report signs of infection: fever, sore throat, flulike symptoms
- To report signs of anemia: fatigue, headache, faintness, shortness of breath, irritability
- To report bleeding; avoid use of razors, commercial mouthwash
- To avoid use of aspirin products or ibuprofen

---

desipramine (R)

(dess-ip′ra-meen)
Apo-Desipramine ✦
desipramine HCl, Norpramin,
Pertofrane ✦
Func. class.: Antidepressant, tricyclic
Chem. class.: Dibenzazepine, secondary amine

Action: Blocks reuptake of norepinephrine, serotonin into nerve endings, increasing action of norepinephrine, serotonin in nerve cells
Uses: Depression
Investigational uses: Chronic pain

DOSAGE AND ROUTES

- *Adult:* PO 100-200 mg/day in a single dose or in divided doses; max 300 mg/day
- *Geriatric:* PO 25-50 mg/day, may increase to 150 mg/day
- *Child >12 yr:* PO 25-50 mg/day in divided doses, max 100 mg/day
- *Child 6-12 yr:* PO 10-30 mg/day or 1-5 mg/kg/day in divided doses

Available forms: Tabs 10, 25, 50, 75, 100, 150 mg; caps 25, 50 mg

SIDE EFFECTS

CNS: Dizziness, drowsiness, confusion, headache, anxiety, tremors, stimulation, weakness, insomnia, nightmares, EPS (elderly), increased psychiatric symptoms, paresthenia
CV: Orthostatic hypotension, ECG changes, tachycardia, hypertension, palpitations
EENT: Blurred vision, tinnitus, mydriasis, ophthalmoplegia
GI: Diarrhea, dry mouth, nausea, vomiting, **paralytic ileus**, increased appetite, cramps, epigastric distress, jaundice, **hepatitis**, stomatitis, constipation
*GU: Retention, **acute renal failure***
*HEMA: **Agranulocytosis, thrombocytopenia, eosinophilia, leukopenia***
INTEG: Rash, urticaria, sweating, pruritus, photosensitivity
Contraindications: Hypersensitivity to tricyclic antidepressants, narrow-angle glaucoma
Precautions: Pregnancy (C), suicidal patients, severe depression, increased intraocular pressure, elderly, lactation, seizure disorder, CV disease, prostatic hypertrophy

PHARMACOKINETICS

Well absorbed, widely distributed, protein binding 92%, extensively metabolized in the liver, excretion is unknown, half-life 12-24 hr
Onset unknown, peak 4-6 hr, duration unknown

INTERACTIONS

Increase: CNS depression—alcohol, barbiturates, opioids, CNS depressants
Increase: desipramine level—cimetidine, fluvoxamine, fluoxetine, paroxetine, sertraline
Increase: life-threatening B/P elevations, do not use concurrently—clonidine
Increase: hypertension—epINEPHrine, norepinephrine

⚠ Safety alert   *"Tall Man" lettering

Increase: hyperpyrexia, seizures, excitation, do not use with 14 days of MAOIs—MAOI inhibitors

Drug/Herb

May lower seizure threshold, do not use concurrently: evening primrose oil
May increase serotonin syndrome, avoid concurrent use: St. John's Wort, SAM-e
Increase: CNS depression—chamomile, hops, kava, valerian

Drug/Lab Test

Increase: Serum bilirubin, blood glucose, alk phosphatase

NURSING CONSIDERATIONS

Assess:

• B/P (lying, standing), pulse q4h; if systolic B/P drops 20 mm Hg, hold drug, notify prescriber; take vital signs q4h in patients with cardiovascular disease
• Blood studies: CBC, leukocytes, differential, cardiac enzymes if patient is receiving long-term therapy
• Hepatic studies: AST, ALT, bilirubin
• Weight qwk; appetite may increase with this drug
• ECG for flattening T wave, bundle branch block, AV block, dysrhythmias in cardiac patients
• EPS primarily in elderly: rigidity, dystonia, akathisia
• Mental status: mood, sensorium, affect, suicidal tendencies, increase in psychiatric symptoms: depression, panic
• Urinary retention, constipation; constipation most likely in children
• Withdrawal symptoms: headache, nausea, vomiting, muscle pain, weakness; not usual unless drug discontinued abruptly
• Alcohol consumption; if consumed, hold dose until morning

Administer:

• Increased fluids, bulk in diet for constipation, especially in elderly
• With food or milk for GI symptoms
• Crushed if patient is unable to swallow medication whole
• Dosage at bedtime if oversedation occurs during day; may take entire dose at bedtime; elderly may not tolerate once a day dosing
• Gum, hard candy, frequent sips of water for dry mouth

Perform/provide:

• Storage at room temperature
• Assistance with ambulation during beginning of therapy for drowsiness/dizziness
• Safety measures, primarily in the elderly
• Check to see that PO medication is swallowed

Evaluate:

• Therapeutic response: decreased depression

Teach patient/family

• That therapeutic effects may take 2-3 wk
• To use caution in driving, other activities requiring alertness because of drowsiness, dizziness, blurred vision
• To avoid alcohol ingestion, other CNS depressants
• Not to discontinue medication quickly after long-term use; may cause nausea, headache, malaise
• To wear sunscreen or large hat, since photosensitivity occurs

Treatment of overdose: ECG monitoring; induce emesis; lavage, activated charcoal; administer anticonvulsant

---

desirudin (℞)
(des-i-rude′in)
Iprivask
Func. class.: Anticoagulant
Chem. class.: Thrombin inhibitor

Action: Inhibits thrombin resulting in prolongation of clotting time
Uses: Prophylaxis for deep vein thrombosis in those undergoing hip replacement

---

DOSAGE AND ROUTES

• *Adult:* SUBCUT 15 mg, 1st dose 5-15 min before surgery, but after regional block anesthesia, then 15 mg q12h, up to 12 days

Available forms: Lyophilized powder 15 mg

SIDE EFFECTS

MISC: Inj site mass, nausea, deep thrombophelibitis, anemia, hypersensitivity

SYST: **Bleeding, hemorrhage**

Contraindications: Hypersensitivity to natural or synthetic hirudins, active bleeding, irreversible coagulation disorders

Precautions: Pregnancy (C), lactation, children, elderly, hepatic and renal impairment, patients with increased risks of hemorrhage

PHARMACOKINETICS

Metabolized and eliminated by the kidney (40-50% unchanged)

INTERACTIONS

Increase: anticoagulant effect—thrombolytics, anticoagulants, antiplatelets (salicylates, NSAIDS, ketorolac, triclopidine, sulfinpyrazone, clopidogrel, abciximab)

NURSING CONSIDERATIONS

Assess:

• APTT daily in those with increased risk for bleeding

⚠ For neurologic changes that may indicate intracranial bleeding

⚠ Retroperitoneal bleeding: back pain, leg weakness, diminished pulses

• For bleeding: gums, petechiae, ecchymosis, black tarry stool, hematuria; notify prescriber

Administer:

• Alone, do not mix with other drugs or solutions

• For 9-12 days

• Only after screening patient for bleeding disorders

• SUBCUT only, do not give IM

• Give to patient recumbent, rotate inj sites (left/right anterolateral, left/right posterolateral abdominal wall)

• Insert whole length of needle into skin fold held with thumb and forefinger

• Give at same time of day to maintain blood level

• Administer only this drug when ordered, not interchangeable with heparin

Perform/provide:

• Bed rest during entire course of treatment

• Avoidance of venous or arterial puncture, inj, rectal temp

• Treatment of fever with acetaminophen

Evaluate:

• Therapeutic response: absence of deep vein thrombosis

Teach patient/family:

• About drug use and expected results; to report adverse reactions; bleeding, bruising

• To avoid all OTC drugs unless prescribed

• To use soft-bristle toothbrush to avoid bleeding gums, to use electric razor

---

desloratadine (℞)

(des′lor-at′ah-deen)
Clarinex, Clarinex Reditabs
Func. class.: Antihistamine, 2nd generation
Chem. class.: Selective histamine (H_1)-receptor antagonist

Action: Binds to peripheral histamine receptors, providing antihistamine action without sedation

Uses: Seasonal allergic rhinitis, chronic idiopathic urticaria

DOSAGE AND ROUTES

• *Adult and child ≥12 yr:* PO 5 mg daily
• *Child 6-11 yr:* PO 2.5 mg daily
• *Child 1-5 yr:* PO 1.25 mg daily
• *Child 6-11 mo:* 1 mg daily

Hepatic/renal dose

• *Adult:* PO 5 mg every other day

Available form: Tabs 5 mg; tabs, orally disintegrating 5 mg (Reditabs); syrup 0.5 mg/ml

SIDE EFFECTS

CNS: Sedation (more common with increased doses), headache

Contraindications: Hypersensitivity, acute asthma attacks, lower respiratory tract disease

Precautions: Pregnancy (C), bronchial asthma, liver or renal impairment

PHARMACOKINETICS

Onset antihistamine effect 1 hr, relief as early as 1 day, duration up to 24 hr, peak 1½ hr, elimination half-life 8½-28 hr; metabolized in liver to active metabolites, excreted in urine

INTERACTIONS

Drug/Food
Food may prolong time to peak with orally disintegrating tabs

NURSING CONSIDERATIONS

Assess:
• Allergy: hives, rash, rhinitis; monitor respiratory status; test interaction, antigen skin test

Administer:
• Without regard to meals
• Do not remove Redi Tabs from blister until ready to use
• Redi Tabs directly on tongue; may take with or without water

Perform/provide:
• Storage in tight container at room temperature

Evaluate:
• Therapeutic response: absence of running or congested nose, other allergy symptoms

Teach patient/family:
• To avoid driving, other hazardous activities if drowsiness occurs; observe caution until drug's effects on the patient are known
• That drug may cause photosensitivity; use sunscreen or stay out of the sun to prevent burns

desmopressin (℞)
(des-moe-press'in)
DDAVP, Stimate
Func. class.: Pituitary hormone
Chem. class.: Synthetic antidiuretic hormone

D

Action: Promotes reabsorption of water by action on renal tubular epithelium; causes smooth muscle constriction, increase in plasma factor VIII levels, which increases platelet aggregation resulting in vasopressor effect, similar to vasopressin

Uses: Hemophilia A, von Willebrand's disease type 1, nonnephrogenic diabetes insipidus, symptoms of polyuria/polydipsia caused by pituitary dysfunction, nocturnal enuresis

DOSAGE AND ROUTES

Primary nocturnal enuresis
• *Adult and child ≥6 yr:* INTRANASAL 20 mcg (10 mcg in each nostril) at bedtime, may increase to 40 mcg; PO 0.2 mg at bedtime, may be increased to max 0.6 mg at bedtime

Diabetes insipidus
• *Adult:* INTRANASAL 0.1-0.4 ml daily in divided doses (1-4 sprays with pump); IV/SUBCUT 0.5-1 ml daily in divided doses
• *Child 3 mo to 12 yr:* INTRANASAL 0.05-0.3 ml daily in divided doses

Hemophilia/von Willebrand's disease
• *Adult and child >3 mo:* IV 0.3 mcg/kg in NaCl over 15-30 min; may repeat if needed

Antihemorrhagic
• *Adult and child >3 mo:* IV 0.3 mcg/kg
• *Adult and child <50 kg:* INTRANASAL 1 spray in one nostril
• *Adult and child >50 kg:* 1 spray each nostril

Available forms: Inj 4, 15 mcg/ml, Rhihal Tube del 2.5 mg/vial (0.1 mg/ml); tabs 0.1, 0.2 mg; nasal spray pump 10 mcg/spray (0.1 mg/ml); nasal sol 1.5 mg/ml (150 mcg/dose)

SIDE EFFECTS

CNS: Drowsiness, headache, lethargy, flushing
CV: Increased B/P
EENT: Nasal irritation, congestion, rhinitis
GI: Nausea, heartburn, cramps
GU: Vulval pain
*SYST: **Anaphylaxis (IV)***
Contraindications: Hypersensitivity, nephrogenic diabetes insipidus
Precautions: Pregnancy (B), CAD, lactation, hypertension

PHARMACOKINETICS

NASAL: Onset 1 hr, peak 1-4 hr, duration 8-20 hr, half-life 8 min, 76 min (terminal)
PO: Onset 1 hr, peak 4-7 hr
IV: Onset 1 min, peak ½ hr, duration more than 3 hr

INTERACTIONS

Increase: antidiuretic action—carbamazepine, chlorpropamide, clofibrate
Decrease: antidiuretic action—lithium, alcohol, demeclocycline, heparin, large doses of epINEPHrine

NURSING CONSIDERATIONS

Assess:
• Pulse, B/P when giving IV or SUBCUT
• I&O ratio, weight daily; check for edema in extremities; if water retention is severe, diuretic may be prescribed
• Water intoxication: lethargy, behavioral changes, disorientation, neuromuscular excitability
• Intranasal use: nausea, congestion, cramps, headache; usually decreased with decreased dose

⚠ For severe allergic reaction including anaphylaxis (IV route)
• For nasal mucosa changes: congestion, edema, discharge, scarring (nasal route)
• Urine vol/osmolality and plasma osmolality (diabetes insipidus)
• Factor VIII coagulant activity before using for hemostasis
Administer:
• Undiluted over 1 min in diabetes insipidus
• Diluted, one single dose/50 ml of 0.9% NaCl (adult and child >10 kg), a single dose/10 ml as an IV inf over 15-30 min in von Willebrand's disease or hemophilia A
Perform/provide:
• Storage in refrigerator or cool environment
Evaluate:
• Therapeutic response: absence of severe thirst, decreased urine output, decreased osmolality
Teach patient/family:
• The proper technique for nasal instillation: to insert tube into nostril to instill drug
• To avoid OTC products: cough, hay fever products, since these preparations may contain epINEPHrine, decrease drug response; do not use with alcohol, adverse reactions may occur
• To wear emergency ID specifying therapy
• That if dose is missed, take when remembered up to 1 hr before next dose; do not double dose
• To report to prescriber upper respiratory infection, nasal congestion

desonide topical
See Appendix C

desoximetasone topical
See Appendix C

desoxyephedrine nasal agent
See Appendix C

---

dexamethasone (Ɍ)
(dex-ah-meth'a-sone)
Decadron, Deronil ✦
Dexasone ✦, Dexon, Hexadrol, Mymethasone

dexamethasone acetate (Ɍ)
Dalalone DP, Dalalone LA, Decadron-LA, Decaject-LA, Dexacen LA-8, Dexasone-LA, Dexone LA, Solurex-LA

dexamethasone sodium phosphate (Ɍ)
Dalalone, Decadron Phosphate, Decaject, Dexacen-4, Dexone, Hexadrol Phosphate, Solurex
Func. class.: Corticosteroid, synthetic
Chem. class.: Glucocorticoid, long-acting

Do not confuse:
Decadron/Percodan
Action: Decreases inflammation by suppression of migration of polymorphonuclear leukocytes, fibroblasts, reversal of increased capillary permeability and lysosomal stabilization
Uses: Inflammation, allergies, neoplasms, cerebral edema, septic shock, collagen disorders

DOSAGE AND ROUTES
Inflammation
• *Adult:* **PO** 0.75-9 mg/day in divided doses q6-12h or phosphate **IM** 0.5-9 mg/day divided q6-12h, or acetate **IM** 4-16 mg q1-3wk
• *Child:* **PO** 0.024-0.34 mg/kg/day in divided doses q6-12h

Shock (Phosphate)
• *Adult:* **IV** single dose 1-6 mg/kg or **IV** 40 mg q2-6h as needed up to 72h
Cerebral edema
• *Adult:* **(Phosphate) IV** 10 mg, then 4-6 mg **IM** q6h × 2-4 days, then taper over 1 wk
• *Child:* Loading dose 1-2 mg/kg (**PO/IM/IV**) then 1-1.5 mg/kg/day, max 16 mg/day divided q4-6hr for 2-4 days, then taper down qwk
Adrenocortical insufficiency
• *Adult:* **PO** 0.5-9 mg/day in divided doses
• *Child:* **PO** 0.03-0.3 mg/kg/day divided in 2-4 doses
Suppression test
• *Adult:* **PO** 1 mg at 11 PM or 0.5 mg q6h × 48 hr

Available forms: Dexamethasone: tabs 0.25, 0.5, 0.75, 1, 1.5, 2, 4, 6 mg; elix 0.5 mg/5 ml; oral sol 0.5 mg/5 ml, 1 mg/1 ml; inj acetate 8, 16 mg/ml; inj phosphate 4, 10, 20, 24 mg/ml

SIDE EFFECTS

CNS: Depression, flushing, sweating, headache, mood changes, euphoria, psychosis, *seizures,* insomnia
*CV: Hypertension, **circulatory collapse, thrombophlebitis, embolism,** tachycardia, edema
EENT: Fungal infections, increased intraocular pressure, blurred vision
ENDO: HPA suppression, hyperglycemia, sodium, fluid retention
*GI: Diarrhea, nausea, abdominal distention, **GI hemorrhage,** increased appetite, **pancreatitis**
*HEMA: **Thrombocytopenia***
INTEG: Acne, poor wound healing, ecchymosis, petechiae, hirsutism
META: Hypokalemia
MS: Fractures, osteoporosis, weakness
Contraindications: Psychosis, hypersensitivity, idiopathic thrombocytopenia, acute glomerulonephritis, amebiasis, fungal infections, nonasthmatic bronchial disease, child <2 yr, AIDS, TB
Precautions: Pregnancy (C), lactation, diabetes mellitus, glaucoma, osteoporo-

---

sis, seizure disorders, ulcerative colitis, CHF, myasthenia gravis, renal disease, peptic ulcer, esophagitis

PHARMACOKINETICS

PO: Onset 1 hr, peak 1-2 hr, duration 2½ days
IM: (acetate) Peak 8 hr, duration 6 days-3 wk
Half-life 36-54 hr

INTERACTIONS

Increase: side effects—alcohol, salicylates, indomethacin, amphotericin B, digitalis, cycloSPORINE, diuretics
Increase: dexamethasone action—salicylates, estrogens, indomethacin, oral contraceptives, ketoconazole, macrolide antiinfectives
Decrease: dexamethasone action—cholestyramine, colestipol, barbiturates, rifampin, epHEDrine, phenytoin, theophylline, antacids
Decrease: effect of anticoagulant effects, anticonvulsants, antidiabetics, ambenonium, neostigmine, isoniazid, toxoids, vaccines, anticholinesterases, salicylates, somatrem
Drug/Herb
Potassium deficiency: aloe, buckthorn, cascara sagrada, Chinese rhubarb, senna
Increase: corticosteroid effect—aloe, licorice, perilla
Drug/Lab Test
Increase: Cholesterol, sodium, blood glucose, uric acid, calcium, urine glucose
Decrease: Calcium, K, T_4, T_3, thyroid ^{131}I uptake test, urine 17-OHCS, 17-KS, PBI
False negative: Skin allergy tests

NURSING CONSIDERATIONS

Assess:

• Potassium, blood, urine glucose while on long-term therapy; hypokalemia and hyperglycemia
• Weight daily; notify prescriber of weekly gain >5 lb
• B/P q4hr, pulse; notify prescriber of chest pain

• I&O ratio; be alert for decreasing urinary output, increasing edema
• Plasma cortisol levels during long-term therapy (normal: 138-635 nmol/L SI units when drawn at 8 AM)
• Infection: fever, WBC even after withdrawal of medication; drug masks infection
• Potassium depletion: paresthesias, fatigue, nausea, vomiting, depression, polyuria, dysrhythmias, weakness
• Edema, hypertension, cardiac symptoms
• Mental status: affect, mood, behavioral changes, aggression
Administer:
• Titrated dose; use lowest effective dose
• IM inj deeply in large muscle mass; rotate sites; avoid deltoid; use 21G needle
• In one dose in AM to prevent adrenal suppression; avoid SUBCUT administration, may damage tissue
• With food or milk to decrease GI symptoms
IV route
• Undiluted direct over 1 min or less or diluted with 0.9% NaCl or D_5W and give as an IV inf at prescribed rate
• After shaking suspension (parenteral); do not give suspension IV
Dexamethasone sodium phosphate
Additive compatibilities: Aminophylline, bleomycin, cimetidine, floxacillin, furosemide, granisetron, lidocaine, meropenem, mitomycin, nafcillin, netilmicin, ondansetron, prochlorperazine, ranitidine, verapamil
Syringe compatibilities: Granisetron, metoclopramide, ranitidine, sufentanil
Y-site compatibilities: Acyclovir, allopurinol, amifostine, amikacin, amphotericin B cholesteryl, amsacrine, aztreonam, cefepime, cefpirome, cisatracurium, cisplatin, cladribine, cyclophosphamide, cytarabine, DOXOrubicin, DOXOrubicin liposome, famotidine, filgrastim, fluconazole, fludarabine, foscarnet, granisetron, heparin, lorazepam, melphalan, meperidine, meropenem, morphine, ondansetron, pacli-

taxel, piperacillin/tazobactam, potassium chloride, propofol, remifentanil, sargramostim, sodium bicarbonate, sufentanil, tacrolimus, teniposide, theophylline, thiotepa, vinorelbine, vit B/C, zidovudine

Perform/provide:

• Assistance with ambulation in patient with bone tissue disease to prevent fractures

Evaluate:

• Therapeutic response: ease of respirations, decreased inflammation

Teach patient/family:

• That ID as steroid user should be carried

• To contact prescriber if surgery, trauma, stress occurs; dose may need to be adjusted

• To notify prescriber if therapeutic response decreases; dosage adjustment may be needed

A Not to discontinue abruptly or adrenal crisis can result

• Symptoms of adrenal insufficiency: nausea, anorexia, fatigue, dizziness, dyspnea, weakness, joint pain

• To avoid OTC products: salicylates, alcohol in cough products, cold preparations unless directed by prescriber

• To teach patient all aspects of drug usage, including cushingoid symptoms; to notify health care provider of infection

• Avoid exposure to chickenpox or measles, persons with infection

dexamethasone ophthalmic
See Appendix C

dexamethasone topical
See Appendix C

dexmedetomidine
Precedex
Func. class.: Sedative, α_2 adrenoceptor agonist

Action: Produces α_2 activity seen at low and moderate doses, also α_1 at high doses

Uses: Sedation in mechanically ventilated, intubated patients ICU

Research note: One study has concluded that more research is needed before wider applications of this drug can be pursued

DOSAGE AND ROUTES

• *Adult:* **IV** loading dose of 1 mcg/kg over 10 min then 0.2-0.7 mcg/kg/hr, do not use for more than 24 hr

Available forms: Inj 100 mcg/ml

SIDE EFFECTS

CV: Bradycardia, hypotension, hypertension, ***atrial fibrillation, infarction***
GI: Nausea, thirst
GU: Oliguria
HEMA: Leukocytosis, anemia
RESP: ***Pulmonary edema, pleural effusion, hypoxia***

Contraindications: Hypersensitivity

Precautions: Pregnancy (C), elderly, respiratory depression, severe respiratory disorders, cardiac dysrhythmias, lactation, children, renal disease

PHARMACOKINETICS

Rapid distribution, excreted in urine; metabolized in liver

INTERACTIONS

Increase: CNS depression—alcohol, opioids, sedative/hypnotics, antipsychotics, skeletal muscle relaxants, inhalational anesthetics

NURSING CONSIDERATIONS

Assess:

• Inj site: phlebitis, burning, stinging

• ECG for changes: atrial fibrillation

• CNS changes: movement, jerking, tremors, dizziness, LOC, pupil reaction
• Respiratory dysfunction: respiratory depression, character, rate, rhythm; notify prescriber if respirations are <10/min

Administer:
• After diluting with D₅W 0.9% NaCl, withdraw 2 ml of drug and add to 48 ml of 0.9% NaCl to a total of 50 ml, shake to mix well
• Only with resuscitative equipment available
• Only by qualified persons trained in ICU sedation

Solution compatibilities: LR, D₅W, 0.9% NaCl, 20% mannitol

Additive compatibilities: Thiopental, etomidate, vecuronium, pancuronium, succinylcholine, atracurium, mivacurium, glycopyrrolate, phenylephrine, atropine, midazolam, morphine, fentanyl

Perform/provide:
• Safety measures: side rails, nightlight, call bell within easy reach

Evaluate:
• Therapeutic response: induction of anesthesia

**dexmethyl-
phenidate** (℞)
(dex′meth-ul-fen′ih-dayt)
Focalin, Focalin XR
Func. class.: Central nervous system (CNS) stimulant, psychostimulant

---

Controlled Substance Schedule II

Action: Increases release of norepinephrine and dopamine into the extraneuronal space, also blocks reuptake of norepinephrine and dopamine into the presynaptic neuron; mode of action in treating attention deficit hyperactivity disorder (ADHD) is unknown

Uses: ADHD, adjunctive treatment

DOSAGE AND ROUTES

• *Child >6 yr:* **PO** 2.5 mg bid with doses at least 4 hr apart, gradually increase to a maximum of 20 mg/day (10 mg bid); for those taking methylphenidate, use ½ of methylphenidate dose initially, then increase as needed to a maximum of 20 mg/day; **EXT REL** 5 mg/day, may adjust to 20 mg/day in 5 mg increments
• *Adult:* **PO EXT REL** 10 mg/day, may adjust to 20 mg/day in 10-mg increments

Available forms: Tabs 2.5, 5, 10 mg; caps ext rel 5, 10, 20 mg (Focalin XR)

SIDE EFFECTS

CNS: Dizziness, headache, drowsiness, **toxic psychosis, neuroleptic malignant syndrome (rare)**, Gilles de la Tourette's syndrome

CV: Palpitations, B/P changes, angina, **dysrhythmias**

GI: Nausea, anorexia, abnormal liver function, **hepatic coma**, abdominal pain

HEMA: **Leukopenia, anemia, thrombocytopenic purpura**

INTEG: **Exfoliative dermatitis**, urticaria, rash, erythema multiforme

MISC: Fever, arthralgia, scalp hair loss

Contraindications: Hypersensitivity to methylphenidate, anxiety, history of Gilles de la Tourette's syndrome, lactation, tics, psychosis; children <6 yr, glaucoma, concurrent treatment with MAOIs or within 14 days of discontinuing treatment with MAOIs

Precautions: Pregnancy (C), hypertension, depression, seizures, drug abuse, cardiovascular disorders, alcoholism

PHARMACOKINETICS

Readily absorbed, peak 1-1½ hr, ext rel 4 hr, elimination half-life 2.2 hr, onset ½-1 hr, ext rel unknown, duration 4 hr, ext rel 8 hr, metabolized by liver, excreted by kidneys

INTERACTIONS

Hypertensive crisis: MAOIs or within 14 days of MAOIs, vasopressors

Increase: sympathomimetic effect—decongestants, vasoconstrictors

Increase: effects of—anticonvulsants,

---

tricyclics, SSRIs, coumarin anticoagulants (warfarin)
Decrease: effects of antihypertensives
Drug/Herb
Synergistic effect: melatonin
Increase: stimulant effect—horsetail, yohimbe

NURSING CONSIDERATIONS
Assess:
• VS, B/P; may reverse antihypertensives; check patients with cardiac disease more often for increased B/P
• CBC, differential platelet counts during long term therapy, urinalysis; in diabetes: blood glucose, urine glucose; insulin changes may have to be made, because eating will decrease
• Height, growth rate q3mo in children; growth rate may be decreased
• Mental status: mood, sensorium, affect, stimulation, insomnia, aggressiveness
⚠ Withdrawal symptoms: headache, nausea, vomiting, muscle pain, weakness
• Appetite, sleep, speech patterns
• For attention span, decreased hyperactivity in persons with ADHD
Administer:
• Twice daily at least 4 hr apart; ext rel once a day
• Without regard to meals
Evaluate:
• Therapeutic response: decreased hyperactivity or ability to stay awake
Teach patient/family:
• To decrease caffeine consumption (coffee, tea, cola, chocolate); may increase irritability, stimulation
• To avoid OTC preparations unless approved by prescriber
• To taper off drug over several wk to avoid depression, increased sleeping, lethargy
• To avoid alcohol ingestion
• To avoid hazardous activities until stabilized on medication
• To get needed rest; patients will feel more tired at end of day
• Notify all health care workers, including school nurse, of medication and schedule
• Discuss information instructions provided in patient information section
Treatment of overdose: Administer fluids; hemodialysis or peritoneal dialysis; antihypertensive for increased B/P; administer short-acting barbiturate before lavage

D

---

dextran 40 (℞)
(deks′tran)
Dextran 40, Gentran 40, LMD 10%, Rheomacrodex
Func. class.: Plasma volume expander
Chem. class.: Low-molecular-weight polysaccharide

Action: Similar to human albumin, which expands plasma volume by drawing fluid from interstitial space to intravascular space
Uses: Expand plasma volume, prophylaxis of embolism, thrombosis

DOSAGE AND ROUTES
Shock
• *Adult:* **IV INF** 500 ml over 15-30 min, total dose in 24 hr not to exceed 20 ml/kg; subsequent doses given slowly; if given >24 hr, not to exceed 10 ml/kg/day; not to exceed therapy >5 days
Thrombosis/embolism
• *Adult:* **IV INF** 500-1000 ml, then 500 ml/day × 3 days, then 500 ml q2-3 days × 2 wk if needed
Available forms: 10% dextran 40/D$_5$W, 10% dextran 40/0.9% NaCl

SIDE EFFECTS
CV: Hypotension, ***cardiac arrest***
GI: Nausea, vomiting, increased AST, ALT
GU: ***Osmotic nephrosis, renal failure, stasis,*** hyponatremia
HEMA: Decreased hematocrit, platelet function; ***increased bleeding/coagulation times***
INTEG: Rash, urticaria, pruritus, ***angioedema,*** chills, fever, flushing

---

RESP: Wheezing, dyspnea, ***bronchospasm, pulmonary edema***
SYST: ***Anaphylaxis***

Contraindications: Hypersensitivity, renal failure, CHF (severe), extreme dehydration

Precautions: Pregnancy (C), active hemorrhage, sodium restriction

PHARMACOKINETICS

IV: Expands blood vol 1-2 × amount infused; excreted in urine and feces

INTERACTIONS

Incompatible with chlortetracycline, phytonadione, promethazine

Drug/Lab Test
False increase: Blood glucose, urinary protein, bilirubin, total protein
Interference: Rh test, blood typing/crossmatching

NURSING CONSIDERATIONS

Assess:
• VS q5min × 30 min; Hgb/Hct, if falling by 30%, notify prescriber
• CVP during infusion (5-10 cm H_2O—normal range)
• Urine output q1h; watch for increase in urinary output (common); if output does not increase, decrease or discontinue infusion
• I&O ratio and specific gravity, urine osmolarity; if specific gravity is very low, renal clearance is low, drug should be discontinued
• Allergy: rash, urticaria, pruritus, wheezing, dyspnea, bronchospasm, drug should be discontinued immediately
⚠ Circulatory overload: increased pulse, respirations, SOB, wheezing, chest tightness, chest pain
• Dehydration after infusion: decreased output, decreased specific gravity of urine, increased temp, poor skin turgor, increased specific gravity, dry skin
Administer:
IV route
• After prescribed dilution; may give

inital 500 mg at 15-30 min; distribute remainder of daily dose over 8-24 hr
• After crossmatch is drawn, if blood is to be given also
• D_5W sol in heart failure patients as ordered

Additive compatibilities: Cloxacillin
Y-site compatibilities: Enalaprilat, famotidine
Perform/provide:
• Storage at constant temperature (15°-30° C [59°-86° F]); discard unused portions, protect from freezing
Evaluate:
• Therapeutic response: increased plasma volume

---

dextran 70/75 (℞)
(deks'tran)
Dextran 75, Gentran 70, Gentran 75, Macrodex
Func. class.: Plasma volume expander
Chem. class.: High-molecular-weight polysaccharide

Action: Similar to human albumin, which expands plasma volume by drawing fluid from interstitial spaces to intravascular space
Uses: Expand plasma volume in hypovolemic shock or impending shock

DOSAGE AND ROUTES

• *Adult:* **IV INF** 500-1000 ml not to exceed 20-40 ml/min, not to exceed 10 ml/kg/24 hr if therapy >24 hr
Available forms: 70/75 dextran in 0.9% NaCl, D_5%

SIDE EFFECTS

CV: Hypotension, ***cardiac arrest***
GI: Nausea, vomiting, increased AST, ALT
GU: ***Osmotic nephrosis, renal failure, stasis,*** hypernatremia
HEMA: Decreased hematocrit, platelet function; ***increased bleeding/coagulation times***
INTEG: Rash, urticaria, pruritus, ***angioedema,*** chills, fever, flushing

---

⚠ Safety alert   *"Tall Man" lettering

RESP: Wheezing, dyspnea, ***bronchospasm, pulmonary edema***
SYST: ***Anaphylaxis***
Contraindications: Hypersensitivity, renal failure, CHF (severe), extreme dehydration
Precautions: Pregnancy (C), active hemorrhage

PHARMACOKINETICS

IV: Onset within mins, duration 12 hr, expands blood vol 1-2 × amount infused; excreted in urine, feces

Drug/Lab Test
False increase: Blood glucose, urinary protein, bilirubin, total protein
Interference: Rh test, blood typing/crossmatching

NURSING CONSIDERATIONS
Assess:
• VS q5min × 30 min; Hgb/Hct, if falling by 30%, notify prescriber
• CVP during infusion (5-10 cm H_2O—normal range)
• Urine output q1h; watch for increase in urinary output (common); if output does not increase, decrease or discontinue infusion
• I&O ratio and specific gravity, urine osmolarity; if specific gravity is very low, renal clearance is low, drug should be discontinued
• Allergy: rash, urticaria, pruritus, wheezing, dyspnea, bronchospasm; drug should be discontinued immediately
⚠ Circulatory overload: increased pulse, respirations, SOB, wheezing, chest tightness, chest pain
• Dehydration after infusion: decreased output, increased temp, poor skin turgor, increased specific gravity, dry skin
Administer:
• After prescribed dilution, may give initial 500 mg at 20-40 ml/min, reduce flow to lowest rate
• After crossmatch is drawn, if blood is to be given also
• D_5W sol in heart failure patients as ordered

Perform/provide:
• Storage at constant temperature (<25° C [77° F]); discard unused portions; do not use unless clear
Evaluate:
• Therapeutic response: increased plasma volume

---

dextroamphetamine (℞)
(dex-troe-am-fet′a-meen)
Dexedrine, dextroamphetamine, Dexedrine Spansule, DextroStat
Func. class.: Cerebral stimulant
Chem. class.: Amphetamine

Controlled Substance Schedule II
Action: Increases release of norepinephrine, dopamine in cerebral cortex to reticular activating system
Uses: Narcolepsy, attention deficit disorder with hyperactivity (ADHD)
Investigational use: Obesity

DOSAGE AND ROUTES
Narcolepsy
• *Adult:* **PO** 5-60 mg daily in divided doses
• *Child >12 yr:* **PO** 10 mg daily increasing by 10 mg/day at weekly intervals
• *Child 6-12 yr:* **PO** 5 mg daily increasing by 5 mg/wk (max 60 mg/day)
ADHD
• *Adult:* **PO** 5-60 mg/day in divided doses
• *Child >6 yr:* **PO** 5 mg daily-bid increasing by 5 mg/day at weekly intervals
• *Child 3-6 yr:* **PO** 2.5 mg daily increasing by 2.5 mg/day at weekly intervals
Available forms: Tabs 5, 10 mg; caps sus rel (Dexedrine Spansule) 5, 10, 15 mg

SIDE EFFECTS
CNS: Hyperactivity, insomnia, restlessness, talkativeness, dizziness, headache, chills, stimulation, dysphoria, irritability,

aggressiveness, tremor, dependence, addiction

CV: Palpitations, tachycardia, hypertension, decrease in heart rate, ***dysrhythmias***

GI: Anorexia, dry mouth, diarrhea, constipation, weight loss, metallic taste

GU: Impotence, change in libido

INTEG: Urticaria

Contraindications: Hypersensitivity to sympathomimetic amines, hyperthyroidism, hypertension, glaucoma, severe arteriosclerosis, drug abuse, cardiovascular disease, anxiety, anorexia nervosa, tartrazine dye hypersensitivity

Precautions: Pregnancy (C), Gilles de la Tourette's disorder, lactation, child <3 yr, depression

PHARMACOKINETICS

PO: Onset 30 min, peak 1-3 hr, duration 4-20 hr; metabolized by liver; urine excretion pH dependent; crosses placenta, breast milk; half-life 10-30 hr

INTERACTIONS

Delayed absorption of barbiturates, phenytoin

⚠ Hypertensive crisis: MAOIs or within 14 days of MAOIs

Increase: dextroamphetamine effect—acetaZOLAMIDE, antacids, sodium bicarbonate

Increase: CNS effect—haloperidol, tricyclics, phenothiazines

Decrease: dextroamphetamine effect—ascorbic acid, ammonium chloride

Decrease: effect of adrenergic blockers, antidiabetics

Drug/Herb

Serotonin syndrome: St. John's wort

Increase: stimulant effect—khat

Decrease: stimulant effect—eucalyptus

Drug/Food

Increase: amine effect—caffeine

NURSING CONSIDERATIONS

Assess:

• VS, B/P; this drug may reverse

antihypertensives; check patients with cardiac disease often

• CBC, urinalysis; in diabetes: blood glucose, urine glucose; insulin changes may be required, since eating will decrease

• Height, growth rate in children; growth rate may be decreased

• Mental status: mood, sensorium, affect, stimulation, insomnia, irritability

• Tolerance or dependency: an increased amount may be used to get same effect; will develop after long-term use

• Overdose: pain, fever, dehydration, insomnia, hyperactivity

Administer:

• Do not break, crush, or chew sus rel forms

• At least 6 hr before bedtime to avoid sleeplessness

Perform/provide:

• Gum, hard candy, frequent sips of water for dry mouth

Evaluate:

• Therapeutic response: increased CNS stimulation, decreased drowsiness

Teach patient/family:

• To decrease caffeine consumption (coffee, tea, cola, chocolate); may increase irritability, stimulation

• To avoid OTC preparations unless approved by prescriber

• To taper drug over several wk; depression, increased sleeping, lethargy

• To avoid alcohol ingestion

• To avoid hazardous activities until stabilized on medication

• To get needed rest; patient will feel more tired at end of day

Treatment of overdose: Administer fluids, hemodialysis, or peritoneal dialysis; antihypertensive for increased B/P, ammonium Cl for increased excretion

---

⚠ Safety alert   *"Tall Man" lettering

dextromethorphan

(otc)

(dex-troe-meth-or′fan)
Balminil DM ✦, Benylin DM ✦, Broncho-Grippol-DM ✦, Children's Hold, Creo-Terpin, Delsym, dextromethorphan, Hold DM, Koffex ✦, Neo-DM ✦, Orex DM ✦, Pertussin, Pertussin ES, Robidex ✦, Robitussin Cough Calmers, Robitussin Pediatric, Sedatuss ✦, St. Joseph Cough Suppressant, Scot-Tussin DM, Sucrets Cough Control, Suppress, Vicks Formula 44

Func. class.: Antitussive, nonopioid
Chem. class.: Levorphanol derivative

Action: Depresses cough center in medulla by direct effect
Uses: Nonproductive cough
Investigational uses: Neuropathy

DOSAGE AND ROUTES

• *Adult and child ≥12 yr:* **PO** 10-20 mg q4h, or 30 mg q6-8h, not to exceed 120 mg/day; **SUS-REL LIQ** 60 mg q12h, not to exceed 120 mg/day
• *Child 6-12 yr:* **PO** 5-10 mg q4h; **SUS-REL LIQ** 30 mg bid, not to exceed 60 mg/day; **LOZ** 5-10 mg q1-4 h, max 60 mg/day
• *Child 2-6 yr:* **PO** 2.5-5 mg q4h, or 7.5 mg q6-8h, not to exceed 30 mg/day
Neuropathy
• *Adult:* **PO** doses vary widely
Available forms: Loz 2.5, 5, 7.5, 15 mg; sol; liq 3.5 mg, 7.5, 15 mg/5 ml, 3.5, 5, 7.5, 10, 15 mg/5 ml; syr 15 mg/15 ml, 10 mg/5 ml; sus action liq equivalent to 30 mg/5 ml; caps 30 mg; ext rel susp 30 mg/5 ml; gel caps 15 mg

SIDE EFFECTS

CNS: Dizziness, sedation
GI: Nausea

Contraindications: Hypersensitivity, asthma/emphysema, productive cough
Precautions: Pregnancy (C), nausea/vomiting, fever, persistent headache

PHARMACOKINETICS

PO: Onset 15-30 min, duration 3-6 hr
SUS: Duration 12 hr

INTERACTIONS

Do not give with MAOIs or within 2 wk of MAOIs
Increase: CNS depression—alcohol, antidepressants, antihistamines, opioids, sedative/hypnotics
Increase: adverse reactions—amiodarone, fluoxetine, quinidine, sibutramine

NURSING CONSIDERATIONS

Assess:
• Cough: type, frequency, character, including sputum
Administer:
• Decreased dose to elderly patients; metabolism may be slowed
Perform/provide:
• Increased fluids to liquefy secretions
• Humidification of patient's room
Evaluate:
• Therapeutic response: absence of cough
Teach patient/family:
• To avoid driving, other hazardous activities until patient is stabilized on this medication
• To avoid smoking, smoke-filled rooms, perfumes, dust, environmental pollutants, cleaners that increase cough
• To avoid alcohol, CNS depressants
• To notify prescriber if cough persists over a few days

dextrose (D-glucose) (℞)
Glucose, Glutose, Insta-Glucose
Func. class.: Caloric

Action: Needed for adequate utilization of amino acids; decreases protein, nitrogen loss; prevents ketosis
Uses: Increases intake of calories; increases fluids in patients unable to take adequate fluids, calories orally; acute hypoglycemia

DOSAGE AND ROUTES
• *Adult and child:* IV depends on individual requirements
Available forms: Inj 2.5%, 5%, 10%, 20%, 30%, 40%, 50%, 60%, 70%; oral gel 40%; chew tab 5 g

SIDE EFFECTS
CNS: Confusion, *loss of consciousness,* dizziness
CV: Hypertension, *CHF, pulmonary edema*
ENDO: Hyperglycemia, rebound hypoglycemia, hyperosmolar syndrome, hyperglycemic nonketotic syndrome
GU: Glycosuria, osmotic diuresis
INTEG: Chills, flushing, warm feeling, rash, urticaria, extravasation necrosis
Contraindications: Hyperglycemia, delirium tremens, hemorrhage (cranial/spinal), CHF
Precautions: Renal, hepatic, cardiac disease, diabetes mellitus

INTERACTIONS
Increase: fluid retention/electrolyte excretion—corticosteroids

NURSING CONSIDERATIONS
Assess:
• Electrolytes (K, Na, Ca, Cl, Mg), blood glucose, ammonia, phosphate
• Inj site for extravasation: redness along vein, edema at site, necrosis, pain; hard, tender area; site should be changed immediately
• Monitor temp q4h for increased fever, indicating infection; if infection suspected, infusion is discontinued, tubing, bottle, catheter tip cultured
• Serum glucose in patients receiving hypotonic glucose 50% and over
• Nutritional status: calorie count by dietitian
Administer:
• Only (4%) protein and dextrose (up to 12.5%) via peripheral vein; stronger sol: central IV administration
• May be given undiluted via prepared sol; give 10% sol, 5 ml/15 sec; 10% sol, 1000 ml/3 hr or more; 20% sol, 500 ml/½-1 hr; 50% sol, 10 ml/min; control rate, rapid infusions may cause fluid shifts
• Oral glucose preparations (gel, chew tabs) are to be used in conscious patients only; check serum blood glucose after first dose
• After changing IV catheter, dressing q24h with aseptic technique
Evaluate:
• Therapeutic response: increased weight
Teach patient/family:
• The reason for dextrose infusion
• To review hypoglycemia/hyperglycemia symptoms
• To review blood glucose monitoring procedure

diazepam (℞)
(dye-az'-e-pam)
Apo-Diazepam ✦, Diazemuls ✦, diazepam, Novodiapam ✦, PMS-Diazepam ✦, Valium, Vivol ✦
Func. class.: Antianxiety, anticonvulsant, skeletal muscle relaxant, central acting
Chem. class.: Benzodiazepine

Controlled Substance Schedule IV
Do not confuse:
diazepam/Ditropan/lorazepam

Action: Potentiates the actions of GABA, especially in limbic system, reticular formation; enhances pre-sympathetic inhibition, inhibits spinal polysynaptic afferent paths

Uses: Anxiety, acute alcohol withdrawal, adjunct in seizure disorders; preoperatively as a relaxant, skeletal muscle relaxation; rectally for acute repetitive seizures

Investigational uses: Panic attacks

DOSAGE AND ROUTES

Anxiety/convulsive disorders
• *Adult:* **PO** 2-10 mg bid-qid
• *Geriatric:* **PO** 1-2 mg daily-bid, increase slowly as needed
• *Child >6 mo:* **PO** 1-2.5 mg tid-qid

Precardioversion
• *Adult:* **IV** 5-15 mg 5-10 min precardioversion

Preendoscopy
• *Adult:* **IV** 2.5-20 mg; **IM** 5-10 mg ½ hr preendoscopy

Muscle relaxation
• *Adult:* **PO** 2-10 mg tid-qid or **EXT REL** 15-30 mg daily; **IV/IM** 5-10 mg repeat in 2-4 hr
• *Geriatric:* **PO** 2-5 mg bid-qid; **IV/IM** 2-5 mg, may repeat in 2-4 hr

Tetanic muscle spasms
• *Child >5 yr:* **IM/IV** 5-10 mg q3-4h prn
• *Infant >30 days:* **IM/IV** 1-2 mg q3-4h prn

Status epilepticus
• *Adult:* **IV/IM** 5-10 mg, 2 mg/min, may repeat q10-15min, not to exceed 30 mg; may repeat in 2-4 hr if seizures reappear
• *Child 1 mo-5 yr:* **IV/IM** 0.2-0.5 mg slowly q2-5min up to 5 mg
• *Child >5 yr:* **IV/IM** 1 mg q2-5min max 10 mg, may repeat in 2-4 hr
• *Adult:* **RECT** 0.2 mg/kg, may repeat 4-12 hr later
• *Child 6-11 yr:* **RECT** 0.3 mg/kg, may repeat 4-12 hr later
• *Child 2-5 yr:* **RECT** 0.5 mg/kg, may repeat 4-12 hr later

Alcohol withdrawal
• *Adult:* **PO** 10 mg tid-qid in 1st 24 hr, then 5 mg tid-qid; **IV/IM** 10 mg, then 5-10 mg after 3 hr

Psychoneurotic reactions
• *Adult:* **IV/IM** 2-10 mg, may repeat in 3-4 hr

Available forms: Tabs 2, 5, 10 mg; inj 5 mg/ml; oral sol 5 mg/5 ml; gel, rectal delivery system 2.5, 5, 10, 15, 20 mg, twin packs

SIDE EFFECTS

CNS: Dizziness, drowsiness, confusion, headache, anxiety, tremors, stimulation, fatigue, depression, insomnia, hallucinations
*CV: Orthostatic hypotension, **ECG changes, tachycardia,*** hypotension
EENT: Blurred vision, tinnitus, mydriasis, nystagmus
GI: Constipation, dry mouth, nausea, vomiting, anorexia, diarrhea
*HEMA: **Neutropenia***
INTEG: Rash, dermatitis, itching
*RESP: **Respiratory depression***
Contraindications: Pregnancy (D), hypersensitivity to benzodiazepines, narrow-angle glaucoma, psychosis, lactation, coma, respiratory depression
Precautions: Elderly, debilitated, hepatic disease, renal disease, addiction, child <6 mo

PHARMACOKINETICS

PO: Rapidly absorbed; onset ½ hr, duration 2-3 hr
IM: Onset 15-30 min, duration 1-1½ hr; absorption slow and erratic
IV: Onset immediate, duration 15 min–1 hr
Metabolized by liver, excreted by kidneys, crosses placenta, excreted in breast milk, crosses the blood-brain barrier; half-life 20-50 hr, more reliable by mouth

INTERACTIONS

Increase: toxicity—barbiturates, SSRIs, cimetidine, CNS depressants, valproic acid

---

Side effects: *italics* = common; **bold italics** = life-threatening

Increase: CNS depression—CNS depressants, alcohol
Decrease: diazepam metabolism—oral contraceptives, valproic acid, disulfiram, isoniazid, propranolol

Drug/Herb
Increase: diazepam action—cowslip, goldenseal, kava, melatonin, mistletoe, pokeweed, poppy, Queen Anne's lace, valerian
Decrease: diazepam effect—cola tree

Drug/Lab Test
Increase: AST/ALT, serum bilirubin
Decrease: RAIU
False increase: 17-OHCS

NURSING CONSIDERATIONS

Assess:
• B/P (lying, standing), pulse; respiratory rate; if systolic B/P drops 20 mm Hg, hold drug, notify prescriber; respirations q5-15min if given IV
• Blood studies: CBC during long-term therapy; blood dyscrasias (rare)
• Degree of anxiety; what precipitates anxiety and whether drug controls symptoms
• For alcohol withdrawal symptoms, including hallucinations (visual, auditory), delirium, irritability, agitation, fine to coarse tremors
• For seizure control and type, duration, intensity of convulsions
• Hepatic studies: AST, ALT, bilirubin, creatinine, LDH, alk phosphatase
• IV site for thrombosis or phlebitis, which may occur rapidly
• Mental status: mood, sensorium, affect, sleeping pattern, drowsiness, dizziness
• Physical dependency, withdrawal symptoms: headache, nausea, vomiting, muscle pain, weakness after long-term use
• Suicidal tendencies

Administer:
• With food or milk for GI symptoms; crushed if patient is unable to swallow medication whole
• Sugarless gum, hard candy, frequent sips of water for dry mouth

• Reduced opioid dose by ⅓ if given concomitantly with diazepam

IV route
• Into large vein; give IV 5 mg or less/1 min or total dose over 3 min or more (children, infants); continuous infusion is not recommended

Additive compatibilities: Netilmicin, verapamil
Syringe compatibilities: Cimetidine
Y-site compatibilities: Cefmetazole, DOBUTamine, nafcillin, quinidine, sufentanil

Rectal route
• Do not use more than 5 ×/mo or for an episode q5d

Perform/provide:
• Assistance with ambulation during beginning therapy, for drowsiness, dizziness, safety measures
• Check to see PO medication has been swallowed

Evaluate:
• Therapeutic response: decreased anxiety, restlessness, insomnia

Teach patient/family:
• That drug may be taken with food
• That drug is not to be used for everyday stress or used longer than 4 mo unless directed by prescriber; no more than prescribed amount; may be habit forming
• To avoid OTC preparations unless approved by prescriber
• To avoid driving, activities that require alertness; drowsiness may occur
• To avoid alcohol, other psychotropic medications unless directed by prescriber; that smoking may decrease diazepam effect, by increasing diazepam metabolism
• Not to discontinue medication abruptly after long-term use
• To rise slowly or fainting may occur, especially in elderly
• That drowsiness may worsen at beginning of treatment
• To avoid use during pregnancy

Treatment of overdose: Lavage, VS, supportive care, flumazenil

diazoxide (℞)
(dye-az-ox′ide)
diazoxide parenteral,
Hyperstat IV
Func. class.: Antihypertensive
Chem. class.: Vasodilator

Action: Vasodilates arteriolar smooth muscle by direct relaxation; a reduction in blood pressure with concomitant increases in heart rate, cardiac output; reduces release of insulin from the pancreas

Uses: Hypertensive crisis when urgent decrease of diastolic pressure required; increase blood glucose levels in hyperinsulinism

DOSAGE AND ROUTES
Hypoglycemia
• *Adult and child:* **PO** 3-8 mg/kg/day in 2-3 divided doses q8-12h
• *Infants and neonates:* **PO** 8-15 mg/kg/day in 2-3 divided doses 8-12h
Hypertension
• *Adult:* **IV BOL** 1-3 mg/kg rapidly up to a max of 150 mg in a single inj; dose may be repeated at 5-15 min intervals until desired response is achieved; give IV in 30 sec or less
• *Child:* **IV BOL** 1-2 mg/kg rapidly; administration same as adult, not to exceed 150 mg
Available forms: Caps 50 mg; oral susp 50 mg/ml; inj 15 mg/ml, 300 mg/20 ml

SIDE EFFECTS
CNS: Headache, sleepiness, euphoria, anxiety, EPS, confusion, tinnitus, blurred vision, dizziness, weakness, *seizures, cerebral ischemia, paralysis*
CV: Hypotension, T-wave changes, angina pectoris, palpitations, *supraventricular tachycardia, edema,* rebound hypertension, *shock, MI*
ENDO: Hyperglycemia in diabetics, transient hyperglycemia in nondiabetics, increased uric acid

GI: Nausea, vomiting, dry mouth
GU: Breast tenderness; increased BUN, fluid, electrolyte imbalances; Na, water retention
HEMA: Decreased Hgb, Hct, *thrombocytopenia*
INTEG: Rash

Contraindications: Hypersensitivity to thiazides, sulfonamides, hypertension of aortic coarctation or AV shunt, pheochromocytoma, dissecting aortic aneurysm

Precautions: Pregnancy (C), tachycardia, fluid, electrolyte imbalances, lactation, impaired cerebral or cardiac circulation, children

PHARMACOKINETICS
IV: Onset 1-2 min, peak 5 min, duration 3-12 hr; **PO:** onset 1 hr, peak 8-12 hr, duration 8 hr, half-life 20-36 hr, excreted slowly in urine, crosses blood-brain barrier, placenta; highly protein bound (>90%)

INTERACTIONS
Hyperglycemia: sulfonylureas
Severe hypotension: antihypertensives
Increase: hyperuricemic, antihypertensive effects of diazoxide—thiazide diuretics
Decrease: anticonvulsant effect—hydantoins
Drug/Herb
Toxicity/death: aconite

NURSING CONSIDERATIONS
Assess:
• B/P q5min until stabilized, then q1h × 2 hr, then q4h
• Pulse, jugular venous distention q4h
• Electrolytes, blood studies: K, Na, Cl, CO_2, CBC, serum glucose
• Weight daily, I&O
• Edema in feet, legs daily
• Skin turgor, mucous membranes for hydration status
• Crackles, dyspnea, orthopnea
• IV site for extravasation

- Signs of CHF: dyspnea, edema, wet crackles
- Postural hypotension, take B/P sitting, standing

Administer:
- Undiluted; give over ½ min or less
- To patient in recumbent position; keep in that position for 1 hr after administration

Syringe compatibilities: Heparin
Perform/provide:
- Store protected from light

Evaluate:
- Therapeutic response: decreased B/P, primarily diastolic pressure

Treatment of overdose: DOPamine, or norepinephrine for hypotension, Trendelenburg maneuver

---

dibucaine topical
See Appendix C

---

diclofenac ophthalmic
See Appendix C

---

diclofenac potassium (R)
(dye-kloe'fen-ak)
Cataflam, Voltaren Rapide ✸
diclofenac sodium
Apo-Dilo ✸, Novo-Difenac ✸, Nu-Diclo, Voltaren, Voltaren-XR

Func. class.: Nonsteroidal antiinflammatory (NSAIDs), nonopioid analgesic
Chem. class.: Phenylacetic acid

Do not confuse:
Cataflam/Catapres
Action: Inhibits prostaglandin synthesis by decreasing enzyme needed for biosynthesis; analgesic, antiinflammatory, antipyretic
Uses: Acute, chronic rheumatoid arthri-tis, osteoarthritis; ankylosing spondylitis, analgesia, primary dysmenorrhea

DOSAGE AND ROUTES
Osteoarthritis
- *Adult:* **PO** 100-150 mg/day in 2-3 divided doses

Rheumatoid arthritis
- *Adult:* **PO** 100-200 mg/day in 2-4 divided doses (potassium); 50 mg tid-qid, then reduce to lowest dose needed (25 mg tid) (sodium)

Ankylosing spondylitis
- *Adult:* **PO** 100-125 mg/day in 4-5 divided doses, give 25 mg qid and 25 mg at bedtime if needed (potassium)

Analgesia/primary dysmenorrhea
- *Adult:* **PO** 50 mg tid, max 150 mg/day (potassium)

Available forms: Potassium: tabs 50, 75 mg; sodium: tabs delayed rel (enteric-coated) 25, 50, 75 mg; ext rel tabs 75, 100 mg; supp 50, 100 mg

SIDE EFFECTS
CNS: Dizziness, headache, drowsiness, fatigue, tremors, confusion, insomnia, anxiety, depression, nervousness, paresthesia, muscle weakness
CV: CHF, tachycardia, peripheral edema, palpitations, *dysrhythmias,* hypotension, hypertension, fluid retention
EENT: Tinnitus, hearing loss, blurred vision, *laryngeal edema*
GI: Nausea, anorexia, vomiting, diarrhea, *jaundice, cholestatic hepatitis,* constipation, flatulence, cramps, dry mouth, peptic ulcer, GI bleeding, *hepatotoxicity*
GU: Nephrotoxicity: dysuria, hematuria, oliguria, azotemia, cystitis, UTI
HEMA: Blood dyscrasias, epistaxis, bruising
INTEG: Purpura, rash, pruritus, sweating, erythema, petechiae, photosensitivity, alopecia
RESP: Dyspnea, hemoptysis, pharyngitis, *bronchospasm,* rhinitis, shortness of breath
SYST: Anaphylaxis

⚠ Safety alert   ✸"Tall Man" lettering

Contraindications: Hypersensitivity to aspirin, iodides, other nonsteroidal antiinflammatory agents, asthma

Precautions: Pregnancy (B) 1st trimester, not recommended in 2nd half of pregnancy, lactation, children, bleeding disorders, GI disorders, cardiac disorders, hypersensitivity to other antiinflammatory agents, CCr <30 ml/min

PHARMACOKINETICS

PO: Peak 2-3 hr, elimination half-life 1-2 hr, 90% bound to plasma proteins, metabolized in liver to metabolite, excreted in urine

INTERACTIONS

Hyperkalemia: potassium-sparing diuretics

Need for dosage adjustment: antidiabetics

Increase: anticoagulant effect—anticoagulants

Increase: toxicity—phenytoin, lithium, cycloSPORINE, methotrexate

Increase: GI side effects—aspirin, other NSAIDs

Decrease: antihypertensive effect—β-blockers, diuretics

Drug/Herb

Severe photosensitivity—St. John's wort

Increase: bleeding risk—bogbean, chondroitin, saw palmetto, turmeric

Increase: gastric irritation—arginine, gossypol

Increase: NSAIDs effect—bearberry, bilberry

NURSING CONSIDERATIONS

Assess:

• For pain: location, character, aggravating, alleviating factors, ROM, before and 1 hr after dose

• Blood counts during therapy; watch for decreasing platelets; if low, therapy may need to be discontinued, restarted after hematologic recovery

• For clients with asthma, aspirin hypersensitivity, nasal polyps; may develop hypersensitivity

• LFTs (may be elevated) and uric acid (may be decreased—serum; increased—urine) periodically; also BUN, creatinine, electrolytes (may be elevated)

⚠ Blood dyscrasias (thrombocytopenia): bruising, fatigue, bleeding, poor healing

Administer:

• Do not break, crush, or chew enteric products

• Take with a full glass of water to enhance absorption, remain upright for ½ hr; if dose is missed, take as soon as remembered within 2 hr if taking 1-2 ×/day, do not double doses

Evaluate:

• Therapeutic response: decreased inflammation in joints, decreased inflammation after cataract surgery

Teach patient/family:

• That drug must be continued for prescribed time to be effective; to contact prescriber prior to surgery as when to discontinue this drug

• To report bleeding, bruising, fatigue, malaise; blood dyscrasias do occur

• To avoid aspirin, alcoholic beverages, NSAIDs, acetaminophen, or other OTC medications unless approved by prescriber

• To take with food, milk, or antacids to avoid GI upset, to swallow whole

• To use caution when driving; drowsiness, dizziness may occur

• To report hepatotoxicity: flulike symptoms, nausea, vomiting, jaundice, pruritus, lethargy

• To use sunscreen to prevent photosensitivity

---

dicloxacillin (℞)
(dye-klox-a-sill′-in)
dicloxacillin sodium, Dycill, Dynapen, Pathocil
Func. class.: Antiinfective
Chem. class.: Penicillinase-resistant penicillin

Do not confuse:
Pathocil/Bactocil

Action: Interferes with cell wall replication of susceptible organisms; osmotically unstable cell wall swells, bursts from osmotic pressure

Uses: Effective for gram-positive cocci (*Staphylococcus aureus, Streptococcus pyogenes, Streptococcus viridans, Streptococcus faecalis, Streptococcus bovis, Streptococcus pneumoniae*), infections caused by penicillinase-producing *Staphylococcus*

DOSAGE AND ROUTES

- *Adult/child ≥40 kg:* **PO** 125-250 mg q6h, max 4 g/day
- *Child ≤40 kg:* **PO** 12.5-25 mg/kg in divided doses q6h, max 4 g/day

Available forms: Caps 250, 500 mg

SIDE EFFECTS

CNS: Lethargy, hallucinations, anxiety, depression, twitching, ***coma, convulsions***

GI: *Nausea, vomiting, diarrhea,* increased AST, ALT, abdominal pain, glossitis, ***pseudomembranous colitis***

GU: *Oliguria, proteinuria, hematuria, vaginitis, moniliasis, **glomerulonephritis***

HEMA: Anemia, increased bleeding time, ***bone marrow depression, granulocytopenia***

SYST: ***Anaphylaxis***

Contraindications: Hypersensitivity to penicillins; neonates

Precautions: Pregnancy (B), hypersensitivity to cephalosporins, lactation, severe renal or hepatic disease

PHARMACOKINETICS

PO: Peak 1 hr, duration 4-6 hr, half-life 30-60 min; metabolized in liver; excreted in urine, bile, breast milk; crosses placenta

INTERACTIONS

Increase: dicloxacillin concentrations—probenecid

Decrease: anticoagulant effect—anticoagulants

Drug/Herb

Do not use acidophilus with antiinfectives

Decrease: absorption—khat, separate by 2 hr

Food/Drug

Citric juices/food decrease absorption of dicloxacillin

Drug/Lab Test

False positive: Urine glucose, urine protein

NURSING CONSIDERATIONS

Assess:

- I&O ratio; report hematuria, oliguria, since penicillin in high doses is nephrotoxic

⚠ Any patient with compromised renal system, since drug is excreted slowly in poor renal system function; toxicity may occur rapidly

- Blood studies: WBC, RBC, Hgb, Hct, bleeding time
- Renal studies: urinalysis, protein, blood
- C&S before drug therapy; drug may be given as soon as culture is taken
- WBC and differential, ALT, AST, BUN, creatinine for patients on long-term therapy
- Bowel pattern before, during treatment
- Anaphylaxis: pruritus, rash, dyspnea, laryngeal edema; have emergency equipment available; skin eruptions after administration of penicillin to 1 wk after discontinuing drug
- For infection: temp, draining wounds, WBC, sputum, urine, stool, before, during treatment

Administer:

- Do not break, crush, or chew caps
- Drug after C&S
- On an empty stomach with a full glass of water
- Susp after shaking well before each dose

Perform/provide:

- Adrenalin, suction, tracheostomy set, endotracheal intubation equipment
- Adequate fluid intake (2 L) during diarrhea episodes

• Scratch test to assess allergy after securing order from prescriber; usually done when penicillin is only drug of choice
• Storage in tight container; after reconstituting, store in refrigerator up to 2 wk

Evaluate:
• Therapeutic response: absence of fever, draining wounds

Teach patient/family:
• All aspects of drug therapy, including need to complete course of medication to ensure organism death (10-14 days); culture may be taken after completed course
• To report sore throat, fever, fatigue; may indicate superinfection
• To wear or carry emergency ID if allergic to penicillins
• To notify prescriber of diarrhea, fever

Treatment of anaphylaxis: Withdraw drug; maintain airway; administer epINEPHrine, aminophylline, O₂, IV corticosteroids

---

Rarely Used

dicyclomine (R̸)
(dye-sye'kloe-meen)
Antispas, Bentyl, Bentylol ✦, Byclomine, Dibent, dicyclomine HCL, Dilomine, Di-Spaz, Formulex ✦, Lomine ✦, Neoquess, Or-Tyl, Spasmoject
Func. class.: Gastrointestinal anticholinergic

Uses: Treatment of peptic ulcer disease in combination with other drugs; infant colic, urinary incontinence, IBS

DOSAGE AND ROUTES
• *Adult:* **PO** 10-20 mg tid-qid; **IM** 20 mg q4-6h
• *Child >2 yr:* **PO** 10 mg tid-qid
• *Child 6 mo-2 yr:* **PO** 5 mg tid-qid
Contraindications: Hypersensitivity to anticholinergics, narrow-angle glaucoma, GI obstruction, myasthenia gravis, paralytic ileus, GI atony, toxic megacolon

---

didanosine (R̸)
(dye-dan'oh-seen)
ddI, dideoxyinosine, Videx, Videx EC
Func. class.: Antiretroviral
Chem. class.: Nucleoside reverse transcriptase inhibitor

D

Action: Nucleoside analog incorporating into cellular DNA by viral reverse transcriptase, thereby terminating the cellular DNA chain
Uses: HIV-1 infection in combination with other antiretrovirals

DOSAGE AND ROUTES
• *Adult:* **PO** >60 kg, 200 mg bid tabs, or 250 mg bid buffered powder; caps, del rel 400 mg daily; <60 kg, 125 mg bid tabs, or 167 mg bid buffered powder; caps, del rel 250 mg daily
• *Child:* **PO** tabs 90-120 mg/m² q12h; buffered powder packets 112.5-150 mg/m² q12h; **PO** (child BSA 1.1-1.4 m²) tab 100 mg q8-12h; recon pedi powder 125 mg q8-12h; **PO** (child BSA 0.8-1 m²) tabs 75 mg q8-12h; recon pedi powder 94 mg q8-12h; **PO** (child BSA 0.5-0.7 m²) tabs 50 mg q8-12h; recon pedi powder 62 mg q8-12h; **PO** (child BSA <0.4 m²) tabs 25 mg q8-12h; recon pedi powder 31 mg q8-12h

Renal dose
• Reduce dosage CCr <60 ml/min
Available forms: Tabs, buffered, chewable/dispersible 25, 50, 100, 150, 200 mg; powder for oral sol 10 mg/ml; caps, del rel 125, 200, 250, 400

SIDE EFFECTS
CNS: **Peripheral neuropathy, seizures,** confusion, *anxiety,* hypertonia, abnormal thinking, asthenia, *insomnia,* **CNS depression,** pain, dizziness, chills, fever
CV: Hypertension, vasodilation, dysrhythmia, syncope, **CHF,** palpitation

---

EENT: Ear pain, otitis, photophobia, visual impairment, retinal depigmentation
*GI: **Pancreatitis**, diarrhea, nausea,* vomiting, *abdominal pain,* constipation, stomatitis, dyspepsia, liver abnormalities, flatulence, taste perversion, dry mouth, oral thrush, melena, increased ALT, AST, alk phosphatase, amylase, *hepatic failure*
GU: Increased bilirubin, uric acid
*HEMA: **Leukopenia, granulocytopenia, thrombocytopenia, anemia***
INTEG: Rash, pruritus, alopecia, ecchymosis, hemorrhage, petechiae, sweating
MS: Myalgia, arthritis, myopathy, muscular atrophy
RESP: Cough, pneumonia, dyspnea, asthma, epistaxis, hypoventilation, sinusitis
*SYST: **Lactic acidosis, anaphylaxis***
Contraindications: Hypersensitivity, lactic acidosis, pancreatitis, phenylketonuria
Precautions: Pregnancy (B), renal, hepatic disease, lactation, children, sodium-restricted diets, elevated amylase, preexisting peripheral neuropathy, hyperuricemia

PHARMACOKINETICS

PO: Peak 0.67 hr; del rel 2 hr; elimination half-life 1.62 hr, extensive metabolism is thought to occur; administration within 5 min of food will decrease absorption, excreted urine/feces

INTERACTIONS

Increase: didanosine level—allopurinol, tenofovir, adjust dose as needed
Increase: side effects from magnesium, aluminum antacids
Decrease: absorption—ketoconazole, dapsone
Decrease: concentrations of fluoroquinolones, other antiretrovirals, itraconazole, tetracyclines
Decrease: didanosine level—methadone
Drug/Food
Any food decreases rate of absorption
Do not use with acidic juices

NURSING CONSIDERATIONS
Assess:
• Peripheral neuropathy: tingling or pain in hands and feet, distal numbness; onset usually occurs 2-6 mo after beginning treatment, may persist if drug is not discontinued
⚠ Pancreatitis: abdominal pain, nausea, vomiting, elevated hepatic enzymes; drug should be discontinued, since condition can be fatal
• For anaphylaxis, lactic acidosis
• Children by dilated retinal exam q6mo to rule out retinal depigmentation
• CBC, differential, platelet count qmo; withhold drug if WBC is <4000 or platelet count is <75,000; notify prescriber of results; alk phosphatase, monitor amylase; viral load, CD4 count
• Renal studies: BUN, serum uric acid, urine CCr before, during therapy
• Temp q4h, may indicate beginning infection
• Hepatic studies before, during therapy (bilirubin, AST, ALT) as needed or qmo
Administer:
• Pediatric powder for oral sol after preparation by pharmacist; dilution is required using purified USP water, then antacid (10 mg/ml), refrigerate, shake before use
• On an empty stomach ≥30 min, ac or 2 hr pc
• Adjust dose in renal impairment
Perform/provide:
• Cleanup of powdered products; use wet mop or damp sponge
• Storage of tabs, caps in tightly closed bottle at room temperature; store oral sol after dissolving at room temperature ≤4 hr
Evaluate:
• Therapeutic response: absence of infection; symptoms of HIV
Teach patient/family:
• To avoid use with alcohol
• To report numbness/tingling in extremities
• To take on an empty stomach; not to take dapsone at same time as ddI; do not

mix powder with fruit juice; chew tab or crush and dissolve in water; drink powder immediately after mixing
• To report signs of infection: increased temp, sore throat, flulike symptoms
• To report signs of anemia: fatigue, headache, faintness, shortness of breath, irritability
• To report bleeding; avoid use of razors, commercial mouthwash
• That hair may be lost during therapy (rare); a wig or hairpiece may make patient feel better

diflorasone topical
See Appendix C

Rarely Used

diflunisal (℞)
(dye-floo'ni-sal)
diflunisal, Dolobid
Func. class.: Nonsteroidal anti-inflammatory/analgesic (nonopioid)

Uses: Mild to moderate pain or fever including arthritis; 3-4 times more potent than aspirin

DOSAGE AND ROUTES
• *Adult:* **PO** loading dose 1 g; then 500-1000 mg/day in 2 divided doses, q12h, not to exceed 1500 mg/day
• *Geriatric:* **PO** ½ adult dose
Contraindications: Hypersensitivity to salicylates, GI bleeding, bleeding disorders, children <12 yr, vit K deficiency

⚠ High Alert

digoxin (℞)
(di-jox'in)
digoxin, Lanoxicaps, Lanoxin
Func. class.: Cardiac glycoside, inotropic, antidysrhythmic
Chem. class.: Digitalis preparation

D

Do not confuse:
Lanoxin/Lasix/Lonox/Lomotil/Xanax/Levoxine
Action: Inhibits the sodium-potassium ATPase, which makes more calcium available for contractile proteins, resulting in increased cardiac output; increases force of contraction (+ inotropic effect); decreases heart rate (chronotropic effect); decreases AV conduction speed
Uses: CHF, atrial fibrillation, atrial flutter, atrial tachycardia, cardiogenic shock, paroxysmal atrial tachycardia, rapid digitalization in these disorders

DOSAGE AND ROUTES
• *Adult:* **IV** *digitalizing dose* 0.6-1 mg given as 50% of the dose initially, additional fractions given at 4-8 hr intervals; **PO digitalizing dose** 0.75-1.25 mg given as 50% of the dose initially, additional fractions given at 4-8 hr intervals; **maintenance** 0.063-0.5 mg/day (tabs), or 0.350-0.5 mg/day (gelatin cap)
• *Child >10 yr:* **IV digitalizing dose** 8-12 mcg/kg given as 50% of the dose initially, additional fractions given at 4-8 hr intervals; **PO digitalizing dose** 0.01-0.015 mg/kg given as 50% of the dose initially, additional fractions given at 6-8 hr intervals; **maintenance** 25%-35% of the loading dose daily as a single dose
• *Child 5-10 yr:* **IV digitalizing dose** 0.015-0.03 mg/kg given as 50% of the dose initially, additional fractions given at 4-8 hr intervals; **PO digitalizing dose** 0.02-0.035 mg/kg given as 50% of the dose initially, additional fractions given at 6-8 hr intervals; **maintenance** 25%-

35% of the loading dose daily in 2 divided doses

- **Child 2-5 yr:** **IV digitalizing dose** 0.025-0.035 mg/kg given as 50% of the dose initially, additional fractions given at 4-8 hr intervals; **PO digitalizing dose** 0.03-0.04 mg/kg given as 50% of the dose initially, additional fractions given at 6-8 hr intervals; **maintenance** 25%-35% of the loading dose daily in 2 divided doses
- **Child 1-2 yr:** **IV digitalizing dose** 0.03-0.05 mg/kg given as 50% of the dose initially, additional fractions given at 4-8 hr intervals; **PO digitalizing dose** 0.035-0.06 mg/kg given as 50% of the dose initially, additional fractions given at 4-8 hr intervals; **maintenance** 25%-35% of the loading dose daily in 2 divided doses
- **Infants:** **IV digitalizing dose** 0.02-0.03 mg/kg given as 50% of the dose initially, additional fractions given at 4-8 hr intervals; **PO digitalizing dose** 0.025-0.035 mg/kg given as 50% of the dose initially, additional fractions given at 6-8 hr intervals; **maintenance** 25%-35% of the loading dose daily in 2 divided doses
- **Infants, premature:** **IV digitalizing dose** 0.015-0.025 mg/kg given as 50% of the dose initially, additional fractions given at 4-8 hr intervals; **PO digitalizing dose** 0.02-0.03 mg/kg given as 50% of the dose initially, additional fractions given at 6-8 hr intervals; **maintenance** 20%-30% of the loading dose daily in 2 divided doses

Available forms: Caps 0.05, 0.1, 0.2 mg; elix 0.05 mg/ml; tabs 0.125, 0.25, 0.5 mg; inj 0.5 ✿, 0.25 mg/ml: pediatric inj 0.1 mg/ml

SIDE EFFECTS

CNS: Headache, drowsiness, apathy, confusion, disorientation, fatigue, depression, hallucinations

*CV: **Dysrhythmias,** hypotension,* bradycardia, ***AV block***

EENT: Blurred vision, yellow-green halos, photophobia, diplopia

GI: Nausea, vomiting, anorexia, abdominal pain, diarrhea

Contraindications: Hypersensitivity to digitalis, ventricular fibrillation, ventricular tachycardia, carotid sinus syndrome, 2nd- or 3rd-degree heart block

Precautions: Pregnancy (C), renal disease, acute MI, AV block, severe respiratory disease, hypothyroidism, elderly, sinus nodal disease, lactation, hypokalemia

PHARMACOKINETICS

PO: Onset ½-2 hr, peak 6-8 hr, duration 3-4 days

IV: Onset 5-30 min, peak 1-5 hr, duration variable

Half-life 1.5 days, excreted in urine

INTERACTIONS

Hypercalcemia, hypomagnesemia, digitalis toxicity: thiazides, parenteral calcium

Hypokalemia, digitalis toxicity: diuretics, amphotericin B, carbenicillin, ticarcillin, corticosteroids

Increase: digoxin levels—propantheline, quinidine, verapamil, amiodarone, anticholinergics, diltiazem, NIFEdipine

Increase: bradycardia—β-adrenergic blockers, antidysrythmics

Increase: cardiac dysrhythmia risk—sympathomimetics

Decrease: digoxin absorption—antacids, kaolin/pectin

Decrease: digoxin level—thyroid agents, cholestyramine, colestipol, metoclopramide

Drug/Herb

Forms insoluble complex: blackroot

Bradycardia: Indian snakeroot

Cardiac toxicity: aconite, hawthorn, horsetail

Increase: digoxin action—aloe, betel palm, broom, buckthorn, cascara sagrada, castor, Chinese rhubarb, figwort, fumitory, hawthorn, khat, kudzu, licorice, lily of the valley, Mayapple, mistletoe, motherwort, night-blooming cereus, oleander, pheasant's eye, purple foxglove, Queen Anne's lace, rhubarb, rue, senna, Siberian ginseng, squill, yellow dock

Increase: hypokalemia—cocoa, coffee, cola, guarana, horsetail, licorice, yerba maté

Decrease: digoxin absorption—psyllium

Decrease: digoxin effect—beth root, goldenseal, St. John's wort

Drug/Lab Test
Increase: CPK

NURSING CONSIDERATIONS
Assess:
• Apical pulse for 1 min before giving drug; if pulse <60 in adult or <90 in an infant, take again in 1 hr; if <60 in adult, call prescriber; note rate, rhythm, character; monitor ECG continuously during parenteral loading dose
• Electrolytes: K, Na, Cl, Mg, Ca; renal function studies: BUN, creatinine; blood studies: ALT, AST, bilirubin, Hct, Hgb before initiating treatment and periodically thereafter
• I&O ratio, daily weights; monitor turgor, lung sounds, edema
• Monitor drug levels (therapeutic level 0.5-2 ng/ml)
• Cardiac status: apical pulse, character, rate, rhythm

Administer:
PO route
• Do not break, crush, or chew caps
• PO with or without food; may crush tabs, only mix with food/fluids
• Potassium supplements if ordered for potassium levels <3, or foods high in potassium: bananas, orange juice

IV route
• Undiluted or 1 ml of drug/4 ml sterile H₂O, D₅, or NS; give >5 min through Y-tube or 3-way stopcock; during digitalization close monitoring is necessary

Additive compatibilities: Bretylium, cimetidine, floxacillin, furosemide, lidocaine, ranitidine, verapamil

Syringe compatibilities: Heparin, milrinone

Y-site compatibilities: Amrinone, cefmetazole, ciprofloxacin, cisatracurium, diltiazem, famotidine, meperidine, meropenem, midazolam, milrinone, morphine, potassium chloride, propofol, remifentanil, tacrolimus, vit B/C

Perform/provide:
• Storage protected from light

Evaluate:
• Therapeutic response: decreased weight, edema, pulse, respiration, crackles; increased urine output; serum digoxin level (0.5-2 ng/ml)

Teach patient/family:
• Not to stop drug abruptly; teach all aspects of drug, to take exactly as ordered; how to monitor heart rate
• To avoid OTC medications, herbal remedies since many adverse drug interactions may occur; do not take antacid at same time
• To notify prescriber of loss of appetite, lower stomach pain, diarrhea, weakness, drowsiness, headache, blurred or yellow vision, rash, depression, toxicity
• The toxic symptoms of this drug and when to notify prescriber
• To maintain a sodium-restricted diet as ordered
• To report shortness of breath, difficulty breathing, weight gain, edema, persistent cough

Treatment of overdose: Discontinue drug; give potassium; monitor ECG; give adrenergic-blocking agent, digoxin immune FAB

---

digoxin immune FAB (ovine) (℞)
(di-jox'in im-myoon' FAB)
Digibind, DigiFab
Func. class.: Antidote—digoxin specific

Action: Antibody fragments bind to free digoxin or digitoxin to reverse toxicity by not allowing digoxin or digitoxin to bind to sites of action

Uses: Life-threatening digoxin toxicity

Side effects: *italics* = common; ***bold italics*** = life-threatening

DOSAGE AND ROUTES

1 (38 mg) vial binds 0.5 mg digoxin

Digoxin toxicity (known amount) (tabs, oral sol, IM)
• *Adult/child:* IV dose (mg) = dose ingested (mg) × 0.8/1000 × 38; if ingested amount is unknown, give 760 mg IV

Toxicity (known amount) (cap, IV)
• *Adult/child:* IV dose = dose ingested (mg)/0.5 × 38

Toxicity (known amount) by serum digoxin concentrations (SDCs)
• *Adult/child:* IV SDC (nanograms/ml) × kg of weight/100 × 38

Digoxin toxicity (unknown amount)
• *Adult/child >20 kg:* IV 228 mg (6 vials)
• *Infant/child <20 kg:* IV 38 mg (1 vial)

Skin test
• *Adult:* ID 9.5 mcg

Available forms: Inj 38 mg/vial (binds 0.5 mg digoxin), 40 mg/vial (binds 0.5 mg digoxin)

SIDE EFFECTS

CV: **CHF,** ventricular rate increase, **atrial fibrillation,** low cardiac output
INTEG: *Hypersensitivity,* allergic reactions, facial swelling, redness
META: **Hypokalemia**
MISC: **Anaphylaxis** (rare)
RESP: **Impaired respiratory function, rapid respiratory rate**

Contraindications: Mild digoxin toxicity, hypersensitivity to this product or papain

Precautions: Pregnancy (C), children, lactation, elderly, cardiac disease, renal disease, allergy to ovine proteins

PHARMACOKINETICS

IV: Peaks after completion of infusion, onset 30 min (variable); not known if crosses placenta, breast milk; half-life biphasic—14-20 hr; prolonged in renal disease; excreted by kidneys

INTERACTIONS

Considered incompatible with all drugs in syringe or sol
Drug/Lab Test
Interference: Immunoassay digoxin

NURSING CONSIDERATIONS

Assess:
• Hypokalemia: ST depression, flat T waves, presence of U wave, ventricular dysrhythmia; potassium levels may decrease rapidly
• CHF: Dyspnea, crackles, peripheral edema, weight gain >5 lb

Administer:
• Test doses have proven to be ineffective in the general population; only use test dose in those with known allergies or those previously treated with digoxin immune FAB
• For test dose dilute 0.1 ml or reconstituted drug (9.5 mg/ml) in 9.9 ml sterile isotonic saline, inj 0.1 ml (1:100 dilution) ID and observe for wheal with erythema; read in 20 min
• For scratch test place 1 gtt of sol on skin and make a scratch through the drop with a sterile needle; read in 20 min
• After diluting 38 mg/4 ml of sterile H_2O for inj 10 mg/ml mix; may be further diluted with normal saline, sol should be clear, colorless
• By bolus if cardiac arrest is imminent or IV over 30 min using a 0.22-μm filter

Perform/provide:
• Storage of reconstituted sol for up to 4 hr in refrigerator
• Do not freeze DigiFab

Evaluate:
• Therapeutic response: correction of digoxin toxicity; check digoxin levels 0.5-2 ng/ml; digitoxin level 9-25 ng/ml

Teach patient/family:
• The purpose of medication; to report delayed hypersensitivity; fever, chills, itching, swelling, dyspnea

---

dihydrotachysterol (R)
(dye-hye-droh-tak-iss′ter-ole)
DHT Intensol ✦, Hytakerol
Func. class.: Parathyroid agent (calcium regulator)
Chem. class.: Vit D analog

Action: Increases intestinal absorption of calcium for bones, increases renal tubular absorption of phosphate; regulates calcium levels by regulating calcitonin, parathyroid hormone

Uses: Renal osteodystrophy, hypoparathyroidism, pseudohypoparathyroidism, familial hypophosphatemia, postoperative tetany

DOSAGE AND ROUTES
Hypophosphatemia
• *Adult/child:* PO 0.5-2 mg daily, maintenance 0.2-1.5 mg daily
Hypoparathyroidism/pseudohypoparathyroidism
• *Adult:* PO 0.8-2.4 mg daily × 4 days, maintenance 0.2-2 mg daily regulated by serum calcium levels
• *Neonates:* PO 0.05-0.1 mg/day
• *Infants, young child:* PO 0.1-0.5 mg/day
• *Older child:* PO 0.5-1 mg/day
Renal osteodystrophy
• *Adult:* PO 0.25-0.375 mg/day
• *Child:* PO 0.125-0.5 mg/day
Rickets (Vit. D—resistant)
• *Child:* PO 0.25-1 mg/day
Available forms: Tabs 0.125, 0.2, 0.4 mg; caps 0.125 mg; oral sol 0.2, 0.25 mg/5 ml, 0.2 mg/ml ✦ (Intensol)

SIDE EFFECTS
CNS: Drowsiness, headache, vertigo, fever, lethargy, depression
CV: **Dysrhythmias,** hypertension
EENT: Tinnitus
GI: Nausea, diarrhea, vomiting, jaundice, anorexia, dry mouth, constipation, cramps, metallic taste, thirst
GU: Polyuria, hypercalciuria, hyperphos-phatemia, hematuria, nocturia, renal calculi
MS: Myalgia, arthralgia, decreased bone development, weakness, ataxia
Contraindications: Hypersensitivity, renal disease, hyperphosphatemia, hypercalcemia
Precautions: Pregnancy (C), renal calculi, lactation, CV disease

PHARMACOKINETICS
PO: Onset 2 wk; readily absorbed from small intestine; metabolized by liver, excreted in feces (active/inactive)

INTERACTIONS
Hypercalcemia: thiazide diuretics, calcium supplements
Cardiac dysrhythmias: cardiac glycosides, verapamil
Decrease: dihydrotachysterol absorption—cholestyramine, colestipol mineral oil
Decrease: dihydrotachysterol effect—corticosteroids, phenytoin, barbiturates
Drug/Lab Test
False increase: Cholesterol

NURSING CONSIDERATIONS
Assess:
• BUN, urinary Ca, AST, ALT, cholesterol, creatinine, alk phosphatase, uric acid, chlorine, magnesium, electrolytes, urine pH, phosphate; may increase calcium, should be kept at 9-10 mg/dl, vit D 50-135 international units/dl, phosphate 70 mg/dl
• Alk phosphatase: may be decreased
• For increased blood level, since toxic reactions may occur rapidly
• For dry mouth, metallic taste, polyuria, bone pain, muscle weakness, headache, fatigue, tinnitus, change in LOC, irregular pulse, dysrhythmias, increased respirations, anorexia, nausea, vomiting, cramps, diarrhea, constipation; may indicate hypercalcemia
• Renal status: decreased urinary output (oliguria, anuria), edema in extremities, weight gain >5 lb, periorbital edema

D

Side effects: *italics* = common; **bold italics** = life-threatening

- Nutritional status, diet for sources of vit D (milk, some seafood), calcium (dairy products, dark green vegetables), phosphates (dairy products) must be avoided

Administer:
- Do not break, crush, or chew caps
- PO, may be increased q4wk depending on blood level

Perform/provide:
- Storage in tight, light-resistant containers at room temperature
- Restriction of sodium, potassium if required
- Restriction of fluids if required for chronic renal failure

Evaluate:
- Therapeutic response: prevention of bone deficiencies

Teach patient/family:
- The symptoms of hypercalcemia
- About foods rich in calcium, vit D

⚠ High Alert

diltiazem (℞)

(dil-tye′a-zem)
Apo-Diltiaz ✦, Cardizem, Cardizem CD, Cardizem LA, Cardizem SR, Dilacor-XR, Diltia XR, diltiazem, Tiazac
Func. class.: Calcium channel blocker
Chem. class.: Benzothiazepine

Do not confuse:
Cardizem CD/Cardizem SR
Cardizem/Cardene
Cardizem SR/Cardene SR

Action: Inhibits calcium ion influx across cell membrane during cardiac depolarization; produces relaxation of coronary vascular smooth muscle, dilates coronary arteries, slows SA/AV node conduction times, dilates peripheral arteries

Uses: **PO:** Angina pectoris due to coronary artery spasm, hypertension, **IV:** atrial fibrillation, flutter, paroxysmal supraventricular tachycardia

DOSAGE AND ROUTES

Hypertension
- *Adult:* **PO** 60-120 mg bid **(SUS REL)** (Cardizem SR), max 540 mg/day, or 180-240 mg **(EXT REL)** daily

Prinzmetal's or variant angina, chronic stable angina
- *Adult:* **PO** 30 mg qid, increasing dose gradually to 180-360 mg/day in divided doses or 60-120 mg bid; may increase to 240-360 mg/day or 120 or 180 mg **EXT REL** (LA, CD, XT, XR products) **PO** daily

Atrial fibrillation/flutter, paroxysmal supraventricular tachycardia
- *Adult:* **IV BOL** 0.25 mg/kg over 2 min initially, then 0.35 mg/kg may be given after 15 min; if no response, may give **CONT INF** 5-15 mg/hr for up to 24 hr

Available forms: Tabs 30, 60, 90, 120 mg; tabs ext rel: 120, 180, 240, 300, 360, 420 mg; caps ext rel 60, 90, 120, 180, 240, 300, 360, 420 mg; sus rel cap 60, 90, 120 mg; inj 5 mg/ml (5, 10 ml); powder for inj 25 mg

SIDE EFFECTS

CNS: Headache, fatigue, drowsiness, dizziness, depression, weakness, insomnia, tremor, paresthesia
*CV: **Dysrhythmia**, edema, **CHF**,* bradycardia, hypotension, palpitations, ***heart block***
GI: Nausea, vomiting, diarrhea, gastric upset, *constipation,* increased LFTs
GU: Nocturia, polyuria, ***acute renal failure***
INTEG: Rash, flushing, photosensitivity, burning, pruritus at inj site
RESP: Rhinitis, dyspnea, pharyngitis

Contraindications: Sick sinus syndrome, 2nd- or 3rd-degree heart block, hypotension less than 90 mm Hg systolic, acute MI, pulmonary congestion, intracranial surgery, bleeding aneurysms, severe hypotension (systolic <90 mm Hg or diastolic <60 mm Hg)

Precautions: Pregnancy (C), CHF, hypotension, hepatic injury, lactation, children, renal disease

---

⚠ Safety alert   *"Tall Man" lettering

PHARMACOKINETICS

Onset 30-60 min; peak 2-3 hr immediate rel; 10-14 hr ext rel, 6-11 hr sus rel; half-life 3½-9 hr; metabolized by liver; excreted in urine (96% as metabolites)

INTERACTIONS

Increase: effect, toxicity—theophylline
Increase: effects of β-blockers, digoxin, lithium, carbamazepine, cyclosporine, anesthetics, HMG CoA reductase inhibitors, benzodiazepines, lovastatin
Increase: effects of diltiazem—cimetidine

Drug/Herb

Increase: diltiazem effect—barberry, betel palm, burdock, goldenseal, khat, khella, lily of the valley, plantain
Decrease: diltiazem effect—yohimbe

Drug/Food

Increase: hypotensive effects—grapefruit juice

NURSING CONSIDERATIONS

Assess:

• Cardiac status: B/P, pulse, respiration, ECG and intervals PR, QRS, QT; if systolic B/P <90 mm Hg or HR <60 bpm, hold dose, notify prescriber

Administer:

PO route

• Do not break, crush, or chew sus rel caps or sus rel tabs
• With a full glass of water before meals, bedtime (PO)
• Give ext rel, sus rel products daily; immediate rel qid
• Dilacor-XR on an empty stomach
• May sprinkle on apple sauce for administration

IV route

• IV undiluted over 2 min or diluted 125 mg/100 ml, 250 mg/250 ml of D_5W, 0.9% NaCl, D_5/0.45% NaCl, give 10 mg/hr, may increase by 5 mg/hr to 15 mg/hr, continue infusion up to 24 hr

Y-site compatibilities: Albumin, amikacin, amphotericin B, aztreonam, bretylium, bumetanide, cefazolin, cefotaxime, cefotetan, cefoxitin, ceftazidime, ceftriaxone, cefuroxime, cimetidine, ciprofloxacin, clindamycin, digoxin, DOBUTamine, DOPamine, doxycycline, epINEPHrine, erythromycin, esmolol, fentanyl, fluconazole, gentamicin, hetastarch, hydromorphone, imipenem-cilastatin, labetalol, lidocaine, lorazepam, meperidine, metoclopramide, metronidazole, midazolam, milrinone, morphine, multivitamins, niCARDipine, nitroglycerin, norepinephrine, oxacillin, penicillin G potassium, pentamidine, piperacillin, potassium chloride, potassium phosphates, ranitidine, sodium nitroprusside, theophylline, ticarcillin, ticarcillin/clavulanate, tobramycin, trimethoprim-sulfamethoxazole, vancomycin, vecuronium

Perform/provide:

• Storage in tight container at room temperature

Evaluate:

• Therapeutic response: decreased anginal pain, decreased B/P

Teach patient/family:

• How to take pulse before taking drug; record or graph should be kept
• To avoid hazardous activities until stabilized on drug, dizziness is no longer a problem
• To limit caffeine consumption
• To avoid OTC drugs unless directed by prescriber
• The importance of complying with all areas of medical regimen: diet, exercise, stress reduction, drug therapy
⚠ To report dizziness, shortness of breath, palpitations
• Not to discontinue abruptly

Treatment of overdose: Atropine for AV block, vasopressor for hypotension

*dimenhyDRINATE

(otc, ℞)

(dye-men-hye'dri-nate)

Apo-Dimenhydrate ✦, Calm-X, Children's Dramamine, dimenhyDRINATE, Dimetabs, Dinate, Dramamine, Dramanate, Dymenate, Gravol ✦, Gravol L/A ✦, Hydrate, Nauseatol ✦, Novo-Dimenate ✦, PMS-Dimenhydrinate ✦, Travamine ✦, Triptone Caplets

Func. class.: Antiemetic, antihistamine, anticholinergic

Chem. class.: H₁-Receptor antagonist, ethanolamine derivative

Do not confuse:

dimenhyDRINATE/diphenhydrAMINE

Action: Vestibular stimulation is decreased

Uses: Motion sickness, nausea, vomiting, vertigo

DOSAGE AND ROUTES

• *Adult:* **PO** 50-100 mg q4h; **IM/IV** 50 mg q4h as needed
• *Child 6-12 yr:* **PO** 25-50 mg q6-8 hr prn, max 150 mg/day
• *Child 2-5 yr:* **PO** 12.5-25 mg q6-8 hr, max 75 mg/day

Available forms: Tabs 50 mg; inj 50 mg/ml; elixir 15 mg/5 ml ✦, chew tabs 50 mg

SIDE EFFECTS

CNS: Drowsiness, restlessness, headache, dizziness, insomnia, confusion, nervousness, tingling, vertigo
CV: Hypertension, *hypotension,* palpitation
EENT: Dry mouth, blurred vision, diplopia, nasal congestion, photosensitivity
GI: Nausea, anorexia, vomiting, *constipation*

INTEG: Rash, urticaria, fever, chills, flushing
*MISC: **Anaphylaxis***

Contraindications: Hypersensitivity to opioids, shock

Precautions: Pregnancy (B), children, cardiac dysrhythmias, elderly, asthma, lactation, prostatic hypertrophy, bladder-neck obstruction, narrow-angle glaucoma, stenosing peptic ulcer, pyloro-duodenal obstruction

PHARMACOKINETICS

IM/PO: Duration 4-6 hr

INTERACTIONS

Increase: effect—alcohol, other CNS depressants
Drug/Herb
Increase: anticholinergic effect—corkwood, henbane
Increase: effect—hops, Jamaican dogwood, khat, senega
Drug/Lab Test
False negative: Allergy skin testing

NURSING CONSIDERATIONS

Assess:
• VS, B/P; check patients with cardiac disease more often
• Signs of toxicity of other drugs or masking of symptoms of disease: brain tumor, intestinal obstruction
• Observe for drowsiness, dizziness
Administer:
• IM inj in large muscle mass; aspirate to avoid IV administration
• Tablets may be swallowed whole, chewed, or allowed to dissolve
IV route
• After diluting 50 mg/10 ml of NaCl inj; give 50 mg or less over 2 min
Additive compatibilities: Amikacin, calcium gluconate, chloramphenicol, corticotropin, erythromycin, heparin, hydrOXYzine, methicillin, norepinephrine, penicillin G potassium, pentobarbital, phenobarbital, potassium chloride, prochlorperazine, vancomycin, vit B/C
Syringe compatibilities: Atropine,

⚠ Safety alert   *"Tall Man" lettering

diphenhydrAMINE, droperidol, fentanyl, heparin, hydromorphone, meperidine, metoclopramide, morphine, pentazocine, perphenazine, ranitidine, scopolamine

Y-site compatibilities: Acyclovir

• Therapeutic response: absence of nausea, vomiting

Teach patient/family:

• That a false-negative result may occur with skin testing; these procedures should not be scheduled for 4 days after discontinuing use

• To avoid hazardous activities, activities requiring alertness; dizziness may occur; instruct patient to request assistance with ambulation

• To avoid alcohol, other depressants

Rarely Used

dimercaprol (℞)
(dye-mer-cap'role)
BAL in Oil, British
Anti-Lewisite ✤,
dimercaptopropanol
Func. class.: Heavy metal antagonist

Uses: Arsenic, gold, mercury, lead poisoning

DOSAGE AND ROUTES

Severe gold/arsenic poisoning

• *Adult:* IM 3 mg/kg q4h × 2 days then qid × 1 day, then bid × 10 days

Mild gold/arsenic poisoning

• *Adult:* IM 2.5 mg/kg qid × 2 days, then bid × 1 day, then daily × 10 days

Acute lead poisoning

• *Adult:* IM 4 mg/kg, then q4h with edetate calcium disodium 12.5 mg/kg IM, not to exceed 5 mg/kg/dose

Mercury poisoning

• *Adult:* IM 5 mg/kg, then 2.5 mg/kg/day or bid × 10 days

Contraindications: Pregnancy (D), hypersensitivity, anuria, hepatic insufficiency, poisoning of other metals (iron, cadmium, selenium), severe renal disease, child <3 yr

dinoprostone (℞)
(dye-noe-prost'one)
Cervidil Vaginal Insert,
Prepidil, Endocervical Gel,
Prostin E Vaginal Suppository
Func. class.: Oxytocic, abortifacient
Chem. class.: Prostaglandin E₂

D

Do not confuse:
Prepidil/bepridil

Action: Stimulates uterine contractions, causing abortion; acts within 30 hr for complete abortion

Uses: Abortion during 2nd trimester, benign hydatidiform mole, expulsion of uterine contents in fetal deaths to 28 wk, missed abortion, to efface and dilate the cervix in pregnancy at term

DOSAGE AND ROUTES

Abortifacient

• *Adult:* VAG SUPP 20 mg, repeat q3-5h until abortion occurs, max dose is 240 mg

Cervical ripening

• *Adult:* GEL warm to room temperature, choose correct length shielded catheter (10 or 20 mm), fill catheter by pushing plunger; patient should remain recumbent for 15-30 min; insert one 10 mg insert

Available forms: Vag supp 20 mg; gel 0.5 mg/3 g (prefilled syringe); 10 mg insert

SIDE EFFECTS

CNS: Headache, dizziness, chills, fever
CV: Hypotension, **dysrhythmias**
EENT: Blurred vision
FETAL: Bradycardia (i.e., deceleration)
GI: Nausea, vomiting, diarrhea
GU: Vaginitis, vaginal pain, vulvitis, vaginismus
INTEG: Rash, skin color changes
MS: Leg cramps, joint swelling, weakness
GEL: Uterine contractile abnormality, GI side effects, back pain, fever
INSERT: Uterine hyperstimulation, fever,

nausea, vomiting, diarrhea, abdominal pain

SUPPOSITORY: **Uterine rupture, anaphylaxis**

Contraindications: Hypersensitivity, uterine fibrosis, cervical stenosis, pelvic surgery, pelvic inflammatory disease, respiratory disease

Precautions: Pregnancy (C), hepatic disease, renal disease, cardiac disease, asthma, anemia, jaundice, diabetes mellitus, convulsive disorders, hypertension, hypotension

INTERACTIONS

Increase: effect—other oxytocics
Decrease: oxytocic effect—alcohol

PHARMACOKINETICS

SUPP: Onset 10 min, duration 2-3 hr; metabolized in spleen, kidney, lungs; excreted in urine

NURSING CONSIDERATIONS

Assess:
• Dilation, effacement of cervix and uterine contraction, fetal heart tones, check for contractions over 1 min
• For fever that occurs ½ hr after suppository insertion (abortion)
• Respiratory rate, rhythm, depth; notify prescriber of abnormalities, pulse, B/P, temp
• Vaginal discharge: check for itching, irritation; indicates vaginal infection
• For fever, chills: increase fluids or give tepid sponge bath or blanket

Administer:
• By gel: after warming to room temp, remove seal from end of syringe, and remove the protective end cap and insert into plunger stopper assembly; make sure plunger is in dorsal position
• Antiemetic/antidiarrheal before administration of this drug

Evaluate:
• Therapeutic response: expulsion of fetus

Teach patient/family:
• To remain supine for 10-15 min after

insertion of supp 2 hr after insert, 15-30 min after gel
• To report excessive cramping, bleeding, chills, fever
• Some methods of pain, comfort control
• Avoid intercourse, tub baths, douches, tampon use for at least 2 wk

---

*diphenhydrAMINE
(OTC, ℞)

(dye-fen-hye′dra-meen)
Allerdryl ✿, AllerMax ✿, Allermed, Banophen, Benadryl, Benadryl 25, Benadryl Kapseals, Benahist 10, Benahist 50, Ben-Allergin-50, Benoject-10, Benoject-50, Benylin Cough, Bydramine, Compoz, Diphenadryl, Diphen Cough, Diphenhist, diphenhydrAMINE HCl, Dormin, Genahist, Hydramine, Hydramyn, Hydril, Hyrexin-50, Insomnal ✿, Nidryl, Nighttime Sleep Aid, Nordryl, Nordryl Cough, Nytol, Phendry, Siladryl, Sleep-Eze 3, Sominex 2, Tusstat, Twilite, Uni-Bent Cough, Wehdryl
Func. class.: Antihistamine (1st generation, nonselective)
Chem. class.: Ethanolamine derivative, H_1-receptor antagonist

---

Do not confuse:
diphenhydrAMINE/dicyclomine
diphenhydrAMINE/dimenhyDRINATE
Action: Acts on blood vessels, GI, respiratory system by competing with histamine for H_1-receptor site; decreases allergic response by blocking histamine
Uses: Allergy symptoms, rhinitis, motion sickness, antiparkinsonism, nighttime sedation, infant colic, nonproductive cough

---

⚠ Safety alert   *"Tall Man" lettering

DOSAGE AND ROUTES

• *Adult and child >12 yr:* **PO** 25-50 mg q4-6h, not to exceed 400 mg/day; **IM/IV** 10-50 mg, not to exceed 400 mg/day

• *Child <12 yr:* **PO/IM/IV** 5 mg/kg/day in 4 divided doses, not to exceed 300 mg/day

Nighttime sleep aid

• *Adult and child ≥12 yr:* **PO** 25-50 mg at bedtime

Antitussive (syrup only)

• *Adult and child ≥12 yr:* 25 mg q4h, max 100 mg/24 hr

• *Child 6-12 yr:* 12.5 mg q4h, max 75 mg/24 hr

• *Child 2-6 yr:* 6.25 mg q4h, max 37.5 mg/24 hr

Renal disease

• CCr >50 ml/min give dose q6h; CCr 10-50 ml/min dose q6-12h; CCr <10 ml/min dose q12-18h

Available forms: Caps 25, 50 mg; tabs 25, 50 mg; chew tabs 12.5 mg; elix 12.5 mg/5 ml; syr 12.5 mg/5 ml; inj 10, 50 mg/ml; orally disintegrating tabs 12.5 mg

SIDE EFFECTS

CNS: Dizziness, drowsiness, poor coordination, fatigue, anxiety, euphoria, confusion, paresthesia, neuritis, *seizures*
EENT: Blurred vision, dilated pupils, tinnitus, nasal stuffiness, dry nose, throat, mouth
GI: Nausea, anorexia, diarrhea
GU: Retention, dysuria, frequency
*HEMA: **Thrombocytopenia, agranulocytosis, hemolytic anemia***
INTEG: Photosensitivity
*MISC: **Anaphylaxis***
RESP: Increased thick secretions, wheezing, chest tightness

Contraindications: Hypersensitivity to H_1-receptor antagonist, acute asthma attack, lower respiratory tract disease
Precautions: Pregnancy (B), increased intraocular pressure, renal disease, cardiac disease, hypertension, bronchial asthma, seizure disorder, stenosed peptic ulcers, hyperthyroidism, prostatic hypertrophy, bladder neck obstruction, lactation

PHARMACOKINETICS

PO: Peak 1-3 hr, duration 4-7 hr
IM: Onset ½ hr, peak 1-4 hr, duration 4-7 hr
IV: Onset immediate, duration 4-7 hr; metabolized in liver, excreted by kidneys; crosses placenta, excreted in breast milk; half-life 2-7 hr

INTERACTIONS

Increase: CNS depression—barbiturates, opiates, hypnotics, tricyclics, alcohol
Increase: diphenhydrAMINE effect—MAOIs
Drug/Herb
Increase: anticholinergic effect—corkwood, henbane
Increase: effect—hops, Jamaican dogwood, khat, senega
Drug/Lab Test
False negative: Skin allergy tests

NURSING CONSIDERATIONS

Assess:

• Be alert for urinary retention, frequency, dysuria; drug should be discontinued

• CBC during long-term therapy; blood dyscrasias may occur

• Respiratory status: rate, rhythm, increase in bronchial secretions, wheezing, chest tightness

Administer:

• With meals for GI symptoms; absorption rate may slightly decrease

• Deep IM in large muscle; rotate site

• hs only if using for sleep aid

IV route

• Undiluted; give 25 mg/1 min

Additive compatibilities: Amikacin, aminophylline, ascorbic acid, bleomycin, cephapirin, erythromycin, hydrocortisone, lidocaine, methicillin, methyldopate, nafcillin, netilmicin, penicillin G potassium, penicillin G sodium, poly-myxin B, vit B/C

Syringe compatibilities: Atropine, butorphanol, chlorproMAZINE, cimetidine, dimenhyDRINATE, droperidol, fentanyl, fluphenazine, glycopyrrolate, hydromorphone, hydrOXYzine, meperidine, metoclopramide, midazolam, morphine, nalbuphine, pentazocine, perphenazine, prochlorperazine, promazine, promethazine, ranitidine, scopolamine, sufentanil, thiothixene

Y-site compatibilities: Acyclovir, aldesleukin, amifostine, amsacrine, aztreonam, ciprofloxacin, cisatracurium, cisplatin, cladribine, cyclophosphamide, cytarabine, DOXOrubicin, DOXOrubicin liposome, famotidine, filgrastim, fluconazole, fludarabine, gallium, granisetron, heparin, hydrocortisone, idarubicin, melphalan, meperidine, meropenem, methotrexate, ondansetron, paclitaxel, piperacillin/tazobactam, potassium chloride, propofol, remifentanil, sargramostim, sufentanil, tacrolimus teniposide, thiotepa, vinorelbine, vit B/C

Perform/provide:

• Hard candy, gum, frequent rinsing of mouth for dryness

• Storage in tight container at room temperature

Evaluate:

• Therapeutic response: absence of running or congested nose or rashes, improved sleep

Teach patient/family:

• All aspects of drug use; to notify prescriber of confusion, sedation, hypotension

• To avoid driving, other hazardous activity if drowsiness occurs

• That photosensitivity may occur

• To avoid concurrent use of alcohol, other CNS depressants

Treatment of overdose: Administer diazepam, vasopressors, barbiturates (short-acting)

---

diphenoxylate/ atropine (Rx)

(dye-fen-ox′ee-late/a′troe-peen)

Logene, Lomanate, Lomotil, Lonox

difenoxin/atropine (Rx)

(dye-fen-ox′in/a′troe-peen)

Motofen

Func. class.: Antidiarrheal

Chem. class.: Phenylpiperidine derivative opiate agonist

Controlled Substance Schedule V

diphenoxylate/atropine; **IV** difenoxin/ atropine (US)

Do not confuse:

Lomotil/Lamictal/Lamasil/Lanoxin/Lasix

Action: Inhibits gastric motility by acting on mucosal receptors responsible for peristalsis

Uses: Acute nonspecific and acute exacerbations of chronic functional diarrhea

DOSAGE AND ROUTES

diphenoxylate/atropine

Adult: **PO** 5 mg qid titrated to patient response needed, not to exceed 8 tabs/24 hr

Child 2-12 yr: **PO** (liquid only) 0.3-0.4 mg/kg/day in divided dose

difenoxin/atropine

• *Adult:* **PO** 2 tabs, then 1 tab after each loose stool or q3-4hr prn, max 8 tabs/ day

Available forms: diphenoxylate/ atropine: tabs 2.5 mg with atropine 0.025 mg; liquid 2.5 mg with atropine 0.025 mg/5 ml; difenoxin/atropine: tabs 1 mg difenoxin/0.025 atropine

SIDE EFFECTS

CNS: Dizziness, drowsiness, lightheadedness, headache, fatigue, nervousness, insomnia, confusion

EENT: Burning eyes, blurred vision

GI: *Nausea, vomiting, dry mouth, epigastric distress,* constipation, ***paralytic ileus***
MISC: ***Anaphylaxis, angioedema***
RESP: ***Respiratory depression***
Contraindications: Hypersensitivity, pseudomembranous enterocolitis, jaundice, glaucoma, child <2 yr, severe electrolyte imbalances, diarrhea associated with organisms that penetrate intestinal mucosa
Precautions: Pregnancy (C), hepatic disease, renal disease, ulcerative colitis, lactation, severe liver disease

PHARMACOKINETICS
PO: Onset 40-60 min, peak 2 hr, duration 3-4 hr, terminal half-life 12-14 hr; metabolized in liver to inactive metabolite; excreted in urine, feces

INTERACTIONS
Do not use with MAOIs; hypertensive crisis may occur
Increase: action of alcohol, opioids, barbiturates, other CNS depressants, anticholinergics
Drug/Herb
Increase: antidiarrheal action—nutmeg

NURSING CONSIDERATIONS
Assess:
• Electrolytes (K, Na, Cl) if on long-term therapy
• Bowel pattern before; for rebound constipation after termination of medication; bowel sounds
• Response after 48 hr; if none, drug should be discontinued
• Abdominal distention, toxic megacolon, which may occur in ulcerative colitis
• Hepatic studies if on long-term therapy
Administer:
• For 48 hr only; if no response, drug should be discontinued
Evaluate:
• Therapeutic response: decreased diarrhea
Teach patient/family:
• To avoid OTC products unless directed

by prescriber (may contain alcohol); do not use alcohol or CNS depressants
• Not to exceed recommended dose
• That drug may be habit forming
• Not to engage in hazardous activities; drowsiness may occur, not to use for longer than 48 hr for acute diarrhea

dipivefrin ophthalmic
See Appendix C

dipyridamole (℞)
(dye-peer-id'a-mole)
Apo-Dipyridamole ✦, dipyridamole ✦, Novo-Dipiradol ✦, Persantine, Persantine IV
Func. class.: Coronary vasodilator, antiplatelet agent
Chem. class.: Nonnitrate

Action: Inhibits adenosine uptake, which produces coronary vasodilation; increases oxygen saturation in coronary tissues, coronary blood flow; acts on small resistance vessels with little effect on vascular resistance; may increase development of collateral circulation; decreases platelet aggregation by the inhibition of phosphodiesterase (an enzyme)
Uses: Prevention of transient ischemic attacks, inhibition of platelet adhesion to prevent myocardial reinfarction, thromboembolism, with warfarin in prosthetic heart valves, prevention of coronary bypass graft occlusion with aspirin; IV form used to evaluate coronary artery disease; used as alternative to exercise in thallium myocardial perfusion imaging to evaluate coronary artery disease

DOSAGE AND ROUTES
TIA
• *Adult:* **PO** 50 mg tid, 1 hr ac, not to exceed 400 mg daily

Inhibition of platelet adhesion
- *Adult:* **PO** 50-75 mg qid in combination with aspirin or warfarin

Thallium myocardial perfusion imaging
- *Adult:* **IV** 570 mcg/kg

Available forms: Tabs 25, 50, 75 mg; inj 10 mg/2 ml

SIDE EFFECTS

CNS: Headache, dizziness, weakness, fainting, syncope; IV: transient cerebral ischemia, weakness
CV: Postural hypotension; IV: *MI*
GI: Nausea, vomiting, anorexia, diarrhea
INTEG: Rash, flushing
RESP: IV: *Bronchospasm*
Contraindications: Hypersensitivity
Precautions: Pregnancy (B), lactation, hypotension

PHARMACOKINETICS

PO: Peak 1.25 hr, duration 6 hr; therapeutic response may take several months; metabolized in liver; excreted in bile; undergoes enterohepatic recirculation

INTERACTIONS

Prevention of coronary vasodilation: theophylline
Increase: bleeding risk—NSAIDs, cefamandole, cefotetan, cefoperazone, plicamycin, valproic acid, sulfinpyrazole, anticoagulants, thrombolytics
Drug/Herb
Gastric irritation: arginine
Increase: antiplatelet effect—bogbean, dong quai, feverfew, ginger, ginkgo
Decrease: antiplatelet effect—bilberry, saw palmetto

NURSING CONSIDERATIONS

Assess:
- B/P, pulse during treatment until stable; take B/P lying, standing; orthostatic hypotension is common
- Cardiac status: chest pain, what aggravates or ameliorates condition

Administer:
PO route
- On an empty stomach: 1 hr before meals or 2 hr after; give with 8 oz water for better absorption
IV route
- IV after diluting to at least 1:2 ratio using D$_5$W, 0.45% NaCl, or 0.9% NaCl to a total vol of 20-50 ml; give over 4 min; do not give undiluted
Perform/provide:
- Storage at room temperature
Evaluate:
- Therapeutic response: decreased platelet adhesion
Teach patient/family:
- That medication is not a cure; may have to be taken continuously in evenly spaced doses only as directed
- To avoid hazardous activities until stabilized on medication; dizziness may occur
- To rise slowly from sitting or lying to prevent orthostatic hypotension
- Not to use alcohol or OTC medications unless approved by prescriber

dirithromycin ($\mathbb{R}$)
(dye-rith-roe-mye′sin)
Dynabac
Func. class.: Antiinfective
Chem. class.: Macrolide

Do not confuse:
Dynabac/DynaCirc
Action: Binds to 50S ribosomal subunits of susceptible bacteria, suppresses protein synthesis
Uses: Infections of the respiratory tract caused by *Moraxella catarrhalis, Streptococcus* sp. *(S. pneumoniae, S. pyogenes, S. agalactiae, S. viridans), Legionella pneumophilia, Mycoplasma pneumoniae, Staphylococcus aureus, Bordetella pertussis*

DOSAGE AND ROUTES
- *Adult:* **PO** 500 mg daily, given for 7-14 days depending on infections

Available forms: Tabs, enteric coated 250 mg

SIDE EFFECTS

CNS: Headache, dizziness, insomnia
GI: Abdominal pain, nausea, diarrhea, vomiting, dyspepsia, GI disorders, flatulence, abnormal stools, anorexia, constipation, **pseudomembranous colitis**
HEMA: Increased platelet count, increased eosinophils
INTEG: Pruritus, urticaria
RESP: Cough, dyspnea

Contraindications: Hypersensitivity to this drug or any other macrolide, or erythromycin, bacteremias
Precautions: Pregnancy (C), lactation, children, hepatic, renal disease

PHARMACOKINETICS

Rapidly absorbed, widely distributed, no hepatic metabolism, excreted in bile, feces (up to 97%), plasma half-life 8 hr, terminal 44 hr

INTERACTIONS

May alter effect of theophylline
Absorption of dirithromycin slightly enhanced: antacids, H$_2$-antagonists
Drug/Herb
Do not use acidophilus with antiinfectives
Drug/Food
Increase: absorption with food

NURSING CONSIDERATIONS

Assess:
• Report hematuria, oliguria
• Hepatic studies: AST, ALT if on long-term therapy
• Renal studies: Urinalysis, protein, blood if on long-term therapy
• C&S before drug therapy; drug may be given as soon as culture is taken; C&S may be repeated after treatment
• Bowel pattern before, during treatment; pseudomembranous colitis may occur
• Skin eruptions, itching
• Respiratory status: rate, character,

wheezing, tightness in chest; discontinue drug
Administer:
• Do not break, crush, or chew tabs
• Adequate intake of fluids (2 L) during diarrhea episodes
• With food or within 1 hr of food at same time each day
Perform/provide:
• Storage at room temperature, in tight container
Evaluate:
• Therapeutic response: C&S negative for infection
Teach patient/family:
• To take with full glass of water; to give with food
• To report sore throat, fever, fatigue; may indicate superinfection
• To notify prescriber of diarrhea stools, dark urine, pale stools, jaundiced eyes or skin, severe abdominal pain
• To take at evenly spaced intervals; complete dosage regimen
Treatment of hypersensitivity:
Withdraw drug, maintain airway, administer epINEPHrine, aminophylline, O$_2$, IV corticosteroids

---

disopyramide (℞)
(dye-soe-peer'a-mide)
disopyramide, Norpace, Norpace CR, Rhythmodan
Func. class.: Antidysrhythmic (Class IA)
Chem. class.: Nonnitrate

Action: Prolongs duration of action potential and effective refractory period; reduces disparity in refractory period between normal and infarcted myocardium; prevents increased myocardial excitability and conduction contractility
Uses: PVCs, ventricular tachycardia, supraventricular tachycardia, atrial flutter, fibrillation
Investigational uses: Supraventricular tachycardia (prevention, treatment)

Side effects: *italics* = common; **bold italics** = life-threatening

DOSAGE AND ROUTES

- *Adult:* PO 100-200 mg q6h, **CONT REL CAPS** 200-400 mg q12h
- *Child 12-18 yr:* PO 6-15 mg/kg/day, in divided doses q6h
- *Child 4-12 yr:* PO 10-15 mg/kg/day in divided doses q6h
- *Child 1-4 yr:* PO 10-20 mg/kg/day in divided doses q6h
- *Child <1 yr:* PO 10-30 mg/kg/day, in divided doses q6h

Renal disease

- CCr 30-40 ml/min dose q8h; CCr 15-30 ml/min dose q12h; CCr <15 ml/min dose q24h

Available forms: Caps 100, 150 mg; ext rel caps (CR) 100, 150 mg; tabs, ext rel 150 mg ✿

SIDE EFFECTS

CNS: Headache, dizziness, psychosis, fatigue, depression, paresthesias, insomnia

CV: Hypotension, bradycardia, angina, PVCs, tachycardia, increased QRS, QT segments, *cardiac arrest,* edema, weight gain, AV block, *CHF,* syncope, chest pain

EENT: Blurred vision; dry nose, throat, eyes; narrow-angle glaucoma

GI: Dry mouth, constipation, nausea, anorexia, flatulence, diarrhea, vomiting

GU: Urinary retention, hesitancy, impotence

*HEMA: **Thrombocytopenia, agranulocytosis,*** anemia (rare), decreased Hgb, Hct

INTEG: Rash, pruritus, urticaria

META: Hypoglycemia, hypokalemia

MS: Weakness, pain in extremities

Contraindications: Hypersensitivity, 2nd- or 3rd-degree block, cardiogenic shock, CHF (uncompensated), sick sinus syndrome, QT prolongation

Precautions: Pregnancy (C), lactation, diabetes mellitus, renal disease, children, hepatic disease, myasthenia gravis, narrow-angle glaucoma, cardiomyopathy, conduction abnormalities, potassium imbalance

PHARMACOKINETICS

PO: Peak 30 min-3 hr, duration 6-12 hr; half-life 4-10 hr; metabolized in liver; excreted in feces, urine, breast milk; crosses placenta

INTERACTIONS

Increase: disopyramide effect—quinidine, procainamide, propranolol, lidocaine, atenolol, other antidysrhythmics, erythromycin

Increase: side effects, urinary retention—anticholinergics

Decrease: disopyramide effect—phenytoin, rifampin, phenobarbital

Drug/Herb

Toxicity/death: aconite

Increase: action—aloe, broom, buckthorn, cascara sagrada, Chinese rhubarb, figwort, fumitory, goldenseal, kudzu, licorice, senna

Increase: serotonin effect—horehound

Decrease: antiarrhythmic action—coltsfoot

Drug/Lab Test

Increase: Hepatic enzymes, lipids, BUN, creatinine

Decrease: Hgb/Hct, blood glucose

NURSING CONSIDERATIONS

Assess:

- Apical pulse for 1 min; if less than 60, check again in 1 hr; if still less than 60, notify prescriber
- ECG; check for increased QT, widening QRS; drug should be discontinued
- Weight daily; a rapid weight gain should be reported
- For dehydration or hypovolemia, I&O ratio, electrolytes (Na, K, Cl)
- Renal, hepatic studies (AST, ALT, bilirubin, BUN, creatinine) during treatment
- Diabetics for signs of hypoglycemia (rare)
- B/P continuously for hypotension, hypertension
- For rebound hypertension after 1-2 hr
- Constipation: increased bulk in diet, water, stool softeners, or laxatives needed

---

⚠ Safety alert   *"Tall Man" lettering

- Cardiac rate, respiration: rate, rhythm, character
- Urinary hesitancy, frequency, or a change in I&O ratio; check for edema daily; check for toxicity

Administer:
- Do not break, crush, or chew sus rel cap; give 1 hr before or 2 hr after meals
- Sugar-free gum, frequent sips of water for dry mouth
- Reduced dosage slowly with ECG monitoring

Evaluate:
- Therapeutic response: decreased dysrhythmias

Teach patient/family:
- To take drug exactly as prescribed; if dose is missed, take within 3-4 hr of next dose; do not double dose
- To avoid alcohol, or severe hypotension may occur; to avoid OTC drugs, or serious drug interactions may occur
- To make position change slowly during early therapy to prevent orthostatic hypotension
- To avoid hazardous activities if dizziness or blurred vision occurs
- The importance of complying with drug regimen; tell patient that this drug does not cure condition

Treatment of overdose: O$_2$, artificial ventilation, ECG, DOPamine for circulatory depression, diazepam or thiopental for convulsions, gastric lavage

Rarely Used

disulfiram (℞)
(dye-sul'fi-ram)
Antabuse, disulfiram
Func. class.: Alcohol deterrent

Uses: Chronic alcoholism (as adjunct)

DOSAGE AND ROUTES
- *Adult:* **PO** 250-500 mg daily × 1-2 wk, then 125-500 mg daily until fully socially recovered
Contraindications: Pregnancy (X),

hypersensitivity, alcohol intoxication, psychoses, CV disease, lactation

*DOBUTamine (℞)
(doe-byoo'ta-meen)
DOBUTamine, Dobutrex
Func. class.: Adrenergic direct-acting β$_1$-agonist, cardiac stimulant
Chem. class.: Catecholamine

Do not confuse:
DOBUTamine/DOPamine
Dobutrex/Diamox
Action: Causes increased contractility, increased cardiac output without marked increase in heart rate by acting on β$_1$-receptors in heart; minor α and β$_2$ effects
Uses: Cardiac decompensation due to organic heart disease or cardiac surgery
Investigational uses: Cardiogenic shock in children; congenital heart disease in children undergoing cardiac cath

DOSAGE AND ROUTES
- *Adult:* **IV INF** 2.5-10 mcg/kg/min; may increase to 40 mcg/kg/min if needed
- *Child:* **IV INF** 5-20 mcg/kg/min over 10 min for cardiac cath
Available forms: Inj 12.5 mg/ml

SIDE EFFECTS
CNS: Anxiety, headache, dizziness
CV: Palpitations, tachycardia, hypertension, hypotension, PVCs, angina
GI: Heartburn, nausea, vomiting
MS: Muscle cramps (leg)
Contraindications: Hypersensitivity, idiopathic hypertrophic subaortic stenosis
Precautions: Pregnancy (B), lactation, children, hypertension

PHARMACOKINETICS
IV: Onset 1-2 min, peak 10 min, half-life 2 min; metabolized in liver (inactive metabolites); excreted in urine

Side effects: *italics* = common; ***bold italics*** = life-threatening

INTERACTIONS

Severe hypertension: guanethidine
Dysrhythmias: general anesthetics, bretylium

Increase: pressor effect, dysrhythmias—tricyclics, MAOIs, oxytocics
Decrease: DOBUTamine action—other β-blockers

NURSING CONSIDERATIONS

Assess:
• Hypovolemia; if present, correct first; administer cardiac glycoside before DOBUTamine
• Oxygenation/perfusion deficit (check B/P, chest pain, dizziness, loss of consciousness)
• Heart failure: S₃ gallop, dyspnea, neck vein distention, bibasilar crackles in patients with CHF, cardiomyopathy
• ECG during administration continuously; if B/P increases, drug is decreased; CVP or PWP, cardiac output during infusion
• Serum electrolytes, urine output
⚠ Sulfite sensitivity, which may be life-threatening

Administer:
• Diluting each 250 mg/10 ml of sterile H₂O or D₅W for inj; may be further diluted in 50 ml or more given at prescribed rate; should be gradually increased to desired rate; use a CVP catheter or large peripheral vein, use inf pump, titrate to patient response
• Give via infusion pump
• Standard concentrations are 250 mcg/ml-1000 mcg/ml, max 5 mg of DOBUTamine/ml

Additive compatibilities: Amiodarone, atracurium, atropine, DOPamine, enalaprilat, epINEPHrine, flumazenil, hydrALAZINE, isoproterenol, lidocaine, meperidine, meropenem, metaraminol, morphine, nitroglycerin, norepinephrine, phentolamine, phenylephrine, procainamide, propranolol, ranitidine

Syringe compatibilities: Heparin, ranitidine

Y-site compatibilities: Amifostine, amiodarone, amrinone, atracurium, aztreonam, bretylium, calcium chloride, calcium gluconate, ciprofloxacin, cisatracurium, cladribine, diazepam, diltiazem, DOPamine, doxorubicin liposome, enalaprilat, epINEPHrine, famotidine, fentanyl, fluconazole, granisetron, haloperidol, hydromorphone, insulin (regular), labetalol, lidocaine, lorazepam, magnesium sulfate, meperidine, milrinone, morphine, niCARdipine, nitroglycerin, norepinephrine, pancuronium, potassium chloride, propofol, ranitidine, remifentanil, sodium nitroprusside, streptokinase, tacrolimus, theophylline, thiotepa, tolazoline, vecuronium, verapamil, zidovudine

Perform/provide:
• Storage of reconstituted solution for 24 hr if refrigerated

Evaluate:
• Therapeutic response: increased B/P with stabilization, increased urine output

Teach patient/family:
• The reason for drug administration; to report dyspnea, chest pain, numbness of extremities, headache, IV site discomfort

Treatment of overdose: Administer a β₁-adrenergic blocker; reduce IV or discontinue, ensure oxygenation/ventilation; for severe tachydysrhythmias (ventricular) give lidocaine or propranolol

---

docetaxel (℞)
(doe-se-tax'el)
Taxotere
Func. class.: Miscellaneous antineoplastic

Do not confuse:
Taxotere/Taxol

Action: Inhibits reorganization of microtubule network needed for interphase and mitotic cellular functions; also causes abnormal bundles of microtubules during cell cycle and multiple esters of microtubules during mitosis

---

⚠ Safety alert   *"Tall Man" lettering

Uses: Locally advanced or metastatic breast cancer, non-small-cell lung cancer, androgen independent metastatic prostate cancer, post-surgery operable node-positive breast cancer

DOSAGE AND ROUTES:
Locally advanced or metastatic breast cancer after failure of other chemotherapy
• *Adult:* **IV** 60-100 mg/m^2 given over 1 hr q3wks; if neutrophil count is < 500/mm^3 for > 1 wk, reduce dose by 25%
Locally advanced or metastatic non-small-cell lung cancer after failure of cisplatin chemotherapy
• *Adult:* **IV** 75 mg/m^2 over 1 hr q3wk; if neutrophil count is <500/mm^3 for >1 wk, reduce dose to 55 mg/m^2; if patient develops grade 3 peripheral neuropathy, stop drug
Unreactable, locally advanced or metastatic non-small-cell lung cancer previously treated with chemotherapy
• *Adult:* **IV** 75 mg/m^2 over 1 hr, then cisplatin 75 mg/m^2 **IV** given over 30-60 min q3wk; reduce dose to 65 mg/m^2 in those with hematologic or non-hematologic toxicities
Androgen-independent metastatic prostate cancer
• *Adult:* **IV** 75 mg/m^2 given over 1 hr q3wk, with 5 mg predniSONE **PO** bid continuously. Give dexamethasone 8 mg **PO** at 12 hr, 3 hr and 1 hr prior to docetaxel; if neutrophil count is <500 cells/mm^3 for more than 1 wk or other toxicities occur, reduce dose to 60 mg/m^2
Adjuvant post-surgery treatment of operable node-positive breast cancer
• *Adult:* **IV** 75 mg/m^2 over 1 hr, given 1 hr after DOXOrubicin 50 mg/m^2, cyclophosphamide 500 mg/m^2 q3wk × 6 cycles
Available forms: Inj 20, 80 mg in single dose vials

SIDE EFFECTS
CV: Hypotension, fluid retention, peripheral edema, flushing

*GI: Nausea, vomiting, diarrhea, **hepatotoxicity***
*HEMA: **Neutropenia, leukopenia, thrombocytopenia, anemia,** bleeding, infections, **myelosuppression***
INTEG: Alopecia, nail pain, rash, skin eruptions
MS: Arthralgia, myalgia, back pain
NEURO: Peripheral neuropathy
RESP: Dyspnea, **pulmonary edema**
*SYST: Hypersensitivity reactions, **death***
Contraindications: Pregnancy (D), hypersensitivity to this drug or other drugs with polysorbate 80, neutropenia of < 1500/mm^3, severe hepatic disease, bilirubin exceeding upper normal limit, or severely elevated ALT, AST, alk phos
Precautions: Children, lactation, cardiovascular disease

PHARMACOKINETICS
Metabolized in liver, excreted in feces; terminal half life 11.1 hr

INTERACTIONS
Altered docetaxel levels metabolism: cycloSPORINE, erythromycin, ketoconazole, troleadomycin
Increase: myelosuppression—other antineoplastics, radiation
Decrease: immune response—live virus vaccines

NURSING CONSIDERATIONS
Assess:
• CBC, differential, platelet count prior to and qwk; withhold drug if WBC is <1500/mm^3 or platelet count is <100,000/mm^3, notify prescriber
• Monitor temp q4h (may indicate beginning of infection)
• Hepatic studies before, during therapy (bilirubin, AST, ALT, LDH) prn or qmo; check for jaundiced skin and sclera, dark urine, clay-colored stools, itchy skin, abdominal pain, fever, diarrhea
• CNS changes: confusion, paresthesias, dysethenia, pain, weakness; if severe, drug should be discontinued

• VS during 1st hr of infusion, check IV site for signs of infiltration

⚠ Hypersensitive reactions, anaphylaxis including hypotension, dyspnea, angioedema, generalized urticaria; discontinue infusion immediately

• Bleeding: hematuria, guaiac, bruising or petechiae, mucosa or orifices q8h; obtain prescription fo viscous lidocaine (Xylocaine)

• Effects of alopecia on body image; discuss feelings about body changes

Administer:

• Antiemetic 30-60 min before giving drug and prn

IV route

• Allow vials to warm to room temperature; withdraw all diluent and inject in vial of docetaxel; rotate gently to mix; allow to stand to decrease foaming, then withdraw the required amount (10 mg/ml) and inject in 250 ml of 0.9% wall or D$_5$W; mix gently; give over 1 hr

Y-site compatibilities:

Acyclovir, amikacin, aminophylline, ampicillin/sulbactam, butorphanol, calcium gluconate, cefepime, cefotetan, ceftazidime, ceftriaxone, cimetidine, diphenhydrAMINE, droperidol, famotidine, fluconazole, furosemide, ganciclovir, gentamicin, granisetron, haloperidol, heparin, hydrocortisone, hydromorphone, lorazepam, magnesium sulfate, mannitol, meperidine, mesna, metoclopramide, morphine, ondansetron, potassium chloride, prochlorperazine, ranitidine, sodium bicarbonate, vancomycin, zidovudine

Perform/provide:

• Confirmation that dexamethasone was given 12 hr and 6 hr before infusion begins

• Storage of prepared sol up to 27 hr in refrigerator

Evaluate:

• Therapeutic response: decreased tumor size, spread of malignancy

Teach patient/family:

• To report signs of infection: fever, sore throat, flulike symptoms

• To report signs of anemia: fatigue, headache, faintness, shortness of breath, irritability

• To report bleeding; avoid use of razors, commercial mouthwash

• To avoid use of aspirin, ibuprofen

• To report any complaints or side effects to nurse or prescriber

• That hair may be lost during treatment; a wig or hairpiece may make patient feel better; new hair may be different in color and texture

• That pain in muscles and joints 2-5 days after infusion is common

• To use nonhormonal type of contraception

• To avoid receiving vaccinations while on this drug

---

docosanol topical
See Appendix C

---

docusate calcium (otc)
(dok'yoo-sate cal'see-um)
DC Softgels, Pro-Cal-Sof, Sulfalax Calcium, Surfak

docusate sodium (otc)
Colace, Correctol Extra Gentle, Dialose, Diocto, Dioeze, Disonate, Di-Sosul, DOK, DOS, D-S-S, Ex-Lax, Modane, Regulax SS, Regulex ✿, Silace
Func. class.: Laxative, emollient; stool softener
Chem. class.: Anionic surfactant

Action: Increases water, fat penetration in intestine; allows for easier passage of stool

Uses: To soften stools

DOSAGE AND ROUTES

• *Adult:* **PO** 50-300 mg daily (sodium) or 240 mg (calcium or potassium) prn; **ENEMA** 5 ml (sodium)

• *Child >12 yr:* **ENEMA** 2 ml (sodium)

• *Child 6-12 yr:* **PO** 40-150 mg daily (sodium) in divided doses
• *Child 3-6 yr:* **PO** 20-60 mg daily (sodium) in divided doses
• *Child <3 yr:* **PO** 10-40 mg daily (sodium) in divided doses

Available forms: *Calcium:* caps 50, 240 mg; *sodium:* caps 50, 100, 240, 250 mg; tabs 50, 100 mg; syr 16.75 mg/5 ml, 20 mg/5 ml, 50, 60/15 ml; liq 150 mg/15 ml; oral sol 10, 50 mg/ml; enema 283 mg/3.9 cap

SIDE EFFECTS

EENT: Bitter taste, throat irritation
GI: Nausea, anorexia, cramps, diarrhea
INTEG: Rash
Contraindications: Hypersensitivity, obstruction, fecal impaction, nausea/vomiting
Precautions: Pregnancy (C), lactation

PHARMACOKINETICS

Onset 24-72 hr

INTERACTIONS

Toxicity: mineral oil
Drug/Herb
Increase: laxative action—flax, senna

NURSING CONSIDERATIONS

Assess:
• Cause of constipation; identify whether fluids, bulk, or exercise are missing from lifestyle, constipating drugs
• Cramping, rectal bleeding, nausea, vomiting; if these symptoms occur, drug should be discontinued
Administer:
• Swallow tabs whole; do not break, crush, or chew
• In milk, fruit juice to decrease bitter taste
• In morning or evening (oral dose)
Perform/provide:
• Storage in cool environment; do not freeze
Evaluate:
• Therapeutic response: decrease in constipation

Teach patient/family:
• That normal bowel movements do not always occur daily
• Not to use in presence of abdominal pain, nausea, vomiting
• To notify prescriber if constipation unrelieved or if symptoms of electrolyte imbalance occur: muscle cramps, pain, weakness, dizziness, excessive thirst
• Inform patient that drug may take up to 3 days to soften stools
• Take oral prep with a full glass of water unless on fluid restrictions and increase fluid intake

---

dofetilide (Ŗ)
Tikosyn
Func. class.: Antidysrhythmic (Class III)

Action: Blocks cardiac ion channel carrying the rapid component of delayed potassium current, no effect on sodium channels
Uses: Atrial fibrillation, flutter, maintenance of normal sinus rhythm

DOSAGE AND ROUTES

• *Adult:* **PO** 125-500 mcg bid depending on CCr, may be adjusted q2-3h to get appropriate increase in QTc
Renal dose
• CCr >60 ml/min 500 mcg bid; CCr 40-60 ml/min 250 mcg bid; CCr 20-40 ml/min 125 mcg bid; CCr <20 ml/min do not use
Available forms: Caps 125, 250, 500 mcg

SIDE EFFECTS

CNS: Syncope, *dizziness,* headache
CV: Hypotension, postural hypotension, bradycardia, angina, PVCs, substernal pressure, transient hypertension, precipitation of angina
GI: Nausea, vomiting, severe diarrhea, anorexia
Contraindications: Hypersensitivity, digitalis toxicity, aortic stenosis, pulmo-

nary hypertension, children, QT syndromes, severe renal disease
Precautions: Pregnancy (C), renal disease, lactation

PHARMACOKINETICS

Well absorbed, max plasma conc 2-3 hr, steady state 2-3 days, half-life 10 hr, metabolized by liver, excreted by kidneys

INTERACTIONS

Do not use with cimetidine, ketoconazole, verapamil, prochlorperazine, trimethoprim-sulfamethizole, amiloride, metformin, megestrol, triamterene
Increase: hypokalemia—potassium-depleting diuretics
Drug/Herb
Increase: toxicity, death—aconite
Increase: serotonin effect—horehound
Increase: effect—aloe, broom, buckthorn (chronic use), cascara sagrada (chronic use), Chinese rhubarb, figwort, fumitory, goldenseal, kudzu, licorice
Decrease: effect—coltsfoot

NURSING CONSIDERATIONS

Assess:
• ECG continuously to determine drug effectiveness, PVCs, other dysrhythmias; renal function, QTc q3mo; this drug is only available to facilities that have been educated in this administration, patient must be hospitalized
• B/P continuously for hypotension, hypertension; orthostatic hypotension; keep supine until hypotension subsides
• Cardiac status: rate, rhythm, character, continuously
Administer:
• For 3 days hospitalized
• Give dofetilide after withholding class I or III antidysrhythmic for 3 half-lives of dofetilide
Perform/provide:
• Place patient in supine position unless otherwise ordered; assist with ambulation

Evaluate:
• Therapeutic response: control in atrial fibrillation
Teach patient/family:
• To make position changes slowly; orthostatic hypotension may occur
• Notify prescriber if fast heartbeats with fainting or dizziness occur
• Notify all prescribers of all medications and supplements taken
• That if dose is missed, do not double, take next dose at usual time
• Avoid breastfeeding

dolasetron (℞)
(do-la′se-tron)
Anzemet
Func. class.: Antiemetic
Chem. class.: 5-HT3 receptor antagonist

Action: Prevents nausea, vomiting by blocking serotonin peripherally, centrally, and in the small intestine
Uses: Prevention of nausea, vomiting associated with cancer chemotherapy, radiotherapy, and prevention of postoperative nausea, vomiting
Investigational uses: Radiotherapy-induced nausea/vomiting

DOSAGE AND ROUTES
Prevention of nausea/vomiting of cancer chemotherapy
• *Adult and child 2-16 yr:* **IV** 1.8 mg/kg as a single dose, ½ hr prior to chemotherapy
• *Adult:* **PO** 100 mg 1 hr prior to chemotherapy
• *Child 2-16 yr:* **PO** 1.8 mg/kg/hr prior to chemotherapy; max 100 mg
Prevention of postoperative nausea/vomiting
• *Adult:* **IV** 12.5 mg as a single dose, 15 min before cessation of anesthesia; **PO** 100 mg 2 hr before surgery (prevention only)
• *Child 2-16 yr:* **IV** 0.35 mg/kg as a single dose, 15 min before cessation of

anesthesia; **PO** 1.2 mg/kg 2 hr before surgery (prevention only)
Available forms: Tabs 50, 100 mg; inj 20 mg/ml (12.5 mg/0.625 ml)

SIDE EFFECTS

CNS: Headache, dizziness, fatigue, drowsiness

CV: **Dysrhythmias,** ECG changes, hypotension, tachycardia, hypertension, bradycardia

GI: Diarrhea, constipation, increased AST, ALT, abdominal pain, anorexia

GU: Urinary retention, oliguria

MISC: Rash, **bronchospasm**

Contraindications: Hypersensitivity

Precautions: Pregnancy (B), lactation, children, elderly, hypokalemia, electrolyte imbalances; granisetron, ondansetron hypersensitivity

PHARMACOKINETICS

Unknown

INTERACTIONS

Dysrhythmias: antidysrhythmics

Increase: dolasetron levels—cimetidine

Increase: QT prolongation—thiazide, loop diuretics

Decrease: dolasetron levels—rifampin

NURSING CONSIDERATIONS

Assess:

• For absence of nausea, vomiting during chemotherapy

• For hypersensitivity reaction: rash, bronchospasm

• For cardiac conduction conditions, electrolyte imbalances, or dysrhythmias

Administer:

• By inj 100 mg/½ min or less or diluted in 50 ml compatible sol; give over 15 min

• Not to mix product for oral administration in juice until immediately before administration; apple or apple-grape diluted can be kept for 2 hr at room temp

Perform/provide:

• Storage at room temperature 48 hr after dilution

Evaluate:

• Therapeutic response: absence of nausea, vomiting during cancer chemotherapy

Teach patient/family:

• To report diarrhea, constipation, nausea, vomiting, rash, or changes in respirations

• May cause headache, use analgesic

donepezil (℞)
(don-ep-ee′zill)
Aricept
Func. class.: Reversible cholinesterase inhibitor

Action: Elevates acetylcholine concentrations (cerebral cortex) by slowing degradation of acetylcholine released in cholinergic neurons; does not alter underlying dementia

Uses: Treatment of mild to moderate dementia in Alzheimer's disease

Investigational uses: Vascular dementia

DOSAGE AND ROUTES

• *Adult:* **PO** 5 mg daily at bedtime; may increase to 10 mg daily after 4-6 wk

Available forms: Tabs 5, 10 mg

SIDE EFFECTS

CNS: Dizziness, *insomnia,* somnolence, *headache,* fatigue, abnormal dreams, syncope, **seizures**

CV: **Atrial fibrillation,** hypotension or hypertension, **sinus bradycardia**

GI: Nausea, vomiting, anorexia; *diarrhea*

GU: Urinary frequency, UTI, incontinence

INTEG: Rash, flushing

MS: Cramps, arthritis

RESP: Rhinitis, URI, cough, pharyngitis

Contraindications: Hypersensitivity to this drug or piperidine derivatives

Precautions: Pregnancy (C), sick sinus syndrome, history of ulcers, GI bleeding, hepatic disease, bladder obstruction, asthma, lactation, children, seizures, asthma, COPD

PHARMACOKINETICS

Well absorbed PO, metabolized to metabolites, elimination half-life 10 hr single dose, 70 hr multiple dosing

INTERACTIONS

Synergistic effect: succinylcholine, cholinesterase inhibitors, cholinergic agonists

Increase: gastric acid secretions—NSAIDs

Decrease: action of anticholinergics

Decrease: donepezil effect—carbamazepine, dexamethasone, phenytoin, phenobarbital, rifampin

NURSING CONSIDERATIONS

Assess:
- B/P: hypotension, hypertension
- Mental status: affect, mood, behavioral changes, depression, complete suicide assessment
- GI status: nausea, vomiting, anorexia, diarrhea
- GU status: urinary frequency, incontinence

Administer:
- Between meals; may be given with meals for GI symptoms
- Dosage adjusted to response no more than q6wk

Perform/provide:
- Assistance with ambulation during beginning therapy; dizziness, ataxia may occur

Evaluate:
- Therapeutic response: decrease in confusion, improved mood

Teach patient/family:
- To report side effects: twitching, nausea, vomiting, sweating; indicates overdose
- To use drug exactly as prescribed; at regular intervals, preferably between meals; may be taken with meals for GI upset
- To notify prescriber of nausea, vomiting, diarrhea (dose increase or beginning treatment), or rash

- Not to increase or abruptly decrease dose; serious consequences may result
- That drug is not a cure, relieves symptoms

Treatment of overdose: Withdraw drug, administer tertiary anticholinergics, provide supportive care

---

> **⚠ High Alert**
>
> *DOPamine (℞)
> (doe′pa-meen)
> DOPamine HCl, Intropin,
> Revimine ✦
> *Func. class.:* Adrenergic
> *Chem. class.:* Catecholamine

Do not confuse:
DOPamine/DOBUTamine

Action: Causes increased cardiac output; acts on β_1- and α-receptors, causing vasoconstriction in blood vessels; low dose causes renal and mesenteric vasodilation; β_1 stimulation produces inotropic effects with increased cardiac output

Uses: Shock; increased perfusion; hypotension

Unlabeled uses: COPD, RDS in infants

DOSAGE AND ROUTES

Shock
- *Adult:* **IV INF** 2-5 mcg/kg/min, not to exceed 50 mcg/kg/min, titrate to patient's response
- *Child:* **IV** 5-20 mcg/kg/min adjust depending on response

COPD
- *Adult:* **IV** 4 mcg/kg/min

CHF
- *Adult:* **IV** 2-5 mcg/kg/min

RDS
- *Infant:* **IV** 5 mcg/kg/min

Available forms: Inj 40 mg, 80 mg, 160 mg/ml conc for IV inf; 0.8, 1.6, 3.2 mg/ml in D_5W

SIDE EFFECTS

CNS: Headache
CV: Palpitations, tachycardia, hyper-

⚠ Safety alert   *"Tall Man" lettering

tension, *ectopic beats, angina, wide QRS complex,* peripheral vasoconstriction
GI: Nausea, vomiting, diarrhea
INTEG: Necrosis, tissue sloughing with extravasation, ***gangrene***
RESP: Dyspnea

Contraindications: Hypersensitivity, ventricular fibrillation, tachydysrhythmias, pheochromocytoma

Precautions: Pregnancy (C), lactation, arterial embolism, peripheral vascular disease

PHARMACOKINETICS

IV: Onset 5 min, duration <10 min; metabolized in liver, kidney, plasma, excreted in urine (metabolites), half-life 2 min

INTERACTIONS

Do not use within 2 wk of MAOIs; hypertensive crisis may result
Bradycardia, hypotension: phenytoin
Dysrhythmias: general anesthetics
Severe hypertension: ergots
Increase: B/P—oxytocics
Increase: pressor effect—tricyclics, MAOIs
Decrease: DOPamine action—β-blockers, α-blockers
Drug/Lab Test
Increase: Urinary catecholamine, serum glucose

NURSING CONSIDERATIONS

Assess:
• Hypovolemia; if present, correct first
• Oxygenation/perfusion deficit (check B/P, chest pain, dizziness, loss of consciousness)
• Heart failure: S₃ gallop, dyspnea, neck vein distention, bibasilar crackles in patients with CHF, cardiomyopathy
• I&O ratio: if urine output decreases, without decrease in B/P, drug may need to be reduced
• ECG during administration continuously; if B/P increases, drug should be decreased

• B/P and pulse q5min
• CVP or PWP during infusion if possible
• Paresthesias and coldness of extremities; peripheral blood flow may decrease
• Injection site: tissue sloughing; if this occurs, administer phentolamine mixed with NS

Administer:
IV route
• IV after diluting 200-400 mg/250-500 ml of D_5W, D_5 0.45% NaCl, D_5 0.9% NaCl, D_5LR, LR
• After reconstituting, use infusion pump; give at rate of 0.5-5 mcg/kg/min, increase by 1-4 mcg/kg/min at 10-30 min intervals, until desired response
Y-site compatibilities: Aldesleukin, amifostine, amiodarone, amrinone, atracurium, aztreonam, cefmetazole, cefpirome, ciprofloxacin, cisatracurium, cladribine, diltiazem, DOBUTamine, doxorubicin liposome, enalaprilat, epINEPHrine, esmolol, famotidine, fentanyl, fluconazole, foscarnet, granisetron, haloperidol, heparin, hydrocortisone, hydromorphone, labetalol, lidocaine, lorazepam, meperidine, methylPREDNISolone, metronidazole, midazolam, milrinone, morphine, niCARdipine, nitroglycerin, norepinephrine, ondansetron, pancuronium, piperacillin/tazobactam, potassium chloride, propofol, ranitidine, remifentanil, sargramostim, sodium nitroprusside, streptokinase, tacrolimus, theophylline, thiotepa, tolazoline, vecuronium, verapamil, vit B/C, warfarin, zidovudine

Perform/provide:
• Storage of reconstituted sol for up to 24 hr if refrigerated
• Do not use discolored sol; protect from light
Evaluate:
• Therapeutic response: increased B/P with stabilization; increased urine output
Teach patient/family:
• The reason for drug administration
Treatment of overdose: Discontinue IV, may give a short-acting α-adrenergic blocker

D

Rarely Used

dornase alfa (℞)
(door'nace alfa)
Pulmozyme
Func. class.: Cystic fibrosis agent
(orphan drug)

Uses: Management of cystic fibrosis

DOSAGE AND ROUTES

• *Adult/child >5 yr:* INH 2.5 mg daily
by nebulizer
Contraindications: Hypersensitivity
to this drug or Chinese hamster ovary cell
products

dorzolamide ophthalmic
See Appendix C

Rarely Used ⚠ High Alert

doxacurium (℞)
(dox-a-cure'ee-um)
Nuromax
Func. class.: Neuromuscular
blocker (nondepolarizing)

Uses: Facilitation of endotracheal intubation, skeletal muscle relaxation during
mechanical ventilation, surgery, or general anesthesia

DOSAGE AND ROUTES

• *Adult:* IV 0.05 mg/kg; 0.08 mg/kg is
used for prolonged neuromuscular
blockade; maintenance 0.005-0.01
mg/kg
• *Child 2-12 yr:* IV 0.03-0.05 mg/kg;
may decrease for maintenance dose
Contraindications: Hypersensitivity,
neonates

doxapram (℞)
(dox'a-pram)
Dopram
Func. class.: Analeptic

Action: Respiratory stimulation through
activation of peripheral carotid
chemoreceptor; with higher doses, medullary respiratory centers are stimulated;
with progressive CNS stimulation
Uses: Chronic obstructive pulmonary
disease (COPD), postanesthesia respiratory depression, prevention of acute
hypercapnia, drug-induced CNS depression
Investigational uses: Neonatal apnea

DOSAGE AND ROUTES

Postanesthesia
• *Adult:* IV inj 0.5-1 mg/kg, not to exceed 1.5 mg/kg total as a single injection;
IV INF 250 mg in 250 ml sol, not to
exceed 4 mg/kg; run at 1-3 mg/min
Drug-induced CNS depression
• *Adult:* IV priming dose of 2 mg/kg,
repeated in 5 min; repeat q1-2h until
patient awakes; IV INF priming dose 2
mg/kg at 1-3 mg/min, not to exceed 3
g/day
COPD (Hypercapnia)
• *Adult:* IV INF 1-2 mg/min, not to
exceed 3 mg/min for no longer than 2 hr
Apnea of premature infant
• *Infant:* IV 1-1.5 mg/kg/hr loading
dose followed by infusion of 0.5-2.5
mg/kg/hr
Available forms: Inj 20 mg/ml

SIDE EFFECTS

CNS: **Convulsions,** (clonus/general-
ized), *headache,* restlessness, dizziness,
confusion, paresthesias, flushing, sweating, bilateral Babinski's sign, rigidity,
depression
*CV: Chest pain, hypertension, change in
heart rate,* lowered T waves, tachycardia,
dysrhythmias
EENT: Pupil dilation, sneezing
*GI: Nausea, vomiting, diarrhea, desire to
defecate*

⚠ Safety alert   *"Tall Man" lettering

GU: Retention, incontinence, elevation of BUN, albuminuria

INTEG: Pruritus, irritation at inj site

RESP: **Laryngospasm, bronchospasm,** rebound hypoventilation, dyspnea, cough, tachypnea, hiccups

Contraindications: Hypersensitivity, seizure disorders, severe hypertension, severe bronchial asthma, severe dyspnea, severe cardiac disorders, flail chest, pneumothorax, pulmonary embolism, severe respiratory disease

Precautions: Pregnancy (B), bronchial asthma, pheochromocytoma, severe tachycardia, dysrhythmias, hypertension, lactation, children

PHARMACOKINETICS

IV: Onset 20-40 sec, peak 1-2 min, duration 5-10 min; metabolized by liver; excreted by kidneys (metabolites); half-life 2.5-4 hr

INTERACTIONS

Synergistic pressor effect: MAOIs, sympathomimetics

Cardiac dysrhythmias: halothane, cyclopropane, enflurane; delay use of doxapram for at least 10 min after inhalation anesthetics

NURSING CONSIDERATIONS
Assess:
• BP, heart rate, deep tendon reflexes, ABGs, LOC before administration, q30min
• Po_2, Pco_2, O_2 saturation during treatment
• Hypertension, dysrhythmias, tachycardia, dyspnea, skeletal muscle hyperactivity; may indicate overdosage; discontinue drug
• Respiratory stimulation: increased rate, abnormal rhythm
• Extravasation; change IV site q48h
Administer:
IV route
• Undiluted or diluted with equal parts of sterile H_2O for inj; may be diluted 250

mg/250 ml of D_5W, $D_{10}W$ and run as infusion
• IV undiluted over 5 min; IV inf at 1-3 mg/min; adjust for desired respiratory response, using infusion pump IV; if an inf is used after initial dose, start at 1-3 mg/min depending on patient response; D/C after 2 hr; wait 1-2 hr and repeat
• Only after adequate airway is established
• After O_2, IV barbiturates, resuscitative equipment available

Syringe compatibilities: Amikacin, bumetadine, chlorproMAZINE, cimetidine, cisplatin, cyclophosphamide, DOPamine, doxycycline, epINEPHrine, hydrOXYzine, imipramine, isoniazid, lincomycin, methotrexate, netilmicin, phytonadione, pyridoxine, terbutaline, thiamine, tobramycin, vinCRIStine

Perform/provide:
• Placing patient in Sims' position to prevent aspiration of vomitus
• Discontinue infusion if side effects occur; narrow margin of safety

Evaluate:
• Therapeutic response: increased breathing capacity

Teach patient/family:
• Purpose of medication

---

doxazosin (R)
(dox-ay'zoe-sin)
Cardura
Func. class.: Peripheral α_1-adrenergic blocker
Chem. class.: Quinazoline

Do not confuse:
Cardura/Coumadin/Cardene/Ridaura
Action: Peripheral blood vessels are dilated, peripheral resistance lowered; reduction in blood pressure results from α_1-adrenergic receptors being blocked
Uses: Hypertension, urinary outflow obstruction, symptoms of benign prostatic hyperplasia
Investigational uses: CHF with digoxin and diuretics

DOSAGE AND ROUTES

BPH

• *Adult:* **PO** 1 mg daily, increase in stepwise manner to 2, 4, 8 mg daily as needed at 1-2 wk intervals, max 8 mg

Hypertension

• *Adult:* **PO** 1 mg daily, increasing up to 16 mg daily if required; usual range 4-16 mg/day

• *Geriatric:* **PO** 0.5 mg nightly, gradually increase

Available forms: Tabs 1, 2, 4, 8 mg

SIDE EFFECTS

CNS: Dizziness, headache, drowsiness, anxiety, depression, vertigo, weakness, fatigue, asthenia

CV: Palpitations, *orthostatic hypotension,* tachycardia, edema, *dysrhythmias,* chest pain

EENT: Epistaxis, tinnitus, dry mouth, red sclera, pharyngitis, rhinitis

GI: Nausea, vomiting, diarrhea, constipation, abdominal pain

GU: Incontinence, polyuria, priapism

Contraindications: Hypersensitivity to quinazolines

Precautions: Pregnancy (C), children, lactation, hepatic disease

PHARMACOKINETICS

PO: Onset 2 hr, peak 2-6 hr, duration 6-12 hr; half-life 22 hr; metabolized in liver; excreted via bile/feces (<63%) and in urine (9%); extensively protein bound (98%)

INTERACTIONS

Increase: hypotensive effects—alcohol, other antihypertensives, sildenafil, vardenafil, nitrates

Decrease: antihypertensive effects of clonidine

Drug/Herb

Toxicity: yohimbe

Increase: doxazosin effect—angelica

Decrease: doxazosin effect—butcher's broom, capsicum peppers

NURSING CONSIDERATIONS

Assess:

• B/P (lying, standing) and pulse 2-6 hr after each dose and with each increase; postural effects may occur, crackles, dyspnea, orthopnea with B/P; pulse; jugular venous distention during beginning treatment

• BUN, uric acid if on long-term therapy

• I&O, weight daily

• Edema in feet, legs daily

• Skin turgor, dryness of mucous membranes for hydration status

Administer:

• Tablets broken, crushed or chewed; if chewed, will be bitter

Perform/provide:

• Storage in tight container in cool environment

Evaluate:

• Therapeutic response: decreased B/P; decreased symptoms of BPH

Teach patient/family:

• That fainting occasionally occurs after first dose; do not drive or operate machinery for 4 hr after first dose or after dosage increase or take first dose at bedtime

• To take 1st dose at bedtime to decrease orthostatic B/P changes, may take 1-2 wk to respond in BPH

Treatment of overdose: Administer volume expanders or vasopressors; discontinue drug; place in supine position

---

doxepin (℞)

(dox′e-pin)

doxepin HCl, Novo-Doxepin ✦, Sinequan, Sinequan Concentrate, Triadapin ✦, Zonolon Topical Cream

Func. class.: Antidepressant, tricyclic

Chem. class.: Dibenzoxepin, tertiary amine

Do not confuse:

Sinequan/Serentil/Sarafem

⚠ Safety alert   *"Tall Man" lettering

Action: Blocks reuptake of norepinephrine, serotonin into nerve endings, increasing action of norepinephrine, serotonin in nerve cells

Uses: Major depression, anxiety

Investigational uses: Chronic pain management, topical pruritus

DOSAGE AND ROUTES
Depression/anxiety
• *Adult:* PO 25-75 mg/day, may increase to 300 mg/day for severely ill
• *Geriatric:* PO 10-25 mg at bedtime, increase qwk by 10-25 mg to desired dose
Pruritus
• *Adult:* PO 10 mg at bedtime, may increase to 25 mg at bedtime; **TOP** apply thin film qid at least 3 hr apart

Available forms: Caps 10, 25, 50, 75, 100, 150 mg; oral conc 10 mg/ml; cream 5%

SIDE EFFECTS
CNS: Dizziness, drowsiness, confusion, headache, anxiety, tremors, stimulation, weakness, insomnia, nightmares, EPS (elderly), increased psychiatric symptoms, paresthesia

CV: Orthostatic hypotension, ECG changes, tachycardia, **hypertension,** palpitations, **dysrhythmias**

EENT: Blurred vision, tinnitus, mydriasis, ophthalmoplegia, glossitis

GI: Diarrhea, dry mouth, nausea, vomiting, **paralytic ileus,** increased appetite, cramps, epigastric distress, jaundice, **hepatitis,** stomatitis, constipation

GU: Urinary retention, **acute renal failure**

HEMA: **Agranulocytosis, thrombocytopenia, eosinophilia, leukopenia**

INTEG: Rash, urticaria, sweating, pruritus, photosensitivity

Contraindications: Hypersensitivity to tricyclics, urinary retention, narrow-angle glaucoma, prostatic hypertrophy

Precautions: Pregnancy (C), suicidal patients, elderly, UK-PO lactation, seizures

PHARMACOKINETICS
PO: Steady state 2-8 days; metabolized by liver; excreted by kidneys; crosses placenta; excreted in breast milk; half-life 8-24 hr

INTERACTIONS
Hyperpyretic crisis, convulsions, hypertensive episode: MAOI

Increase: hypertensive action—clonidine, epINEPHrine, norepinephrine

Increase: doxepin effect—cimetidine, fluoxetine, sertraline

Increase: CNS depression—other CNS depressants

Drug/Herb
Serotonin syndrome: SAM-e, St. John's wort

Increase: anticholinergic effect—belladonna, corkwood, jimsonweed, henbane

Increase: doxepin action—hops, kava, lavender, scopolia

Increase: hypertension—yohimbe

Drug/Lab Test
Increase: Serum bilirubin, blood glucose, alk phosphatase

NURSING CONSIDERATIONS
Assess:
• B/P (lying, standing), pulse q4h; if systolic B/P drops 20 mm Hg, hold drug, notify prescriber; take vital signs q4h in patients with cardiovascular disease
• Blood studies: CBC, leukocytes, differential, cardiac enzymes if patient is receiving long-term therapy
• Hepatic studies: AST, ALT, bilirubin
• Weight qwk; appetite may increase with drug
• ECG for flattening of T wave, bundle branch block, AV block, dysrhythmias in cardiac patients; drug should be discontinued gradually several days before surgery
• EPS primarily in elderly: rigidity, dystonia, akathisia
• Mental status: mood, sensorium, affect, suicidal tendencies, increase in psychiatric symptoms: depression, panic

• Urinary retention, constipation; constipation most likely in children, elderly
• Withdrawal symptoms: headache, nausea, vomiting, muscle pain, weakness; not usual unless drug is discontinued abruptly
• Alcohol consumption; if alcohol is consumed, hold dose until morning

Administer:

• Oral conc should be diluted with 120 ml of water, milk, orange, grapefruit juice, tomato, prune, pineapple juice; do not mix with grape juice
• Increased fluids, bulk in diet for constipation
• With food, milk for GI symptoms, do not give with carbonated beverages
• Dosage at bedtime for oversedation during day; may take entire dose at bedtime; elderly may not tolerate daily dosing
• Gum, hard candy, or frequent sips of water for dry mouth
• Topically by applying to affected area, rub slightly

Perform/provide:

• Storage in tight container protected from direct sunlight
• Assistance with ambulation during beginning therapy, since drowsiness/dizziness occurs
• Safety measures primarily for elderly
• Checking to see PO medication swallowed

Evaluate:

• Therapeutic response: decreased anxiety, depression

Teach patient/family:

• That therapeutic effect (depressions) may take 2-3 wk, antianxiety effects sooner
• To use caution in driving, other activities requiring alertness, because of drowsiness, dizziness, blurred vision
• To avoid alcohol ingestion, other CNS depressants, may potentiate effects
• Not to discontinue medication quickly after long-term use; may cause nausea, headache, malaise
• To wear sunscreen or large hat, since photosensitivity occurs

• To report immediately urinary retention

Treatment of overdose: ECG monitoring; lavage, activated charcoal; administer anticonvulsant, sodium bicarbonate

---

doxercalciferol (℞)

Hectorol
Func. class.: Parathyroid agent (calcium regulator)
Chem. class.: Vit D hormone

Action: Synthetic vit D analog, reduces parathyroid hormone

Uses: To lower high parathyroid hormone levels in patients undergoing chronic kidney dialysis and those in stages 3/4 of chronic renal disease prior to dialysis; postmenopausal osteoporosis, prostate cancer

DOSAGE AND ROUTES

• *Adult:* **PO** 10 mcg 3×/wk at dialysis
• *Adult:* **IV** 4 mcg 3×/wk at end of dialysis, max 18 mcg/dose

Available forms: Caps 2.5 mcg; inj 2 mcg/ml

SIDE EFFECTS

CNS: Drowsiness, headache, lethargy
GI: Nausea, diarrhea, vomiting, anorexia, dry mouth, constipation, cramps, metallic taste
GU: Polyuria, hypercalciuria, hyperphosphatemia, hematuria
MS: Myalgia, arthralgia, decreased bone development
RESP: SOB

Contraindications: Hypersensitivity, hyperphosphatemia, hypercalcemia, vit D toxicity

Precautions: Pregnancy (C), renal calculi, lactation, CV disease

PHARMACOKINETICS

Metabolism in liver, terminal half-life 96 hr

INTERACTIONS

Decrease: absorption of doxercalci-ferol—cholestyramine, magnesium antacids, mineral oil, do not use together

NURSING CONSIDERATIONS
Assess:

• BUN, urinary calcium, AST, ALT, cholesterol, creatinine, albumin, uric acid, chloride, magnesium, electrolytes, urine pH, phosphate; may increase calcium, should be kept at 9-10 mg/dl, vit D 50-135 international units/dl, phosphate 70 mg/dl
• Alk phosphatase; may be decreased
• For increased drug level, since toxic reactions may occur rapidly
• For dry mouth, metallic taste, polyuria, bone pain, muscle weakness, headache, fatigue, change in LOC, dysrhythmias, increased respirations, anorexia, nausea, vomiting, cramps, diarrhea, constipation; may indicate hypercalcemia
• Renal status: decreased urinary output (oliguria, anuria), edema in extremities, weight gain 5-7 lb, periorbital edema
• Nutritional status, diet for sources of vit D (milk, some seafood); calcium (dairy products, dark green vegetables), phosphates (dairy products) must be avoided

Administer:

• Do not break, crush, or chew caps

Perform/provide:

• Storage protected from light, heat, moisture
• Restriction of sodium, potassium if required
• Restriction of fluids if required for chronic renal failure

Evaluate:

• Therapeutic response: calcium 9-10 mg/dl, decreasing symptoms of hypocalcemia, hypoparathyroidism

Teach patient/family:

• The symptoms of hypercalcemia
• About foods rich in calcium
• To avoid products with sodium in chronic renal failure: cured meats, dairy products, cold cuts, olives, beets, pickles, soups, meat tenderizers
• To avoid products with potassium in chronic renal failure: oranges, bananas, dried fruit, peas, dark green leafy vegetables, milk, melons, beans
• To avoid OTC products containing calcium, potassium, or sodium in chronic renal failure
• To avoid all preparations containing vit D
• To monitor weight weekly

D

⚠ High Alert

***DOXOrubicin** (℞)
(dox-oh-roo'bi-sin)
Adriamycin PFS, Adriamycin RDF, Rubex
***DOXOrubicin liposome** (℞)
Doxil
Func. class.: Antineoplastic, antibiotic
Chem. class.: Anthracycline glycoside

Do not confuse:
Adriamycin/Aredia/Indamycin
DOXOrubicin/idamycin/DAUNOrubicin

Action: Inhibits DNA synthesis primarily; derived from *Streptomyces peucetius;* replication is decreased by binding to DNA, which causes strand splitting; active throughout entire cell cycle; a vesicant

Uses: Wilms' tumor; bladder, breast, liver, lung, ovarian, stomach, testicular, thyroid cancer; Hodgkin's disease; acute lymphoblastic leukemia; myeloblastic leukemia; neuroblastomas; lymphomas; sarcomas; Doxil: AIDs-related Kaposi's sarcoma, metastatic ovarian carcinoma

DOSAGE AND ROUTES
DOXOrubicin
• *Adult:* IV 60-75 mg/m^2 q3wk, or 30

Side effects: *italics* = common; ***bold italics*** = life-threatening

mg/m^2 on days 1-3 of 4-wk cycle, not to exceed 550 mg/m^2 cumulative dose
• *Child:* IV 30 mg/m^2/day × 3 days, may repeat q4wk

DOXOrubicin liposome
• *Adult:* IV 20 mg/m^2 q3wk
Ovarian cancer
• *Adult:* IV 50 mg/m^2 (DOXOrubicin equivalent) given 1 mg/min; if no adverse reactions, may increase to finish infusion in 1 hr
Available forms: Inj 10, 20, 50, 100, 150 mg; Doxil: liposomal dispersion for inj: 20 mg/10 ml, 50 mg/30 ml

SIDE EFFECTS

CV: Increased B/P, *sinus tachycardia, PVCs,* chest pain, *bradycardia, extrasystoles*
GI: Nausea, vomiting, anorexia, *mucositis, hepatotoxicity*
GU: Impotence, sterility, amenorrhea, gynecomastia, hyperuricemia
HEMA: Thrombocytopenia, leukopenia, anemia
INTEG: Rash, necrosis at inj site, dermatitis, reversible *alopecia,* cellulitis, thrombophlebitis at inj site
Contraindications: Pregnancy (D) 1st trimester, hypersensitivity, lactation, systemic infections, cardiac disorders
Precautions: Renal, hepatic, cardiac disease; gout, bone marrow depression (severe)

PHARMACOKINETICS

Triphasic pattern of elimination; half-life 12 min, 3⅓ hr, 29⅔ hr; metabolized by liver; crosses placenta; excreted in urine, bile, breast milk

INTERACTIONS

Hypersensitivity: mercaptopurine
Increase: toxicity—other antineoplastics or radiation, mercaptopurine
Increase: hemorrhagic cystitis risk, cardiac toxicity—cyclophosphamide
Decrease: antibody response—live virus vaccine

Drug/Lab Test
Increase: Uric acid

NURSING CONSIDERATIONS
Assess:
• CBC, differential, platelet count weekly; withhold drug if WBC is <4000/mm^3 or platelet count is <75,000/mm^3; notify prescriber of these results
• Blood, urine uric acid levels
• Renal studies: BUN, serum uric acid, urine CCr, electrolytes before, during therapy
• I&O ratio; report fall in urine output to <30 ml/hr
• Monitor temp q4h; fever may indicate beginning infection
• Hepatic studies before, during therapy: bilirubin, AST, ALT, alk phosphatase as needed or monthly; check for jaundice of skin and sclera, dark urine, clay-colored stools, itchy skin, abdominal pain, fever, diarrhea
• ECG; watch for ST-T wave changes, low QRS and T, possible dysrhythmias (sinus tachycardia, heart block, PVCs); signs of irreversible cardiomyopathy
• Bleeding: hematuria, guaiac, bruising, or petechiae, mucosa or orifices q8h
• Effects of alopecia on body image; discuss feelings about body changes
• Inflammation of mucosa, breaks in skin
• Buccal cavity q8h for dryness, sores, ulceration, white patches, oral pain, bleeding, dysphagia
• Alkalosis if severe vomiting is present
• Local irritation, pain, burning at inj site
• GI symptoms: frequency of stools, cramping
• Acidosis, signs of dehydration: rapid respirations, poor skin turgor, decreased urine output, dry skin, restlessness, weakness
• Cardiac status: B/P, pulse, character, rhythm, rate, ABGs, ECG
Administer:
• Antiemetic 30-60 min before giving drug to prevent vomiting
• Allopurinol or sodium bicarbonate to

maintain uric acid levels, alkalinization of urine

- Topical or systemic analgesics for pain
- Transfusion for anemia
- Antispasmodic for GI symptoms

IV route

⚠ Do not interchange DOXOrubicin with DOXOrubicin liposome

- Hydrocortisone, dexamethasone, or sodium bicarbonate (1 mEq/1 ml) for extravasation; apply ice compresses
- IV after diluting 10 mg/5 ml of NaCl for inj; another 5 ml of diluent/10 mg is recommended; shake; give over 3-5 min; give through Y-tube of free-flowing 5% dextrose INF or NS
- IV liposome inj (Doxil): dilute dose up to 90 mg/250 ml D_5W, give over ½ hr; do not admix with other sol or meds
- Dose modifications for toxicity: Grade 1, redose unless patient has experienced previous grade 3 or 4; Grade 2, delay dosing up to 2 wk or until resolved to grades 0 or 1; Grade 3 delay dosing up to 2 wk or until resolved to grades 0 or 1, resume dose at 25% decrease, return to original dose after interval; Grade 4 delay dosing up to 2 wk or until grade 0 or 1, resume dose at 25% decrease then return to original dose, if after 2 wk there is no resolution, discontinue

Additive compatibilities: Ondansetron

Syringe compatibilities: Bleomycin, cisplatin, cyclophosphamide, droperidol, leucovorin, methotrexate, metoclopramide, mitomycin, vinCRIStine

Y-site compatibilities: Amifostine, aztreonam, bleomycin, chlorproMAZINE, cimetidine, cisplatin, cladribine, cyclophosphamide, dexamethasone, diphenhydrAMINE, droperidol, famotidine, filgrastim, fludarabine, fluorouracil, granisetron, hydromorphone, leucovorin, lorazepam, melphalan, methotrexate, methylPREDNISolone, metoclopramide, mitomycin, morphine, ondansetron, paclitaxel, prochlorperazine, promethazine, propofol, ranitidine, sargramostim, sodium bicarbonate,

teniposide, thiotepa, vinBLAStine, vinCRIStine, vinorelbine

Perform/provide:

- Liquid diet: carbonated beverages, geletin may be added if patient is not nauseated or vomiting
- Increased fluid intake to 2-3 L/day to prevent urate, calculi formation
- Rinsing of mouth tid-qid with water, club soda; brushing of teeth bid-tid with soft brush or cotton-tipped applicators for stomatitis; use unwaxed dental floss
- Storage at room temperature for 24 hr after reconstituting or 48 hr refrigerated

Evaluate:

- Therapeutic response: decreased tumor size, spread of malignancy

Teach patient/family:

- To add 2-3 L of fluids unless contraindicated prior to and for 24-48 hr after, to decrease possible hemorrhagic cystitis
- To report any complaints, side effects to nurse or prescriber
- That hair may be lost during treatment and wig or hairpiece may make patient feel better; tell patient that new hair may be different in color, texture
- To avoid foods with citric acid, hot or rough texture
- To report any bleeding, white spots, ulcerations in mouth to prescriber; tell patient to examine mouth daily
- That urine and other body fluids may be red-orange for 48 hr
- To avoid crowds and persons with infections when granulocyte count is low
- That contraceptive measures are recommended during therapy and 4 mo after
- To avoid vaccinations; reactions may occur

Side effects: *italics* = common; ***bold italics*** = life-threatening

doxycycline (R)

(dox-i-sye'kleen)
Apo-Doxy ✦, Doryx, Doxy,
Doxycin ✦, doxycycline,
Monodox, Novodoxycin ✦,
Periostat, Vibramycin,
Vibra-Tabs
Func. class.: Antiinfective
Chem. class.: Tetracycline

Do not confuse:

doxycycline/doxepin

Action: Inhibits protein synthesis, phosphorylation in microorganisms by binding to 30S ribosomal subunits, reversibly binding to 50S ribosomal subunits; bacteriostatic

Uses: Syphilis, *Chlamydia trachomatis*, gonorrhea, *Rickettsia*, lymphogranuloma venereum, uncommon gram-negative/positive organisms, malaria prophylaxis, chronic periodontitis, acne, anthrax

Investigational uses: Traveler's diarrhea, Lyme disease, prevention of chronic bronchitis

DOSAGE AND ROUTES

• *Adult:* **PO/IV** 100 mg q12h on day 1, then 100 mg/day; **IV** 200 mg in 1-2 inf on day 1, then 100-200 mg/day
• *Child >8 yr:* **PO/IV** 2.2-4.4 mg/kg/day in divided doses q12h

Gonorrhea (uncomplicated) in patients allergic to penicillin
• *Adult:* **PO** 100 mg q12h × 7 days or 300 mg followed 1 hr later by another 300 mg

Malaria prophylaxis
• *Adult:*
• 100 mg daily 1-2 days prior to travel and daily during travel

C. trachomatis
• *Adult:* **PO** 100 mg bid × 7 days

Syphilis
• *Adult:* **PO** 300 mg/day in divided doses × 10 days

Anthrax
• *Adult/child >45 kg:* **IV** 100 mg q12h change to **PO** when able × 60 days
• *Child ≤45 kg:* **PO** 2.2 mg/kg bid × 60 days; **IV** 100 mg q12h, change to **PO** when able × 60 days

Periodontitis
• *Adult:* 20 mg bid after scaling and root planing for ≤9 mo; give close to meal time AM or PM

Available forms: Tabs 100 mg; caps 50, 100 mg; syr 50 mg/5 ml; inj 100, 200 mg; powder for oral susp 25 mg/5 ml; mouth products: tabs 20 mg; inj 42.5 mg

SIDE EFFECTS

CNS: Fever
CV: Pericarditis
EENT: Dysphagia, glossitis, decreased calcification of deciduous teeth, oral candidiasis
GI: Nausea, abdominal pain, vomiting, diarrhea, anorexia, enterocolitis, **hepatotoxicity,** flatulence, abdominal cramps, gastric burning, stomatitis
GU: Increased BUN
*HEMA: **Eosinophilia, neutropenia, thrombocytopenia, hemolytic anemia***
*INTEG: Rash, urticaria, photosensitivity, increased pigmentation, **exfoliative dermatitis,** pruritus, **angioedema***

Contraindications: Pregnancy (D), hypersensitivity to tetracyclines, children <8 yr

Precautions: Hepatic disease, lactation

PHARMACOKINETICS

PO: Well absorbed, widely distributed peak 1½-4 hr, half-life 14-17 hr; excreted in urine, feces, bile, 90% protein bound, crosses placenta, enters breast milk

INTERACTIONS

Increase: effect—warfarin
Decrease: doxycycline effect—antacids, NaHCO₃, dairy products, alkali products, iron, kaolin/pectin, barbitu-

rates, carbamazepine, phenytoin, cimetidine sucralfate, cholestyramine, colestipol, rifampin, bismuth
Decrease: effects—penicillins, oral contraceptives, digoxin
Drug/Herb
Do not use acidophilus with antiinfectives
Increase: action—bromelain
Drug/Lab Test
False increase: Urinary catecholamines; ALT, AST

NURSING CONSIDERATIONS
Assess:
• I&O ratio
• Blood studies: PT, CBC, AST, ALT, BUN, creatinine
• Signs of infection
• Allergic reactions: rash, itching, pruritus, angioedema
• Nausea, vomiting, diarrhea; administer antiemetic, antacids as ordered
• Overgrowth of infection: fever, malaise, redness, pain, swelling, drainage, perineal itching, diarrhea, changes in cough or sputum
• IV site for phlebitis/thrombosis; drug is highly irritating
Administer:
• Do not break, crush, or chew caps
• After C&S
• An empty stomach, or with a full glass of water 2 hr before or after meals; avoid dairy products, antacids, laxatives, iron-containing products; if these must be taken, give 2 hr before or after this agent
IV route
• After diluting 100 mg or less/10 ml of sterile H_2O or NS for inj; further dilute with 100-1000 ml of NaCl, D_5, Ringer's LR D_5LR, Normosol-M, Normosol-R in D_5W; run 100 mg or less over 1-4 hr; do not give IM/SUBCUT; inf must be completed in 6 hr, when diluted in LR sol, or 12 hr in other sol
Additive compatibilities: Ranitidine
Syringe compatibilities: Doxapram
Y-site compatibilities: Acyclovir, amifostine, amiodarone, aztreonam, cisatracurium, cyclophosphamide, diltiazem, filgrastim, fludarabine, granis-

etron, hydromorphone, magnesium sulfate, melphalan, meperidine, morphine, ondansetron, perphenazine, propofol, remifentanil, sargramostim, tacrolimus, teniposide, theophylline, thiotepa, vinorelbine
Perform/provide:
• Storage in tight, light-resistant container at room temperature; IV stable for 12 hr at room temperature, 72 hr refrigerated; discard if precipitate forms
Evaluate:
• Therapeutic response: decreased temp, absence of lesions, negative C&S
Teach patient/family:
• To avoid sun, since burns may occur; sunscreen does not seem to decrease photosensitivity
• That all prescribed medication must be taken to prevent superinfection

---

⚠ High Alert

droperidol (℞)
(droe-per′i-dole)
droperidol, Inapsine
Func. class.: Neuroleptic
Chem. class.: Butyrophenone

Action: Acts on CNS at subcortical levels, produces tranquilization, sleep; antiemetic; mild α-blockade
Uses: Premedication for surgery; induction, maintenance in general anesthesia; postoperatively for nausea, vomiting

DOSAGE AND ROUTES
Induction, adjunct
• *Adult:* **IV/IM** 1.25-2.5 mg, may give additional 1.25 mg
• *Child 2-12 yr:* **IV** 0.05-0.1 mg/kg, titrate to response
Premedication
• *Adult:* **IM** 2.5-10 mg ½-1 hr before surgery, may give 1.25-2.5 mg additionally
• *Child 2-12 yr:* **IM** 0.05-0.1 mg/kg
Available forms: Inj 2.5 mg/ml

SIDE EFFECTS

CNS: EPS (dystonia, akathisia, flexion of arms, fine tremors); dizziness, anxiety, drowsiness, restlessness, hallucination, depression, *seizures*, extrapyramidal symptoms, *neuroleptic malignant syndrome*
CV: *Tachycardia, hypotension,* prolonged QT
EENT: Upward rotation of eyes, oculogyric crisis
INTEG: Chills, facial sweating, shivering
RESP: Laryngospasm, bronchospasm

Contraindications: Hypersensitivity, child <2 yr, lactation
Precautions: Pregnancy (C), elderly, cardiovascular disease (hypotension, bradydysrhythmias), renal disease, hepatic disease, Parkinson's disease, pheochromocytoma

PHARMACOKINETICS

IM/IV: Onset 3-10 min, peak ½ hr, duration 3-6 hr; metabolized in liver; excreted in urine as metabolites; crosses placenta, half-life 2-3 hr

INTERACTIONS

Increase: CNS depression—alcohol, opiates, barbiturates, antihistamines, antipsychotics, or other CNS depressants
Increase: hypotension—nitrates, antihypertensives
Increase: side effects of lithium
Drug/Herb
Increase: action—kava

NURSING CONSIDERATIONS

Assess:
• VS q10min during IV administration, q30min after IM dose
• EPS: dystonia, akathisia
⚠ For increasing heart rate or decreasing B/P, notify prescriber at once; do not place patient in Trendelenburg position, or sympathetic blockade may occur, causing respiratory arrest
• EKG prior to and 2-3 hr after administration for serious arrhythmias

Administer:
• Protect solution from light
• Anticholinergics (benztropine, diphenhydramine) for EPS
• Only with crash cart, resuscitative equipment nearby
• IM deep in large muscle mass
IV, direct route
• Undiluted; give through Y-tube at 10 mg or less/min; titrate to patient response
Intermittent INF route
• May be given as an infusion by adding dose to 250 ml LR, D₅W, 0.9% NaCl; give slowly, titrate to patient response
Syringe compatibilities: Atropine, bleomycin, butorphanol, chlorproMAZINE, cimetidine, cisplatin, cyclophosphamide, dimenhyDRINATE, diphenhydrAMINE, DOXOrubicin, fentanyl, glycopyrrolate, hydrOXYzine, meperidine, metoclopramide, midazolam, mitomycin, morphine, nalbuphine, pentazocine, perphenazine, prochlorperazine, promazine, promethazine, scopolamine, vinBLAStine, vinCRIStine
Y-site compatibilities: Amifostine, aztreonam, bleomycin, cisatracurium, cisplatin, cladribine, cyclophosphamide, cytarabine, DOXOrubicin, DOXOrubicin liposome, famotidine, filgrastim, fluconazole, fludarabine, granisetron, hydrocortisone, idarubicin, melphalan, meperidine, metoclopramide, mitomycin, ondansetron, paclitaxel, potassium chloride, propofol, remifentanil, sargramostim, teniposide, thiotepa, vinBLAStine, vinCRIStine, vinorelbine, vit B/C
Evaluate:
• Therapeutic response: decreased anxiety, absence of vomiting during and after surgery
Teach patient/family:
• To rise slowly from sitting or standing to minimize orthostatic hypotension
• To avoid ambulation without assistance

⚠ Safety alert   *"Tall Man" lettering

drotrecogin alfa (℞)

(droh'treh-koh-jin al'fah)

Xigris

Func. class.: Thrombolytic agent

Chem. class.: Recombinant human activated protein C

Action: Activated protein C exerts an antithrombotic effect by inhibiting factor Va/VIIIa

Uses: Severe sepsis associated with organ dysfunction

DOSAGE AND ROUTES

• *Adult:* IV INF 24 mcg/kg/hr × 96 hr

Available forms: Powder for inj, lyophilized, 5, 20 mg

SIDE EFFECTS

HEMA: Decreased Hct, ***bleeding***

SYST: ***GI, GU, intracranial, intraabdominal, intrathoracic, retroperitoneal bleeding; surface bleeding***

Contraindications: Hypersensitivity, internal active bleeding, intraspinal surgery, CNS neoplasms, ulcerative colitis, enteritis, hepatic disease, hypocoagulation, hemorrhagic stroke, epidural catheter in place, cerebral embolism/thrombosis/hemorrhage, recent major surgery, trauma

Precautions: Pregnancy (C), recent GI bleeding, prothrombin time − INR >3, lactation, children, use >96 hr

PHARMACOKINETICS

Inactivated by endogenous plasma protease inhibitors

INTERACTIONS

Bleeding potential: aspirin, indomethacin, phenylbutazone, anticoagulants, thrombolytics, glycoprotein IIb/IIIa inhibitors

NURSING CONSIDERATIONS

Assess:

⚠ For bleeding during treatment; hematuria, hematemesis, bleeding from mucous membranes, epistaxis, ecchymosis; may require transfusion (rare), continue to assess for bleeding

• Blood studies (Hct, platelets, PTT, PT, TT, aPTT) before starting therapy; PT or aPTT must be less than 2× control before starting therapy; PTT or PT q3-4h during treatment

• VS, B/P, pulse, respirations, neurologic signs, temp at least q4h; temp >104° F (40° C) indicates internal bleeding; systolic pressure increase >25 mm Hg should be reported to prescriber

⚠ For neurologic changes that may indicate intracranial bleeding

⚠ Retroperitoneal bleeding: back pain, leg weakness, diminished pulses

Administer:

IV route

• Reconstitute 5 mg vial/2.5 ml; 20 mg vial/10 ml sterile water for inj to a concentration of 2 mg/ml; slowly add sterile water for inj, do not shake or invert, gently swirl until dissolved

• Further dilute with 0.9% NaCl, slowly withdraw prescribed amount and add to bag of 0.9% NaCl, direct stream to side of bag, gently invert bag; do not transport infusion bag between locations using mechanical delivery systems

• Use immediately after reconstituting, may be held for only 3 hr at controlled room temperature 59°-86° F; must complete infusion within 12 hr after preparation

• Do not use if discolored or if particulate is present

• If using an infusion pump, usual concentration is 100-200 mcg/ml; if using a syringe pump, usual concentration is 100-1000 mcg/ml

• Use a dedicated IV line, or dedicated lumen of central venous catheter; may use only 0.9% NaCl, LR, dextrose, or dextrose/saline mixtures through same line

• Do not expose to heat or direct sunlight

• Discontinue 2 hr prior to invasive surgery or procedures introducing risk of bleeding

Side effects: *italics* = common; ***bold italics*** = life-threatening

Perform/provide:

- Refrigerated storage at 2° to 8° C (36° to 46° F); do not freeze
- Protect unreconstituted vials from light; keep in carton until time of use

Evaluate:

- Therapeutic response: Decreasing symptoms of sepsis, lack of mortality

Teach patient/family:

- Reason for therapy and expected results
- That bleeding may occur for up to 1 month after therapy; signs, symptoms of bleeding

---

duloxetine (℞)

(du-lox′uh-teen)

Cymbalta

Func. class.: Antidepressant—miscellaneous

Chem. class.: Serotonin, norepinephrine reuptake inhibitor

Action: Unknown, may potentiate serotonergic, nonadrenergic activity in the CNS; in studies duloxetine is a potent inhibitor of neuronal serotonin and norepinephrine reuptake

Uses: Major depressive disorder (MDD), neuropathic pain associated with diabetic neuropathy

DOSAGE AND ROUTES

Depression
- *Adult:* **PO** 20 mg bid, may increase to 30 mg bid if needed

Diabetic neuropathy
- *Adult:* **PO** 60 mg daily

Available forms: Caps 20, 30, 60 mg

SIDE EFFECTS

CNS: Insomnia, anxiety, dizziness, tremor, fatigue, decreased appetite, decreased weight

CV: Thrombophlebitis, peripheral edema

EENT: Abnormal vision

GI: Constipation, diarrhea, dysphagia, nausea, vomiting, anorexia, dry mouth, colitis, gastritis

GU: Abnormal ejaculation, urinary hesitation, ejaculation delayed, erectile dysfunction

INTEG: Photosensitivity, bruising, sweating

Contraindications: Hypersensitivity, narrow-angle glaucoma

Precautions: Pregnancy (C), mania, lactation, children, elderly, hypertension, cardiac disease, narrow-angle glaucoma, renal disease, hepatic disease, seizures

PHARMACOKINETICS

Well absorbed, extensively metabolized (CYP2D6, CYP1A2) in the liver to an active metabolite; 70% of drug recovered in urine, 20% in feces; 90% protein binding; half-life 12 hr

INTERACTIONS

Narrow therapeutic index: CYP2D6 extensively metabolized drugs (flecainide, phenothiazines, propafenone, tricyclics, thioridazine)

⚠ Hyperthermia, rigidity, rapid fluctuations of vital signs, mental status changes, neuroleptic malignant syndrome—MAOIs, coadministration is contraindicated or within 14 days of MAOIs use

Increase: CNS depression—opioids, antihistamines, sedative/hypnotics

Increase: action of duloxetine—CYP1A2 inhibitors (fluvoxamine, quinolone antiinfectives); CYP2D6 (fluoxetine, quinidine, paroxetine)

Increase: ALT, bilirubin—alcohol

Drug/Herb

Serotonin syndrome: SAM-e, St. John's wort

Increase: CNS depression—chamomile, hops, kava, lavender, skullcap, valerian

Increase: anticholinergic effect—corkwood, jimsonweed

Increase: hypertension—yohimbe

NURSING CONSIDERATIONS

Assess:

- B/P lying, standing; pulse q4h; if systolic B/P drops 20 mm Hg, hold drug, notify prescriber; take VS q4h in patients with cardiovascular disease

---

⚠ Safety alert   *"Tall Man" lettering

- Hepatic studies: AST, ALT, bilirubin
- Weight qwk; weight loss or gain; appetite may increase; peripheral edema may occur
- Sugarless gum, hard candy, frequent sips of water for dry mouth
- Mental status: mood, sensorium, affect, suicidal tendencies, increase in psychiatric symptoms; depression, panic
- Withdrawal symptoms: headache, nausea, vomiting, muscle pain, weakness; not usual unless drug is discontinued abruptly

Administer:
- Swallow cap whole; do not break, crush, or chew; do not sprinkle on food or mix with liquid

Perform/provide:
- Storage in tight container at room temperature; do not freeze
- Assistance with ambulation during beginning therapy since drowsiness, dizziness occur
- Checking to see if PO medication swallowed

Evaluate:
- Therapeutic response; decreased depression

Teach patient/family:
- To dispense in small amounts because of suicide potential, especially in the beginning of therapy
- To use with caution when driving or other activities requiring alertness because of drowsiness, dizziness, blurred vision
- To avoid alcohol ingestion, MAOIs, other CNS depressants
- Not to discontinue medication quickly after long-term use; may cause nausea, headache, malaise
- To wear sunscreen or large hat, since photosensitivity may occur
- To notify prescriber if pregnancy is planned or suspected, or if breastfeeding
- Improvement may occur in 1-4 wk

dutasteride (R)
(doo-tass'ter-ide)
Duagen
Func. class.: Sex hormone 5α-reductase inhibitor
Chem. class.: Synthetic 4-azasteroid compound

D

Action: Inhibits both types 1 and 2 forms of a steroid enzyme that converts testosterone to 5α-dihydrotestosterone (DHT), which is responsible for the initial growth of prostatic tissue
Uses: Treatment of benign prostatic hyperplasia (BPH) in men with an enlarged prostate gland
Investigational uses: Alopecia

DOSAGE AND ROUTES
- *Adult:* **PO** 0.5 mg daily
Available form: Caps 0.5 mg

SIDE EFFECTS
GU: Decreased libido, impotence, gynecomastia, ejaculation disorders (rare), mastalgia, teratogenesis
Contraindications: Pregnancy (X), hypersensitivity, lactation, women, children
Precautions: Hepatic disease

PHARMACOKINETICS
Peak 2-3 hr, protein binding 99%; metabolized in liver by CYP3A4, excreted in feces; half-life 5 wk at steady state

INTERACTIONS
Increase: dutasteride concentrations—ritonavir, ketoconazole, verapamil, diltiazem, cimetidine, ciprofloxacin, antiretroviral protease inhibitors, or other drugs metabolized by the CYP3A4 pathway

Drug/Lab Test
Increase: TSH
Decrease: PSA

NURSING CONSIDERATIONS

Assess:
- For decreasing symptoms in BPH: decreasing urinary retention, frequency, urgency, nocturia
- PSA levels, digital rectal, urinary obstruction; determine the absence of urinary cancer before starting treatment
- Hepatic studies: ALT, AST, bilirubin

Administer:
- Swallow caps whole; do not break, crush, or chew
- Without regard to meals

Evaluate:
- Therapeutic response: Decreasing symptoms of BPH—decreased urinary frequency, retention, urgency, nocturia

Teach patient/family:
- To read patient information leaflet before starting therapy and reread it upon prescription renewal
- To notify prescriber if therapeutic response decreases; if edema occurs
- Not to discontinue drug abruptly
- About changes in sex characteristics
- That men taking dutasteride should not donate blood for at least 6 mo after last dose, to prevent blood administration to pregnant female
- That caps should not be handled by a pregnant woman because this drug can be absorbed through the skin
- That ejaculate volume may decrease during treatment; that drug rarely interferes with sexual function

---

dyphylline (R)

(dye'fi-lin)

Dilor, Dyflex-200, Dylline, dyphylline, Lufyllin, Neothylline

Func. class.: Bronchodilator

Chem. class.: Xanthine, theophylline derivative

Action: Relaxes smooth muscle of respiratory system by blocking phosphodiesterase, which increases cyclic AMP; cyclic AMP results in positive inotropic, chronotropic effects, bronchodilation, stimulation of CNS

Uses: Bronchial asthma, bronchospasm in chronic bronchitis and emphysema, COPD

DOSAGE AND ROUTES

- *Adult:* **PO** 200-800 mg q6h; **IM** 250-500 mg q6h injected slowly, max 15 mg/kg q6h
- *Child >6 yr:* **PO** 4-7 mg/kg/day in 4 divided doses

Available forms: Tabs 200, 400 mg; elix 33.3, 53.3 mg/5 ml; inj 250 mg/ml

SIDE EFFECTS

*CNS: Anxiety, restlessness, insomnia, dizziness, **convulsions,** headache,* light-headedness, muscle twitching

*CV: Palpitations, **circulatory failure,** sinus tachycardia, hypotension, flush-ing, **dysrhythmias***

GI: Nausea, diarrhea, vomiting, anorexia, dyspepsia, epigastric pain, rectal irritation, bleeding, reflux

INTEG: Flushing, urticaria

OTHER: Fever, dehydration, **albuminuria,** hyperglycemia, increased diuresis

RESP: Tachypnea, **respiratory arrest**

Contraindications: Hypersensitivity to xanthines, seizure disorder, peptic ulcer

Precautions: Pregnancy (C), elderly, CHF, cor pulmonale, hepatic disease, diabetes mellitus, hypertension, children, renal disease, lactation, glaucoma, hyperthyroidism

PHARMACOKINETICS

Well absorbed, peak 1 hr, duration 6 hr, half-life 2 hr, excreted in urine (85%) unchanged, and in breast milk

INTERACTIONS

Cardiotoxicity: β-blockers

Increase: action of dyphylline—cimetidine, propranolol, erythromycin, probenecid

Increase: dyphylline metabolism—barbiturates, phenytoin

Decrease: dyphylline elimination—
uricosurics
Decrease: phenytoin levels

NURSING CONSIDERATIONS
Assess:
• Dyphylline blood levels; toxicity may
occur with small increase above 20 mcg/
ml; assess for drug toxicity: nausea, vomiting, anorexia, cramping, diarrhea,
confusion, dysrhythmias, seizures, diuresis, flushing, headache
• Monitor I&O; diuresis occurs; dehydration may be the result in elderly or
children
• Whether theophylline was given recently
• Auscultate lung fields bilaterally; notify
prescriber of abnormalities, monitor
pulmonary function studies baseline and
periodically
• Allergic reactions: rash, urticaria; drug
should be discontinued
Administer:
• Give around the clock to maintain
blood levels, give daily dose each AM
• PO after meals to decrease GI
symptoms; absorption may be affected
• Avoid IM inj, do not give IV; pain occurs, do not use if precipitate occurs
Perform/provide:
• Storage protected from light, at room
temperature
Evaluate:
• Therapeutic response: decreased
dyspnea, respiratory rate, rhythm
Teach patient/family:
• To check OTC medications, current
prescription medications for epHEDrine;
will increase stimulation; not to drink
alcohol, caffeine, or other xanthine
products; not to change brands
• To avoid hazardous activities; dizziness, drowsiness, blurred vision may
occur
• For GI upset, to take drug with 8 oz
water and food
• To avoid smoking, condition may
worsen
• To obtain blood levels 6-12 mo

econazole topical
See Appendix C

ecothiophate ophthalmic
See Appendix C

Rarely Used

edetate calcium disodium (℞)
(ee'de-tate)
calcium disodium versenate,
calcium EDTA, edathamil
calcium disodium, sodium
calcium edetate
Func. class.: Heavy metal antagonist
(antidote)

Uses: Lead poisoning, acute lead encephalopathy

DOSAGE AND ROUTES
Acute lead encephalopathy
• *Adult and child:*
• 1.5 g/m²/day × 3-5 days in 2-3 divided
doses **IM** or slow **IV** with dimercaprol;
may be given again after 4 days off drug
Lead poisoning
• *Adult:* **IV** 1 g/250-500 ml D₅W or
0.9% NaCl over 1-2 hr or q12h × 3-5
days; may repeat after 2 days; not to exceed 50 mg/kg/day; may be given as
CONT INF over 8-24 hr
• *Adult:* **IM** 35 mg/kg bid
• *Child:* **IM** 35 mg/kg/day in divided
doses q8-12h, not to exceed 50 mg/kg/
day; may give for 3-5 days, off 4 days
before next course
Contraindications: Hypersensitivity,
anuria, poisoning of other metals, severe
renal disease, child <3 yr

Rarely Used

edetate disodium (℞)

(ee′de-tate)
Chealamide, Disodium EDTA,
Disotate, Endrate
Func. class.: Metal antagonist

Uses: Hypercalcemic crisis, control of ventricular dysrhythmias associated with digitalis toxicity

DOSAGE AND ROUTES

• *Adult and child:* **IV INF** 15-50 mg/kg/day in 2 divided doses, diluted in 500 ml D₅W or 0.9% NaCl, given over 3-4 hr, not to exceed 3 g/day (adult) or 70 mg/kg/day (child); allow 5 days between courses (child), 2 days (adult)

Contraindications: Hypersensitivity, anuria, hepatic insufficiency, poisoning of other metals, severe renal disease, child <3 yr, seizure disorders, active/inactive TB

edrophonium (℞)

(ed-roh-fone′ee-um)
Enlon, Reversol, Tensilon
Func. class.: Cholinergics, anticholinesterase
Chem. class.: Quaternary ammonium compound

Action: Inhibits breakdown of acetylcholine, which increases concentration at sites where acetylcholine is released; this facilitates transmission of impulses across myoneural junction

Uses: To diagnose myasthenia gravis; curare antagonist; differentiation of myasthenic crisis from cholinergic crisis

DOSAGE AND ROUTES

Tensilon test (myasthenia gravis diagnosis)
• *Adult:* **IV** 1-2 mg over 15-30 sec, then 8 mg if no response; **IM** 10 mg; if cholinergic reaction occurs, retest after ½ hr with 2 mg **IM**

• *Child >34 kg:* **IV** 2 mg; if no response in 45 sec, then 1 mg q45sec, not to exceed 10 mg; **IM** 5 mg
• *Child <34 kg:* **IV** 1 mg; if no response in 45 sec, then 1 mg q45sec, not to exceed 5 mg; **IM** 2 mg
• *Infant:* **IV** 0.5 mg
Reversal of nondepolarizing neuromuscular blockers
• *Adult:* **IV** 10 mg over 30-45 sec, may repeat, not to exceed 40 mg
Differentiation of myasthenic crisis from cholinergic crisis
• *Adult:* **IV** 1 mg, if no response in 1 min, may repeat
Available forms: Inj 10 mg/ml

SIDE EFFECTS

CNS: Dizziness, headache, sweating, weakness, ***convulsions,*** incoordination, ***paralysis,*** drowsiness, ***loss of consciousness***
CV: Dysrhythmias, bradycardia, hypotension, ***AV block,*** ECG changes, ***cardiac arrest,*** syncope
EENT: Miosis, blurred vision, lacrimation, visual changes
GI: Nausea, *diarrhea, vomiting, cramps, increased salivary and gastric secretions, dysphagia, increased peristalsis*
GU: Urinary frequency, incontinence, urgency
INTEG: Rash, urticaria
RESP: ***Respiratory depression, bronchospasm, constriction, laryngospasm, respiratory arrest,*** dyspnea, increased bronchial secretions
Contraindications: Obstruction of intestine, renal system, hypersensitivity
Precautions: Pregnancy (C), seizure disorders, bronchial asthma, coronary occlusion, hyperthyroidism, dysrhythmias, peptic ulcer, megacolon, poor GI motility, bradycardia, hypotension

PHARMACOKINETICS

IV: Onset 30-60 sec, duration 6-15 min
IM: Onset 2-10 min, duration 12-45 min

INTERACTIONS

Bradycardia: digitalis
Prolonged action of: depolarizing muscle relaxants
Decrease: action of edrophonium—procainamide, quinidine, atropine, anesthetics, phenothiazines, antihistamines, haloperidol, magnesium, corticosteroids, antidysrhythmics

NURSING CONSIDERATIONS

Assess:
• VS, respiration during test; muscle strength
• Diabetic patient carefully, since this drug lowers blood glucose

Administer:
⚠ Only with atropine sulfate available for cholinergic crisis
• Only after all other cholinergics have been discontinued

IV, direct route
• 2 mg or less over 15-30 sec; as a curare antagonist, over 30-45 sec; or given as continuous infusion in myasthenic crisis

Y-site compatibilities: Heparin, hydrocortisone, potassium chloride, vit B/C

Perform/provide:
• Storage at room temperature

Evaluate:
• Therapeutic response: increased muscle strength, hand grasp; improved gait; absence of labored breathing (if severe)

Teach patient/family:
• To wear emergency ID specifying myasthenia gravis, drugs taken

Treatment of overdose: Respiratory support, atropine 1-4 mg (IV)

Rarely Used

efalizumab (℞)
(eh-fah-lih′zyoo-mab)
Raptiva
Func. class.: Immunosuppressive

Uses: Adults 18 years of age and older with moderate to severe plaque psoriasis

---

DOSAGE AND ROUTES

• *Adult:* **SUBCUT** 0.7 mg/kg as a conditioning dose, then **SUBCUT** 1 mg/kg qwk, max single dose 200 mg

Contraindications: Hypersensitivity

---

efavirenz (℞)
(ef-ah-veer′enz)
Sustiva
Func. class.: Antiretroviral
Chem. class.: Nonnucleoside reverse transcriptase inhibitor (NNRTI)

E

Action: Binds directly to reverse transcriptase and blocks RNA, DNA causing a disruption of the enzyme's site

Uses: HIV-1 in combination with other antivirals

DOSAGE AND ROUTES

Given in combination with protease inhibitor or nucleoside analog reverse transcriptase inhibitors (NARTIs)

• *Adult and child >40 kg:* **PO** 600 mg daily at bedtime
• *Child: 10-15 kg:* **PO** 200 mg daily at bedtime
• *Child: 15-20 kg:* **PO** 250 mg daily at bedtime
• *Child: 20-25 kg:* **PO** 300 mg daily at bedtime
• *Child: 25-32.5 kg:* **PO** 350 mg daily at bedtime
• *Child: 32.5-40 kg:* **PO** 400 mg daily at bedtime

Available forms: Caps 50, 100, 200 mg; 600 mg tabs

SIDE EFFECTS

CNS: Fatigue, impaired concentration, insomnia, abnormal dreams, depression, headache, dizziness, anxiety, drowsiness
GI: Diarrhea, abdominal pain, *nausea,* hyperlipidemia
GU: Hematuria, kidney stones
INTEG: Rash, ***erythema multiforme, Stevens-Johnson syndrome, toxic epidermal necrolysis***

Contraindication: Pregnancy (D), hypersensitivity

Precautions: Hepatic disease, lactation, children <3 yr, renal disease, myelosuppression, depression, seizures

PHARMACOKINETICS

Peak 3–5 hr, well absorbed, metabolized by liver, terminal half-life 52-76 hr, >99% protein binding, metabolized by liver, excreted in urine/feces

INTERACTIONS

Do not give together with benzodiazepines, ergots, midazolam, triazolam, cisapride

Increase: CNS depression—alcohol, antidepressants, antihistamines, opioids

Increase: levels of both drugs—ritonavir, estrogens, anticonvulsants

Increase: levels of warfarin, ergots, midazolam, triazolam, statins (except pravastatin, fluvastatin)

Decrease: efavirenz levels—rifamycins

Decrease: levels of indinavir, saquinavir, clarithromycin, methadone

Drug/Herb

Decrease: efavirenz level—St. John's wort, do not use together

Drug/Food

Increase: absorption—high-fat foods

Drug/Lab Test

Increase: ALT

False positive: cannibinoids

NURSING CONSIDERATIONS

Assess:

• Signs of infection, anemia

• Hepatic studies: ALT, AST: renal studies

• Bowel pattern before, during treatment; if severe abdominal pain with bleeding occurs, drug should be discontinued; monitor hydration

• Skin eruptions; rash, urticaria, itching

• Allergies before treatment, reaction to each medication

• CBC, blood chemistry, plasma HIV RNA, absolute CD4+/CD8+ cell counts/%, serum β_2 microglobulin, serum ICD+24 antigen levels, cholesterol, hepatic enzymes

• Signs of toxicity: severe nausea/vomiting, maculopapular rash

Administer:

• Give on empty stomach; at bedtime to decrease CNS side effects

Evaluate:

• Therapeutic response: increased CD4 cell counts; decreased viral load; slowing progression of HIV

Teach patient/family:

• To take as prescribed; if dose is missed, take as soon as remembered; do not double dose; take with water, juice; taken on empty stomach at bedtime

• To make sure health care provider knows all the medications, supplements, or OTC drugs taken

• That if severe rash occurs, to notify health care provider; that adverse reactions (rash, dizziness, abnormal dreams, insomnia) lessen after a month

• Not to breastfeed or become pregnant if taking this drug, use nonhormonal contraception, serious birth defects have occurred

• To avoid hazardous activities if dizziness/drowsiness occur

• That drug does not cure disease, but controls symptoms, HIV can be transmitted to others even while taking this drug, to continue with safe-sex practices

---

eletriptan (R)

(el-ee-trip′tan)

Relpax

Func. class.: Antimigraine agent

Chem. class.: 5-HT$_1$-1B/1D receptor agonist

Action: Binds selectively to the vascular 5-HT$_1$-receptor subtype; causes vasoconstriction in cranial arteries

Uses: Acute treatment of migraine with or without aura

DOSAGE AND ROUTES

• *Adult:* **PO** 20 mg, may increase if needed, max 40 mg (single dose); may

---

repeat in 2 hr if headache improves but returns, max 80 mg/day
Available forms: Tabs 20, 40 mg

SIDE EFFECTS

CNS: Dizziness, headache, anxiety, paresthesia, asthenia, somnolence, flushing, fatigue, hot/cold sensation
CV: Chest pain, palpitations, hypertension
GI: Nausea, dry mouth
MS: Weakness
RESP: Chest tightness, pressure
Contraindications: Hypersensitivity, coronary artery vasospasm, peripheral vascular disease, hemiplegic/basilar migraine, concurrent use of ergotamine-containing preparations, uncontrolled hypertension; ischemic bowel, heart disease; severe hepatic disease
Precautions: Pregnancy (C), postmenopausal women, men >40 yr, risk factors of CAD, MI, or other cardiac disease, hypercholesterolemia, obesity, diabetes, impaired hepatic or renal function, lactation, children, elderly

PHARMACOKINETICS

Onset of pain relief 2 hr; metabolized in the liver; excreted in urine, feces

INTERACTIONS

Increase: plasma concentration of eletriptan—CYP3A4 inhibitors (clarithromycin, ketoconazole, erythromycin, itraconazole, ritonavir, nelfinavir); also propranolol
Drug/Herb
Increase: effect—butterbur

NURSING CONSIDERATIONS

Assess:
• B/P; signs/symptoms of coronary vasospasms
• Tingling, hot sensation, burning, feeling of pressure, numbness, flushing
• For stress level, activity, recreation, coping mechanisms
• Neurologic status: LOC, blurring vision, nausea, vomiting, tingling in extremities preceding headache

• Ingestion of tyramine foods (pickled products, beer, wine, aged cheese), food additives, preservatives, colorings, artificial sweeteners, chocolate, caffeine, which may precipitate these types of headaches
Administer:
• Swallow tabs whole; do not break, crush, or chew
Perform/provide:
• Quiet, calm environment with decreased stimulation from noise, bright light, excessive talking
Evaluate:
• Therapeutic response: decrease in severity of migraine
Teach patient/family:
• To report any side effects to prescriber
• To use contraception while taking drug
• To provide dark, quiet environment
• That drug does not prevent or reduce number of migraine attacks

---

emedastine ophthalmic
See Appendix C

---

emtricitabine (R)
(em-tri-sit'uh-bean)
Emtriva
Func. class.: Antiretroviral
Chem. class.: Nucleoside reverse transcriptase inhibitor (NRTI)

Action: A synthetic nucleoside analog of cytosine. Inhibits replication of HIV virus by competing with the natural substrate and then becoming incorporated into cellular DNA by viral reverse transcriptase, thereby terminating cellular DNA chain.
Uses: HIV-1 infection with other antiretrovirals.

DOSAGE AND ROUTES

• *Adult:* **PO** 200 mg daily
Renal dose
• *Adult:* **PO** CCr 30-49 ml/min 200 mg

---

q48h; 15-29 ml/min 200 mg q72h; <15 ml/min 200 mg q96h
Available forms: Cap 200 mg

SIDE EFFECTS

CNS: Headache, abnormal dreams, depression, dizziness, insomnia, neuropathy, paresthesia
GI: Nausea, vomiting, diarrhea, anorexia, abdominal pain, dyspepsia
INTEG: Rash, skin discolorization
MS: Arthralgia, myalgia
RESP: Cough
SYST: Change in body fat distribution
Contraindications: Hypersensitivity
Precautions: Pregnancy (B), lactation, children, elderly, renal disease, hepatic insufficiency, chronic hepatitis B

PHARMACOKINETICS

Rapidly, extensively absorbed, peak 1-2 hr, protein binding <4%, excreted unchanged in urine (86%), feces (14%); half-life 10 hr

INTERACTIONS

None known

NURSING CONSIDERATIONS

Assess:
• Renal, hepatic function tests: AST, ALT, bilirubin, amylase, lipase, triglycerides periodically during treatment
⚠ For lactic acidosis, severe hepatomegaly with steatosis; if lab reports confirm these conditions, discontinue treatment
Administer:
• Give without regard to meals
Perform/provide:
• Storage at 25° C (77° F)
Evaluate:
• Therapeutic response: Decrease in signs/symptoms of HIV
Teach patient/family:
• That GI complaints resolve after 3-4 wk of treatment
• Not to breastfeed while taking this drug

• That drug must be taken at same time of day to maintain blood level
• That drug will control symptoms, but is not a cure for HIV; patient is still infectious, may pass HIV virus on to others
• That other drugs may be necessary to prevent other infections
• That changes in body fat distribution may occur

**enalapril/
enalaprilat (Ɓ)**
(e-nal′a-pril)/(e-nal′a-pril-at)
Vasotec, Vasotec IV
Func. class.: Antihypertensive
Chem. class.: Angiotensin-converting enzyme (ACE) inhibitor

Do not confuse:
enalapril/ramipril/Anafranil
enalapril/Eldepryl
Action: Selectively suppresses renin-angiotensin-aldosterone system; inhibits ACE; prevents conversion of angiotensin I to angiotensin II, dilation of arterial, venous vessels
Uses: Hypertension, CHF, left ventricular dysfunction

DOSAGE AND ROUTES

Hypertension
• *Adult:* **PO** 5 mg/day, may increase or decrease to desired response, range 10-40 mg/day; **IV** 1.25 mg q6h over 5 min
• *Child:* **PO** 0.08 mg/kg/day in 1-2 divided doses, max 0.58 mg/kg/day
• *Child:* **IV** 5-10 mcg/kg/dose q8-24h
Patients on diuretics
• *Adult:* **IV** 0.625 mg over 5 min, may give additional doses of 1.25 mg q6h
Renal impairment
• *Adult:* **PO** 2.5 mg daily (CCr <30 ml/min) increase gradually; **IV** CCr >30 ml/min 1.25 mg q6h; CCr <30 ml/min 0.625 mg as one-time dose, increase as per B/P

⚠ Safety alert   *"Tall Man" lettering

CHF
• *Adult:* **PO** 2.5-20 mg/day in 2 divided doses, max 40 mg daily in divided doses
Available forms: enalapril: tabs 2.5, 5, 10, 20 mg; enalaprilat: inj 1.25 mg/ml

SIDE EFFECTS

CNS: Insomnia, dizziness, paresthesias, headache, fatigue, anxiety
CV: Hypotension, chest pain, tachycardia, *dysrhythmias,* syncope, angina, *MI,* orthostatic hypotension
EENT: Tinnitus, visual changes, sore throat, double vision, dry burning eyes
GI: Nausea, vomiting, colitis, cramps, diarrhea, constipation, flatulence, dry mouth, loss of taste
GU: Proteinuria, renal failure, increased frequency of polyuria or oliguria
HEMA: Agranulocytosis, neutropenia
INTEG: Rash, purpura, alopecia, hyperhidrosis, photosensitivity
META: Hyperkalemia
RESP: Dyspnea, dry cough, crackles, angioedema
Contraindications: Pregnancy (D) 2nd/3rd trimester, hypersensitivity, history of angioedema
Precautions: Renal disease, hyperkalemia, pregnancy (C) 1st trimester, lactation, hepatic failure, dehydration, bilateral renal artery stenosis

PHARMACOKINETICS

Enalapril:
PO: Onset 1 hr, peak 4-6 hr, duration ≥24 hr; half-life 1½ hr; metabolized by liver to active metabolite, excreted in urine
Enalaprilat:
IV: Onset 5-15 min, peak up to 4 hr

INTERACTIONS

Hypersensitivity: allopurinol
Increase: hypotension—diuretics, other antihypertensives, phenothiazines, nitrates, acute alcohol ingestion, general anesthesia
Increase: potassium levels—salt substitutes, potassium-sparing diuretics, potassium supplements, cycloSPORINE, indomethacin
Increase: levels of lithium, digoxin
Decrease: effects of enalapril—antacids, rifampin
Drug/Herb
Severe photosensitivity: St. John's wort
Fatal hypokalemia: arginine
Increase: effect—pill-bearing spurge
Decrease: effect—pineapple, yohimbe
Drug/Lab Test
Increase: ALT, AST, bilirubin, alk phosphatase, glucose, uric acid
False positive: ANA titer

NURSING CONSIDERATIONS

Assess:
• Blood studies: neutrophils, decreased platelets; WBC with diff baseline and q3mo, if neutrophils <1000/mm^3, discontinue treatment (recommended in collagen-vascular disease)
• B/P, peak/trough level, orthostatic hypotension, syncope when used with diuretic, pulse q4h; note rate, rhythm, quality
• Electrolytes: K, Na, Cl during 1st 2 wk of therapy
• Baselines in renal, hepatic studies before therapy begins and 1 wk into therapy
• Edema in feet, legs daily
• Skin turgor, dryness of mucous membranes for hydration status
• Symptoms of CHF: edema, dyspnea, wet crackles
Administer:
IV direct/Intermittent INF route
• Undiluted over 5 min, use diluent provided or 50 ml D$_5$W, 0.9% NaCl, 0.9% NaCl in D$_5$W or LR, Isolyte E, give through Y-tube of free-flowing inf of 0.9% NaCl, D$_5$W, LR, Isolyte E
Additive compatibilities: DOBUTamine, DOPamine, heparin, meropenem, nitroglycerin, nitroprusside, potassium chloride

Y-site compatibilities: Allopurinol, amifostine, amikacin, aminophylline, ampicillin, ampicillin/sulbactam, aztreonam, butorphanol, calcium gluconate, cefazolin, cefoperazone, ceftazidime, ceftizoxime, chloramphenicol, cimetidine, cisatracurium, cladribine, clindamycin, dextran 40, DOBUTamine, DOPamine, doxorubicin liposome, erythromycin, esmolol, famotidine, fentanyl, filgrastim, ganciclovir, gentamicin, granisetron, heparin, hetastarch, hydrocortisone, labetalol, lidocaine, magnesium sulfate, melphalan, meropenem, methylPREDNISolone, metronidazole, morphine, nafcillin, niCARdipine, nitroprusside, penicillin G potassium, phenobarbital, piperacillin, piperacillin/tazobactam, potassium chloride, potassium phosphate, propofol, ranitidine, remifentanil, teniposide, thiotepa, tobramycin, trimethoprim-sulfamethoxazole, vancomycin, vinorelbine

Evaluate:
• Therapeutic response: decreased B/P

Teach patient/family:
• Not to use OTC (cough, cold, or allergy) products unless directed by prescriber; to avoid potassium, salt substitutes
• To avoid sunlight or wear sunscreen for photosensitivity
• To comply with dosage schedule, even if feeling better
• To notify prescriber of mouth sores, sore throat, fever, swelling of hands or feet, irregular heartbeat, chest pain, signs of angioedema
• That excessive perspiration, dehydration, vomiting, diarrhea may lead to fall in blood pressure; consult prescriber if these occur
• That drug may cause dizziness, fainting; light-headedness may occur during 1st few days of therapy
• That drug may cause skin rash, impaired perspiration or angioedema; discontinue if angioedema occurs
• Not to discontinue drug abruptly
• That CV adverse reactions may reoccur
• To rise slowly to sitting or standing

position to minimize orthostatic hypotension

Treatment of overdose: Lavage, IV atropine for bradycardia, IV theophylline for bronchospasm, digitalis, O_2, diuretic for cardiac failure

---

enfuvirtide (Ŗ)
(en-fyoo'vir-tide)
Fuzeon
Func. class.: Antiretroviral
Chem. class.: Fusion Inhibitor

Action: Inhibitor of the fusion of HIV-1 with CD4+ cells
Uses: Treatment of HIV-1 infection in combination with other antiretrovirals

DOSAGE AND ROUTES
• *Adult:* **SUBCUT** 90 mg (1 ml) bid
• *Child 6-16 yr:* **SUBCUT** 2 mg/kg bid, max 90 mg bid
Available forms: Powder for inj, lyophilized 108 mg (90 mg/ml when reconstituted)

SIDE EFFECTS
CNS: Anxiety, peripheral neuropathy, taste disturbance, *Gullain-Barré syndrome*, insomnia, depression
GI: Abdominal pain, anorexia, constipation, pancreatitis
GU: *Glomerulonephritis, renal failure*
HEMA: *Thrombocytopenia, neutropenia*
INTEG: Inj site reactions
MISC: Influenza, cough, conjunctivitis, lymphadenopathy, myalgia, hyperglycemia, pneumonia, rhinitis, fatigue
Contraindications: Hypersensitivity
Precautions: Pregnancy (B), liver disease, lactation, children <6 yr, myelosuppression, infections

PHARMACOKINETICS
Peak 8 hr, terminal half-life 3.8 hr, well absorbed, undergoes catabolism, 92% protein binding

---

INTERACTIONS
None known

NURSING CONSIDERATIONS
Assess:
• Signs of infection, inj site reactions
• Renal studies: BUN, creatinine, renal failure may occur
• Bowel pattern before, during treatment; if severe abdominal pain or constipation occurs, notify prescriber; monitor hydration
• Skin eruptions, rash, urticaria, itching
• Allergies before treatment, reaction to each medication
• CBC, blood chemistry, plasma HIV RNA, absolute CD4+/CD8+ cell counts/%, serum β_2 microglobulin, serum ICD+24 antigen levels, cholesterol
Administer:
• SUBCUT, give bid, rotate sites
Evaluate:
• Therapeutic response: increased CD4 cell counts; decreased viral load; slowing progression of HIV-1 infection
Teach patient/family:
• To notify prescriber if pregnancy is suspected, or if breastfeeding
• That pneumonia may occur, to contact prescriber if cough, fever occur
• That hypersensitive reactions may occur, rash, pruritus; stop drug, contact prescriber
• That this drug is not a cure for HIV-1 infection but controls symptoms, HIV-1 can still be transmitted to others
• This drug is to be used in combination only with other antiretrovirals

---

enoxacin (℞)
(e-nox′a-sin)
Penetrex
Func. class.: Antiinfective
Chem. class.: Fluoroquinolone

Do not confuse:
enoxacin/enoxaparin
Action: Inhibits the enzyme that repairs bacterial DNA, thereby preventing bacterial replication; DNA-gyrase inhibitor
Uses: Uncomplicated urethral or cervical gonorrhea, uncomplicated and complicated UTI; effective against staphylococci, *Aeromonas* sp., *Citrobacter* sp., *Enterobacter* sp., *Escherichia coli*, *Haemophilus ducreyi*, *Klebsiella* sp., *Morganella morganii*, *Neisseria gonorrhoeae*, *Proteus vulgaris*, *Proteus mirabilis*, *Providencia* sp., *Pseudomonas aeruginosa*, *Serratia*

DOSAGE AND ROUTES
Gonorrhea
• *Adult:* **PO** 400 mg as a single dose
Uncomplicated UTI
• *Adult:* **PO** 200 mg q12h × 7 days
Complicated UTI
• *Adult:* **PO** 400 mg q12h × 14 days
Renal disease
• CCr <30 ml/min give initial dose, then give 50% of dose q12h
Available forms: Tabs 200, 400 mg

SIDE EFFECTS
CNS: Dizziness, headache, fatigue, somnolence, depression, insomnia, anxiety, ***seizures***
EENT: Visual disturbances, dizziness
GI: Diarrhea, nausea, vomiting, anorexia, flatulence, heartburn, abdominal pain, dry mouth, increased AST, ALT, ***pseudomembranous colitis***
INTEG: Rash, pruritus, photosensitivity
*SYST: **Anaphylaxis, Stevens-Johnson syndrome***
Contraindications: Hypersensitivity to quinolones
Precautions: Pregnancy (C), lactation, children, elderly, renal disease, seizure disorders

PHARMACOKINETICS
PO: Peak 1 hr, half-life 3-6 hr, steady state 2 days; excreted in urine as unchanged drug, metabolites

---

INTERACTIONS

Increase: levels of aminophylline, cimetidine, cycloSPORINE, warfarin, use cautiously

Increase: levels toxicity—theophylline; do not use together

Increase: digoxin levels—digoxin, monitor for toxicity

Decrease: absorption of enoxacin—antacids with magnesium, aluminum; iron salts, sucralfate, bismuth subsalicylate

Drug/Herb
Do not use acidophilus with antiinfectives

Drug/Food
Decrease: absorption with food, dairy products

NURSING CONSIDERATIONS

Assess:
• Renal, hepatic studies: BUN, creatinine, AST, ALT, alk phosphatase
• I&O ratio, urine pH; <5.5 is ideal
• CNS symptoms: insomnia, vertigo, headache, agitation, confusion
• Allergic reactions and anaphylaxis: rash, flushing, urticaria, pruritus; may occur a few days after therapy begins, emergency equipment should be available

Administer:
• After clean-catch urine for C&S
• 2 hr before or 2 hr after antacids, zinc, iron, calcium

Perform/provide:
• Limited intake of alkaline foods, drugs; milk, dairy products, peanuts, vegetables, alkaline antacids, sodium bicarbonate

Evaluate:
• Therapeutic response: negative C&S, absence of symptoms of infection

Teach patient/family:
• That fluids must be increased to 2 L/day to avoid crystallization in kidneys
• If dizziness occurs, to ambulate, perform activities with assistance, do not perform hazardous activities
• Not to take within 2 hr of antacids, calcium, iron, milk, sucralfate; not to double or miss doses
• To use sunscreen, protective clothing for photosensitivity
• To complete full course of drug therapy, take 1 hr ac or 2 hr pc
• To contact prescriber if adverse reactions occur or if inflammation or pain of tendon occurs
• To avoid use with OTC medications unless approved by prescriber

---

⚠ High Alert

enoxaparin (℞)
(ee-nox′a-par-in)
Lovenox
Func. class.: Anticoagulant, antithrombotic
Chem. class.: Low-molecular-weight heparins (LMWH)

Do not confuse:
enoxaparin/enoxacin
Lovenox/Lotronex

Action: Prevents conversion of fibrinogen to fibrin and prothrombin to thrombin by enhancing inhibitory effects of antithrombin III; produces higher ratio of anti–factor Xa to IIa

Uses: Prevention of deep-vein thrombosis, pulmonary emboli in hip and knee replacement, abdominal surgery at risk for thrombosis; unstable angina/non–Q-wave MI

DOSAGE AND ROUTES

DVT prevention before hip/knee surgery
• *Adult:* SUBCUT 30 mg bid given 12-24 hr postop for 7-10 days, provided that hemostasis has been established

DVT prevention before hip replacement
• *Adult:* SUBCUT 40 mg daily started 12 hr preop or 30 mg q12hr, started 12-24 hr postop

DVT prophylaxis before abdominal surgery
• *Adult:* SUBCUT 40 mg daily × 7-10

days to prevent thromboembolic complications, start 24 hr before surgery

Treatment of DVT/PE
- *Adult:* **SUBCUT** (Outpatient) (without PE) 1 mg/kg q12h or 1.5 mg/kg daily (outpatient and inpatient)

Prevention of ischemic complications in unstable angina/non−Q-wave MI
- *Adult:* **SUBCUT** 1 mg/kg q12h until stable with aspirin 100-325 mg daily × 2-8 days

Available forms: Inj 30 mg/0.3 ml, 40 mg/0.4 ml, 60 mg/0.6 ml, 80 mg/0.8 ml, 100 mg/1 ml, 120 mg/0.8 ml, 150 mg/ml, 300 mg/3 ml

SIDE EFFECTS

CNS: Fever, confusion
GI: Nausea
HEMA: **Hemorrhage, hypochromic anemia, thrombocytopenia,** bleeding
INTEG: Ecchymosis, inj site hematoma
SYST: Edema, peripheral edema

Contraindications: Hypersensitivity to this drug, heparin, or pork; hemophilia, leukemia with bleeding, peptic ulcer disease, thrombocytopenic purpura, heparin-induced thrombocytopenia, increased risk of bleeding

Precautions: Pregnancy (B), alcoholism, elderly, hepatic disease (severe), renal disease (severe), blood dyscrasias, severe hypertension, subacute bacterial endocarditis, acute nephritis, lactation, children, recent burn, spinal surgery

PHARMACOKINETICS

SUBCUT: 90% absorbed, maximum antithrombin activity (3-5 hr), elimination half-life 4½ hr, excreted in urine

INTERACTIONS

Increase: enoxaparin action—anticoagulants, salicylates, NSAIDs, antiplatelets, thrombolytics

Drug/Herb
Increase: risk of bleeding—agrimony, alfalfa, angelica, anise, basil, bay, bilberry, black haw, bogbean, bromelain, buchu, chondroitin, cinchona bark, dong quai, fenugreek, feverfew, garlic, ginger, ginkgo, ginseng, horse chestnut, Irish moss, kelp, kelpware, khella, lovage, lungwort, meadowsweet, motherwort, mugwort, nettle, papaya, parsley (large amts), pau d'arco, pineapple, poplar, prickly ash, safflower, saw palmetto, tonka bean, turmeric, wintergreen, yarrow
Decrease: anticoagulant effect—chamomile, coenzyme Q10, flax, glucomannan, goldenseal, guar gum

Drug/Lab Test
Increase: AST, ALT
Decrease: Platelet count

NURSING CONSIDERATIONS

Assess:
- Blood studies (Hct, CBC, coagulation studies, platelets, occult blood in stools), anti–factor Xa; thrombocytopenia may occur
- For bleeding: gums, petechiae, ecchymosis, black tarry stools, hematuria; notify prescriber
- For neurologic symptoms in patients who have received spinal anesthesia

Administer:
- Only after screening patient for bleeding disorders
- SUBCUT only; do not give IM, begin 1 hr prior to surgery, do not aspirate, rotate sites, do not expel bubble from syringe before administration
- To recumbent patient; give SUBCUT; rotate inj sites (left/right anterolateral, left/right posterolateral abdominal wall)
- Insert whole length of needle into skin fold held with thumb and forefinger
- Do not mix with other drugs or infusion fluids
- **A** Only this drug when ordered; not interchangeable with heparin or other LMWHs
- At same time each day to maintain steady blood levels
- Leave vascular access sheath in place for 6 hr after dose, then give next dose 6 hr after sheath removal

- Avoid all IM inj that may cause bleeding

Perform/provide:
- Storage at 77° F (25° C); do not freeze

Evaluate:
- Therapeutic response: prevention of deep vein thrombosis

Teach patient/family:
- To use soft-bristle toothbrush to avoid bleeding gums, to use electric razor
- To report any signs of bleeding: gums, under skin, urine, stools
- To avoid OTC drugs containing aspirin unless approved by prescriber

Treatment of overdose: Protamine SO$_4$ 1% sol; dose should equal dose of enoxaparin

---

entacapone (R)
(en'ta-kah-pone)
Comtan
Func. class.: Antiparkinson agent
Chem. class.: COMT inhibitor

Action: Inhibits COMT (catechol *O*-methyltransferase) and alters the plasma pharmacokinetics of levodopa. Given with levodopa/carbidopa
Uses: Parkinson's disease in those experiencing end of dose, decreased effect as adjunct to levodopa/carbidopa

DOSAGE AND ROUTES
- *Adult:* **PO** 200 mg given with carbidopa/levodopa, max 1600 mg/day
Available forms: Tabs 200 mg film coated

SIDE EFFECTS

CNS: Involuntary choreiform movements, hand tremors, fatigue, headache, anxiety, twitching, numbness, dyskinesia, hypokinesia, hyperkinesia, weakness, confusion, agitation, nightmares, psychosis, hallucination, hypomania, severe depression, dizziness, ***neuroleptic malignant syndrome***
CV: Orthostatic hypotension
GI: Nausea, vomiting, anorexia, abdominal distress, dry mouth, flatu-
lence, bitter taste, diarrhea, constipation, dyspepsia, gastritis, GI disorder
INTEG: Rash, sweating, alopecia
MISC: Dark urine and other body fluids, back pain, dyspnea, purpura, fatigue, asthenia, infection-bacterial, ***rhabdomyolysis***

Contraindications: Hypersensitivity
Precautions: Pregnancy (C), renal disease, hepatic disease, affective disorders, psychosis, lactation, children

PHARMACOKINETICS

Duration up to 8 hr; excreted in urine, feces; well absorbed, protein binding 98%, metabolized in liver extensively, enters breast milk; half-life of levodopa is extended, half-life 0.5 hr initial, 2.5 hr second

INTERACTIONS

Prevents catecholamine metabolism, do not use together—MAOIs
Increase: B/P, tachycardia, dysrhythmias, avoid use—bitolterol, DOPamine, DOBUTamine, epINEPHrine, methyldopa, isoetharine, norepinephrine
Decrease: excretion of entacapone—ampicillin, chloramphenicol, probenecid, erythromycin, rifampin
Drug/Herb
Decrease: effect—kava

NURSING CONSIDERATIONS
Assess:
⚠ Neuroleptic malignant syndrome: high temp, increased CPK, rigidity, change in consciousness
- Involuntary movements in Parkinson's disease: akinesia, tremors, staggering gait, muscle rigidity, drooling when given with levodopa/carbidopa
- B/P, respiration during initial treatment
- Mental status: affect, mood, behavioral changes, depression; complete suicide assessment

Administer:
- Only after MAOIs have been discontinued for 2 wk

⚠ Safety alert   *"Tall Man" lettering

• Give with a dose of levodopa/carbidopa, this drug has no effect on its own

Perform/provide:
• Assistance with ambulation during beginning therapy

Evaluate:
• Therapeutic response: decrease in akathisia, increased mood when given with levodopa/carbidopa

Teach patient/family:
• That hallucinations, mental changes, nausea, dyskinesia can occur and may mean patient is overmedicated
• To change positions slowly to prevent orthostatic hypotension; not to drive or operate machinery until stabilized on medication and mental performance is not affected
• To use drug exactly as prescribed
• That urine, sweat may darken
• To notify prescriber if pregnancy is suspected; or if lactating, drug is excreted in breast milk

---

entecavir
See Appendix A—Selected New Drugs

⚠ High Alert

epHEDrine (℞)
(e-fed'rin)
epHEDrine sulfate, Pretz-D (OTC)
Func. class.: Bronchodilator, nonselective adrenergic, mixed direct and indirect effects
Chem. class.: Phenylisopropylamine

Do not confuse:
epHEDrine/epINEPHrine
Action: Causes increased contractility and heart rate by acting on β-receptors in the heart; also acts on α-receptors, causing vasoconstriction in blood vessels
Uses: Shock; increased perfusion; hypotension, bronchodilation

DOSAGE AND ROUTES
Hypotension
• *Adult:* **PO** 25 mg daily-qid; **IM/SUBCUT** 25-50 mg; **IV** 10-25 mg, max 150 mg/24 hr
• *Child:* **SUBCUT/IV** 25-100 mg/m^2/day in 4-6 divided doses
Bronchodilator
• *Adult/child >12 yr:* **PO** 12.5-50 mg q3-4h prn, max 150 mg/24 hr; **NASAL** 2-3 sprays in each nostril q4h
• *Child 2-12 yr:* **PO** 2-3 mg/kg or 100 mg/m^2/day in 4-6 divided doses
• *Child 6-12 yr:* **PO** 6.25-12.5 mg q4h, max 75 mg/24 hr, **NASAL** 1-2 sprays in each nostril q4h
Available forms: Inj 25, 30, 50 mg/ml; caps 25, 50 mg

SIDE EFFECTS
CNS: Tremors, anxiety, insomnia, sweating, headache, dizziness, confusion, hallucinations, ***convulsions, CNS depression, cerebral hemorrhage*** weakness drowsiness
CV: Palpitations, tachycardia, hypertension, chest pain, ***dysrhythmias***
GI: Anorexia, nausea, vomiting
GU: Dysuria, urinary retention
*RESP: **Dyspnea***

Contraindications: Hypersensitivity to sympathomimetics, narrow-angle glaucoma, nonanaphylactic shock during general anesthesia
Precautions: Pregnancy (C), lactation, cardiac disorders, hyperthyroidism, diabetes mellitus, prostatic hypertrophy, hypertension

PHARMACOKINETICS
PO: Onset 15-60 min, duration 2-4 hr
IM: Onset 10-20 min, duration 1 hr
IV: Onset 5 min, duration 2 hr
Metabolized in liver; excreted in urine (unchanged), breast milk; crosses blood-brain barrier, placenta

INTERACTIONS
Severe hypertension: oxytocics
Do not use with MAOIs; hypertensive crisis may occur

Dysrhythmia: halothane anesthetics, cardiac glycosides, levodopa
Increase: effect of epHEDrine—urinary alkalizers
Decrease: effect of guanethidine
Decrease: effect of epHEDrine—methyldopa, urinary acidifiers, rauwolfia alkaloids, α-adrenergic blockers, diuretics, tricyclics

NURSING CONSIDERATIONS
Assess:
• I&O ratio
• ECG continuously during administration; if B/P increases, drug is decreased; B/P and pulse q5min after parenteral route; CVP or PWP during infusion if possible
• For paresthesias and coldness of extremities; peripheral blood flow may decrease; long-term use may produce a pseudoanxiety state requiring sedative; increased lactic acid with severe metabolic acidosis can occur
• Inj site: tissue sloughing; if this occurs, administer phentolamine mixed with 0.9% NaCl
Administer:
IV, direct route
• Through Y-tube or 3-way stopcock; give 10-25 mg slowly; may repeat in 5-10 min, protect from light
Additive compatibilities: Chloramphenicol, lidocaine, metaraminol, nafcillin, penicillin G potassium
Solution compatibilities: D_5W, $D_{10}W$, LR, 0.9% NaCl, 0.45% NaCl, Ringer's
Syringe compatibilities: Pentobarbital
Y-site compatibilities: Etomidate, propofol
Perform/provide:
• Storage of reconstituted sol refrigerated no longer than 24 hr
• Do not use discolored sol
Evaluate:
• Therapeutic response: increased B/P with stabilization
Teach patient/family:
• The reason for drug administration

*ePHEDrine nasal agent
See Appendix C

epinastine ophthalmic
See Appendix C

⚠ High Alert

epINEPHrine (Ⓡ)
(ep-i-nef′rin)
Adrenalin Ana-Guard, AsthmaHaler Mist, AsthmaNefrin (racepinephrine), Bronitin Mist, Bronkaid Mist, Epinal, epINEPHrine, EpINEPHrine Pediatric, EpiPen, EpiPen Jr., Epitrate, Eppy/N, Medihaler microNefrin, Nephron, Primatene Mist, S-2, Sus-Phrine, Vaponefrin (racepinephrine)
Func. class.: Bronchodilator nonselective adrenergic agonist, vasopressor
Chem. class.: Catecholamine

Do not confuse:
epINEPHrine/epHEDrine
Action: β_1- and β_2-agonist causing increased levels of cAMP producing bronchodilation, cardiac, and CNS stimulation; high doses cause vasoconstriction via α-receptors; low doses can cause vasodilation via β_2-vascular receptors
Uses: Acute asthmatic attacks, hemostasis, bronchospasm, anaphylaxis, allergic reactions, cardiac arrest, adjunct in anesthesia, shock

DOSAGE AND ROUTES
Asthma
• *adult and child:* **INH** 1-2 puffs of 1:100 or 2.25% racemic q15min

---

⚠ Safety alert   *"Tall Man" lettering

Bronchodilator
• *Adult:* SUBCUT/IM 0.1-0.5 mg
(1:1000 sol) q10-15min-4h, max 1 mg/
dose

Anaphylactic reaction/asthma
• *Adult:* SUBCUT/IM 0.1-0.5 mg, repeat
q10-15min, max 1 mg/dose; epINEPH-
rine susp 0.5 mg SUBCUT, may repeat
0.5-1.5 mg q6h
• *Child:* SUBCUT 0.01 mg/kg, repeat
q15min, × 2 doses, then q4h, max 0.5
mg/dose; epINEPHrine susp 0.025 mg/kg
SUBCUT, may repeat q6h, max 0.75 mg
in child ≤30 kg

Cardiac arrest (ACLS)
• *Adult:* IV 1 mg q3-5min; ENDOTRA-
CHEAL 2-2.5 mg IC 0.3-0.5 mg

Symptomatic bradycardia/pulseless arrest (PALS)
• *Child:* IV 0.1 mg/kg, may repeat
q3-5min; ENDOTRACHEAL give 2-10 ×
IV dose diluted to a volume of 3-5 ml of
0.9% NaCl, followed by positive pressure
ventilation

Available forms: Aerosol 0.16 mg/
spray, 0.2 mg/spray, 0.25 mg/spray; inj
1:1000 (1 mg/ml), 1:200 (5 mg/ml),
0.01 mg/ml (1:100,000), 0.1 mg/ml
(1:10,000), 0.5 mg/ml (1:2000); sol for
nebulization 1:100, 1.25%, 2.25%
(base)

SIDE EFFECTS

CNS: Tremors, anxiety, insomnia, headache, *dizziness,* confusion, hallucinations, *cerebral hemorrhage,* weakness, drowsiness
CV: Palpitations, tachycardia, hypertension, *dysrhythmias,* increased T wave
GI: Anorexia, nausea, vomiting
RESP: Dyspnea

Contraindications: Hypersensitivity
to sympathomimetics, narrow-angle
glaucoma, nonanaphylactic shock during
general anesthesia, organic brain syndrome, local anesthesia of certain areas,
labor, cardiac dilation, coronary insufficiency, cerebral arteriosclerosis, organic
heart disease

Precautions: Pregnancy (C), lactation,
cardiac disorders, hyperthyroidism,
diabetes mellitus, prostatic hypertrophy,
hypertension

PHARMACOKINETICS

SUBCUT: Onset 3-5 min, duration 20
min-4 hr
INH: Onset 3 min
Crosses placenta; metabolized in liver

INTERACTIONS

Do not use with MAOIs or tricyclics;
hypertensive crisis may occur
Toxicity: other sympathomimetics
Decrease: hypertensive effects—
α-adrenergic blockers

NURSING CONSIDERATIONS
Assess:
• ECG during administration
continuously; if B/P increases, decrease
dose; B/P and pulse q5min after parenteral route; CVP, ISVR, PCWP during infusion if possible; inadvertent high arterial
B/P can result in angina, aortic rupture,
cerebral hemorrhage
• Injection site: tissue sloughing; administer phentolamine with NS
• Sulfite sensitivity, which may be life-
threatening
Administer:
• Increased dose of insulin in diabetic
patients if glucose is elevated
• Check for correct concentration,
route, dosage before administering
IM/SUBCUT route
• Rotate inj sites, massage after inj,
shake before using
IV route
• Parenteral dose slowly, after reconstituting 1 mg (1:1000 sol)/10 ml or more
0.9% NaCl; to prepare a 1:10,000 sol for
maintenance, may be further diluted in
500 ml D₅W; give 1 mg or less over 1 min
or more through Y-tube or 3-way
stopcock; 1 mg = 1 ml of 1:1000 or 10
ml of 1:10,000; protect from light, use
large vein
Additive compatibilities: Cimetidine, DOBUTamine, floxacillin, furosemide, metaraminol, ranitidine, verapamil

Syringe compatibilities: Doxapram, heparin, milrinone

Y-site compatibilities: Atracurium, calcium chloride, calcium gluconate, cisatracurium, diltiazem, DOBUTamine, DOPamine, famotidine, fentanyl, furosemide, heparin, hydrocortisone sodium succinate, hydromorphone, labetalol, lorazepam, midazolam, milrinone, morphine, niCARdipine, nitroglycerin, norepinephrine, pancuronium, phytonadione, potassium chloride, propofol, ranitidine, remifentanil, vecuronium, vit B/C, warfarin

Endotracheal route
• Give directly via endrotracheal tube, use 1:10,000 sol; for small dose further dilute dose prior to administration, follow with quick insufflations

Inhalation route
• Place in nebulizer (10 gtt of a 1% base sol)
• Dilute racepinephrine 2.25% sol

Perform/provide:
• Storage of reconstituted sol refrigerated no longer than 24 hr
• Do not use discolored sol

Evaluate:
• Therapeutic response: increased B/P with stabilization or ease of breathing

Teach patient/family:
• The reason for drug administration
• To rinse mouth after use to prevent dryness after inhalation
• Not to take OTC preparations

Treatment of overdose: Administer an α-blocker and a β-blocker

---

*epINEPHrine/ epinephryl borate ophthalmic
See Appendix C

---

*epINEPHrine nasal agent
See Appendix C

> ### ⚠ High Alert
>
> ## epirubicin (℞)
> (ep-ih-roo'bi-sin)
> Ellence
> *Func. class.:* Antineoplastic, antibiotic
> *Chem. class.:* Anthracycline

Action: Inhibits DNA synthesis primarily; replication is decreased by binding to DNA, which causes strand splitting; maximum cytotoxic effects at S and G_2 phases, a vesicant

Uses: Breast cancer as an adjuvant therapy, with axillary node involvement following resection

Investigational uses: Used in combination for treatment of advanced forms of cancer

DOSAGE AND ROUTES

• *Adult:* IV INF 100-120 mg/m^2 initially, given with other antineoplastics (cyclophosphamide, 5-fluorouracil); given in repeated cycles; 3-4 wk cycles

Epirubicin dosage adjustments
• *Adult:* IV 100 mg/m^2 on day 1 of each cycle; toxicity nadir platelet counts <50,000 mm^3, ANC 250 mm^3, neutropenic fever or grade 3 or 4 nonhematologic toxicity; next cycle give 75% of day 1 dose; delay next cycle until platelets are ≥100,000 mm^3, ANC ≥1500 mm^3, and nonhematologic toxicities have recovered to < grade 1

Hepatic dose
• *Adult:* IV bilirubin 1.2-3 mg/dl or AST 2-4 × normal upper limit 50% of starting dose; bilirubin >3 mg/dl or AST >4 × normal upper limit 25% of starting dose

Available forms: Inj 2 mg/ml

SIDE EFFECTS

CV: Increased B/P, **sinus tachycardia, PVCs,** chest pain, **bradycardia, extrasystoles; CHF confirm for doses >900 mg/m^2**
GI: Nausea, vomiting, anorexia, mucositis, diarrhea

⚠ Safety alert   *"Tall Man" lettering

GU: Amenorrhea, hot flashes, hyperuricemia

HEMA: **Thrombocytopenia, leukopenia, anemia, neutropenia, secondary AML**

INTEG: Rash, **necrosis, pain at inj site,** *reversible alopecia*

MISC: Infection, febrile neutropenia, lethargy, fever, conjunctivitis

Contraindications: Pregnancy (D), hypersensitivity to this drug, anthracyclines, anthracenediones, severe hepatic disease, baseline neutrophil count <1500 cell/mm^3, severe myocardial insufficiency, recent MI, lactation, systemic infections

Precautions: Renal, hepatic, cardiac disease; gout, bone marrow depression (severe), elderly, children

PHARMACOKINETICS

Triphasic pattern of elimination; half-life 3 min, 2.5 hr, 33 hr; metabolized by liver; crosses placenta; excreted in urine, bile, breast milk

INTERACTIONS

Increase: toxicity—other antineoplastics or radiation, cimetidine

Decrease: antibody response—live virus vaccine

NURSING CONSIDERATIONS
Assess:

• Bone marrow depression, infection: increased temp

• CBC, differential, platelet count weekly; withhold drug if baseline neutrophil ≤1500/mm^3; leukocyte nadir occurs 10-14 days after administration, recovery by 21st day; notify prescriber of these results

• Blood, urine uric acid levels; swelling, joint pain primarily in extremities, patient should be well hydrated to prevent urate deposits

• Renal studies: BUN, serum uric acid, urine CCr, electrolytes before, during therapy; I&O ratio; report fall in urine

output to <30 ml/hr; dosage adjustment is needed if serum creatinine >5 mg/dl

• Hepatic studies before, during therapy: bilirubin, AST, ALT, alk phosphatase as needed or monthly

• Cardiac status: B/P, pulse, character, rhythm, rate, ABGs, ECG, LVEF, MUGA scan, or ECHO; watch for ST-T wave changes, low QRS and T, possible dysrhythmias (sinus tachycardia, heart block, PVCs)

• Bleeding: hematuria, guaiac, bruising, or petechiae, mucosa or orifices q8h

• Effects of alopecia on body image; discuss feelings about body changes

• Local irritation, pain, burning, necrosis at inj site

• GI symptoms: frequency of stools, cramping

Administer:

• Antiemetic 30-60 min before giving drug to prevent vomiting

• Allopurinol or sodium bicarbonate to maintain uric acid levels, alkalinization of urine

IV route

• Hydrocortisone, dexamethasone, or sodium bicarbonate (1 mEq/1 ml) for extravasation; apply ice compresses

• Given into tubing of free-flowing IV infusion (0.9% NaCl or D$_5$) give over 3-5 min; do not mix with other drugs in syringe

Perform/provide:

• Strict hand-washing technique, gloves, protective clothing

• Liquid diet: carbonated beverages, gelatin may be added if patient is not nauseated or vomiting

• Increased fluid intake to 2-3 L/day to prevent urate, calculi formation

Evaluate:

• Therapeutic response: decreased tumor size, spread of malignancy

Teach patient/family:

• To report any complaints, side effects to nurse or prescriber

• That hair may be lost during treatment and wig or hairpiece may make patient feel better; tell patient that new hair may be different in color, texture

Side effects: *italics* = common; **bold italics** = life-threatening

• To avoid crowds and persons with infections when granulocyte count is low
• That contraceptive measures are recommended during therapy and 4 mo thereafter for men and women
• To avoid vaccinations, reactions may occur; to avoid cimetidine during therapy
• That urine may appear red for 2 days
• To avoid OTC medications, supplements unless approved by prescriber
• That irreversible myocardial damage, leukopenia, menopause may occur

---

eplerenone (℞)
(ep-ler-ee'known)
Inspra
Func. class.: Antihypertensive
Chem. class.: Selective aldosterone receptor antagonist

Action: Binds to mineralocorticoid receptor and blocks the binding of aldosterone, a component of the renin-angiotensin aldosterone system (RAAS)
Uses: Hypertension, alone or in combination with thiazide diuretics, CHF post-MI

DOSAGE AND ROUTES

• *Adult:* **PO** 50 mg daily, initially, may increase to 50 mg bid after 4 wk; start dose at 25 mg daily if patient is taking CYP3A4 inhibitors
Available forms: Tabs 25, 50, 100 mg

SIDE EFFECTS

CNS: Headache, dizziness, fatigue
CV: angina, ***MI***
GI: Increased GGT diarrhea, abdominal pain, increased ALT
GU: Increased BUN, creatinine, gynecomastia, mastodynia (males), abnormal vaginal bleeding
META: Hyperkalemia, hyponatremia, hypercholesteremia, hypertriglyceridemia, increased uric acid
RESP: Cough
Contraindications: Hypersensitivity, lactation, children, increased serum creatinine >2 mg/dl (male), >1.8 mg/dl

(female), potassium >5.5 mEq/L, type 2 diabetes with microalbuminuria, hepatic disease, CCr <30 ml/min; <50 ml/min in hypertension
Precautions: Pregnancy (B), impaired renal, hepatic function, elderly, hyperkalemia, lactation

PHARMACOKINETICS

PO: Peak 1½ hr, serum protein binding 50%, half-life 4-6 hr, metabolized by liver (CYP3A4 inhibitor), excreted in urine

INTERACTIONS

Increase: hyperkalemia—ACE inhibitors, angiotensin II antagonists, NSAIDs, potassium supplements
Increase: serum levels of lithium
Increase: levels of eplerenone—CYP3A4 inhibitors (ketoconazole, itraconazole, saquinavir, erythromycin, verapamil, fluconazole), reduce dose of eplerenone
Decrease: antihypertensive effect—NSAIDs
Drug/Herb
Increase: toxicity, death—aconite
Increase: antihypertensive effect—barberry, betony, black catechu, black cohosh, bloodroot, broom, burdock, cat's claw, dandelion, goldenseal, Irish moss, Jamaican dogwood, kelp, khella, mistletoe, parsley
Increase or decrease: antihypertensive effect—astragalus, cola tree
Decrease: antihypertensive effect—coltsfoot, guarana, khat, licorice
Decrease: levels of eplerenone—St. John's wort
Drug/Food
Grapefruit juice increased drug level by 25%

NURSING CONSIDERATIONS

Assess:
• B/P at peak/trough level of drug, orthostatic hypotension, syncope when used with diuretic; monitor lithium level in those also taking lithium

---

⚠ Safety alert   *"Tall Man" lettering

- Renal studies: protein, BUN, creatinine; increased LFTs, uric acid may be increased
- Potassium levels, hyperkalemia may occur

Perform/provide:
- Storage in tight container at 86° F (30° C) or less

Evaluate:
- Therapeutic response: decreased B/P

Teach patient/family:
- Not to discontinue drug abruptly
- Not to use OTC products (cough, cold, allergy) unless directed by prescriber; do not use salt substitutes containing potassium without consulting prescriber
- Important to comply with dosage schedule, even if feeling better
- That drug may cause dizziness, fainting, light-headedness; may occur during first few days of therapy
- How to take B/P, and normal readings for age-group

---

epoetin (℞)
(ee-poe′e-tin)
EPO, Epogen, Eprex ✦, Procrit
Func. class.: Antianemic, biologic modifier, hormone
Chem. class.: Amino acid polypeptide

Action: Erythropoietin is one factor controlling rate of red cell production; drug is developed by recombinant DNA technology
Uses: Anemia caused by reduced endogenous erythropoietin production, primarily end-stage renal disease; to correct hemostatic defect in uremia; anemia due to AZT treatment in HIV patients or chemotherapy; reduction of allogenic blood transfusion in surgery patients
Investigational uses: Pruritus; anemia in: premature preterm infants, myelodysplastic syndrome, chronic inflammatory disorders

DOSAGE AND ROUTES
Anemia related to chemotherapy
- *Adult:* SUBCUT 150 units/kg 3 ×/wk, may increase after 2 mo up to 300 units/kg 3 ×/wk
Anemia in chronic renal failure
- *Adult:* SUBCUT/IV 50-100 units/kg 3 ×/wk, then adjust to maintain target Hct of 30%-36%
- *Child:* IV/SUBCUT 50 units/kg 3 ×/wk
Anemia secondary to zidovudine treatment
- *Adult:* SUBCUT/IV 100 units/kg 3 ×/wk × 2 mo, may increase by 50-100 units/kg q1-2mo, up to 300 units/kg 3 ×/wk
Surgery
- *Adult:* SUBCUT 300 units/kg/day × 10 days prior to surgery, the day of surgery, and for 4 days postsurgery or 600 units/kg at 3 wk, 2 wk, 1 wk, prior to and on day of surgery
Available forms: Inj 2000, 3000, 4000, 10,000, 20,000, 40,000 units/ml

SIDE EFFECTS
CNS: **Seizures,** coldness, sweating, headache
CV: Hypertension, **hypertensive encephalopathy**
MS: Bone pain

Contraindications: Hypersensitivity to mammalian cell–derived products, or human albumin, uncontrolled hypertension
Precautions: Pregnancy (C), seizure disorder, porphyria, children <1 mo, lactation, multidose preserved formulation contains benzyl alcohol and should not be used in premature infants

PHARMACOKINETICS
IV: Metabolized in body; extent of metabolism unknown; onset of increased reticulocyte count 2-6 wk; peak, immediate

INTERACTIONS
Need for increased anticoagulant during hemodialysis

NURSING CONSIDERATIONS
Assess:

• Renal studies: urinalysis, protein, blood, BUN, creatinine; I&O, report drop in output <50 ml/hr

• Blood studies: ferritin, transferrin monthly; transferrin sat ≥20%, ferritin ≥100 ng/ml; Hct 2 ×/wk until stabilized in target range (30%-36%) then at regular intervals; those with endogenous erythropoietin levels of <500 units/L respond to this agent; monitor Hct 2 ×/wk in chronic renal failure; patients treated with zidovudine or cancer patients should be monitored wk, then periodically after stabilization

• B/P; check for rising B/P as Hct rises, antihypertensives may be needed; hypertension may occur rapidly leading to hypertensive encephalopathy

• CNS symptoms: coldness, sweating, pain in long bones; for seizures if Hct is increased within 2 wk by 4 pts

• For hypersensitivity reactions: skin rashes, urticaria (rare), antibody development does not occur

🅰 For pure cell aplasia (PRCA) in absence of other causes, evaluate by testing sera for recombinant erythropoetin antibodies; any loss of response to epoetin should be evaluated

• Dialysis patients: thrill, bruit of shunts, monitor for circulation impairment

Administer:

• Do not shake vial

SUBCUT route

• Before injecting preservative free-, single-dose formulation may be admixed using 0.9% NaCl with benzyl alcohol 0.9% at a 1:1 ratio to reduce injection site discomfort

IV route

• Additional heparin to lower chance of clots

• By direct inj or bolus into IV tubing or venous line at end of dialysis

• Decrease dose by 25 units/kg, if Hct increases by 4% in 2 wk; increase dose if Hct does not increase by 5-6 pts after 8 wk of therapy, suggested target Hct range 30%–36%

Solution compatibilities: Do not dilute or administer with other solutions

Evaluate:

• Therapeutic response: increase in reticulocyte count in 2-6 wk, Hgb/Hct; increased appetite, enhanced sense of well-being

Teach patient/family:

• To avoid driving or hazardous activity during beginning of treatment

• To monitor B/P

• To take iron supplements, vitamin B_{12}, folic acid as directed

---

eprosartan (℞)
(ep-roh-sar′tan)
Teveten
Func. class.: Antihypertensive
Chem. class.: Angiotensin II–receptor antagonist (Subtype AT_1)

Action: Blocks the vasoconstrictor and aldosterone-secreting effects of angiotensin II; selectively blocks the binding of angiotensin II to the AT_1 receptor found in tissues

Uses: Hypertension, alone or with other antihypertensives

DOSAGE AND ROUTES

• *Adult:* **PO** 600 mg daily; dose may be divided and given bid with total daily doses from 400-800 mg

Available forms: 400, 600 mg

SIDE EFFECTS

CNS: Dizziness, depression, fatigue, headache
CV: Chest pain
EENT: Sinusitis
GI: Diarrhea, dyspepsia, abdominal pain
GU: UTI
META: Hypertriglyceridemia
MS: Myalgia, arthralgia
RESP: Cough, upper respiratory infection, rhinitis, pharyngitis, viral infection

Contraindications: Pregnancy (D) 2nd/3rd trimesters, hypersensitivity

---

🅰 Safety alert   *"Tall Man" lettering

Precautions: Pregnancy (C) 1st trimester, hypersensitivity to ACE inhibitors; lactation, children, elderly; renal, hepatic disease

PHARMACOKINETICS

Peak 1-2 hr, food delays absorption, protein binding 98%, moderate renal impairment increases drug levels by 30%, hepatic impairment increases levels by 40%, excreted in urine and feces

INTERACTIONS
Drug/Herb
Increase: toxicity, death—aconite
Increase: antihypertensive effect—barberry, betony, black catechu, black cohosh, bloodroot, broom, burdock, cat's claw, dandelion, goldenseal, Irish moss, Jamaican dogwood, kelp, khella, mistletoe, parsley
Increase or decrease: antihypertensive effect—astragalus, cola tree
Decrease: antihypertensive effect—coltsfoot, guarana, khat, licorice
Drug/Lab Test
Increase: ALT, AST, alk phosphatase
Decrease: Hgb

NURSING CONSIDERATIONS
Assess:
• B/P with position changes, pulse q4h; note rate, rhythm, quality
• Electrolytes (K, Na, Cl)
• Baselines in renal, hepatic studies before therapy begins
• Edema in feet, legs daily
• Skin turgor, dryness of mucous membranes for hydration status
Administer:
• Without regard to meals
Evaluate:
• Therapeutic response: Decrease B/P
Teach patient/family:
• To comply with dosage schedule, even if feeling better
• To notify prescriber of fever, swelling of hands or feet, chest pain

• That excessive perspiration, dehydration, diarrhea may lead to fall in blood pressure; consult prescriber if these occur
• That drug may cause dizziness, avoid hazardous activities until effect is known
• Not to take this medication if pregnant or breastfeeding, or have had an allergic reaction to this drug
• To take missed dose as soon as possible, unless within 1 hr before next dose

⚠ High Alert

eptifibatide (℞)
(ep-tih-fib′ah-tide)
Integrilin
Func. class.: Antiplatelet agent
Chem. class.: Glycoprotein IIb/IIIa inhibitor

Action: Platelet glycoprotein antagonist. this agent reversibly prevents fibrinogen, von Willebrand's factor from binding to the glycoprotein IIb/IIIa receptor, inhibiting platelet aggregation
Uses: Acute coronary syndrome including those undergoing PCI (percutaneous coronary intervention)

DOSAGE AND ROUTES
Acute coronary syndrome
• *Adult:* **IV BOL** 180 mcg/kg as soon as diagnosed, max 22.6 mg, then **IV CONT** 2 mcg/kg/min until discharge or CABG up to 72 hr, max 15 mg/hr
PCI in patients without acute coronary syndrome
• *Adult:* **IV BOL** 180 mcg/kg given immediately before PCI; then 2 mcg/kg/min × 18 hr and a second 180-mcg/kg bolus, 10 min after 1st bolus; continue inf for up to 18-24 hr
Renal dose
• CCr <50 ml/min: 2-4 mg/dl same loading dose, then ½ usual inf dose
Available forms: Sol for inj 2 mg/ml (10 ml), 0.75 mg/ml (100 ml)

Side effects: *italics* = common; ***bold italics*** = life-threatening

SIDE EFFECTS

CV: **Stroke,** hypotension
GU: Hematuria
HEMA: **Thrombocytopenia**
SYST: **Bleeding, anaphylaxis**

Contraindications: Hypersensitivity, active internal bleeding; history of bleeding, stroke within 1 mo; major surgery with severe trauma, severe hypertension, history of intracranial bleeding, current or planned use of another parenteral GP IIb/IIIa inhibitor, dependence on renal dialysis, coagulopathy

Precautions: Pregnancy (B), bleeding, lactation, children, elderly, renal function impairment

PHARMACOKINETICS

Half-life 2.5 hr, steady state 4-6 hr, metabolism limited, excretion via kidneys

INTERACTIONS

Do not give with glycoprotein inhibitors IIb, IIIa

Increase: bleeding—aspirin, heparin, NSAIDs, anticoagulants, ticlopidine, clopidogrel, dipyridamole, thrombolytics, valproate, abciximab

NURSING CONSIDERATIONS

Assess:

⚠ Platelets, Hgb, Hct, creatinine, PT/APTT baseline INR within 6 hr of loading dose and daily theralter, patients undergoing PCI should have ACT monitored; maintain APTT 50-70 sec unless PCI is to be performed; during PCI, ACT should be 200-300 sec; if platelets drop <100,000/mm³, obtain additional platelet counts; if thrombocytopenia is confirmed, discontinue drug; also, draw Hct, Hgb, serum creatinine

⚠ For bleeding: gums, bruising, ecchymosis, petechiae; from GI, GU tract, cardiac cath sites, IM inj sites

Administer:

• Aspirin and heparin may be given with this drug

• D/C heparin before removing femoral artery sheath, after PCI

IV route

• After withdrawing bolus dose from 10-ml vial, give IV push over 1-2 min; follow bolus dose with continuous inf using pump, give drug undiluted directly from 100-ml vial, spike 100-ml vial with vented infusion set, use caution when centering spike on circle of stopper top

Y-site compatabilities: alteplase, atropine, DOBUTamine, heparin, lidocaine, meperidine, metoprolol, midazolam, morphine, nitroglycerin, verapamil

Solution compatibilities: 0.9% NaCl, D₅/0.9% NaCl

Perform/provide:

• Do not give discolored solutions or those with particulates, discard unused amount

• Discontinue drug prior to CABG

• All medications PO if possible, avoid IM inj and all catheters

Teach patient/family:

• Reason for medication and expected results

• To report bruising, bleeding, chest pain immediately

---

ergonovine (℞)
(er-goe-noe'veen)
ergonovine, Ergotrate
Func. class.: Oxytocic
Chem. class.: Ergot alkaloid

Action: Stimulates uterine contractions and vascular smooth muscle, decreases bleeding

Uses: Postpartum or postabortion hemorrhage

Investigational uses: To induce a coronary artery spasm for diagnostic purposes

DOSAGE AND ROUTES

Oxytocic

• *Adult:* **PO/SL** 0.2-0.4 mg q6-12h; **IM** 0.2 mg q2-4h, not to exceed 5 doses; **IV** 0.2 mg given over 1 min

---

⚠ Safety alert   *"Tall Man" lettering

E

Induced coronary artery spasm

• **Adult:** **IV** 50 mcg q5min up to 400 mcg or when chest pain occurs
Available forms: Inj 0.2, 0.25 mg/ml; tab 0.2 mg

SIDE EFFECTS

CNS: Headache, dizziness, fainting
CV: Hypertension, chest pain
EENT: Tinnitus
GI: Nausea, vomiting, diarrhea
GU: Cramping
INTEG: Sweating
RESP: Dyspnea
Contraindications: Hypersensitivity to ergot medication, augmentation of labor, before delivery of placenta, spontaneous abortion (threatened), PID
Precautions: Hepatic, renal, cardiac disease, asthma, anemia, convulsive disorders, hypertension, glaucoma, obliterative vascular disease

PHARMACOKINETICS

IM: Onset 2-5 min, duration 3 hr
IV: Onset immediate, duration 45 min
Metabolized in liver, excreted in urine

INTERACTIONS

Hypertension: sympathomimetics, ergots
Drug/Herb
Increase: serotonin effect—horehound

NURSING CONSIDERATIONS

Assess:
• Ergotism: nausea, vomiting, weakness, muscular pain, insensitivity to cold, paresthesias of extremities; drug should be discontinued
• B/P, pulse; watch for change that may indicate hemorrhage
• Respiratory rate, rhythm, depth; notify prescriber of abnormalities
• Fundal tone, nonphasic contractions; check for relaxation
Administer:
• IM inj deep in large muscle mass; rotate inj sites if additional doses are given
• With emergency equipment available

IV, direct route

• Dilute with 5 ml 0.9% NaCl, give through Y-tube or 3-way stopcock over 1 min
Additive compatibilities: Amikacin, cephapirin, sodium bicarbonate
Evaluate:
• Therapeutic response: decreased blood loss, severe cramping
Teach patient/family:
• To report increased blood loss, increased temp, or foul-smelling lochia; that cramping is normal
• The importance of pad count
• To avoid nicotine products
Treatment of overdose: Stop drug, give vasodilators, heparin, dextran

---

ergotamine (R)
(er-got′a-meen)
Ergomar ✦, Ergostat, Gynergen ✦
dihydroergotamine
(dye-hye-droe-er-got′a-meen)
DHE45, Dihydroergotamine-Sandoz ✦, Migranal
Func. class.: α-Adrenergic blocker, vascular headache suppressant
Chem. class.: Ergot alkaloid— amino acid

Action: Constricts smooth muscle in peripheral, cranial blood vessels, relaxes uterine muscle; blocks serotonin release
Uses: Vascular headache (migraine, cluster histamine)

DOSAGE AND ROUTES

ergotamine

• **Adult:** **SL** 1 tab (2 mg), may use q30min, max 3 tabs (6 mg)/24 hr or 10 mg/wk
dihydroergotamine
• **Adults:** **SUBCUT/IM** 1 mg, may repeat in 1 hr to 3 mg, max 3 mg/day or 6 mg/wk; **IV** 0.5-1 mg, may repeat in 1 hr, max 2 mg/day or 6 mg/wk; **INTRANASAL** 1 spray in each nostril, repeat in 15 min, max 3 mg/24 hr, 4 mg/wk

---

• *Child ≥6 yr:* **SUBCUT/IM** 0.5 mg, may repeat in 1 hr; **IV:** 0.25 mg, may repeat in 1 hr

Severe acute migraine

• *Child 12-16 yr:* **IV** 0.25-0.5 mg, may repeat q20min for 1-2 doses

Available forms: ergotamine: SL tabs 2 mg; tabs 1 mg; dihydroergotamine: inj 1 mg/ml; nasal spray 4 mg/ml

SIDE EFFECTS

CNS: Numbness in fingers, toes, headache, weakness

CV: Transient tachycardia, chest pain, bradycardia, edema, claudication, increase or decrease in B/P, *MI,* peripheral vascular ischemia

GI: Nausea, vomiting, diarrhea, abdominal cramps

MS: Muscle pain

Contraindications: Pregnancy (X), hypersensitivity to ergot preparations, occlusion (peripheral, vascular), CAD, hepatic disease, renal disease, peptic ulcer, hypertension, Raynaud's disease, peripheral vascular disease, intermittent claudication, glaucoma, angina

Precautions: Lactation, children, anemia, elderly, basilar/hemiplagic migraine

PHARMACOKINETICS

IM/SUBCUT: Peak (IM) 30 min, (SUBCUT) 15-45 min; duration 8 hr

IV: Peak 3 min, duration 8 hr

PO: Peak 30 min-3 hr; metabolized in liver; excreted as metabolites in feces; crosses blood-brain barrier; excreted in breast milk

INTERACTIONS

Increase: toxicity—CYP4503A4 inhibitors (protease inhibitors, some macrolides, azole antifungals); do not use together

Increase: vasoconstriction—β-blockers, oral contraceptives, nicotine, vasoconstrictors, other migraine agents

Drug/Herb

Increase: serotonin effect—horehound

NURSING CONSIDERATIONS

Assess:

• Migraine characteristics: duration, nausea, vomiting, change in vision, frequency before and at least 1 hr after administration

• Ergotism: nausea, vomiting, weakness, muscular pain, insensitivity to cold, paresthesia of extremities; drug should be discontinued

• Toxicity: dyspnea, hypotension or hypertension, rapid, weak pulse, delirium, nausea, vomiting

Administer:

• At beginning of headache; dose must be titrated to patient response

• Not to pregnant women; harm to fetus may occur

Intranasal route

• Prime nasal sprayer 4 × before dose, use 1 spray in each nostril, wait 15 min, use another spray in each nostril, use nasal applicator for 4 treatments only, discard

IV route

• Give dihydroergotamine undiluted over 1 min

Perform/provide:

• Quiet, calm environment with decreased stimulation for noise, bright light, or excessive talking

Evaluate:

• Therapeutic response: decrease in frequency, severity of headache

Teach patient/family:

• Not to use OTC medications; serious drug interactions may occur

• To maintain dose at approved level; not to increase even if drug does not relieve headache

• To report side effects including increased vasoconstriction starting with cold extremities, then paresthesia, weakness

• That an increase in headaches may occur when this drug is discontinued after long-term use

⚠ To keep drug out of reach of children; death may occur

Treatment of overdose: Induce

emesis or gastric lavage if orally ingested; administer saline cathartic; keep warm

erlotinib (℞)

(er-loe'tye-nib)

Tarceva

Func. class.: Antineoplastic—miscellaneous

Chem. class.: Epidermal growth factor receptor inhibitor

Action: Not fully understood; inhibits intracellular phosphorylation of cell surface receptors associated with epidermal growth factor receptors

Uses: Non–small cell lung cancer (NSCLC)

DOSAGE AND ROUTES

• *Adult:* PO 150 mg daily taken at least 1 hr before or 2 hr after food

CYP3A4 inducers concurrently (such as rifampin or phenytoin)

• Dosage increase is advised

CYP3A4 inhibitors (atazanavir, clarithromycin, indinavir, itraconazole, ketoconazole, telithromycin, ritonavir, saquinavir, troleandomycin, nelfinavir)

• Dosage reduction may be needed

Available forms: Tabs 25, 100, 150 mg

SIDE EFFECTS

GI: Nausea, diarrhea, vomiting, anorexia, mouth ulceration

INTEG: Rash

MISC: Conjunctivitis, eye pain, fatigue, infection

RESP: **Interstitial lung disease,** *cough, dyspnea*

Contraindications: Pregnancy (D), hypersensitivity

Precautions: Renal, hepatic, ocular, pulmonary disorders, lactation, children, elderly

PHARMACOKINETICS

Slowly absorbed, peak 3-7 hr, excreted in feces (86%), urine (<4%), metabolized by CYP3A4, terminal half-life 36 hours

INTERACTIONS

Increase: erlotinib concentrations—(CYP3A4 inhibitors) ketoconazole, itraconazole, erythromycin, clarithromycin, telithromycin

Increase: plasma concentration of warfarin, metoprolol

Decrease: erlotinib levels—(CYP3A4 inducers) phenytoin, rifampin, carbamazepine, phenobarbital, St. John's wort

NURSING CONSIDERATIONS

Assess:

⚠ Pulmonary changes: lung sounds, cough, dyspnea; interstitial lung disease may occur, may be fatal; discontinue therapy if confirmed

• Ocular changes: eye irritation, corneal erosion/ulcer, aberrant eyelash growth

• GI symptoms: frequency of stools; if diarrhea is poorly tolerated, therapy may be discontinued for up to 14 days

Administer:

• 1 hr before or 2 hr after food

Evaluate:

• Therapeutic response: decrease non–small cell lung cancer cells

Teach patient/family:

⚠ To report adverse reactions immediately: shortness of breath, severe abdominal pain, persistent diarrhea or vomiting, ocular changes, skin eruptions

• Reason for treatment, expected results

• Use contraception during treatment, pregnancy (D)

ertapenem (℞)

(er-tah-pen'em)

Invanz

Func. class.: Antiinfective—miscellaneous

Chem. class.: Carbapenem

Do not confuse:

Invanz/Avinza

Action: Interferes with cell wall replication of susceptible organisms; osmotically unstable cell wall swells, bursts from osmotic pressure

Uses: Adult patients with moderate to severe infections caused by the following organisms: intraabdominal infections—*Escherichia coli, Clostridium clostridioforme, Eubacterium lentum, Peptostreptococcus* sp., *Bacteroides fragilis, Bacteroides distasonis, Bacteroides ovatus, Bacteroides thetaiotaomicron, Bacteroides uniformis;* complicated skin/skin structure infections—*Staphylococcus aureus* (methicillin-susceptible), *Streptococcus pyogenes, E. coli, Peptostreptococcus* sp.; community-acquired pneumonia—*Streptococcus pneumoniae* (penicillin-susceptible), *Haemophilus influenzae* (β-lactamase–negative), *Moraxella catarrhalis;* complicated UTI—*E. coli, Klebsiella pneumoniae;* acute pelvic infections—*Streptococcus agalactiae, E. coli, B. fragilis, Porphyromonas asaccharolytica, Peptostreptococcus* sp., *Prevotella bivia*

DOSAGE AND ROUTES

Complicated intraabdominal infections
• *Adult:* **IV/IM** 1 g daily × 5-14 days
Complicated skin/skin structure infections
• *Adult:* **IV/IM** 1 g daily × 7-14 days
Community-acquired pneumonia
• *Adult:* **IV/IM** 1 g daily × 10-14 days
Complicated UTI
• *Adult:* **IV/IM** 1 g daily × 10-14 days
Acute pelvic infections
• *Adult:* **IV/IM** 1 g daily × 3-10 days
Available form: Powder, lyophilized, 1 g

SIDE EFFECTS

CNS: Insomnia, *seizures*, dizziness, *headache*
GI: Diarrhea, nausea, vomiting, *pseudomembranous colitis*
GU: Vaginitis
INTEG: Rash, urticaria, *pruritus*, pain at inj site, *infused vein complication, phlebitis/thrombophlebitis*, erythema at inj site

RESP: Dyspnea, cough, pharyngitis, crackles, respiratory distress
SYST: **Anaphylaxis**
Contraindications: Hypersensitivity to this drug or its components, to amide-type local anesthetics (IM only); anaphylactic reactions to β-lactams
Precautions: Pregnancy (B), lactation, elderly, children, renal disease

PHARMACOKINETICS

IV: Onset immediate, peak dose dependent, half-life 4 hr, metabolized by liver, excreted in urine, feces, breast milk

INTERACTIONS

Increase: ertapenem levels—probenecid; do not coadminister
Drug/Herb
Do not use acidophilus with antiinfectives

NURSING CONSIDERATIONS
Assess:
• Sensitivity to carbapenem antibiotics, other β-lactam antibiotics, penicillins
• Renal disease: lower dose may be required
• Bowel pattern daily: if severe diarrhea occurs, drug should be discontinued; may indicate pseudomembranous colitis
• For infection: temp, sputum, characteristics of wound before, during, after treatment
⚠ Allergic reactions, anaphylaxis; rash, urticaria, pruritus; may occur a few days after therapy begins
• Overgrowth of infection: perineal itching, fever, malaise, redness, pain, swelling, drainage, rash, diarrhea, change in cough or sputum
Administer:
• By IV or IM
• After C&S is taken
IM route
• Reconstitute 1 g vial of ertapenem with 3.2 ml of 1% lidocaine HCl without epiNEPHrine, shake well

---

⚠ Safety alert   *"Tall Man" lettering

• Withdraw contents, administer deep IM in large muscle mass, use within 1 hr

IV route

• Do not coinfuse or mix with other medications; do not use diluents containing dextrose

• Reconstitute 1 g vial of ertapenem with either 10 ml of water for inj, 0.9% NaCl, or bacteriostatic water for inj

• Shake well to dissolve, transfer contents of reconstituted vial to 50 ml 0.9% NaCl inj

• Complete inf within 6 hr

Evaluate:

• Therapeutic response: negative C&S, absence of signs and symptoms of infection

Teach patient/family:

• To report severe diarrhea; may indicate pseudomembranous colitis

• To report overgrowth of infection: black, furry tongue, vaginal itching, foul-smelling stools

• To avoid breastfeeding; drug is excreted in breast milk

Treatment of overdose: EpINEPHrine, antihistamines; resuscitate if needed (anaphylaxis)

---

erythromycin base (℞)

(eh-rith-roh-my'sin)

Apo-Erythro ✦, E-Mycin, Eramycin, Erybid ✦, Eryc, Ery-Tab, E-Base, Erythromid ✦, Erythromycin Base Filmtab, Erythromycin Delayed-Release, Novo-Rythro Encap ✦, PCE

erythromycin estolate (℞)

Ilosone, Novo-Rythro ✦

erythromycin ethylsuccinate (℞)

Apo-Erythro-Es ✦, E.E.S., Ery Ped, Novo-Rythro ✦

erythromycin gluceptate erythromycin lactobionate (℞)

Erythrocin

erythromycin stearate (℞)

Apo-Erythro-S ✦, Novo-Rythro ✦

Func. class.: Antiinfective
Chem. class.: Macrolide

Do not confuse:

erythromycin/azithromycin

Action: Binds to 50S ribosomal subunits of susceptible bacteria and suppresses protein synthesis

Uses: Infections caused by *Neisseria gonorrhoeae;* mild to moderate respiratory tract, skin, soft tissue infections caused by *Bordetella pertussis, Borrelia burgdorferi, Chlamydia trachomatis; Corynebacterium diphtheriae, Haemophilus influenzae* (when used with sulfonamides); *Legionella pneumophila,* Legionnaire's disease, *Listeria monocytogenes; Mycoplasma pneumoniae, Streptococcus pneumoniae,* syphilis: *Treponema pallidum*

Research note: Grapefruit juice increased erythromycin concentrations in a study of 6 people

---

✦ Canada only

Side effects: *italics* = common; ***bold italics*** = life-threatening

DOSAGE AND ROUTES

Soft tissue infections
• *Adult:* **PO** 250-500 mg q6h (base, estolate, stearate); **PO** 400-800 mg q6h (ethylsuccinate); **IV INF** 15-20 mg/kg/day (lactobionate) divided q6h
• *Child:* **PO** 30-50 mg/kg/day in divided doses q6h (salts); **IV** 20-40 mg/kg/day in divided doses q6h (lactobionate), max adult dose

Neisseria gonorrhoeae/PID
• *Adult:* **IV** 500 mg q6h × 3 days (gluceptate, lactobionate), then **PO** 250 mg (base, estolate, stearate) or 400 mg (ethylsuccinate) q6h × 1 wk

Syphilis
• *Adult:* **PO** 20-40 g in divided doses over 15 days (base, estolate, stearate)

Chlamydia
• *Adult:* **PO** 500 mg q6h × 1 wk or 250 mg qid × 2 wk
• *Infant:* **PO** 50 mg/kg/day in 4 divided doses × 3 wk or more
• *Newborn:* **PO** 50 mg/kg/day in 4 divided doses × 2 wk or more

Intestinal amebiasis
• *Adult:* **PO** 250 mg q6h × 10-14 days (base, estolate, stearate)
• *Child:* **PO** 30-50 mg/kg/day in divided doses q6h × 10-14 days (base, estolate, stearate)

Available forms: Base: tabs, enteric-coated 250, 333, 500 mg; tabs, film-coated 250, 500 mg; caps, enteric-coated 250, 333 mg; estolate: tabs 500 mg; caps 125, 250 mg; drops 100 mg/ml; susp 125, 250 mg/5 ml; stearate: tabs, film-coated 250 mg; ethylsuccinate: tabs, chewable 200 mg; susp 100 mg/2.5 ml, 200, 400 mg/5 ml; powder for inj: 500 mg and 1 g (lactobionate), 1 g (as gluceptate)

SIDE EFFECTS

CV: **Dysrhythmias**
EENT: Hearing loss, tinnitus
GI: Nausea, vomiting, diarrhea, **hepatotoxicity,** abdominal pain, stomatitis, heartburn, anorexia, pruritus ani
GU: Vaginitis, moniliasis
INTEG: Rash, urticaria, pruritus, thrombophlebitis (IV site)
SYST: **Anaphylaxis**

Contraindications: Hypersensitivity, preexisting hepatic disease (estolate), hepatic disease

Precautions: Pregnancy (B), hepatic disease, lactation

PHARMACOKINETICS

Peak 4 hr (base): ½–2½ hr (ethylsuccinate), duration 6 hr, half-life 1-2 hr; metabolized in liver; excreted in bile, feces, protein binding 75%-90%

INTERACTIONS

⚠ Serious dysrhythmias—pimozide, sparfloxacin; do not use together
Increase: action, toxicity of bromocriptine, clindamycin, cycloSPORINE, digoxin, diazepam, disopyramide, ergots, HMG-CoA reductase inhibitors, lovastatin, methylPREDNISolone, midazolam, simvastatin, theophylline, triazolam, warfarin
Drug/Herb
Do not use acidophilus with antiinfectives
Drug/Lab Test
Increase: AST/ALT
Decrease: Folate assay
False increase: 17-OHCS/17-KS

NURSING CONSIDERATIONS

Assess:
• For infection: temp, characteristics of wounds, urine, stools, sputum, WBCs, baseline and periodically
• I&O ratio; report hematuria, oliguria in renal disease
• Hepatic studies: AST, ALT, if patient is on long-term therapy
• Renal studies: urinalysis, protein, blood
• C&S before drug therapy; drug may be given as soon as culture is taken; C&S may be repeated after treatment
• Bowel pattern before, during treatment
• Skin eruptions, itching
• Respiratory status: rate, character,

⚠ Safety alert   *"Tall Man" lettering

wheezing, tightness in chest; discontinue drug if these occur

• Allergies before treatment, reaction of each medication

Administer:

• Do not break, crush, or chew time-rel cap or tab; chew only chewable tabs

• Do not give by IM or IV push

• Enteric-coated tablets may be given with food

• Oral drug with full glass of water; do not give with fruit juice

• Oral drug with food for GI symptoms

IV route

• After diluting 500 mg or less/10 ml sterile H_2O without preservatives; dilute further in 80-250 ml of 0.9% NaCl, LR, Normosol-R; may be further diluted to 1 mg/ml and given as cont inf; run 1 g or less/100 ml over ½-1 hr; cont inf over 6 hr, may require buffers to neutralize pH if dilution is <250 ml, use inf pump

Additive compatibilities:

Gluceptate: Calcium gluconate, hydrocortisone, methicillin, penicillin G potassium, potassium chloride, sodium bicarbonate

Lactobionate: Aminophylline, ampicillin, cimetidine, diphenhydrAMINE, hydrocortisone, lidocaine, methicillin, penicillin G potassium or sodium, pentobarbital, polymyxin B, potassium chloride, prednisoLONE, prochlorperazine, promazine, ranitidine, sodium bicarbonate, verapamil

Syringe compatibilities:

Lactobionate: Methicillin

Y-site compatibilities: Acyclovir, amiodarone, cyclophosphamide, diltiazem, enalaprilat, esmolol, famotidine, foscarnet, heparin, hydromorphone, idarubicin, labetalol, lorazepam, magnesium sulfate, meperidine, midazolam, morphine, multivitamins, perphenazine, tacrolimus, theophylline, vit B/C, zidovudine

Perform/provide:

• Storage at room temperature; store susp in refrigerator

• Adequate intake of fluids (2 L) during diarrhea episodes

Evaluate:

• Therapeutic response: decreased symptoms of infection

Teach patient/family:

• To report sore throat, fever, fatigue (could indicate superinfection)

• To notify nurse of diarrhea stools, dark urine, pale stools, jaundice of eyes or skin, and severe abdominal pain

• To take at evenly spaced intervals; complete dosage regimen

Treatment of hypersensitivity:
Withdraw drug; maintain airway; administer epINEPHrine, aminophylline, O_2, IV corticosteroids

erythromycin ophthalmic
See Appendix C

erythromycin topical
See Appendix C

escitalopram (R)
(es-sit-tal′oh-pram)
Lexapro
Func. class.: Antidepressant, SSRI (selective serotonin reuptake inhibitor)

Action: Inhibits CNS neuron uptake of serotonin but not of norepinephrine

Uses: General anxiety disorder, major depressive disorder

Investigational uses: Panic disorder

DOSAGE AND ROUTES

• *Adult:* **PO** 10 mg daily in AM or PM; after 1 wk if no clinical improvement is noted, dose may be increased to 20 mg daily PM; maintenance 10-20 mg/day, reassess to determine need for treatment

Hepatic dose/geriatric

• *Adult:* **PO** 10 mg/day

Available forms: Tabs 5, 10, 20 mg; oral sol 5 mg (as base)/5 ml

Side effects: *italics* = common; ***bold italics*** = life-threatening

SIDE EFFECTS

*CNS: Headache, nervousness, insomnia, drowsiness, anxiety, tremor, dizziness, fatigue, sedation, poor concentration, abnormal dreams, agitation, **sei-zures,** apathy, euphoria, hallucinations, delusions, psychosis*

*CV: Hot flashes, palpitations, angina pectoris, **hemorrhage,** hypertension, **tachycardia,** 1st-degree AV block, **bradycardia, MI, thrombophlebi-tis,** postural hypotension*

EENT: Visual changes, ear/eye pain, pho-tophobia, tinnitus

GI: Nausea, diarrhea, dry mouth, anorexia, dyspepsia, constipation, cramps, vomiting, taste changes, flatu-lence, decreased appetite

GU: Dysmenorrhea, decreased libido, urinary frequency, UTI, amenorrhea, cystitis, impotence, urine retention

INTEG: Sweating, rash, pruritus, acne, alopecia, urticaria, photosensitivity

MS: Pain, arthritis, twitching

RESP: Infection, pharyngitis, nasal congestion, sinus headache, sinusitis, cough, dyspnea, bronchitis, asthma, hyperventilation, pneumonia

SYST: Asthenia, viral infection, fever, allergy, chills

Contraindications: Hypersensitivity

Precautions: Pregnancy (C), lactation, children, elderly, renal disease, history of seizures

PHARMACOKINETICS

PO: Metabolized in liver; excreted in urine

INTERACTIONS

Paradoxical worsening of OCD: busPIRone

Serotonin syndrome: tryptophan, am-phetamines, antidepressants, busPIRone, lithium, amantadine, bromocriptine

⚠ Do not use MAOIs with or 14 days before escitalopram

Increase: CNS depression—alcohol, antidepressants, opioids, sedatives

Increase: side effects of escitalopram—highly protein-bound drugs

Increase: effect—haloperidol

Increase: half-life of diazepam

Increase: levels or toxicity of carbamaz-epine, lithium, warfarin, phenytoin

Increase: levels of tricyclics, phenothi-azines

Decrease: escitalopram effect—cyproheptadine

Drug/Herb

SAM-e, St. John's wort: do not use together

Increase: anticholinergic effect—corkwood, jimsonweed

Increase: CNS effect—hops, kava, lav-ender

Increase: hypertension—yohimbe

Drug/Lab Test

Increase: Serum bilirubin, blood glu-cose, alk phosphatase

Decrease: VMA, 5-HIAA

False increase: Urinary catecholamines

NURSING CONSIDERATIONS

Assess:

• Mental status: mood, sensorium, af-fect, suicidal tendencies, increase in psychiatric symptoms, depression, panic

• Appetite in bulimia nervosa, weight daily, increase nutritious foods in diet, watch for bingeing and vomiting

• Allergic reactions: itching, rash urti-caria, drug should be discontinued, may need to give antihistamine

• B/P (lying/standing), pulse q4h; if systolic B/P drops 20 mm Hg, hold drug, notify prescriber; take VS q4h in patients with cardiovascular disease

• Blood studies: CBC, leukocytes, differ-ential, cardiac enzymes if patient is re-ceiving long-term therapy; check platelets; bleeding can occur

• Hepatic studies: AST, ALT, bilirubin, creatinine

• Weight qwk; appetite may decrease with drug

• ECG for flattening of T wave, bundle branch, AV block, dysrhythmias in car-diac patients

• Alcohol consumption; if alcohol is consumed, hold dose until AM

Administer:
- With food or milk for GI symptoms
- Crushed if patient is unable to swallow medication whole
- Dosage at bedtime if oversedation occurs during the day
- Gum, hard candy, frequent sips of water for dry mouth

Perform/provide:
- Storage at room temperature; do not freeze
- Assistance with ambulation during therapy, since drowsiness, dizziness occur
- Safety measures primarily in elderly
- Checking to see if PO medication swallowed

Evaluate:
- Therapeutic response: decreased depression

Teach patient/family:
- That therapeutic effect may take 1-4 wk
- To use caution in driving, other activities requiring alertness because of drowsiness, dizziness, blurred vision
- To use sunscreen to prevent photosensitivity
- To avoid alcohol ingestion, other CNS depressants
- To notify prescriber if pregnant or plan to become pregnant or breast-feed
- To change positions slowly, orthostatic hypotension may occur
- To avoid all OTC drugs unless approved by prescriber
- To report immediately signs of urinary retention

---

esmolol (℞)

(ez′moe-lole)
Brevibloc
Func. class.: β-Adrenergic blocker (antidysrhythmic II)

Do not confuse:
Brevibloc/Brevital -
esmolol/Osmitrol

Action: Competitively blocks stimulation of β₁-adrenergic receptors in the myocardium; produces negative chronotropic, inotropic activity (decreases rate of SA node discharge, increases recovery time), slows conduction of AV node, decreases heart rate, decreases O_2 consumption in myocardium; also decreases renin-aldosterone-angiotensin system at high doses; inhibits β₂-receptors in bronchial system at higher doses

Uses: Supraventricular tachycardia, noncompensatory sinus tachycardia, hypertensive crisis, intraoperative and postoperative tachycardia and hypertension

DOSAGE AND ROUTES

- *Adult:* **IV** loading dose 500 mcg/kg/min over 1 min; maintenance 50 mcg/kg/min for 4 min; if no response in 5 min, give 2nd loading dose; then increase inf to 100 mcg/kg/min for 4 min; if no response, repeat loading dose, then increase maintenance inf by 50 mcg/kg/min (max of 200 mcg/kg/min), titrate to patient response
- *Child:* **IV** 50 mcg/kg/min, may increase q10min (max 300 mcg/kg/min)

Available forms: Inj 10 mg, 250 mg/ml

SIDE EFFECTS

CNS: Confusion, light-headedness, paresthesia, somnolence, fever, dizziness, fatigue, headache, depression, anxiety, **seizures**

CV: Hypotension, bradycardia, chest pain, peripheral ischemia, shortness of breath, **CHF,** conduction disturbances, 1st, 2nd, 3rd degree heart block

GI: Nausea, vomiting, anorexia, gastric pain, flatulence, constipation, heartburn, bloating

GU: Urinary retention, impotence, dysuria

INTEG: Induration, inflammation at site, discoloration, edema, erythema, burning pallor, flushing, rash, pruritus, dry skin, alopecia

*RESP: **Bronchospasm,*** dyspnea, cough, wheeziness, nasal stuffiness

Contraindications: 2nd- or 3rd-

---

degree heart block, cardiogenic shock, CHF, cardiac failure, hypersensitivity

Precautions: Pregnancy (C), hypotension, peripheral vascular disease, diabetes, hypoglycemia, thyrotoxicosis, renal disease, lactation

PHARMACOKINETICS

Onset very rapid, duration short, half-life 9 min; metabolized by hydrolysis of the ester linkage; excreted via kidneys

INTERACTIONS

Avoid use with MAOIs

Increase: digoxin levels—digoxin

Increase: α-adrenergic stimulation—epHEDrine, epINEPHrine, amphetamine, norepinephrine, phenylephrine, pseudoephedrine

Decrease: action of thyroid hormones

Decrease: action of esmolol—thyroid hormone

Drug/Herb

Potassium deficiency: aloe, buckthorn, cascara sagrada, senna

Increase: β-blocking effect—betel palm, butterbur, cola tree, figwort, fumitory, guarana, hawthorn, lily of the valley, motherwort, plantain

Increase: CV reactions—jaborandi tree

Decrease: β-blocking effect—coenzyme Q10, yohimbe

Drug/Lab Test

Interference: Glucose/insulin tolerance test

NURSING CONSIDERATIONS

Assess:
- I&O ratio, weight daily, watch for signs of CHF (jugular vein distention, weight gain, crackles, edema)
- B/P, pulse q4h; note rate, rhythm, quality; rapid changes can cause shock; if systolic <100 or diastolic <60, notify prescriber before giving drug
- ECG continuously during inf, hypotension is common
- Baselines in renal, hepatic studies before therapy begins
- Breath sounds and respiratory pattern: wheezing from bronchospasm

Administer:
- Reduced dosage in cool environment

IV route
- IV diluted 5 g/20 ml of D_5W, D_5R, D_5 0.9% NaCl, 0.45% NaCl, LR, D_5 0.45% NaCl, 0.9% NaCl further dilute in the remaining 480 ml (10 mg/ml) and give as infusion; give loading dose over 1 min, then maintenance over 4 min; may repeat loading dose q5min with increased maintenance dose; maintenance dose should not be >200 mcg/kg/min and be given up to 48 hr; dose should be tapered at 25 mcg/kg/min; use infusion pump

Additive compatibilities: Aminophylline, atracurium, bretylium, heparin

Y-site compatibilities: Amikacin, aminophylline, amiodarone, ampicillin, atracurium, butorphanol, calcium chloride, cefazolin, cefmetazole, cefoperazone, ceftazidime, ceftizoxime, chloramphenicol, cimetidine, cisatracurium, clindamycin, diltiazem, DOPamine, enalaprilat, erythromycin, famotidine, fentanyl, gentamicin, heparin, hydrocortisone, insulin (regular), labetalol, magnesium sulfate, methyldopate, metronidazole, midazolam, morphine, nafcillin, nitroglycerin, nitroprusside, norepinephrine, pancuronium, penicillin G potassium, phenytoin, piperacillin, polymyxin B, potassium chloride, potassium phosphate, propofol, ranitidine, remifentanil, streptomycin, tacrolimus, tobramycin, trimethoprim-sulfamethoxazole, vancomycin, vecuronium

Perform/provide:
- Storage protected from light, moisture; in cool environment

Evaluate:
- Therapeutic response: lower B/P immediately, lower heart rate

Teach patient/family:
- To notify prescriber if pain, swelling occurs at IV site

Treatment of overdose: Discontinue drug

esomeprazole (℞)
(es'oh-mep'rah-zohl)
Nexium
Func. class.: Antiulcer, proton pump inhibitor
Chem. class.: Benzimidazole

Action: Suppresses gastric secretion by inhibiting hydrogen/potassium ATPase enzyme system in gastric parietal cell; characterized as gastric acid pump inhibitor, because it blocks final step of acid production

Uses: Gastroesophageal reflux disease (GERD), severe erosive esophagitis; treatment of active duodenal ulcers in combination with antiinfectives for *Helicobacter pylori* infection

DOSAGE AND ROUTES
Active duodenal ulcers associated with H. pylori
• *Adult:* **PO** 40 mg daily × 10 days in combination with clarithromycin 500 mg bid × 10 days and amoxicillin 1000 mg bid × 10 days

GERD
• *Adult:* **PO** 20 or 40 mg daily × 4-8 wk; no adjustment needed in renal, liver failure, elderly

Available forms: Caps 20, 40 mg

SIDE EFFECTS
CNS: Headache, dizziness
GI: Diarrhea, flatulence, abdominal pain, constipation, dry mouth
INTEG: Rash, dry skin
MISC: Dizziness
RESP: Cough

Contraindications: Hypersensitivity
Precautions: Pregnancy (B), lactation, children, elderly

PHARMACOKINETICS
Eliminated in urine as metabolites and in feces; in elderly, elimination rate decreased, bioavailability increased

INTERACTIONS
Increase: effect toxicity of diazepam, digoxin, penicillins
Decrease: effect—dapsone, iron, itraconazole, ketoconazole

NURSING CONSIDERATIONS
Assess:
• GI system: bowel sounds q8h, abdomen for pain, swelling, anorexia
• Hepatic enzymes: AST, ALT, alk phosphatase during treatment
Administer:
• Swallow caps whole; do not crush or chew; cap may be opened and sprinkled over tbsp of applesauce
• Same time daily
• At least 1 hr before eating
Evaluate:
• Therapeutic response: absence of epigastric pain, swelling, fullness
Teach patient/family:
• To report severe diarrhea; drug may have to be discontinued
• That diabetic patient should know hypoglycemia may occur
• To avoid hazardous activities; dizziness may occur
• To avoid alcohol, salicylates, ibuprofen; may cause GI irritation

E

estradiol
(es-tra-dye'ole)
Estrace

estradiol cypionate
depGynogen, Depo-Estradiol, Depogen, Dura-Estrin, E-Cypionate, Estragyn LA5, Estro-Cyp, Estrofem, Estroject-LA, Estrol-L.A.

estradiol topical emulsion
Estrasorb

estradiol valerate
Clinigen LA, Delestrogen, Dioval, Duragen, Estra-L, Estro-span, Femogex ✤, Gynogen LA, Menaval, Valergen

estradiol transdermal system
Alora, Climara, Esclim, Estraderm, FemPatch, Vivelle

estradiol vaginal tablet
Vagifem

estradiol vaginal ring
Estring

Func. class.: Estrogen, progestins

Action: Needed for adequate functioning of female reproductive system; affects release of pituitary gonadotropins, inhibits ovulation, adequate calcium use in bone

Uses: Symptoms associated with menopause, inoperable breast cancer (selected cases), prostatic cancer, atrophic vaginitis, kraurosis vulvae, hypogonadism, primary ovarian failure, prevention of osteoporosis

DOSAGE AND ROUTES
Hormone replacement
• *Adult:* **TD** 0.05-0.1 mg/24 hr, apply 2 ×/wk
Menopause/hypogonadism/castration/ovarian failure
• *Adult:* **PO** 1-2 mg daily, 3 wk on, 1 wk off or 5 days on, 2 days off; **IM** 1-5 mg

q3-4wk (cypionate); 10-20 mg q4wk (valerate)
• *Adult:* **TOP** Estraderm 0.05 mg/24 hr applied 2 ×/wk Climara 0.05 mg/hr applied 1 ×/wk in a cyclic regimen; women with hysterectomy may use continuously
Prostatic cancer
• *Adult:* **IM** 30 mg q1-2wk (valerate); **PO** 1-2 mg tid (oral estradiol)
Breast cancer
• *Adult:* **PO** 10 mg tid × 3 mo or longer
Atropic vaginitis/kraurosis vulvae
• *Adult:* **VAG CREAM** 2-4 g daily × 1-2 wk, then 1 g 1-3 ×/wk cycled; vag tab 1 daily × 2 wk, maintenance 1 tab 2 ×/wk; **VAG RING** inserted and left in place continuously for 3 mo
Vasomotor symptoms
• *Adult:* **TOP** After cleaning and drying skin on left thigh, calf, rub in contents of pouch using both hands until completely absorbed; wash hands
Available forms: Estradiol tabs 0.5, 1, 2 mg; valerate inj 10, 20, 40 mg/ml; transderm 0.025, 0.0375, 0.05, 0.075, 0.1 mg/24 hr release rate; vag cream 100 mcg/g; vag tab 25 mcg; vag ring 2 mg/90 days; topical emulsion 2.5 mg

SIDE EFFECTS
CNS: Dizziness, headache, migraines, depression, *seizures*
CV: Hypotension, thrombophlebitis, edema, *thromboembolism, stroke, pulmonary embolism, myocardial infarction*
EENT: Contact lens intolerance, increased myopia, astigmatism
GI: Nausea, vomiting, diarrhea, anorexia, pancreatitis, cramps, constipation, increased appetite, increased weight, *cholestatic jaundice, hepatic adenoma*
GU: Amenorrhea, cervical erosion, breakthrough bleeding, dysmenorrhea, vaginal candidiasis, breast changes, *gynecomastia, testicular atrophy, impotence, increased risk of breast cancer, endometrial cancer,* changes in libido
INTEG: Rash, urticaria, acne, hirsutism,

alopecia, oily skin, seborrhea, purpura, melasma
META: Folic acid deficiency, hypercalcemia, hyperglycemia
Contraindications: Pregnancy (X), breast cancer, thromboembolic disorders, reproductive cancer, genital bleeding (abnormal, undiagnosed), lactation
Precautions: Hypertension, asthma, blood dyscrasias, gallbladder disease, CHF, diabetes mellitus, bone disease, depression, migraine headache, seizure disorders, hepatic disease, renal disease, family history of cancer of breast or reproductive tract, smoking

PHARMACOKINETICS

PO/INJ/TD: Degraded in liver; excreted in urine; crosses placenta; excreted in breast milk

INTERACTIONS

Increase: action of corticosteroids
Increase: toxicity—cycloSPORINE, dantrolene
Decrease: action of anticoagulants, oral hypoglycemics, tamoxifen
Decrease: estradiol action—anticonvulsants, barbiturates, phenylbutazone, rifampin, calcium

Drug/Herb
Altered estrogen effect: black cohosh, DHEA
Increase: estrogen effect—alfalfa, hops
Decrease: estrogen effect—saw palmetto

Drug/Food
Increase: estrogen level—grapefruit juice

Drug/Lab Test
Increase: BSP retention test, PBI, T_4, serum sodium, platelet aggregation, thyroxine-binding globulin (TBG), prothrombin, factors VII, VIII, IX, X, triglycerides
Decrease: Serum folate, serum triglyceride, T_3 resin uptake test, glucose tolerance test, antithrombin III, pregnanediol, metyrapone test

False positive: LE prep, antinuclear antibodies

NURSING CONSIDERATIONS

Assess:
• Blood glucose of diabetic patient, hyperglycemia may occur
• Weight daily, notify prescriber of weekly weight gain >5 lb; if increase, diuretic may be ordered
• B/P q4h, watch for increase caused by H_2O and sodium retention
• I&O ratio; decreasing urinary output, increasing edema, report changes
• Hepatic studies, including AST, ALT, bilirubin, alk phosphatase baseline, periodically
• Hypertension, cardiac symptoms, jaundice, hypercalcemia
• Mental status: affect, mood, behavioral changes, aggression
• Female patient for intact uterus, if so, progesterone should be added to estrogen therapy to decrease risk of endometrial cancer

Administer:
• Titrated dose; use lowest effective dose
• IM inj deeply in large muscle mass

PO route
• With food or milk to decrease GI symptoms

Transdermal route
• Apply to trunk of body 2 ×/wk; press firmly and hold in place for 10 sec to ensure good contact
• On intermittent cycle schedule: 3 wk on, then 1 wk off; if patch falls off, reapply

Vaginal route
• Use applicator provided

Evaluate:
• Therapeutic response: reversal of menopause symptoms or decrease in tumor size in prostatic, breast cancer

Teach patient/family:
• To weigh weekly, report gain >5 lb
⚠ To report breast lumps, vaginal bleeding, edema, jaundice, dark urine, clay-colored stools, dyspnea, headache, blurred vision, abdominal pain, numbness or stiffness in legs, chest pain, ten-

derness, redness, and swelling in extremities; male to report impotence or gynecomastia

estramustine
(ess-tra-muss'teen)
Emcyt
Func. class.: Antineoplastic

Uses: Metastatic prostate cancer

DOSAGE AND ROUTES

• *Adult:* **PO** 10-16 mg/kg in 3-4 divided doses/day; treatment may continue for ≥3 mo or 600 mg/m^2/day in 3 divided doses

Contraindications: Pregnancy (D), hypersensitivity to estradiol, thromboembolic disorders

estrogens, conjugated
Cenestin, C.E.S. ✦, Congest, Premarin

estrogens, conjugated synthetic B
Enjuvia
Func. class.: Estrogen, hormone

Do not confuse:
Premarin/Provera

Action: Needed for adequate functioning of female reproductive system; affects release of pituitary gonadotropins, inhibits ovulation, adequate calcium use in bone

Uses: Symptoms associated with menopause, inoperable breast cancer, prostatic cancer, abnormal uterine bleeding, hypogonadism, primary ovarian failure, prevention of osteoporosis

DOSAGE AND ROUTES

Estrogens conjugated

Menopause
• *Adult:* **PO** 0.3-1.25 mg daily 3 wk on, 1 wk off

Prevention of osteoporosis
• *Adult:* **PO** 0.625 mg daily or in cycle
Atrophic vaginitis
• *Adult:* **VAG CREAM** 2-4 g ml daily × 21 days, off 7 days, repeat
Prostatic cancer
• *Adult:* **PO** 1.25-2.5 mg tid
Advanced inoperable breast cancer
• *Adult:* **PO** 10 mg tid × 3 mo or longer
Abnormal uterine bleeding
• *Adult:* **IV/IM** 25 mg, repeat in 6-12 hr
Castration/primary ovarian failure
• *Adult:* **PO** 1.25 mg daily, 3 wk on, 1 wk off
Hypogonadism
• *Adult:* **PO** 2.5 mg bid-tid × 20 days/mo
Estrogens conjugated synthetic B menopause
• *Adult:* **PO** 0.625 mg daily initially; may increase based on response

Available forms: Tabs 0.3, 0.625, 0.9, 1.25, 2.5 mg; inj 25 mg/vial; vag cream 0.625 mg/g; synthetic B, tabs 0.625, 1.25 mg

SIDE EFFECTS

CNS: Dizziness, headache, migraine, depression, *seizures*
CV: Hypotension, thrombophlebitis, edema, *thromboembolism, stroke, pulmonary embolism, myocardial infarction*
EENT: Contact lens intolerance, increased myopia, astigmatism
GI: Nausea, vomiting, diarrhea, anorexia, pancreatitis, cramps, constipation, increased appetite, increased weight, *cholestatic jaundice, hepatic adenoma*
GU: Amenorrhea, cervical erosion, breakthrough bleeding, dysmenorrhea, vaginal candidiasis, breast changes, *gynecomastia, testicular atrophy, impotence, increased risk of breast cancer, endometrial cancer,* libido changes
INTEG: Rash, urticaria, acne, hirsutism, alopecia, oily skin, seborrhea, purpura, melasma

META: Folic acid deficiency, hypercalcemia, hyperglycemia

Contraindications: Pregnancy (X), thromboembolic disorders, reproductive cancer, genital bleeding (abnormal, undiagnosed), lactation

Precautions: Hypertension, asthma, blood dyscrasias, gallbladder disease, CHF, diabetes mellitus, bone disease, depression, migraine headache, convulsive disorders, hepatic disease, renal disease, family history of cancer of breast or reproductive tract, smoking

PHARMACOKINETICS

PO/IV/IM: Degraded in liver, excreted in urine, crosses placenta, excreted in breast milk

INTERACTIONS

Increase: toxicity—cycloSPORINE, dantrolene

Increase: action of corticosteroids

Decrease: action of estrogens—anticonvulsants, barbiturates, phenylbutazone, rifampin

Decrease: action of anticoagulants, oral hypoglycemics, tamoxifen

Drug/Herb

Altered estrogen effect—black cohosh, DHEA

Increase: estrogen effect—alfalfa, hops

Decrease: estrogen effect—saw palmetto

Drug/Food

Increase: estrogen level—grapefruit juice

Drug/Lab Test

Increase: BSP retention test, PBI, T_4, serum sodium, platelet aggregation, thyroxine-binding globulin (TBG), prothrombin, factors VII, VIII, IX, X, triglycerides

Decrease: Serum folate, serum triglyceride, T_3 resin uptake test, glucose tolerance test, antithrombin III, pregnanediol, metyrapone test

False positive: LE prep, antinuclear antibodies

NURSING CONSIDERATIONS

Assess:

• Blood glucose if diabetic patient, hyperglycemia may occur

• Weight daily; notify prescriber of weekly weight gain >5 lb; if increase, diuretic may be ordered

• B/P q4h; watch for increase caused by H_2O and Na retention

• I&O ratio; be alert for decreasing urinary output, increasing edema

• Hepatic studies: AST, ALT, bilirubin, alk phosphatase

• Hypertension, cardiac symptoms, jaundice, hypercalcemia

• Mental status: affect, mood, behavioral changes, aggression

• Female patient for intact uterus, if so, progesterone should be added to estrogen therapy to decrease risk of endometrial cancer

Administer:

• Titrated dose, use lowest effective dose

IM route

• IM reconstitute after withdrawing >5 ml of air from container and inject sterile diluent on vial side, rotate to dissolve; give inj deep in large muscle mass

• With food or milk to decrease GI symptoms (PO)

Vaginal route

• Use applicator provided

IV, direct route

• IV, after reconstituting as for IM, inject into distal port of running IV line of D_5W, 0.9% NaCl, LR at 5 mg/min or less

Y-site compatibilities: Heparin/hydrocortisone, potassium chloride, vit B/C

Evaluate:

• Therapeutic response: absence of breast engorgement, reversal of menopause symptoms, or decrease in tumor size in prostatic cancer

Teach patient/family:

• To avoid breastfeeding, since drug is excreted in breast milk

• To weigh weekly, report gain >5 lb

Side effects: *italics* = common; ***bold italics*** = life-threatening

⚠ To report breast lumps, vaginal bleeding, edema, jaundice, dark urine, clay-colored stools, dyspnea, headache, blurred vision, abdominal pain, leg pain and redness, numbness or stiffness in legs, chest pain; male to report impotence or gynecomastia

• To avoid sunlight or wear sunscreen; burns may occur

• To notify prescriber if pregnancy is suspected

---

etanercept (℞)
(eh-tan'er-sept)
Enbrel
Func. class.: Antirheumatic agent (disease modifying)

Action: Binds tumor necrosis factor (TNF), which is involved in immune and inflammatory reactions

Uses: Acute, chronic rheumatoid arthritis that has not responded to other disease-modifying agents, polyarticular course juvenile rheumatoid arthritis (JRA)

Investigational uses: CHF, psoriasis/psoriatic arthritis

DOSAGE AND ROUTES

Osteoarthritis

• *Adult:* **SUBCUT** 25 mg 2 ×/wk, may be given with other drugs for rheumatoid arthritis

• *Child 4-17 yr:* **SUBCUT** 0.4 mg/kg 2 ×/wk, max 25 mg 1 dose

CHF

• *Adult:* **SUBCUT** 5-12 mg/m² 2 ×/wk × 3 mo

Psoriasis/psoriatic arthritis

• *Adult:* **SUBCUT** 25 mg 2 ×/wk × 12 wk

Available forms: Powder for inj: 25 mg

SIDE EFFECTS

CNS: Headache, asthenia, dizziness
GI: Abdominal pain, dyspepsia
INTEG: Rash, *inj site reaction*

RESP: Pharyngitis, cough, URI, non-URI, sinusitis, *rhinitis*

Contraindications: Hypersensitivity, sepsis

Precautions: Pregnancy (B), lactation, children <4 yr, elderly

PHARMACOKINETICS

Elimination half-life 115 hr, 60% absorbed SUBCUT

INTERACTIONS

Do not give concurrently with vaccines, immunizations should be brought up to date before treatment

NURSING CONSIDERATIONS

Assess:
• Pain, stiffness, ROM, swelling of joints during treatment

• For inj site pain, swelling, usually occurs after 2 inj (4-5 days)

Administer:
• After reconstituting 1 ml of supplied diluent, slowly inject diluent into vial, swirl contents, do not shake, sol should be clear/colorless, do not use if cloudy or discolored

• Do not admix with other sol or medications, do not use filter

• May be injected SUBCUT into upper arm, abdomen, or thigh, rotate inj sites

Evaluate:
• Therapeutic response: decreased inflammation, pain in joints

Teach patient/family:
• That drug must be continued for prescribed time to be effective

• To use caution when driving; dizziness may occur

• About self-administration if appropriate: inj should be made in thigh, abdomen, upper arm; rotate sites at least 1 in from old site

---

⚠ Safety alert   *"Tall Man" lettering

ethambutol (R)
(e-tham'byoo-tole)
Etibi ✤, Myambutol
Func. class.: Antitubercular
Chem. class.: Diisopropylethylene
diamide derivative

Do not confuse:
ethambutol/Ethmozine
Action: Inhibits RNA synthesis, decreases tubercle bacilli replication
Uses: Pulmonary tuberculosis, as an adjunct, other mycobacterial infections

DOSAGE AND ROUTES

• *Adult and child >13 yr:* **PO** 15-25 mg/kg/day as a single dose or 50 mg/kg 2 ×/wk or 25-30 mg/kg 3 ×/wk
Renal disease
• CCr 10-50 ml/min dose q24-36h; CCr <10 ml/min dose q48h
Retreatment
• *Adult:* **PO** 25 mg/kg/day as single dose × 2 mo with at least 1 other drug, then decrease to 15 mg/kg/day as single dose, max 2.5 g/day
• *Child:* **PO** 15 mg/kg/day
Available forms: Tabs 100, 400 mg

SIDE EFFECTS

CNS: Headache, confusion, fever, malaise, dizziness, *disorientation,* hallucinations
EENT: Blurred vision, optic neuritis, photophobia, decreased visual acuity
GI: Abdominal distress, anorexia, nausea, vomiting
INTEG: Dermatitis, pruritus, ***toxic epidermal necrolysis***
META: Elevated uric acid, acute gout, liver function impairment
*MISC: **Thrombocytopenia,*** joint pain, bloody sputum, ***anaphylaxis***
Contraindications: Hypersensitivity, optic neuritis, child <13 yr
Precautions: Pregnancy (B), lactation, renal disease, diabetic retinopathy, cataracts, ocular defects, hepatic and hematopoietic disorders

PHARMACOKINETICS

PO: Peak 2-4 hr, half-life 3 hr; metabolized in liver; excreted in urine (unchanged drug/inactive metabolites, unchanged drug in feces)

INTERACTIONS

Delayed absorption of ethambutol: aluminum salts
Neurotoxicity: other neurotoxics

NURSING CONSIDERATIONS

Assess:
• Hepatic studies qwk × 2 wk, then q2mo: ALT, AST, bilirubin
• Signs of anemia: Hct, Hgb, fatigue
• Mental status often: affect, mood, behavioral changes; psychosis may occur
• Hepatic status: decreased appetite, jaundice, dark urine, fatigue
• C&S, including sputum, before treatment
• Visual status: decreased activity, altered color perception
Administer:
• With meals to decrease GI symptoms
• Antiemetic if vomiting occurs
• After C&S is completed; qmo to detect resistance
• 2 hr before antacids
Evaluate:
• Therapeutic response: decreased symptoms of TB, decrease in acid-fast bacteria
Teach patient/family:
• To avoid alcohol products
• That compliance with dosage schedule, duration is necessary
• That scheduled appointments must be kept or relapse may occur
• To report any visual changes, rash, hot, swollen, painful joints, numbness or tingling of extremities to prescriber

E

ethosuximide (Ŗ)
(eth-oh-sux′i-mide)
Zarontin
Func. class.: Anticonvulsant

Uses: Absence seizures, partial seizures, tonic-clonic seizures

DOSAGE AND ROUTES
• *Adult and child >6 yr:* **PO** 250 mg bid initially; may increase by 250 mg q4-7d, max 2 g/day
• *Child 3-6 yr:* **PO** 250 mg/day or 125 mg bid; may increase by 250 mg q4-7d
Contraindications: Hypersensitivity

---

etidronate (Ŗ)
(eh-tih-droe′nate)
Didronel, Didronel IV
Func. class.: Bone resorption inhibitor
Chem. class.: Bisphosphonate

Do not confuse:
etidronate/etretinate/etomidate
Action: Decreases bone resorption and new bone development (accretion)
Uses: Paget's disease, heterotopic ossification, hypercalcemia of malignancy

DOSAGE AND ROUTES
Paget's disease
• *Adult:* **PO** 5-10 mg/kg/day, 2 hr ac with H_2O, not to exceed 20 mg/kg/day, max 6 mo or 11-20 mg/kg/day for max of 3 mo
Heterotopic ossification
• *Adult:* **PO** 20 mg/kg daily × 2 wk, then 10 mg/kg/day for 10 wk, total 12 wk
Hypercalcemia
• *Adult:* **IV** 7.5 mg/kg/day × 3 days, then **PO** 20 mg/kg/day
Heterotopic ossification/hip replacement
• *Adult:* **PO** 20 mg/kg/day × 4 wk before and 3 mo after surgery (4 mo total)

Available forms: Tabs 200, 400 mg; inj 50 mg/ml

SIDE EFFECTS
GI: Nausea, constipation; metallic taste (IV), diarrhea
GU: **Nephrotoxicity**
MISC: Dyspnea, low magnesium, phosphorus, alopecia
MS: Bone pain, hypocalcemia, decreased mineralization of nonaffected bones
Contraindications: Pathologic fractures, clinically overt osteomalacia, severe renal disease with creatinine >5 mg/dl
Precautions: Pregnancy (C), renal disease, lactation, restricted vit D, calcium for children, enterocolitis

PHARMACOKINETICS
Absorbed poorly (PO), not metabolized; excreted in urine/feces; therapeutic response: 1-3 mo

INTERACTIONS
Increase: protime—warfarin
Decrease: absorption—calcium, aluminum, magnesium antacids/supplements, iron products
Drug/Food
Dairy products: decreased absorption

NURSING CONSIDERATIONS
Assess:
• I&O ratio; check for decreased output in renal patients
• BUN, creatinine, uric acid, phosphate chloride, albumin, pH, urine calcium, magnesium, alk phosphatase, urinalysis; calcium should be kept at 9-10 mg/dl, vit D 50-135 international units/dl
• Muscle spasm, laryngospasm, paresthesias, facial twitching, colic; may indicate hypocalcemia
• Nutritional status, diet for sources of vit D (milk, some seafood), calcium (dairy products, dark green vegetables), phosphates—adequate intake is necessary
• Persistent nausea or diarrhea

Administer:
PO route
- Drug therapy should not last longer than 6 mo
- On empty stomach with H_2O 2 hr ac
IV route
- IV after diluting in 250 ml or more 0.9% NaCl; give over 2 hr or longer
- Food, especially high in calcium; vitamins with mineral supplements or antacids high in metals should not be given within 2 hr of dose

Evaluate:
- Therapeutic response: management of bone deficiencies, Paget's disease

Teach patient/family:
- To avoid OTC products
- That therapeutic response may take 1-3 mo; effects persist for months after drug is discontinued
- That adequate intake of calcium, vit D is necessary
- To report sudden onset of unexplained pain, restricted mobility, heat over bone; hypercalcemic relapse

---

etodolac (Ŗ)
(ee-toe'doe-lak)
Lodine, Lodine XL
Func. class.: Nonsteroidal antiinflammatory/nonopioid analgesic

Do not confuse:
Lodine/codeine/iodine
Action: Inhibits prostaglandin synthesis by decreasing an enzyme needed for biosynthesis; analgesic, antiinflammatory, antipyretic
Uses: Mild to moderate pain, osteoarthritis

DOSAGE AND ROUTES
Osteoarthritis
- *Adult:* **PO** 800-1200 mg/day in divided doses q6-8h initially, then adjust dose to 600-1200 mg/day in divided doses; do not exceed 1200 mg/day; patients <60 kg not to exceed 20 mg/kg
Analgesia
- *Adult:* **PO** 200-400 mg q6-8h prn for acute pain; do not exceed 1200 mg/day; patients <60 kg, not to exceed 20 mg/kg
Available forms: Caps 200, 300 mg; tabs 400, 500 mg; ext rel tabs (XL) 400, 600 mg

SIDE EFFECTS
CNS: Dizziness, headache, drowsiness, fatigue, tremors, confusion, insomnia, anxiety, depression, light-headedness, vertigo
CV: Tachycardia, peripheral edema, fluid retention, palpitations, dysrhythmias, CHF
EENT: Tinnitus, hearing loss, blurred vision, photophobia
GI: Nausea, anorexia, vomiting, diarrhea, jaundice, ***cholestatic hepatitis,*** constipation, flatulence, cramps, dry mouth, peptic ulcer, dyspepsia, ***GI bleeding***
*GU: **Nephrotoxicity:** dysuria, **hematuria,** oliguria, azotemia,* cystitis, urinary tract infection
*HEMA: **Blood dyscrasias***
INTEG: Erythema, urticaria, purpura, rash, pruritus, sweating, ***Stevens-Johnson syndrome***
*SYST: **Angioedema, anaphylaxis***
Contraindications: Hypersensitivity; patients in whom aspirin, iodides, or other nonsteroidal antiinflammatories have produced asthma; rhinitis, urticaria, nasal polyps, angioedema, bronchospasm
Precautions: Pregnancy (C), avoid in 2nd half of pregnancy, lactation; children; bleeding; GI, cardiac disorders; elderly; renal, hepatic disorders

PHARMACOKINETICS
PO: Peak 1-2 hr, serum protein binding >90%, half-life 7 hr; metabolized by liver (metabolites excreted in urine)

INTERACTIONS
Increase: toxicity—cycloSPORINE, digoxin, lithium, methotrexate, phenytoin
Increase: GI toxicity—aspirin
Decrease: effect of etodolac—antacids

Side effects: *italics* = common; ***bold italics*** = life-threatening

Decrease: effect of β-blockers, diuretics

Drug/Herb
Severe photosensitivity: St. John's wort
Increase: gastric irritation—arginine, gossypol
Increase: NSAIDs effect—bearberry, bilberry
Increase: bleeding risk—bogbean, chondroitin, saw palmetto, turmeric

NURSING CONSIDERATIONS

Assess:
• Pain: location, frequency, characteristics; relief after med
• Blood, renal, hepatic studies: BUN, creatinine, AST, ALT, Hgb, before treatment, periodically thereafter
• For GI bleeding: black stools, hematemesis
• Audiometric, ophthalmic examination before, during, after treatment
• For eye, ear problems: blurred vision, tinnitus; may indicate toxicity
• For asthma, aspirin hypersensitivity, nasal polyps that may be hypersensitive to etodolac

Administer:
• Do not break, crush, or chew ext rel tabs
• With food to decrease GI symptoms, since extent of absorption is not affected by food

Perform/provide:
• Storage at room temperature

Evaluate:
• Therapeutic response: decreased pain, stiffness, swelling in joints, ability to move more easily

Teach patient/family:
• To report blurred vision or ringing, roaring in ears; may indicate toxicity
• To avoid driving, other hazardous activities if dizziness or drowsiness occurs
⚠ To report change in urine pattern, weight increase, edema, pain increase in joints, fever, blood in urine; indicates nephrotoxicity
• That therapeutic effects may take up to 1 mo

• To avoid aspirin, NSAIDs, acetaminophen, alcoholic beverages while taking this medication

---

Rarely Used

etomidate (℞)
(e-tom'i-date)
Amidate
Func. class.: General anesthetic

Uses: Induction of general anesthesia

DOSAGE AND ROUTES
• *Adult and child >10 yr:* **IV** 0.2-0.6 mg/kg over ½-1 min
Contraindications: Hypersensitivity, labor/delivery

⚠ High Alert

etoposide (℞)
(e-toe-poe'side)
VePesid, VP-16
Func. class.: Antineoplastic—miscellaneous
Chem. class.: Semisynthetic podophyllotoxin

Do not confuse:
VePesid/Versed
Action: Inhibits mitotic activity through metaphase to mitosis; also inhibits cells from entering mitosis, depresses DNA, RNA synthesis, cell cycle specific S and G_2
Uses: Leukemias, testicular cancer, lymphomas, small cell carcinoma of the lung

DOSAGE AND ROUTES
Testicular cancer
• *Adult:* **IV** 50-100 mg/m²/day × 3-5 days given q3-5wk or 200-250 mg/m²/wk, or 125-140 mg/m²/day 3 × wk, q5wk
Small cell carcinoma of the lung
• *Adult:* **PO** 70 mg/m²/day × 4 days, given q3-4wk, **IV** 35 mg/m²/day × 4 days, up to 50 mg/m² daily × 5 day q3-4 wk

---

⚠ Safety alert   *"Tall Man" lettering

Available forms: Inj 20 mg/ml; caps 50 mg

SIDE EFFECTS

CNS: Headache, *fever,* peripheral neuropathy, paresthesias, confusion
CV: Hypotension, **MI, dysrhythmias**
*GI: Nausea, vomiting, anorexia, **hepatotoxicity,*** dyspepsia, diarrhea, constipation
GU: **Nephrotoxicity**
HEMA: **Thrombocytopenia, leukopenia, myelosuppression, anemia**
INTEG: Rash, alopecia, phlebitis at IV site, radiation recall
RESP: **Bronchospasm,** pleural effusion
SYST: **Anaphylaxis**
Contraindications: Pregnancy (D), hypersensitivity, bone marrow depression, severe hepatic disease, severe renal disease, bacterial infection, viral infection
Precautions: Renal disease, hepatic disease, lactation, children, gout

PHARMACOKINETICS

Half-life 7 hr, metabolized in liver; excreted in urine; crosses placental barrier

INTERACTIONS

Increase: bone marrow depression—other antineoplastics, radiation
Increase: adverse reactions—live virus vaccines

NURSING CONSIDERATIONS
Assess:

• CBC, differential, platelet count weekly; withhold drug if WBC is <1000 or platelet count is <50,000; notify prescriber
• Renal studies: BUN, serum uric acid, urine CCr, electrolytes before, during therapy
• I&O ratio; report fall in urine output to <30 ml/hr; check blood pressure bid and report any significant decrease
• Monitor temp q4h; may indicate beginning infection

• Hepatic studies before, during therapy (bilirubin, AST, ALT, LDH) as needed or monthly
• RBC, Hct, Hgb; may be decreased
• Bleeding: hematuria, guaiac stools, bruising or petechiae, mucosa or orifices q8h
• Effects of alopecia on body image; discuss feelings about body changes
• Jaundice of skin and sclera, dark urine, clay-colored stools, itchy skin, abdominal pain, fever, diarrhea
• B/P q15 min during inf, if systolic reading <90 mm Hg, discontinue inf and notify prescriber
• Buccal cavity q8h for dryness, sores or ulceration, white patches, oral pain, bleeding, dysphagia
• Local irritation, pain, burning, discoloration at inj site
⚠ Symptoms indicating severe allergic reaction: rash, pruritus, urticaria, purpuric skin lesions, itching, flushing
⚠ Symptoms of anaphylaxis: flushing, restlessness, coughing, difficulty breathing
• Frequency of stools, characteristics: cramping, acidosis; signs of dehydration: rapid respirations, poor skin turgor, decreased urine output, dry skin, restlessness, weakness
Administer:
• Antiemetic 30-60 min before giving drug and prn to prevent vomiting
• Allopurinol or sodium bicarbonate to maintain uric acid levels, alkalinization of urine
• Antispasmodic, epINEPHrine, corticosteroids, antihistamines for reactions
IV route (VePesid)
• After diluting 100 mg/250 ml or more D_5W or NaCl to 0.2-0.4 mg/ml, infuse over 30-60 min; phosphate may be given over 5 min-3½ hr; may dilute further to 0.1 mg/ml in 0.9% NaCl, D_5W
Additive compatibilities: Carboplatin, cisplatin, cytarabine, floxuridine, fluorouracil, hydrOXYzine, ifosfamide, ondansetron
Y-site compatibilities: Allopurinol, amifostine, aztreonam, cladribine,

DOXOrubicin liposome, fludarabine, granisetron, melphalan, ondansetron, paclitaxel, piperacillin/tazobactam, sargramostim, sodium bicarbonate, teniposide, thiotepa, vinorelbine

Perform/provide:

• Liquid diet: carbonated beverages, Jell-O; dry toast or crackers may be added if patient is not nauseated or vomiting

• Increase fluid intake to 2-3 L/day to prevent urate deposits, calculi formation

• Diet low in purines: organ meats (kidney, liver), dried beans, peas to maintain alkaline urine

• Nutritious diet with iron, vitamin supplements

Evaluate:

• Therapeutic response: decreased tumor size, spread of malignancy

Teach patient/family:

• To report any complaints or side effects to nurse or prescriber

• To report any changes in breathing or coughing

• That hair may be lost during treatment; a wig or hairpiece may make patient feel better; tell patient that new hair may be different in color, texture

• That metallic taste may occur

---

exemestane (℞)

(ex-em'eh-stane)
Aromasin
Func. class.: Antineoplastic
Chem. class.: Aromatase inhibitor

Action: Lowers serum estradiol concentrations; many breast cancers have strong estrogen receptors

Uses: Advanced breast carcinoma not responsive to other therapy (postmenopausal)

DOSAGE AND ROUTES

• *Adult:* **PO** 25 mg daily pc

Available forms: Tabs 25 mg

SIDE EFFECTS

CNS: Headache, depression, insomnia, anxiety, fatigue
CV: Hypertension
GI: Nausea, vomiting, diarrhea, constipation, abdominal pain, *hot flashes,* increased appetite
HEMA: Lymphopenia
RESP: Cough, *dyspnea*

Contraindications: Pregnancy (D), hypersensitivity, premenopausal women

Precautions: Lactation, children, elderly, hepatic disease, renal disease

INTERACTIONS

Decrease: exemestane action—CYP3A4 inducers, estrogens

PHARMACOKINETICS

Half-life 24 hr, excreted in feces, urine

NURSING CONSIDERATIONS

Assess:

• B/P, hypertension may occur

Perform/provide:

• Liquid diet, if needed, including cola, gelatin; dry toast or crackers may be added if patient is not nauseated or vomiting

• Nutritious diet with iron, vitamin supplements as ordered

Evaluate:

• Therapeutic response: decreased tumor size, spread of malignancy

Teach patient/family:

• To report any complaints, side effects to prescriber

• That hot flashes are reversible after discontinuing treatment

---

exenatide

See Appendix A—Selected New Drugs

---

ezetimibe (℞)
(ehz-eh-tim'bee)
Zetia
Func. class.: Antilipemic

Action: Inhibits absorption of cholesterol by the small intestine
Uses: Hypercholesterolemia, homozygous familial hypercholesterolemia (HoFH), homozygous sitosterolemia

DOSAGE AND ROUTES
• *Adult:* **PO** 10 mg daily; may be given with HMG-CoA reductase inhibitor at same time; may be given with bile acid sequestrant; give ezetimibe 2 hr before or 4 hr after the bile acid sequestrant
Available forms: Tabs 10 mg

SIDE EFFECTS
CNS: Fatigue, dizziness, headache
GI: Diarrhea, abdominal pain
MISC: Chest pain
MS: Myalgias, arthralgias, back pain
RESP: Pharyngitis, sinusitis, cough, URI
Contraindications: Hypersensitivity, severe hepatic disease
Precautions: Pregnancy (C), lactation, children, hepatic disease

PHARMACOKINETICS
Metabolized in small intestine, liver, excreted in feces 78%, urine 11%

INTERACTIONS
Increase: action of ezetimibe—fibric acid derivatives, cycloSPORINE
Decrease: action of ezetimibe—antacids, cholestyramine
Drug/Herb
Increase: effect—glucomannan
Decrease: effect—gotu kola

NURSING CONSIDERATIONS
Assess:
• Lipid levels, LFTs baseline and periodically during treatment
Administer:
• Without regard to meals

Evaluate:
• Therapeutic response: decreased cholesterol
Teach patient/family:
• That compliance is needed
• That risk factors should be decreased: high-fat diet, smoking, alcohol consumption, absence of exercise
• To notify prescriber if pregnancy is suspected or planned

⚠ High Alert

factor IX complex (human)/factor IV (℞)
Alpha-Nine SD, Benefix, Konyne 80, Mononine, Profilnine/Alpha Nine, Proplex SX-T, Proplex T
Func. class.: Hemostatic
Chem. class.: Factors II, VII, IX, X

Action: Causes an increase in blood levels of clotting factors II, VII, IX, X; factor IX (human) has IX activity
Uses: Hemophilia B (Christmas disease), factor IX deficiency, anticoagulant reversal, control of bleeding in patients with factor VIII inhibitors, reversal of overdose of anticoagulants in emergencies

DOSAGE AND ROUTES
Factor IX complex (human) bleeding in hemophilia B
• *Adult and child:* **IV** establish 25% of normal factor IX or 60-75 units/kg, then 10-20 units/kg/day 1-2 ×/wk
Prophylaxis for bleeding in hemophilia B
• *Adult and child:* **IV** 10-20 units/kg 1-2 ×/wk
Bleeding in hemophilia A/inhibitors of factor VIII (Proplex T, Konyne 80)
• *Adult and child:* **IV** 75 units/kg, repeat in 12 hr
Oral anticoagulant reversal
• *Adult and child:* **IV** 15 units/kg

Factor VII deficiency (use Proplex T only)
• *Adult and child:* IV 0.5 units/kg × weight (kg) × desired factor IX increase (% of normal); repeat q4-6h if needed
Factor IX (human) minor-moderate hemorrhage
Use only Alpha Nine, Alpha-Nine SD
• *Adult and child:* IV dose to increase factor IX level to 20%-30% in one dose
Serious hemorrhage
• *Adult and child:* IV dose to increase factor IX to 30%-50% as daily inf
Minor hemorrhage (mononine only)
• *Adult and child:* IV dose to increase factor IX to 15%-25% (20-30 units/kg), repeat in 24 hr if needed
Major hemorrhage
• *Adult and child:* IV dose to increase factor IX to 25%-50% (75 units/kg) q18-30h × 10 days or less
Available forms: Inj (number of units noted on label)

SIDE EFFECTS

CNS: Headache, dizziness, malaise, paresthesia, *lethargy, chills, fever, flushing*
CV: Hypotension, tachycardia, *MI, venous thrombosis, pulmonary embolism*
GI: Nausea, vomiting, abdominal cramps, jaundice, *viral hepatitis*
HEMA: Thrombosis, hemolysis, AIDS, DIC
INTEG: Rash, flushing, *urticaria*
RESP: Bronchospasm
Contraindications: Hypersensitivity to mouse/hamster protein, hepatic disease, DIC, elective surgery, mild factor IX deficiency
Precautions: Pregnancy (C), neonates/infants

PHARMACOKINETICS

IV: Half-life factor VII–3-6 hr, factor IX–24-36 hr; rapidly cleared from plasma

INTERACTIONS

Incompatible with protein products

⚠ Increase: thrombosis risk—aminocaproic acid; do not administer
Decrease: effect of warfarin

NURSING CONSIDERATIONS

Assess:
• Blood studies (coagulation factors assays by % normal: 5% prevents spontaneous hemorrhage, 30%-50% for surgery, 80%-100% for severe hemorrhage)
• Increased B/P, pulse
• For bleeding q15-30min, immobilize and apply ice to affected joints
• I&O; if urine becomes orange or red, notify prescriber
• Allergic or pyrogenic reaction: fever, chills, rash, itching, slow inf rate if not severe
⚠ DIC: bleeding, ecchymosis, hypersensitivity, changes in coagulation tests
Administer:
• Hepatitis B vaccine before administration
• IV after warming to room temperature 3 ml/min or less, with plastic syringe only; do not admix
• After dilution with provided diluent, 50 units/ml or 25 units/ml; do not exceed 10 ml/min; decrease rate if fever, headache, flushing, tingling occur
• After crossmatch if patient has blood type A, B, AB, to determine incompatibility with factor
Perform/provide:
• Storage of reconstituted sol for 3 hr at room temperature or up to 2 yr refrigeration (powder); check expiration date
Evaluate:
• Therapeutic response: prevention of hemorrhage
Teach patient/family:
• To report any signs of bleeding: gums, under skin, urine, stools, emesis
• The risk of viral hepatitis, AIDS; to be tested q2-3mo for HIV, even though risk is low
• That immunization for hepatitis B may be given first
• To carry emergency ID identifying disease; avoid salicylates, NSAIDs; inform other health professionals of condition

famciclovir (R)

(fam-cy´clo-veer)
Famvir
Func. class.: Antiviral
Chem. class.: Guanosine nucleoside

Action: Inhibits DNA polymerase and viral DNA synthesis by conversion of this guanosine nucleoside to penciclovir
Uses: Treatment of acute herpes zoster (shingles), genital herpes; recurrent mucocutaneous herpes simplex virus (HSV) in HIV patients
Investigational uses: Initial episodes of herpes genitalis

DOSAGE AND ROUTES

Herpes zoster
• *Adult:* **PO** 500 mg q8h for 7 days
Renal dose
• CCr ≥60 ml/min, 500 mg q8h; 40-59 ml/min, 500 mg q12h; 20-39 ml/min, 500 mg q24h
Recurrent mucocutaneous herpes simplex
• *Adult:* **PO** 500 mg q12h × 1 wk
Recurrent herpes simplex virus
• *Adult:* **PO** 125 mg q12h × 5 days
Suppression of recurrent herpes simplex virus
• *Adult:* **PO** 250 mg q12h up to 1 yr
Genital herpes (recurrent)
• *Adult:* **PO** 125 mg bid × 5 day; begin treatment at first sign of recurrence
Suppression of recurrent genital herpes
• *Adult:* **PO** 250 mg bid for up to a year
Herpes genitalis initial episodes (off-label)
• *Adult:* **PO** 25 mg tid × 7-10 days
Available forms: Tabs 125, 250, 500 mg

SIDE EFFECTS

CNS: Headache, fatigue, dizziness, paresthesia, somnolence, fever
GI: Nausea, vomiting, diarrhea, constipation, abdominal pain, anorexia
GU: Decreased sperm count
INTEG: Pruritus
MS: Back pain, arthralgia
RESP: Pharyngitis, sinusitis
Contraindications: Hypersensitivity to this drug, penciclovir
Precautions: Pregnancy (B), renal disease, hypersensitivity to acyclovir, ganciclovir, lactation

PHARMACOKINETICS

Unknown

INTERACTIONS

Decrease: renal excretion—theophylline, probenecid, digoxin
Decrease: metabolism—cimetidine

NURSING CONSIDERATIONS

Assess:
• For number, distribution of lesions; burning, itching, pain, which are early symptoms of herpes infection
• Renal studies: urine CCr, BUN before and during treatment if decreased renal function; dose may have to be lowered
• Bowel pattern before, during treatment; diarrhea may occur
• Posttherapeutic neuralgia during and after treatment
Administer:
• With or without meals; absorption does not appear to be lowered when taken with food
• Within 72 hr of the appearance of rash in herpes zoster
Evaluate:
• Therapeutic response: decreased size, spread of lesions
Teach patient/family:
• How to recognize beginning infection
• How to prevent spread of infection; that this medication does not prevent the spread to others, that condoms should be used
• The reason for medication, expected results
• That women with genital herpes should have yearly Pap smears, cervical cancer is more likely

famotidine (OTC, ℞)

(fa-moe′ti-deen)

Mylanta AR, Pepcid, Pepcid AC, Pepcid IV, Pepcid RPD ✿

Func. class.: H₂-histamine receptor antagonist

Action: Competitively inhibits histamine at histamine H₂-receptor site, decreasing gastric secretion while pepsin remains at a stable level

Uses: Short-term treatment of active duodenal ulcer, maintenance therapy for duodenal ulcer, Zollinger-Ellison syndrome, multiple endocrine adenomas, gastric ulcers; gastroesophageal reflux disease, heartburn

Investigational uses: GI disorders in those taking NSAIDs; urticaria; prevention of stress ulcers, aspiration pneumonitis, inactivation of oral pancreatic enzymes in pancreatic disorders, prevention of paclitaxel hypersensitivity reactions

DOSAGE AND ROUTES

Active ulcer

• *Adult:* **PO** 40 mg daily at bedtime × 4-8 wk, then 20 mg daily at bedtime if needed (maintenance); **IV** 20 mg q12h if unable to take **PO**

• *Child 1-16 yr:* 0.5 mg/kg/day at bedtime or divided bid, max 40 mg daily

Hypersecretory conditions

• *Adult:* **PO** 20 mg q6h; may give 160 mg q6h if needed; **IV** 20 mg q12h if unable to take **PO**

• *Child* 1-16 yr: 1 mg/kg/day divide bid, max 40 mg bid

Heartburn relief/prevention

• *Adult:* **PO** 10 mg with water or 1 hr before eating

Paclitaxel hypersensitivity reactions

• *Adult:* **IV** 20 mg ½ hr prior to infusion

Renal disease

• CCr <10 ml/min 20 mg at bedtime or dose q36-48h

Available forms: Tabs 10, 20, 40 mg; powder for oral susp 40 mg/5 ml; inj 10

mg/ml, 20 mg/50 ml 0.9% NaCl; orally disintegrating tabs (RPD) 20, 40 mg; chew tabs 10 mg

SIDE EFFECTS

CNS: Headache, dizziness, paresthesia, depression, anxiety, somnolence, insomnia, fever

CV: Dysrhythmias

EENT: Taste change, tinnitus, orbital edema

GI: Constipation, nausea, vomiting, anorexia, cramps, abnormal hepatic enzymes, diarrhea

HEMA: Thrombocytopenia, aplastic anemia

INTEG: Rash

MS: Myalgia, arthralgia

Contraindications: Hypersensitivity

Precautions: Pregnancy (B), lactation, children <12 yr, severe renal disease, severe hepatic disease, elderly

PHARMACOKINETICS

Absorption 50% (PO)

PO: Onset 30-60 min, duration 6-12 hr, peak 1-3 hr

IV: Onset immediate, peak 30-60 min, duration 8-15 hr, plasma protein-binding 15%-20%; metabolized in liver 30% (active metabolites), 70% excreted by kidneys, half-life 2½-3½ hr

INTERACTIONS

Decrease: absorption—ketoconazole

Decrease: famotidine absorption—antacids

NURSING CONSIDERATIONS

Assess:

• For epigastric pain, adominal pain, frank or occult blood in emesis, stools

• Blood counts during therapy; watch for decreasing platelets; if low, therapy may have to be discontinued and restarted after hematologic recovery

• For bleeding, hematuria, hematuresis, occult blood in stools; abdominal pain

• Blood dyscrasias (thrombocytopenia): bruising, fatigue, bleeding, poor healing
Administer:
• Antacids 1 hr before or 2 hr after famotidine; may be given with foods or liquids
• After shaking oral suspension
IV, direct route
• After diluting 2 ml of drug (10 mg/ml) in 0.9% NaCl to total volume of 5-10 ml; inject over 2 min to prevent hypotension
IV Intermittent INF route
• After diluting 20 mg (2 ml) of drug in 100 ml of LR, 0.9% NaCl, D_5W, $D_{10}W$; run over 15-30 min
Additive compatibilities: Cefazolin, cefmetazole, flumazenil, vancomycin
Y-site compatibilities: Acyclovir, allopurinol, amifostine, aminophylline, amphotericin, ampicillin, ampicillin/sulbactam, amrinone, amsacrine, atropine, aztreonam, bretylium, calcium gluconate, cefazolin, cefoperazone, cefotaxime, cefotetan, cefoxitin, ceftazidime, ceftizoxime, ceftriaxone, cefuroxime, cephalothin, cephapirin, chlorproMAZINE, cisatracurium, cisplatin, cladribine, cyclophosphamide, cytarabine, dexamethasone, dextran 40, digoxin, diphenhydrAMINE, DOBUTamine, DOPamine, DOXOrubicin, DOXOrubicin liposome, droperidol, enalaprilat, epINEPHrine, erythromycin, esmolol, filgrastim, fluconazole, fludarabine, folic acid, gentamicin, granisetron, haloperidol, heparin, hydrocortisone, hydromorphone, hydrOXYzine, imipenem/cilastatin, insulin (regular), isoproterenol, labetalol, lidocaine, lorazepam, magnesium sulfate, melphalan, meperidine, methotrexate, methylPREDNISolone, metoclopramide, mezlocillin, midazolam, morphine, nafcillin, nitroglycerin, nitroprusside, norepinephrine, ondansetron, oxacillin, paclitaxel, perphenazine, phenylephrine, phenytoin, phytonadione, piperacillin, potassium chloride/phosphate, procainamide, propofol, remifentanil, sargramostim, sodium bicarbonate, teniposide, theophylline, thiamine, thiotepa, ticarcillin, ticarcillin/clavulanate, verapamil, vinorelbine
Perform/provide:
• Storage in cool environment (oral); IV sol is stable for 48 hr at room temperature; do not use discolored sol; discard unused oral sol after 1 mo
• To increase bulk and fluids in the diet to prevent constipation
Evaluate:
• Therapeutic response: decreased abdominal pain
Teach patient/family:
• That drug must be continued for prescribed time in prescribed method to be effective; do not double dose
• To report bleeding, bruising, fatigue, malaise, since blood dyscrasias occur
• About possibility of decreased libido, reversible after discontinuing therapy
• To avoid irritating foods, alcohol, aspirin, and extreme temperature of foods that may irritate GI system
• That smoking should be avoided; diminishes effectiveness of drug
• To avoid tasks requiring alertness; dizziness, drowsiness may occur

---

fat emulsions (℞)

Intralipid 10%, Intralipid 20%, Liposyn II 10%, Liposyn II 20%, Liposyn III 10%, Liposyn III 20%, Soyacal 20%
Func. class.: Caloric
Chem. class.: Fatty acid, long chain

Action: Needed for energy, heat production; consist of neutral triglycerides, primarily unsaturated fatty acids
Uses: Increase calorie intake, fatty acid deficiency, prevention

DOSAGE AND ROUTES
Deficiency
• *Adult and child:* **IV** 8%-10% of required calorie intake (intralipid)
Adjunct to TPN
• *Adult:* **IV** 1 ml/min over 15-30 min (10%) or 0.5 ml/min over 15-30 min

(20%); may increase to 500 ml over 4-8 hr if no adverse reactions occur; not to exceed 2.5 g/kg

• *Child:* **IV** 0.1 ml/min over 10-15 min (10%) or 0.05 ml/min over 10-15 min (20%); may increase to 1 g/kg over 4 hr if no adverse reactions occur; not to exceed 4 g/kg

Prevention of deficiency

• *Adult:* **IV** 500 ml 2 ×/wk (10%), given 1 ml/min for 30 min, not to exceed 500 ml over 6 hr

• *Child:* **IV** 5-10 ml/kg/day (10%), given 0.1 ml/min for 30 min, not to exceed 100 ml/hr

Available forms: Inj 10% (50, 100, 200, 250, 500 ml), 20% (50, 100, 200, 250, 500 ml)

SIDE EFFECTS

CNS: Dizziness, headache, drowsiness, *focal seizures*
CV: Shock
GI: Nausea, vomiting, *hepatomegaly*
HEMA: Hyperlipemia, hypercoagulation, thrombocytopenia, leukopenia, leukocytosis
RESP: Dyspnea, *fat in lung tissue*
Contraindications: Hypersensitivity, hyperlipemia, lipid necrosis, acute pancreatitis accompanied by hyperlipemia, hyperbilirubinemia of the newborn
Precautions: Pregnancy (C), severe hepatic disease, diabetes mellitus, thrombocytopenia, gastric ulcers, premature/term newborns, sepsis

NURSING CONSIDERATIONS

Assess:

• Triglycerides, free fatty acid levels, platelet counts daily to prevent fat overload, thrombocytopenia

• Hepatic studies: AST, ALT, Hct, Hgb; notify prescriber if abnormal

• Nutritional status: calorie count by dietitian; monitor weight daily

Administer:

IV Intermittent INF route

• At 10% (1 ml/min); 20% (0.5 ml/min) initially × 15-30 min, may increase 10% (120 ml/hr); 20% (62.5 ml/hr) if no

adverse reaction; do not give more than 500 ml on first day

• After changing IV tubing at each infusion: infection may occur with old tubing

• With inf pump at prescribed rate; do not use in-line filter sized for lipid emulsion; clogging will occur

Additive compatibilities: Cefamandole, chloramphenicol, cimetidine, cycloSPORINE, diphenhydrAMINE, famotidine, heparin, hydrocortisone, multivitamins, nizatidine, penicillin G potassium

Y-site compatibilities: Ampicillin, cefamandole, cefazolin, cefoxitin, cephapirin, clindamycin, digoxin, DOPamine, erythromycin, furosemide, gentamicin, IL-2, isoproterenol, kanamycin, lidocaine, norepinephrine, oxacillin, penicillin G potassium, ticarcillin, tobramycin

Perform/provide:

• Do not use mixed sol if separated or oily looking

Evaluate:

• Therapeutic response: increased weight

Teach patient/family:

• The reason for use of lipids

Rarely Used

felbamate (℞)
(fell′ba-mate)
Felbatol
Func. class.: Anticonvulsant

Uses: Partial seizures, with or without generalization in adults; partial and generalized seizures in children with Lennox-Gastaut syndrome

DOSAGE AND ROUTES

Adjunctive therapy

• *Adult or child >14 yr:* **PO** add 1.2 g/day in 3-4 divided doses; reduce other anticonvulsants (valproic acid, phenytoin, carbamazepine and derivatives) by 20% to control plasma concentrations; may increase felbamate 1.2 g/day increments qwk, up to 3.6 g/day

Monotherapy
• *Adult:* **PO** 1.2 g/day in 3-4 divided doses; titrate with close supervision; increase dose by 600-mg increments q2wk to 3.6 g/day if needed
Lennox-Gastaut syndrome adjunctive therapy
• *Child 2-14 yr:* **PO** add 15 mg/kg/day in 3-4 divided doses; reduce other anticonvulsants (valproic acid, phenytoin, carbamazepine and derivatives) by 20% to control plasma concentrations; may increase felbamate 15 mg/kg/day qwk up to 45 mg/day

Contraindications: Hypersensitivity to this drug, other carbamates, history of blood dyscrasia, aplastic anemia, hepatic disease

---

felodipine (℞)

(fe-loe′-di-peen)
Plendil, Renedil ✦
Func. class.: Antihypertensive, calcium channel blocker, antianginal
Chem. class.: Dihydropyridine

Do not confuse:
Plendil/pindolol/Pletal/Prilosec
Plendil/Prinivil
Action: Inhibits calcium ion influx across cell membrane, resulting in inhibition of excitation/contraction
Uses: Essential hypertension, alone or with other antihypertensives, angina pectoris, Prinzmetal's angina (vasospastic)

DOSAGE AND ROUTES
• *Adult:* **PO** 5 mg daily initially, usual range 5-10 mg daily; max 10 mg daily; do not adjust dosage at intervals of <2 wk
• *Geriatric:* **PO** 2.5 mg daily
Hepatic disease
• **PO** 2.5-5 mg, max 10 mg/day
Available forms: Ext rel tabs 2.5, 5, 10 mg

SIDE EFFECTS
CNS: Headache, fatigue, drowsiness, dizziness, anxiety, depression, nervousness, insomnia, light-headedness, paresthesia, tinnitus, psychosis, somnolence
CV: ***Dysrhythmia,*** edema, ***CHF,*** hypotension, palpitations, ***MI, pulmonary edema,*** tachycardia, syncope, AV block, angina
GI: Nausea, vomiting, diarrhea, gastric upset, constipation, increased LFTs, dry mouth
GU: Nocturia, polyuria
HEMA: Anemia
INTEG: Rash, pruritus
MISC: Flushing, sexual difficulties, cough, nasal congestion, shortness of breath, wheezing, epistaxis, respiratory infection, chest pain, ***Stevens-Johnson syndrome,*** gingival hyperplasia
Contraindications: Hypersensitivity, sick sinus syndrome, 2nd- or 3rd-degree heart block, hypotension <90 mm Hg systolic
Precautions: Pregnancy (C), CHF, hepatic injury, lactation, children, renal disease, elderly

PHARMACOKINETICS

Peak plasma levels 2.5-5 hr; highly protein bound, >99% metabolized in liver, 0.5% excreted unchanged in urine; elimination half-life 11-16 hr

INTERACTIONS

Bradycardia, CHF: β-blockers, digoxin, phenytoin, disopyramide
Increase: toxicity—ketoconazole, erythromycin, itraconazole, propranolol
Increase: hypotension—fentanyl, nitrates, alcohol, quinidine
Decrease: antihypertensive effects—NSAIDs
Drug/Herb
Increase: toxicity, death—aconite
Increase: antihypertensive effect—barberry, betony, black catechu, black cohosh, bloodroot, broom, burdock, cat's claw, dandelion, goldenseal, Irish moss, Jamaican dogwood, kelp, khella, mistletoe, parsley
Increase or decrease: antihypertensive effect—astragalus, cola tree

---

Side effects: *italics* = common; ***bold italics*** = life-threatening

Decrease: antihypertensive effect—coltsfoot, guarana, khat, licorice

Drug/Food

Increase: felodipine level—grapefruit juice

NURSING CONSIDERATIONS

Assess:

• I&O, weight daily; for CHF: weight gain, crackles, dyspnea, edema, jugular venous distention

• Renal, hepatic studies

• Cardiac status: B/P, pulse, respiration; ECG periodically

• For angina pain: location, duration, intensity; ameliorating, aggravating factors

Administer:

• Swallow whole; do not break, crush, or chew sus rel products

• Once daily without regard to meals

Evaluate:

• Therapeutic response: decreased B/P, decreased anginal attacks, increase in activity tolerance

Teach patient/family:

• To avoid hazardous activities until stabilized on drug, dizziness is no longer a problem

• To avoid OTC drugs, alcohol, unless directed by a prescriber, to limit caffeine consumption

• The importance of complying with all areas of medical regimen: diet, exercise, stress reduction, drug therapy

• That tablets may appear in stools, but are insignificant

• To report dyspnea, palpitations, irregular heart beat, swelling of extremities, nausea, vomiting, severe dizziness, severe headache

• To change positions slowly to prevent orthostatic hypotension

• To obtain correct pulse, to contact prescriber if pulse is <50 bpm

• To use protective clothing, sunscreen to prevent photosensitivity

Treatment of overdose: Atropine for AV block, vasopressor for hypotension

---

fenofibrate (R)
(fen-oh-fee′brate)
Tricor
Func. class.: Antilipemic
Chem. class.: Fibric acid derivative

Action: Increases lipolysis and elimination of triglyceride rich particles from plasma by activating lipoprotein lipase, resulting in triglyceride change in size and composition of LDL leading to rapid breakdown of LDL; mobilizes triglycerides from tissue; increases excretion of neutral sterols

Uses: Hypercholesterolemia, types IV, V hyperlipidemia that do not respond to other treatment and are at risk for pancreatitis, Fredrickson type IIa, IIb, hypertriglyceridemia

Investigational uses: Polymetabolic syndrome X

DOSAGE AND ROUTES

Hypertriglyceridemia

• *Adult:* PO 54-160 mg/day, may increase q4-8wk, max 160 mg/day

Primary hypercholesterolemia/ mixed hyperlipidemia

• *Adult:* PO 160 mg/day

Renal dose

• *Adult:* PO 54 mg/day (CCr <50 ml/min)

Available forms: Tabs 54, 160 mg

SIDE EFFECTS

CNS: Fatigue, weakness, drowsiness, dizziness, insomnia, depression, vertigo

CV: Angina, ***dysrhythmias,*** hypertension

GI: Nausea, vomiting, dyspepsia, increased liver enzymes, flatulence, hepatomegaly, gastritis

GU: Dysuria, proteinuria, oliguria, urinary frequency

HEMA: Anemia, leukopenia, ecchymosis

INTEG: Rash, urticaria, pruritus

MISC: Polyphagia, weight gain

MS: Myalgias, arthralgias, myopathy

RESP: Pharyngitis, bronchitis, cough

Contraindications: Hypertensivity, severe hepatic disease, severe renal disease, primary biliary cirrhosis, preexisting gallbladder disease

Precautions: Pregnancy (C), peptic ulcer, lactation, pancreatitis, renal, hepatic disease, elderly

PHARMACOKINETICS

Peak 6-8 hr; protein binding 99%, converted to fenofibric acid, metabolized in liver, excreted in urine (60%), half-life 20 hr

INTERACTIONS

Nephrotoxicity: cycloSPORINE

Avoid use with HMG-CoA reductase inhibitors, rhabdomyolysis may occur

Increase: anticoagulant effects—oral anticoagulants

Decrease: absorption of fenofibrate—bile acid sequestrants

Drug/Herb

Increase: effect—glucomannan

Decrease: effect—gotu kola

Drug/Food

Increase: absorption

NURSING CONSIDERATIONS

Assess:
• Lipid levels, LFTs baseline and periodically during treatment, CPK if muscle pain occurs, CBC, Hct, Hgb; PT with anticoagulant therapy
• Pancreatitis, cholelithiasis renal failure, rhabdomyolyis (when combined with HMG Co-A reductase inhibitors), myositis, drug should be discontinued

Administer:
• Drug with meals; may increase q4-8wk

Evaluate:
• Therapeutic response: decreased triglycerides

Teach patient/family:
• That compliance is needed
• That risk factors should be decreased: high-fat diet, smoking, alcohol consumption, absence of exercise
• To notify prescriber if pregnancy is suspected or planned

• To report GU symptoms: decreased libido, impotence, dysuria, proteinuria, oliguria, hematuria
• To notify prescriber of muscle pain, weakness, fever, fatigue; epigastric pain

---

fenoldopam (℞)
(feh-nahl'doh-pam)
Corlopam
Func. class.: Antihypertensive, vasodilator

Action: Agonist at D_1-like dopamine receptors; binds to α_2-adrenoceptors; increases renal blood flow

Uses: Hypertensive crisis, malignant hypertension

DOSAGE AND ROUTES

• *Adult:* **IV** 0.01-1.6 mcg/kg/min

Available forms: Inj conc 10 mg/ml in single-use ampules

SIDE EFFECTS

CNS: Headache, anxiety, dizziness

CV: **Hypotension,** ST-T-wave changes, angina pectoris, palpitations, **MI, ischemic heart disease, flushing**

GI: Nausea, vomiting, constipation, diarrhea

HEMA: **Leukocytosis,** bleeding

META: Increased BUN, glucose, LDH, creatinine, hypokalemia

Contraindications: Hypersensitivity, sulfite sensitivity

Precautions: Pregnancy (B), tachycardia, lactation, children, intraocular pressure, hypokalemia

PHARMACOKINETICS

Elimination half-life 5 min, steady state 20 min

INTERACTIONS

Increase: hypotension—avoid use with β-blockers

Drug/Herb

Increase: toxicity, death—aconite

Increase: antihypertensive effect—barberry, betony, black catechu, black cohosh, bloodroot, broom, burdock, cat's claw, dandelion, goldenseal, Irish moss, Jamaican dogwood, kelp, khella, mistletoe, parsley

Increase or decrease antihypertensive effect—astragalus, cola tree

Decrease: antihypertensive effect—coltsfoot, guarana, khat, licorice

NURSING CONSIDERATIONS

Assess:

• B/P q5min until stabilized, then q1h × 2 hr, then q4h; pulse, jugular venous distention q4h

• Electrolytes, blood studies: K, Na, Cl, CO_2, CBC, serum glucose

• Skin turgor, dryness of mucous membranes for hydration status

• IV site for extravasation, rate

Administer:

• After diluting contents of ampules in 0.9% NaCl, or 5% dextrose inj (40 mcg/ml); then add 4 ml of conc (40 mg of drug/1000 ml); 2 ml of conc (20 mg of drug/500 ml); 1 ml of conc (10 mg of drug/250 ml); do not admix

• To patient in recumbent position; keep in that position for 1 hr after administration

Perform/provide:

• Diluted sol is stable in normal light/temperature for 24 hr

Evaluate:

• Therapeutic response: decreased B/P

Teach patient/family:

• To report dyspnea, chest pain, bleeding

• Reason for medication and expected results

Rarely Used

fenoprofen (Ŗ)

(fen-oh-proe'fen)

Fenoprofen, Nalfon

Func. class.: Nonsteroidal antiinflammatory/nonopioid analgesic

Uses: Mild to moderate pain, osteoarthritis, rheumatoid arthritis, acute gout, arthritis, inflammation

DOSAGE AND ROUTES

Pain

• *Adult:* **PO** 200 mg q4-6h prn

Arthritis

• *Adult:* **PO** 300-600 mg qid, not to exceed 3.2 g/day

Contraindications: Hypersensitivity, asthma, severe renal disease, severe hepatic disease

⚠ High Alert

fentanyl (Ŗ)

(fen'ta-nill)

Actiq, Fentanyl, Fentanyl Oralet, Sublimaze

Func. class.: Opioid analgesic

Chem. class.: Synthetic phenylpiperidine

Controlled Substance Schedule II

Do not confuse:

fentanyl/Sufenta

Action: Inhibits ascending pain pathways in CNS, increases pain threshold, alters pain perception by binding to opiate receptors

Uses: Preoperatively, postoperatively; adjunct to general anesthetic, adjunct to regional anesthesia; Fentanyl Oralet—anesthesia as premedication, conscious sedation; Actiq—breakthrough cancer pain

DOSAGE AND ROUTES

Anesthetic

• *Adult:* **IV** 25-100 mcg (0.7-2 mcg/kg) q2-3 min prn

Anesthesia supplement
• *Adult:* IV 2-20 mcg/kg IV INF 0.025-0.25 mcg/kg/min
Induction and maintenance
• *Adult:* IV BOL 5-40 mcg/kg
• *Child 2-12 yr:* IV 2-3 mcg/kg
Preoperatively
• *Adult:* IM 0.05-0.1 mg q30-60min before surgery
Postoperatively
• *Adult:* IM 0.05-0.1 mg q1-2h prn
Fentanyl Oralet
• *Adult:* Transmucosal 5 mcg/kg = fentanyl IM 0.75-1.25 mcg/kg, do not exceed 5 mcg/kg
• *Child:* Transmucosal may need doses of 5-15 mcg/kg; must be watched continuously for hypoventilation
Actiq
• *Adult:* Transmucosal 200 mcg, redose if needed 15 min after completion of 1st dose, do not give more than 2 doses during titration period
Available forms: Inj 0.05 mg/ml; lozenges 100, 200, 300, 400 mcg; lozenges on a stick 200, 400, 600, 800, 1200, 1600 mcg

SIDE EFFECTS

CNS: Dizziness, delirium, euphoria
CV: **Bradycardia, arrest,** hypotension or hypertension
EENT: Blurred vision, miosis
GI: Nausea, vomiting
GU: Urinary retention
INTEG: Rash, diaphoresis
MS: Muscle rigidity
RESP: **Respiratory depression, arrest, laryngospasm**
Contraindications: Hypersensitivity to opiates, myasthenia gravis
Precautions: Pregnancy (C), elderly, respiratory depression, increased intracranial pressure, seizure disorders, severe respiratory disorders, cardiac dysrhythmias, lactation

PHARMACOKINETICS

IM: Onset 7-8 min, peak 30 min, duration 1-2 hr
IV: Onset 1 min, peak 3-5 min, duration ½-1 hr; metabolized by liver; excreted by kidneys; crosses placenta; excreted in breast milk; half-life 1½-6 hr; 80% bound to plasma proteins

INTERACTIONS

Increase: with other CNS depressants—alcohol, opioids, sedative/hypnotics, antipsychotics, skeletal muscle relaxants
Drug/Herb
Increase: anticholinergic effect—corkwood
Increase: action—Jamaican dogwood, kava, lavender, mistletoe, nettle, pokeweed, poppy, senega, valerian

NURSING CONSIDERATIONS
Assess:
• VS after parenteral route; note muscle rigidity, drug history, hepatic and renal function tests
• CNS changes: dizziness, drowsiness, hallucinations, euphoria, LOC, pupil reaction
• Allergic reactions: rash, urticaria
• Respiratory dysfunction: respiratory depression, character, rate, rhythm; notify prescriber if respirations are <10/min
Administer:
• By inj (IM, IV); give slowly to prevent rigidity
• Only with resuscitative equipment available
Transmucosal
• Remove foil just before administration, instruct patient to place under tongue and suck, not chew (Oralet); place between cheek and lower gum, moving it back and forth and suck, not chew (Actiq); all products not used or partially used should be flushed down the toilet
IV route
• IV undiluted by anesthesiologist or diluted with 5 ml or more sterile H_2O or 0.9% NaCl given through Y-tube or 3-way stopcock at 0.1 mg or less/1-2 min
Additive compatibilities: Bupivacaine

Solution compatibilities: D_5W, 0.9% NaCl

Syrine compatibilities: Atracurium, atropine, bupivacaine/ketamine, butorphanol, chlorproMAZINE, cimetidine, clonidine/lidocaine, diphenhyDRINATE, diphenhydrAMINE, droperidol, heparin, hydromorphone, hydrOXYzine, meperidine, metoclopramide, midazolam, morphine, pentazocine, perphenazine, prochlorperazine, promazine, promethazine, ranitidine, scopolamine

Y-site compatibilities: Amphotericin B cholesteryl, atracurium, cisatracurium, diltiazem, DOBUTamine, DOPamine, enalaprilat, epINEPHrine, esmolol, etomidate, furosemide, heparin, hydrocortisone, hydromorphone, labetalol, lorazepam, midazolam, milrinone, morphine, nafcillin, niCARdipine, nitroglycerin, norepinephrine, pancuronium, potassium chloride, propofol, ranitidine, remifentanil, sargramostim, thiopental, vecuronium, vit B/C

Perform/provide:
• Storage in light-resistant area at room temperature

Teach patient/family:
• Coughing, turning, deep breathing for postoperative patients
• Safety measures: side rails, night-light, call bell within reach

Evaluate:
• Therapeutic response: induction of anesthesia, breakthrough cancer pain

---

⚠ High Alert

fentanyl transdermal (℞)

Duragesic
Func. class.: Opioid analgesic
Chem. class.: Synthetic phenylpiperidine

Controlled Substance Schedule II
Action: Inhibits ascending pain pathways in CNS, increases pain threshold, alters pain perception by binding to opiate receptors

Uses: Management of chronic pain for those requiring opioid analgesia

DOSAGE AND ROUTES

• *Adult:* 25 mcg/hr; may increase until pain relief occurs; apply patch to flat surface on upper torso and wear for 72 hr; apply new patch on different site for continued relief
Available forms: Patch 12, 25, 50, 75, 100 mcg/hr

SIDE EFFECTS

CNS: Dizziness, delirium, euphoria, lightheadedness, sedation, dysphoria, agitation, anxiety, confusion, headache, depression
CV: Bradycardia, ***cardiac arrest,*** hypotension or hypertension, facial flushing, chills, chest pain, dysrhythmias
EENT: Blurred vision, miosis
GI: Nausea, vomiting, diarrhea, cramps, anorexia, constipation, dyspepsia
GU: Urinary retention, urgency, dysuria, frequency, oliguria
INTEG: Sweating, pruritus, rash, erythema, papules
MS: Asthenia
RESP: ***Respiratory depression, laryngospasm, bronchospasm,*** depresses cough, hypoventilation, dyspnea, hiccups, apnea
Contraindications: Hypersensitivity to opiates, myasthenia gravis, children <12 yr, patient <18 yr with weight <110 lb
Precautions: Pregnancy (C), elderly, respiratory depression, increased intracranial pressure, seizure disorders, severe respiratory disorders, cardiac dysrhythmias, fever

INTERACTIONS

Increase: with other CNS depressants—alcohol, opioids, sedative/hypnotics, antipsychotics, skeletal muscle relaxants
Drug/Herb
Increase: anticholinergic effect—corkwood

⚠ Safety alert   *"Tall Man" lettering

Increase: action—Jamaican dogwood, kava, lavender, mistletoe, nettle, pokeweed, poppy, senega, valerian

Drug/Lab Test
Increase: Amylase, lipase

NURSING CONSIDERATIONS

Assess:
• Pain control; check for duration, site, character of pain, fever; use pain and sedation scoring
• CNS changes: dizziness, drowsiness, hallucinations, euphoria, LOC, pupil reaction
• Allergic reactions: rash, urticaria
• Respiratory dysfunction: respiratory depression, character, rate, rhythm; notify prescriber if respirations are <10/min

Administer:
• q72h for continuous pain relief; dosage is adjusted after at least two applications, apply to clean, dry skin, press firmly
• Give short-acting analgesics until patch takes effect (8-12 hr); when reducing dosage or switching to alternate IV treatment, withdraw gradually; serum levels drop gradually, give ½ the equianalgesic dose of new analgesic 12-18 hr after removal as ordered

Perform/provide:
• Safety measures: side rails, night-light, call bell within reach

Evaluate:
• Therapeutic response: decreased pain

Teach patient/family:
• To avoid activities that require alertness
• That excessive heat may increase absorption
• That excessive perspiration may alter adhesiveness
• To dispose of patch by placing sticky sides together and flushing in toilet
• That patient may need to clip hair before applying to ensure adhesion

---

ferrous fumarate (Ⓡ)
Femiron, Feostat, Feostat Drops, Hemocyte, Ircon, Nephro-Fer, Novofumar ✤, Palafer ✤, Span-FF

ferrous gluconate (Ⓡ)
Fergon, Fertinic ✤, Novoferrogluc ✤

ferrous sulfate (Ⓡ)
Apo-Ferrous Sulfate ✤, ED-IN-SOL, Feosol, Fer-gen-sol, Fer-Iron Drops, Fero-Grad, Mol-Iron

ferrous sulfate, dried (Ⓡ)
Fe⁵⁰, Feosol, Feratab, Novoferrosulfa ✤, PMS-Ferrous Sulfate, Slow Fe

ferric gluconate complex (Ⓡ)
Ferrlecit

carbonyl iron
(kar′bo-nil)
Feosol

iron polysaccharide
Hytinic, Niferex, Nu-Iron, Nu-Iron 150
Func. class.: Hematinic
Chem. class.: Iron preparation

Action: Replaces iron stores needed for red blood cell development, energy and O_2 transport, utilization; fumarate contains 33% elemental iron; gluconate, 12%; sulfate, 20%; iron, 30%; ferrous sulfate exsiccated

Uses: Iron deficiency anemia, prophylaxis for iron deficiency in pregnancy

DOSAGE AND ROUTES

Fumarate
• *Adult:* **PO** 200 mg daily-qid
• *Child 2-12 yr:* **PO** 3 mg/kg/day (elemental iron) tid-qid
• *Child 6 mo-2 yr:* **PO** up to 6 mg/kg/day (elemental iron) tid-qid
• *Infant:* **PO** 10-25 mg/day (elemental

---

iron) in 3-4 divided doses, max 15 mg/day

Gluconate
- *Adult:* **PO** 200-600 mg daily-tid
- *Child 6-12 yr:* **PO** 300-900 mg daily
- *Child <6 yr:* **PO** 100-300 mg daily

Sulfate
- *Adult:* **PO** 0.75-1.5 g/day in divided doses tid
- *Child 6-12 yr:* **PO** 600 mg/day in divided doses

Pregnancy
- *Adult:* **PO** 300-600 mg/day in divided doses

Complex
- *Adult:* **IV INF** (125 mg) 10 ml/100 ml of NaCl for inj given over 1 hr

Iron polysaccharide
- *Adult:* **PO** 100-200 mg tid
- *Child:* **PO** 4-6 mg/kg/day in 3 divided doses

Available forms:

Fumarate
Tabs 63, 195, 200, 324, 325 mg; tabs chewable 100 mg; tabs cont rel 300 mg; oral susp 100 mg/5 ml, 45 mg/0.6 ml

Gluconate
Tabs 300, 320, 325 mg; caps 86, 325, 435 mg; tabs film-coated 300 mg; elix 300 mg/5 ml

Sulfate
Tabs, 195, 300, 325 mg; tabs enteric-coated 325 mg; tabs ext rel, time-rel caps, 525 mg

Dried
Tabs, 200 mg; tabs ext rel 160 mg; caplets ext rel 160 mg

Complex
Inj. 62.5 mg/5 ml (12.5 mg/ml)

Iron polysaccharide
Tabs 50 mg, caps 150 mg, sol 100 mg/5 ml

SIDE EFFECTS

GI: Nausea, constipation, epigastric pain, black and red tarry stools, vomiting, diarrhea
INTEG: Temporarily discolored tooth enamel and eyes
Contraindications: Hypersensitivity, ulcerative colitis/regional enteritis, hemo-

siderosis/hemochromatosis, peptic ulcer disease, hemolytic anemia, cirrhosis
Precautions: Pregnancy (B) (ferric gluconate complex), (C) (iron dextran, oral products), anemia (long-term)

PHARMACOKINETICS

PO: Excreted in feces, urine, skin, breast milk; enters bloodstream; bound to transferrin; crosses placenta

INTERACTIONS

Increase: action of iron preparation—ascorbic acid, chloramphenicol
Decrease: absorption of penicillamine, levodopa, methyldopa, fluoroquinolones, L-thyroxine, tetracycline
Decrease: absorption of iron preparations—antacids, H$_2$-antagonists, proton pump inhibitors, cholestyramine, vit E

Drug/Herb
Forms insoluble complex: black catechu
Increase: iron effect—anise
Decrease: iron absorption—allspice, bilberry, condurango, elderberry, eyebright (PO), gentian, ground ivy, hawthorn, horse chestnut, lady mantle, lemon balm, marshmallow, meadowsweet, mistletoe, motherwort, nettle, oak bark, plantain, poplar, prickly ash, raspberry, sage, tea made with artichoke, valerian

Drug/Food
Decrease: absorption—dairy products, caffeine, eggs

Drug/Lab Test
False positive: Occult blood

NURSING CONSIDERATIONS

Assess:
- Blood studies: Hct, Hgb, reticulocytes, bilirubin before treatment, at least monthly; iron studies (Fe, TIBC, ferritin)
- ⚠ Toxicity: nausea, vomiting, diarrhea (green, then tarry stools), hematemesis, pallor, cyanosis, shock, coma
- Elimination; if constipation occurs, increase water, bulk, activity

---

⚠ Safety alert   *"Tall Man" lettering

• Nutrition: amount of iron in diet (meat, dark green leafy vegetables, dried beans, dried fruits, eggs)
• Cause of iron loss or anemia, including salicylates, sulfonamides, antimalarials, quinidine

Administer:
• Swallow tabs whole; not to break, crush, or chew unless labeled as chewable
• Between meals for best absorption; may give with juice; do not give with antacids or milk, delay at least 1 hr; if GI symptoms occur, give pc even if absorption is decreased; eggs, milk products, chocolate, caffeine interfere with absorption
• Liquid through plastic straw to avoid discoloration of tooth enamel; dilute thoroughly
• At least 1 hr before bedtime, since corrosion may occur in stomach; ferrous gluconate is less GI irritating than ferrous sulfate
• For <6 mo for anemia

Perform/provide:
• Storage in tight, light-resistant container

Evaluate:
• Therapeutic response: improvement in Hct, Hgb, reticulocytes; decreased fatigue, weakness

Teach patient/family:
• That iron will change stools black or dark green
• That iron poisoning may occur if increased beyond recommended level
• To keep out of reach of children
• Not to substitute one iron salt for another; elemental iron content differs (e.g., 300 mg ferrous fumarate contains about 100 mg elemental iron; 300 mg ferrous gluconate contains only about 30 mg elemental iron)
• To avoid reclining position for 15-30 min after taking drug to avoid esophageal corrosion
• To follow diet high in iron

Treatment of overdose: Induce vomiting; give eggs, milk until lavage can be done

---

fexofenadine (R)

(fex-oh-fi′na-deen)
Allegra
Func. class.: Antihistamine
Chem. class.: Piperidine, peripherally selective

F

Do not confuse:
Allegra/Viagra

Action: Acts on blood vessels, GI, respiratory system by competing with histamine for H_1-receptor site; decreases allergic response by blocking pharmacologic effects of histamine

Uses: Rhinitis, allergy symptoms, chronic idiopathic urticaria

DOSAGE AND ROUTES

• *Adult and child >12 yr:* 60 mg bid
• *Child 6-11 yr:* **PO** 30 mg bid
Renal dose
• *Adult and child ≥12 yr:* **PO** CCr <80 ml/min 60 mg daily

Available forms: Caps 60 mg; ext rel tab 180 mg; tab 30, 60, 180 mg

SIDE EFFECTS

CNS: Headache, stimulation, drowsiness, sedation, fatigue, confusion, blurred vision, tinnitus, restlessness, tremors, paradoxical excitation in children or elderly
CV: Hypotension, palpitations, bradycardia, tachycardia, *dysrhythmias* (rare)
GI: Nausea, diarrhea, abdominal pain, vomiting, constipation
GU: Frequency, dysuria, urinary retention, impotence
HEMA: **Hemolytic anemia, thrombocytopenia, leukopenia, agranulocytosis, pancytopenia**
INTEG: Rash, eczema, photosensitivity, urticaria
RESP: Thickening of bronchial secretions, dry nose, throat

Contraindications: Hypersensitivity, newborn or premature infants, lactation, severe hepatic disease

Precautions: Pregnancy (C), elderly,

---

children, respiratory disease, narrow-angle glaucoma, prostatic hypertrophy, bladder neck obstruction, asthma

PHARMACOKINETICS

Well absorbed; onset 1 hr, peak 2-3 hr, duration 12-24 hr

INTERACTIONS

Increase: sedation—alcohol, other CNS depressants
Decrease: effect—magnesium-aluminum-containing antacids
Drug/Herb
Increase: sedation—hops, Jamaican dogwood, khat, senega
Increase: anticholinergic effect—corkwood, henbane leaf
Drug/Food
Decrease: absorption—apple, orange, grapefruit juice
Drug/Lab Test
False negative: Skin allergy tests

NURSING CONSIDERATIONS

Assess:
• I&O ratio: be alert for urinary retention, frequency, dysuria, especially elderly; drug should be discontinued if these occur
• Respiratory status: rate, rhythm, increase in bronchial secretions, wheezing, chest tightness
Administer:
• Do not break, crush, or chew caps, ext rel tabs
• With food or milk to decrease GI symptoms; caps/tabs should not be given with juice
Perform/provide:
• Hard candy, gum, frequent rinsing of mouth for dryness
• Storage in tight, light-resistant container
Evaluate:
• Therapeutic response: absence of running or congested nose or rashes
Teach patient/family:
• All aspects of drug use; to notify pre-

scriber if confusion, sedation, hypotension occur
• To avoid driving, other hazardous activity if drowsiness occurs
• To avoid alcohol, other CNS depressants
• Not to exceed recommended dose; dysrhythmias may occur
Treatment of overdose: Lavage, diazepam, vasopressors, barbiturates (short-acting)

---

filgrastim (℞)
(fill-grass'stim)
G-CSF, granulocyte colony stimulator, Neupogen
Func. class.: Biologic modifier
Chem. class.: Granulocyte colony-stimulating factor

Action: Stimulates proliferation and differentiation of neutrophils
Uses: To decrease infection in patients receiving antineoplastics that are myelosuppressive; to increase WBC in patients with drug-induced neutropenia; bone marrow transplantation
Investigational uses: Neutropenia in HIV infection, aplastic anemia, ganciclovir- induced neutropenia, zidovudine-induced neutropenia

DOSAGE AND ROUTES

After myelosuppressive chemotherapy
• *Adult and child:* **IV/SUBCUT** 5 mcg/kg/day in a single dose × 14 days; may increase by 5 mcg/kg in each cycle; give daily for up to 2 wk until the absolute neutrophil count (ANC) is 10,000/mm^3; response to G-CSF is much greater with **SUBCUT** than IV therapy
After bone marrow transplantation
• **IV/SUBCUT** 10 mcg/kg/day as an **INF (IV)** over 4 hr or 24 hr, begin 24 hr after chemotherapy and 24 hr after bone marrow transplantation
Peripheral blood progenitor cell collection/therapy
• 10 mcg/kg/day as a bolus or **CONT**

INF × 4 days or more before leukapheresis, continue to last leukapheresis; may alter dose if WBC >100,000 cells/mm^3

Severe neutropenia (chronic)
• *Adult:* SUBCUT 5 mcg/kg daily-bid
Available forms: Inj 300 mcg/ml

SIDE EFFECTS

CNS: Fever
GI: Nausea, vomiting, diarrhea, mucositis, anorexia
*HEMA: **Thrombocytopenia***
INTEG: Alopecia, exacerbation of skin conditions, urticaria
MS: Osteoporosis, skeletal pain
OTHER: Chest pain
RESP: Respiratory distress syndrome, wheezing

Contraindications: Hypersensitivity to proteins of *E. coli*
Precautions: Pregnancy (C), lactation, cardiac conditions, children, myeloid malignancies, radiation therapy, sepsis, sickle cell disease

PHARMACOKINETICS

IV: Onset 5-60 min, peak 24 hr, duration up to a week
SUBCUT: Onset 5-60 min, peak 2-8 hr, duration up to a week

INTERACTIONS

Do not use this drug concomitantly with antineoplastics

Drug/Lab Test
Increase: Uric acid, lactate dehydrogenase, alk phosphatase

NURSING CONSIDERATIONS

Assess:
• Blood studies: CBC, platelet count before treatment and twice weekly; neutrophil counts may be increased for 2 days after therapy
• B/P, respirations, pulse before and during therapy
• Bone pain, give mild analgesics
Administer:
• Using single-use vials; after dose is withdrawn, do not reenter vial

• For 2 wk or until ANC is 10,000/mm^3 after the expected chemotherapy neutrophil nadir
CONT IV INF route
• Dilute in D$_5$W to a conc of >15 mcg/ml, vial is for one-time use; give over 15-30 min (chemotherapy); over 4-24 hr (bone marrow transplantation); do not use 0.9% NaCl to dilute drug
Y-site compatibilities: Acyclovir, allopurinol, amikacin, aminophylline, ampicillin, ampicillin/sulbactam, aztreonam, bleomycin, bumetanide, buprenorphine, butorphanol, calcium gluconate, carboplatin, carmustine, cefazolin, cefotetan, ceftazidime, chlorproMAZINE, cimetidine, cisplatin, cyclophosphamide, cytarabine, dacarbazine, DAUNOrubicin, dexamethasone, diphenhydrAMINE, DOXOrubicin, doxycycline, droperidol, enalaprilat, famotidine, floxuridine, fluconazole, fludarabine, gallium, ganciclovir, granisetron, haloperidol, hydrocortisone, hydromorphone, hydrOXYzine, idarubicin, ifosfamide, leucovorin, lorazepam, mechlorethamine, melphalan, meperidine, mesna, methotrexate, metoclopramide, miconazole, minocycline, mitoxantrone, morphine, nalbuphine, netilmicin, ondansetron, plicamycin, potassium chloride, promethazine, ranitidine, sodium bicarbonate, streptozocin, ticarcillin, ticarcillin/clavulanate, tobramycin, trimethoprim-sulfamethoxazole, vancomycin, vinBLAStine, vinCRIStine, vinorelbine, zidovudine
Perform/provide:
• Storage in refrigerator; do not freeze; may store at room temperature up to 6 hr
• Avoid shaking
Evaluate:
• Therapeutic response: absence of infection
Teach patient/family:
• The technique for self-administration: dose, side effects, disposal of containers and needles; provide instruction sheet

F

finasteride (℞)

(fin-ass´te-ride)
Propecia, Proscar
Func. class.: Hormone, androgen inhibitor, hair stimulant
Chem. class.: 5-α-Reductase inhibitor

Do not confuse:
Proscar/Prosom
Proscar/Prozac
Action: Inhibits 5-α-reductase and reduction in DHT; DHT induces androgenic effects by binding to androgen receptors in the cell nuclei of the prostate gland, liver, skin; prevents development of BHP
Uses: Symptomatic benign prostatic hyperplasia (Proscar); male-pattern baldness (Propecia)

DOSAGE AND ROUTES

BPH
• *Adult:* **PO** 5 mg daily × 6-12 mo
Male pattern baldness
• *Adult:* **PO** 1 mg daily
Available forms: Tabs 1, 5 mg

SIDE EFFECTS

GU: Impotence, decreased libido, decreased volume of ejaculate
Contraindications: Pregnancy (X), hypersensitivity, children, women who are pregnant or may become pregnant should not handle tabs
Precautions: Large residual urinary volume, severely diminished urinary flow, hepatic function abnormalities

PHARMACOKINETICS

Bioavailability 63%, readily absorbed from GI tract, plasma protein binding 90%; metabolized in the liver; excreted in urine (metabolites) 39%, feces (57%); crosses blood-brain barrier; peak 1-2 hr, duration 24 hr

INTERACTIONS

Decrease: finasteride effect—theophylline, adrenergic bronchodilators, anticholinergics

NURSING CONSIDERATIONS

Assess:
• Urinary patterns, residual urinary volume, severely diminished urinary flow
• PSA levels and digital rectal exam prior to initiating therapy and periodically thereafter
• Hepatic studies prior to treatment; extensively metabolized in liver
Administer:
• Without regard to meals
• For a minimum of 6 mo; not all patients will respond
Perform/provide:
• Storage <86° F (30° C); protect from light; keep container tightly closed
Evaluate:
• Therapeutic response: increased urinary flow, decreased postvoiding dribbling, frequency, nocturia or hair growth within 3-6 mo
Teach patient/family:
⚠ Pregnant women or women who may become pregnant should not touch crushed tabs or come into contact with semen of a patient taking this drug; may adversely affect developing male fetus
• That volume of ejaculate may be decreased during treatment; impotence and decreased libido may also occur
• Propecia results may not occur for 3 mo
• Proscar results may not occur for 6-12 mo

flavocoxid (℞)

(flav-uh-kox´id)
Limbrel
Func. class.: Oral nutritional supplement

Action: Exhibits antiinflammatory, analgesic properties, thought to be due to inhibition of prostaglandin synthesis via inhibition of cyclooxygenase
Uses: For dietary management of osteoarthritis

⚠ Safety alert   *"Tall Man" lettering

DOSAGE AND ROUTES
• *Adult:* **PO** 250 mg q12h
Available forms: Cap 250 mg

SIDE EFFECTS
MISC: Hypertension, increase in varicose veins, psoriasis
MS: Fluid accumulation in the knees
Contraindications: Hypersensitivity
Precautions: Pregnancy (UK), lactation, children <18 yr, history of stomach ulcers
Pharmacokinetics: Metabolism primarily via glucuronidation and sulfation

INTERACTIONS
Unknown

NURSING CONSIDERATIONS
Assess:
• For pain of rheumatoid arthritis, osteoarthritis; check ROM, inflammation of joints, characteristics of pain
Administer:
• 1 hr before or after meals
Evaluate:
• Therapeutic response: decreased pain, inflammation in arthritic conditions
Teach patient/family:
• That drug does not take the place of other drugs, including corticosteroids for osteoarthritis
• To notify prescriber if pregnancy is planned or suspected

Rarely Used
flavoxate (℞)
(fla-vox'ate)
Func. class.: Spasmolytic

Uses: Relief of nocturia, incontinence, suprapubic pain, dysuria, frequency associated with urologic conditions (symptomatic only)

DOSAGE AND ROUTES
• *Adult and child >12 yr:* **PO** 100-200 mg tid-qid
Contraindications: Hypersensitivity, GI obstruction, GI hemorrhage, GU obstruction

flecainide (℞)
(flek-ay'nide)
Tambocor
Func. class.: Antidysrhythmic (Class IC)

F

Action: Decreases conduction in all parts of the heart, with greatest effect on His-Purkinje system, which stabilizes cardiac membrane
Uses: Life-threatening ventricular dysrhythmias, sustained ventricular tachycardia, supraventricular tachydysrhythmias, paroxysmal atrial fibrillation/flutter associated with disabling symptoms

DOSAGE AND ROUTES
PSVTT/PAF
• *Adult:* **PO** 50 mg q12h; may increase q4d by 50 mg q12h to desired response, max 300 mg/day
Life-threatening ventricular dysrhythmias
• *Adult:* **PO** 100 mg q12h; may increase by 50 mg q12h q4d, max 400 mg/day
Renal disease
• *Adult:* **PO** CCr <35 ml/min dose 50%-75%
Available forms: Tabs 50, 100, 150 mg

SIDE EFFECTS
CNS: Headache, dizziness, involuntary movement, confusion, psychosis, restlessness, irritability, paresthesias, ataxia, flushing, somnolence, depression, anxiety, malaise, fatigue, asthenia, tremors
CV: Hypotension, bradycardia, angina, PVCs, **heart block, cardiovascular collapse, arrest,** dysrhythmias, **CHF, fatal ventricular tachycardia**
EENT: Tinnitus, *blurred vision,* hearing loss
GI: Nausea, vomiting, anorexia, constipation, abdominal pain, flatulence, change in taste

---

GU: Impotence, decreased libido, polyuria, urinary retention

HEMA: Leukopenia, thrombocytopenia

INTEG: Rash, urticaria, edema, swelling

RESP: Dyspnea, ***respiratory depression***

Contraindications: Hypersensitivity, severe heart block, cardiogenic shock, nonsustained ventricular dysrhythmias, frequent PVCs, non–life-threatening dysrhythmias

Precautions: Pregnancy (C), lactation, children, renal disease, hepatic disease, CHF, respiratory depression, myasthenia gravis

PHARMACOKINETICS

PO: Peak 3 hr; half-life 12-27 hr; metabolized by liver; excreted unchanged by kidneys (10%); excreted in breast milk

INTERACTIONS

Increase: of both drugs—propranolol

Increase: CV depressant action—β-blockers, disopyramide, verapamil

Increase: flecainide level—amiodarone, cimetidine, ritonavir

Increase: digoxin level—digoxin

Increase or decrease effect: urinary, alkalinizing agents, acidifying agents

Drug/Herb

Increase: toxicity, death—aconite

Increase: effect—aloe, broom, chronic buckthorn use, cascara sagrada (chronic use), Chinese rhubarb, figwort, fumitory, goldenseal, kudzu, licorice

Increase: serotonin effect—horehound

Decrease: effect—coltsfoot

Drug/Lab Test

Increase: CPK

NURSING CONSIDERATIONS

Assess:

• I&O, daily weight

• CHF: edema, weight gain, dyspnea, jugular vein distention, crackles

• For hypokalemia, hyperkalemia before administration; correct electrolytes

• Blood levels: trough (0.2-1 mcg/ml)

• B/P, ECG continuously for fluctuations, watch for QRS widening, prolongation of QT and PR

• CNS effects: dizziness, confusion, psychosis, paresthesias, convulsions; drug should be discontinued

• Increased respiration, increased pulse; drug should be discontinued

Administer:

• Reduced dosage as soon as dysrhythmia is controlled

• May give with meals for GI upset

• May adjust dose q4 day

Evaluate:

• Therapeutic response: decreased dysrhythmias

Teach patient/family:

• To change position slowly from lying or sitting to standing to minimize orthostatic hypotension

• To take as prescribed, not to skip or double dose

• To avoid hazardous activities that require alertness until response is known

• To carry emergency ID with disorder, medications taken

• To notify all health care providers of treatment

Treatment of overdose: O₂, artificial ventilation, ECG, DOPamine for circulatory depression, diazepam or thiopental for convulsions, treat ventricular dysrhythmias

Rarely Used

floxuridine (℞)

(flox-yoor′i-deen)

Floxuridine, FUDR

Func. class.: Antineoplastic, antimetabolite

Uses: GI adenocarcinoma metastatic to liver; cancer of breast, head, neck, liver, brain, gallbladder, bile duct

DOSAGE AND ROUTES

• *Adult:* **INTRAARTERIAL** by cont inf 0.1-0.6 mg/kg/day × 1-6 wk; **HEPATIC**

ARTERY INJ 0.4-0.6 mg/kg/day × 1-6 wk

Contraindications: Pregnancy (D), hypersensitivity, myelosuppression, poor nutritional status, serious infections

fluconazole (R)

(floo-kon′a-zole)
Diflucan
Func. class.: Antifungal, systemic
Chem class: Triazole derivative

Do not confuse:
Diflucan/Diprivan
Action: Inhibits ergosterol biosynthesis, causes direct damage to fungal membrane phospholipids
Uses: Oropharyngeal candidiasis in AIDS patients, chronic mucocutaneous candidiasis, systemic, vaginal, urinary candidiasis, cryptococcal meningitis

DOSAGE AND ROUTES

Vaginal candidiasis
• *Adult:* **PO** 150 mg as a single dose
Serious fungal infections
• *Adult:* **PO/IV** 50-400 mg initially, then 200 mg daily for 4 wk
• *Child:* 6-12 mg/kg/day
Oropharyngeal candidiasis
• *Adult:* **PO/IV** 200 mg initially, then 100 mg daily for at least 2 wk
• *Child:* 3 mg/kg/day
Renal disease
• CCr 11-50 ml/min dose 50%
Available forms: Tabs 50, 100, 150, 200 mg; inj 2 mg/ml; powder for oral susp 50, 200 mg/ml

SIDE EFFECTS

CNS: Headache
GI: Nausea, vomiting, diarrhea, cramping, flatus, increased AST, ALT, **hepatotoxicity**
INTEG: **Stevens-Johnson syndrome**
Contraindications: Hypersensitivity to azoles
Precautions: Pregnancy (C), renal disease, hepatic disease, lactation

PHARMACOKINETICS

Peak 2-4 hr, bioavailability (PO) >90%, excreted unchanged in urine 80%

INTERACTIONS

Hypoglycemia: oral antidiabetics
Increase: anticoagulation—warfarin
Increase: plasma concentrations—cycloSPORINE, phenytoin, theophylline, rifabutin, tacrolimus
Increase: effect of zidovudine
Decrease: effect of: oral contraceptives
Drug/Herb
Increase: nephrotoxicity—gossypol

NURSING CONSIDERATIONS

Assess:
• For infection: clearing of CSF and other culture during treatment, obtain C&S baseline and throughout, drug may be started as soon as culture is taken
A For hepatotoxicity: increasing AST, ALT, periodically alk phosphatase, bilirubin
Administer:
PO route
• Shake oral susp before each use
IV route
• After diluting according to package directions; run at 200 mg/hr or less; do not use plastic containers in connections; check for bag leaks
• Using an infusion pump check for extravasation and necrosis q2h
• Do not use if cloudy or precipitated
• Do not admix
Y-site compatibilities: Acyclovir, aldesleukin, allopurinol, amifostine, amikacin, aminophylline, ampicillin/sulbactam, aztreonam, benztropine, cefazolin, cefepime, cefotetan, cefoxitin, chlorproMAZINE, cimetidine, cisatracurium, dexamethasone, diphenhydrAMINE, DOBUTamine, DOPamine, DOXOrubicin liposome, droperidol, famotidine, filgrastim, fludarabine, foscarnet, gallium, ganciclovir, gentamicin, granisetron, heparin, hydrocortisone,

F

immune globulin, leucovorin, loraze-pam, melphalan, meperidine, mero-penem, metoclopramide, metronidazole, midazolam, morphine, nafcillin, nitro-glycerin, ondansetron, oxacillin, pacli-taxel, pancuronium, penicillin G potas-sium, phenytoin, piperacillin/tazobactam, prochlorperazine, promethazine, propofol, ranitidine, remifentanil, sargramostim, tacrolimus, teniposide, theophylline, thiotepa, ticarcillin/clavulanate, tobramycin, van-comycin, vecuronium, vinorelbine, zido-vudine

Perform/provide:
• Storage protected from moisture and light, diluted sol is stable 24 hr, do not freeze

Evaluate:
• Therapeutic response: decreasing oral candidiasis, fever, malaise, rash; negative C&S for infection organism

Teach patient/family:
• That long-term therapy may be needed to clear infection
• That medication may be taken with food to reduce GI effects
• To notify prescriber of nausea, vomiting, diarrhea, jaundice, anorexia, clay-colored stools, dark urine
• Use alternative method of contraception while taking this drug

---

Rarely Used

fludarabine (℞)
(floo-dar'a-been)
Fludara
Func. class.: Antineoplastic, antimetabolite

Uses: Chronic lymphocytic leukemia, non-Hodgkin's lymphoma

DOSAGE AND ROUTES
• *Adult:* IV 25 mg/m² over 30 min daily × 5 days, may repeat q28d; reconstitute with 2 ml of sterile water for inj; dissolution should occur in <15 sec

Contraindications: Pregnancy (D), hypersensitivity, lactation

---

fludrocortisone (℞)
(floo-droe-kor'ti-sone)
Florinef
Func. class.: Corticosteroid, synthetic
Chem. class.: Mineralocorticoid

Action: Promotes increased reabsorption of sodium and loss of potassium, water, hydrogen from distal renal tubules
Uses: Adrenal insufficiency, salt-losing adrenogenital syndrome
Investigational uses: Renal tubular acidosis (type IV) idiopathic orthostatic hypotension

DOSAGE AND ROUTES
• *Adult:* PO 0.1-0.2 mg daily
• *Child:* PO 0.05-0.1 mg/day
Available forms: Tabs 0.1 mg

SIDE EFFECTS
CNS: Flushing, sweating, headache, paralysis, dizziness
*CV: Hypertension, **circulatory collapse, thrombophlebitis, embolism,** tachycardia, **CHF,** edema
ENDO: Weight gain, adrenal suppression
META: Hypokalemia
MISC: Hypersensitivity
MS: Fractures, osteoporosis, weakness
Contraindications: Hypersensitivity, acute glomerulonephritis, amebiasis, psychoses, Cushing's syndrome, fungal infections, child <2 yr
Precautions: Pregnancy (C), osteoporosis, CHF, lactation, child >2 yr, hypertension, diabetes

PHARMACOKINETICS
PO: Peak 1.5 hr, half-life 3.5 hr, metabolized by liver, excreted in urine

INTERACTIONS
Increase: B/P—sodium-containing food or medication

⚠ Safety alert   *"Tall Man" lettering

Decrease: fludrocortisone action—
barbiturates, rifampin, phenytoin
Decrease: potassium levels—thiazides,
potassium-wasting drugs, loop diuretics,
amphotericin B, piperacillin, mezlocillin
Drug/Herb
Increase: Hypokalemia—aloe, buck-
thorn, cascara sagrada, Chinese rhubarb,
senna
Increase: Corticosteroid effect—aloe,
licorice, perilla
Drug/Lab Test
Increase: Potassium, sodium
Decrease: Hct

NURSING CONSIDERATIONS

Assess:

• Weight daily; notify prescriber of
weekly gain >5 lb
• I&O ratio; be alert for decreasing urinary output, increasing edema
• B/P q4h, pulse; notify prescriber if
chest pain occurs
• Potassium depletion: paresthesias,
fatigue, nausea, vomiting, depression,
polyuria, dysrhythmias, weakness
• Electrolytes: sodium, potassium, chloride, hypokalemia is common

Administer:

• Titrated dose; use lowest effective dose
• With food or milk to decrease GI
symptoms

Perform/provide:

• Assistance with ambulation in patient
with bone tissue disease to prevent fractures

Evaluate:

• Therapeutic response: correction of
adrenal insufficiency

Teach patient/family:

• That emergency ID as steroid user
should be carried
• Not to discontinue this medication
abruptly
• To notify health care provider of muscle cramps, weight gain, edema, nausea,
infection, trauma, stress
• Not to breastfeed while taking this
medication

---

flumazenil (R)
(flu-maz′e-nill)
Anexate ✤ Romazicon
Func. class.: Antidote: Benzodiazepine receptor antagonist
Chem. class.: Imidazobenzodiaz-
epine derivative

F

Do not confuse:
Mazicon/Mivacron

Action: Antagonizes actions of benzodiazepines on CNS, competitively inhibits
activity at benzodiazepine recognition
site on GABA/benzodiazepine receptor
complex

Uses: Reversal of sedative effects of
benzodiazepines

DOSAGE AND ROUTES

*Reversal of conscious sedation or in
general anesthesia*

• *Adult:* **IV** 0.2 mg given over 15 sec;
wait 45 sec, then give 0.2 mg if consciousness does not occur; may be repeated at 60-sec intervals prn (max 3
mg/hr)
• *Child:* **IV** 10 mcg (0.01 mg)/kg; cumulative dose of 1 mg or less

*Management of suspected benzodi-
azepine overdose*

• *Adult:* **IV** 0.2 mg given over 30 sec;
wait 30 sec, then give 0.3 mg over 30 sec
if consciousness does not occur; further
doses of 0.5 mg can be given over 30 sec
at intervals of 1 min up to cumulative
dose of 3 mg
• *Child:* **IV** 100 mcg (0.1 mg)/kg; cumulative dose of 1 mg or less
Available forms: Inj 0.1 mg/ml

SIDE EFFECTS

CNS: Dizziness, agitation, emotional lability, confusion, *seizures,* somnolence
CV: Hypertension, palpitations, cutaneous
vasodilation, *dysrhythmias,* bradycardia, tachycardia, chest pain
EENT: Abnormal vision, blurred vision,
tinnitus
GI: Nausea, vomiting, hiccups

✤ Canada only   Side effects: *italics* = common; ***bold italics*** = life-threatening

SYST: Headache, inj site pain, increased sweating, fatigue, rigors

Contraindications: Hypersensitivity to this drug or benzodiazepines, serious cyclic antidepressant overdose, patients given benzodiazepine for control of life-threatening condition

Precautions: Pregnancy (C), lactation, children, elderly, status epilepticus, head injury, labor/delivery, renal disease, hepatic disease, hypoventilation, panic disorder, drug and alcohol dependency, ambulatory patients

PHARMACOKINETICS

Terminal half-life 41-79 min; metabolized in liver

INTERACTIONS

Toxicity: mixed drug overdosage
Antagonize action of benzodiazepines, zaleplon, zolpidem

NURSING CONSIDERATIONS
Assess:
• Cardiac status using continuous monitoring
• For seizures; protect patient from injury; most likely those that have withdrawals from sedatives
• GI symptoms: nausea, vomiting; place in side-lying position to prevent aspiration
• Allergic reactions: flushing, rash, urticaria, pruritus
Administer:
• Check airway and IV access before administration
IV, direct route
• Give undiluted or diluted with 0.9% NaCl, D₅W, LR, give over 15 sec into running IV
Additive compatibilities: Aminophylline, cimetidine, DOBUTamine, DOPamine, famotidine, heparin, lidocaine, procainamide, ranitidine
Solution compatibilities: D₅W
Evaluate:
• Therapeutic response: decreased sedation, respiratory depression, toxicity

Teach patient/family:
• That amnesia may continue
• Not to engage in hazardous activities for 18-24 hr after discharge
• Not to take any alcohol or non-prescription drugs for 18-24 hr

flunisolide nasal agent
See Appendix C

fluocinolone topical
See Appendix C

fluoride (PO) (℞)
(floor′ide)
Fluor-A-Day ✦, Fluoride Loz, Fluoritab, Flura-Loz, Karidium, Luride, Pediaflor, Pharmaflur, Phos-Flur, Solu-Flur ✦

fluoride (TOP) (℞)
ACT, Fluorigard, Fluorinse, Gel Kam, Gel-Tin, Karigel, MouthKote, Stop, Thera-Flur
Func. class.: Trace elements
Chem. class.: Fluoride ion

Action: Needed for hard tooth enamel and for resistance to periodontal disease; reduces acid production by dental bacteria

Uses: Prevention of dental caries, osteoporosis

DOSAGE AND ROUTES
Prevention of dental caries
• *Adult and child >12 yr:* **TOP** 10 ml 0.2% sol daily after brushing teeth, rinse mouth for >1 min with sol
• *Child 6-12 yr:* **TOP** 5 ml 0.2% sol
• *Child >3 yr:* **PO** 1 mg daily
• *Child <3 yr:* **PO** 0.5 mg daily
Mild-moderate osteoporosis
• *Adult:* **PO** slow rel fluoride 25 mg, given as calcium citrate 400 mg bid
Available forms: Tabs chewable 0.5,

1 mg; tabs 1 mg, tabs effervescent 10 mg; drops 0.125, 0.25, 0.5 mg/drop; rinse supplements 0.2 mg/ml, rinse 0.01%, 0.02%, 0.04%, 0.09%; gel 0.1%, 0.5%; lozenges 1 mg; sol 0.2 mg/ml; honey-wax, slow rel sodium fluoride tab

SIDE EFFECTS

*ACUTE OVERDOSE: **Black tarry stools, bloody vomit, diarrhea, decreased respiration, increased salivation, watery eyes***

*CHRONIC OVERDOSE: **Hypocalcemia and tetany, respiratory arrest, sores in mouth, constipation, loss of appetite, nausea, vomiting, weight loss, discoloration of teeth*** (white, black, brown)

Contraindications: Pregnancy (UK), hypersensitivity
Precautions: Child <6 yr

PHARMACOKINETICS

PO: Excreted in urine and feces; crosses placenta, breast milk

INTERACTIONS

Drug/Food
Avoid use with dairy products

NURSING CONSIDERATIONS

Assess:
• For mottling of teeth, during treatment
Administer:
• Drops after meals with fluids or undiluted tabs; may be chewed; do not swallow whole; may be given with water or juice; avoid milk
Evaluate:
• Therapeutic response: absence of dental caries
Teach patient/family:
• To monitor children using gel or rinse; not to be swallowed
• Not to drink, eat, or rinse mouth for at least ½ hr
• Not to use during pregnancy
• To apply after brushing and flossing at bedtime
• To store out of children's reach

---

fluorometholone ophthalmic
See Appendix C

⚠ High Alert

fluorouracil (℞)
(flure-oh-yoor'a-sil)
Adrucil, Efudex, 5-FU
Func. class.: Antineoplastic, antimetabolite
Chem. class.: Pyrimidine antagonist

Do not confuse:
fluorouracil/flucytosine
Action: Inhibits DNA, RNA synthesis; interferes with cell replication by competitively inhibiting thymidylate production, S phase of cell cycle–specific, a vesicant
Uses: Systemic: Cancer of breast, colon, rectum, stomach, pancreas; Topical: Multiple actinic keratoses, superficial basal cell carcinomas

DOSAGE AND ROUTES

• *Adult:* **IV** 12 mg/kg/day × 4 days, not to exceed 800 mg/day; may repeat with 6 mg/kg on day 6, 8, 10, 12; maintenance is 10-15 mg/kg/wk as a single dose, not to exceed 1 g/wk
Actinic/solar keratoses
• *Adult:* **TOP** 1% cream/sol 1-2 ×/day
Superficial basal cell carcinoma
• *Adult:* **TOP** 5% sol or cream 2 ×/day × 3-12 wk
Available forms: Inj 50 mg/ml; cream 1%, 5%; sol 1%, 2%, 5%

SIDE EFFECTS

Systemic use

CNS: Lethargy, malaise, weakness, acute cerebellar dysfunction
CV: Myocardial ischemia, angina
EENT: Epistaxis
GI: Anorexia, stomatitis, diarrhea, nausea, vomiting, ***hemorrhage,*** enteritis glossitis

HEMA: **Thrombocytopenia, leukopenia, myelosuppression, anemia, agranulocytosis**

INTEG: Rash, fever, photosensitivity

Contraindications: Pregnancy (D), hypersensitivity, myelosuppression, poor nutritional status, serious infections, major surgery within 1 month

Precautions: Renal disease, hepatic disease, bone marrow depression, angina, lactation, children

PHARMACOKINETICS

Half-life 20 hr terminal; metabolized in the liver; excreted in the urine; crosses blood-brain barrier

INTERACTIONS

Increase: toxicity, bone marrow depression—radiation or other antineoplastics

Increase: toxicity—irinotecan

Decrease: antibody response—live virus vaccines

Drug/Lab Test

Increase: LFTs, 6-HIAA

Decrease: Albumin

NURSING CONSIDERATIONS

Assess:

• CBC, differential, platelet count daily (IV); withhold drug if WBC is <3500/ mm^3 or platelet count is <100,000/mm^3; notify prescriber of these results; drug should be discontinued; nadir of leukopenia within 2 wk, recovery 1 mo

• Renal studies: BUN, serum uric acid, urine CCr, electrolytes before, during therapy

• Hepatic studies before, during therapy: bilirubin, alk phosphatase, AST, ALT, LDH; before and during therapy

• Bleeding: hematuria, guaiac, bruising or petechiae, mucosa or orifices q8h

• Inflammation of mucosa, breaks in skin; buccal cavity q8h for dryness, sores or ulceration, white patches, oral pain, bleeding, dysphagia

• GI symptoms: frequency of stools, cramping, intractable vomiting, stomatitis

Administer:

• Antiemetic 30-60 min before giving drug to prevent vomiting and for several days thereafter

Topical

• Wear gloves when applying; may use with a loose dressing; use a plastic or wooden applicator

IV route

• Prepared in biologic cabinet using gloves, gown, mask

• Undiluted; may inject through Y-tube or 3-way stopcock; give over 1-3 min; may be diluted in NS, D$_5$W, given over 2-8 hr as IV INF

Additive compatibilities: Bleomycin, cephalothin, cyclophosphamide, etoposide, floxuridine, hydromorphone, ifosfamide, methotrexate, mitoxantrone, prednisoLONE, vinCRIStine

Solution compatibilities: Amino acids 4.25%/D$_{25}$, D$_5$/LR, D$_{3.3}$/0.3 NaCl, D$_5$W, 0.9% NaCl, TPN #23

Syringe compatibilities: Bleomycin, cisplatin, cyclophosphamide, furosemide, heparin, leucovorin, methotrexate, metoclopramide, mitomycin, vinBLAStine, vinCRIStine

Y-site compatibilities: Allopurinol, amifostine, aztreonam, bleomycin, cefepime, cisplatin, cyclophosphamide, DOXOrubicin, DOXOrubicin liposome, fludarabine, furosemide, granisetron, heparin, hydrocortisone, leucovorin, mannitol, melphalan, methotrexate, metoclopramide, mitomycin, paclitaxel, piperacillin/tazobactam, potassium chloride, propofol, sargramostim, teniposide, thiotepa, vinBLAStine, vinCRIStine, vit B/C

Perform/provide:

• Strict asepsis, protective isolation if WBC levels are low

• Changing of IV site q48h

• Rinsing of mouth tid-qid with water, club soda; brushing of teeth bid-tid with soft brush or cotton-tipped applicator for stomatitis; use unwaxed dental floss, give ice chips for mucositis

• Nutritious diet with iron, vitamin

⚠ Safety alert   *"Tall Man" lettering

supplements, low fiber, few dairy products, especially when combined with radiotherapy as ordered

Evaluate:
• Therapeutic response: decreased tumor size, spread of malignancy

Teach patient/family:
• To avoid crowds, persons with known infections
• To avoid foods with citric acid, hot or rough texture if stomatitis is present; to drink adequate fluids
• To report stomatitis: any bleeding, white spots, ulcerations in mouth; tell patient to examine mouth daily, report symptoms; viscous lidocaine may be used
• To report signs of infection: fever, sore throat, flulike symptoms
• To report signs of anemia: fatigue, headache, faintness, shortness of breath, irritability
• To report bleeding: avoid use of razors, commercial mouthwash
• To avoid use of aspirin products or NSAIDs
• To use contraception during therapy (men and women)
• Not to receive vaccinations during therapy
• To use sunscreen or stay out of the sun to prevent photosensitivity
• About hair loss, explore use of wigs or other products until hair regrowth occurs

---

fluoxetine (R)

(floo-ox'eh-teen)
Prozac, Prozac Weekly, Sarafem
Func. class.: Antidepressant, SSRI (selective serotonin reuptake inhibitor)

Do not confuse:
Prozac/Proscar/Prosom
Sarafem/Serophene
Prozac/Prilosec
Action: Inhibits CNS neuron uptake of serotonin but not of norepinephrine
Uses: Major depressive disorder,

obsessive-compulsive disorder (OCD), bulimia nervosa; *Sarafem:* premenstrual dysphoric disorder (PMDD)
Investigational uses: Alcoholism, anorexia nervosa, ADHD, bipolar II affective disorder, borderline personality disorder, cataplexy, narcolepsy, kleptomania, migraine, obesity, posttraumatic stress disorder, schizophrenia, Tourette's syndrome, trichotillomania, levodopa-induced dyskinesia, social phobia, premenstrual dysphoric disorder

DOSAGE AND ROUTES
ADHD (unlabeled)
• *Adult:* **PO** 20-60 mg/day
Alcoholism (unlabeled)
• *Adult:* **PO** 20-80 mg/day
Anorexia nervosa (unlabeled)
• *Adult:* **PO** 10 mg every other day-20 mg/day
Bipolar II affective disorder (unlabeled)
• *Adult:* **PO** 10 mg every other day-20 mg/day
Borderline personality disorder (unlabeled)
• *Adult:* **PO** 20 mg/day
Bulimia nervosa
• *Adult:* **PO** 60 mg/day in AM
Depression/obsessive-compulsive disorder
• *Adult:* **PO** 20 mg daily in AM; after 4 wk if no clinical improvement is noted, dose may be increased to 20 mg bid in AM, PM, not to exceed 80 mg/day; **PO** weekly
• *Geriatric:* **PO** 5-10 mg/day, increase as needed
• *Child 5-18 yr:* **PO** 5-10 mg/day, max 20 mg/day
Kleptomania (unlabeled)
• *Adult:* **PO** 60-80 mg/day
Migraine, chronic daily headaches (unlabeled)
• *Adult:* **PO** 10-80 mg/day
Narcolepsy (unlabeled)
• *Adult:* **PO** 20-40 mg/day
Posttraumatic stress disorder (unlabeled)
• *Adult:* **PO** 10-80 mg/day

Side effects: *italics* = common; ***bold italics*** = life-threatening

Premenstrual dysphoric disorder (Sarafem)
• *Adult:* **PO** 20 mg daily, may be taken daily week before menses
Schizophrenia (unlabeled)
• *Adult:* **PO** 20-60 mg/day
Available forms: Caps 10, 20, 40 mg; tabs 10, 20 mg; oral sol 20 mg/5 ml; caps, del rel (Prozac Weekly) 90 mg

SIDE EFFECTS

*CNS: Headache, nervousness, insomnia, drowsiness, anxiety, tremor, dizziness, fatigue, sedation, poor concentration, abnormal dreams, agitation, **seizures,** apathy, euphoria, hallucinations, delusions, psychosis*
*CV: Hot flashes, palpitations, angina pectoris, **hemorrhage,** hypertension, **tachycardia,** first-degree AV block, **bradycardia, MI, thrombophlebitis***
EENT: Visual changes, ear/eye pain, photophobia, tinnitus
GI: Nausea, diarrhea, dry mouth, anorexia, dyspepsia, constipation, cramps, vomiting, taste changes, flatulence, decreased appetite
GU: Dysmenorrhea, decreased libido, urinary frequency, UTI, amenorrhea, cystitis, impotence, urine retention
INTEG: Sweating, rash, pruritus, acne, alopecia, urticaria
MS: Pain, arthritis, twitching
RESP: Infection, pharyngitis, nasal congestion, sinus headache, sinusitis, cough, dyspnea, bronchitis, asthma, hyperventilation, pneumonia
SYST: Asthenia, viral infection, fever, allergy, chills
Contraindications: Hypersensitivity
Precautions: Pregnancy (B), lactation, children, elderly, diabetes mellitus

PHARMACOKINETICS

PO: Peak 6-8 hr; metabolized in liver; excreted in urine; terminal half-life 2-3 days; steady state 28-35 days, protein binding 94%

INTERACTIONS

Paradoxical worsening of OCD: busPIRone
Do not use with thioridazine, or within 5 wk of discontinuing fluoxetine
⚠ Do not use MAOIs with or 14 days prior to fluoxetine
Increase: side effects—highly protein-bound drugs
Increase: effect—haloperidol
Increase: half-life of diazepam
Increase: levels or toxicity of carbamazepine, lithium, digoxin, warfarin, phenytoin
Increase: levels of tricyclics, phenothiazines
Increase: CNS depression—alcohol, antidepressants, opioids, sedatives
Decrease: fluoxetine effect—cyproheptadine
Drug/Herb
⚠ Do not use together; increased risk of serotonin syndrome: St. John's wort, SAM-e
Increase: anticholinergic effect—corkwood, jimsonweed
Increase: CNS effect—hops, kava, lavender
Drug/Lab Test
Increase: Serum bilirubin, blood glucose, alk phosphatase
Decrease: VMA, 5-HIAA
False increase: Urinary catecholamines

NURSING CONSIDERATIONS
Assess:
• Mental status: mood, sensorium, affect, suicidal tendencies, increase in psychiatric symptoms, depression, panic; monitor for seizures, seizure potential is increased
• Appetite in bulimia nervosa, weight daily, increase nutritious foods in diet, watch for binging and vomiting
• Allergic reactions: itching, rash urticaria, drug should be discontinued, may need to give antihistamine
• B/P (lying/standing), pulse q4h; if systolic B/P drops 20 mm Hg, hold drug,

notify prescriber; take vital signs q4h in patients with cardiovascular disease

• Blood studies: CBC, leukocytes, differential, cardiac enzymes if patient is receiving long-term therapy; check platelets; bleeding can occur

• Hepatic studies: AST, ALT, bilirubin, creatinine

• Weight qwk; appetite may decrease with drug

• ECG for flattening of T wave, bundle branch, AV block, dysrhythmias in cardiac patients

• Alcohol consumption; if alcohol is consumed, hold dose until AM

Administer:

• With food or milk for GI symptoms

• Crushed if patient is unable to swallow medication whole (tab only)

• Dosage at bedtime if oversedation occurs during the day; may take entire dose at bedtime; elderly may not tolerate once/day dosing

• Gum, hard candy, frequent sips of water for dry mouth

• Prozac weekly on the same day each week

Perform/provide:

• Storage at room temperature; do not freeze

• Assistance with ambulation during therapy, since drowsiness, dizziness occur

• Safety measures primarily in elderly

• Checking to see if PO medication swallowed

Evaluate:

• Therapeutic response: decreased depression, symptoms of OCD

Teach patient/family:

• That therapeutic effect may take 1-4 wk

• To use caution in driving, other activities requiring alertness because of drowsiness, dizziness, blurred vision

• To use sunscreen to prevent photosensitivity

• To avoid alcohol ingestion, other CNS depressants

• To notify prescriber if pregnant or plan to become pregnant or breast-feed

• To change positions slowly, orthostatic hypotension may occur

• To avoid all OTC drugs unless approved by prescriber

---

fluphenazine decanoate (℞)

(floo-fen′a-zeen)
Modecate ✤, Modecate Concentrate ✤, Prolixin Decanoate

fluphenazine hydrochloride (℞)

Apo-Fluphenazine ✤, Moditen HCL ✤, Moditen HCl-H.P. ✤, Permitil ✤, Prolixin
Func. class.: Antipsychotic
Chem. class.: Phenothiazine, piperazine

Do not confuse:
Prolixin/Proloid

Action: Depresses cerebral cortex, hypothalamus, limbic system, which control activity and aggression; blocks neurotransmission produced by dopamine at synapse; exhibits strong α-adrenergic and anticholinergic blocking action; mechanism for antipsychotic effects is unclear

Uses: Psychotic disorders, schizophrenia

DOSAGE AND ROUTES

Decanoate

• *Adult and child >16 yr:* **SUBCUT/IM** 12.5-25 mg q1-3wk, may increase slowly

• *Child 12-16 yr:* **IM/SUBCUT** 6.25-18.75 mg, then repeat q1-3wk, then increase slowly, max 25 mg

• *Child 5-12 yr:* **IM/SUBCUT** 3.125-12.5 mg, then repeat q1-3wk, increase slowly

HCl

• *Adult:* **PO** 2.5-10 mg, in divided doses q6-8h, not to exceed 20 mg daily; **IM** initially 1.25 mg then 2.5-10 mg in divided doses q6-8h

---

• *Child:* **PO** 0.25-3.5 mg daily in divided doses q4-6h, max 10 mg/daily
Available forms: HCl tabs 1, 2.5, 5, 10 mg; elix 2.5 mg/5 ml; inj 2.5 ml; decanoate inj 25 mg/ml

SIDE EFFECTS

CNS: EPS: pseudoparkinsonism, akathisia, dystonia, tardive dyskinesia, drowsiness, headache, seizures, neuroleptic malignant syndrome
CV: Orthostatic hypotension, hypertension, *cardiac arrest,* ECG changes, *tachycardia*
EENT: Blurred vision, glaucoma, dry eyes
GI: Dry mouth, nausea, vomiting, anorexia, constipation, diarrhea, jaundice, weight gain, *paralytic ileus, hepatitis,* cholecystic jaundice
GU: Urinary retention, urinary frequency, enuresis, impotence, amenorrhea, gynecomastia
HEMA: Anemia, *leukopenia, leukocytosis, agranulocytosis, aplastic anemia, thrombocytopenia*
INTEG: Rash, photosensitivity, dermatitis
RESP: Laryngospasm, dyspnea, *respiratory depression*
Contraindications: Hypersensitivity, circulatory collapse, liver damage, cerebral arteriosclerosis, coronary disease, severe hypertension/hypotension, blood dyscrasias, coma, brain damage, narrow-angle glaucoma, bone marrow depression, alcohol and barbiturate withdrawal
Precautions: Pregnancy (C), lactation, seizure disorders, hypertension, hepatic disease, cardiac disease, elderly, child <12 yr

PHARMACOKINETICS

PO/IM (HCl): Onset 1 hr, peak 2-4 hr, duration 6-8 hr, half-life 3.5-4 days
Decanoate: onset 1-3 days, peak 1-2 days, duration over 4 wk, single-dose half-life 6.8-9.6 days; multiple dose, 14.3 days
Metabolized by liver; excreted in urine (metabolites); crosses placenta; enters breast milk

INTERACTIONS

Oversedation: other CNS depressants, alcohol, barbiturate anesthetics
Toxicity: epINEPHrine
Increase: anticholinergic effects—anticholinergics
Decrease: effects of levodopa, lithium
Decrease: fluphenazine effects—smoking, barbiturates
Drug/Herb
Increase: EPS—betel palm, kava
Increase: anticholinergic effect—henbane leaf
Increase: action—cola tree, hops, kava, nettle, nutmeg
Drug/Lab Test
Increase: LFTs, cardiac enzymes, cholesterol, blood glucose, prolactin, bilirubin, PBI, cholinesterase
Decrease: Hormones (blood and urine)
False positive: Pregnancy tests, PKU urinary steroids, 17-OHCS

NURSING CONSIDERATIONS

Assess:
• Swallowing of PO medication; check for hoarding, giving of medication to other patients
• I&O ratio; palpate bladder if low urinary output occurs, urinary retention may be the cause
• Bilirubin, CBC, LFTs monthly
• Urinalysis is recommended before and during prolonged therapy
• Affect, orientation, LOC, reflexes, gait, coordination, sleep pattern disturbances
• B/P standing and lying; take pulse and respirations q4h during initial treatment; establish baseline before starting treatment; report drops of 30 mm Hg
• Dizziness, faintness, palpitations, tachycardia on rising
• EPS including akathisia (inability to sit still, no pattern to movements), tardive dyskinesia (bizarre movements of jaw, mouth, tongue, extremities), pseudoparkinsonism (rigidity, tremors, pill rolling, shuffling gait)
• Skin turgor daily

- Constipation, urinary retention daily; if these occur, increase bulk, H_2O in diet

Administer:
- Elixir with juice, milk, or uncaffeinated drinks
- Antiparkinsonian agent if EPS occur
- IM inj into large muscle mass; to minimize postural hypotension, give inj and have patient remain seated or recumbent for ½ hr
- Use dry needle, or solution will become cloudy; use 21G or larger due to viscosity

Syringe compatibilities: Benztropine, diphenhydrAMINE, hydrOXYzine

Perform/provide:
- Decreased sensory input by dimming lights, avoiding loud noises
- Supervised ambulation until stabilized on medication; do not involve in strenuous exercise; fainting is possible; patient should not stand still for long periods
- Increased fluids to prevent constipation
- Sips of water, candy, gum for dry mouth
- Storage in tight, light-resistant container in cool environment

Evaluate:
- Therapeutic response: decrease in emotional excitement, hallucinations, delusions, paranoia, reorganization of patterns of thought, speech

Teach patient/family:
- That orthostatic hypotension occurs often; to rise from sitting or lying position gradually; avoid hazardous activities until stabilized on medication
- To avoid hot tubs, hot showers, tub baths, since hypotension may occur; that in hot weather, heat stroke may occur; take extra precautions to stay cool
- ⚠ To avoid abrupt withdrawal of this drug, or EPS may result; drug should be withdrawn slowly
- To avoid OTC preparations (cough, hay fever, cold) unless approved by prescriber; serious drug interactions may occur; avoid use with alcohol, CNS depressants; increased drowsiness may occur
- To use a sunscreen to prevent burns
- About importance of compliance with drug regimen
- About EPS and necessity for meticulous oral hygiene, since oral candidiasis may occur
- To report sore throat, malaise, fever, bleeding, mouth sores; if these occur, CBC should be drawn and drug discontinued
- That urine may turn pink to reddish-brown

Treatment of overdose: Lavage; if orally ingested, provide an airway; *do not induce vomiting*

---

flurandrenolide topical
See Appendix C

---

flurazepam (℞)
(flure-az'e-pam)
Apo-Flurazepam ✹, Dalmane, flurazepam, Novoflupam ✹, Somnol ✹
Func. class.: Sedative/hypnotic
Chem. class.: Benzodiazepine derivative

Controlled Substance Schedule IV (USA), Targeted (CDSA IV) (Canada)

Do not confuse:
flurazepam/temazepam

Action: Produces CNS depression at the limbic, thalamic, hypothalamic levels of CNS; may be mediated by neurotransmitter γ-aminobutyric acid (GABA); results are sedation, hypnosis, skeletal muscle relaxation, anticonvulsant activity, anxiolytic action

Uses: Insomnia

DOSAGE AND ROUTES
- *Adult:* **PO** 15-30 mg at bedtime; may repeat dose once if needed
- *Elderly:* **PO** 15 mg at bedtime; may increase if needed

Available forms: Caps 15, 30 mg

SIDE EFFECTS

CNS: *Lethargy, drowsiness, daytime sedation,* dizziness, confusion, light-headedness, headache, anxiety, irritability
CV: Chest pain, pulse changes, palpitations
GI: Nausea, vomiting, diarrhea, heartburn, abdominal pain, constipation
HEMA: **Leukopenia, granulocytopenia** (rare)
MISC: Physical, psychological dependence

Contraindications: Pregnancy (UK), hypersensitivity to benzodiazepines, lactation, intermittent porphyria, uncontrolled pain

Precautions: Anemia, hepatic disease, renal disease, suicidal individuals, drug abuse, elderly, psychosis, child <15 yr

PHARMACOKINETICS

PO: Onset 15-45 min, duration 7-8 hr; metabolized by liver; excreted by kidneys (inactive/active metabolites); crosses placenta; excreted in breast milk; half-life 47-100 hr

INTERACTIONS

Increase: flurazepam effects—cimetidine, disulfiram, probenicid, isoniazid, oral contraceptives, fluoxetine, ketoconazole, propranolol, valproic acid
Increase: CNS depression—alcohol, CNS depressants
Decrease: flurazepam effect—rifampin, barbiturates, theophylline

Drug/Herb
Increase: sedative effect—catnip, chamomile, clary, cowslip, kava, lavender, mistletoe, nettle, pokeweed, poppy, Queen Anne's lace, senega, valerian
Increase: hypotension—black cohosh

Drug/Lab Test
Increase: AST, ALT, serum bilirubin
Decrease: RAI uptake
False increase: Urinary 17-OHCS

NURSING CONSIDERATIONS

Assess:
• Blood studies: Hct, Hgb, RBC (if on long-term therapy)

• Hepatic studies: AST, ALT, bilirubin
• Mental status: mood, sensorium, affect, memory (long, short), physical, psychological dependence or tolerance
• Type of sleep problem: falling asleep, staying asleep

Administer:
• After removal of cigarettes to prevent fires
• After trying conservative measures for insomnia
• ½-1 hr before bedtime for sleeplessness
• Caps may be opened and mixed with food

Perform/provide:
• Assistance with ambulation after receiving dose
• Safety measures: night-light, call bell within easy reach
• Checking to see if PO medication has been swallowed
• Storage in tight container in cool environment

Evaluate:
• Therapeutic response: ability to sleep at night, decreased amount of early morning awakening if taking drug for insomnia

Teach patient/family:
• To avoid driving or other activities requiring alertness until drug is stabilized
• To avoid alcohol ingestion or CNS depressants; serious CNS depression may result
• That effects may take 2 nights for benefits to be noticed
• Alternative measures to improve sleep: reading, exercise several hr before bedtime, warm bath, warm milk, TV, self-hypnosis, deep breathing
• That hangover is common in elderly

Treatment of overdose: Lavage, activated charcoal; monitor electrolytes, VS

flurbiprofen ophthalmic
See Appendix C

A Safety alert   *"Tall Man" lettering

flutamide (Ⴥ)
(floo′-ta-mide)
Eulexin
Func. class.: Antineoplastic, hormone
Chem. class.: Antiandrogen

Action: Interferes with androgen uptake in the nucleus or androgen activity in target tissues; arrests tumor growth in androgen-sensitive tissue (i.e., prostate gland)
Uses: Metastatic prostatic carcinoma, stage D_2 in combination with LHRH agonistic analogs (leuprolide)

DOSAGE AND ROUTES
• *Adult:* **PO** 250 mg q8h, for a daily dosage of 750 mg
Available forms: Caps 125, 250 ✦mg

SIDE EFFECTS
CNS: Hot flashes, drowsiness, confusion, depression, anxiety, paresthesia
GI: Diarrhea, nausea, vomiting, increased levels in hepatic studies, ***hepatitis,*** anorexia, ***hepatotoxicity***
GU: Decreased libido, impotence, gynecomastia
HEMA: ***Leukopenia, thrombocytopenia, hemolytic anemia***
INTEG: Irritation at site, rash, photosensitivity
MISC: Edema, neuromuscular and pulmonary symptoms, hypertension
Contraindications: Pregnancy (D), hypersensitivity

PHARMACOKINETICS
Rapidly and completely absorbed; excreted in urine and feces as metabolites; half-life 6 hr, geriatric half-life 8 hr; 94% bound to plasma proteins

INTERACTIONS
Increase: PT—warfarin
Decrease: flutamide action—LHRH analog (leuprolide)

NURSING CONSIDERATIONS
Assess:
⚠ Hepatic studies: AST, ALT, alk phosphatase, which may be elevated; if LFTs are elevated, drug may need to be discontinued; monitor CBC, bilirubin, creatinine
• For CNS symptoms including: drowsiness, confusion, depression, anxiety
Administer:
• Do not break, crush, or chew caps
• Flutamide must be taken with leuprolide, do not change dosing
Evaluate:
• Therapeutic response: decrease in prostatic tumor size, decrease in spread of cancer
Teach patient/family:
• To report side effects: decreased libido, impotence, breast enlargement, hot flashes, diarrhea
• To report nausea, vomiting, yellow eyes or skin, dark urine, clay-colored stools, hepatotoxicity may be the cause
• Notify of yellow, green urine discoloration

fluticasone (Ⴥ)
(floo-tic′a-sone)
Flonase, Flovent HFA, Flovent Diskus ✦
Func. class: Corticosteroids, inhalation; antiasthmatic

Action: Decreases inflammation by inhibiting mast cells, macrophages, and leukotrienes. Anti-inflammatory, and vasoconstrictor properties.
Uses: Prevention of chronic asthma during maintenance treatment in those requiring oral corticosteroids; nasal symptoms of seasonal/ perennial, and allergic/non-allergic rhinitis

DOSAGE AND ROUTES
Prevention of chronic asthma during maintenance treatment in those requiring oral corticosteroids
Flovent HFA
• *Adult and child ≥12 yr:* **INH** 88-440 mcg bid (in those previously taking bron-

chodilators, alone); **INH** 88-220 mcg bid, max 440 mcg bid (in those previously taking inhaled corticosteroids); **INH** 440 mcg bid, max 880 mcg bid (in those previously taking oral corticosteroids)

Flovent Diskus ✿
• *Adult and child ≥12 yr:* **INH** 100 mcg bid, max 500 mcg (in those previously taking bronchodilators, alone); **INH** 100-250 mcg bid, max 500 mcg bid (in those previously taking inhaled corticosteroids); **INH** 500-1000 mcg bid, max 1000 mcg bid (in those previously taking oral corticosteroids)
• *Child 4-11 yrs:* **INH** Initially 50 mcg bid, max 100 mcg bid (in those previously taking bronchodilators alone or inhaled corticosteroids)

Nasal symptoms of seasonal/perennial rhinitis
Flonase
• *Adult:* **NASAL SPRAY** 2 sprays (100 mcg) in each nostril daily or 1 spray (50 mcg) in each nostril bid; when symptoms are controlled, decrease to 1 spray (50 mcg) in each nostril every day
• *Adolescents and child ≥4 yr:* **NASAL SPRAY** 1 spray (50 mcg) in each nostril daily; may increase to 2 sprays (100 mcg) in each nostril daily; max 2 sprays in each nostril, daily

Available forms: Nasal spray 50 mcg/metered spray; oral inhalation aerosol 44, 110, 220 mcg; oral inhalation powder 50, 100, 250 mcg

SIDE EFFECTS

CNS: Fever, headache, nervousness, dizziness, migraines
EENT: Pharyngitis, sinusitis, rhinitis, laryngitis, hoarseness, dry eyes, cataracts, nasal discharge, epistaxis
GI: Diarrhea, abdominal pain, nausea, vomiting, *oral candidiasis*, gastroenteritis
GU: UTI
INTEG: Urticaria, dermatitis
META: Hyperglycemia, growth retardation in children, cushingoid features
MISC: Influenza, *eosinophilic condi-*

tions, angioedema, Churg-Strauss syndrome
MS: Osteoporosis, muscle soreness, joint pain
RESP: Upper respiratory infection, dyspnea, cough, bronchitis, *bronchospasm*

Contraindications: Hypersensitivity, primary treatment in status asthmaticus
Precautions: Pregnancy (C), lactation, active infections, glaucoma, diabetes, immunocompromised patients

PHARMACOKINETICS

Absorption 30% aerosol, 13.5% powder; protein binding 91%, metabolized in the liver after absorption in lung, half-life 7.8 hrs, < 5% excreted in urine and feces.
Nasal INH: Onset 12 hr, peak several days, duration 1-2 wks
Oral INH: Onset 24 hrs, peak several days, duration 1-2 wks

INTERACTIONS

Increase: fluticasone levels—P450 3A4 inhibitors (ketoconazole)
Drug/Lab Test
Increase: urine/serum glucose

NURSING CONSIDERATIONS

Assess:
• Respiratory status: lung sounds, pulmonary function tests during and several months after change from systemic to inhalation corticosteroids
• Withdrawal symptoms from oral corticosteroids: depression, pain in joints, fatigue
⚠ Adrenal insufficiency: nausea, weakness, fatigue, hypotension, hypoglycemia, anorexia; may occur when changing from systemic to inhalation corticosteroids; may be life-threatening
• Growth rate in children
• Adrenal function tests periodically: HPA (hypothalamic–pituitary-adrenal) axis suppression in long term treatment
Administer:
• Give at 1 min intervals

⚠ Safety alert   *"Tall Man" lettering

• Decrease dose to lowest effective dose after desired effect, decrease dose at 2-4 wk intervals

Teach patient/family:

• To use bronchodilator first before using inhalation, if taking both

• Not to use for acute asthmatic attack; for acute asthma, may require oral corticosteroids

• To avoid smoking, smoke filled rooms, those with URIs, those not immunized against chickenpox or measles

---

fluticasone nasal agent
See Appendix C

---

fluticasone topical
See Appendix C

---

fluvastatin (℞)

(flu'vah-stay-tin)
Lescol
Func. class.: Antilipidemic
Chem. class.: HMG-CoA reductase inhibitor

Action: Inhibits HMG-CoA reductase enzyme, which reduces cholesterol synthesis
Uses: As an adjunct in primary hypercholesterolemia (types Ia, Ib), coronary atherosclerosis in CAD; to reduce the risk of undergoing coronary revascularization in patients with CAD

DOSAGE AND ROUTES

• *Adult:* **PO** 20-40 mg daily in PM initially, usual range 20-80 mg, max 80 mg; may be given in 2 doses (40 mg AM, 40 mg PM); dosage adjustments may be made in 4 wk intervals or more
Available forms: Caps 20, 40 mg; ext rel tab 80 mg

SIDE EFFECTS

CNS: Headache, dizziness, insomnia
EENT: Lens opacities
GI: Abdominal pain, cramps, nausea, constipation, diarrhea, dyspepsia, flatus, hepatic dysfunction, pancreatitis
*HEMA: **Thrombocytopenia, hemolytic anemia, leukopenia***
INTEG: Rash, pruritus
MISC: Fatigue, influenza, photosensitivity
MS: Myalgia, ***myositis, rhabdomyolysis,*** *arthritis, arthralgia*
RESP: Upper respiratory infection, rhinitis, cough, pharyngitis, sinusitis
Contraindications: Pregnancy (X), hypersensitivity, lactation, active liver disease
Precautions: Past hepatic disease, alcoholism, severe acute infections, trauma, hypotension, uncontrolled seizure disorders, severe metabolic disorders, electrolyte imbalance

PHARMACOKINETICS

Metabolized in liver, highly protein bound, excreted primarily in feces, half-life <1 hr

INTERACTIONS

Increase: effects of warfarin, digoxin
Increase: myalgia, myositis—cycloSPORINE, gemfibrozil, niacin, erythromycin, clofibrate; azole antiinfectives
Increase: effects of fluvastatin—alcohol, cimetidine, ranitidine, omeprazole, saquinavir
Decrease: fluvastatin effect—rifampin
Drug/Herb
Increase: effect—glucomannan
Decrease: effect—gotu kola
Drug/Food
Grapefruit juice: possible increased toxicity

NURSING CONSIDERATIONS
Assess:
• Fasting lipid profile (cholesterol, LDL, HDL, TG) q8wk, then q3-6mo when stable
• Hepatic studies q1-2mo during the first 1½ yr of treatment; AST, ALT, LFTs may be increased

- Renal studies in patients with compromised renal system: BUN, I&O ratio, creatinine
- For muscle pain, tenderness; obtain baseline CPK and if these occur, drug may need to be discontinued

Administer:
- Do not break, crush, or chew ext rel tabs
- Bile acid sequestrant should be given at least 2 hr before or after fluvastatin

Perform/provide:
- Storage in cool environment in tight container protected from light

Evaluate:
- Therapeutic response: decrease in LDL, VLDL, total cholesterol; increased HDL, decreased triglycerides

Teach patient/family:
- That blood work will be necessary during treatment, to take as prescribed
- To report severe GI symptoms, headache, muscle pain, weakness, tenderness
- That previously prescribed regimen will continue: low-cholesterol diet, exercise program, smoking cessation
- To report suspected pregnancy, not to use during pregnancy
- To use sunscreen or stay out of sun to prevent photosensitivity
- To notify all health care providers of drugs taken

---

fluvoxamine (℞)

(flu-vox′a-meen)
Luvox
Func. class.: Antidepressant SSRI (selective serotonin reuptake inhibitor)

Do not confuse:
Luvox/Levoxyl

Action: Inhibits CNS neuron uptake of serotonin but not of norepinephrine

Uses: Obsessive-compulsive disorder

Investigational uses: Depression, bulimia nervosa, panic disorder, social phobia

DOSAGE AND ROUTES

- *Adult:* **PO** 50 mg at bedtime, increase by 50 mg at 4-7 day intervals, max 300 mg, doses over 100 mg should be divided
- *Child 8-17 yr:* **PO** 25 mg at bedtime, increase by 25 mg/day q4-7d, max 200 mg/day, doses over 50 mg should be divided

Hepatic dose/elderly
- Reduce dose

Available forms: Tabs 25, 50, 100 mg

SIDE EFFECTS

CNS: Headache, drowsiness, dizziness, convulsions, sleep disorders, insomnia
*GI: Nausea, anorexia, constipation, **hepatotoxicity**, vomiting, diarrhea,* dry mouth
GU: Decreased libido
INTEG: Rash, sweating

Contraindications: Hypersensitivity
Precautions: Pregnancy (C), lactation, children, elderly

PHARMACOKINETICS

Crosses blood-brain barrier, 77% protein binding, metabolism by the liver, terminal half-life 16.9 hr, peak 2-8 hr

INTERACTIONS

⚠ Fatal reaction—MAO inhibitors
Increase: CNS depression—alcohol, barbiturates, benzodiazepines
Increase: fluvoxamine, toxicity levels—tricyclics, clozapine
Increase: metabolism, decrease effects—smoking
Decrease: metabolism, increase action of propranolol, diazepam, lithium, theophylline, carbamazepine, warfarin

Drug/Herb
⚠ *Increase:* effect, possible fatal reaction—St. John's wort
Increase: anticholinergic effect—corkwood, jimsonweed
Increase: CNS effect—hops, kava, lavender

⚠ Safety alert   *"Tall Man" lettering

NURSING CONSIDERATIONS
Assess:
- Hepatic studies: AST, ALT, bilirubin
- Mental status: mood, sensorium, affect, suicidal tendencies; increase in psychiatric symptoms: depression, panic, obsessive-compulsive symptoms
- Constipation; most likely in elderly
- ⚠ For toxicity: nausea, vomiting, diarrhea, syncope, increased pulse, seizures

Administer:
- With food, milk for GI symptoms

Perform/provide:
- Storage at room temperature; do not freeze

Evaluate:
- Therapeutic response: decrease in depression

Teach patient/family:
- That therapeutic effects may take 2-3 wk
- To use caution in driving, other activities requiring alertness because of drowsiness, dizziness that may occur
- Not to use other CNS depressants, alcohol, barbiturates, benzodiazepines, St. John's wort, kava
- To notify prescriber if pregnancy is suspected or planned
- To notify prescriber of allergic reaction
- To increase bulk in diet if constipation occurs, especially elderly

---

folic acid (vit B₉) (otc)
(foe'lik a'sid)
Apo-Folic ✦, Folate, Folvite, Novofolacid ✦, Vitamin B₉
Func. class.: Vit B complex group

Action: Needed for erythropoiesis; increases RBC, WBC, platelet formation in megaloblastic anemias
Uses: Megaloblastic or macrocytic anemia caused by folic acid deficiency; hepatic disease, alcoholism, hemolysis, intestinal obstruction, pregnancy

DOSAGE AND ROUTES
RDA
- *Adult/child ≥14 yr:* 400 mcg
- *Child 9-13 yr:* 300 mcg
- *Child 4-8 yr:* 200 mcg
- *Child 1-3 yr:* 150 mcg
- *Infant 6 mo-1 yr:* 80 mcg
- *Neonates/infants <6 mo:* 65 mcg

Megaloblastic/macrocytic anemia due to folic acid or nutritional deficiency
- *Pregnant:* 600 mcg
- *Lactating:* 500 mcg

Therapeutic dose
- *Adult and child:* **PO/IM/SUBCUT/IV** up to 1 mg daily

Maintenance dose
- *Adult and child >4 yr:* **PO/IM/IV/SUBCUT** 0.4 mg/day
- *Pregnant and lactating:* **PO/IM/IV/SUBCUT** 0.8 mg/day
- *Child <4 yr:* **PO/IM/IV/SUBCUT** up to 0.3 mg/day
- *Infants:* **PO/IM/IV/SUBCUT** up to 0.1 mg/day

Prevention of neural tube defects during pregnancy
- *Adult:* **PO** 0.4 mg daily

Prevention of megaloblastic anemia during pregnancy
- *Adult:* **PO/IM/SUBCUT** up to 1 mg/day during pregnancy

Tropical sprue
- *Adult:* **PO** 3-15 mg daily

Available forms: Tabs 0.1, 0.4, 0.8, 1, 5 mg; inj 5, 10 mg/ml

SIDE EFFECTS
INTEG: Flushing
RESP: ***Bronchospasm***
Contraindications: Hypersensitivity, anemias other than megaloblastic/macrocytic anemia, vit B₁₂ deficiency anemia, uncorrected pernicious anemia
Precautions: Pregnancy (A)

Side effects: *italics* = common; ***bold italics*** = life-threatening

F

PHARMACOKINETICS

PO: Peak ½-1 hr; bound to plasma proteins; excreted in breast milk; metabolized by liver; excreted in urine (small amounts)

INTERACTIONS

Increase: need for folic acid—estrogen, hydantoins, carbamazepine, glucocorticoids

Decrease: folate levels—methotrexate, sulfonamides, sulfasalazine

Decrease: phenytoin levels, fosphenytoin, may increase seizures

NURSING CONSIDERATIONS

Assess:

• For fatigue, dyspnea, weakness, dyspnea that are signs of megaloblastic anemia

• Hgb, Hct, and reticulocyte count

• Nutritional status: bran, yeast, dried beans, nuts, fruits, fresh vegetables, asparagus

• Drugs currently taken: estrogen, carbamazepine, glucocorticoids, hydantoins; these drugs may cause increased folic acid use by body and contribute to a deficiency

Administer:

IV route

• Direct undiluted 5 mg or less/1 min or more; or may be added to most IV sol or TPN

Solution compatibilities: $D_{20}W$
Y-site compatibilities: Famotidine
Perform/provide:

• Storage in light-resistant container

Evaluate:

• Therapeutic response: increased weight, oriented, well-being; absence of fatigue; increase in reticulocyte count within 5 days of beginning treatment

Teach patient/family:

• To take drug exactly as prescribed; periodic lab work is required

• To alter nutrition to include high-folic-acid foods: organ meats, vegetables, fruit

• That urine will turn bright yellow

• To notify prescriber of allergic reaction

---

fomivirsen ophthalmic
See Appendix C

---

fondaparinux (℞)
(fon-dah-pair′ih-nux)
Arixtra
Func. class.: Anticoagulant, antithrombotic
Chem. class.: Synthetic, selective factor Xa inhibitor

Do not confuse:
Arixtra/Anti-Xa

Action: Acts by antithrombin III (ATIII)-mediated selective inhibition of factor Xa; neutralization of factor Xa interrupts blood coagulation and inhibits thrombin formation; does not inactivate thrombin (activated factor II) or affect platelets

Uses: Prevention of deep-vein thrombosis, pulmonary emboli in hip and knee replacement, hip fracture surgery

DOSAGE AND ROUTES

• *Adult:* **SUBCUT** 2.5 mg daily; after hemostasis established, initial dose is given 6-8 hr after surgery, usual duration 5-9 days

Available forms: Inj 2.5 mg/0.5 ml single-dose syringe

SIDE EFFECTS

CNS: Fever, confusion, headache, dizziness, *insomnia*
GI: Nausea, vomiting, diarrhea, dyspepsia, *constipation,* increased AST, ALT
GU: UTI, urinary retention
HEMA: Anemia, minor bleeding, purpura, hematoma, ***thrombocytopenia, major bleeding (intracranial, cerebral, retroperitoneal hemorrhage), postoperative hemorrhage***
INTEG: Increased wound drainage, bul-

---

lous eruption, local reaction—*rash,*
pruritus, inj site bleeding
META: Hypokalemia
OTHER: Hypotension, pain, *edema*
Contraindications: Hypersensitivity
to this drug; hemophilia, leukemia with
bleeding, peptic ulcer disease, hemorrhagic stroke, surgery, thrombocytopenic
purpura, weight <50 kg, severe renal
disease (CCr <30 ml/min)
Precautions: Pregnancy (B), alcoholism, hepatic disease (severe), blood
dyscrasias, heparin-induced thrombocytopenia, uncontrolled, severe hypertension, subacute bacterial endocarditis,
acute nephritis, lactation, elderly, children, mild to moderate renal disease

PHARMACOKINETICS

Rapidly, completely absorbed; peak
steady state 3 hr; distributed primarily
in blood, does not bind to plasma proteins except 94% to ATIII; metabolism
unknown; eliminated unchanged in
urine in 72 hr in normal renal function

INTERACTIONS

Discontinue use of other drugs that may
increase the risk of hemorrhage before
starting fondaparinux; monitor closely if
coadministration is essential
Do not mix with other drugs or infusion
fluids

Drug/Herb
Increase: risk of bleeding—agrimony,
alfalfa, angelica, anise, basil, bay, bilberry, black haw, bogbean, bromelain,
buchu, chondroitin, cinchona bark,
dong quai, fenugreek, feverfew, garlic,
ginger, ginkgo, ginseng, horse chestnut,
Irish moss, kelp, kelpware, khella, lovage, lungwort, meadowsweet, motherwort, mugwort, nettle, papaya, parsley
(large amts), pau d'arco, pineapple,
poplar, prickly ash, safflower, saw palmetto, tonka bean, turmeric, wintergreen, yarrow

Drug/Herb
Decrease: anticoagulant effect—
chamomile, coenzyme Q10, flax, glucomannan, goldenseal, guar gum

NURSING CONSIDERATIONS

Assess:
• Blood studies (Hct, CBC, coagulation
studies, platelets, occult blood in stools),
anti-Xa; thrombocytopenia may occur
• For bleeding: gums, petechiae, ecchymosis, black tarry stools, hematuria;
notify prescriber
• For neurologic symptoms in patients
who have received spinal anesthesia
• For risk of hemorrhage if coadministering with other drugs that may cause
bleeding

Administer:
• Alone; do not mix with other drugs or
solutions; cannot be used interchangeably (unit to unit) with other anticoagulants
• For 5-9 days
• Only after screening patient for bleeding disorders
• SUBCUT only; do not give IM; do not
give earlier than 6 hr after surgery
SUBCUT route
• Check for discolored sol or sol with
particulate; if present, do not give
• Administer 6-8 hr after surgery
• Administer to recumbent patient, rotate inj sites (left/right anterolateral,
left/right posterolateral abdominal wall)
• Wipe surface of inj site with alcohol
swab, twist plunger cap and remove,
remove rigid needle guard by pulling
straight off needle, do not aspirate, do
not expel air bubble from surface
• Insert whole length of needle into
skinfold held with thumb and forefinger
• When drug is injected, a soft click may
be felt or heard
• Give at same time each day to maintain
steady blood levels
• Avoid all IM inj that may cause bleeding
⚠ Administer only this drug when
ordered; not interchangeable with heparin

Perform/provide:

• Storage at 25° C (77° F); do not freeze

Evaluate:

• Therapeutic response: Prevention of deep vein thrombosis

Teach patient/family:

• To use soft-bristle toothbrush to avoid bleeding gums, to use electric razor

• To report any signs of bleeding: gums, under skin, urine, stools

• To avoid OTC drugs containing aspirin

---

formoterol (Ⓡ)

(for-moh'ter-ahl)

Foradil Aerolizer

Func. class.: Bronchodilator

Chem. class.: β-Adrenergic agonist

Do not confuse:

Foradil/Toradol

Action: Has β_1 and β_2 action; relaxes bronchial smooth muscle and dilates the trachea and main bronchi by increasing levels of cAMP, which relaxes smooth muscles; causes increased contractility and heart rate by acting on β-receptors in heart

Uses: Maintenance, treatment of asthma, COPD, prevention of exercise-induced bronchospasm

DOSAGE AND ROUTES

Maintenance, treatment of asthma

• *Adult/child ≥5 yr:* **INH** AM and PM long term 1 cap (12 mcg) q12h using aerolizer inhaler

Maintenance of COPD

• *Adult:* **INH** 12 mcg q12h

Prevention of exercise-induced bronchospasm

• *Adult/child ≥12 yr:* **INH** prn occasionally 1 cap (12 mcg) at least 15 min before exercise

Available form: INH powder in cap 12 mcg

SIDE EFFECTS

CNS: Tremors, anxiety, insomnia, headache, dizziness, stimulation

CV: Palpitations, tachycardia, hypertension

GI: Nausea, vomiting

RESP: Bronchial irritation, dryness of oropharynx, ***bronchospasms*** (overuse)

Contraindications: Hypersensitivity to sympathomimetics, narrow-angle glaucoma

Precautions: Pregnancy (C), cardiac disorders, hyperthyroidism, diabetes mellitus, prostatic hypertrophy, elderly

PHARMACOKINETICS

INH: Onset 15 min, peak 1-3 hr, duration 12 hr

Metabolized in liver, lungs, GI tract

INTERACTIONS

Serious dysrhythmias: MAOIs, tricyclics

Increase: effects of both drugs—other sympathomimetics

Decrease: action when used with β-blockers

NURSING CONSIDERATIONS

Assess:

• Respiratory function: B/P, pulse, lung sounds

• I&O ratio; check for urinary retention, frequency, hesitancy

• For paresthesias and coldness of extremities; peripheral blood flow may decrease

Perform/provide:

• Storage at room temperature, protection from heat, moisture

Evaluate:

• Therapeutic response: ease of breathing

Teach patient/family:

• To rinse mouth after use

• Correct use of inhaler; review package insert with patient; to avoid getting aerosol in eyes; to wash inhaler in warm water and dry daily

• About all aspects of drug; to avoid smoking, smoke-filled rooms, persons with respiratory infections

---

Treatment of overdose: Administration of a β-blocker

---

fosamprenavir (Ꝝ)
(fos-am-pren'a-veer)
Lexiva
Func. class.: Antiretroviral
Chem. class.: Protease inhibitor

Action: A prodrug of amprenavir. Inhibits human immunodeficiency virus (HIV) protease, which prevents maturation of the infectious virus

Uses: HIV-1 infection in combination with antiretrovirals

DOSAGE AND ROUTES
Therapy-naïve patients
• *Adult:* **PO** 1400 mg bid without ritonavir or fosamprenavir 1400 mg daily and ritonavir 200 mg daily or fosamprenavir 700 mg bid and ritonavir 100 mg bid
Protease experienced patients (PI)
• *Adult:* **PO** 700 mg bid and ritonavir 100 mg bid
Combination with efavirenz
• *Adult:* **PO** Add another 100 mg/day of ritonavir for a total of 300 mg/day when all three drugs are given
Hepatic dose
• *Adult:* **PO** (Child-Pugh 5-8) 700 mg bid, (Child-Pugh 9-12) do not use
Available forms: Tabs 700 mg (equivalent to 600 mg amprenavir)

SIDE EFFECTS
CNS: Headache, fatigue, depression, oral paresthesia
GI: Nausea, diarrhea, vomiting, abdominal pain
INTEG: Rash, pruritus
MISC: Redistribution or accumulation of body fat, hyperglycemia
Contraindications: Hypersensitivity to protease inhibitors
Precautions: Pregnancy (C), liver disease, hemolytic anemia, diabetes, sulfa sensitivity, lactation, elderly

PHARMACOKINETICS
A prodrug of amprenavir, peak 1½-4 hr., 90% protein binding, metabolized in the liver by cytochrome P450 3AY (CYP3A4), excretion of unchanged drug is minimal

INTERACTIONS
Do not use with pimozide, ergots, midazolam, triazolam, flecainide, propafenone
May affect coagulation: warfarin
Avoid use with St. John's wort, rifampin, delavirdine, H₂ receptor antagonists, proton-pump inhibitors, carbamazepine, phenobarbital, phenytoin because may lose virologic response and possibly lead to resistance to fosamprenavir
⚠ Serious dysrhythmias: amiodarone, calcium channel blockers, lidocaine
Increase: effect—rifbutin, ketoconazole, itraconazole, sildenafil, vardenafil
Increase: toxicity—HMG-CoA reductase inhibitors
Decrease: effect of oral contraceptives, methadone
Decrease: fosamprenavir levels—nevirapine, antacids, efavirenz, saquinavir, ranitidine, carbamazepine, phenytoin

NURSING CONSIDERATIONS
Assess:
• Bowel pattern before, during treatment, monitor hydration
• Skin eruptions, rash, urticaria, itching
• Viral load, CD4 cell counts baseline and throughout treatment
Administer:
• Without regard to food
Teach patient/family:
• To avoid taking with other medications unless directed by provider
• That drug does not cure, but does manage symptoms and does not prevent transmission of HIV to others
• To use nonhormonal form of birth control while taking this drug
• If dose is missed, take as soon as remembered up to 1 hr before next dose, do not double dose

---

- Not to alter dose or stop therapy without talking to physician
- Advise physician if they have sulfa allergy
- To report all medications including herbal supplements to physician
- That patients receiving phosphodiesterase type 5 inhibitors may be at increased risk for PDE5 inhibitor adverse effects

foscarnet (R)

(foss-kar′net)
Foscavir
Func. class.: Antiviral
Chem. class.: Inorganic pyrophosphate organic analog

Action: Antiviral activity is produced by selective inhibition at the pyrophosphate binding site on virus-specific DNA polymerases and reverse transcriptases at concentrations that do not affect cellular DNA polymerases

Uses: Treatment of CMV retinitis, HSV infections, used with ganciclovir for relapsing patients

DOSAGE AND ROUTES

CMV retinitis

- *Adult:* **IV INF** 60 mg/kg given over at least 1 hr, q8h × 2-3 wk initially, then 90-120 mg/kg/day over 2 hr, usually give with at least 750-1000 ml **NS** daily

HSV

- *Adult:* **IV** 40 mg/kg q8-12h × 2-3 wk

In renal abnormalities:

- *Adult:* **IV**

Male:

$$\frac{140 - age}{serum\ creatinine \times 72} = CCr$$

Female: $0.85 \times$ above value
Dose based on table provided in package insert

Available forms: Inj 24 mg/ml

SIDE EFFECTS

CNS: Fever, dizziness, *headache,* *seizures,* *fatigue,* neuropathy, tremor, ataxia, dementia, stupor, EEG abnormalities, vertigo, *coma,* abnormal gait, hypertonia, EPS, hemiparesis, *paralysis,* hyperreflexia, paraplegia, *tetany,* hyporeflexia, neuralgia, neuritis, *cerebral edema,* *paresthesia,* depression, *confusion,* *anxiety,* insomnia, somnolence, amnesia, hallucinations, agitation

CV: Hypertension, palpitations, ECG abnormalities, 1st-degree AV block, nonspecific ST-T segment changes, hypotension, cerebrovascular disorder, cardiomyopathy, *cardiac arrest,* bradycardia, dysrhythmias

EENT: Visual field defects, vocal cord paralysis, speech disorders, taste perversion, eye pain, conjunctivitis, tinnitus, otitis

GI: Nausea, *vomiting, diarrhea, anorexia,* abdominal pain, constipation, dysphagia, rectal hemorrhage, dry mouth, melena, flatulence, ulcerative stomatitis, pancreatitis, enteritis, enterocolitis, glossitis, proctitis, stomatitis, increased amylases, gastroenteritis, *pseudomembranous colitis,* duodenal ulcer, *paralytic ileus, esophageal ulceration,* abnormal A-G ratio, increased AST, ALT, cholecystitis, *hepatitis,* dyspepsia, tenesmus, hepatosplenomegaly, jaundice

GU: *Acute renal failure,* decreased CCr and increased serum creatinine, *glomerulonephritis, toxic nephropathy, nephrosis, renal tubular disorders, pyelonephritis, uremia, hematuria, albuminuria,* dysuria, polyuria

HEMA: Anemia, *granulocytopenia, leukopenia, thrombocytopenia,* platelet abnormalities, *thrombosis, pulmonary embolism, coagulation disorders, decreased prothrombin, hypochromic anemia, pancytopenia, hemolysis, leukocytosis,* lymphadenopathy, epistaxis, lymphopenia

INTEG: *Rash,* sweating, pruritus, skin ulceration, seborrhea, skin discoloration, alopecia, acne, dermatitis, pain/

⚠ Safety alert   *"Tall Man" lettering

inflammation at inj site, facial edema, dry skin, urticaria

MS: Arthralgia, myalgia

RESP: *Coughing, dyspnea,* pneumonia, sinusitis, pharyngitis, *pulmonary infiltration,* stridor, *pneumothorax, hemoptysis, bronchospasm,* bronchitis, *respiratory depression, pleural effusion, pulmonary hemorrhage,* rhinitis

SYST: *Hypokalemia, hypocalcemia, hypomagnesemia;* increased alk phosphatase, LDH, BUN; acidosis, hypophosphatemia, hyperphosphatemia, dehydration, glycosuria, increased CPK, hypervolemia, infection, *sepsis, death, ascites,* hyponatremia, hypochloremia, hypercalcemia

Contraindications: Hypersensitivity, CCr <0.4 ml/min/kg

Precautions: Pregnancy (C), lactation, children, elderly, renal disease, seizure disorders, electrolyte/mineral imbalances, severe anemia

PHARMACOKINETICS

14%-17% plasma protein bound, half-life 2-8 hr in normal renal function

INTERACTIONS

Nephrotoxicity: aminoglycosides, amphotericin B

Hypocalcemia: pentamidine

NURSING CONSIDERATIONS

Assess:

General

• Renal, hepatic studies: BUN, creatinine, AST, ALT

• I&O ratio, urine pH, serum creatinine baseline, 3 ×/wk during initial therapy, then 2 ×/wk thereafter; CCr baseline, throughout treatment; if CCr <0.4 ml/min/kg, discontinue

• Blood counts q2wk; watch for decreasing granulocytes, Hgb; if low, therapy may have to be discontinued and restarted after hematologic recovery; blood transfusions may be required

• Electrolytes and minerals (Ca, P, Mg,

Na, K); watch closely for tetany during first administration

• GI symptoms: nausea, vomiting, diarrhea; severe symptoms may necessitate discontinuing drug

Ⓐ Blood dyscrasias (anemia, granulocytopenia); bruising, fatigue, bleeding, poor healing

• Allergic reactions: flushing, rash, urticaria, pruritus

CMV retinitis

• Culture should be done prior to treatment (blood, urine, throat)

• Ophthalmic exam should confirm diagnosis

Administer:

• Increased fluids before and during drug administration to induce diuresis and minimize renal toxicity

IV Intermittent INF route

• Using inf device, at no more than 1 mg/kg/min; do not give by rapid or bolus IV; give by CVP or peripheral vein; standard 24 mg/ml sol may be used without dilution if using by CVP; dilute the 24 mg/ml sol to 12 mg/ml with D_5W or NS if using peripheral vein

Y-site compatibilities: Aldesleukin, amikacin, aminophylline, ampicillin, aztreonam, benzquinamide, cefazolin, cefoperazone, cefoxitin, ceftazidime, ceftizoxime, ceftriaxone, cefuroxime, chloramphenicol, cimetidine, clindamycin, dexamethasone, DOPamine, erythromycin, fluconazole, flucytosine, furosemide, gentamicin, heparin, hydrocortisone, hydromorphone, hydrOXYzine, imipenem-cilastatin, metoclopramide, metronidazole, miconazole, morphine, nafcillin, oxacillin, penicillin G potassium, phenytoin, piperacillin, ranitidine, ticarcillin/clavulanate, tobramycin

Perform/provide:

• Regular ophthalmologic exams

• Close monitoring during therapy for tingling, numbness, paresthesias; if these occur, stop infusion, obtain lab sample for electrolytes

F

Side effects: *italics* = common; ***bold italics*** = life-threatening

Evaluate:

• Therapeutic response: improvement in CMV retinitis

Teach patient/family:

• To call prescriber if sore throat, swollen lymph nodes, malaise, fever occur, since other infections may occur

• To report perioral tingling, numbness in extremities, and paresthesias

• That serious drug interactions may occur if OTC products are ingested; check first with prescriber

• That drug is not a cure but will control symptoms

---

fosinopril (℞)
(foss'in-oh-pril)
Monopril
Func. class.: Antihypertensive
Chem. class.: Angiotensin-converting enzyme (ACE) inhibitor

Do not confuse:

Monopril/minoxidil/Accupril/Monoket

Action: Selectively suppresses renin-angiotensin-aldosterone system; inhibits ACE; prevents conversion of angiotensin I to angiotensin II; results in dilation of arterial, venous vessels

Uses: Hypertension, alone or in combination with thiazide diuretics, systolic CHF

DOSAGE AND ROUTES

CHF

• *Adult:* PO 10 mg daily, then up to 40 mg/day increased over several wk; use lower dose in those diuresed before fosinopril

Hypertension

• *Adult:* PO 10 mg daily initially, then 20-40 mg/day divided bid or daily, max 80 mg/day

Available forms: Tabs 10, 20, 40 mg

SIDE EFFECTS

CNS: Insomnia, paresthesia, headache, dizziness, fatigue, memory disturbance, tremor, mood change
CV: Hypotension, chest pain, palpita-

tions, angina, orthostatic hypotension, dysrhythmias, tachycardia
GI: Nausea, constipation, vomiting, diarrhea
*GU: **Proteinuria,*** increased BUN, creatinine, decreased libido
HEMA: Decreased Hct, Hgb; ***eosinophilia, leukopenia, neutropenia***
*INTEG: **Angioedema,*** rash, flushing, sweating, photosensitivity, pruritus
META: Hyperkalemia
MS: Arthralgia, myalgia
RESP: Cough, sinusitis, dyspnea, ***bronchospasm***

Contraindications: Pregnancy (D) 2nd/3rd trimester, hypersensitivity to ACE inhibitors, lactation, children
Precautions: Impaired hepatic function, hypovolemia, blood dyscrasias, CHF, COPD, asthma, elderly

PHARMACOKINETICS

PO: Peak 2-6 hr; serum protein binding 97%; half-life 12 hr; metabolized by liver (metabolites excreted in urine, feces)

INTERACTIONS

Hypersensitivity reactions: allopurinol
Increase: hypotension—diuretics, other antihypertensives, ganglionic blockers, adrenergic blockers, phenothiazines, nitrates, acute alcohol ingestion
Increase: toxicity—vasodilators, hydrALAZINE, prazosin, potassium-sparing diuretics, sympathomimetics, digoxin, lithium
Decrease: absorption—antacids
Decrease: antihypertensive effect—indomethacin

Drug/Herb

Severe photosensitivity: St. John's wort
Fatal hypokalemia: arginine
Increase: antihypertensive effect—pill-bearing spurge
Decrease: antihypertensive effect—pineapple, yohimbe

Drug/Lab Test

Increase: AST, ALT, alk phosphatase, glucose, bilirubin, uric acid

---

False-positive: Urine acetone
Positive: ANA titer

NURSING CONSIDERATIONS
Assess:

• Blood studies: neutrophils, decreased platelets; obtain WBC with diff baseline and qmo × 6 mo, then q2-3 mo × 1 yr; if neutrophils <1000/mm³, discontinue (recommended in collagen-vascular disease)
• B/P, orthostatic hypotension, syncope
• Renal studies: protein, BUN, creatinine; increased levels may indicate nephrotic syndrome
• Baselines in renal, hepatic studies before therapy begins
• Potassium levels, although hyperkalemia rarely occurs
• Edema in feet, legs daily, weigh daily in CHF
• Allergic reactions: rash, fever, pruritus, urticaria; drug should be discontinued if antihistamines fail to help

Administer:
• May be taken without regard to meals
Perform/provide:
• Storage in tight container at 86° F (30° C) or less
• Supine position for severe hypotension
Evaluate:
• Therapeutic response: decrease in B/P
Teach patient/family:
• Not to discontinue drug abruptly
• Not to use OTC products (cough, cold, allergy) unless directed by prescriber; not to use salt substitutes containing potassium without consulting prescriber
• The importance of complying with dosage schedule, even if feeling better
• To rise slowly to sitting or standing position to minimize orthostatic hypotension
• To notify prescriber of mouth sores, sore throat, fever, swelling of hands or feet, irregular heartbeat, chest pain
• To report excessive perspiration, dehydration, vomiting, diarrhea; may lead to fall in B/P

• That drug may cause dizziness, fainting, light-headedness during first few days of therapy
• That drug may cause skin rash or impaired perspiration
• How to take B/P; normal readings for age-group
• To notify prescriber if pregnancy is planned or suspected
Treatment of overdose: 0.9% NaCl IV inf, hemodialysis

fosphenytoin (℞)
(foss-fen'i-toy-in)
Cerebyx
Func. class.: Anticonvulsant
Chem. class.: Hydantoin

Action: Inhibits spread of seizure activity in motor cortex by altering ion transport; increases AV conduction
Uses: Generalized tonic-clonic seizures; status epilepticus

DOSAGE AND ROUTES
Status epilepticus
• *Adult and child:* **IV** loading dose 15-20 mg PE/kg given at 100-150 mg PE/min (PE = phenytoin equivalent)
Nonemergent/maintenance dosing
• *Adult and child:* **IV/IM** loading dose 10-20 mg PE/kg; maintenance dosing 4-6 mg PE/kg/day given at a rate of <150 mg PE/min
Available forms: Inj 150 mg (100 mg phenytoin equiv), 750 mg (500 mg phenytoin equiv)

SIDE EFFECTS
CNS: Drowsiness, dizziness, insomnia, paresthesias, depression, suicidal tendencies, aggression, headache, confusion
CV: Hypotension, ***ventricular fibrillation***
EENT: Nystagmus, diplopia, blurred vision
GI: Nausea, vomiting, diarrhea, constipation, anorexia, weight loss, hepatitis, jaundice, gingival hyperplasia
HEMA: ***Agranulocytosis, leukope-***

nia, aplastic anemia, thrombocy-topenia, megaloblastic anemia
INTEG: Rash, lupus erythematosus, *Stevens-Johnson syndrome*, hirsutism
SYST: Hyperglycemia
Contraindications: Pregnancy (D), hypersensitivity, psychiatric conditions, bradycardia, SA and AV block, Stokes-Adams syndrome
Precautions: Allergies, hepatic disease, renal disease, lactation, myocardial insufficiency

PHARMACOKINETICS

Metabolized by liver, excreted by kidneys

INTERACTIONS

Increase: fosphenytoin level—cimetidine, amiodarone, chloramphenicol, estrogens, H_2 antagonists, phenothiazines, salicylates, sulfonamides, tricyclics
Decrease: fosphenytoin effects—alcohol (chronic use), antihistamines, antacids, antineoplastics, rifampin, folic acid, carbamazepine, theophylline
Drug/Herb
Increase: anticonvulsant effect—ginkgo
Decrease: anticonvulsant effect—ginseng, santonica, valerian
Drug/Lab Test
Increase: Glucose, alk phosphatase
Decrease: Dexamethasone, metyrapone test serum, PBI, urinary steroids

NURSING CONSIDERATIONS
Assess:
• Drug level: toxic level 30-50 mcg/ml, wait at least 2 hr after dose before testing
• Blood studies: CBC, platelets q2wk until stabilized, then qmo × 12 mo, then q3mo; discontinue drug if neutrophils <1600/mm³, serum calcium albumin, phosphorus
• Mental status: mood, sensorium, affect, memory (long, short)
• Seizure activity including type, location, duration, and character; provide seizure precaution
• Renal studies; urinalysis, BUN, urine creatinine
• Hepatic studies: ALT, AST, bilirubin, creatinine
• Allergic reaction: red raised rash; if this occurs, drug should be discontinued
• For toxicity: bone marrow depression, nausea, vomiting, ataxia, diplopia, cardiovascular collapse, slurred speech, confusion
• Respiratory depression; rate, depth, character of respirations
⚠ Blood dyscrasias: fever, sore throat, bruising, rash, jaundice
• Continuous monitoring of ECG, B/P, respiratory function
• Rash, discontinue as soon as rash develops, serious adverse reactions such as Stevens-Johnson syndrome can occur
Administer:
IV route
• Dilute in D_5 or 0.9% NaCl to 1.5-25 mg PE/ml, give <150 mg PE/min
Y-site compatibilities: Esmolol, famotidine, foscarnet
Additive compatibilities: Potassium chloride
Solution compatibilities: D_5W, $D_{10}W$, amino acid inj 10%, D_5LR, D_5/0.9% NaCl, Plasmalyte A, LR, sterile water for inj
Evaluate:
• Therapeutic response: decrease in severity of seizures
Teach patient/family:
• The reason for and expected outcome of treatment
• Not to use machinery or engage in hazardous activity, as drowsiness, dizziness may occur
• To carry emergency ID denoting drug use, name of prescriber
• To notify prescriber of rash, bleeding, bruising, slurred speech, jaundice of skin or eyes, joint pain, nausea, vomiting, severe headaches
• To keep all medical appointments, including lab work, physical assessment

---

⚠ Safety alert   *"Tall Man" lettering

- To notify prescriber if pregnancy is planned, suspected
- To use contraception while using this product

frovatriptan (Ŗ)
(froh-vah-trip′tan)
Frova
Func. class.: Antimigraine agent
Chem. class.: 5-HT$_1$-Receptor agonist

Action: Binds selectively to the vascular 5-HT$_{1B}$, 5-HT$_{1D}$ receptor subtypes, exerts antimigraine effect; binds to benzodiazepine receptor sites, causes vasoconstriction in cranium

Uses: Acute treatment of migraine with or without aura

DOSAGE AND ROUTES

- *Adult:* **PO** 2.5 mg, a 2nd dose may be taken after ≥2 hr; max 3 tabs (7.5 mg/day)

Available form: Tabs 2.5 mg

SIDE EFFECTS

CNS: Hot/cold sensation, paresthesia, *dizziness,* headache, fatigue
CV: Flushing, chest pain, palpitation
GI: Dry mouth, dyspepsia, abdominal pain, diarrhea, vomiting
MS: Skeletal pain

Contraindications: Hypersensitivity, angina pectoris, history of MI, documented silent ischemia, Prinzmetal's angina, ischemic heart disease; concurrent ergotamine-containing preparations; uncontrolled hypertension; basilar or hemiplegic migraine; ischemic bowel disease; peripheral vascular disease, severe hepatic disease, prophylactic migraine treatment

Precautions: Pregnancy (C), postmenopausal women, men >40 yr, risk factors for CAD, hypercholesterolemia, obesity, diabetes, impaired hepatic function, lactation, children, elderly, seizure disorder

PHARMACOKINETICS

Onset of pain relief 10 min-2 hr, terminal half-life 25-29 hr, protein binding 15%

INTERACTIONS

Increase: frovatriptan levels—CYP1A2 inhibitors (cimetidine, ciprofloxacin, erythromycin); estrogen, propranolol
Increase: toxicity—SSRIs, other serotonin agonists (dextromethorphan, tramadol, antidepressants)
Drug/Herb
Increase: effect—butterbur

NURSING CONSIDERATIONS
Assess:
- B/P; signs/symptoms of coronary vasospasms
- For stress level, activity, recreation, coping mechanisms
- Neurologic status: LOC, paresthesia, hot/cold sensations, dizziness, headache, fatigue
- Ingestion of tyramine-containing foods (pickled products, beer, wine, aged cheese), food additives, preservatives, colorings, artificial sweeteners, chocolate, caffeine, which may precipitate these types of headaches

Administer:
- Swallow tabs whole; do not break, crush, or chew

Perform/provide:
- Quiet, calm environment with decreased stimulation from noise, bright light, excessive talking

Evaluate:
- Therapeutic response: decrease in frequency, severity of migraine

Teach patient/family:
- To report any side effects to prescriber
- To use contraception while taking drug; inform prescriber if pregnant or intend to become pregnant
- To have dark, quiet environment available
- Consult prescriber if breastfeeding

fulvestrant (℞)

(full-vess'trant)
Faslodex
Func. class.: Antineoplastic
Chem. class.: Antiestrogen hormone

Action: Inhibits cell division by binding to cytoplasmic estrogen receptors
Uses: Advanced breast carcinoma in estrogen-receptor-positive patients (usually postmenopausal)

DOSAGE AND ROUTES

• *Adult:* **IM** 250 mg qmo
Available forms: Inj 50 mg/ml

SIDE EFFECTS

CNS: Headache, depression, dizziness, insomnia, paresthesia, anxiety
GI: Nausea, vomiting, anorexia, constipation, diarrhea, abdominal pain
INTEG: Rash, sweating, hot flashes, inj site pain
MS: Bone pain, arthritis, back pain
RESP: Pharyngitis, dyspnea, cough
Contraindications: Pregnancy (D), hypersensitivity
Precautions: Lactation, children, hepatic disease

PHARMACOKINETICS

Half-life 40 days, metabolized by CYP3A4, excretion feces 90%

NURSING CONSIDERATIONS

Assess:
• For side effects, report to prescriber
Administer:
• IM 5 ml as a single inj or 2, 2.5 ml inj; give slowly in buttock
• Antiemetic 30-60 min before giving drug to prevent vomiting prn
Perform/provide:
• Liquid diet, if needed, including cola, gelatin; dry toast or crackers may be added if patient is not nauseated or vomiting
• Nutritious diet with iron, vitamin supplements as ordered
• Store in refrigerator, protect from light

Evaluate:
• Therapeutic response: decreased tumor size, spread of malignancy
Teach patient/family:
• To report any complaints, side effects to prescriber
• To report vaginal bleeding immediately
• That tumor flare—increase in size of tumor, increased bone pain—may occur and will subside rapidly; may take analgesics for pain
• That premenopausal women must use mechanical birth control because ovulation may be induced

furosemide (℞)

(fur-oh'se-mide)
Apo-Furosemide ✦,
Furoside ✦, Lasix, Lasix
Special ✦, Myrosemide ✦,
Novosemide ✦, Uritol ✦
Func. class.: Loop diuretic
Chem. class.: Sulfonamide derivative

Do not confuse:
furosemide/torsemide
Lasix/Luvox/Lomotil
Lasix/Lanoxin
Action: Inhibits reabsorption of sodium and chloride at proximal and distal tubule and in the loop of Henle
Uses: Pulmonary edema; edema in CHF, hepatic disease, nephrotic syndrome, ascites, hypertension
Investigational uses: Hypercalcemia in malignancy

DOSAGE AND ROUTES

• *Adult:* **PO** 20-80 mg/day in AM; may give another dose in 6 hr up to 600 mg/day; **IM/IV** 20-40 mg, increased by 20 mg q2h until desired response
• *Child:* **PO/IM/IV** 2 mg/kg; may increase by 1-2 mg/kg/q6-8h up to 6 mg/kg
Pulmonary edema
• *Adult:* **IV** 40 mg given over several min, repeated in 1 hr; increase to 80 mg if needed

⚠ Safety alert   *"Tall Man" lettering

Hypertensive crisis/acute renal failure
• *Adult:* **IV** 100-200 mg over 1-2 min
Antihypercalcemia
• *Adult:* **IM/IV** 80-100 mg q1-4h or **PO** 120 mg daily or divided bid
• *Child:* **IM/IV** 25-50 mg, repeat q4h if needed

Available forms: Tabs 20, 40, 80 mg; oral sol 10 mg/ml, 40 mg/5 ml; inj 10 mg/ml

SIDE EFFECTS

CNS: Headache, fatigue, weakness, vertigo, paresthesias
CV: Orthostatic hypotension, chest pain, ECG changes, ***circulatory collapse***
EENT: ***Loss of hearing,*** ear pain, tinnitus, blurred vision
ELECT: Hypokalemia, hypochloremic alkalosis, hypomagnesemia, hyperuricemia, hypocalcemia, hyponatremia, metabolic alkalosis
ENDO: Hyperglycemia
GI: Nausea, diarrhea, dry mouth, vomiting, anorexia, cramps, oral, gastric irritations, pancreatitis
GU: Polyuria, ***renal failure,*** glycosuria
HEMA: ***Thrombocytopenia, agranulocytosis, leukopenia, neutropenia, anemia***
INTEG: Rash, pruritus, purpura, ***Stevens-Johnson syndrome,*** sweating, photosensitivity, urticaria
MS: Cramps, stiffness

Contraindications: Hypersensitivity to sulfonamides, anuria, hypovolemia, infants, lactation, electrolyte depletion
Precautions: Pregnancy (C), diabetes mellitus, dehydration, severe renal disease, cirrhosis, ascites

PHARMACOKINETICS

PO: Onset 1 hr, peak 1-2 hr, duration 6-8 hr; absorbed 70%
IV: Onset 5 min, peak ½ hr, duration 2 hr (metabolized by the liver 30%); excreted in urine, some as unchanged drug, feces; crosses placenta; excreted in breast milk; half-life ½-1 hr

INTERACTIONS

Increase: toxicity—lithium, nondepolarizing skeletal muscle relaxants, digitalis
Increase: hypotensive action of antihypertensives, nitrates
Increase: ototoxicity—aminoglycosides, cisplatin, vancomycin
Drug/Herb
Severe photosensitivity: St. John's wort
Increase: diuretic effect—aloe, cucumber, dandelion, khella, horsetail, pumpkin, Queen Anne's lace
Drug/Lab Test
Interference: GTT

NURSING CONSIDERATIONS
Assess:
• Signs of metabolic alkalosis: drowsiness, restlessness
• Signs of hypokalemia: postural hypotension, malaise, fatigue, tachycardia, leg cramps, weakness
• Rashes, temp elevation daily
• Confusion, especially in elderly; take safety precautions if needed
• Hearing, including tinnitus and hearing loss, when giving high doses for extended periods
• Weight, I&O daily to determine fluid loss; effect of drug may be decreased if used daily
• Rate, depth, rhythm of respiration, effect of exertion, lung sounds
• B/P lying, standing; postural hypotension may occur
• Electrolytes (K, Na, Cl); include BUN, blood glucose, CBC, serum creatinine, blood pH, ABGs, uric acid, calcium, magnesium
• Skin turgor, edema, condition of mucous membranes in mouth and nose
• Glucose in urine if patient is diabetic
• Allergies to sulfonamides, thiazides
Administer:
• In AM to avoid interference with sleep if using drug as a diuretic
• Potassium replacement if potassium <3 mg/dl
• PO with food if nausea occurs; absorp-

tion may be decreased slightly; tabs may be crushed

IV route

• Undiluted; may be given through Y-tube or 3-way stopcock; give 20 mg or less/min; may be added to NS or D₅W if large doses are required and given as IV inf, not to exceed 4 mg/min; use infusion pump

Additive compatibilities: Amikacin, aminophylline, ampicillin, atropine, bumetanide, calcium gluconate, cefamandole, cefoperazone, cefuroxime, cimetidine, cloxacillin, dexamethasone, diamorphine, digoxin, epINEPHrine, heparin, isosorbide, kanamycin, lidocaine, meropenem, morphine, nitroglycerin, penicillin G, potassium chloride, ranitidine, scopolamine, sodium bicarbonate, theophylline, tobramycin, verapamil

Syringe compatibilities: Bleomycin, cisplatin, cyclophosphamide, fluorouracil, heparin, leucovorin, methotrexate, mitomycin

Y-site compatibilities: Allopurinol, amifostine, amikacin, amphotericin B cholesteryl, aztreonam, bleomycin, cefepime, cefmetazole, cisplatin, cladribine, cyclophosphamide, cytarabine, DOXOrubicin liposome, epINEPHrine, fentanyl, fludarabine, fluorouracil, foscarnet, gallium, granisetron, heparin, hydrocortisone, hydromorphone, indomethacin, kanamycin, leucovorin, lorazepam, melphalan, meropenem, methotrexate, mitomycin, nitroglycerin, norepinephrine, paclitaxel, piperacillin/tazobactam, potassium chloride, propofol, ranitidine, remifentanil, sargramostim, tacrolimus, teniposide, thiotepa, tobramycin, tolazoline, vit B/C

Perform/provide:

• Increased fluid intake 2-3 L/day unless contraindicated

Evaluate:

• Therapeutic response: improvement in edema of feet, legs, sacral area daily if medication is being used for CHF

Teach patient/family:

• To discuss the need for a high-potassium diet or potassium replacement with prescriber

• To rise slowly from lying or sitting position; orthostatic hypotension may occur

• To recognize adverse reactions that may occur: muscle cramps, weakness, nausea, dizziness

• Regarding entire regimen, including exercise, diet, stress relief for hypertension

• To take with food or milk for GI symptoms

• To use sunscreen or protective clothing to prevent photosensitivity

• To take early in day to prevent sleeplessness

• To avoid OTC medication unless directed by prescriber

Treatment of overdose: Lavage if taken orally; monitor electrolytes; administer dextrose in saline; monitor hydration, CV, renal status

---

gabapentin (℞)

(gab′a-pen-tin)
Neurontin
Func. class.: Anticonvulsant

Do not confuse:
Neurontin/Noroxin/Neoral

Action: Mechanism unknown; may increase seizure threshold; structurally similar to GABA; gabapentin binding sites in neocortex, hippocampus

Uses: Adjunct treatment of partial seizures, with or without generalization in patients >12 yr; adjunct in partial seizures in children 3-12 yr, postherpetic neuralgia

Investigational uses: Tremors in multiple sclerosis, neuropathic pain, bipolar disorder, migraine prophylaxis, diabetic neuropathy

DOSAGE AND ROUTES

• *Adult and child >12 yr:* **PO** 900-1800 mg/day in 3 divided doses; may titrate by

---

giving 300 mg on first day, 300 mg bid on second day, 300 mg tid on third day; may increase to 1800 mg/day by adding 300 mg on subsequent days

• *Child 5-12 yr:* **PO** 10-15 mg/kg/day in 3 divided doses, initially titrate dose upward over approximately 3 days; 25-35 mg/kg/day; all given in 3 divided doses; rect 200 mg as single dose

• *Child 3-4 yr:* **PO** 10-15 mg/kg/day in 3 divided doses, initially titrate dose upward over approximately 3 days; 40 mg/kg/day; all given in 3 divided doses; rect 200 mg as single dose

Postherpetic neuralgia

• *Adult:* **PO** 300 mg on day 1, 600 mg/ day divided bid on day 2, 900 mg/day divided tid, may titrate to 1800 mg divided tid if needed

Renal dose

• *Adult and child >12 yr:* CCr 30-60 ml/min 300 mg bid, CCr 15-30 ml/min 300 mg daily, CCr <15 ml/min 125 mg daily

Available forms: Caps 100, 300, 400 mg; tabs 600, 800 mg; oral sol 250 mg/5 ml

SIDE EFFECTS

CNS: Dizziness, fatigue, anxiety, somnolence, ataxia, amnesia, abnormal thinking, unsteady gait, depression; 3-12 yr old, emotional lability, aggression, thought disorder, hyperkinesia
CV: Vasodilation, peripheral edema, hypotension
EENT: Dry mouth, blurred vision, *diplopia,* nystagmus
GI: Constipation, increased appetite, dental abnormalities, nausea, vomiting
GU: Impotence, bleeding, *UTI*
HEMA: **Leukopenia,** decreased WBC
INTEG: Pruritus, abrasion
MS: Myalgia
RESP: *Rhinitis,* pharyngitis, cough
Contraindications: Hypersensitivity to this drug
Precautions: Pregnancy (C), renal disease, lactation, children <12 yr, elderly, hemodialysis

PHARMACOKINETICS

Largely unbound to plasma proteins; not metabolized; excreted in urine (unchanged); elimination half-life 5-7 hr; prolonged to 130 hr in ESRD

INTERACTIONS

Increase: CNS depression—alcohol, sedatives, antihistamines, all other CNS depressants
Decrease: gabapentin levels—antacids
Drug/Herb
Increase: CNS depression—chamomile, hops, kava, skullcap, valerian
Drug/Lab Test
False-positive: Urinary protein using Ames N-multistix SG

NURSING CONSIDERATIONS

Assess:
• Seizures: aura, location, duration, activity at onset
• Pain: location, duration, characteristics if using for chronic pain
• Renal studies: urinalysis, BUN, urine creatinine q3mo
• Description of seizures; location, duration, characteristics
• Mental status: mood, sensorium, affect, behavioral changes; if mental status changes, notify prescriber
• Eye problems, need for ophthalmic exam before, during, after treatment (slit lamp, funduscopy, tonometry)
Administer:
• Do not crush or chew caps; caps may be opened and contents put in applesauce or dissolved in juice
• 2 hr apart when giving antacids
• Give without regard to meals
• Gradually withdraw over 7 days, abrupt withdrawal may precipitate seizures
Perform/provide:
• Storage at room temperature away from heat and light
• Hard candy, frequent rinsing of mouth, gum for dry mouth
• Assistance with ambulation during early part of treatment; dizziness occurs

---

- Seizure precautions: padded side rails; move objects that may harm patient
- Increased fluids, bulk in diet for constipation

Evaluate:
- Therapeutic response: decreased seizure activity; decrease in chronic pain

Teach patient/family:
- To carry emergency ID stating patient's name, drugs taken, condition, prescriber's name and phone number
- To avoid driving, other activities that require alertness: dizziness, drowsiness may occur
- Not to discontinue medication quickly after long-term use, taper over ≥1 wk; withdrawal-precipitated seizures may occur, not to double doses if dose is missed, take if 2 hr or more before next dose
- To notify prescriber if pregnancy planned or suspected, avoid breastfeeding

Treatment of overdose: Lavage, VS

---

galantamine (℞)
(gah-lan'tah-meen)
Razadyne
Func. class.: Anti-Alzheimer agent, cholinesterase inhibitor

Action: May enhance cholinergic functioning by increasing acetylcholine
Uses: Mild to moderate dementia of Alzheimer's disease

DOSAGE AND ROUTES

- *Adult:* **PO** 4 mg bid with morning and evening meals; after 4 wk or more may increase to 8 mg bid; may increase to 12 mg bid after another 4 wk, usual dose 16-24 mg/day in 2 divided doses

Hepatic dose
- *Child-Pugh 7-9:* max 16 mg/day
- *Child-Pugh 10-15:* avoid use

Renal dose
- *Moderate renal impairment:* max 16 mg/day
- *CCr <9 ml/min:* avoid use

Available forms: Tabs 4, 8, 12 mg; oral sol 4 mg/ml

SIDE EFFECTS

CNS: Tremors, insomnia, depression, dizziness, headache, somnolence, fatigue
CV: Bradycardia, anemia, hematuria, chest pain
GI: Nausea, vomiting, anorexia, abdominal distress, flatulence, diarrhea
GU: Urinary incontinence, bladder outflow obstruction, hematuria
META: Weight decrease
MS: Asthenia, anemia
RESP: URI, rhinitis

Contraindications: Hypersensitivity to this drug
Precautions: Pregnancy (B), renal disease, hepatic disease, respiratory disease, seizure disorder, peptic ulcer, asthma, lactation, children

PHARMACOKINETICS

Rapidly and completely absorbed, metabolized by CYP450 enzyme, excreted via kidneys; clearance is lower in the elderly, hepatic disease; clearance is 20% lower in females, elimination half-life 7 hr

INTERACTIONS

Synergistic effect: cholinomimetics, other cholinesterase inhibitors
Increase: galantamine bioavailability—cimetidine, paroxetine, ketoconazole, erythromycin, quinidine, amitriptyline, fluvoxamine

Drug/Herb
Cholinergic antagonism: jimsonweed, scopolia
Increase: effect—pill-bearing spurge

NURSING CONSIDERATIONS

Assess:
- Hepatic studies: AST, ALT, alk phosphatase, LDH, bilirubin, CBC
- For severe GI effects: nausea, vomiting, anorexia, weight loss
- B/P, respiration during initial treatment

• Mental status: affect, mood, behavioral changes, depression

Administer:
• With meals; take with morning and evening meal
• Dose increase after minimum of 4 wk at prior dose

Perform/provide:
• Assistance with ambulation during beginning therapy
• Complete suicide assessment

Evaluate:
• Therapeutic response: decreased confusion

Teach patient/family:
• Correct procedure for giving oral solution, using instruction sheet provided
• To notify prescriber of severe GI effects
• To report hypo/hypertension

---

gallium (℞)
(gal'ee-um)
Ganite
Func. class.: Electrolyte modifier
Chem. class.: Hypocalcemic drug

Action: Lowers serum calcium levels by inhibiting calcium resorption from bone
Uses: Cancer-related hypercalcemia

DOSAGE AND ROUTES
• *Adult:* **IV** 100-200 mg/m² daily × 5 days; infuse over 24 hr, rest period of 2-4 wk between courses
Available forms: 25 mg/ml inj

SIDE EFFECTS
CV: Tachycardia, hypotension
EENT: Blurred vision, optic neuritis, hearing loss
GI: Nausea, vomiting, diarrhea, constipation, mucositis, metallic taste
GU: **Nephrotoxicity,** increased BUN, creatinine
HEMA: **Anemia, leukopenia, thrombocytopenia**
META: **Hypophosphatemia,** hypocalcemia, decreased serum bicarbonate
Contraindications: Hypersensitivity,

hypocalcemia, renal failure, severe renal disease (specific gravity >2.5 mg/dl)
Precautions: Pregnancy (C), lactation, children, mild renal disease, dehydration

PHARMACOKINETICS
IV: Onset 12-48 hr, peak 5 days, duration 4-14 days, excreted by kidneys

INTERACTIONS
Increase: nephrotoxicity—aminoglycosides, amphotericin B, cisplatin, foscarnet, ganciclovir, vancomycin

NURSING CONSIDERATIONS
Assess:
• Renal status: BUN, creatinine, urine output; if creatinine level is 2.5 mg/dl or more, drug should be discontinued
• Monitor calcium, phosphate, bicarbonate, since all levels may be decreased and supplements of phosphate may be needed
• For hypercalcemia: nausea, vomiting, fatigue, weakness, thirst, dehydration, dysrhythmias, change in mental status
• For hypocalcemia: dysrhythmias; paresthesia; twitching; colic; laryngospasm; Trousseau's, Chvostek's sign; tremors
• For hypophosphatemia: confusion, decreased reflexes, joint stiffness and pain, portal hypotension
Administer:
• Adequate hydration with IV saline, 2 L/day during treatment
• After dilution of dose/1 L 0.9% NaCl or D₅W, run over 24 hr, use infusion pump
Y-site compatibilities: Acyclovir, allopurinol, amifostine, aminophylline, ampicillin/sulbactam, aztreonam, cefazolin, ceftazidime, ceftriaxone, cimetidine, ciprofloxacin, cladribine, cyclophosphamide, dexamethasone, diphenhydrAMINE, filgrastim, fluconazole, furosemide, granisetron, heparin, hydrocortisone, ifosfamide, magnesium sulfate, mannitol, melphalan, meperidine, mesna, methotrexate, metoclopramide, ondansetron, piperacillin, piperacillin/tazobactam,

potassium chloride, ranitidine, sodium bicarbonate, teniposide, thiotepa, ticarcillin/clavulanate, trimethoprim-sulfamethoxazole, vancomycin, vinorelbine

Perform/provide:
• Storage of solution 48 hr at room temperature, 1 wk in refrigerator

Evaluate:
• Therapeutic response: decreased serum calcium levels

Teach patient/family:
• To follow dietary guidelines given by prescriber, including avoiding calcium (dairy products, broccoli) and vit D (fortified milk, grain products, fish oil)

galsulfase
See Appendix A—Selected New Drugs

ganciclovir (R)
(gan-sye'kloe-vir)
Cytovene, Vitrasert
Func. class.: Antiviral
Chem. class.: Synthetic nucleoside analog

Do not confuse:
Cytovene/Cytosar

Action: Inhibits replication of herpesviruses, competitively inhibits human CMV DNA polymerase and is incorporated resulting in termination of DNA elongation

Uses: Cytomegalovirus (CMV) retinitis in immunocompromised persons, including those with AIDS, after indirect ophthalmoscopy confirms diagnosis, prophylaxis CVM in transplantation

Investigational uses: CMV pneumonia in organ transplant patients, CMV gastroenteritis in patients with IBS, CMV pneumonitis

DOSAGE AND ROUTES

Renal dose
• Reduce dose in CCr <70 ml/min

Prevention of CMV
• *Adult:* **IV** 5 mg/kg/dose over 1 hr q12h × 1-2 wk, then 5 mg/kg/day 7 day/wk, then 6 mg/kg/day × 5 days/wk; **PO** 1000 mg tid

Induction treatment
• *Adult:* **IV** 5 mg/kg per dose given over 1 hr, q12h × 2-3 wk

Maintenance treatment
• *Adult:* **IV INF** 5 mg/kg daily given over 1 hr, daily × 7 days/wk; or 6 mg/kg daily × 5 days/wk; **PO** 1000 mg tid with food or 500 mg q3h while awake for 6 doses; **INTRAVITREAL:** 4.5 mg implant

Available forms: Powder for inj 500 mg/vial; caps 250, 500 mg; implant, intraviteral 4.5 mg

SIDE EFFECTS

CNS: Fever, chills, **coma, confusion,** abnormal thoughts, dizziness, bizarre dreams, *headache,* psychosis, tremors, somnolence, *paresthesia, weakness, seizures*
CV: Dysrhythmia, hyper/hypotension
EENT: Retinal detachment in CMV retinitis
GI: Abnormal LFTs, nausea, vomiting, anorexia, diarrhea, *abdominal pain, hemorrhage*
*GU: **Hematuria,** increased creatinine,* BUN
*HEMA: **Granulocytopenia, thrombocytopenia, irreversible neutropenia, anemia, eosinophilia***
INTEG: Rash, alopecia, *pruritus,* urticaria, pain at site, phlebitis, **Stevens-Johnson syndrome**
RESP: Dyspnea

Contraindications: Hypersensitivity to acyclovir or ganciclovir, absolute neutrophil count <500, platelet count <25,000

Precautions: Pregnancy (C), preexisting cytopenias, renal function impairment, lactation, children <6 mo, elderly

PHARMACOKINETICS

Half-life 3-4½ hr; excreted by kidneys (unchanged); crosses blood-brain barrier, CSF

INTERACTIONS

⚠ Severe granulocytopenia: zidovudine, antineoplastics, radiation; do not give together

Increase: ganciclovir toxicity—adriamycin, amphotericin B, cycloSPORINE, dapsone, DOXOrubicin, flucytosine, pentamidine, probenecid, trimethoprim-sulfamethoxazole combinations, vinBLASTine, vinCRIStine, or other nucleoside analogs

Increase: seizures—imipenem/cilastatin

Decrease: ganciclovir renal clearance—probenecid

Decrease: didanosine effect—ganciclovir

NURSING CONSIDERATIONS

Assess:

• For leukopenia/neutropenia/thrombocytopenia: WBCs, platelets q2d during 2 ×/day dosing and then q1wk
• For leukopenia with daily WBC count in patients with prior leukopenia with other nucleoside analogs or for whom leukopenia counts are <1000 cells/mm³ at start of treatment
• Serum creatinine or CCr ≥q2wk

Administer:

PO route

• With food

IV route

• Mixed in biologic cabinet, using gown, gloves, mask

Intermittent INF route

• IV after diluting 500 mg/10 ml sterile H₂O for inj (50 mg/ml); shake; further dilute in 100 ml D₅W, 0.9% NaCl, LR, Ringer's and run over 1 hr; use infusion pump, in-line filter
• Slowly; do not give by bolus IV, IM, SUBCUT inj
• Using reconstituted sol within 12 hr; do not refrigerate or freeze; infusion solution is stable for 14 days when refrigerated

Y-site compatibilities: Allopurinol, amphotericin B cholesteryl, cisplatin, cyclophosphamide, DOXOrubicin liposome, enalaprilat, etoposide, filgrastim, fluconazole, gatifloxacin, granisetron, linezolid, melphalan, methotrexate, paclitaxel, propofol, remifentanil, tacrolimus, teniposide, thiotepa

Evaluate:

• Therapeutic response: decreased symptoms of CMV

Teach patient/family:

• That drug does not cure condition, that regular blood tests, ophthalmologic exams are necessary
• That major toxicities may necessitate discontinuing drug
• To use contraception during treatment and that infertility may occur; should use barrier contraception for 90 days after treatment
• To take PO with food
⚠ To report infection: fever, chills, sore throat; blood dyscrasias: bruising, bleeding, petechiae
• To avoid crowds, persons with respiratory infections
• To use sunscreen to prevent burns

---

ganciclovir ophthalmic
See Appendix C

---

ganirelix (℞)
Antagon
Func. class.: Gonadotropin-releasing hormone antagonist
Chem. class.: Synthetic decapeptide

Action: Inhibitor of pituitary gonadotropin secretion; initially increases LH and FSH, induces a rapid suppression of gonadotropin secretion
Uses: For inhibition of premature LH surges in women undergoing controlled ovarian hyperstimulation

DOSAGE AND ROUTES

• *Adult:* SUBCUT 250 mcg daily during early to mid-follicular phase, continue until the day of hCG administration
Available forms: Inj 250 mcg/0.5 ml

SIDE EFFECTS

CNS: Headache

ENDO: Ovarian hyperstimulation syndrome, abdominal pain (gyn)

GI: Nausea

GU: Spotting, breakthrough bleeding

INTEG: Pain on inj

SYST: Fetal death

Contraindications: Pregnancy (X), hypersensitivity, latex allergy, lactation

PHARMACOKINETICS

Excreted in feces/urine, half-life 13-16 hr, metabolized to metabolites, protein binding 82%

NURSING CONSIDERATIONS

Assess:

• For suspected pregnancy, drug should not be used

• For latex allergy, drug should not be used

Administer:

• SUBCUT using abdomen, around navel or upper thigh, swab inj area with disinfectant, clean a 2-in circle and allow to dry, pinch up area between thumb and finger, insert needle at 45°-90° to surface, if positioned correctly, no blood will be drawn back into syringe, if blood is drawn into syringe, reposition needle without removing it

Perform/provide:

• Protection from light

Evaluate:

• Therapeutic response: pregnancy

Teach patient/family:

• To report abdominal pain, vaginal bleeding

---

gatifloxacin (℞)

(gat-ih-floks′ah-sin)

Tequin

Func. class.: Broad-spectrum antiinfective

Chem. class.: Fluoroquinolone

Action: Interferes with conversion of intermediate DNA fragments into high–molecular weight DNA in bacteria; DNA gyrase inhibitor

Uses: Infection caused by susceptible *Escherichia coli, Staphylococcus aureus, Haemophilus influenzae, Haemophilus parainfluenzae, Klebsiella pneumoniae, Moraxella catarrhalis, Neisseria gonorrhoeae, Proteus mirabilis,* and other microorganisms: *Chlamydia pneumoniae, Legionella pneumophila, Mycoplasma pneumoniae* causing acute bacterial exacerbation of chronic bronchitis, acute sinusitis, community-acquired respiratory tract infections, gonorrhea

Investigational uses: Multidrug-resistant *Streptococcus pneumoniae* in children with acute otitis media, sinusitis; *Mycobacterium leprae,* atypical pneumonia, uncomplicated skin, soft tissue infections, chronic prostatitis

DOSAGE AND ROUTES

Renal dose

• CCr ≥40 ml/min 400 mg daily; <40 ml/min 200 mg daily after 400 mg initially; hemodialysis 200 mg daily after 400 mg initially

Uncomplicated urinary tract infections

• *Adult:* **PO/IV** 400 mg single dose

Complicated/severe urinary tract infections

• *Adult:* **PO/IV** 400 mg × 7-10 days

Chronic bronchitis

• *Adult:* **PO/IV** 400 mg × 5 days

Acute sinusitis

• *Adult:* **PO/IV** 400 mg × 10 days

Community-acquired pneumonia

• *Adult:* **PO/IV** 400 mg × 7-14 days

Gonorrhea

• *Adult:* **PO/IV** 400 mg single dose

Available forms: Tabs 200, 400 mg; inj 20 ml (200 mg), 40 ml (400 mg); inj premix 200, 400 mg

SIDE EFFECTS

CNS: Headache, dizziness, insomnia, paresthesia, tremor, vasodilation

ENDO: Increased blood glucose

GI: Nausea, diarrhea, increased ALT,

AST, *pseudomembranous colitis, hepatotoxicity*
INTEG: Rash, pruritus, urticaria, photosensitivity, flushing, fever, chills
RESP: Dyspnea, pharyngitis
SYST: Anaphylaxis, Stevens-Johnson syndrome
Contraindications: Hypersensitivity to quinolones, severe hepatic disease
Precautions: Pregnancy (C), lactation, children, renal disease

PHARMACOKINETICS

Half-life 6½-14 hr; excreted in urine unchanged, protein binding 20%, peak 1-2 hr (PO) depending on dose, duration 24 hr

INTERACTIONS

Increase: gatifloxacin serum levels— probenecid, cimetidine
Increase: warfarin level
Increase: nephrotoxicity risk— cycloSPORINE
Decrease: gatifloxacin absorption— magnesium antacids, aluminum hydroxide, sucralfate, calcium

NURSING CONSIDERATIONS
Assess:
• CNS symptoms: headache, dizziness, insomnia
• Renal, hepatic studies, blood glucose: BUN, creatinine, AST, ALT
• I&O ratio, urine pH <5.5 is ideal
• Allergic reactions and anaphylaxis: fever, flushing, rash, urticaria, pruritus, emergency equipment should be nearby
Administer:
PO route
• 2 hr before or 4 hr after aluminum or magnesium antacids, zinc, iron
IV route
• Do not use flexible containers in series connections, air embolism may occur
• Do not use if particulate matter is present
• Do not admix with other drugs
• Dilute with compatible sol to 2 mg/ml

before administration, give over 1 hr; do not give by bolus or rapid IV
Solution compatibilities: D$_5$, 0.9% NaCl, D$_5$/0.9% NaCl, LR/D$_5$, water for inj
Perform/provide:
• Limited intake of aluminum, magnesium containing antacids; iron
• Increase fluid intake to 2 L/day to prevent crystalluria
Evaluate:
• Therapeutic response: decreased pain, frequency, urgency, C&S; absence of infection
Teach patient/family:
• Not to take any products containing magnesium or aluminum (such as antacids) or iron with this drug or within 4 hr of drug
• That photosensitivity may occur; patient should avoid sunlight or use sunscreen to prevent burns
• If dizziness occurs, to ambulate, perform activities with assistance
• To contact prescriber if adverse reaction occurs or if inflammation or pain in tendon occurs
• To use frequent rinsing of mouth, sugarless candy, or gum for dry mouth
• To avoid other medications unless approved by prescriber
• To take as prescribed, not to double or miss doses, to take all medications

---

gatifloxacin ophthalmic
See Appendix C

---

gefitinib (℞)
(ge-fi'tye-nib)
Iressa
Func. class.: Antineoplastic— miscellaneous
Chem. class.: Epidermal growth factor receptor inhibitor

Action: Not fully understood. Inhibits intracellular phosphorylation of cell surface receptors associated with epidermal growth factor receptors.

Uses: Advanced/metastatic non–small cell lung cancer (NSCLC) in those that have not responded to platinum or docetaxel products

DOSAGE AND ROUTES
• *Adult:* **PO** 250 mg daily
CYP3A4 inducers concurrently (such as rifampin or phenytoin)
• *Adult:* **PO** 500 mg daily
Available forms: Tabs 250 mg

SIDE EFFECTS
GI: Nausea, diarrhea, vomiting, anorexia, ***pancreatitis,*** mouth ulceration
INTEG: Rash, pruritus, *acne, dry skin,* ***toxic epidermal neurolysis, angioedema***
MISC: Peripheral edema, amblyopia, conjunctivitis, eye pain, corneal erosion/ulcer
*RESP: **Interstitial lung disease,*** cough, dyspnea
Contraindications: Pregnancy (D), hypersensitivity
Precautions: Renal, hepatic, ocular, pulmonary disorders, lactation, children, elderly

PHARMACOKINETICS
Slowly absorbed, excreted in feces (86%), urine (<4%); elimination half-life 48 hr, metabolism by CYP3A4

INTERACTIONS
Increase: Gefitinib concentrations—ketoconazole, itraconazole, erythromycin, clarithromycin
Increase: plasma concentration of warfarin, metoprolol
Decrease: Gefitinib levels—phenytoin, rifampin, cimetidine, ranitidine, sodium bicarbonate

NURSING CONSIDERATIONS
Assess:
⚠ Pulmonary changes: lung sounds, cough, dyspnea; interstitial lung disease may occur, may be fatal; discontinue therapy if confirmed

• Ocular changes: eye irritation, corneal erosion/ulcer, aberrant eyelash growth
⚠ Pancreatitis: abdominal pain, levels of amylase, lipase
⚠ Toxic epidermal necrosis, angioedema
• GI symptoms: frequency of stools, if diarrhea is poorly tolerated, therapy may be discontinued for up to 14 days
Administer:
• Without regard to food
Evaluate:
• Therapeutic response: decreased non–small cell lung cancer cells
Teach patient/family:
⚠ To report adverse reactions immediately: SOB, severe abdominal pain, ocular changes, skin eruptions
• Reason for treatment, expected results
• Use contraception during treatment

---

gemcitabine (℞)
(jem-sit′a-been)
Gemzar
Func. class.: Antineoplastic—miscellaneous
Chem. class.: Nucleoside analog

Do not confuse:
Gemzar/Zinecard
Action: Exhibits antitumor activity by killing cells undergoing DNA synthesis (S-phase) and blocking G1/S-phase boundary
Uses: Adenocarcinoma of the pancreas (nonresectable stage II, III, or metastatic stage IV); non–small cell lung cancer (stage IIIA or B, IV); in combination with cisplatin for inoperable, advanced, or metastatic non–small cell lung cancer

DOSAGE AND ROUTES
Pancreatic carcinoma
• *Adult:* **IV** 1000 mg/m² given over ½ hr qwk × 7 wk, then 1 wk rest period; subsequent cycles should be infused once qwk × 3 wk out of every 4 wk
Non–small cell lung cancer
4-wk schedule:
• *Adult:* **IV** 1000 mg/m² given over ½ hr

on days 1, 8, 15, of each 28-day cycle. Give cisplatin **IV** 100 mg/m² on day 1 after gemcitabine

3-wk schedule:

• *Adult:* **IV** 1250 mg/m² given over ½ hr on days 1, 8 of each 21-day cycle. Give cisplatin 100 mg/m² after the inf of gemcitabine on day 1

Available forms: Lyophilized powder for inj 20 mg/ml

SIDE EFFECTS

GI: Diarrhea, nausea, vomiting, anorexia, constipation, stomatitis

GU: Proteinuria, hematuria

HEMA: **Leukopenia, anemia, neutropenia, thrombocytopenia**

INTEG: Irritation at site, rash, alopecia

OTHER: Dyspnea, fever, **hemorrhage,** infection, flulike symptoms, paresthesia

Contraindications: Pregnancy (D), hypersensitivity, lactation

Precautions: Children, elderly, myelosuppression, irradiation, renal/hepatic disease

PHARMACOKINETICS

Half-life 42-79 min, crosses placenta

INTERACTIONS

Increase: bleeding—NSAIDs, alcohol, salicylates

Increase: myelosuppression, diarrhea—other antineoplastics, radiation

Decrease: antibody response—live virus vaccines

NURSING CONSIDERATIONS

Assess:

• CBC, differential, platelet count before each dose; absolute granulocyte count >1000, platelets >100,000, give complete dose; absolute granulocyte count 500-1000, platelets 50,000-100,000, give 75%; absolute granulocyte count <500, platelets <50,000, do not give

• Blood dyscrasias: bruising, bleeding, petechiae

• I&O, nutritional intake; food preferences: list likes, dislikes

• Renal, hepatic studies before and during treatment; may increase AST, ALT, alk phosphatase, bilirubin, BUN, creatinine

• Buccal cavity q8h for dryness, sores/ulceration, white patches, oral pain, bleeding, dysphagia

• GI symptoms: frequency of stools; cramping

• Signs of dehydration: rapid respirations, poor skin turgor, decreased urine output, dry skin, restlessness, weakness

Administer:

• Prepare in biologic cabinet using gown, mask, gloves

• After reconstituting with 0.9% NaCl 5 ml/200 mg vial of drug or 25 ml/1 g of drug, shake = 40 mg/ml may be further diluted with 0.9% NaCl to conc as low as 0.1 mg/ml; discard unused portions, give over ½ hr, do not admix

Perform/provide:

• Increased fluid intake to 2-3 L/day to prevent dehydration, unless contraindicated

• Changing of IV site q48h

• Rinsing of mouth tid-qid with water, club soda; brushing of teeth bid-tid with soft brush or cotton-tipped applicator for stomatitis; use unwaxed dental floss

• Nutritious diet with iron, vitamin supplement, low fiber, few dairy products

Evaluate:

• Therapeutic response: decrease in tumor size, decrease in spread of cancer

Teach patient/family:

• To avoid foods with citric acid or hot or rough texture if stomatitis is present; to drink adequate fluids

• To avoid use with NSAIDs, alcohol, salicylates

• To report stomatitis; any bleeding, white spots, ulcerations in mouth; tell patient to examine mouth daily, report symptoms

• To report signs of anemia: fatigue, headache, faintness, shortness of breath, irritability; hematuria, dysuria

• To use contraception during therapy and for 4 mo after
• Not to receive vaccinations during treatment

gemfibrozil (R)

(jem-fi'broe-zil)
gemfibrozil, Lopid
Func. class.: Antilipemic
Chem. class.: Fibric acid derivative

Do not confuse:
Lopid/Levbid/Slo-bid
Action: Inhibits biosynthesis of VLDL, decreases triglycerides, increases HDL
Uses: Type IIb, IV, V hyperlipidemia as adjunct with diet therapy

DOSAGE AND ROUTES

• *Adult:* **PO** 1200 mg in divided doses bid 30 min before AM, PM meal
Available forms: Tabs 600 mg

SIDE EFFECTS

CNS: Fatigue, vertigo, headache, paresthesia, dizziness, somnolence
GI: *Dyspepsia, diarrhea, abdominal pain,* nausea, vomiting
HEMA: **Leukopenia, anemia, eosinophilia, thrombocytopenia**
INTEG: Rash, urticaria, pruritus
MISC: Taste perversion
Contraindications: Severe hepatic disease, preexisting gallbladder disease, severe renal disease, primary biliary cirrhosis, hypersensitivity
Precautions: Pregnancy (C), monitor hematologic and hepatic function, lactation

PHARMACOKINETICS

PO: Peak 1-2 hr; plasma protein binding >90%; half-life 1½ hr; 70% excreted in urine as conjugate; <2% excreted unchanged; metabolized in liver (minimal)

INTERACTIONS

Increase: hypoglycemic effect—sulfonylureas

Increase: anticoagulant properties—oral anticoagulants
Increase: risk of myositis, myalgia—HMG-CoA reductase inhibitors
Decrease: effect of cycloSPORINE
Drug/Herb
Increase: effect—glucomannan
Decrease: effect—gotu kola
Drug/Lab Test
Increase: LFTs, CPK, BSP, thymol turbidity, glucose
Decrease: Hgb, Hct, WBC

NURSING CONSIDERATIONS

Assess:
• Triglycerides, cholesterol; if lipids increase, drug should be discontinued; LDL, VLDL baseline and periodically
• Renal, hepatic studies, CBC, blood glucose if patient is on long-term therapy; if LFTs increase, therapy should be discontinued
• Bowel pattern daily; watch for increasing diarrhea (common)
Administer:
• 30 min before morning and evening meals
Evaluate:
• Therapeutic response: decreased cholesterol, triglyceride levels, HDL, cholesterol ratios improved
Teach patient/family:
• That compliance is needed for positive results; do not double or skip dose
• That risk factors should be decreased: high-fat diet, smoking, alcohol consumption, absence of exercise
• To notify prescriber of diarrhea, nausea, vomiting, chills, fever, sore throat, muscle cramps, abdominal cramps, severe flatulence
• That drug may be discontinued if no improvement in 3 mo

A Safety alert　　*"Tall Man" lettering

gemifloxacin (R)

(gem-ah-flox′a-sin)
Factive
Func. class.: Antiinfective
Chem. class.: Fluoroquinolone

Action: Inhibits DNA gyrase which is an enzyme involved in replication, transcription and repair of bacterial DNA

Uses: Acute bacterial exacerbation of chronic bronchitis caused by *Streptococcus pneumoniae, Haemophilus influenzae, Haemophilus parainfluenzae, Moraxella catarrhalis*; community acquired pneumonia caused by *Streptococcus pneumoniae* including multidrug resistant strains, *H. influenzae, M. catarrhalis, Mycoplasma pneumoniae, Chlamydia pneumoniae, Klebsiella pneumoniae*

DOSAGE AND ROUTES

• *Adult:* **PO** 320 mg/day × 5-7 days depending on type of infection
Renal dose
• *Adult:* **PO** CCr ≤40 ml/min 160 mg q24hr
Available forms: Tabs 320 mg

SIDE EFFECTS

CNS: Dizziness, headache, somnolence, depression, insomnia, nervousness, confusion, agitation, ***seizures***
EENT: Visual disturbances
GI: Diarrhea, *nausea,* vomiting, anorexia, flatulence, heartburn, dry mouth; increased AST, ALT; constipation, abdominal pain, oral thrush, glossitis, stomatitis, ***pseudomembranous colitis***
INTEG: Rash, pruritus, urticaria, *photosensitivity*
SYST: ***Anaphylaxis, Stevens-Johnson syndrome***

Contraindications: Hypersensitivity to quinolones
Precautions: Pregnancy (C), hypokalemia, hypomagnesium, lactation, children, elderly, renal disease, seizure disorders, excessive exposure to sunlight, psychosis, increased intracranial pressure, history of arrhythmias, history of QT interval prolongation, dysrhythmias

PHARMACOKINETICS

PO: Peak 1-2 hr, half-life 6-8 hr; excreted in urine as active drug, metabolites

INTERACTIONS

May increase toxicity of gemifloxacin: probenecid
May decrease effect of antidysrhythmias (amiodarone, procainamide, quinidine, sotalol, disopyramide), result in life-threatening arrhythmias
Decrease: absorption antacids containing aluminum, magnesium, sucralfate, zinc, iron, give 4 hr ac or 2 hr pc

NURSING CONSIDERATIONS

Assess:
• Renal, hepatic studies: BUN, creatinine, AST, ALT
• I&O ratio
• CNS symptoms: insomnia, vertigo, headache, agitation, confusion
⚠ Allergic reactions and anaphylaxis: rash, flushing, urticaria, pruritus, chills, fever, joint pain; may occur a few days after therapy begins; epINEPHrine and resuscitation equipment should be available for anaphylactic reaction
• Bowel pattern daily, if severe diarrhea occurs, drug should be discontinued
• For overgrowth of infection: perineal itching, fever, malaise, redness, pain, swelling, drainage, rash, diarrhea, change in cough, sputum
Administer:
• 4 hr before or 2 hr after antacids, iron, calcium, zinc products
Evaluate
• Therapeutic response: negative C&S, absence of signs/symptoms of infection
Teach patient/family:
• May take with or without food
• That fluids must be increased to 2 L/day to avoid crystallization in kidneys

---

- That if dizziness or light-headedness occurs, perform activities with assistance
- To complete full course of drug therapy
- To contact prescriber if adverse reactions occur
- To avoid iron- or mineral-containing supplements or antacids within 4 hr before and 2 hr after dosing
- That photosensitivity may occur and sunscreen should be used
- To use frequent rinsing of mouth, sugarless candy or gum for dry mouth
- To avoid other medication unless approved by prescriber

⚠ High Alert

gemtuzumab (℞)

(gem-tue-zue′mab)
Mylotarg
Func. class.: Antineoplastic—miscellaneous
Chem. class.: Monoclonal antibody

Action: Composed of recombinant humanized IgG$_4$ kappa antibody, binds to CD33 antigen that is released in myeloid cells

Uses: Acute myeloid leukemia (AML) in patients with first relapse who are 60 yr or older

DOSAGE AND ROUTES

- *Adult:* **IV** 9 mg/m^2 as a 2 hr inf; before giving inf, give diphenhydrAMINE 50 mg **PO**, acetaminophen 650-1000 mg **PO** 1 hr prior to inf; then use acetaminophen 650-1000 mg q1-4h prn

Available forms: Powder for inj, lyophilized 5 mg

SIDE EFFECTS

CNS: Dizziness, insomnia, depression
CV: Hypertension, hemorrhage, tachycardia, hypotension
GI: Anorexia, diarrhea, constipation, nausea, stomatitis, vomiting
GU: Hematuria, *vaginal hemorrhage*

INTEG: Rash, herpes simplex, local reaction, petechiae
META: Hypokalemia, hypomagnesemia
MISC: Fever, myalgias, headache, chills
RESP: Cough, pneumonia, epistaxis, rhinitis

Contraindications: Pregnancy (D), hypersensitivity, severe myelosuppression, lactation
Precautions: Children, severe renal or hepatic disease

PHARMACOKINETICS

Half-life 45 and 100 hr, respectively

NURSING CONSIDERATIONS

Assess:
- For symptoms of infection; chills, fever, headache, may be masked by drug fever
- CNS reaction: LOC, mental status, dizziness, confusion
- Cardiac status: Lung sounds; ECG before and during treatment, especially in those with cardiac disease
- Bone marrow depression: bruising, bleeding, blood in stools, urine, sputum, emesis

Administer:
- Do not give IV push or bolus
- Protect from light, use biologic safety hood, allow to come to room temp
- Reconstitute each vial with 5 ml sterile water for inj using sterile syringes, swirl each vial, check for discoloration or particulate matter, give over 2 hr, use a separate line with 1.2 micron terminal filter

Perform/provide:
- Storage of reconstituted sol for ≤8 hr in refrigerator

Evaluate:
- Therapeutic response: decrease in size, number of lesions

Teach patient/family:
- To take acetaminophen for fever
- To avoid hazardous tasks, since confusion, dizziness may occur; avoid prolonged sunlight, use sunscreen

---

⚠ Safety alert   *"Tall Man" lettering

- To report signs of infection: sore throat, fever, diarrhea, vomiting
- To avoid immunizations
- To avoid crowds, people with known infections

---

gentamicin (R)

(jen-ta-mye'sin)
Cidomycin ✖, Garamycin, gentamicin sulfate, G-Mycin, Jenamicin

Func. class.: Antiinfective
Chem. class.: Aminoglycoside

Do not confuse:
Garamycin/kanamycin

Action: Interferes with protein synthesis in bacterial cell by binding to ribosomal subunit, causing misreading of genetic code; inaccurate peptide sequence forms in protein chain, causing bacterial death

Uses: Severe systemic infections of CNS, respiratory, GI, urinary tract, bone, skin, soft tissues caused by susceptible strains of *Pseudomonas aeruginosa, Proteus, Klebsiella, Serratia, Escherichia coli, Enterobacter, Citrobacter, Staphylococcus, Shigella, Salmonella, Acinetobacter,* acute PID

DOSAGE AND ROUTES
Severe systemic infections
- *Adult:* **IV INF** 3-5 mg/kg/day in 3 divided doses q8h; dilute in 50-200 ml 0.9% NaCl or D₅W given over 30 min-1 hr; **IM** 3 mg/kg/day in divided doses q8h
- *Child:* **IV/IM** 2-2.5 mg/kg q8h
- *Neonate and infant:* **IV/IM** 2.5 mg/kg q8-12h
- *Neonate <1 wk:* 2.5 mg/kg q12-24h
Once daily dosing/extended interval dosing (unlabeled)
- *Adult:* **IV** 4-7 mg/kg/q24h, adjust according to levels
Renal dose
- *Adult:* **IV/IM** 1-1.7 mg/kg initially, then adjust according to levels
Available forms: Inj 10, 40 mg/ml; premixed inj 40, 60, 70, 80, 100 mg/50 ml; 40, 60, 80, 90, 100, 120, 160, 180 mg/ml

SIDE EFFECTS
CNS: Confusion, depression, numbness, tremors, ***convulsions,*** muscle twitching, ***neurotoxicity,*** dizziness, vertigo
CV: Hypotension, hypertension, palpitations
EENT: ***Ototoxicity, deafness,*** visual disturbances, tinnitus
GI: Nausea, vomiting, anorexia; increased ALT, AST, bilirubin; hepatomegaly, ***hepatic necrosis,*** splenomegaly
GU: ***Oliguria, hematuria, renal damage, azotemia, renal failure, nephrotoxicity***
HEMA: ***Agranulocytosis, thrombocytopenia, leukopenia, eosinophilia,*** anemia
INTEG: *Rash,* burning, urticaria, dermatitis, alopecia

Contraindications: Severe renal disease, hypersensitivity

Precautions: Pregnancy (C), neonates, mild renal disease, hearing deficits, myasthenia gravis, lactation, elderly, Parkinson's disease

PHARMACOKINETICS
IM: Onset rapid, peak 1-2 hr
IV: Onset immediate, peak 1-2 hr; plasma half-life 1-2 hr, infants 6-7 hr; duration 6-8 hr; not metabolized; excreted unchanged in urine; crosses placental barrier; poor penetration into CSF

INTERACTIONS
Increase: ototoxicity, neurotoxicity, nephrotoxicity—other aminoglycosides, amphotericin B, polymyxin, vancomycin, ethacrynic acid, furosemide, mannitol, methoxyflurane, cisplatin, cephalosporins, penicillins
Increase: effects—nondepolarizing neuromuscular blockers

NURSING CONSIDERATIONS
Assess:
- Weight before treatment; calculation of dosage is usually based on ideal body

---

weight, but may be calculated on actual body weight

• I&O ratio, urinalysis daily for proteinuria, cells, casts; report sudden change in urine output; toxicity is increased in patients with decreased renal function if high doses are given

• VS during infusion; watch for hypotension, change in pulse

• IV site for thrombophlebitis, including pain, redness, swelling, q30min, change site if needed; discontinue, apply warm compresses to site

• Serum peak, drawn at 30-60 min after IV inf or 60 min after IM inj, and trough level drawn just before next dose; blood level should be 2-4 times bacteriostatic level; peak = 4-12 mcg/ml, trough = 1-2 mcg/ml

• Urine pH if drug is used for UTI; urine should be kept alkaline

• Renal impairment by securing urine for CCr testing, BUN, serum creatinine; lower dosage should be given in renal impairment (CCr <80 ml/min)

• Deafness by audiometric testing, ringing, roaring in ears, vertigo; assess hearing before, during, after treatment

• Dehydration: high specific gravity, decrease in skin turgor, dry mucous membranes, dark urine

• Overgrowth of infection including fever, malaise, redness, pain, swelling, perineal itching, diarrhea, stomatitis, change in cough or sputum

• C&S before starting treatment to identify infecting organism

• Vestibular dysfunction: nausea, vomiting, dizziness, headache; drug should be discontinued if severe

• Injection sites for redness, swelling, abscesses; use warm compresses at site

Administer:
• IM inj in large muscle mass; rotate inj sites

• Drug in evenly spaced doses to maintain blood level

IV route
• After diluting in 50-200 ml NS or D$_5$W; sol concentration should be 1 mg/ml or less; decrease vol of diluent in child;

maintain 0.1% sol run over ½-1 hr (adults) or up to 2 hr (children); flush IV line with NS or D$_5$W after administration

Additive compatibilities: Atracurium, aztreonam, bleomycin, cefoxitin, cimetidine, ciprofloxacin, fluconazole, meropenem, methicillin, metronidazole, ofloxacin, penicillin G sodium, ranitidine, verapamil

Syringe compatibilities: Clindamycin, methicillin, penicillin G sodium

Y-site compatibilities: Acyclovir, amifostine, amiodarone, amsacrine, atracurium, aztreonam, cefpirome, ciprofloxacin, cyclophosphamide, cytarabine, diltiazem, enalaprilat, esmolol, famotidine, filgrastim, fluconazole, fludarabine, foscarnet, granisetron, hydromorphone, IL-2, insulin, labetalol, lorazepam, magnesium sulfate, melphalan, meperidine, meropenem, midazolam, morphine, multivitamins, ondansetron, paclitaxel, pancuronium, perphenazine, sargramostim, tacrolimus, teniposide, theophylline, thiotepa, tolazine, vecuronium, vinorelbine, vit B/C, zidovudine

Perform/provide:
• Adequate fluids of 2-3 L/day, unless contraindicated, to prevent irritation of tubules

• Supervised ambulation, other safety measures with vestibular dysfunction

Evaluate:
• Therapeutic response: absence of fever, draining wounds, negative C&S after treatment

Teach patient/family:
• To report headache, dizziness, symptoms of overgrowth of infection, renal impairment

• To report loss of hearing, ringing, roaring in ears, or feeling of fullness in head

---

gentamicin ophthalmic
See Appendix C

---

gentamicin topical
See Appendix C

glatiramer (℞)
(glah-tear′a-meer)
Copaxone
Func. class.: Multiple sclerosis agent

Action: Unknown, may modify the immune responses responsible for multiple sclerosis (MS)
Uses: Reduction of the frequency of relapses in patients with relapsing-remitting MS

DOSAGE AND ROUTES
- *Adult:* **SUBCUT** 20 mg/day

Available forms: Inj, *premixed* 20 mg/ml

SIDE EFFECTS
CNS: Anxiety, hypertonia, tremor, vertigo, speech disorder, *agitation,* confusion
CV: Migraine, palpitations, syncope, tachycardia, vasodilation, chest pain
EENT: Ear pain, blurred vision
GI: Nausea, vomiting, diarrhea, anorexia, gastroenteritis
GU: Urinary urgency, dysmenorrhea, vaginal moniliasis
HEMA: Ecchymosis, lymphadenopathy
INTEG: Pruritus, rash, sweating, urticaria, erythema
META: Edema, weight gain
MS: Arthralgia, back pain, neck pain
RESP: Bronchitis, dyspnea, laryngismus, rhinitis
Contraindications: Hypersensitivity to this drug or mannitol
Precautions: Pregnancy (B), immune disorders, renal disease, lactation, child <18 yr

PHARMACOKINETICS
May be hydrolyzed locally, may reach regional lymph nodes

NURSING CONSIDERATIONS
Assess:
- Blood, renal, hepatic studies: prior to treatment
- For CNS symptoms: anxiety, confusion, vertigo
- GI status: diarrhea, vomiting, abdominal pain, gastroenteritis
- Cardiac status: tachycardia, palpitations, vasodilation, chest pain

Administer:
SUBCUT route
- Using a sterile syringe/needle to transfer the supplied diluent into the vial, rotate vial gently, do not shake; withdraw medication using a syringe with 27G needle; administer SUBCUT into hip, thigh, arm; discard unused portion
- Use SUBCUT route only; do not give IM or IV
- Do not use sol that contains precipitate or is discolored
- Use immediately

Evaluate:
- Therapeutic response: decreased symptoms of MS

Teach patient/family:
- Give written, detailed instructions about the drug; provide initial and return demonstrations on inj procedure; give information on use and disposal of drug, inj site reaction (hives, rash, irritation, severe pain, flushing, chest pain)
- That blurred vision, sweating may occur
- That irregular menses, dysmenorrhea, or metrorrhagia as well as breast pain may occur; use contraception during treatment
- That if pregnancy is suspected, or if nursing, notify prescriber
- Not to change dosing or to stop taking drug without advice of prescriber
- Immediate post inj reaction: flushing, chest pain, palpitations, anxiety, dyspnea, laryngeal constriction, urticaria, does not usually require treatment

G

glimepiride
(glye-me'pi-ride)
Amaryl
* **glipiZIDE** (℞)
(glip-i'zide)
Glucotrol, Glucotrol XL
Func. class.: Antidiabetic
Chem. class.: Sulfonylurea (2nd generation)

Do not confuse:

glipiZIDE/ Glucotrol/glyBURIDE

Action: Causes functioning β-cells in pancreas to release insulin, leading to drop in blood glucose levels; may improve insulin binding to insulin receptors or increase the number of insulin receptors with prolonged administration; may also reduce basal hepatic glucose secretion; not effective if patient lacks functioning β-cells

Uses: Type 2 diabetes mellitus

DOSAGE AND ROUTES

Glimepiride
• *Adult:* PO 1-2 mg daily, then increase q1-2wk up to 8 mg/day
Renal dose
• *Adult:* PO CCr <20 ml/min, 1 mg daily with breakfast, may titrate upward as needed
GlipiZIDE
• *Adult:* PO 5 mg initially, then increase to desired response; max 40 mg/day in divided doses or 15 mg/dose
Hepatic disease/elderly
• PO 2.5 mg initially, then increase to desired response; max 40 mg/day in divided doses or 15 mg/dose

Available forms: *glimepiride:* tabs 1, 2, 4 mg; *glipiZIDE:* tabs 5, 10 mg scored; ext rel tab (XL) 5, 10 mg

SIDE EFFECTS

CNS: Headache, weakness, dizziness, drowsiness, tinnitus, fatigue, vertigo
ENDO: Hypoglycemia
GI: Hepatotoxicity, cholestatic jaundice, nausea, vomiting, diarrhea, heartburn
HEMA: Leukopenia, thrombocytopenia, agranulocytosis, aplastic anemia; increased AST, ALT, alk phosphatase; *pancytopenia, hemolytic anemia*
INTEG: Rash, allergic reactions, pruritus, urticaria, eczema, photosensitivity, erythema

Contraindications: Hypersensitivity to sulfonylureas, type 1/juvenile diabetes, diabetic ketoacidosis

Precautions: Pregnancy (C), elderly, cardiac disease, severe renal disease, severe hepatic disease, thyroid disease

PHARMACOKINETICS

PO: Completely absorbed by GI route, onset 1-1½ hr, peak 1-3 hr, duration 10-24 hr, half-life 2-4 hr; metabolized in liver; excreted in urine; 90%-95% is plasma protein bound

INTERACTIONS

Effect may be decreased: thiazide diuretics, rifampin, isoniazid, cholestyramine, diazoxide, hydantoins, urinary alkalinizers, charcoal
May mask symptoms of hypoglycemia: β-blockers
Increase: action of digitalis, glycosides
Increase: hypoglycemic effects—insulin, MAOIs, cimetidine, chloramphenicol, guanethidine, methyldopa, NSAIDs, salicylates, probenecid, androgens, anticoagulants, clofibrate, fenfluramine, fluconazole, gemfibrozil, histamine H_2 antagonists, magnesium salts, phenylbutazone, sulfinpyrazone, sulfonamides, tricyclics, urinary acidifiers
Drug/Herb
Increase: antidiabetic effect—alfalfa, aloe, basil, bay, bilberry, bitter melon, black catechu, buchu, burdock, coriander, dandelion, eyebright (po), garlic, glucomannan, glucosamine, goat's rue, gymnema, horehound, horse chestnut, jambul, myrrh, myrtle
Increase: glucose tolerance—karela

Increase or decrease: hypoglycemic effect—chromium, fenugreek, ginseng, coenzyme Q-10

Decrease: hypoglycemic effect—broom, buchu, dandelion, glucosamine, juniper

Decrease: antidiabetic effect—bee pollen, blue cohosh, broom, chromium, elecampane, eucalyptus, gotu kola

NURSING CONSIDERATIONS

Assess:
• Blood, A1c levels during treatment to determine diabetes control
• CBC baseline and throughout treatment
• Hypo/hyperglycemic reaction that can occur soon after meals; for severe hypoglycemia give IV $D_{50}W$, then IV dextrose solution

Administer:
• Do not break, crush, or chew ext rel tabs
• Drug 30 min before meals; if patient is NPO, may need to hold dose to prevent hypoglycemia
• May crush tabs and mix with fluids, if unable to swallow whole

Perform/provide:
• Storage in tight, light-resistant container at room temperature

Evaluate:
• Therapeutic response: decrease in polyuria, polydipsia, polyphagia, clear sensorium, absence of dizziness, stable gait

Teach patient/family:
• Not to drink alcohol; explain disulfiram reaction (nausea, headache, cramps, flushing, hypoglycemia)
• To check for symptoms of cholestatic jaundice: dark urine, pruritus, yellow sclera; prescriber should be notified
• The symptoms of hypo/hyperglycemia, what to do about each; to have glucagon emergency kit available, carry sugar packets
• That drug must be continued on daily basis; explain consequences of discontinuing drug abruptly
• To take drug in morning to prevent hypoglycemic reactions at night

• To use sunscreen or stay out of the sun to prevent photosensitivity
• To avoid OTC medications unless ordered by prescriber
• That diabetes is a lifelong illness; drug will not cure disease
• That all food in diet plan must be eaten to prevent hypoglycemia
• To carry emergency ID with prescriber and medications
• To test using blood glucose meter while on this drug
• To continue weight control, dietary restrictions, exercise, hygiene
• Ext rel tab may appear in stool

Treatment of overdose: Glucose 25 g IV via dextrose 50% solution 50 ml or 1 mg glucagon

---

*glyBURIDE (℞)
(glye′byoor-ide)
Apo-Glyburide ✤, DiaBeta ✤, Euglucon ✤, Gen-Glybe ✤, Glynase PresTab, Micronase, Novo-Glyburide ✤, Nu-Glyburide ✤
Func. class.: Antidiabetic
Chem. class.: Sulfonylurea (2nd generation)

Do not confuse:
glyBURIDE/Glucotrol/glipiZIDE
DiaBeta/Zebeta

Action: Causes functioning β-cells in pancreas to release insulin, leading to drop in blood glucose levels; may improve insulin binding to insulin receptors and increase number of insulin receptors with prolonged administration; may also reduce basal hepatic glucose secretion; not effective if patient lacks functioning β-cells

Uses: Type 2 diabetes mellitus

DOSAGE AND ROUTES

DiaBeta/Micronase
• *Adult:* **PO** 1.25-5 mg initially, then increased to desired response at weekly intervals up to 20 mg/day

---

✤ Canada only   Side effects: *italics* = common; ***bold italics*** = life-threatening

- *Elderly:* **PO** 1.25 mg initially, then increased to desired response; max 20 mg/day, maintenance 1.25-20 mg/daily

Glynase PresTab (micronized)

- *Adult:* **PO** 1.5-3 mg/day initially, may increase by 1.5 mg/wk, max 12 mg/day
- *Elderly:* **PO** 0.75-3 mg/day, may increase by 1.5 mg/wk

Available forms: (Diabeta) Tabs 1.25, 2.5, 5 mg; (Glynase PresTab) 1.5, 3, 6 mg

SIDE EFFECTS

CNS: Headache, weakness, paresthesia, tinnitus, fatigue, vertigo

ENDO: **Hypoglycemia**

GI: Nausea, fullness, heartburn, **hepatotoxicity, cholestatic jaundice,** vomiting, diarrhea

HEMA: **Leukopenia, thrombocytopenia, agranulocytosis, aplastic anemia,** increased AST, ALT, alk phosphatase

INTEG: Rash, allergic reactions, pruritus, urticaria, eczema, photosensitivity, erythema

MS: Joint pain

Contraindications: Hypersensitivity to sulfonylureas, juvenile or type 1 diabetes, diabetic ketoacidosis

Precautions: Pregnancy (B), elderly, cardiac disease, severe renal disease, severe hepatic disease, thyroid disease, severe hypoglycemic reactions

PHARMACOKINETICS

PO: Completely absorbed by GI route; onset 2-4 hr, peak 4 hr, duration 24 hr; half-life 10 hr; metabolized in liver; excreted in urine, feces (metabolites); crosses placenta; 99% is plasma protein bound

INTERACTIONS

Both drugs' effects may be decreased: diazoxide

Mask symptoms of hypoglycemia: decrease-blockers

Increase: level—digoxin

Increase: hypoglycemic effects—

insulin, MAOIs, oral anticoagulants, chloramphenicol, guanethidine, methyldopa, NSAIDs, salicylates, probenecid, androgens, fenfluramine, fluconazole, gemfibrozil, histamine H_2 antagonists, magnesium salts, phenylbutazone, sulfinpyrazone, sulfonamides, tricyclics, urinary acidifiers

Decrease: glyBURIDE action—thiazide diuretics, rifampin, isoniazid, cholestyramine, hydantoins, urinary alkalinizers, charcoal

Drug/Herb

Increase: antidiabetic effect—alfalfa, aloe, basil, bay, bilberry, bitter melon, black catechu, buchu, burdock, coriander, dandelion, eyebright (po), garlic, glucomannan, glucosamine, goat's rue, gymnema, horehound, horse chestnut, jambul, myrrh, myrtle

Increase: glucose tolerance: karela

Increase or decrease: hypoglycemic effect—chromium, coenzyme Q10, fenugreek, ginseng

Decrease: antidiabetic effect—bee pollen, blue cohosh, broom, chromium, elecampane, eucalyptus, gotu kola

Decrease: hypoglycemic effect—broom, buchu, dandelion, glucosamine, juniper

NURSING CONSIDERATIONS

Assess:

- Hypo/hyperglycemic reaction that can occur soon after meals; for severe hypoglycemia, give IV $D_{50}W$, then IV dextrose sol
- Blood glucose; A1c levels during treatment
- CBC baseline and throughout treatment

Administer:

- With breakfast, hold dose if NPO to avoid hypoglycemia

Perform/provide:

- Storage in tight container in cool environment

Evaluate:

- Therapeutic response: decrease in polyuria, polydipsia, polyphagia, clear sensorium, absence of dizziness, stable gait

Teach patient/family:

• To check for symptoms of cholestatic jaundice: dark urine, pruritus, jaundiced sclera; if these occur, notify prescriber

• To use a blood glucose meter for testing while on this drug

• The symptoms of hypo/hyperglycemia, what to do about each

• That drug must be continued on daily basis; explain consequences of discontinuing drug abruptly

• To take drug in morning to prevent hypoglycemic reactions at night

• To avoid OTC medications unless ordered by prescriber

• That diabetes is a lifelong illness; drug will not cure disease

• That all food included in diet plan must be eaten to prevent hypoglycemia; to have glucagon emergency kit, sugar packets available

• To use sunscreen or stay out of the sun to prevent photosensitivity

• To carry an emergency ID with prescriber and medications

Treatment of overdose: Glucose 25 g IV via dextrose 50% sol, 50 ml or 1 mg glucagon

Rarely Used

glycerin (OTC)
(gli′ser-in)
Fleet Babylax, Glycerin USP, Glycerol, Osmoglyn, Sani-Supp
Func. class.: Laxative, hyperosmotic

Uses: Constipation, intraocular pressure reduction

DOSAGE AND ROUTES

Laxative

• *Adult and child >6 yr:* **RECT SUPP** 3 g; **ENEMA** 5-15 ml

• *Child <6 yr:* **RECT SUPP** 1-1.5 g; **ENEMA** 2-5 ml

Intraocular pressure reduction

• *Adult:* **PO** 1-1.5 g/kg once, then may be given 500 mg/kg q6h

• *Child:* **PO** 1-1.5 g/kg once, then 500 mg/kg 4-8 hr after first dose

Contraindications: Hypersensitivity

glycopyrrolate (℞)
(glye-koe-pye′roe-late)
glycopyrrolate, Robinul, Robinul-Forte
Func. class.: Cholinergic blocker
Chem. class.: Quaternary ammonium compound

Action: Inhibits the action of acetylcholine at receptor sites in autonomic nervous system, which controls secretions, free acids in stomach

Uses: Decreased secretions before surgery, reversal of neuromuscular blockade, peptic ulcer disease, irritable bowel syndrome, bradycardia

Investigational uses: Drooling, hypersalivation

DOSAGE AND ROUTES

Preoperatively

• *Adult:* **IM** 4.4 mcg/kg ½-1 hr before surgery, max 0.1 mg

• *Child:* **IM** 4.4-8.8 mcg/kg

Reversal of neuromuscular blockade

• *Adult and child:* **IV** 200 mcg for each 1 mg of neostigmine or 5 mg **IV** of pyridostigmine simultaneously

GI disorders

• *Adult:* **PO** 1-2 mg bid-tid; **IM/IV** 100-200 mcg tid-qid, titrated to patient response

Antidysrhythmic

• *Adult:* **IV** 100 mcg, may repeat q2min

• *Child:* **IV** 4.4 mcg/kg, may repeat q2min, max 100 mcg

Drooling

• *Adult:* **PO** doses vary widely

Available forms: Tabs 1, 2 mg; inj 200 mcg (0.2 mg)/ml

SIDE EFFECTS

CNS: Confusion, anxiety, restlessness, irritability, delusions, hallucinations, headache, sedation, depression, incoherence, dizziness, lethargy, flushing, weakness

CV: Palpitations, tachycardia, postural hypotension, paradoxical bradycardia

EENT: Blurred vision, photophobia, dilated pupils, difficulty swallowing, increased intraocular pressure, mydriasis, cycloplegia

GI: Dryness of mouth, constipation, nausea, vomiting, abdominal distress, paralytic ileus, altered taste perception

GU: Urinary hesitancy, retention, impotence

INTEG: Urticaria, allergic reactions

MISC: Suppression of lactation, nasal congestion, decreased sweating

*SYST: **Anaphylaxis***

Contraindications: Hypersensitivity, narrow-angle glaucoma, myasthenia gravis, GI/GU obstruction, child <3 yr, tachycardia, myocardial ischemia, hepatic disease, ulcerative colitis, toxic megacolon, prostatic hypertrophy

Precautions: Pregnancy (B), elderly, lactation, renal disease, CHF, pulmonary disease, hyperthyroidism

PHARMACOKINETICS

PO: Peak 1 hr, duration 8-12 hr
IM: Peak 30-45 min, duration 2-7 hr
IV: Peak 10-15 min, duration 2-7 hr; excreted in urine (50%) (unchanged); half-life 1-2 hr

INTERACTIONS

Increase: anticholinergic effect—alcohol, antihistamines, phenothiazines, amantadine, tricyclics

Decrease: glycopyrrolate absorption—antacids, antidiarrheals

NURSING CONSIDERATIONS

Assess:

• I&O ratio; retention commonly causes decreased urinary output

• Urinary hesitancy, retention: palpate bladder if retention occurs

• Constipation; increase fluids, bulk, exercise if this occurs

• Mental status: affect, mood, CNS depression, worsening of mental symptoms during early therapy

Administer:

• Parenteral dose with patient recumbent to prevent postural hypotension

• Parenteral dose slowly; keep in bed for at least 1 hr after dose; monitor VS

• After checking dose carefully; even slight overdose may lead to toxicity

• With or after meals to prevent GI upset; may give with fluids other than water

IV route

• Undiluted, give through a Y-tube or 3-way stopcock; give 0.2 mg or less over 1-2 min

Syringe compatibilities: Atropine, benz quinamide, chlorproMAZINE, cimetidine, codeine, diphenhydrAMINE, droperidol, droperidol/fentanyl, hydromorphone, hydrOXYzine, levorphanol, lidocaine, meperidine, meperidine/promethazine, midazolam, morphine, nalbuphine, neostigmine, oxymorphone, procaine, prochlorperazine, promazine, promethazine, pyridostigmine, ranitidine, scopolamine, triflupromazine, trimethobenzamide

Solution compatibilities: D$_5$W, 0.9% NaCl, Ringer's, D$_5$/0.45% NaCl

Perform/provide:

• Storage at room temperature

Evaluate:

• Therapeutic response: decreased secretions; decreased pain in GI disorders; reversal of neuromuscular blockers

Teach patient/family:

• Hard candy, frequent drinks, sugarless gum to relieve dry mouth, use good oral hygiene

• Not to discontinue this drug abruptly; to taper off over 1 wk; to take PO ½-1 hr ac

• To avoid driving, other hazardous activities; drowsiness, blurred vision may occur

• To avoid OTC medication: cough, cold preparations with alcohol, antihistamines unless directed by prescriber
• To avoid hot temperatures, since sweating is decreased, heat stroke is possible
• To change positions slowly to prevent orthostatic hypotension
• To notify prescriber of eye pain, blurred vision, light sensitivity

---

goserelin (℞)
(goe'se-rel-lin)
Zoladex
Func. class.: Gonadotropin-releasing hormone, antineoplastic (hormone)
Chem. class.: Synthetic decapeptide analog of LHRH

Action: Inhibitor of pituitary gonado-tropin secretion; initially increases LH and FSH, with increases in testosterone, reduction in sex steroid levels (substitute serum testosterone levels)
Uses: Advanced prostate cancer stage B2-C (10.8 mg), endometriosis, advanced breast cancer, endometrial thinning (3.6 mg)

DOSAGE AND ROUTES
• *Adult:* SUBCUT 3.6 mg q28days or 10.8 mg q12wk
Endometrial thinning
• *Adult:* SUBCUT 1-2 depot inj, usually 1 depot, surgery performed at 4 wk, if 2 depots, surgery performed 2-4 wk after 2nd depot
Available forms: Depot inj 3.6, 10.8 mg

SIDE EFFECTS
*CNS: Headaches, **spinal cord compression**, anxiety, depression, dizziness, insomnia, lethargy*
*CV: **Dysrhythmia, cerebrovascular accident**, hypertension, **MI**, chest pain, **CHF***
ENDO: Gynecomastia, breast tenderness, hot flashes

GI: Nausea, vomiting, constipation, diarrhea, ulcer
GU: Spotting, breakthrough bleeding, decreased libido, renal insufficiency, urinary obstruction, urinary tract infection, impotence
INTEG: Rash, pain on inj
MS: Osteoneuralgia
RESP: COPD, URI
Contraindications: Pregnancy (D) (breast cancer), (X)-endometriosis; lactation, nondiagnosed vaginal bleeding; hypersensitivity to LHRH, LHRH-agonist analogs, children

PHARMACOKINETICS
Peak serum concentrations in 14-28 days; half-life 4½ hr

Drug/Lab Test
Increase: Alk phosphatase, estradiol, FSH, LH, testosterone levels
Decrease: Testosterone levels, progesterone

NURSING CONSIDERATIONS
Assess:
• I&O ratios; palpate bladder for distention in urinary obstruction
• For relief of bone pain (back pain), change in motor function
• Acid phosphatase PSA baseline and periodically
Administer:
Depot
• SUBCUT using implant, inserted by qualified person into upper subcutaneous tissue in abdominal wall q28d or q12wk (10.8 mg)
Evaluate:
• Therapeutic response: more normal levels of prostate-specific antigen, acid phosphatase, alk phosphatase; testosterone level of <25 ng/dl
Teach patient/family:
• That gynecomastia and postmenopausal symptoms may occur but will decrease after treatment is discontinued
• That bone pain may increase, then decrease

Side effects: *italics* = common; ***bold italics*** = life-threatening

- To notify prescriber of difficulty urinating, hot flashes
- To keep appointments
- Not to breastfeed, use effective nonhormonal contraception

granisetron (R)
(grane-iss'e-tron)
Kytril
Func. class.: Antiemetic
Chem. class.: 5-HT$_3$ receptor antagonist

Action: Prevents nausea, vomiting by blocking serotonin peripherally, centrally, and in the small intestine

Uses: Prevention of nausea, vomiting associated with cancer chemotherapy including high-dose cisplatin

Investigational uses: Acute nausea, vomiting following surgery

DOSAGE AND ROUTES

Nausea, vomiting in chemotherapy
- *Adult and child ≥2 yr:* **IV** 10 mcg/kg over 5 min, 30 min before the start of cancer chemotherapy
- *Adult:* **PO** 1 mg bid, give first dose 1 hr before chemotherapy and next dose 12 hr after first

Nausea, vomiting in radiation therapy
- *Adult:* **PO** 2 mg daily 1 hr prior to radiation

Available forms: Inj 1 mg/ml; tab 1 mg

SIDE EFFECTS

CNS: Headache, asthenia, anxiety, dizziness
CV: Hypertension
GI: Diarrhea, *constipation,* increased AST, ALT, *nausea*
HEMA: **Leukopenia,** anemia, ***thrombocytopenia***
MISC: Rash, ***bronchospasm***
Contraindications: Hypersensitivity
Precautions: Pregnancy (B), lactation, children, elderly, ondansetron hypersensitivity

PHARMACOKINETICS

Metabolized in liver to an active metabolite, half-life 10-12 hr

NURSING CONSIDERATIONS

Assess:
- For absence of nausea, vomiting during chemotherapy
- Hypersensitive reaction: rash, bronchospasm

Administer:
IV, direct route
- Dilute in 0.9% NaCl for inj or D$_5$W (20-50 ml); give over 5-15 min; ½ hr before chemotherapy

Additive compatibilities: Dexamethasone, methylPREDNISolone
Solution compatibilities: D$_5$W, 0.9% NaCl
Y-site compatibilities: Acyclovir, allopurinol, amifostine, amikacin, aminophylline, amphotericin B cholesteryl, ampicillin, ampicillin/sulbactam, amsacrine, aztreonam, bleomycin, bumetanide, buprenorphine, butorphanol, calcium gluconate, carboplatin, carmustine, cefazolin, cefepime, cefonicid, cefoperazone, cefotaxime, cefotetan, cefoxitin, ceftazidime, ceftizoxime, ceftriaxone, cefuroxime, chlorproMAZINE, cimetidine, ciprofloxacin, cisplatin, cladribine, clindamycin, cyclophosphamide, cytarabine, dacarbazine, dactinomycin, DAUNOrubicin, dexamethasone, diphenhydrAMINE, DOBUTamine, DOPamine, DOXOrubicin, DOXOrubicin liposome, doxycycline, droperidol, enalaprilat, etoposide, famotidine, filgrastim, fluconazole, fluorouracil, floxuridine, fludarabine, furosemide, gallium, ganciclovir, gentamicin, haloperidol, heparin hydrocortisone, hydromorphone, hydrOXYzine, idarubicin, ifosfamide, imipenem-cilastatin, leucovorin, lorazepam, magnesium sulfate, melphalan, meperidine, mesna, methotrexate, methylPREDNISolone, metoclopramide, metronidazole, mezlocillin, miconazole, minocycline, mitomycin, mitoxantrone, morphine, nalbu-

phine, netilmicin, ofloxacin, paclitaxel, piperacillin, piperacillin/tazobactam, plicamycin, potassium chloride, prochlorperazine, promethazine, propofol, ranitidine, sargramostim, sodium bicarbonate, streptozocin, teniposide, thiotepa, ticarcillin, ticarcillin/clavulanate, tobramycin, trimethoprim - sulfamethoxazole, vancomycin, vinBLAStine, vinCRIStine, vinorelbine, zidovudine

Perform/provide:
• Storage at room temperature for 24 hr after dilution

Evaluate:
• Therapeutic response: absence of nausea, vomiting during cancer chemotherapy

Teach patient/family:
• To report diarrhea, constipation, rash, changes in respirations

---

Rarely Used

griseofulvin microsize (℞)
(gris-ee-oh-ful'vin)
Fulvicin-U/F, Grifulvin V, Grisactin, Grisovin-FP ✤

griseofulvin ultramicrosize (℞)
Fulvicin P/G, Grisactin Ultra, Gris-PEG
Func. class.: Antifungal

Uses: Mycotic infections: tinea corporis, tinea pedis, tinea cruris, tinea barbae, tinea capitis, tinea unguium if caused by *Epidermophyton, Microsporum, Trichophyton*

DOSAGE AND ROUTES

• *Adult:* **PO** 500-1000 mg daily in single or divided doses (microsize), 125-165 mg bid (ultramicrosize) or 250-330 mg daily; may need 500-660 mg in divided doses for severe infections
• *Child:* **PO** 10 mg/kg/day or 30 mg/m²/day (microsize) or 5 mg/kg/day (ultramicrosize)

Contraindications: Hypersensitivity, porphyria, hepatic disease, lupus erythematosus

---

guaifenesin (OTC, ℞)
(gwye-fen'e-sin)
Altarussin, Benylin-E ✤, Calmylin Expectorant ✤, Diabetic Tussin, Ganidin NR, guaifenesin, Guaifenesin NR, Guiatuss, Hytuss, Hytuss 2X, Mucinex, Naldecon Senior EX, Organidin NR, Respa-GF, Resyl ✤, Robitussin, Scot-Tussin Expectorant, Siltussin DAS, Siltussin SA
Func. class.: Expectorant

Action: Acts as an expectorant by stimulating a gastric mucosal reflex to increase the production of lung mucus

Uses: Productive and nonproductive cough

DOSAGE AND ROUTES

• *Adult and child ≥12 yr:* **PO** 200-400 mg q4h, not to exceed 2.4 g/day; **EXT REL** (Mucinex) 600-1200 mg q12h, not to exceed 2.4 g/day
• *Child 6-12 yr:* **PO** 100-200 mg q4h; 600 mg q12h
• *Child 2-6 yr:* **PO** 50-100 mg q4h; not to exceed 600 mg/day
• *Child 6 mo-<2 yr:* **PO** 25-50 mg q4h, max 300 mg/day, individualized

Available forms: Tabs 100, 200, 400 mg; tabs, ext rel 600 mg; caps 200 mg; liquid 100, 200 mg/5 ml; ext rel tabs (Mucinex) 600, 1200 mg

SIDE EFFECTS

CNS: Drowsiness, headache, dizziness
GI: Nausea, anorexia, vomiting
Contraindications: Hypersensitivity; chronic, persistent cough
Precautions: Pregnancy (C)

PHARMACOKINETICS

Half-life 1 hr

NURSING CONSIDERATIONS

Assess:

• Cough: type, frequency, character, including sputum; fluids should be increased to 2 L/day

Administer:

• Do not break, crush, chew ext rel tabs
• Scot-Tussin is not recommended for child <2 yr, Naldecon Senior EX, Mucinex is not recommended in child <12 yr

Perform/provide:

• Storage at room temperature
• Increased fluids, room humidification to liquefy secretions

Evaluate:

• Therapeutic response: absence of cough

Teach patient/family:

• To avoid driving, other hazardous activities if drowsiness occurs (rare)
• To avoid smoking, smoke-filled room, perfumes, dust, environmental pollutants, cleansers
• To consult health provider if cough lasts >7 days

Rarely Used

guanfacine (℞)
(gwahn′fa-seen)
Func. class.: Antihypertensive

Uses: Hypertension in individual using a thiazide diuretic or other antihypertensive

Investigational uses: Heroin withdrawal

DOSAGE AND ROUTES

• *Adult:* **PO** 1 mg/day at bedtime; may increase dose in 3-4 wk to 2 mg/day, max 4 mg daily

Contraindications: Hypersensitivity

Rarely Used

halcinonide (℞)
(hal-sin′oh-nide)
Func. class.: Corticosteroid, synthetic

Uses: Inflammation of corticosteroid-responsive dermatoses

DOSAGE AND ROUTES

• *Adult:* **TOP** apply to affected area bid-tid (not around eyes)

Contraindications: Hypersensitivity, viral infections, fungal infections

halcinonide topical
See Appendix C

halobetasol topical
See Appendix C

haloperidol (℞)
(hal-oh-pehr′ih-dol)
Apo-Haloperidol ✤, Haldol, Novo-Peridol ✤, Peridol ✤

haloperidol decanoate (℞)
Haldol Decanoate, Haldol LA ✤

haloperidol lactate (℞)
Haldol, Haldol Concentrate, Haloperidol Intensol
Func. class.: Antipsychotic, neuroleptic
Chem. class.: Butyrophenone

Do not confuse:
haloperidol/Halotestin
Haldol/Stadol

Action: Depresses cerebral cortex, hypothalamus, limbic system, which control activity and aggression; blocks neurotransmission produced by dopamine at synapse; exhibits strong

---

α-adrenergic, anticholinergic blocking action; mechanism for antipsychotic effects unclear

Uses: Psychotic disorders, control of tics, vocal utterances in Gilles de la Tourette's syndrome, short-term treatment of hyperactive children showing excessive motor activity, prolonged parenteral therapy in chronic schizophrenia, control of severe nausea and vomiting in chemotherapy, organic mental syndrome with psychotic features, hiccups (short-term), emergency sedation of severely agitated or delirious patients

Investigational uses: Nausea, vomiting in chemotherapy, surgery

DOSAGE AND ROUTES

Psychosis
• *Adult:* **PO** 0.5-5 mg bid or tid initially depending on severity of condition; dose is increased to desired dose, max 100 mg/day; **IM** (lactate) 2-5 mg q4-8h or bid-tid
• *Geriatric:* 0.25-0.5 mg daily-bid, titrate q3-4 days by 0.25-0.5 mg/dose
• *Child 3-12 yr:* **PO/IM** (lactate) 0.05-0.15 mg/kg/day
• *Decanoate: Adult:* Initial dose **IM** is 10-15 mg × daily oral dose at 4 wk interval; do not administer **IV**; not to exceed 100 mg

Chronic schizophrenia
• *Decanoate: Adult:* **IM** 50-100 mg q4wk
• *Child 3-12 yr:* **PO/IM** 0.05-0.15 mg/kg/day

Tics/vocal utterances
• *Adult:* **PO** 0.5-5 mg bid or tid, increased until desired response occurs
• *Child 3-12 yr:* **PO** 0.05-0.075 mg/kg/day

Hyperactive children
• *Child 3-12 yr:* **PO** 0.05-0.075 mg/kg/day

Available forms: Tabs 0.5, 1, 2, 5, 10, 20 mg; lactate conc 2 mg/ml; inj 5 mg/ml, decanoate 50 mg base/ml, 100 mg base/ml

SIDE EFFECTS

CNS: EPS: pseudoparkinsonism, akathisia, dystonia, tardive dyskinesia, drowsiness, headache, **seizures, neuroleptic malignant syndrome,** confusion

CV: Orthostatic hypotension, hypertension, **cardiac arrest,** ECG changes, **tachycardia**

EENT: Blurred vision, glaucoma, dry eyes

GI: Dry mouth, nausea, vomiting, anorexia, constipation, diarrhea, jaundice, weight gain, **ileus, hepatitis**

GU: Urinary retention, dysuria, urinary frequency, enuresis, impotence, amenorrhea, gynecomastia

INTEG: Rash, photosensitivity, dermatitis

RESP: **Laryngospasm,** dyspnea, **respiratory depression**

Contraindications: Hypersensitivity, blood dyscrasias, coma, child <3 yr, brain damage, bone marrow depression, alcohol and barbiturate withdrawal states, Parkinson's disease, angina, epilepsy, urinary retention, narrow-angle glaucoma

Precautions: Pregnancy (C), lactation, seizure disorders, hypertension, hepatic disease, cardiac disease, elderly

PHARMACOKINETICS

PO: Onset erratic, peak 2-6 hr, half-life 24 hr
IM: Onset 15-30 min, peak 15-20 min, half-life 21 hr
IM (Decanoate): Peak 4-11 days, half-life 3 wk
Metabolized by liver; excreted in urine, bile; crosses placenta; enters breast milk

INTERACTIONS

Oversedation: other CNS depressants, alcohol, barbiturate anesthetics
Toxicity: epINEPHrine, lithium
Increase: both drugs' effects—β-adrenergic blockers, alcohol
Increase: anticholinergic effects—anticholinergics
Decrease: effects—lithium, levodopa

Decrease: haloperidol effects—phenobarbital, carbamazepine

Drug/Herb

Antagonist action: jimsonweed, scopolia

Increase: action—chamomile, cola tree, hops, kava, nettle, nutmeg, skullcap, valerian

Increase: EPS—betel palm, kava

Drug/Lab Test

Increase: LFTs, cardiac enzymes, cholesterol, blood glucose, prolactin, bilirubin, PBI, cholinesterase, alk phosphatase

Decrease: Hormones (blood, urine), PT

False positive: Pregnancy tests, PKU

False negative: Urinary steroids

NURSING CONSIDERATIONS

Assess:

• Swallowing of PO medication; check for hoarding or giving of medication to other patients

• I&O ratio; palpate bladder if low urinary output occurs

• Bilirubin, CBC, LFTs monthly

• Urinalysis is recommended before and during prolonged therapy

• Affect, orientation, LOC, reflexes, gait, coordination, sleep pattern disturbances

• B/P standing and lying; take pulse and respirations q4h during initial treatment; establish baseline before starting treatment; report drops of 30 mm Hg

• Dizziness, faintness, palpitations, tachycardia on rising

• EPS including akathisia (inability to sit still, no pattern to movements), tardive dyskinesia (bizarre movements of jaw, mouth, tongue, extremities), pseudoparkinsonism (rigidity, tremors, pill rolling, shuffling gait)

• Skin turgor daily

⚠ For neuroleptic malignant syndrome: hyperthermia, muscle rigidity, altered mental status, increased CPK, seizures, hyper/hypotension, tachycardia, notify prescriber immediately

• Constipation, urinary retention daily; if these occur, increase bulk, water in diet

Administer:

• Reduced dose to elderly

• Antiparkinsonian agent, to be used if EPS occurs

• Avoid use with CNS depressants

PO route

• Oral liquid: use calibrated dropper; do not mix in coffee or tea

• PO with food or milk

IM route

• IM inj into large muscle mass, use 21G, 2-in needle; give no more than 3 ml/inj site; patient should remain recumbent for ½ hr

IV route

• Give undiluted for psychotic episode at 5 mg/min

• Give by intermittent inf after dilution in 30-50 ml of D_5W, run over ½ hr

Solution compatibilities: D_5W

Syringe compatibilities: Hydromorphone, sufentanil

Y-site compatibilities: Amifostine, amsacrine, aztreonam, cimetidine, cisatracurium, cladribine, DOBUTamine, DOPamine, DOXOrubicin liposome, famotidine, filgrastim, fludarabine, granisetron, lidocaine, lorazepam, melphalan, midazolam, nitroglycerin, norepinephrine, ondansetron, paclitaxel, phenylephrine, propofol, remifentanil, sufentanil, tacrolimus, teniposide, theophylline, thiotepa, vinorelbine

Perform/provide:

• Decreased sensory input by dimming lights, avoiding loud noises

• Supervised ambulation until stabilized on medication; do not involve in strenuous exercise program because fainting is possible; patient should not stand still for long periods

• Increased fluids, roughage to prevent constipation

• Sips of water, sugarless candy, gum for dry mouth

• Storage in tight, light-resistant container

Evaluate:

• Therapeutic response: decrease in emotional excitement, hallucinations, delusions, paranoia, reorganization of patterns of thought, speech, improvement in specific behaviors

---

⚠ Safety alert   *"Tall Man" lettering

Teach patient/family:
• That orthostatic hypotension occurs often and to rise from sitting or lying position gradually
• To avoid hazardous activities until stabilized on medication
• To remain lying down after IM inj for at least 30 min
• To avoid hot tubs, hot showers, tub baths, since hypotension may occur
• To avoid abrupt withdrawal of this drug, or EPS may result; drug should be withdrawn slowly
• To avoid OTC preparations (cough, hay fever, cold) unless approved by prescriber, since serious drug interactions may occur; avoid use with alcohol; increased drowsiness may occur
• To use a sunscreen to prevent burns
• Regarding compliance with drug regimen
• About EPS and necessity for meticulous oral hygiene, since oral candidiasis may occur
• To report impaired vision, jaundice, tremors, muscle twitching
• That in hot weather, heat stroke may occur; take extra precautions to stay cool
Treatment of overdose: Activated charcoal, lavage if orally ingested; provide an airway; do not induce vomiting

---

haloprogin topical
See Appendix C

▲ High Alert

heparin (℞)
(hep′a-rin)
Calcilean ✦, Calciparine ✦,
Hepalean ✦, Heparin Leo ✦,
heparin sodium, Hep-Lock,
Hep-Lock U/P
Func. class.: Anticoagulant, antithrombotic

Do not confuse:
heparin/Hespan
Action: Prevents conversion of fibrinogen to fibrin and prothrombin to thrombin by enhancing inhibitory effects of antithrombin III
Uses: Prevention of deep-vein thrombosis, pulmonary emboli, myocardial infarction, open heart surgery, disseminated intravascular clotting syndrome, atrial fibrillation with embolization, as an anticoagulant in transfusion and dialysis procedures, prevention of DVT/PE, to maintain patency of indwelling venipuncture devices; diagnosis, treatment of disseminated intravascular coagulation (DIC)

DOSAGE AND ROUTES
Deep-vein thrombosis/MI
• *Adult:* **IV BOL** 5000-7000 units q4h then titrated to PTT or ACT level; **IV INF** after bolus dose, then 1000 units/hr titrated to PTT or ACT level
• *Child:* **IV INF** 50 units/kg, maintenance 100 units/kg q4h or 20,000 units/m² daily
Anticoagulation
• *Adult:* **SUBCUT** 500 units IV then 10,000-20,000 units, then 8,000-10,000 units q8h or 15,000-20,000 units q12h
Pulmonary embolism
• *Adult:* **IV BOL** 7500-10,000 units q4h then titrated to PTT or ACT level; **IV INF** after bolus dose, then 1000 units/hr titrated to PTT or ACT level
• *Child:* **IV INF** 50 units/kg, maintenance 100 units/kg q4h or 20,000 units/m² daily
Cardiovascular surgery
• *Adult:* **IV INF** 150-300 units/kg
Prophylaxis for DVT/PE
• *Adult:* **SUBCUT** 5000 units q8-12h
Heparin flush
• *Adult and child:* **IV** 10-100 units
Available forms:
Sodium carpaject: 5000 units/ml; disposable inj: 1000, 2500, 5000, 7500, 10,000, 15,000, 20,000, 40,000 units/ml; unit dose: 1000, 5000, 10,000, 20,000, 40,000 units/ml; vials: 1000, 2000, 2500, 5000, 7500, 10,000, 20,000, 40,000 units/ml; disposable syringes flush: 10 units/ml; vials: 100 units/ml; Ca inj: 5000 units/0.2 ml;

H

---

ampules: 12,500 units/0.5 ml; 20,000 units/0.8 ml

SIDE EFFECTS

CNS: Fever, chills

GU: Hematuria

HEMA: Hemorrhage, thrombocytopenia, anemia

INTEG: Rash, dermatitis, urticaria, pruritus, delayed transient alopecia, hematoma, cutaneous necrosis (SUBCUT)

SYST: Anaphylaxis

Contraindications: Hypersensitivity, hemophilia, leukemia with bleeding, peptic ulcer disease, severe thrombocytopenic purpura, hepatic disease (severe), renal disease (severe), blood dyscrasias, severe hypertension, subacute bacterial endocarditis, acute nephritis

Precautions: Pregnancy (C), alcoholism, elderly, children, hyperlipidemia, diabetes, renal disease

PHARMACOKINETICS

Well absorbed (SUBCUT)

IV: Peak 5 min, duration 2-6 hr

SUBCUT: Onset 20-60 min, duration 8-12 hr

Half-life 1½ hr, excreted in urine, 95% bound to plasma proteins, does not cross placenta or alter breast milk; removed from the system via the lymph and spleen, partially metabolized in kidney, liver, excreted in urine (<50% unchanged)

INTERACTIONS

Resistance to heparin: streptokinase

Increase: diazepam action

Increase: heparin action—oral anticoagulants, salicylates, dextran, NSAIDs, platelet inhibitors, cephalosporins, penicillins, ticlopidine, dipyridamole

Decrease: corticosteroids action

Decrease: heparin action—digitalis, tetracyclines, antihistamines

Drug/Herb

Increase: risk of bleeding—agrimony, alfalfa, angelica, anise, basil, bay, bilberry, black haw, bogbean, bromelain, buchu, chondroitin, cinchona bark, dong quai,

fenugreek, feverfew, garlic, ginger, ginkgo, ginseng, horse chestnut, Irish moss, kelp, kelpware, khella, lovage, lungwort, meadowsweet, motherwort, mugwort, nettle, papaya, parsley (large amts), pau d'arco, pineapple, poplar, prickly ash, safflower, saw palmetto, tonka bean, turmeric, wintergreen, yarrow

Decrease: anticoagulant effect: chamomile, coenzyme Q10, flax, glucomannan, goldenseal, guar gum

Drug/Lab Test

Increase: ALT, AST, INR, PT, PTT

Decrease: Platelets

NURSING CONSIDERATIONS

Assess:

• Blood studies (Hct, occult blood in stools) q3mo

• Partial prothrombin time, which should be 1.5-2 × control, PTT often done daily, also APTT, ACT

• Platelet count q2-3d; thrombocytopenia may occur on 4th day of treatment

⚠ Bleeding gums, petechiae, ecchymosis, black tarry stools, hematuria, epistaxis, decrease in Hct, B/P; may indicate bleeding, hemorrhage

• Fever, skin rash, urticaria

• Needed dosage change q1-2wk

Administer:

• Cannot be used interchangeably (unit for unit) with LMWHS or heparinoids

• At same time each day to maintain steady blood levels

• SUBCUT deep with 25G ⅜-in needle; do not massage area or aspirate when giving SUBCUT inj; give in abdomen between pelvic bones, rotate sites; do not pull back on plunger, leave in for 10 sec; apply gentle pressure for 1 min

• Changing needles is not recommended

• Avoiding all IM inj that may cause bleeding, hematoma

IV route

• Diluted in 0.9% NaCl, dextrose, Ringer's sol and given by direct, intermittent, or continuous infusion; give 1000 units or less over 1 min; then 5000 units or less over 1 min; infusion may run from 4-24 hr; use infusion pump

---

⚠ Safety alert   *"Tall Man" lettering

• When drug is added to inf sol for cont IV, invert container at least 6 times to ensure adequate mixing

• Blood after adding 7500 units/100 ml NaCl inj, add 6-8 ml of this sol/100 ml of whole blood

Additive compatibilities: Aminophylline, amphotericin, ascorbic acid, bleomycin, calcium gluconate, cefepime, cephapirin, chloramphenicol, clindamycin, cloxacillin, colistimethate, dimenhyDRINATE, DOPamine, enalaprilat, erythromycin gluceptate, esmolol, floxacillin, fluconazole, flumazenil, furosemide, hydrocortisone, isoproterenol, lidocaine, lincomycin, magnesium sulfate, meropenem, methyldopate, methylPREDNISolone, metronidazole/sodium bicarbonate, nafcillin, norepinephrine, octreotide, penicillin G, potassium chloride, prednisoLONE, promazine, ranitidine, sodium bicarbonate, verapamil, vit B/C

Syringe compatibilities: Aminophylline, amphotericin B, ampicillin, atropine, azlocillin, bleomycin, cefamandole, cefazolin, cefoperazone, cefotaxime, cefoxitin, chloramphenicol, cimetidine, cisplatin, clindamycin, cyclophosphamide, diazoxide, digoxin, dimenhyDRINATE, DOBUTamine, DOPamine, epINEPHrine, fentanyl, fluorouracil, furosemide, leucovorin, lidocaine, lincomycin, methotrexate, metoclopramide, mezlocillin, mitomycin, moxalactam, nafcillin, naloxone, neostigmine, nitroglycerin, norepinephrine, pancuronium, penicillin G, phenobarbital, piperacillin, sodium nitroprusside, succinylcholine, trimethoprim-sulfamethoxazole, verapamil

Y-site compatibilities: Acyclovir, aldesleukin, allopurinol, amifostine, aminophylline, ampicillin, ampicillin/sulbactam, atracurium, atropine, aztreonam, betamethasone, bleomycin, calcium gluconate, cefazolin, cefotetan, cefotiam, ceftazidime, ceftriaxone, cephalothin, cephapirin, chlordiazepoxide, chlorproMAZINE, cimetidine, cisplatin, cladribine, clindamycin, conjugated estrogens, cyanocobalamin, cyclophosphamide, cytarabine, dexamethasone, digoxin, diphenhydrAMINE, DOPamine, DOXOrubicin liposome, edrophonium, enalaprilat, epINEPHrine, erythromycin, esmolol, ethacrynate, famotidine, fentanyl, fluconazole, fludarabine, fluorouracil, foscarnet, furosemide, gallium, granisetron, hydrALAZINE, hydrocortisone, hydromorphone, insulin (regular), isoproterenol, kanamycin, leucovorin, lidocaine, lorazepam, magnesium sulfate, melphalan, menadiol, meperidine, meropenem, methicillin, methotrexate, methoxamine, methyldopate, methylergonovine, metoclopramide, metronidazole, midazolam, milrinone, minocycline, mitomycin, morphine, nafcillin, neostigmine, nitroglycerin, nitroprusside, norepinephrine, ondansetron, oxacillin, oxytocin, paclitaxel, pancuronium, penicillin G potassium, pentazocine, phytonadione, piperacillin, piperacillin/tazobactam, potassium chloride, prednisoLONE, procainamide, prochlorperazine, propofol, propranolol, pyridostigmine, ranitidine, remifentanil, sargramostim, scopolamine, sodium bicarbonate, streptokinase, succinylcholine, tacrolimus, teniposide, theophylline, thiopental, thiotepa, ticarcillin, ticarcillin/clavulanate, trimethobenzamide, vecuronium, vinBLAStine, vinorelbine, warfarin, zidovudine

Perform/provide:
• Storage in tight container

Evaluate:
• Therapeutic response: decrease of deep-vein thrombosis, PTT 1.5-2.5 × control, free flowing IV

Teach patient/family:
• To avoid OTC preparations that may cause serious drug interactions unless directed by prescriber
• That drug may be held during active bleeding (menstruation), depending on condition
• To use soft-bristle toothbrush to avoid bleeding gums, avoid contact sports, use electric razor, avoid IM inj
• To carry emergency ID identifying drug taken

H

• To report any signs of bleeding: gums, under skin, urine, stools

Treatment of overdose: Withdraw drug, protamine 1 mg protamine/100 units heparin

---

hepatitis B immune globulin (Ⓡ)

Bay Hep B, Nabi-HB

Func. class.: Immune globulin

Action: Provides passive immunity to hepatitis B

Uses: Prevention of hepatitis B virus in exposed patients, including passive immunity in neonates born to HBsAg-positive mother

DOSAGE AND ROUTES

Acute exposure to blood with HBsAg
• *Adult:* **INJ** 2 doses, given after exposure and 1 mo later

Perinatal exposure of infants born to HBsAg-positive mothers
• *Infant:* 1 dose at birth, then start hepatitis B vaccine series soon after birth

Sexual exposure to HBsAg
• *Adult:* Administer 1 dose within 2 wk of exposure

Available forms: Bay Hep B: Sol for inj 15%-18% protein; Nabi-HB: Sol for inj 5% ± 1% protein

SIDE EFFECTS

CNS: Headache, dizziness, fever
GI: Nausea, vomiting
INTEG: Soreness at inj site, urticaria, erythema, swelling
SYST: Induration, ***anaphylaxis, angioedema***

Contraindications: Hypersensitivity to immune globulins, coagulation disorders
Precautions: Pregnancy (C), hemophilia, elderly, lactation, children; active infection, IgA deficiency

INTERACTIONS

Do not use within 3 months of hepatitis B immune globulin: MMR, varicella, or rotavirus vaccines

NURSING CONSIDERATIONS

Assess:
• For history of allergies, skin conditions (eczema, psoriasis, dermatitis), reactions to vaccinations
• For skin reactions: rash, induration, urticaria
🅐 For anaphylaxis: inability to breathe, bronchospasm, hypotension, wheezing, diaphoresis, fever, flushing

Administer:
• After rotating vial; do not shake
• Only with epINEPHrine 1:1000 on unit to treat laryngospasm
• In deltoid for better absorption (adult)

Perform/provide:
• Written record of immunization
• Comfort measures

Evaluate:
• Prevention of hepatitis B

Teach patient/family:
• That discomfort may occur at site
• To report any rash, wheezing, inability to breathe immediately

---

hetastarch (Ⓡ)

(het′a-starch)
Hespan

Func. class.: Plasma expander
Chem. class.: Synthetic polymer

Do not confuse:
Hespan/heparin

Action: Similar to human albumin, which expands plasma volume by colloidal osmotic pressure

Uses: Plasma volume expander, leukapheresis, hypovolemia

DOSAGE AND ROUTES

• *Adult:* **IV INF** 500-1000 ml (30-60 g), total dose not to exceed 1500 ml/day, not to exceed 20 ml/kg/hr (hemorrhagic shock)

Leukapheresis
• *Adult:* **IV INF** 250-700 ml infused at 1:8 ratio with whole blood, may be repeated 2/wk up to 10 treatments

---

Renal dose
• *Adult:* **IV** CCr <10 ml/min give initial dose, but reduce subsequent doses by 25%-50%

Available forms: 6% hetastarch/0.9% NaCl inj

SIDE EFFECTS

CNS: Headache
EENT: Periorbital edema
GI: Nausea, vomiting
HEMA: Decreased Hct, platelet function, increased bleeding/coagulation times, increased sed rate, DIC
INTEG: Rash, urticaria, pruritus, chills, fever, flushing, peripheral edema
RESP: Wheezing, dyspnea, ***bronchospasm, pulmonary edema***
SYST: ***Anaphylaxis, angioedema***
Contraindications: Hypersensitivity, severe bleeding disorders, renal failure, CHF (severe), anuria, oliguria, intracranial bleeding
Precautions: Pregnancy (C), hepatic disease, pulmonary edema

PHARMACOKINETICS

IV: Expands blood volume 1-2 × amount infused, excreted in urine

INTERACTIONS

Increase: sodium, water retention—fludrocortisone

Drug/Lab Test
False increase: Bilirubin

NURSING CONSIDERATIONS

Assess:
• VS q5min × 30 min; CVP during infusion (5-10 cm H_2O normal range), PCWP
• Monitor CBC with differential, Hgb, Hct, PT, PTT, platelet count, clotting time during treatment; Hct may drop; do not allow to drop >30% by vol
• Urine output q1h, watch for increase in urinary output (common); if output does not increase, decrease or discontinue infusion
• I&O ratio and specific gravity, urine osmolarity; if specific gravity is very low,

renal clearance is low; drug should be discontinued
• Allergy: rash, urticaria, pruritus, wheezing, dyspnea, bronchospasm; drug should be discontinued immediately
A For circulatory overload: increased pulse, respirations, dyspnea, wheezing, chest tightness, chest pain
• For dehydration after infusion: decreased output, fever, poor skin turgor, increased specific gravity, dry skin

Administer:
IV route
• INF undiluted, run at 20 ml/kg/hr (1.2 g/kg); reduced rate in septic shock, burns

Additive compatibilities: Cloxacillin, fosphenytoin
Y-site compatibilities: Cimetidine, diltiazem, enalaprilat
• Storage at room temperature; discard unused portion, do not freeze, do not use if turbid or deep brown or if precipitate forms

Evaluate:
• Therapeutic response: increased plasma volume

Teach patient/family:
• When to notify prescriber

homatropine ophthalmic
See Appendix C

Rarely Used

hyaluronidase (℞)
(hye-al-yoor-on'i-dase)
Wydase
Func. class.: Enzyme

Uses: Hypodermoclysis, subcutaneous urography; adjunct to dispersion of other drugs

DOSAGE AND ROUTES
Adjunct
• *Adult and child:* **INJ** 150 units with other drug

Urography
• *Adult and child:* **SUBCUT** 75 units over scapula, then contrast medium injected at same site

Hypodermoclysis
• *Adult and child >3 yr:* **SUBCUT** 150 units/L of lysis sol

Contraindications: Hypersensitivity to bovine products, CHF, hypoproteinemia, around infected/inflamed or cancerous area

---

*hydrALAZINE (℞)

(hye-dral′a-zeen)
Alazine, Apresoline, hydrALAZINE HCl, Novo-Hylazin ✿, Pralzine, Rolzine, Supres ✿
Func. class.: Antihypertensive, direct-acting peripheral vasodilator
Chem. class.: Phthalazine

Do not confuse:
Apresoline/allopurinol
hydrALAZINE/hydrOXYzine
Action: Vasodilates arteriolar smooth muscle by direct relaxation; reduction in blood pressure with reflex increases in heart rate, stroke volume, cardiac output
Uses: Essential hypertension; severe essential hypertension
Investigational uses: CHF

DOSAGE AND ROUTES

Hypertension
• *Adult:* **PO** 10 mg qid 2-4 days, then 25 mg for rest of first wk, then 50 mg qid individualized to desired response, not to exceed 300 mg daily
• *Child:* **PO** 0.75-3 mg/kg/day in 4 divided doses, max 7.5 mg/kg/24 hr

Hypertensive crisis
• *Adult:* **IV BOL/IM** 10-20 mg q4-6h, administer **PO** as soon as possible; **IM** 10-50 mg q4-6h
• *Child:* **IV BOL** 0.1-0.2 mg/kg q4-6h; **IM** 0.1-0.2 mg/kg q4-6h

CHF
• *Adult:* **PO** 10-25 mg bid, max 75 mg tid
Available forms: Inj 20 mg/ml; tabs 10, 25, 50, 100 mg

SIDE EFFECTS

CNS: Headache, tremors, dizziness, anxiety, peripheral neuritis, depression, fever, chills
*CV: Palpitations, reflex tachycardia, angina, **shock,** rebound hypertension*
GI: Nausea, vomiting, anorexia, diarrhea, constipation, paralytic ileus
GU: Urinary retention
*HEMA: **Leukopenia, agranulocytosis,** anemia, **thrombocytopenia***
INTEG: Rash, pruritus, urticaria
MISC: Nasal congestion, muscle cramps, lupuslike symptoms, flushing, edema, dyspnea
Contraindications: Hypersensitivity to hydrALAZINEs, mitral valvular rheumatic heart disease
Precautions: Pregnancy (C), CVA, advanced renal disease, elderly, coronary artery disease, lactation

PHARMACOKINETICS

PO: Onset 20-30 min, peak 1-2 hr, duration 6-12 hr
IM: Onset 5-10 min, peak 1 hr, duration 2-4 hr
IV: Onset 5-20 min, peak 10-80 min, duration 2-6 hr
Half-life 2-8 hr; metabolized by liver; 12%-14% excreted in urine

INTERACTIONS

Severe hypotension: MAOIs
Increase: tachycardia, angina—sympathomimetics (epINEPHrine, norepinephrine)
Increase: effects of β-blockers
Decrease: hydrALAZINE effects—indomethacin
Drug/Herb
Increase: toxicity, death—aconite
Increase: antihypertensive effect—barberry, betony, black catechu, black cohosh, bloodroot, broom, burdock, cat's claw, dandelion, goldenseal, Irish

---

moss, Jamaican dogwood, kelp, khella, mistletoe, parsley

Increase or decrease: antihypertensive effect—astragalus, cola tree

Decrease: antihypertensive effect—coltsfoot, guarana, khat, licorice

NURSING CONSIDERATIONS

Assess:
• B/P q5min × 2 hr, then q1h × 2 hr, then q4h
• Pulse, jugular venous distention q4h
• Electrolytes, blood studies: K, Na, Cl, CO_2, CBC, serum glucose
• Weight daily, I&O
• LE prep, ANA titer before starting therapy and during treatment; assess for fever, joint pain, rash, sore throat (lupus-like symptoms); notify prescriber
• Edema in feet, legs daily
• Skin turgor, dryness of mucous membranes for hydration status
• Crackles, dyspnea, orthopnea
• IV site for extravasation, rate
• Fever, joint pain, tachycardia, palpitations, headache, nausea
• Mental status: affect, mood, behavior, anxiety; check for personality changes

Administer:
• Give with meals (PO) to enhance absorption
• To recumbent patient, keep for 1 hr after administration

IV route
• IV undiluted; give through Y-tube or 3-way stopcock, give each 10 mg ≤min

Additive compatibilities: DOB-UTamine

Y-site compatibilities: Heparin, hydrocortisone, potassium chloride, verapamil, vit B/C

Evaluate:
• Therapeutic response: decreased B/P

Teach patient/family:
• To take with food to increase bioavailability (PO)
• To avoid OTC preparations unless directed by prescriber
• To notify prescriber if chest pain, severe fatigue, fever, muscle or joint pain occurs
• To rise slowly to prevent orthostatic hypotension
• To notify prescriber if pregnancy is suspected

Treatment of overdose: Administer vasopressors, volume expanders for shock; if PO, lavage or give activated charcoal, digitalization

hydrochlorothia-zide (R)

(hye-droe-klor-oh-thye'a-zide)
Apo-Hydrol ✦, Esidrix, HCTZ, Hydro-Chlor, hydrochlorothiazide, HydroDIURIL, Microzide, Neo-Codema ✦, Novohydrazide ✦, Oretic, Urozide ✦

Func. class.: Thiazide diuretic, antihypertensive
Chem. class.: Sulfonamide derivative

Action: Acts on distal tubule and ascending limb of loop of Henle by increasing excretion of water, sodium, chloride, potassium

Uses: Edema, hypertension, diuresis, CHF; edema in corticosteroid, estrogen, NSAIDs, idiopathic lower extremity edema therapy

DOSAGE AND ROUTES
• *Adult:* **PO** 25-100 mg/day
• *Geriatric:* **PO** 12.5 mg/day, initially
• *Child >6 mo:* **PO** 2 mg/kg/day in divided doses
• *Child <6 mo:* **PO** up to 4 mg/kg/day in divided doses

Available forms: Tabs 25, 50, 100 mg; caps 12.5 mg; oral sol 10 mg/5 ml, 100 mg/ml

SIDE EFFECTS

CNS: Drowsiness, paresthesia, depression, headache, *dizziness, fatigue, weakness,* fever
CV: Irregular pulse, orthostatic hypotension, palpitations, volume depletion, allergic myocarditis

---

EENT: Blurred vision
ELECT: Hypokalemia, hypercalcemia, hyponatremia, hypochloremia, hypomagnesemia
GI: Nausea, vomiting, anorexia, constipation, diarrhea, cramps, pancreatitis, GI irritation, **hepatitis**
GU: Urinary frequency, polyuria, **uremia, glucosuria,** hyperuricemia
*HEMA: **Aplastic anemia, hemolytic anemia, leukopenia, agranulocytosis, thrombocytopenia, neutropenia***
INTEG: Rash, urticaria, purpura, photosensitivity, alopecia, erythema multiforme
META: Hyperglycemia, hyperuricemia, increased creatinine, BUN

Contraindications: Hypersensitivity to thiazides or sulfonamides, anuria, renal decompensation, hypomagnesemia

Precautions: Pregnancy (B), hypokalemia, renal disease, lactation, hepatic disease, gout, COPD, LE, diabetes mellitus, hyperlipidemia, CCr <25 ml/min

PHARMACOKINETICS

PO: Onset 2 hr, peak 4 hr, duration 6-12 hr, half-life 6-15 hr; excreted unchanged by kidneys; crosses placenta; enters breast milk

INTERACTIONS

Hyperglycemia, hyperuricemia, increased antihypertensives: diazoxide
Hypokalemia: glucocorticoids, amphotericin B
Increase: toxicity—lithium, nondepolarizing skeletal muscle relaxants, cardiac glycosides
Increase: renal failure risk—NSAIDs
Increase: effects—loop diuretics
Decrease: antidiabetics effects
Decrease: thiazides absorption—cholestyramine, colestipol

Drug/Herb

Severe photosensitivity: St. John's wort
Increase: hypokalemia—aloe, buckthorn, cascara sagrada, Chinese rhubarb, gossypol, licorice, nettle, senna
Increase: diuretic effect—cucumber, dandelion, ginkgo, horsetail, khella,
licorice, nettle, pumpkin, Queen Anne's lace

Drug/Lab Test

Increase: BSP retention, amylase, parathyroid test
Decrease: PBI, PSP

NURSING CONSIDERATIONS

Assess:

• Weight, I&O daily to determine fluid loss; effect of drug may be decreased if used daily
• Rate, depth, rhythm of respiration, effect of exertion
• B/P lying, standing; postural hypotension may occur
• Electrolytes: K, Mg, Na, Cl; include BUN, blood glucose, CBC, serum creatinine, blood pH, ABGs, uric acid, Ca; renal function
• Glucose in urine if patient is diabetic
• Signs of metabolic alkalosis: drowsiness, restlessness
• Signs of hypokalemia: postural hypotension, malaise, fatigue, tachycardia, leg cramps, weakness, dehydration
• Rashes, temp daily
• Confusion, especially in elderly; take safety precautions if needed

Administer:

• In AM to avoid interference with sleep if using drug as a diuretic
• Potassium replacement if potassium <3 mg/dl
• With food; if nausea occurs, absorption may be decreased slightly

Evaluate:

• Therapeutic response: improvement in edema of feet, legs, sacral area daily, decreased B/P

Teach patient/family:

• To increase fluid intake to 2-3 L/day unless contraindicated; to rise slowly from lying or sitting position
• To notify prescriber of muscle weakness, cramps, nausea, dizziness
• That drug may be taken with food or milk
• To use sunscreen for photosensitivity
• That blood glucose may be increased in diabetics

⚠ Safety alert   *"Tall Man" lettering

- To take early in day to avoid nocturia
- To avoid alcohol; avoid OTC meds unless approved by prescriber

Treatment of overdose: Lavage if taken orally; monitor electrolytes; administer dextrose in saline; monitor hydration, CV, renal status

---

hydrocodone (℞)
(hye-droe-koe′done)
Hycodan, Robidone ✤,
Tussigon

hydrocodone/ acetaminophen
Allay, Anexsia, Anolor DH, Bancap HC, Co-Gesic, Dolacet, Dolagesic, Duocet, Hycomed, Hyco-Pap, Hydrocet, Hydrogesic, Lorcet, Lortab, Onset, Pancet, Panlor, Polygesic, Stagesic, T-Gesic, Ugesic, Vanacet, Vandone, Vicodin, Zydone

hydrocodone/aspirin
Azdone, Damason-P, Lortab ASA, Panasal

hydrocodone/ ibuprofen
Vicoprofen
Func. class.: Antitussive opioid analgesic, nonopioid analgesic

---

Controlled Substance Schedule III
Do not confuse:
hydrocodone/hydrocortisone
Hycodan/Vicodan
Action: Acts directly on cough center in medulla to suppress cough; binds to opiate receptors in CNS to reduce pain
Uses: Hyperactive and nonproductive cough, mild pain

DOSAGE AND ROUTES

Analgesic
- *Adult:* **PO** 2.5-10 mg q3-6h prn
- *Child:* **PO** 0.15-0.2 mg/kg q3-6h

Antitussive
- *Adult:* **PO** 5 mg q4-6 hr prn

Available forms: Hydrocodone: tabs 5 mg (Hycodan); syr 5 mg/ml (Hycodan, Robidone ✤); hydrocodone/ acetaminophen: tabs 2.5 mg hydrocodone/500 mg acetaminophen (Lortabs 2.5/500), 5 mg hydrocodone/ 400 mg acetaminophen (Zydone), 5 mg hydrocodone/500 mg acetaminophen (Anexsia 5/500, Co-Gesic, Dolacet, Hydrocet, Hydrogesic, Hy-Phen, Loracet, Loratab 5/500, Maragesic-H, Panacet 5/500, Stagesic, T-Gesic, Vicodin); 7.5 mg hydrocodone/400 mg acetaminophen (Zydone), 7.5 mg hydrocodone/500 mg acetaminophen (Loratab 7.5/500, 7.5 mg hydrocodone/650 mg acetaminophen (Anexsia 7.5/650, Loracet Plus), 7.5 mg hydrocodone/750 mg acetaminophen (Vicodin ES), 10 mg hydrocodone/325 acetaminophen (Norco), 10 mg hydrocodone/500 mg acetaminophen (Lortab 10/500), 10 mg hydrocodone/ 650 mg acetaminophen (Loracet 10/650, Vicodin HP), 10 mg hydrocodone/660 acetaminophen (Anexia 10/660); caps 5 mg hydrocodone/500 mg acetaminophen (Bancap-HC, Dolacet, Hydrocet, Hydrogesic, Loracet-HD, Maragesic-H, Stragesic, T-Gesic, Zydone); elixir or oral solution 2.5 mg hydrocodone/167 mg acetaminophen/5 ml; hydrocodone/ aspirin: tabs 5 mg hydrocodone/500 mg aspirin (Alor 5/500, Azdone, Damason-P, Loratab ASA, Panasal 5/500); hydrocodone/ibuprofen: tabs 7.5 mg hydrocodone/200 mg ibuprofen (Vicoprofen)

SIDE EFFECTS

CNS: Drowsiness, dizziness, lightheadedness, confusion, headache, sedation, euphoria, dysphoria, weakness, hallucinations, disorientation, mood changes, dependence, ***convulsions***
CV: Palpitations, tachycardia, bradycardia, change in B/P, ***circulatory depression,*** syncope
EENT: Tinnitus, blurred vision, miosis, diplopia
GI: Nausea, vomiting, anorexia, constipation, cramps, dry mouth

---

GU: Increased urinary output, dysuria, urinary retention

INTEG: Rash, urticaria, flushing, pruritus

RESP: **Respiratory depression**

Contraindications: Hypersensitivity, addiction (opioid)

Precautions: Pregnancy (C), addictive personality, lactation, increased intracranial pressure, MI (acute), severe heart disease, respiratory depression, hepatic disease, renal disease

PHARMACOKINETICS

Onset 10-20 min, duration 4-6 hr, half-life 3½-4½ hr; metabolized in liver; excreted in urine; crosses placenta

INTERACTIONS

Increase: CNS depression—alcohol, opioids, sedative/hypnotics, phenothiazines, skeletal muscle relaxants, general anesthetics, tricyclics

Drug/Herb

Increase: CNS depression—Jamaican dogwood, lavender, mistletoe, nettle, pokeweed, poppy, senega, valerian

Increase: anticholinergic effect—corkwood

Drug/Lab Test

Increase: Amylase, lipase

NURSING CONSIDERATIONS

Assess:

• Pain: intensity, type, location, and other characteristics

• CNS changes: dizziness, drowsiness, hallucinations, euphoria, LOC, pupil reaction

• Allergic reactions: rash, urticaria

• Cough and respiratory dysfunction: respiratory depression, character, rate, rhythm; notify prescriber if respirations are <10/min

• Need for pain medication, physical dependence

Administer:

• Do not break, crush, or chew tabs; only scored tabs can be broken

• With antiemetic after meals if nausea or vomiting occurs

Perform/provide:

• Storage in light-resistant area at room temperature

• Assistance with ambulation

• Safety measures: night-light, call bell within easy reach

Evaluate:

• Therapeutic response: decrease in pain or cough

Teach patient/family:

• To report any symptoms of CNS changes, allergic reactions

• That physical dependency may result when used for extended periods

• That withdrawal symptoms may occur: nausea, vomiting, cramps, fever, faintness, anorexia

• To avoid driving, other hazardous activities, drowsiness occurs

• To avoid other CNS depressants, will enhance sedating properties of this drug

Treatment of overdose: Naloxone HCl (Narcan) 0.2-0.8 mg IV, O_2, IV fluids, vasopressors

---

hydrocortisone (℞)

(hy-dro-kor'tih-sone)

Cortef, Cortenema, Hydrocortone

hydrocortisone acetate (℞)

Cortifoam, Hydrocortone Acetate

hydrocortisone cypionate (℞)

Cortef

hydrocortisone sodium phosphate (℞)

Hydrocortone Phosphate

hydrocortisone sodium succinate (℞)

A-hydroCort, Solu-Cortef

Func. class.: Corticosteroid

Chem. class.: Short-acting glucocorticoid

Do not confuse:

hydrocortisone/hydrocodone

Action: Decreases inflammation by suppression of migration of polymorphonuclear leukocytes, fibroblasts, reversal of increased capillary permeability, and lysosomal stabilization

Uses: Severe inflammation, septic shock, adrenal insufficiency, ulcerative colitis, collagen disorders

DOSAGE AND ROUTES

Adrenal insufficiency/inflammation
• *Adult:* **PO** 5-30 mg bid-qid; **IM/IV** 100-250 mg (succinate), then 50-100 mg **IM** as needed; **IM/IV** 15-240 mg q12h (phosphate)

Shock
• *Adult:* 500 mg-2 g q2-6h (succinate)
• *Child:* **IM/IV** 0.186-1 mg/kg bid-tid (succinate)

Colitis
• *Adult:* **ENEMA** 100 mg nightly for 21 days

Available forms: Tabs 5, 10, 20 mg; inj 25, 50 mg/ml; enema 100 mg/60 ml; acetate—inj 25 ✦, 50 mg/ml ✦, enema 10% aerosol foam; supp 25 mg; cypionate—oral susp 10 mg/5 ml; phosphate—inj 50 mg/ml; succinate inj 100 mg ✦, 250 mg ✦, 500 mg ✦, 1000 mg/vial ✦

SIDE EFFECTS

CNS: Depression, flushing, sweating, headache, mood changes
*CV: Hypertension, **circulatory collapse**, **thrombophlebitis**, **embolism**,* tachycardia, edema
EENT: Fungal infections, increased intraocular pressure, blurred vision
GI: Diarrhea, nausea, abdominal distention, ***GI hemorrhage***, increased appetite, ***pancreatitis***
*HEMA: **Thrombocytopenia***
INTEG: Acne, poor wound healing, ecchymosis, petechiae
MS: Fractures, osteoporosis, weakness
Contraindications: Psychosis, hypersensitivity, idiopathic thrombocytopenia (IM), acute glomerulonephritis, amebiasis, fungal infections, nonasthmatic bronchial disease, child <2 yr, AIDS, TB

Precautions: Pregnancy (C), lactation, diabetes mellitus, glaucoma, osteoporosis, seizure disorders, ulcerative colitis, CHF, myasthenia gravis, renal disease, esophagitis, peptic ulcer

PHARMACOKINETICS

PO: Onset 1-2 hr, peak 1 hr, duration 1-1½ days
IM/IV: Onset 20 min, peak 4-8 hr, duration 1-1½ days
RECT: Onset 3-5 days
Metabolized by liver, excreted in urine (17-OHCS, 17-KS), crosses placenta

INTERACTIONS

Risk of GI bleeding: salicylates, NSAIDs
Increase: side effects—alcohol, amphotericin B, digitalis, cycloSPORINE, diuretics
Decrease: hydrocortisone action—cholestyramine, colestipol, barbiturates, rifampin, epHEDrine, phenytoin, theophylline
Decrease: anticoagulant effects, anticonvulsants, antidiabetics, toxoids, vaccines
Drug/Herb
Increase: hypokalemia—aloe, buckthorn, cascara sagrada, Chinese rhubarb, senna
Increase: corticosteroid effect—aloe, licorice, perilla
Drug/Lab Test
Increase: Cholesterol, sodium, blood glucose, uric acid, calcium, urine glucose
Decrease: Ca, K, T_4, T_3, thyroid ^{131}I uptake test, urine 17-OHCS, 17-KS
False negative: Skin allergy tests

NURSING CONSIDERATIONS
Assess:
• Potassium, blood glucose, urine glucose while on long-term therapy; hypokalemia and hyperglycemia
• Weight daily, notify prescriber of weekly gain >5 lb
• B/P q4h, pulse; notify prescriber of chest pain
• I&O ratio; be alert for decreasing urinary output, increasing edema
• Plasma cortisol levels during long-

term therapy (normal level: 138-635 nmol/L SI units when drawn at 8 AM)

- Infection: increased temp, WBC, even after withdrawal of medication; drug masks infection
- Potassium depletion: paresthesias, fatigue, nausea, vomiting, depression, polyuria, dysrhythmias, weakness
- Edema, hypertension, cardiac symptoms
- Mental status: affect, mood, behavioral changes, aggression

Administer:

- Daily dose in AM for better results
- IM inj deep in large muscle mass; rotate sites; avoid deltoid; use 21G needle
- In one dose in AM to prevent adrenal suppression; avoid SUBCUT administration; may damage tissue
- With food or milk for GI symptoms (PO)
- Rectal: telling patient to retain for 20 min if possible

IV route

- Phosphate: IV undiluted or added to dextrose or saline inj and given by inf; give 25 mg or less/min
- Succinate: IV in mix-o-vial, or reconstitute 250 mg or less/2 ml bacteriostatic H_2O for inj; mix gently; give direct IV over 1 min or more; may be further diluted in 100, 250, 500, or 1000 ml of D_5W, D_5 0.9%, NaCl 0.9% given over ordered rate

Sodium phosphate preparations

Additive compatibilities: Amikacin, amphotericin B, bleomycin, cephapirin, metaraminol, sodium bicarbonate, verapamil

Syringe compatibilities: Metoclopramide

Y-site compatibilities: Allpurinol, amifostine, aztreonam, cefepime, cladribine, famotidine, filgrastim, fluconazole, fludarabine, granisetron, melphalan, ondansetron, paclitaxel, piperacillin/tazobactam, teniposide, thiotepa, vinorelbine

Sodium succinate preparations

Additive compatibilities: Amikacin, aminophylline, amphotericin B, calcium chloride, calcium gluconate, cephalothin, cephapirin, chloramphenicol, clindamycin, cloxacillin, corticotropin, DAUNOrubicin, diphenhydrAMINE, DOPamine, erythromycin, floxacillin, lidocaine, magnesium sulfate, mephentermine, metronidazole/sodium bicarbonate, mitomycin, mitoxantrone, netilmicin, netilmicin/potassium chloride, norepinephrine, penicillin G potassium/sodium, piperacillin, polymyxin B, potassium chloride, sodium bicarbonate, theophylline, thiopental, vancomycin, verapamil, vit B/C

Syringe compatibilities: Metoclopramide, thiopental

Y-site compatibilities: Acyclovir, allopurinol, amifostine, aminophylline, amphotericin B cholesteryl, ampicillin, amrinone, amsacrine, atracurium, atropine, aztreonam, betamethasone, calcium gluconate, cefepime, cefmetazole, cephalothin, cephapirin, chlordiazepoxide, chlorproMAZINE, cisatracurium, cladribine, cyanocobalamin, cytarabine, dexamethasone, digoxin, diphenhydrAMINE, DOPamine, DOXOrubicin liposome, droperidol, edrophonium, enalaprilat, epINEPHrine, esmolol, estrogens conjugated, ethacrynate, famotidine, fentanyl, fentanyl/droperidol, filgrastim, fludarabine, fluorouracil, foscarnet, furosemide, gallium, granisetron, heparin, hydrALAZINE, insulin (regular), isoproterenol, kanamycin, lidocaine, lorazepam, magnesium sulfate, melphalan, menadiol, meperidine, methicillin, methoxamine, methylergonovine, minocycline, morphine, neostigmine, norepinephrine, ondansetron, oxacillin, oxytocin, paclitaxel, pancuronium, penicillin G potassium, pentazocine, phytonadione, piperacillin/tazobactam, prednisolone, procainamide, prochlorperazine, propofol, propranolol, pyridostigmine, remifentanil, scopolamine, sodium bicarbonate, succinylcholine, tacrolimus, teniposide, theophylline, thiotepa, trimethaphan, trimethobenzamide, vecuronium, vinorelbine

Perform/provide:

- Assistance with ambulation in patient with bone tissue disease to prevent fractures

Evaluate:

• Therapeutic response: ease of respirations, decreased inflammation

Teach patient/family:

• That emergency ID as steroid user should be carried

• To notify prescriber if therapeutic response decreases; dosage adjustment may be needed; of signs of infection

• Not to discontinue abruptly, or adrenal crisis can result; drug should be tapered off

• To avoid OTC products: salicylates, alcohol in cough products, cold preparations unless directed by prescriber

• About cushingoid symptoms of adrenal insufficiency: nausea, anorexia, fatigue, dizziness, dyspnea, weakness, joint pain

---

hydrocortisone topical
See Appendix C

⚠ High Alert

hydromorphone (℞)
(hye-droe-mor'fone)
Dilaudid, Dilaudid HP,
hydromorphone HCl,
Hydrostat IR,
PMS-Hydromorphone
Func. class.: Opiate analgesic
Chem. class.: Semisynthetic phenanthrene

Controlled Substance Schedule II
Do not confuse:
Dilaudid/Demerol
hydromorphone/meperidine
hydromorphone/morphine
Action: Inhibits ascending pain pathways in CNS, increases pain threshold, alters pain perception
Uses: Moderate to severe pain, nonproductive cough

DOSAGE AND ROUTES

Analgesic
• *Adult:* **PO** 1-6 mg q4-6h prn; **IM/** **SUBCUT/IV** 2-4 mg q4-6h; **RECT** 3 mg q4-6h prn
• *Geriatric:* **PO** 1-2 mg q4-6h
• *Child:* 0.03-0.08 mg/kg q4-6h, max 5 mg/dose
Antitussive
• *Adult:* **PO** 1 mg q3-4h prn
Available forms: Inj 1, 2, 3, 4, 10 mg/ml; tabs 1, 2, 3, 4, 8 mg; supp 3 mg; oral sol 5 mg/5 ml; syrup 1 mg/5 ml

SIDE EFFECTS

CNS: Drowsiness, dizziness, confusion, headache, sedation, euphoria, mood changes, **seizures**
CV: Palpitations, bradycardia, change in B/P, hypotension, tachycardia
EENT: Tinnitus, blurred vision, miosis, diplopia
GI: Nausea, vomiting, anorexia, constipation, cramps, dry mouth
GU: Increased urinary output, dysuria, urinary retention
INTEG: Rash, urticaria, bruising, flushing, diaphoresis, pruritus
RESP: **Respiratory depression**
Contraindications: Hypersensitivity, addiction (opiate)
Precautions: Pregnancy (C), addictive personality, lactation, increased intracranial pressure, MI (acute), severe heart disease, respiratory depression, hepatic disease, renal disease, child <18 yr

PHARMACOKINETICS

Onset 15-30 min, peak ½-1 hr, duration 4-5 hr; metabolized by liver; excreted by kidneys; crosses placenta; excreted in breast milk, half-life 2-3 hr

INTERACTIONS

Increase: with other CNS depressants—alcohol, opiates, sedative/hypnotics, antipsychotics, skeletal muscle relaxants
Drug/Herb
Increase: action—chamomile, hops, Jamaican dogwood, kava, lavender, mistletoe, nettle, pokeweed, poppy, senega, skullcap, valerian
Increase: anticholinergic effect—corkwood

Side effects: *italics* = common; ***bold italics*** = life-threatening

Drug/Lab Test
Increase: Amylase

NURSING CONSIDERATIONS
Assess:
- I&O ratio; check for decreasing output; may indicate urinary retention
- CNS changes: dizziness, drowsiness, hallucinations, euphoria, LOC, pupil reaction
- Bowel function, constipation
- Allergic reactions: rash, urticaria
- Respiratory dysfunction: respiratory depression, character, rate, rhythm; notify prescriber if respirations are <10/min
- Need for pain medication, physical dependence
- Pain control, sedation by scoring on 0-10 scale, ATC dosing is best for pain control

Administer:
- With antiemetic if nausea, vomiting occur
- When pain is beginning to return; determine interval by response
- Rotate inj sites when giving SUBCUT

IV route
- Direct, diluted with 5 ml sterile H_2O or NS; give through Y-connector or 3-way stopcock; give 2 mg or less/3-5 min
- IV INF: Dilute each 0.1-1 mg/ml NS (0.1-1 mg/ml), deliver by opioid syringe infusor; may be diluted in D_5W, D_5/NaCl, 0.45% NaCl, or NS for larger amounts and delivery through an infusion pump

Additive compatibilities: Bupivacaine, fluorouracil, midazolam, ondansetron, promethazine, verapamil

Solution compatibilities: D_5W, D_5/0.45% NaCl, D_5/0.9% NaCl, D_5/LR, D_5/Ringer's sol, 0.45% NaCl, 0.9% NaCl, Ringer's and lactated Ringer's sol

Syringe compatibilities: Atropine, bupivacaine, ceftazidime, chlorproMAZINE, cimetidine, dimenhyDRINATE, diphenhydrAMINE, fentanyl, glycopyrrolate, haloperidol, hydrOXYzine, lorazepam, midazolam, pentazocine, pentobarbital, prochlorperazine, promethazine, ranitidine, scopolamine, tetracaine, thiethylperazine, trimethobenzamide

Y-site compatibilities: Acyclovir, allopurinol, amifostine, amikacin, amsacrine, aztreonam, cefamandole, cefazolin, cefepime, cefmetazole, cefoperazone, cefotaxime, cefoxitin, ceftazidime, ceftizoxime, cefuroxime, cephalothin, cephapirin, chloramphenicol, cisatracurium, cisplatin, cladribine, clindamycin, cyclophosphamide, cytarabine, diltiazem, DOBUTamine, DOPamine, DOXOrubicin, DOXOrubicin liposome, doxycycline, epINEPHrine, erythromycin lactobionate, famotidine, fentanyl, filgrastim, fludarabine, foscarnet, furosemide, gentamicin, granisetron, heparin, kanamycin, labetalol, lorazepam, magnesium sulfate, melphalan, methotrexate, metronidazole, mezlocillin, midazolam, milrinone, morphine, moxalactam, nafcillin, niCARdipine, nitroglycerin, norepinephrine, ondansetron, oxacillin, paclitaxel, penicillin G potassium, piperacillin, piperacillin/tazobactam, propofol, ranitidine, remifentanil, teniposide, thiotepa, ticarcillin, tobramycin, trimethoprimsulfamethoxazole, vancomycin, vecuronium, vinorelbine

Perform/provide:
- Storage in light-resistant area at room temperature
- Assistance with ambulation
- Safety measures: side rails, night-light, call bell within easy reach

Evaluate:
- Therapeutic response: decrease in pain

Teach patient/family:
- To report any symptoms of CNS changes, allergic reactions
- That physical dependency may result when used for extended periods
- That withdrawal symptoms may occur: nausea, vomiting, cramps, fever, faintness, anorexia
- To avoid driving, other hazardous activities, drowsiness occurs

Treatment of overdose: Naloxone HCl (Narcan) 0.2-0.8 mg IV, O_2, IV fluids, vasopressors

---

⚠ Safety alert   *"Tall Man" lettering

hydromorphone/ guaifenesin/ alcohol (℞)

(hye-droe-mor'fone)
Dilaudid Cough Syrup
Func. class.: Antitussive, opioid
Chem. class.: Phenanthrene derivative

Controlled Substance Schedule II
Do not confuse:
hydromorphone/meperidine/morphine
Action: Increases respiratory tract fluid by decreasing surface tension, adhesiveness, which increases removal of mucus; analgesic, antitussive suppresses the cough reflex by a direct central action
Uses: Cough

DOSAGE AND ROUTES

• *Adult:* **PO** 1 mg q3-4h prn
Available forms: Syr 1 mg/5 ml

SIDE EFFECTS

CNS: Dizziness, drowsiness
CV: Hypotension
GI: Nausea, constipation, vomiting, anorexia
INTEG: Urticaria, rash
RESP: ***Respiratory depression***
Contraindications: Hypersensitivity, increased intracranial pressure, status asthmaticus
Precautions: Pregnancy (C), hypothyroidism, Addison's disease, CNS depression, brain tumor, asthma, hepatic disease, renal disease, COPD, psychosis, alcoholism, convulsive disorders, lactation

PHARMACOKINETICS

Metabolized by liver; half-life 2-4 hr

INTERACTIONS

Increase: CNS depression—barbiturates, opioids, antipsychotics, antidepressants
Drug/Herb
Increase: anticholinergic effect—corkwood
Increase: sedative effect—chamomile, hops, Jamaican dogwood, lavender, mistletoe, nettle, pokeweed, poppy, senega, skullcap, valerian

NURSING CONSIDERATIONS
Assess:
• VS, cardiac status, including hypotension
• Respiratory rate, depth
• Cough: type, frequency, character, including sputum
Administer:
• Decreased dose to elderly patients; metabolism may be slowed
Perform/provide:
• Storage at room temperature
• Increased fluids, bulk, exercise to decrease constipation
Evaluate:
• Therapeutic response: absence of cough
Teach patient/family:
• To avoid driving, other hazardous activities until patient stabilized on medication if drowsiness occurs
• To avoid alcohol, other CNS depressants; will enhance sedating properties of this drug
• May be taken with food for GI upset
• Physical dependency may result when used for extended periods of time

hydroxyamphetamine HBr ophthalmic

See Appendix C

hydroxychloro- quine (℞)

(hye-drox-ee-klor'oh-kwin)
Plaquenil
Func. class.: Antimalarial, antirheumatic (DMARDs)
Chem. class.: 4-Aminoquinoline derivative

Action: Inhibits parasite replications, transcription of DNA to RNA by forming complexes with DNA in parasite

Uses: Malaria caused by *Plasmodium vivax, P. malariae, P. ovale, P. falciparum* (some strains); LE, rheumatoid arthritis

DOSAGE AND ROUTES

Malaria
• *Adult:* PO suppression or prevention 200 mg qwk, begin 1-2 wk before travel, continue 4 wk after returning; treatment 400 mg, then 200 mg at 6, 24, 48 hr after 1st dose
• *Child:* PO suppression or prevention 5 mg/kg qwk, begin 1-2 wk before travel, continue 4 wk after returning; treatment 10 mg/kg, then 5 mg/kg at 6, 24, 48 hr after 1st dose

Lupus erythematosus
• *Adult:* PO 400 mg daily-bid; length depends on patient response; maintenance 200-400 mg daily

Rheumatoid arthritis
• *Adult:* PO 400-600 mg daily for 4-12 wk; then 200-300 mg daily after good response
• *Child:* PO 3-5 mg/kg/day max 400 mg/day

Available forms: Tabs 200 mg

SIDE EFFECTS

CNS: Headache, stimulation, fatigue, irritability, *seizures,* bad dreams, dizziness, confusion, psychosis, decreased reflexes
CV: Hypotension, heart block, *asystole with syncope*
EENT: Blurred vision, corneal changes, retinal changes, difficulty focusing, tinnitus, vertigo, deafness, photophobia, corneal edema
GI: Nausea, vomiting, anorexia, diarrhea, cramps
HEMA: Thrombocytopenia, agranulocytosis, leukopenia, aplastic anemia
INTEG: Pruritus, pigmentation changes, skin eruptions, lichen planus–like eruptions, eczema, *exfoliative dermatitis,* alopecia

Contraindications: Hypersensitivity, retinal field changes, children (long-term)

Precautions: Pregnancy (C), blood dyscrasias, severe GI disease, neurologic disease, alcoholism, hepatic disease, G6PD deficiency, psoriasis, eczema, lactation

PHARMACOKINETICS

PO: Peak 1-2 hr, half-life 3-5 days; metabolized in liver; excreted in urine, feces, breast milk; crosses placenta

INTERACTIONS

Increase: digoxin levels
Increase: antibody titer—rabies vaccine
Decrease: hydroxychloroquine action—Mg or Al compounds

NURSING CONSIDERATIONS

Assess:
• For LE, malaria symptoms
• For rheumatoid arthritis: pain, swelling, ROM, temperature of joints
• Ophthalmic exam baseline and q6mo if long-term treatment or drug dosage >150 mg/day
• Hepatic studies qwk: AST, ALT, bilirubin
• Blood studies: CBC, platelets; WBC, RBC, platelets may be decreased; if severe, drug should be discontinued
• For decreased reflexes: knee, ankle
• ECG during therapy
• Watch for depression of T waves, widening of QRS complex
• Allergic reactions: pruritus, rash, urticaria
• Blood dyscrasias: malaise, fever, bruising, bleeding (rare)
• For ototoxicity (tinnitus, vertigo, change in hearing); audiometric testing should be done before, after treatment
⚠ For toxicity: blurring vision, difficulty focusing, headache, dizziness, knee, ankle reflexes; drug should be discontinued immediately

Administer:
• Before or after meals or with milk; at same time each day to maintain drug level
• Tabs may be crushed and mixed with food, fluids

⚠ Safety alert   *"Tall Man" lettering

• For malaria prophylaxis should be started 2 wk prior to exposure and 4-6 wk after leaving exposure area

Perform/provide:

• Storage in tight, light-resistant container at room temperature; keep inj in cool environment

Evaluate:

• Therapeutic response: decreased symptoms of malaria, LE, rheumatoid arthritis

Teach patient/family:

• To use sunglasses in bright sunlight to decrease photophobia

• That urine may turn rust or brown

• To report hearing, visual problems, fever, fatigue, bruising, bleeding, which may indicate blood dyscrasias

Treatment of overdose: Induce vomiting; gastric lavage; administer barbiturate (ultrashort-acting), vasopressor, ammonium chloride; tracheostomy may be necessary

---

hydroxyurea (℞)

(hye-drox'ee-yoo-ree-ah)
Droxia, Hydrea
Func. class.: Antineoplastic, antimetabolite
Chem. class.: Synthetic urea analog

Action: Acts by inhibiting DNA synthesis without interfering with RNA or protein synthesis; incorporates thymidine into DNA, causing direct damage to DNA strands; S phase specific of cell cycle

Uses: Melanoma, chronic myelocytic leukemia, recurrent or metastatic ovarian cancer, squamous cell carcinoma of the head and neck, sickle cell anemia, psoriasis

DOSAGE AND ROUTES

Solid tumors

• *Adult:* **PO** 80 mg/kg as a single dose q3d or 20-30 mg/kg as a single dose daily

In combination with radiation

• *Adult:* **PO** 80 mg/kg as a single dose q3d; should be started 7 days before irradiation

Resistant chronic myelocytic leukemia

• *Adult:* **PO** 20-30 mg/kg/day as a single daily dose

Sickle cell anemia

• *Adult:* **PO** 15 mg/kg/day, may increase by 5 mg/kg/day, max 35 mg/kg/day

Renal disease

• CCr 10-50 ml/min dose 50%; CCr <10 ml/min dose 20%

Available forms: Caps 200, 300, 400, 500 mg

SIDE EFFECTS

CNS: Headache, confusion, hallucinations, dizziness, ***convulsions***

CV: Angina, ischemia

GI: Nausea, vomiting, anorexia, diarrhea, stomatitis, constipation

GU: Increased BUN, uric acid, creatinine, temporary renal function impairment

*HEMA: **Leukopenia, anemia, thrombocytopenia, megaloblastic erythropoiesis***

INTEG: Rash, urticaria, pruritus, dry skin, facial erythema

MISC: Fever, chills, malaise

Contraindications: Pregnancy (D), hypersensitivity, leukopenia (<2500/mm^3), thrombocytopenia (<100,000/mm^3), anemia (severe), lactation

Precautions: Renal disease (severe)

PHARMACOKINETICS

Readily absorbed when taken orally, peak level in 2 hr; degraded in liver; excreted in urine, almost totally eliminated in 24 hr; readily crosses blood-brain barrier, eliminated as CO_2

INTERACTIONS

Increase: toxicity—radiation or other antineoplastics

Drug/Lab Test

Increase: Renal studies

NURSING CONSIDERATIONS

Assess:

• CBC, differential, platelet count qwk; withhold drug if WBC is <2500/mm^3 or platelet count is <100,000/mm^3; notify

prescriber; drug should be discontinued
- Renal studies: BUN, serum uric acid, urine CCr, electrolytes before, during therapy
- I&O ratio; report fall in urine output to <30 ml/hr
- Monitor temp q4h; fever may indicate beginning infection
- Hepatic studies before, during therapy: bilirubin, alk phosphatase, AST, ALT, LDH; prn or qmo
- B/P q3-4h; check for chest pain; angina, ischemia may occur
- Bleeding: hematuria, guaiac, bruising or petechiae, mucosa or orifices q8h
- Food preferences; list likes, dislikes
- Inflammation of mucosa, breaks in skin
- Buccal cavity q8h for dryness, sores or ulceration, white patches, oral pain, bleeding, dysphagia
- Symptoms indicating severe allergic reaction: rash, urticaria, itching, flushing
- Neurotoxicity: headaches, hallucinations, convulsions, dizziness

Administer:
- Do not crush or chew caps; caps can be opened and contents mixed with water.
- Allopurinol or NaHCO$_3$ concurrently to prevent high uric acid levels; extra fluids
- Antiemetic 30-60 min before giving drug and prn
- Antibiotics for prophylaxis of infection
- Transfusion for anemia

Perform/provide:
- Rinsing of mouth tid-qid with water, club soda; brushing of teeth bid-tid with soft brush or cotton-tipped applicators for stomatitis; use unwaxed dental floss
- Nutritious diet with iron, vitamin supplements as ordered

Evaluate:
- Therapeutic response: decreased tumor size, spread of malignancy

Teach patient/family:
- To report signs of infection: elevated temp, sore throat, flulike symptoms
- To report signs of anemia: fatigue, headache, faintness, shortness of breath, irritability
- To report bleeding: avoid use of razors, commercial mouthwash

- To avoid use of aspirin products, ibuprofen
- To avoid foods with citric acid, hot or rough texture if stomatitis is present
- To report stomatitis: any bleeding, white spots, ulcerations in the mouth; tell patient to examine mouth daily, report symptoms
- That contraceptive measures are recommended during therapy
- To notify prescriber of fever, chills, sore throat, nausea, vomiting, anorexia, diarrhea, bleeding, bruising; may indicate blood dyscrasias

---

*hydrOXYzine (R)

(hye-drox'i-zeen)
Apo-Hydroxyzine ✲, Atarax, hydroxyzine, Multi-pax ✲, Novohydroxyzine ✲, Vistaril
Func. class.: Antianxiety/antihistamine/sedative-hypnotic, antiemetic
Chem. class.: Piperazine derivative

Do not confuse:
Atarax/amoxicillin/Ativan
Vistaril/Versed
hydrOXYzine/hydrALAZINE

Action: Depresses subcortical levels of CNS, including limbic system, reticular formation; competes with H$_1$-receptor sites

Uses: Anxiety preoperatively, postoperatively to prevent nausea, vomiting, to potentiate opioid analgesics; sedation; pruritus

DOSAGE AND ROUTES
- *Adult:* **PO** 25-100 mg tid-qid, max 600 mg/day
- *Geriatric:* **PO** 10 mg tid-qid (pruritus)
- *Child >6 yr:* 50-100 mg/day in divided doses
- *Child <6 yr:* 50 mg/day in divided doses

Preoperatively/postoperatively
- *Adult:* **IM** 25-100 mg q4-6h
- *Child:* **IM** 0.5-1.1 mg/kg q4-6h

Pruritus
- *Adult:* **PO** 25 mg tid-qid

Antiemetic
- *Adult:* **IM** 25-100 mg/dose q4-6h prn

Available forms: Tabs 10, 25, 50, 100 mg; caps 10, 25, 50, 100 mg; oral susp 25 mg/5 ml; inj 25, 50 mg/ml

SIDE EFFECTS

CNS: Dizziness, drowsiness, confusion, headache, tremors, fatigue, depression, ***seizures***
CV: Hypotension
GI: Dry mouth, increased appetite, nausea, diarrhea, weight gain

Contraindications: Pregnancy (1st trimester), hypersensitivity to this drug or cetirizine, lactation, acute asthma
Precautions: Pregnancy (C) (2nd/3rd trimester), elderly, debilitated, hepatic disease, renal disease, narrow-angle glaucoma, COPD, prostatic hypertrophy

PHARMACOKINETICS

PO: Onset 15-30 min, duration 4-6 hr, half-life 3 hr, metabolized by liver, excreted by kidneys

INTERACTIONS

Increase: CNS depressant effect—barbiturates, opioids, analgesics, alcohol
Increase: anticholinergic effects—phenothiazines, quinidine, disopyramide, antihistamines, antidepressants, atropine, haloperidol

Drug/Herb
Increase: anticholinergic effect—corkwood, henbane leaf, jimsonweed, scopolia
Increase: sedative action—chamomile, cowslip, hops, Jamaican dogwood, kava, khat, Queen Anne's lace, senega, skullcap, valerian

NURSING CONSIDERATIONS

Assess:
- B/P (lying, standing), pulse; if systolic B/P drops 20 mm Hg, hold drug, notify prescriber
- Mental status: mood, sensorium, affect, anxiety, behavior, increased sedation

Administer:

PO route
- With food or milk for GI symptoms (PO)
- Crushed if patient is unable to swallow medication whole
- Gum, hard candy, frequent sips of water for dry mouth

IM route
- By Z-track inj in large muscle for IM to decrease pain, chance of necrosis, never give IV/SUBCUT

Additive compatibilities: Cisplatin, cyclophosphamide, cytarabine, dimenhyDRINATE, etoposide, lidocaine, mesna, methotrexate, nafcillin

Syringe compatibilities: Atropine, atropine/meperidine, benzquinamide, bupivacaine, butorphanol, chlorproMAZINE, cimetidine, codeine, diphenhydrAMINE, doxapram, droperidol, fentanyl, fluphenazine, glycopyrrolate, hydromorphone, lidocaine, meperidine, meperidine/atropine, methotrimeprazine, metoclopramide, midazolam, morphine, nalbuphine, oxymorphone, pentazocine, perphenazine, procaine, prochlorperazine, promazine, promethazine, scopolamine, sufentanil, thiothixene

Perform/provide:
- Assistance with ambulation during beginning therapy, since drowsiness/dizziness occurs
- Safety measures, including side rails
- Checking to see if PO medication has been swallowed

Evaluate:
- Therapeutic response: decreased anxiety

Teach patient/family:
- That medication is not to be used for everyday stress or used longer than 4 mo
- To avoid OTC preparations (cold, cough, hay fever) unless approved by prescriber
- To avoid driving, activities that require alertness

H

- To avoid alcohol ingestion, psychotropic medications
- Not to discontinue medication quickly after long-term use
- To rise slowly or fainting may occur

Treatment of overdose: Lavage if orally ingested; VS, supportive care; IV norepinephrine for hypotension

---

hyoscyamine (℞)

(hye-oh-sye′a-meen)
Anaspaz, A-Spas S/L,
Cystospaz, Cystospaz-M,
Donnamar, ED-SPAZ,
Gastrosed, Levsin, Levsinex,
NuLev Timecaps
Func. class.: Anticholinergic/antispasmodics
Chem. class.: Belladonna alkaloid

Action: Inhibits muscarinic actions of acetylcholine at postganglionic parasympathetic neuroeffector sites, reduces rigidity, tremors, hyperhidrosis of Parkinsonism

Uses: Treatment of peptic ulcer disease in combination with other drugs; other GI disorders, other spastic disorders, IBS, urinary incontinence

DOSAGE AND ROUTES

- *Adult:* **PO/SL** 0.125-0.25 mg tid-qid ac, at bedtime; **TIME REL** 0.375 q12h; **IM/SUBCUT/IV** 0.25-0.5 mg q6h
- *Child 2-12 yr:* **PO** (orally disintegrating tabs) 0.0625-0.125 mg (½-1 tab) q4h, max 6×/day
- *Child 34-36 kg:* **PO** 125-187 mcg q4h prn
- *Child 22.7-33 kg:* **PO** 94-125 mcg q4h prn
- *Child 13.6-22.6 kg:* **PO** 63 mcg q4h prn
- *Child 9.1-13.5 kg:* **PO** 31.3 mcg q4h prn
- *Child 6.8-9 kg:* **PO** 25 mg q4h prn
- *Child 4.5-6.7 kg:* **PO** 18.8 mcg q4h prn
- *Child 3.4-4.4 kg:* **PO** 15.6 mcg q4h prn

- *Child 2.3-3.3 kg:* **PO** 12.5 mcg q4h prn

Available forms: Tabs 0.125, 0.13, 0.15 mg; caps time rel 0.375 mg; sol 0.125 mg/ml; elix 0.125 mg/5 ml; inj 0.5 mg/ml

SIDE EFFECTS

CNS: Confusion, stimulation in elderly, headache, insomnia, dizziness, drowsiness, anxiety, weakness, hallucination
CV: Palpitations, tachycardia
EENT: Blurred vision, photophobia, mydriasis, cycloplegia, increased ocular tension
GI: Dry mouth, constipation, paralytic ileus, heartburn, nausea, vomiting, dysphagia, absence of taste
GU: Urinary hesitancy, retention, impotence
INTEG: Urticaria, rash, pruritus, anhidrosis, fever, allergic reactions

Contraindications: Hypersensitivity to anticholinergics, narrow-angle glaucoma, GI obstruction, myasthenia gravis, paralytic ileus, GI atony, toxic megacolon, prostatic hypertrophy

Precautions: Pregnancy (C), hyperthyroidism, coronary artery disease, dysrhythmias, CHF, ulcerative colitis, hypertension, hiatal hernia, hepatic disease, renal disease, urinary retention, elderly

PHARMACOKINETICS

PO: Duration 4-6 hr; metabolized by liver; excreted in urine; half-life 3.5 hr

INTERACTIONS

Increase: anticholinergic effect—amantadine, tricyclics, MAOIs, H_1-antihistamines
Decrease: hyoscyamine effect—antacids
Decrease: effect of phenothiazines, levodopa, ketoconazole
Drug/Herb
Increase: constipation—black catechu
Increase: anticholinergic effect—butterbur, jimsonweed

Decrease: anticholinergic effect—jaborandi tree, pill-bearing spurge

NURSING CONSIDERATIONS
Assess:
• VS, cardiac status: checking for dysrhythmias, increased rate, palpitations
• I&O ratio; check for urinary retention or hesitancy
• GI complaints: pain, bleeding (frank or occult), nausea, vomiting, anorexia

Administer:
• Do not break, crush, or chew time rel caps
• ½ hr ac for better absorption
• Decreased dose to elderly patients; metabolism may be slowed
• Gum, hard candy, frequent rinsing of mouth for dryness of oral cavity

Perform/provide:
• Storage in tight container protected from light
• Increased fluids, bulk, exercise to decrease constipation

Evaluate:
• Therapeutic response: absence of epigastric pain, bleeding, nausea, vomiting

Teach patient/family:
• To avoid driving, other hazardous activities until stabilized on medication
• To avoid alcohol or other CNS depressants; will enhance sedating properties of this drug
• To avoid hot environments; heat stroke may occur; drug suppresses perspiration
• To use sunglasses when outside to prevent photophobia; may cause blurred vision

---

ibritumomab
tiuxetan (℞)
(ee-brit-u-moe′mab)
Zevalin
Func. class.: Miscellaneous antineoplastic
Chem. class.: Monoclonal antibody

Action: High affinity for indium-111, yttrium-90; induces CD20 + B-cell lines

Uses: Non-Hodgkin's lymphoma, B-cell NHL

DOSAGE AND ROUTES
• *Adult:* **IV INF** 250 mg/m² at a rate of 50 mg/hr; if hypersensitivity does not occur, increase rate by 50 mg/hr q^1/$_2$h, max 400 mg/hr; slow/interrupt inf if hypersensitivity occurs
Available forms: Inj 3.2 mg/2 ml

SIDE EFFECTS
CV: ***Cardiac dysrhythmias***
GI: Nausea, vomiting, anorexia, abdominal pain, diarrhea
GU: ***Renal failure***
HEMA: ***Leukopenia, neutropenia, thrombocytopenia,*** anemia
*INTEG: Irritation at site, rash, **fatal mucocutaneous infections (rare)***
OTHER: Fever, chills, asthenia, headache, angioedema, hypotension, myalgia, ***bronchospasm, hemorrhage,*** infections, cough, dyspnea, dizziness, anxiety
SYST: ***Stevens-Johnson syndrome***
Contraindications: Pregnancy (D), hypersensitivity to this agent or murine proteins
Precautions: Lactation, children, elderly, cardiac conditions, immunizations after therapy

PHARMACOKINETICS
Half-life 30 hr

NURSING CONSIDERATIONS
Assess:
⚠ For signs of fatal infusion reaction: hypoxia, pulmonary infiltrates, ARDS, MI, ventricular fibrillation, cardiogenic shock; most fatal infusion reactions occur with first infusion; potentially fatal
• Biodistribution: 1st image 2-24 hr, 2nd image 48-72 hr, 3rd image 90-120 hr (optimal)
⚠ For signs of severe mucocutaneous reactions: Stevens-Johnson syndrome, lichenoid dermatitis, toxic epidermal lysis; occur 1-13 wk after drug was given
⚠ Tumor lysis syndrome: acute renal

Side effects: *italics* = common; ***bold italics*** = life-threatening

failure requiring hemodialysis, hyperkalemia, hypocalcemia, hyperuricemia, hyperphosphatemia

• CBC, differential, platelet count weekly; withhold drug if WBC is <3500/mm³, or platelet count <100,000/mm³; notify prescriber of these results; drug should be discontinued

• GI symptoms: frequency of stools

• Signs of dehydration: rapid respirations, poor skin turgor, decreased urine output, dry skin, restlessness, weakness

Administer:

• Do not use as bolus or IV direct

IV INF route

• See manufacturer's product labeling for preparation

Perform/provide:

• Increased fluid intake to 2-3 L/day to prevent dehydration, unless contraindicated

• Emergency equipment nearby with epINEPHrine, antihistamines, corticosteroids

• Changing of IV site q48h

• Nutritious diet with iron, vitamin supplement, low fiber, few dairy products

• Storage of vials at 36°-46° F, do not freeze

Evaluate:

• Therapeutic response: decrease in tumor size, decrease in spread of cancer

Teach patient/family:

• To report adverse reactions

• To use contraception during and for 12 months after therapy

ibuprofen (otc, ℞)

(eye-byoo-proe′fen)

Actiprofen ✦, Advil, Advil Migraine ✦, Apo-Ibuprofen ✦, Bayer Select Ibuprofen Pain Relief, Children's Advil, Children's Motrin, Excedrin IB, Genpril, Haltran, ibuprofen, Medipren, Menadol, Midol Maximum Strength Cramp Formula, Motrin, Motrin IB, Motrin Junior Strength, Motrin Migraine Pain, Novoprofen ✦, Nuprin, Nu-Ibuprofen, PediaCare Children's Fever

Func. class.: Nonsteroidal antiinflammatory, antipyretic, nonopioid analgesics

Chem. class.: Propionic acid derivative

Do not confuse:

Nuprin/Lupron

Action: Inhibits prostaglandin synthesis by decreasing enzyme needed for biosynthesis; analgesic, antiinflammatory, antipyretic

Uses: Rheumatoid arthritis, osteoarthritis, primary dysmenorrhea, gout, dental pain, musculoskeletal disorders, fever

DOSAGE AND ROUTES

Analgesic

• *Adult:* **PO** 200-400 mg q4-6h, not to exceed 3.2 g/day

• *Child:* **PO** 4-10 mg/kg/dose q6-8h

Antipyretic

• *Child 6 mo-12 yr:* **PO** 5 mg/kg (temp <102.5° F or 39.2° C), 10 mg/kg, (temp >102.5° F), may repeat q4-6h, max 40 mg/kg/day

Antiinflammatory

• *Adult:* **PO** 300-800 mg tid-qid, max 3.2 g/day

• *Child:* **PO** 30-40 mg/kg/day in 3-4 divided doses, max 50 mg/kg/day

Available forms: Tabs 100, 200, 300, 400, 600, 800 mg; cap, liq gels 200 mg;

oral susp 100 mg/2.5 ml, 100 mg/5 ml;
liq 100 mg/5 ml; tabs, chew 50, 100 mg;
drops 50 mg/1.25 ml

SIDE EFFECTS

CNS: Headache, dizziness, drowsiness,
fatigue, tremors, confusion, insomnia,
anxiety, depression
CV: Tachycardia, peripheral edema, palpitations, dysrhythmias
EENT: Tinnitus, hearing loss, blurred
vision
GI: Nausea, *anorexia,* vomiting, diarrhea, jaundice, ***hepatitis,*** constipation,
flatulence, cramps, dry mouth, peptic
ulcer, ***GI bleeding***
GU: ***Nephrotoxicity:***
dysuria, hematuria, oliguria, azotemia
HEMA: ***Blood dyscrasias,*** increased
bleeding time
INTEG: Purpura, rash, pruritus, sweating,
urticaria, ***nectrotizing fasciitis***
SYST: ***Anaphylaxis, Stevens Johnson
syndrome***
Contraindications: Hypersensitivity,
asthma, severe renal disease, severe
hepatic disease, avoid in 2nd/3rd trimester of pregnancy
Precautions: Pregnancy (B) 1st trimester, lactation, children, bleeding
disorders, GI disorders, cardiac disorders, hypersensitivity to other antiinflammatory agents, elderly, CHF, CCr <25
ml/min

PHARMACOKINETICS

Well absorbed (PO)
PO: Onset ½ hr; peak 1-2 hr, half-
life 2-4 hr, metabolized in liver (inactive metabolites), excreted in urine
(inactive metabolites), 90%-99%
plasma protein binding, does not
enter breast milk

INTERACTIONS

Increase: bleeding risk—cefamandole,
cefotetan, cefoperazone, valproic acid,
thrombolytics, antiplatelets, warfarin
Increase: blood dyscrasias possibility—antineoplastics, radiation

Increase: toxicity—digoxin, lithium,
oral anticoagulants, cycloSPORINE, probenecid
Increase: GI reactions—aspirin, corticosteroids, NSAIDs, alcohol
Increase: hypoglycemia—oral antidiabetics, insulin
Decrease: effect of antihypertensives,
thiazides, furosemide
Decrease: ibuprofen action—aspirin
Drug/Herb
Increase: bleeding risk—arnica, chamomile, clove, dong quai, fenugreek, feverfew, garlic, ginger, ginkgo, ginseng
(Panax)
Increase: gastric irritation—arginine,
gossypol
Increase: NSAID effect—bearberry,
bilberry
Increase: bleeding risk—bogbean,
chondroitin

NURSING CONSIDERATIONS
Assess:
• Renal, hepatic, blood studies: BUN,
creatinine, AST, ALT, Hgb, before treatment, periodically thereafter
• Pain: note type, duration, location, and
intensity with ROM 1 hr after administration
• Audiometric, ophthalmic exam before,
during, after treatment; for eye, ear
problems: blurred vision, tinnitus; may
indicate toxicity
• Fever: temp before and 1 hr after administration
• Cardiac status: edema (peripheral),
tachycardia, palpitations; monitor B/P,
pulse for character, quality, rhythm especially in patients with cardiac disease/
elderly
• For history of peptic ulcer disorder;
asthma, aspirin, hypersensitivity, check
closely for hypersensitivity reactions
Administer:
• With food, milk, or antacid to decrease
GI symptoms; however, taking on empty
stomach best facilitates absorption; if
nausea and vomiting occur/persist, notify
prescriber

Side effects: *italics* = common; ***bold italics*** = life-threatening

Perform/provide:
• Storage at room temperature

Evaluate:
• Therapeutic response: decreased pain, stiffness in joints; decreased swelling in joints; ability to move more easily; reduction in fever or menstrual cramping

Teach patient/family:
• To report blurred vision, ringing, roaring in ears; may indicate toxicity; eye and hearing tests should be done during long-term therapy
• To avoid driving, other hazardous activities if dizziness or drowsiness occurs
⚠ To report change in urinary pattern, increased weight, edema, increased pain in joints, fever, blood in urine; indicate nephrotoxicity
• That therapeutic inflammatory effects may take up to 1 mo
⚠ To avoid alcohol, NSAIDs, salicylates; bleeding may occur
• To use sunscreen to prevent photosensitivity

⚠.High Alert

ibutilide (Ŗ)
(eye-byoo'tih-lide)
Corvert
Func. class.: Antidysrhythmic (Class III)

Action: Prolongs duration of action potential and effective refractory period
Uses: For rapid conversion of atrial fibrillation/flutter occurring within 1 wk of coronary artery bypass or valve surgery

DOSAGE AND ROUTES

• *Adult:* **IV INF** (≥60 kg) 1 vial (1 mg) given over 10 min, may repeat same dose in 10 min; **IV INF** (<60 kg) 0.01 mg/kg given over 10 min, may repeat same dose in 10 min
Available forms: Inj 0.1 mg/ml

SIDE EFFECTS

CNS: Headache
*CV: Hypotension, bradycardia, **sinus arrest, CHF, dysrhythmias,** hyper-tension, extrasystoles, ventricular tachycardia, bundle branch block, AV block, palpitations, supraventricular extrasystoles, syncope*
GI: Nausea

Contraindications: Hypersensitivity
Precautions: Pregnancy (C), sinus node dysfunction, 2nd- or 3rd-degree AV block, electrolyte imbalances, bradycardia, lactation, children <18 yr, renal/hepatic disease, elderly

PHARMACOKINETICS

Elimination half-life in 6 hr; metabolized by liver, excreted by kidneys

INTERACTIONS

Prodysrhythmia: phenothiazines, tricyclics, tetracyclics, antidepressants, H_1-receptor antagonists, antihistamines
Masking of cardiotoxicity: digoxin
Do not use within 4 hr of ibutilide: Class Ia antidysrhythmics (disopyramide, quinidine, procainamide), Class III agents (amiodarone, sotalol)

Drug/Herb
Increase: toxicity, death—aconite
Increase: effect—aloe, broom, chronic buckthorn use, cascara sagrada (chronic use), Chinese rhubarb, figwort, fumitory, goldenseal, kudzu, licorice
Increase: serotonin effect—horehound
Decrease: effect—coltsfoot

NURSING CONSIDERATIONS

Assess:
• I&O ratio; electrolytes: K, Na, Cl
• Hepatic studies: AST, ALT, bilirubin, alk phosphatase
• ECG continuously to determine drug effectiveness, measure PR, QRS, QT intervals, check for PVCs, other dysrhythmias, discontinue if atrial fibrillation/flutter ceases
• For dehydration or hypovolemia
• For rebound hypertension after 1-2 hr

⚠ Safety alert   *"Tall Man" lettering

• Cardiac rate, respiration: rate, rhythm, character, chest pain

Administer:
• Undiluted or diluted in 50 ml 0.9% NaCl, or D$_5$W (0.017 mg/ml) give over 10 min
• Solution is stable for 48 hr refrigerated or 24 hr, room temperature
• Do not admix with other solution, drugs
• Reduce dosage slowly with ECG monitoring

Evaluate:
• Therapeutic response: decrease in atrial fibrillation/flutter

Teach patient/family:
• To report side effects immediately
• Reason for medication

⚠ High Alert

idarubicin (℞)
(eye-dah-roob'ih-sin)
Idamycin, Idamycin PFS
Func. class.: Antineoplastic, antibiotic
Chem. class.: Anthracycline glycoside

Do not confuse:
Idamycin/Adriamycin
idarubicin/DOXOrubicin

Action: Inhibits DNA synthesis by binding to DNA, a vesicant derived from daunorubicin by binding to DNA, which causes strand splitting; cell cycle specific (S phase)

Uses: Used in combination with other antineoplastics for acute myelocytic leukemia in adults

Investigational uses: Breast cancer, solid tumors

DOSAGE AND ROUTES

• *Adult:* **IV** 12 mg/m^2/day × 3 days in combination with extarabine (induction)
Renal/hepatic dose
• *Adult:* **IV** Reduce dose, if bilirubin is >5 mg/dl, do not administer
Available forms: Inj 1 mg/ml

SIDE EFFECTS

CNS: Fever, chills, *headache*
CV: ***Dysrhythmias, CHF, pericarditis, myocarditis,*** peripheral edema, angina, ***MI***
GI: *Nausea, vomiting, abdominal pain, mucositis, diarrhea,* ***hepatotoxicity***
GU: ***Nephrotoxicity***
HEMA: ***Thrombocytopenia, leukopenia, anemia***
INTEG: Rash, extravasation, dermatitis, *reversible alopecia,* urticaria, thrombophlebitis and tissue necrosis at inj site
Contraindications: Pregnancy (D), hypersensitivity, lactation, myelosuppression
Precautions: Renal and hepatic disease, gout, bone marrow depression, children, preexisting CV disease

PHARMACOKINETICS

Half-life 22 hr; metabolized by liver; crosses placenta; excreted in bile, urine (primarily as metabolites)

INTERACTIONS

Increase: toxicity—other antineoplastics or radiation
Decrease: antibody response—live virus vaccines
Drug/Lab Test
Increase: Uric acid

NURSING CONSIDERATIONS

Assess:
• CBC, differential, platelet count weekly; withhold drug if WBC is <4000/mm^3 or platelet count is <75,000/mm^3; notify prescriber of these results
• Blood, urine, uric acid levels
• Renal studies: BUN, serum uric acid, urine CCr, electrolytes before, during therapy
• I&O ratio; report fall in urine output to <30 ml/hr
• Monitor temp q4h; fever may indicate beginning infection
• Hepatic studies before, during therapy: bilirubin, AST, ALT, alk phosphatase prn or qmo; check for jaundice of skin,

sclera, dark urine, clay-colored stools, itchy skin, abdominal pain, fever, diarrhea

• Cardiac toxicity: CHF, dysrhythmias, cardiomyopathy; cardiac studies should be done before and periodically during treatment: ECG, chest x-ray

• ECG: watch for ST-T wave changes, low QRS and T, possible dysrhythmias (sinus tachycardia, heart block, PVCs)

• Bleeding: hematuria, guaiac stools, bruising or petechiae, mucosa or orifices q8h

• Effects of alopecia on body image; discuss feelings about body changes

• Inflammation of mucosa, breaks in skin

• Buccal cavity q8h for dryness, sores, ulceration, white patches, oral pain, bleeding, dysphagia

• Local irritation, pain, burning at inj site

• GI symptoms: frequency of stools, cramping

• Acidosis, signs of dehydration: rapid respirations, poor skin turgor, decreased urine output, dry skin, restlessness, weakness

Administer:

• Allopurinol or sodium bicarbonate to reduce uric acid levels, alkalinization of urine

• Transfusion for anemia

• Hydrocortisone for extravasation; apply ice compress after stopping infusion

IV, direct route

• Do not give IM/SUBCUT

• After preparing in biologic cabinet wearing gown, gloves, mask

• Antiemetic 30-60 min before giving drug and 6-10 hr after treatment to prevent vomiting

• After reconstituting 5 mg vial with 5 ml 0.9% NaCl (1 mg/1 ml); give over 10-15 min through Y-tube or 3-way stopcock of inf of D_5 or NS; discard unused portion

Solution compatibilities: $D_{3.3}$/0.3% NaCl, D_5/0.9% NaCl, D_5W, LR, 0.9% NaCl

Y-site compatibilities: Amifostine, amikacin, aztreonam, cimetidine, cladribine, cyclophosphamide, cytarabine, diphenhydrAMINE, droperidol, erythromycin, filgrastim, granisetron, imipenem/cisplatin, magnesium sulfate, mannitol, melphalan, metoclopramide, potassium chloride, ranitidine, sargramostim, thiotepa, vinorelbine

Perform/provide:

• Strict hand-washing technique, gloves, protective clothing

• Liquid diet: carbonated beverages, gelatin may be added if patient is not nauseated or vomiting

• Increase fluid intake to 2-3 L/day to prevent urate and calculi formation

• Rinsing of mouth tid-qid with water, club soda; brushing of teeth tid-qid with soft brush or cotton-tipped applicators for stomatitis; use unwaxed dental floss

• Storage at room temperature for 3 days after reconstituting or 7 days refrigerated

Evaluate:

• Therapeutic response: decreased tumor size, spread of malignancy

Teach patient/family:

• To report any complaints, side effects to nurse or prescriber

• That hair may be lost during treatment and wig or hairpiece may make patient feel better; tell patient that new hair may be different in color, texture

• To avoid foods with citric acid, hot or rough texture

• To report any bleeding, white spots, ulcerations in mouth; tell patient to examine mouth daily

• That urine may be red-orange for 48 hr

• To use contraception during treatment with this drug and for ≥4 mo after treatment

---

idoxuridine-IDU ophthalmic
See Appendix C

A High Alert

ifosfamide (R)
(i-foss'fa-mide)
Ifex
Func. class.: Antineoplastic alkylating agent
Chem. class.: Nitrogen mustard

Action: Alkylates DNA, RNA, inhibits enzymes that allow synthesis of amino acids in proteins; also responsible for cross-linking DNA strands; activity is not cell cycle stage specific

Uses: Testicular cancer, soft tissue sarcoma, Ewing's sarcoma, non-Hodgkin's lymphoma, lung, pancreatic sarcoma

DOSAGE AND ROUTES
• *Adult:* **IV** 1.2 g/m^2/day × 5 days, repeat course q3wk, given with mesna
Available forms: Inj 1, 3 g

SIDE EFFECTS
CNS: Facial paresthesia, fever, malaise, somnolence, confusion, depression, hallucinations, dizziness, disorientation, *seizures, coma,* cranial nerve dysfunction
GI: Nausea, vomiting, anorexia, *hepatotoxicity,* stomatitis, constipation, diarrhea
GU: **Hematuria, nephrotoxicity, hemorrhagic cystitis,** dysuria, urinary frequency
HEMA: **Thrombocytopenia, leukopenia, anemia**
INTEG: Dermatitis, alopecia, pain at inj site
Contraindications: Pregnancy (D), hypersensitivity, bone marrow suppression
Precautions: Renal disease, lactation, children

PHARMACOKINETICS
Metabolized by liver; saturation occurs at high doses; excreted in urine; half-life 7-15 hr

INTERACTIONS
Increase: myelosuppression—other antineoplastics, radiation
Increase: toxicity—barbiturates, allopurinol
Decrease: antibody response—live virus vaccines

NURSING CONSIDERATIONS
Assess:
• Hepatic studies before, during therapy (bilirubin, AST, ALT, LDH) as needed or monthly
• CBC, differential, platelet count weekly; withhold drug if WBC <2000 or platelet count <50,000; notify prescriber
• Monitor temp q4h (may indicate beginning infection)
• Blood dyscrasias (anemia, granulocytopenia); bruising, fatigue, bleeding, poor healing
• Allergic reactions: dermatitis, exfoliative dermatitis, pruritus, urticaria
• I&O ratio; monitor for hematuria; hemorrhagic cystitis can occur; increase fluids to 3 L/day
• Neurologic symptoms: hallucinations, confusion, disorientation, drug should be discontinued
• Bleeding: hematuria, guaiac, bruising or petechiae, mucosa or orifices q8h
• Jaundice of skin, sclera, dark urine, clay-colored stools, itchy skin, abdominal pain, fever, diarrhea
Administer:
• Antiemetic 30-60 min before giving drug to prevent vomiting
• Antibiotics for prophylaxis of infection
• Always give with mesna to prevent ifosfamide-induced hemorrhagic cystitis
IV route
• After diluting 1 g/20 ml sterile or bacteriostatic H$_2$O for inj with parabens or benzyl only; shake; may be diluted further with D$_5$W, LR, NS, sterile H$_2$O for inj; 1 g/20 ml = 50 mg/ml; 1 g/50 ml = 20 mg/ml; 1 g/200 ml = 5 mg/ml; give over ≥30 min; may also give as cont inf over 72 hr
Additive compatibilities: Carbopl-

atin, cisplatin, etoposide, fluorouracil, mesna

Syringe compatibilities: Mesna
Y-site compatibilities: Allopurinol, amifostine, amphotericin B cholesteryl, aztreonam, DOXOrubicin liposome, filgrastim, fludarabine, gallium, granisetron, melphalan, ondansetron, paclitaxel, piperacillin/tazobactam, propofol, sargramostim, sodium bicarbonate, teniposide, thiotepa, vinorelbine

Perform/provide:

• Storage of powder at room temperature

• Increase fluid intake to 3 L/day to prevent hemorrhagic cystitis

• Warm compresses at inj site for inflammation

Evaluate:

• Therapeutic response: decrease in size and spread of tumor

Teach patient/family:

• To notify prescriber of sore throat, swollen lymph nodes, malaise, fever; other infections may occur

• Not to have vaccinations during treatment

• That hair may be lost during treatment; a wig or hairpiece may make the patient feel better; new hair may be different in color, texture

• To report signs of anemia: fatigue, headache, faintness, shortness of breath, irritability

• To report bleeding; avoid use of razors, commercial mouthwash

• To avoid use of aspirin products, NSAIDs, ibuprofen, hemorrhage can occur

• To use contraceptive measures during therapy

• To avoid crowds, those with infections

• To report confusion, hallucinations, extreme drowsiness, numbness, tingling; avoid alcohol use for ≥4 mo after treatment

---

imatinib (R)

(im-ah-tin′ib)
Gleevec
Func. class.: Miscellaneous antineoplastic
Chem. class.: Protein-tyrosine kinase inhibitor

Action: Inhibits Bcr-Abl tyrosine kinase created in chronic myeloid leukemia (CML)

Uses: Treatment of chronic myeloid leukemia (CML) in blast cell crisis or chronic failure after treatment failure with interferon alfa; gastrointestinal stromal tumors (GIST)

DOSAGE AND ROUTES

CML, chronic phase
• *Adult:* PO 400 mg/day
• *Child:* PO 260 mg/m^2/day

CML, accelerated phase/blast crisis
• *Adult:* PO 600 mg/day

GIST
• *Adult:* PO 400 or 600 mg/day

Available form: Tabs 100, 400 mg

SIDE EFFECTS

CNS: **CNS hemorrhage,** headache, dizziness, insomnia
CV: Hemorrhage
GI: Nausea, **hepatotoxicity, vomiting, dyspepsia,** GI hemorrhage, *anorexia, abdominal pain*
HEMA: **Neutropenia, thrombocytopenia, bleeding**
INTEG: Rash, pruritus
META: Fluid retention, hypokalemia, edema
MISC: Fatigue, epistaxis, pyrexia, night sweats, increased weight
MS: Cramps, pain, arthralgia, myalgia
RESP: Cough, dyspnea, nasopharyngitis, pneumonia, URI

Contraindications: Pregnancy (D), hypersensitivity
Precautions: Lactation, children, elderly

PHARMACOKINETICS

Well absorbed (98%) (PO), protein binding 95%, metabolized by CYP3A4, excreted in feces, small amount in urine; peak 2-4 hr, duration 24 hr (imatinib), 40 hr (metabolite), half-life 18 hr

INTERACTIONS

Increase: hepatotoxicity—acetaminophen

Increase: imatinib concentrations—ketoconazole, itraconazole, erythromycin, clarithromycin

Increase: plasma concentrations of simvastatin, calcium channel blockers

Increase: plasma concentration of warfarin; avoid use with warfarin, use low-molecular-weight anticoagulants instead

Decrease: imatinib concentrations—dexamethasone, phenytoin, carbamazepine, rifampin, phenobarbital

Drug/Herb
Decrease: imatinib concentration—St. John's wort

NURSING CONSIDERATIONS
Assess:
• ANC and platelets; in chronic phase if ANC <1×10^9/L and/or platelets <50×10^9/L, stop until ANC >1.5×10^9/L and platelets >75×10^9/L; in accelerated phase/blast crisis if ANC <0.5×10^9/L and/or platelets <10×10^9/L, determine whether cytopenia is related to biopsy/aspirate, if not, reduce dose by 200 mg, if cytopenia continues, reduce dose by another 100 mg; if cytopenia continues for 4 wk, stop drug until ANC ≥1×10^9/L
• For renal toxicity: if bilirubin >$3 \times$ IULN, withhold imatinib until bilirubin levels return to <$1.5 \times$ IULN
• For hepatotoxicity: monitor LFTs, before treatment and qmo; if liver transaminases >$5 \times$ IULN, withhold imatinib until transaminase levels return to <$2.5 \times$ IULN
• CBC, differential, platelet count weekly; withhold drug if WBC is <3500/

mm^3, or platelet count <100,000/mm^3; notify prescriber of these results; drug should be discontinued
• Signs of fluid retention, edema: weigh, monitor lung sounds, assess for edema, some fluid retention is dose dependent

Administer:
• With meal and large glass of water, to decrease GI symptoms, doses of 800 mg should be given 400 mg bid

Perform/provide:
• Nutritious diet with iron, vitamin supplement, low fiber, few dairy products
• Storage at 25° C (77° F)

Evaluate:
• Therapeutic response: decrease in leukemic cells or size of tumor

Teach patient/family:
• To report adverse reactions immediately: SOB, swelling of extremities, bleeding
• Reason for treatment, expected result

---

imipenem/cilastatin (Ʀ)
(i-me-pen′em sye-la-stat′in)
Primaxin IM, Primaxin IV
Func. class.: Antiinfective—miscellaneous
Chem. class.: Carbapenem

Do not confuse:
imipenem/Omnipen
Primaxin/Premarin

Action: Interferes with cell wall replication of susceptible organisms; osmotically unstable cell wall swells, bursts from osmotic pressure; addition of cilastatin prevents renal inactivation that occurs with high urinary concentrations of imipenem

Uses: Serious infections caused by gram-positive: *Streptococcus pneumoniae,* group A β-hemolytic streptococci, *Staphylococcus aureus,* enterococcus; gram-negative: *Klebsiella, Proteus, Escherichia coli, Acinetobacter, Serratia, Pseudomonas aeruginosa, Salmonella, Shigella*

Side effects: *italics* = common; ***bold italics*** = life-threatening

DOSAGE AND ROUTES

• *Adult:* **IV** 250-500 mg q6-8h; severe infections may require 1 g q8h; may give **IM** q12h (total daily **IM** dosage >1500 mg not recommended); mild to moderate infections

• *Child:* **IV** 60-100 mg/kg/day in divided doses, max 4 g/day

Renal dose

• *Adult:* **IV** CCr 30-70 ml/min give 50% dose q6-8h; CCr 20-30 ml/min give 40% dose q8-12h; CCr 5-20 ml/min give 25% dose q12h

Available forms: Inj 250, 500 mg (IV); inj 500, 750 mg (IM)

SIDE EFFECTS

CNS: Fever, somnolence, *seizures,* confusion, dizziness, weakness, myoclonia
CV: Hypotension, palpitations
GI: Diarrhea, nausea, vomiting, pseudomembranous colitis, hepatitis, glossitis
HEMA: Eosinophilia, neutropenia, decreased Hgb, Hct
INTEG: Rash, urticaria, pruritus, pain at injection site, phlebitis, erythema at injection site
RESP: Chest discomfort, dyspnea, hyperventilation
SYST: Anaphylaxis

Contraindications: Hypersensitivity, IM hypersensitivity to local anesthetics of the amide type

Precautions: Pregnancy (C), lactation, elderly, hypersensitivity to penicillins, seizure disorders, renal disease, children

PHARMACOKINETICS

IV: Onset immediate, peak ½-1 hr, half-life 1 hr; 70%-80% excreted unchanged in urine

INTERACTIONS

Increase: imipenem plasma levels—probenecid
Increase: antagonistic effect—β-lactam antibiotics
Increase: seizure risk—ganciclovir

Drug/Lab Test

Increase: AST, ALT, LDH, BUN, alk phosphatase, bilirubin, creatinine
False-positive: Direct Coombs' test

NURSING CONSIDERATIONS

Assess:

• For infection: increased temp, WBC, characteristics of wounds, sputum, urine culture or stool culture
• Sensitivity to penicillin—may have sensitivity to this drug
• Renal disease: lower dose may be required
• Bowel pattern daily; if severe diarrhea occurs, drug should be discontinued; may indicate pseudomembranous colitis
A Allergic reactions, anaphylaxis: rash, urticaria, pruritus, wheezing, laryngeal edema; may occur few days after therapy begins; have epINEPHrine, antihistamine, emergency equipment available
• Overgrowth of infection: perineal itching, fever, malaise, redness, pain, swelling, drainage, rash, diarrhea, change in cough, sputum

Administer:

• After C&S is taken

IV route

• After reconstitution of 250 or 500 mg with 10 ml of diluent and shake; add to at least 100 ml of same inf sol
• 250-500 mg over 20-30 min; 1 g over 40-60 min; give through Y-tube or 3-way stopcock; do not give by IV bolus or if cloudy

Y-site compatibilities: Acyclovir, amifostine, aztreonam, cefepime, cisatracurium, diltiazem, famotidine, fludarabine, foscarnet, granisetron, idarubicin, insulin (regular), melphalan, methotrexate, ondansetron, propofol, remifentanil, tacrolimus, teniposide, thiotepa, vinorelbine, zidovudine

Evaluate:

• Therapeutic response: negative C&S; absence of signs and symptoms of infection

Teach patient/family:

A To report severe diarrhea; may indicate pseudomembranous colitis

---

A Safety alert　＊"Tall Man" lettering

To report sore throat, bruising, bleeding, joint pain; may indicate blood dyscrasias (rare)

Treatment of anaphylaxis: EpINEPHrine, antihistamines; resuscitate if needed

---

imipramine (R)

(im-ip′ra-meen)
Apo-Imipramine ✤, imipramine HCl ✤, Impril ✤, Norfranil, Novo Pramine ✤, Tipramine, Tofranil, Tofranil PM
Func. class.: Antidepressant, tricyclic
Chem. class.: Dibenzazepine, tertiary amine

Do not confuse:
imipramine/desipramine

Action: Blocks reuptake of norepinephrine, serotonin into nerve endings, increasing action of norepinephrine, serotonin in nerve cells

Uses: Depression, enuresis in children

Investigational uses: Chronic pain, migraine headaches, cluster headaches as adjunct, incontinence

DOSAGE AND ROUTES

• *Adult:* **PO/IM** 75-100 mg/day in divided doses, may increase by 25-50 mg to 200 mg, not to exceed 300 mg/day; may give daily dose at bedtime
• *Geriatric:* **PO** 25 mg at bedtime, may increase to 100 mg/day in divided doses
• *Child:* **PO** 25-75 mg/day
Enuresis
• *Child 6-12 yr:* **PO** 10 mg at bedtime, max 50 mg
Available forms: Tabs 10, 25, 50, 75 mg; inj 25 mg/2 ml; caps 75, 100, 125, 150 mg

SIDE EFFECTS

CNS: Dizziness, drowsiness, confusion, ***seizures,*** headache, anxiety, tremors, stimulation, weakness, insomnia, nightmares, EPS (elderly), increased psychiatric symptoms, paresthesia
CV: Orthostatic hypotension, ECG changes, tachycardia, hypertension, palpitations, ***dysrhythmias***
EENT: Blurred vision, tinnitus, mydriasis
GI: Diarrhea, dry mouth, nausea, vomiting, ***paralytic ileus;*** increased appetite; cramps, epigastric distress, jaundice, ***hepatitis,*** stomatitis, constipation, taste change
GU: Retention, ***acute renal failure***
HEMA: ***Agranulocytosis, thrombocytopenia, eosinophilia, leukopenia***
INTEG: Rash, urticaria, sweating, pruritus, photosensitivity

Contraindications: Hypersensitivity to tricyclics, recovery phase of MI, convulsive disorders, prostatic hypertrophy
Precautions: Pregnancy (C), suicidal patients, severe depression, increased intraocular pressure, narrow-angle glaucoma, urinary retention, cardiac disease, hepatic disease, hyperthyroidism, electroshock therapy, elective surgery, elderly, lactation

PHARMACOKINETICS

PO: Steady state 2-5 days; metabolized by liver; excreted in urine, breast milk, feces; crosses placenta; half-life 6-20 hr

INTERACTIONS

Hyperpyretic crisis, convulsions, hypertensive episode: MAOIs, clonidine
Increase: toxicity: SSRIs, avoid concurrent use
Increase: effects of direct-acting sympathomimetics (epINEPHrine), alcohol, barbiturates, benzodiazepines, CNS depressants
Decrease: effects of guanethidine, clonidine, indirect-acting sympathomimetics (epHEDrine)
Drug/Herb
Increase: anticholinergic effect—belladonna, corkwood, henbane, jimsonweed, scopolia

---

Side effects: *italics* = common; ***bold italics*** = life-threatening

Increase: imipramine action—chamomile, hops, kava, lavender, skullcap, valerian

Increase: hypertension—yohimbe

Increase: serotonin syndrome—SAM-e, St. John's wort

Drug/Lab Test

Increase: Serum bilirubin, alk phosphatase, blood glucose

Decrease: 5-HIAA, VMA, urinary catecholamines

NURSING CONSIDERATIONS

Assess:

• B/P (lying, standing), pulse q4h; if systolic B/P drops 20 mm Hg, hold drug, notify prescriber; take vital signs q4h in patients with cardiovascular disease

• Blood studies: CBC, leukocytes, differential, cardiac enzymes if patient is receiving long-term therapy

• Hepatic studies: AST, ALT, bilirubin

• Weight qwk; appetite may increase with drug

⚠ ECG for flattening of T wave, bundle branch block, AV block, dysrhythmias in cardiac patients

• EPS primarily in elderly: rigidity, dystonia, akathisia

• Mental status: mood, sensorium, affect, suicidal tendencies, increase in psychiatric symptoms: depression, panic

• Urinary retention, constipation; constipation is more likely to occur in children, elderly

⚠ Withdrawal symptoms: headache, nausea, vomiting, muscle pain, weakness, diarrhea, insomnia, restlessness; not usual unless drug is discontinued abruptly

• Alcohol consumption; if alcohol is consumed, hold dose until morning

Administer:

• Not to break, crush, or chew caps

• Increased fluids, bulk in diet for constipation, urinary retention

• With food or milk for GI symptoms

• Dosage at bedtime if oversedation occurs during day; may take entire dose at bedtime; elderly may not tolerate once/day dosing

• Sugarless gum, hard candy, or frequent sips of water for dry mouth

• In IM route after running warm water over ampule to dissolve crystals

Syringe compatibilities: Doxapram

Y-site compatibilities: Cladribine

Perform/provide:

• Storage in tight container at room temperature; do not freeze

• Assistance with ambulation during beginning therapy, since drowsiness/dizziness, orthostatic hypotension occurs

• Safety measures, primarily in elderly

Evaluate:

• Therapeutic response: decreased depression, enuresis, pain

Teach patient/family:

• That therapeutic effects may take 2-3 wk

• That drug is dispensed in small amounts because of suicide potential, especially in beginning of therapy

• To use caution in driving, other activities requiring alertness because of drowsiness, dizziness, blurred vision

• To report urinary retention immediately

• To avoid alcohol ingestion, other CNS depressants during treatment

• Not to discontinue medication quickly after long-term use; may cause nausea, headache, malaise

• To wear sunscreen or large hat, since photosensitivity occurs

• To rise slowly, orthostatic hypotension may occur

Treatment of overdose: ECG

monitoring; induce emesis; lavage, activated charcoal; administer anticonvulsant

---

⚠ Safety alert   *"Tall Man" lettering

immune globulin IM
gamma globulin, IG, IGIM Bay Gam

immune globulin IV (IGIV) (℞)
Carimune NF, Flebogamma 5%, Gamimune N, Gammagard S/D, gamma globulin, Gammar-P IV, Gamunex, Iveegam, Octagam, Panglobulin NF, Polygam, Polygam S/D, Sandoglobulin, Venoglobulin-I, Venoglobulin-S

Func. class.: Immune serum
Chem. class.: IgG

Action: Provides passive immunity to hepatitis A, measles, varicella, rubella, immune globulin deficiency; contains gamma globulin antibodies (IgG)

Uses: Immunodeficiency syndrome, B-cell chronic lymphocytic leukemia, Kawasaki syndrome, bone marrow transplantation, pediatric HIV infection, agammaglobulinemia, hepatitis A, B exposure, measles exposure, measles vaccine complications, purpura, rubella exposure, chickenpox exposure

Investigational uses: IV posttransfusion purpura, Guillain-Barré syndrome, chronic inflammatory demyelinating polyneuropathy

DOSAGE AND ROUTES
Primary immunodeficiency
• *Adult and child:* IV (Carimune, Panglobulin NF) 200 mg/kg qmo, max 300 mg/kg qmo or give more frequently if needed; IV (Gamimune N) 100-200 mg/kg qmo, max 400 mg/kg; IV (Gammagard S/D) 200-400 mg qmo, minimum 100 mg/kg qmo

Hepatitis A exposure
• *Adult and child:* IM 0.02-0.04 ml/kg or 0.1 mg/kg if treatment is delayed

Hepatitis B exposure
• *Adult and child:* IM 0.06 ml/kg within 1 wk, qmo

Rubella exposure in pregnancy (1st trimester)
• *Women:* IM 0.55 ml/kg as soon as possible, within 72 hr

Chickenpox exposure
• *Adult and child:* IM 0.6-1.2 ml/kg as soon as exposed

Measles (postexposure)
• *Adult and child:* IM 0.25 ml/kg within 6 days

B-cell chronic lymphocytic leukemia (CLL) (Gammagard S/D, Polygam S/D)
• *Adult:* IV 400 mg/kg q3-4wk

Immunoglobulin deficiency
• *Adult and child:* IM 1.3 ml/kg, then 0.66 ml/kg after 2-4 wk and q2-4wk thereafter

Idiopathic thrombocytopenia, purpura
• *Adult and child:* IV 0.4 g/kg/day × 5 days or 1 g/kg/day × 1-2 days

Kawasaki syndrome (Iveegam, Venoglobulin-S, Gammagard S/D, Polygam S/D)
• *Adult and child:* IV (Iveegam, Venglobulin-S 5% or 10%) 2000 mg/kg over 10-12 hr, may repeat; IV (Gammagard S/D, Polygam S/D) 1 g/kg as single dose

Bone marrow transplantation (BMT) (Gamimune N)
• *Adults >20 yr:* IV 500 mg/kg 5% or 10% sol on days 2, 7 before transplant, then qwk for 90 days thereafter

Pediatric HIV (Gamimune N)
• *Child:* IV 400 mg/kg 5% or 10% sol q28days

Available forms: IM: Inj 2, 10 ml vial (Bay Gam); IV: 5%, 10% sol (Gamimune N, Venoglobulin-S); powder for inj 1-, 3-, 6-, 12-g vials (Carimune NF; 50 mg protein/ml in 2.5-, 5-, 10-g vials (Gammagard S/D); 1-, 2.5-, 5-, 10-g vials (Gammar-P IV); 500 mg, 1-, 2.5-, 5-g vials (Iveegam); 6-, 12-g vials (Panglobulin); 2.5-, 5-, 10-g vials (Polygam S/D); sol for inj 1-, 2.5-, 5-, 10-, 20-g vials (Gamunex)

SIDE EFFECTS

CNS: Headache, fatigue, malaise
GI: Abdominal pain
INTEG: Pain at inj site, rash, pruritus, chills
MS: Arthralgia, chest pain
SYST: Lymphadenopathy, **anaphylaxis**
Contraindications: Hypersensitivity
Precautions: Pregnancy (C)

INTERACTIONS

Do not administer live virus vaccines within 3 mo of this drug

NURSING CONSIDERATIONS
Assess:

• For exposure date: this drug should be given within 6 days of measles, 7 days of hepatitis B, 14 days of hepatitis A
• For anaphylaxis: diaphoresis, wheezing, chest tightness, hypotension
Administer:

• IM ≤3 ml in one site, use large muscle mass
• Only with epINEPHrine 1:1000, resuscitative equipment available
• Only within 2 wk of exposure to hepatitis A
IV route

• Gamimune N: IV undiluted or dilute with D₅; give 0.01 ml/kg/min; may increase to 0.02-0.04 ml/kg/min
• Sandoglobulin: IV diluted with provided diluent; give 0.5-1 ml/min × 15-30 min; may increase to 1.5-2.5 ml/min
• Venoglobulin-I: (50 mg/ml sol) give 0.01-0.02 ml/kg/min; if no adverse reaction in ½ hr, increase to 0.04 ml/kg/min, store at room temperature
• Gammagard: reconstitute with sterile H₂O for inj (50 mg protein/ml); give 0.5 ml/kg/hr, may increase to 4 ml/kg/hr, use infusion set provided
• Gammar-IV: give 0.01 ml/kg/min (50 mg/ml sol) × 15-30 min, may increase to 0.02 ml/kg/min, may increase to 0.03-0.06 ml/kg/min
Y-site compatibilities: Fluconazole, sargramostim

Perform/provide:

• Storage at 36°-46° F (2°-8° C)
Evaluate:

• Prevention of infection, increased platelets
Teach patient/family:

• That passive immunity is temporary
• The treatment of anaphylaxis: epINEPHrine, diphenhydrAMINE, O₂, vasopressors, corticosteroids

---

⚠ High Alert

inamrinone (℞)
(in-am′rih-nohn)
Inocor
Func. class.: Inotropic
Chem. class.: Bipyrimidine derivative

Do not confuse:
inamrinone/amiodarone
Action: Positive inotropic agent with vasodilator properties; reduces preload and afterload by direct relaxation of vascular smooth muscle, increases cardiac output
Uses: Short-term management of CHF that has not responded to other medication (diuretics, other vasodilators); can be used with digitalis

DOSAGE AND ROUTES

• *Adult and child:* **IV BOL** 0.75 mg/kg given over 2-3 min; start inf of 5-10 mcg/kg/min; may give another bol 30 min after start of therapy, max 10 mg/kg total daily dose
• *Infant:* **IV** 3-4.5 mg/kg in divided doses, then give by inf 10 mcg/kg/min
• *Neonate:* **IV** 3-4.5 mg/kg in divided doses, then give by inf 3-5 mcg/kg/min
Available forms: Inj 5 mg/ml

SIDE EFFECTS

CV: **Dysrhythmias,** *hypotension,* chest pain
GI: *Nausea, vomiting, anorexia,* abdominal pain, **hepatotoxicity (rare)**, **ascites,** jaundice, hiccups

---

HEMA: **Thrombocytopenia**
INTEG: Allergic reactions, burning at inj site
RESP: Pleuritis, **pulmonary densities, hypoxemia**

Contraindications: Hypersensitivity to this drug or bisulfites, severe aortic disease, severe pulmonic valvular disease, acute MI

Precautions: Pregnancy (C), lactation, children, renal disease, hepatic disease, atrial flutter/fibrillation, elderly, asthma

PHARMACOKINETICS

IV: Onset 2-5 min, peak 10 min, duration variable; half-life 4-6 hr, metabolized in liver, excreted in urine as drug and metabolites 60%-90%

INTERACTIONS

Excessive hypotension: antihypertensives, disopyramide
Additive effect: cardiac glycosides

Drug/Herb
Increase: amrinone action—aloe, buckthorn, cascara sagrada, senna

Drug/Lab Test
Increase: Hepatic enzymes
Decrease: Serum K

NURSING CONSIDERATIONS

Assess:
• B/P and pulse q5min during infusion; if B/P drops 30 mm Hg, stop infusion and call prescriber
• Electrolytes: K, S, Cl, Ca; renal studies: BUN, creatinine; blood studies: platelet count; monitor fluid status (CVP) in elderly
• ALT, AST, bilirubin daily
• I&O ratio and weight daily; diuresis should increase with continuing therapy
⚠ If platelets are <150,000/mm³, drug is usually discontinued and another drug started
• Extravasation; change site q48h

Administer:
• Do not mix directly with dextrose solutions; chemical reaction occurs over 24 hr; precipitate forms if inamrinone and furosemide come in contact
• May inject into running dextrose infusion through Y-connector or directly into tubing; may give undiluted over 2-3 min or dilute with 0.9%, 0.45% NaCl to 1-3 mg/ml, run at prescribed rate by continuous infusion
• By infusion pump for doses other than bolus
• Potassium supplements if ordered for potassium levels <3.0, correct before using amrinone

Syringe compatibilities: Propranolol, verapamil

Y-site compatibilities: Aminophylline, atropine, bretylium, calcium chloride, cimetidine, cisatracurium, digoxin, DOBUTamine, DOPamine, epINEPHrine, famotidine, hydrocortisone, isoproterenol, lidocaine, metaraminol, methylPREDNISolone, nitroglycerin, nitroprusside, norepinephrine, phenylephrine, potassium chloride, propofol, propranolol, remifentanil, verapamil

Evaluate:
• Therapeutic response: increased cardiac output, decreased PCWP, adequate CVP, decreased dyspnea, fatigue, edema, ECG

Teach patient/family:
• That burning may occur at IV site
• To report adverse reactions promptly
• Not to breastfeed unless approved by prescriber

Treatment of overdose: Discontinue drug, support circulation

indapamide (℞)
(in-dap′a-mide)
indapamide, Lozide ✦, Lozol
Func. class.: Diuretic—thiazide-like, antihypertensive
Chem. class.: Indoline

Action: Acts on proximal section of distal renal tubule and thick ascending loop of Henle by inhibiting reabsorption dfum; may act by direct vasodilation so-caused by blocking of calcium channel

Uses: Edema of CHF, hypertension, diuresis

DOSAGE AND ROUTES
Edema
• *Adult:* **PO** 2.5 mg daily in AM; may be increased to 5 mg daily if needed
Antihypertensive
• *Adult:* **PO** 1.25-5 mg daily; may increase to 5 mg/day over 8 wk
Available forms: Tabs 1.25, 2.5 mg

SIDE EFFECTS

CNS: Headache, dizziness, fatigue, weakness, nervousness, agitation, extremity numbness, depression
CV: Orthostatic hypotension, volume depletion, palpitations, dysrhythmias, PVCs
EENT: Blurred vision, nasal congestion, increased intraocular pressure
ELECT: Hypochloremic alkalosis, hypomagnesemia, hyperuricemia, hypercalcemia, hyponatremia, hypokalemia, hyperglycemia
GI: Nausea, diarrhea, dry mouth, vomiting, anorexia, cramps, constipation, abdominal pain
GU: Polyuria, nocturia, urinary frequency, impotence
INTEG: Rash, pruritus
MS: Cramps
Contraindications: Hypersensitivity, anuria, hepatic coma
Precautions: Pregnancy (B), hypokalemia, dehydration, ascites, hepatic disease, severe renal disease, lactation, CCr <25 ml/min (not effective)

PHARMACOKINETICS

Well absorbed (PO), widely distributed, metabolized by liver, excreted by kidney (small amounts); onset 1-2 hr, peak 2 hr, duration up to 36 hr; excreted in urine, feces; half-life 14-18 hr

INTERACTIONS

Hyperglycemia: diazoxide
Increase: toxicity of muscle relaxants, steroids, lithium, digitalis

Decrease: hypokalemia—steroids, amphotericin B, other diuretics
Decrease: effects—antidiabetics, antigout agents, anticoagulants
Decrease: absorption—cholestyramine, colestipol
Decrease: hypotensive effect—indomethacin, NSAIDs
Drug/Herb
Severe photosensitivity: St. John's wort
Increase: hypokalemia—aloe, buckthorn, cascara sagrada, Chinese cucumber, licorice, senna
Increase: diuretic effect—aloe, cucumber, dandelion, horsetail, pumpkin, Queen Anne's lace
Drug/Lab Test
Increase: Calcium, parathyroid test glucose, uric acid

NURSING CONSIDERATIONS
Assess:
• Weight daily, I&O daily to determine fluid loss; effect of drug may be decreased if used daily
• Rate, depth, rhythm of respiration, effect of exertion
• B/P lying, standing; postural hypotension may occur
• Electrolytes: K, Mg, Na, Cl: include BUN, CBC, serum creatinine, blood pH, ABGs, uric acid, Ca, glucose
• Signs of metabolic alkalosis, hypokalemia
• Rashes, fever daily
• Confusion, especially in elderly; take safety precautions if needed
• Hydration: skin turgor, thirst, dry mucous membranes
Administer:
• In AM to avoid interference with sleep
• With food; if nausea occurs, absorption may be decreased slightly
Evaluate:
• Therapeutic response: improvement in edema of feet, legs, sacral area daily, decreased B/P

A Safety alert   *"Tall Man" lettering

Teach patient/family:
• Diet high in potassium; to rise slowly from lying or sitting position
• To recognize adverse reactions: muscle cramps, weakness, nausea, dizziness
• To take with food or milk for GI symptoms
• To use sunscreen for photosensitivity
• To take early in day to prevent nocturia
• To notify prescriber if urinary output decreases; daily weight
Treatment of overdose: Lavage if taken orally; monitor electrolytes, administer IV fluids; monitor hydration, CV, renal status

---

indinavir (R)
(en-den'a-veer)
Crixivan
Func. class.: Antiretroviral
Chem. class.: Protease inhibitor

Do not confuse:
indinavir/Denavir
Action: Inhibits human immunodeficiency virus (HIV-1) protease; this prevents maturation of virus
Uses: HIV-1 in combination with other antiretrovirals
Investigational uses: Prevention of HIV-1 after exposure

DOSAGE AND ROUTES
• Reduce dose in mild/moderate hepatic impairment and ketoconazole coadministration
• *Adult:* **PO** 800 mg q8h; if given with ddI, give 1 hr apart on empty stomach
Available forms: Caps 100, 200, 333, 400 mg

SIDE EFFECTS
CNS: Headache, insomnia, dizziness, somnolence
GI: Diarrhea, abdominal pain, nausea, vomiting, anorexia, dry mouth
GU: Nephrolithiasis
INTEG: Rash
MS: Pain
OTHER: Asthenia, ***insulin-resistant***

hyperglycemia, hyperlipidemia, ***keto-acidosis,*** lipodystrophy
Contraindications: Hypersensitivity
Precautions: Pregnancy (C), hepatic disease, lactation, children, renal disease, history of renal stones, diabetes, hypercholesterolemia

PHARMACOKINETICS
Terminal half-life 1-2 hr, 60% protein binding, metabolized liver, excreted 20% unchanged in urine

INTERACTIONS
A Life-threatening dysrhythmias: ergots, midazolam, rifampin, triazolam
Increase: myopathy—atorvastatin, lovastatin, simvastatin
Increase: indinavir levels—ketoconazole, delavirdine, itraconazole
Increase: levels of both drugs—clarithromycin, zidovudine
Increase: levels of isoniazid, oral contraceptives
Decrease: indinavir levels—rifamycins, fluconazole, nevirapine, efavirenz
Decrease: of both drugs—anticonvulsants
Drug/Herb
Decrease: indinavir levels—St. John's wort; avoid concurrent use
Drug/Food
Decrease: indinavir absorption—grapefruit juice, high-fat, high-protein foods

NURSING CONSIDERATIONS
Assess:
• For complaints of lower back, flank pain, indicates kidney stones
• Signs of infection, anemia, the presence of other sexually transmitted diseases
• Hepatic studies: ALT, AST; total bilirubin, amylase, all may be elevated
• Viral load, CD4 during treatment
• Bowel pattern before, during treatment; if severe abdominal pain with bleeding occurs, drug should be discontinued; monitor hydration

---

• Skin eruptions; rash, urticaria, itching
• Allergies before treatment, reaction of each medication; place allergies on chart

Administer:

• Do not break, crush, or chew caps
• With water, 1 hr ac or 2 hr pc; may be given with other liquids or small meal; do not give with high-fat, high-protein meals
• Dosage adjustment will need to be considered when given with efavirenz
• Water to 1.5 L/day minimum to prevent nephrolithiasis

Teach patient/family:

• To take as prescribed; if dose is missed, take as soon as remembered up to 1 hr before next dose; do not double dose
• That drug must be taken in equal intervals around the clock to maintain blood levels for duration of therapy
⚠ That hyperglycemia may occur; watch for increased thirst, weight loss, hunger, dry, itchy skin; notify prescriber
• To increase fluids to prevent kidney stones, if stone formation occurs, treatment may need to be interrupted
• That drug does not cure AIDS, only controls symptoms; not to donate blood

---

indomethacin (℞)

(in-doe-meth′a-sin)
Apo-Indomethacin ✿,
Indameth ✿, Indocid ✿,
Indocin, Indocin IV, Indocin
PDA ✿, Indocin SR,
indomethacin, Indochron
E-R, Novomethacin ✿,
Nu-Indo ✿

Func. class.: Nonsteroidal antiinflammatory (NSAID), antirheumatic
Chem. class.: Propionic acid derivative

Action: Inhibits prostaglandin synthesis by decreasing enzyme needed for biosynthesis; analgesic, antiinflammatory, antipyretic

Uses: Rheumatoid arthritis, ankylosing rheumatoid spondylitis, acute gouty arthritis; closure of patent ductus arteriosus in premature infants (IV)

Research note: Indomethacin reduces the antihypertensive effects of captopril and losartan; monitor carefully

DOSAGE AND ROUTES

Arthritis/antiinflammatory
• *Adult:* **PO/RECT** 25-50 mg bid; may increase by 25 mg/day qwk, not to exceed 200 mg/day; **SUS REL** 75 mg daily, may increase to 75 mg bid

Acute arthritis
• *Adult:* **PO/RECT** 100/mg intially, then 50 mg tid; use only for acute attack, then reduce dose

Patent ductus arteriosus
Longer or repeated treatment courses may be necessary for very premature infants
• *Infant <2 days:* **IV** 0.2 mg/kg, then 0.1 mg/kg × 2 doses after 12, 24 hr
• *Infant 2-7 days:* **IV** 0.2 mg/kg, then 0.2 mg/kg × 2 doses after 12, 24 hr
• *Infant >7 days:* **IV** 0.2 mg/kg, then 0.25 mg/kg × 2 doses after 12, 24 hr

Available forms: Caps 25, 50 mg; caps sus rel 75 mg; susp 25 mg/5 ml; rec supp 50, 100 mg; inj 1 mg vial

SIDE EFFECTS

CNS: Dizziness, drowsiness, fatigue, tremors, confusion, insomnia, anxiety, depression, headache
CV: Tachycardia, peripheral edema, palpitations, dysrhythmias, hypertension
EENT: Tinnitus, hearing loss, blurred vision
GI: Nausea, anorexia, *vomiting,* diarrhea, jaundice, ***cholestatic hepatitis,*** *constipation,* flatulence, cramps, dry mouth, peptic ulcer, ***ulceration, perforation, GI bleeding***
*GU: **Nephrotoxicity: dysuria, hematuria, oliguria, azotemia***
*HEMA: **Blood dyscrasias,*** prolonged bleeding
INTEG: Purpura, rash, pruritus, sweating
Contraindications: Pregnancy (X) 2nd/3rd trimester, hypersensitivity,

---

⚠ Safety alert   ✿ "Tall Man" lettering

asthma, severe renal disease, severe hepatic disease, ulcer disease

Precautions: Pregnancy (B) 1st trimester, lactation, children, bleeding disorders, GI disorders, cardiac disorders, hypersensitivity to other antiinflammatory agents, depression

PHARMACOKINETICS

PO: Onset 1-2 hr, peak 3 hr, duration 4-6 hr; metabolized in liver, kidneys; excreted in urine, bile, feces; crosses placenta; excreted in breast milk; 99% plasma protein binding

INTERACTIONS

Hyperkalemia: potassium-sparing diuretics

Toxicity: lithium, methotrexate, cyclo-SPORINE, zidovudine

Increase: effect of digoxin, penicillamine, phenytoin, aminoglycosides

Increase: bleeding risk—anticoagulants, abciximab, cefamandole, cefoperazone, cefotetan, clopidogrel, eptifibatide, plicamycin, ticlopidine, tirofiban, valproic acid, thrombolytics, aspirin

Decrease: effect of antihypertensives

Drug/Herb

Increase: bleeding risk—anise, arnica, bogbean, chamomile, chondroitin, clove, dong quai, feverfew, garlic, ginger, ginkgo, ginseng (*Panax*)

Increase: gastric irritation—arginine, gossypol

Increase: NSAIDs effect—bearberry, bilberry

NURSING CONSIDERATIONS

Assess:

• Arthritis symptoms: ROM, pain, swelling before and 2 hr after treatment

• Patent ductus arteriosus: respiratory rate, character, heart sounds

• Renal, hepatic, blood studies: BUN, creatinine, AST, ALT, Hgb, before treatment, periodically thereafter; if renal function has decreased, do not give subsequent doses

• For eye, ear problems: blurred vision, tinnitus; may indicate toxicity; audiometric, ophthalmic exam before, during, after treatment if on long-term therapy

• For confusion, mood changes, hallucinations, especially in elderly

• For asthma, nasal polyps, aspirin sensitivity, may develop hypersensitivity to indomethacin

Administer:

PO route

• Do not break, crush, or chew sus rel cap or reg caps.

• With food to decrease GI symptoms and prevent ulcerations

• Shake susp, do not mix with other liquids

Rectal route

• Have patient retain for 1 hr

IV route

• After diluting 1-2 mg/ml or more NS or sterile H_2O for inj without preservative; 5-10 sec to avoid dramatic shift in cerebral blood flow

Y-site compatibilities: Furosemide, insulin (regular), potassium chloride, sodium bicarbonate, sodium nitroprusside

Perform/provide:

• Storage at room temperature

Evaluate:

• Therapeutic response: decreased pain, stiffness in joints, decreased swelling in joints, ability to move more easily

Teach patient/family:

• To report blurred vision, ringing, roaring in ears; may indicate toxicity

• To avoid driving, other hazardous activities if dizziness, drowsiness occurs

• To report change in urine pattern, increased weight, edema, increased pain in joints, fever, blood in urine; indicate nephrotoxicity; to report mood changes: anxiety, depression

• That therapeutic antiinflammatory effects may take up to 1 mo

• To avoid alcohol, NSAIDs, salicylates; bleeding may occur

infliximab
(in-fliks′ih-mab)
Remicade
Func. class.: Monoclonal antibody

Action: Monoclonal antibody that neutralizes the activity of tumor necrosis factor alpha (TNF α) found in Crohn's disease; decreased infiltration of inflammatory cells

Uses: Crohn's disease, fistulizing (moderate-severe); rheumatoid arthritis given with methotrexate

Investigational uses: Plaque psoriasis, ankylosing spondylitis, ulcerative colitis, psoriatic arthritis, psoriasis, Behçet's syndrome, uveitis, juvenile arthritis

DOSAGE AND ROUTES
Crohn's disease (moderate-severe)
• *Adult:* **IV INF** 5 mg/kg × 1
Crohn's disease (fistulizing)
• *Adult:* **IV INF** 5 mg/kg initially, then repeat dose 2 wk, 6 wk after 1st dose
Rheumatoid arthritis
• *Adult:* **IV** 3 mg/kg initially and q2, 6, 8wk thereafter given with methotrexate
Available forms: Powder for inj 100 mg

SIDE EFFECTS
*CNS: Headache, dizziness, depression, vertigo, fatigue, anxiety, fever, **seizures***
CV: Chest pain, hyper/hypotension, ***tachycardia***
GI: Nausea, vomiting, abdominal pain, stomatitis, constipation, dyspepsia, flatulence
GU: Dysuria, urinary frequency
*HEMA: **Anemia***
INTEG: Rash, dermatitis, urticaria, dry skin, sweating, flushing, hematoma, pruritus
MS: Myalgia, back pain, arthralgia
RESP: URI, pharyngitis, bronchitis, cough, dyspnea, sinusitis
*SYST: **Anaphylaxis, fatal infections, sepsis, malignancies, immunogenicity***

Contraindications: Hypersensitivity to murines, moderate to severe CHF (NYHA Class III/IV)
Precautions: Pregnancy (B), lactation, children, elderly

PHARMACOKINETICS
Distributed to vascular compartment, half-life 9.5 days

INTERACTIONS
Do not administer live vaccines concurrently

NURSING CONSIDERATIONS
Assess:
• GI symptoms: nausea, vomiting, abdominal pain
• Periodic blood counts (CBC)
• CV status: B/P, pulse, chest pain
⚠ Allergic reaction, anaphylaxis: rash, dermatitis, urticaria, dyspnea, hypotension, fever, chills; discontinue if severe, administer epINEPHrine, corticosteroids, antihistamines; assess for allergies to murine proteins before starting therapy
⚠ Fatal infections: discontinue if infection occurs, do not administer to patients with active infections
• Identify TB before beginning treatment, a TB test should be obtained, if present, TB should be treated prior to receiving infliximab
Administer:
IV INF route
• Give immediately after reconstitution; reconstitute each vial with 10 ml of sterile water for inj, further dilute total dose/250 ml of 0.9% NaCl inj to a total conc of 0.4-4 mg/ml; use 21G or smaller needle for reconstitution, direct sterile water at glass wall of vial, gently swirl
• Give over ≥2 hr, use polyethylene-lined infusion with in-line, sterile, low-protein-bind filter
• Do not admix
Perform/provide:
• Refrigerated storage, do not freeze

⚠ Safety alert   *"Tall Man" lettering

Evaluate:
• Therapeutic response: absence of fever, mucus in stools
Teach patient/family:
• Not to breastfeed while taking this drug
• To notify prescriber of GI symptoms, hypersensitivity reactions
• Not to operate machinery, drive if dizziness, vertigo occur

⚠ High Alert

INSULINS

Rapid Acting
insulin glulisine (℞)
Apidra
insulin aspart
Novolog
insulin lispro (℞)
Humalog

Short Acting
insulin, regular (℞)
Humulin R ✤, Novolin ge Toronto ✤, Iletin II Regular, Novolin R, Velosulin BR
insulin, regular concentrated (℞)
regular (concentrated), Iletin II U-500

Intermediate Acting
insulin, isophane suspension (NPH) (℞)
Humulin N, Iletin NPH ✤, Iletin II NPH ✤, Novolin N
insulin, zinc suspension (Lente) (℞)
Humulin L, Lente Iletin II, Lente L, Novolin ge Lente ✤, Novolin L

Long Acting
insulin, zinc suspension extended (Ultralente) (℞)
Humulin U Ultralente, Novolin ge Ultralente ✤, Novolin U, Ultralente U
insulin detemir (℞)
Levemir
insulin glargine (℞)
Lantus

Mixtures
insulin, isophane suspension and regular insulin (℞)
Humulin 70/30, Humalin 30/70 ✤, Novolin 70/30, Novolin 70/30 PenFill, Novolin 70/30 Prefilled, Novolin ge 30/70 ✤
isophane insulin suspension (NPH) and insulin mixtures (℞)
Humulin 50/50, Novolin 50/50
Func. class.: Antidiabetic, pancreatic hormone
Chem. class.: Exogenous unmodified insulin

Do not confuse:
Lantus/lente
Novolin 70/30 Penfill/Novolin 70/30 Prefilled
Action: Decreases blood glucose; by transport of glucose into cells and the conversion of glucose to glycogen, indirectly increases blood pyruvate and lactate, decreases phosphate and potassium; insulin may be beef, pork, human (processed by recombinant DNA technologies)
Uses: Type 1 diabetes mellitus, type 2 diabetes mellitus, insulin lispro may be

used in combination with sulfonylureas in children >3 yr

DOSAGE AND ROUTES

Insulin glulisine
• *Adult:* **SUBCUT** dosage individualized, give within 15 min before or 20 min after starting a meal

Insulin aspart
• *Adult and child* ≥6 yr: 0.5-1 unit/kg/day divided in treatment, meal-related, highly individualized

Insulin lispro
• *Adult:* **SUBCUT** 15 min ac

Human regular
• *Adult:* **SUBCUT** ½-1 ac

Insulin, isophane suspension
• *Adult:* **SUBCUT** dosage individualized by blood, urine glucose; usual dose 7-26 units; may increase by 2-10 units/day if needed

Insulin detemir
• *Adult:* **SUBCUT** 1 or 2 times daily; if 1 time, give with evening meal

Insulin glargine
• *Adult and child* ≥ 6 yr: **SUBCUT** 10 international units daily, range 2-100 international units/day

Regular insulin (ketoacidosis)
• *Adult:* **IV** 5-10 units, then 5-10 units/hr until desired response, then switch to **SUBCUT** dose; **IV**/inf 2-12 units (50 units/500 ml of normal saline)
• *Child:* **IV** 0.1 units/kg

Replacement
• *Adult and child:* **SUBCUT** 0.5-1 units/kg/day qid given 30 min ac
• *Adolescent:* **SUBCUT** 0.8-1.2 mg/kg/day; this dosage is used during rapid growth

Available forms: *NPH* Inj 100 units/ml; *regular* inj 100 units/ml; *zinc susp* 100 units/ml; *insulin analog* inj 100 units/ml; *insulin zinc susp,* ext (Ultralente) 100 units/ml; *isophane insulin/insulin* inj 100 units/ml; *insulin lispro* 100 units/ml, 1.5-ml cartridges; *insulin glulisine* inj 100 units/ml; *insulin glargine* inj 100 units/ml insulin detemir inj 100 units/ml

SIDE EFFECTS

EENT: Blurred vision, dry mouth
INTEG: Flushing, rash, urticaria, warmth, *lipodystrophy,* lipohypertrophy, swelling, redness
META: Hypoglycemia, rebound hyperglycemia (Somogyi effect 12-72 hr or longer)
SYST: **Anaphylaxis**
Contraindications: Hypersensitivity to protamine
Precautions: Pregnancy (C) glargine, (B) all others

PHARMACOKINETICS

Rapid acting
Insulin glulisine: Onset 15-30 min, peak ½-1½ hr, duration, 3-4 hr
Insulin aspart: Onset 15-30 min, peak ½-1½ hr, duration 3-4 hr
Insulin lispro: Onset 15-30 min, peak ½-1½ hr, duration 3-4 hr

Short acting
Insulin regular: Onset ½-1 hr, peak 2-3 hr, duration 3-6 hr

Intermediate acting
Insulin, isophane suspension (NPH): Onset 2-4 hr, peak 6-10 hr, duration 10-16 hr
Insulin, zinc suspension (Lente): Onset 3-4 hr, peak 6-12 hr, duration 12-18 hr

Long acting
Insulin, zinc suspension extended (Ultralente): Onset 6-10 hr, peak 10-16, duration 18-20 hr
Insulin glargine: Onset 5 hr, no peak identified, duration ≥24 hr

Mixtures
Insulin, isophane suspension and regular insulin (70/30): Onset ½-1 hr, peak dual, duration 10-16 hr
Insophane insulin suspension (NPH) and insulin mixtures (50/50): Onset ½-1 hr, peak dual, duration 10-16 hr

---

INTERACTIONS

Increase: hypoglycemia—salicylate, alcohol, β-blockers, anabolic steroids, fenfluramine, phenylbutazone, sulfinpyrazone, guanethidine, oral hypoglycemics, MAOIs, tetracycline

Decrease: hypoglycemia—thiazides, thyroid hormones, oral contraceptives, corticosteroids, estrogens, DOBUTamine, epINEPHrine

Drug/Herb

Increase: antidiabetic effect—alfalfa, aloe, basil, bay, bilberry, bitter melon, black catechu, buchu, burdock, coriander, dandelion, eyebright (po), fenugreek, garlic, ginseng, glucomannan, glucosamine, goat's rue, gymnema, horehound, horse chestnut, jambul, myrrh, myrtle

Increase: glucose tolerance—karela

Increase: hypoglycemics—aceitilla, adiantum agrimony, aloe gel, banana flowers/roots, banyan stembark, bilberry, bitter melon, broom, bugleweed, burdock, carob, cumin, damiana, dandelion, eucalyptus, fenugreek, fo-ti, garlic, goat's rue, guar gum, horse chestnut, jambue, juniper, konjac, maitake, onion, psyllium, reishi

Decrease or increase: hypoglycemic effect—chromium

Decrease: hypoglycemic effect—annato, cocoa seeds, coffee seeds, cola seeds, guarana, ma huang, yerba maté, rosemary

Decrease: antidiabetic effect—bee pollen, blue cohosh, broom, chromium, elecampane, eucalyptus, gotu kola

Drug/Lab Test

Increase: VMA

Decrease: Potassium, calcium

Interference: LFTs, thyroid function studies

NURSING CONSIDERATIONS

Assess:

• Fasting blood glucose, 2 hr PP (80-150 mg/dl, normal fasting level; 70-130 mg/dl, normal 2 hr level); also A1c may be drawn to identify treatment effectiveness

• Urine ketones during illness; insulin requirements may increase during stress, illness, surgery

• For hypoglycemic reaction that can occur during peak time (sweating, weakness, dizziness, chills, confusion, headache, nausea, rapid weak pulse, fatigue, tachycardia, memory lapses, slurred speech, staggering gait, anxiety, tremors, hunger)

• For hyperglycemia: acetone breath, polyuria, fatigue, polydipsia, flushed, dry skin, lethargy

Administer:

SUBCUT route

• After warming to room temperature by rotating in palms to prevent injecting cold insulin; use only insulin syringes with markings or syringe matching units/ml; rotate inj sites within one area: abdomen, upper back, thighs, upper arm, buttocks; keep record of sites

• Increased dosages if tolerance occurs; give human insulin to those allergic to beef or pork

• Do not use if cloudy, thick, or discolored

• Lispro: 15 min ac

IV route

• IV direct, undiluted via vein, Y-site, 3-way stopcock; give at 50 units/min or less

• By cont inf after diluting with IV sol and run at prescribed rate; use IV inf pump for correct dosing; give reduced dose at serum glucose level of 250 mg/100 ml

Additive compatibilities: Bretylium, cimetidine, lidocaine, meropenem, ranitidine, verapamil

Syringe compatibilities: Metoclopramide

Y-site compatibilities: Amiodarone, ampicillin, ampicillin/sulbactam, aztreonam, cefazolin, cefotetan, DOBUTamine, esmolol, famotidine, gentamicin, heparin, heparin/hydrocortisone, imipenem/cilastatin, indomethacin, magnesium sulfate, meperidine, meropenem, midazolam, morphine, nitroglycerin, oxytocin, pentobarbital, potassium chloride, propofol, ritodrine, sodium

---

bicarbonate, sodium nitroprusside, tacrolimus, terbutaline, ticarcillin,
ticarcillin/clavulanate, tobramycin, vancomycin, vit B/C

Perform/provide:
• Store at room temperature for <1 mo;
keep away from heat and sunlight; refrigerate all other supply; do not use if
discolored; do not freeze—IV route,
regular only

Evaluate:
• Therapeutic response: decrease in
polyuria, polydipsia, polyphagia, clear
sensorium, absence of dizziness, stable
gait

Teach patient/family:
• That blurred vision occurs; not to
change corrective lens until vision is
stabilized 1-2 mo
• To keep insulin, equipment available at
all times
• That drug does not cure diabetes but
controls symptoms
• To carry emergency ID as diabetic
• To recognize hypoglycemia reaction:
headache, tremors, fatigue, weakness
• The dosage, route, mixing instructions, if any diet restrictions, disease
process
• To carry candy or lump sugar to treat
hypoglycemia
• The symptoms of ketoacidosis: nausea,
thirst, polyuria, dry mouth, decreased
B/P, dry, flushed skin, acetone breath,
drowsiness, Kussmaul respirations
• That a plan is necessary for diet,
exercise; all food on diet should be
eaten; exercise routine should not vary
• About blood glucose testing; make sure
patient is able to determine glucose level
• To avoid OTC drugs unless directed by
prescriber

Treatment of overdose: Glucose 25
g IV, via dextrose 50% sol, 50 ml or glucagon 1 mg

insulin, inhaled
See Appendix A—Selected
New Drugs

interferon alfa-2a/
interferon alfa-2b (℞)
(in-ter-feer′on)
Roferon-a/Intron-a
Func. class.: Antineoplastic—
miscellaneous
Chem. class.: Protein product

Do not confuse:
Roferon-A/Imferon

Action: Antiviral action inhibits viral
replication by reprogramming virus;
antitumor action suppresses cell
proliferation; immunomodulating action
phagocytizes target cells; may also inhibit
virus replication in virus-infested cells

Uses: Hairy cell leukemia in persons
>18 yr, condylomata acuminata, malig-
nant melanoma, AIDS (use phase II with
zidovudine), chronic hepatitis B, C

Investigational uses: Bladder tumors, carcinoid tumors, non-Hodgkin's
lymphoma, essential thrombocytopenia,
cytomegaloviruses, herpes simplex, Kaposi's sarcoma, HPV-associated diseases

DOSAGE AND ROUTES
alfa-2a
Hairy cell leukemia
• *Adult:* **SUBCUT/IM** 3 million international units/day × 16-24 wk, then 3 million international units 3 ×/wk maintenance

Condylomata acuminata
• 1 million international units/lesion 3
×/wk × 3 wk

alfa-2b
Chronic hepatitis B
• 3 million international units/3 ×/wk ×
18-24 mo **SUBCUT/IM** as 5 million
international units/day or 10 million
international units/3 ×/wk × 16 wk

Hairy cell leukemia
• 2 million international units/m² 3
×/wk; if severe adverse reactions occur,
dose should be skipped or reduced by ½

Kaposi's sarcoma
• *Adult:* **SUBCUT/IM** 30 million international units/m² 3 ×/wk

Available forms:
alfa-2a inj 3, 6, 36 million international units/ml; alfa-2b inj 3, 5, 10, 18, 25 million units/vial, powder for inj 5, 10, 18, 25, 50 million units/vial

SIDE EFFECTS

CNS: Dizziness, confusion, numbness, paresthesias, hallucinations, **seizures, coma,** amnesia, anxiety, mood changes, depression, somnolence, paranoia, irritability
CV: Edema, hypotension, hypertension, chest pain, palpitations, dysrhythmias, **CHF, MI, CVA,** tachycardia, syncope
GI: Weight loss, taste changes, nausea, anorexia, diarrhea, xerostomia
GU: Impotence
HEMA: **Neutropenia, thrombocytopenia**
INTEG: Rash, dry skin, itching, alopecia, flushing, photosensitivity
MISC: Flulike syndrome; fever, fatigue, myalgias, headache, chills
Contraindications: Hypersensitivity
Precautions: Pregnancy (C), severe hypotension, dysrhythmia, tachycardia, lactation, children, severe renal or hepatic disease, convulsion disorder

PHARMACOKINETICS

Half-life (interferon alfa-2a) 3.7-8.5 hr, peak 3-4 hr; half-life (interferon alfa-2b) 2-7 hr, peak 6-8 hr

INTERACTIONS

Increase: theophylline levels—aminophylline
Increase: neutropenia—zidovudine
Drug/Lab Test
Interference: AST, ALT, LDH, alk phosphatase, WBC, platelets, granulocytes, creatinine

NURSING CONSIDERATIONS
Assess:
• For symptoms of infection; chills, fever, headache; may be masked by drug fever
• CNS reaction: LOC, mental status, dizziness, confusion, paresthesia, slurred speech

• Cardiac status: lung sounds; ECG before and during treatment, especially in those with cardiac disease
• Bone marrow depression: bruising, bleeding, blood in stools, urine, sputum, emesis
• Mental status: depression, suicidal thoughts, hallucinations, amnesia
Administer:
alfa-2a
• SUBCUT/IM after reconstituting 18 million units/3 ml of diluent provided (6 million units/ml)
• 36 million units/ml is used for Kaposi's sarcoma only
alfa-2b
• IM/SUBCUT after reconstituting 3-5 million international units/1 ml, 10 million international units/2 ml, 25 million international units/5 ml, of diluent provided, mix gently
• Intralesional after reconstituting 10 million international units/1 ml bacteriostatic water for inj; no more than 5 lesions can safely be treated at a time
• At bedtime to minimize side effects
• Acetaminophen as ordered to alleviate fever and headache
Perform/provide:
• Reconstituted sol must be used within 30 days
• Increased fluid intake to 2-3 L/day
Evaluate:
• Therapeutic response: decrease in size, number of lesions
Teach patient/family:
• To take acetaminophen for fever
• To avoid hazardous tasks, since confusion, dizziness may occur; avoid prolonged sunlight, use sunscreen
• That brands of this drug should not be changed; each form is different, with different doses
• That fatigue is common; activity may have to be altered; to take at bedtime to minimize flulike symptoms
• Not to become pregnant while taking drug; possible mutagenic effects
• To report signs of infection: sore throat, fever, diarrhea, vomiting, sore or white patches in mouth

• That impotence may occur during treatment but is temporary
• That emotional lability is common; notify prescriber if severe or incapacitating

interferon alfacon-1 (℞)

(in-ter-feer'on al'fa-kon)
Infergen
Func. class.: Recombinant type 1 interferon

Action: Induces biologic responses and has antiviral, antiproliferative, and immunomodulatory effects

Uses: Chronic hepatitis C infections in those 18 yr and older with compensated liver disease who have anti-HCV antibodies or HCV RNA

Investigational uses: Hairy cell leukemia when used with G-CSF

DOSAGE AND ROUTES

• *Adult:* SUBCUT 9 mcg as a single inj 3 ×/wk × 24 wk
Available forms: Inj 9 mcg/0.3 ml, 15 mcg/0.5 ml

SIDE EFFECTS

CNS: Headache, fatigue, fever, rigors, insomnia, dizziness
CV: Hypertension, palpitation
EENT: Tinnitus, earache, conjunctivitis, eye pain
GI: Abdominal pain, nausea, diarrhea, anorexia, dyspepsia, vomiting, constipation, flatulence, hemorrhoids, decreased salivation
GU: Dysmenorrhea, vaginitis, menstrual disorders
HEMA: **Granulocytopenia, thrombocytopenia, leukopenia,** ecchymosis
INTEG: Alopecia, pruritus, rash, erythema, dry skin
MS: Back, limb, neck skeletal pain
PSYCH: Nervousness, depression, anxiety, lability, abnormal thinking
RESP: Pharyngitis, upper respiratory infection, cough, sinusitis, rhinitis, respiratory tract congestion, epistaxis, dyspnea, bronchitis

Contraindications: Hypersensitivity to alpha interferons, or products from *Escherichia coli*

Precautions: Pregnancy (C), thyroid disorders, myelosuppression, hepatic, cardiac disease, lactation, children <18 yr

PHARMACOKINETICS

Peak 24-36 hr

INTERACTIONS

None known

NURSING CONSIDERATIONS

Assess:
• Platelet counts, heme concentration, ANC, serum creatinine concentration, albumin, bilirubin, TSH, T_4
• For myelosuppression: hold dose if neutrophil count is $<500 \times 10^6$/L or if platelets are $<50 \times 10^9$/L
• For hypersensitivity: discontinue immediately if hypersensitivity occurs

Administer:

Evaluate:
• Therapeutic response: decreased chronic hepatitis C signs/symptoms

Teach patient/family:
• Provide patient or family member with written, detailed information about drug

interferon alfa-n 3 (℞)

(in-ter-feer'on)
Alferon N
Func. class.: Antineoplastic, antiviral
Chem. class.: Human interferon α-protein

Action: Binds interferon to membrane receptors on cell surface with high specificity; this produces protein synthesis, inhibition of virus replication, suppression of cell proliferation, increased phagocytosis

Uses: Condylomata acuminata (venereal/genital warts), papillomavirus

Investigational uses: Adenovirus, coronavirus, encephalomyocarditis virus, hepatitis B virus, hepatitis C infection/virus, hepatitis D, herpes simplex type 1 and 2, HIV, HTLV-I, poliovirus, rhinovirus, varicella-zoster virus, variola virus, vesicular stomatitis virus

DOSAGE AND ROUTES
External condylomata acuminata
• *Adult:* 0.05 ml (250,000 international units) per wart, given 2 ×/wk × 8 wk; not to exceed 0.5 ml (2.5 million international units); inject into base of wart
Chronic hepatitis C (off label)
• *Adult:* **SUBCUT/IM** 3-6 million international units 3 ×/wk

Available forms: Inj 5 m international units/L ml vial with 3.3 mg/ml phenol and 1 mg/ml human albumin

SIDE EFFECTS
CNS: Fever, headache, sweating, vasovagal reaction, chills, fatigue, dizziness, insomnia, sleepiness, depression
CV: Chest pain, hypotension
GI: Nausea, vomiting, heartburn, diarrhea, constipation, anorexia, stomatitis, dry mouth
INTEG: Pain at inj site, pruritus
MS: Myalgias, arthralgia, back pain, flulike symptoms

Contraindications: Hypersensitivity to this product, egg protein, IgG, neomycin, murine protein

Precautions: Pregnancy (C), lactation, children, CHF, angina (unstable), COPD, diabetes mellitus with ketoacidosis, hemophilia, pulmonary embolism, thrombophlebitis, bone marrow depression, seizure disorder

PHARMACOKINETICS
Unable to detect

Drug/Lab Test
Interference: AST, ALT, LDH, alk phosphatase, WBC, platelets, granulocytes, creatinine

NURSING CONSIDERATIONS
Assess:
• For symptoms of infection; may be masked by drug fever

• CNS reaction: LOC, mental status, dizziness, confusion
• For body image disturbance
Administer:
• Acetaminophen to alleviate fever and headache
Perform/provide:
• Storage of reconstituted sol for 1 mo in refrigerator
• Increased fluid intake to 2-3 L/day
Evaluate:
• Therapeutic response: decrease in wart size
Teach patient/family:
• To avoid hazardous tasks, since confusion, dizziness may occur
• That brands of this drug should not be changed; each form is different, with different doses
• That fatigue is common; activity may have to be altered
• Not to become pregnant while taking drug; possible mutagenic effects
• To report signs of infection: sore throat, fever, diarrhea, vomiting
• To recognize the signs of hypersensitivity: liver, urticaria, wheezing, dyspnea; notify prescriber immediately

---

interferon beta-1a
(in-ter-feer'on)
Avonex
interferon beta-1b (℞)
Betaseron
Func. class.: Multiple sclerosis agent, immune modifier
Chem. class.: Interferon, *Escherichia coli* derivative

Action: Antiviral, immunoregulatory; action not clearly understood; biologic response modifying properties mediated through specific receptors on cells, inducing expression of interferon-induced gene products
Uses: Ambulatory patients with relapsing-remitting multiple sclerosis
Investigational uses: May be useful in treatment of AIDS, AIDS-related Kaposi's sarcoma, malignant melanoma,

---

metastatic renal cell carcinoma, cutaneous T cell lymphoma, acute non-A, non-B hepatitis

DOSAGE AND ROUTES

Interferon beta-1a
• *Adult:* **IM** 30 mcg qwk
Interferon beta-1b
Relapsing-remitting multiple sclerosis
• *Adult:* **SUBCUT** 0.25 mg (8 international units) every other day
Available forms: beta-1a 33 mcg (6.6 million international units/vial); beta-1b powder for inj 0.3 mg (9.6 m international units)

SIDE EFFECTS

CNS: Headache, fever, pain, chills, mental changes, hypertonia, ***suicide attempts, seizures***
CV: Migraine, palpitations, hypertension, tachycardia, peripheral vascular disorders
EENT: Conjunctivitis, blurred vision
GI: Diarrhea, constipation, vomiting, abdominal pain
GU: Dysmenorrhea, irregular menses, metrorrhagia, cystitis, breast pain
*HEMA: **Decreased lymphocytes, ANC, WBC;** lymphadenopathy*
INTEG: Sweating, inj site reaction
*MS: Myalgia, **myasthenia***
RESP: Sinusitis, dyspnea
Contraindications: Hypersensitivity to natural or recombinant interferon-β or human albumin, hamster protein
Precautions: Pregnancy (C), lactation, child <18 yr, chronic progressive MS, depression, mental disorders, seizure disorder, latex allergy

PHARMACOKINETICS

beta-1a: Onset up to 12 hr, peak 48 hr, duration 4 days, half-life 8-6 hr
beta-1b: Onset rapid, peak 2-8 hr, duration unknown, half-life 8 min-4.3 hr

INTERACTIONS

Decrease: clearance of zidovudine

NURSING CONSIDERATIONS

Assess:
• Blood, renal, hepatic studies: CBC, differential, platelet counts, BUN, creatinine ALT, urinalysis; if absolute neutrophil count < 750/mm^3, or if AST/ALT is 10 × normal, drug is discontinued
• CNS symptoms: headache, fatigue, depression
• GI status: diarrhea or constipation, vomiting, abdominal pain
• Cardiac status: increased B/P, tachycardia
• Mental status: depression, depersonalization, suicidal thoughts, insomnia
• For multiple sclerosis symptoms
Administer:
• Acetaminophen for fever, headache
• SUBCUT only; products are not interchangeable
Interferon beta-1a
• Reconstitute with 1.1-ml diluent, swirl, give within 6 hr
Interferon beta-1b
• Reconstitute by injecting diluent provided (1.2 ml) into vial, swirl (8 m international units/ml), use 27G needle for inj
Perform/provide:
• Storage in refrigerator; do not freeze
Evaluate:
• Therapeutic response: decreased symptoms of multiple sclerosis
Teach patient/family:
• To provide patient or family member with written, detailed information about the drug
• That blurred vision, sweating may occur
• That female patients may experience irregular menses, dysmenorrhea, or metrorrhagia as well as breast pain
• To use sunscreen to prevent photosensitivity
• To notify prescriber if pregnancy is suspected
• Inj technique and care of equipment
• To notify prescriber of increased temp, chills, muscle soreness, fatigue

interferon gamma-1b (℞)

(in-ter-feer'on)

Actimmune

Func. class.: Biologic response modifier

Chem. class.: Lymphokine, interleukin type

Action: Species-specific protein synthesized in response to viruses, effects; can mediate killing of *Staphylococcus aureus, Toxoplasma gondii, Leishmania donovani, Listeria monocytogenes, Mycobacterium avium-intracellulare;* enhances oxidative metabolism of macrophages, enhances antibody-dependent cellular cytotoxicity

Uses: Serious infections associated with chronic granulomatous disease, osteoporosis

Investigational uses: Osteoporosis, *Mycobacterium avium* complex (MAC), ovarian cancer, pulmonary fibrosis

DOSAGE AND ROUTES

• *Adult:* **SUBCUT** 50 mcg/m^2 (1.5 million units/m^2) for patients with surface area >0.5 m^2; 1.5 mcg/kg/dose for patient with surface area <0.5 m^2; give Monday, Wednesday, Friday for 3 ×/wk dosing

Available forms: Inj 100 mcg (3 million units)/single-dose vial

SIDE EFFECTS

CNS: Headache, fatigue, depression, fever, chills

GI: Nausea, anorexia, abdominal pain, weight loss, diarrhea, vomiting

INTEG: Rash, pain at inj site

MS: Myalgia, arthralgia

Contraindications: Hypersensitivity to interferon-γ, *Escherichia coli*-derived products

Precautions: Pregnancy (C), cardiac disease, seizure disorders, CNS disorders, myelosuppression, lactation, children

PHARMACOKINETICS

SUBCUT: Dose absorbed 89%, elimination half-life 5.9 hr, peak 7 hr

INTERACTIONS

May interfere with fosphenytoin, phenytoin, warfarin

Increase: myelosuppression—other myelosuppressive agents

Increase: level of theophylline, aminophylline

NURSING CONSIDERATIONS

Assess:

• Blood, renal, hepatic studies: CBC, differential, platelet counts, BUN, creatinine, ALT, urinalysis

• CNS symptoms: headache, fatigue, depression

Administer:

• At bedtime to minimize adverse reactions; administer acetaminophen for fever, headache

• 50% of dose if severe reactions occur or discontinue treatment until reactions subside

• In right and left deltoid and anterior thigh

• Warm to room temperature before use; do not leave at room temperature over 12 hr (unopened vial)

Perform/provide:

• Storage in refrigerator upon receipt; do not freeze; do not shake

Evaluate:

• Therapeutic response: decreased serious infections, improvement in existing infections and inflammatory conditions

Teach patient/family:

• The method of administration if family members will be giving medication

• Provide patient or family member with written, detailed information about drug

ipratropium (℞)

(i-pra-troe´pee-um)
Atrovent
Func. class.: Anticholinergic, bronchodilator
Chem. class.: Synthetic quaternary ammonium compound

Do not confuse:
Atrovent/Alupent

Action: Inhibits interaction of acetylcholine at receptor sites on the bronchial smooth muscle, resulting in decreased cGMP and bronchodilation

Uses: COPD; rhinorrhea in children 6-11 yr (nasal spray)

DOSAGE AND ROUTES

• *Adult:* 2 **INH** 4 × day, not to exceed 12 **INH**/24 hr; sol 500 mcg (1 unit dose) given 3-4 ×/day
• *Child 6-11 yr:* **NASAL** 1 spray in each nostril

Available forms: Aerosol 18 mcg/actuation; nasal spray 0.03%, 0.06%; sol for inh 0.02%

SIDE EFFECTS

CNS: Anxiety, dizziness, headache, nervousness
CV: Palpitation
EENT: Dry mouth, blurred vision
GI: Nausea, vomiting, cramps
INTEG: Rash
RESP: Cough, worsening of symptoms, ***bronchospasms***

Contraindications: Hypersensitivity to this drug, atropine, soya lecithin
Precautions: Pregnancy (B), lactation, children <12 yr, narrow-angle glaucoma, prostatic hypertrophy, bladder neck obstruction

PHARMACOKINETICS

Half-life 2 hr; does not cross blood-brain barrier

INTERACTIONS

Drug/Herb
Increase: constipation—black catechu
Increase: anticholinergic effect—butterbur, jimsonweed
Increase: bronchodilator effect—green tea (large amts), guarana
Decrease: anticholinergic effect—jaborandi tree, pill-bearing spurge

NURSING CONSIDERATIONS

Assess:
• For palpitations; if severe, drug may have to be changed
• For tolerance over long-term therapy; dose may have to be increased or changed

Administer:
Nebulizer
• Use sol in nebulizer with a mouthpiece rather than a face mask
Nasal spray
• Priming pump initially requires 7 actuations of the pump, priming again is not necessary if used regularly

Perform/provide:
• Storage at room temperature
• Hard candy, frequent drinks, sugarless gum to relieve dry mouth

Evaluate:
• Therapeutic response: ability to breathe adequately

Teach patient/family:
• That compliance is necessary with number of inhalations/24 hr or overdose may occur; spacer device in the elderly
• To shake before using
• The correct method of inhalation and cleaning of equipment daily

irbesartan (℞)

(er-be-sar´tan)
Avapro
Func. class.: Antihypertensive
Chem. class.: Angiotensin II receptor blocker (Type AT₁)

Do not confuse:
Avapro/Anaprox

Action: Blocks the vasoconstrictor and aldosterone-secreting effects of angiotensin II; selectively blocks the binding of angiotensin II to the AT_1 receptor found in tissues

Uses: Hypertension, alone or in combination; nephropathy in type 2 diabetic patients

Investigational uses: Heart failure

DOSAGES AND ROUTES

Hypertension
- *Adult:* **PO** 150 mg daily; may be increased to 300 mg daily

Neuropathy in type 2 diabetic patients
- *Adult:* **PO** maintenance dose 300 mg daily, start 75 mg daily
- *Child 13-16 yr:* **PO** 150 mg daily, may increase to 300 mg daily
- *Child 6-12 yr:* **PO** 75 mg daily, may increase to 150 mg daily

Volume- and salt-depleted patients
- *Adult:* **PO** 75 mg daily

Available forms: 75, 150, 300 mg

SIDE EFFECTS

CNS: Dizziness, anxiety, headache, fatigue
GI: Diarrhea, dyspepsia
MISC: Edema, chest pain, rash, tachycardia, UTI, ***angioedema,*** hyperkalemia
RESP: Cough, upper respiratory infection, sinus disorder, pharyngitis, rhinitis
Contraindications: Pregnancy (D) 2nd/3rd trimester, hypersensitivity
Precautions: Pregnancy (C) 1st trimester, hypersensitivity to ACE inhibitors; lactation, children, elderly, renal disease

PHARMACOKINETICS

Extensively metabolized, half-life 11-15 hr, highly bound to plasma proteins, excreted in urine and feces

INTERACTIONS

Increase: hyperkalemia: potassium-sparing diuretics, potassium salt substitutes

Decrease: antihypertensive effect—NSAIDs
Drug/Herb
Increase: toxicity, death—aconite
Increase: antihypertensive effect—barberry, betony, black catechu, black cohosh, bloodroot, broom, burdock, cat's claw, dandelion, goldenseal, Irish moss, Jamaican dogwood, kelp, khella, mistletoe, parsley
Increase or decrease: antihypertensive effect—astragalus, cola tree
Decrease: antihypertensive effect—coltsfoot, guarana, khat, licorice

NURSING CONSIDERATIONS

Assess:
- B/P, pulse q4h; note rate, rhythm, quality
- Electrolytes: K, Na, Cl
- Baselines in renal, hepatic studies before therapy begins
- Edema in feet, legs daily
- Skin turgor, dryness of mucous membranes for hydration status

Administer:
- Without regard to meals

Evaluate:
- Therapeutic response: decreased B/P

Teach patient/family:
- To comply with dosage schedule, even if feeling better
- That drug may cause dizziness, fainting; light-headedness may occur
- To rise slowly to sitting or standing position to minimize orthostatic hypotension
- To notify prescriber if pregnancy is suspected

⚠ High Alert

irinotecan (Ŗ)
(ear-een-oh-tee'kan)
Camptosar
Func. class.: Antineoplastic hormone
Chem. class.: Topoisomerase inhibitor

Action: Cytotoxic by producing damage to double-strand DNA during DNA synthesis

Uses: Metastatic carcinoma of the colon or rectum, or 1st-line treatment in combination with 5-FU and leucovorin for metastatic colon or rectal carcinomas

DOSAGE AND ROUTES
Single agent
• *Adult:* IV 125 mg/m^2 given over 1½ hr qwk × 4 wk, then 2-wk rest period, may be repeated; 4 wk or 2 wk off; dosage adjustments may be made to 150 mg/m^2 (high) or 50 mg/m^2 (low); adjustments should be made in increments of 25-50 mg/m^2 depending on patient's tolerance
Combination dosage schedules
• *Regimen 1:* irinotecan 75-125 mg/m^2, leucovorin 20 mg/m^2, 5-FU 300-500 mg/m^2 depending on dosing levels
• *Regimen 2:* irinotecan 120-180 mg/m^2, leucovorin 200 mg/m^2, 5-FU BOL 240-400 mg/m^2, 5-FU infusion 360-600 mg/m^2
Hepatic impairment
• *Adult:* IV 100 mg/m^2 qwk × 4 wk, then 2-wk rest, may repeat cycle or 300 mg/m^2 q3wk, dose may be adjusted up or down
Available forms: Inj 20 mg/ml

SIDE EFFECTS
CNS: Fever, headache, chills, dizziness
CV: Vasodilation
*GI: **Severe diarrhea,** nausea, vomiting, anorexia, constipation, cramps, flatus, stomatitis, dyspepsia, **hepatotoxicity**
*HEMA: **Leukopenia, anemia, neutropenia***

INTEG: Irritation at site, rash, sweating, alopecia
MISC: Edema, asthenia, weight loss
RESP: Dyspnea, increased cough, rhinitis
Contraindications: Pregnancy (D), hypersensitivity
Precautions: Lactation, children, elderly, myelosuppression, irradiation

PHARMACOKINETICS
Rapidly and completely absorbed; excreted in urine and bile as metabolites; half-life 10 hr, bound to plasma proteins 30%-68%

INTERACTIONS
Increase: myelosuppression, diarrhea—other antineoplastics, radiation
Increase: lymphocytopenia—dexamethasone
Increase: akathisia—prochlorperazine
Increase: dehydration—diuretics

NURSING CONSIDERATIONS
Assess:
• For CNS symptoms: fever, headache, chills, dizziness
• CBC, differential, platelet count weekly; withhold drug if WBC is <2000/mm^3, or platelet count <100,000/mm^3, Hgb ≤9 g/dl, neutrophil ≤1000/mm^3; notify prescriber of these results; drug should be discontinued and colony-stimulating factor given
• Buccal cavity q8h for dryness, sores or ulceration, white patches, oral pain, bleeding, dysphagia
⚠ GI symptoms: frequency of stools; cramping; severe life-threatening diarrhea may occur with fluid and electrolyte imbalances
• Signs of dehydration: rapid respirations, poor skin turgor, decreased urine output, dry skin, restlessness, weakness
• Bone marrow depression: bruising, bleeding, blood in stools, urine, sputum, emesis
Administer:
• Antiemetics and dexamethasone 10 mg at least ½ hr before antineoplastics

---

⚠ Safety alert   *"Tall Man" lettering

• After preparing in biologic cabinet using gloves, mask, gown

• Early diarrhea and other cholinergic symptoms can be treated with atropine

• Late diarrhea must be treated promptly with loperimide; late diarrhea can be life-threatening

IV route

• By intermittent inf after diluting with 0.9% NaCl or D_5 (0.12-1.1 mg/ml) give over 1½ hr

• Do not admix with other solutions or medications

• Stable for 24 hr at room temperature; 48 hr, refrigerated

Perform/provide:

• Increased fluid intake to 2-3 L/day to prevent dehydration, unless contraindicated

• Changing of IV site q48h

• Rinsing of mouth tid-qid with water, club soda; brushing of teeth bid-tid with soft brush or cotton-tipped applicator for stomatitis; use unwaxed dental floss

• Nutritious diet with iron, vitamin supplement, low fiber, few dairy products

Evaluate:

• Therapeutic response: decrease in tumor size, decrease in spread of cancer

Teach patient/family:

• To avoid foods with citric acid or hot or rough texture if stomatitis is present; to drink adequate fluids

• To report stomatitis; any bleeding, white spots, ulcerations in mouth; tell patient to examine mouth daily, report symptoms

• To report signs of anemia: fatigue, headache, faintness, shortness of breath, irritability

• To use contraception during therapy

• To avoid salicylates, NSAIDs, alcohol; bleeding may occur

• About alopecia, that when hair grows back, it will be different texture, thickness

• To avoid vaccinations while taking this drug

⚠ To report diarrhea that occurs 24 hr after administration, severe dehydration can occur rapidly

Treatment of overdose: Induce vomiting, provide supportive care, prevent dehydration

---

iron dextran (℞)

DexFerrum, Imferon, InFeD
Func. class.: Hematinic
Chem. class.: Ferric hydroxide complex with dextran

Do not confuse:

Imferon/Imuran
Imferon/Roferon-A

Action: Iron is carried by transferrin to the bone marrow, where it is incorporated into hemoglobin

Uses: Iron deficiency anemia

DOSAGE AND ROUTES

• *Adult and child:* **IM** 0.5 ml as a test dose by Z-track, then no more than the following per day:

• *Adult <50 kg:* **IM** 100 mg

• *Adult >50 kg:* **IM** 250 mg

• *Infant <5 kg:* **IM** 25 mg

• *Child <5-9 kg:* **IM** 50 mg

• *Adult:* **IV** 0.5 ml (25 mg) test dose, then 100 mg daily after 2-3 days; give 25 mg test dose, wait 5 min, then infuse over 6-12 hr or use equation that follows:

$$0.3 \times wt\ (lb) \times \frac{100\text{-Hgb (g/dl)} \times 100}{14.8} = mg\ iron$$

<30 lb (66 kg) should be given 80% of above formula dose

Available forms: Inj 50 mg/ml (2 ml, 10 ml vials)

SIDE EFFECTS

CNS: Headache, paresthesia, dizziness, shivering, weakness, ***seizures***

CV: Chest pain, ***shock,*** hypotension, tachycardia

GI: Nausea, vomiting, metallic taste, abdominal pain

*HEMA: **Leukocytosis***

INTEG: Rash, pruritus, urticaria, fever, sweating, chills, brown skin discolor-

---

ation, pain at inj site, necrosis, sterile abscesses, phlebitis

OTHER: **Anaphylaxis**

RESP: Dyspnea

Contraindications: Hypersensitivity, all anemias excluding iron deficiency anemia, hepatic disease

Precautions: Pregnancy (C), acute renal disease, children, asthma, lactation, rheumatoid arthritis (IV), infants <4 mo

PHARMACOKINETICS

IM: Excreted in feces, urine, bile, breast milk; crosses placenta; most absorbed through lymphatics; can be gradually absorbed over weeks/months from fixed locations

INTERACTIONS

Increase: toxicity—oral iron; do not use

Decrease: reticulocyte response—chloramphenicol

Drug/Lab Test

False increase: Serum bilirubin

False decrease: Serum calcium

False positive: ^{99m}Tc diphosphate bone scan, iron test (large doses >2 ml)

NURSING CONSIDERATIONS

Assess:

• Observe for 1 hr after test dose

• Blood studies: Hct, Hgb, reticulocytes, transferrin, plasma iron concentrations, ferritin, total iron-binding, bilirubin before treatment, at least monthly

• Allergy: anaphylaxis, rash, pruritus, fever, chills, wheezing; notify prescriber immediately, keep emergency equipment available

• Cardiac status: anginal pain, hypotension, tachycardia

• Nutrition: amount of iron in diet (meat, dark green leafy vegetables, dried beans, dried fruits, eggs)

• Cause of iron loss or anemia, including use of salicylates, sulfonamides

• Toxicity: nausea, vomiting, diarrhea, fever, abdominal pain (early symptoms),

cyanotic-looking lips, nailbeds, seizures, CV collapse (late symptoms)

Administer:

• D/C oral iron before parenteral; give only after test dose of 25 mg by preferred route; wait at least 1 hr before giving remaining portion

• IM deeply in large muscle mass; use Z-track method and a 19-20G 2-3-in needle; ensure needle is long enough to place drug deep in muscle, change needles after withdrawing drug and before injecting to prevent skin, tissue staining

A Only with epINEPHrine available in case of anaphylactic reaction during dose

IV route

• IV after flushing with 10 ml 0.9% NaCl; give undiluted; may be diluted in 50-250 ml NS for infusion; give 1 ml (50 mg) or less over 1 min or more; flush line after use with 10 ml 0.9% NaCl; patient should remain recumbent for ½-1 hr

• IV injection requires single-dose vial without preservative; verify on label IV use is approved

Additive compatibilities: Netilmicin

Solution compatibility: TPN #211

Perform/provide:

• Storage at room temperature in cool environment

• Recumbent position 30 min after IV inj to prevent orthostatic hypotension

• Therapeutic response: increased serum iron levels, Hct, Hgb

Teach patient/family:

• That iron poisoning may occur if increased beyond recommended level; not to take oral iron preparation

• That delayed reaction may occur 1-2 days after administration and last 3-4 days (IV), 3-7 days (IM); report fever, chills, malaise, muscle, joint aches, nausea, vomiting, backache

Treatment of overdose: Discontinue drug, treat allergic reaction, give diphenhydramine or epINEPHrine as needed, give iron-chelating drug in acute poisoning

---

iron sucrose (℞)

Venofer
Func. class.: Hematinic
Chem. class.: Ferric hydroxide complex with dextran

Action: Iron is carried by transferrin to the bone marrow, where it is incorporated into hemoglobin
Uses: Iron deficiency anemia
Investigational uses: Dystrophic epidermolysis bullosa (DEB)

DOSAGE AND ROUTES

• *Adult:* **IV** 5 ml (100 mg of elemental iron) given during dialysis, most will need 1000 mg of elemental iron over 10 dialysis sessions
Available forms: Inj 20 mg/ml

SIDE EFFECTS

CNS: Headache, dizziness
CV: Chest pain, hypotension, hypertension, hypervolemia
GI: Nausea, vomiting, abdominal pain
INTEG: Rash, pruritus, urticaria, fever, sweating, chills
*OTHER: **Anaphylaxis***
RESP: Dyspnea, pneumonia, cough
Contraindications: Hypersensitivity, all anemias excluding iron deficiency anemia, iron overload
Precautions: Pregnancy (B), lactation, elderly, children

PHARMACOKINETICS

Excreted in urine, half-life 6 hr

INTERACTIONS

Increase: toxicity—oral iron; do not use

NURSING CONSIDERATIONS

Assess:
• Blood studies: Hct, Hgb, reticulocytes, transferrin, plasma iron concentrations, ferritin, total iron-binding, bilirubin before treatment, at least monthly

• Allergy: anaphylaxis, rash, pruritus, fever, chills, wheezing; notify prescriber immediately, keep emergency equipment available
• Cardiac status: hypotension, hypertension, hypervolemia
• Toxicity: nausea, vomiting, diarrhea, fever, abdominal pain (early symptoms), cyanotic-looking lips, nailbeds, seizures, CV collapse (late symptoms)
Administer:
⚠ Only with epINEPHrine available in case of anaphylactic reaction during dose
IV route
• Give directly in dialysis line by slow inj or inf; give by slow inj at 1 ml/min (5 min/vial); inf dilute each vial exclusively in a maximum of 100 ml of 0.9% NaCl, give at rate of 100 mg of iron/15 min, discard unused portions
Perform/provide:
• Storage at room temperature in cool environment, do not freeze
• Therapeutic response: increased serum iron levels, Hct, Hgb
Teach patient/family:
• That iron poisoning may occur if increased beyond recommended level; not to take oral iron preparation
Treatment of overdose: Discontinue drug, treat allergic reaction, give diphenhydrAMINE or epINEPHrine as needed, give iron-chelating drug in acute poisoning

isoniazid (R)

(eye-soe-nye′a-zid)
INH, isoniazid, Isotamine ✤,
Laniazid, Nydrazid,
PMS-Isoniazid ✤
Func. class.: Antitubercular
Chem. class.: Isonicotinic acid hydrazide

Action: Bactericidal interference with lipid, nucleic acid biosynthesis
Uses: Treatment, prevention of TB

DOSAGE AND ROUTES

Treatment
• *Adult:* **PO/IM** 300 mg/day or 15 mg/kg 2-3 ×/wk, max 900 mg 2-3 ×/wk
• *Child and infant:* **PO/IM** 10-20 mg/kg daily in 1-2 divided doses max 300 mg/day or 20-40 mg/kg, max 900 mg 2-3 ×/wk
Available forms: Tabs 50, 100, 300 mg; inj 100 mg/ml; powder, syr 50 mg/5 ml

SIDE EFFECTS

CNS: Peripheral neuropathy, dizziness, memory impairment, ***toxic encephalopathy, convulsions,*** psychosis, slurred speech
EENT: Blurred vision, optic neuritis
*GI: **Nausea,** vomiting,* epigastric distress, ***jaundice, fatal hepatitis***
*HEMA: **Agranulocytosis, hemolytic, aplastic anemia, thrombocytopenia, eosinophilia, methemoglobinemia***
HyperSENsitivity: Fever, skin eruptions, lymphadenopathy, vasculitis
MISC: Dyspnea, B_6 deficiency, pellagra, hyperglycemia, metabolic acidosis, gynecomastia, rheumatic syndrome, SLE-like syndrome
Contraindications: Hypersensitivity, acute hepatic disease
Precautions: Pregnancy (C), renal disease, diabetic retinopathy, cataracts, ocular defects, hepatic disease, child <13 yr

PHARMACOKINETICS

PO: Peak 1-2 hr, duration 6-8 hr
IM: Peak 45-60 min
Metabolized in liver; excreted in urine (metabolites); crosses placenta; excreted in breast milk

INTERACTIONS

Increase: toxicity—tyramine foods, alcohol, cycloSERINE, ethionamide, rifampin, carbamazepine, warfarin, phenytoin, benzodiazepines, meperidine
Decrease: absorption—aluminum antacids
Decrease: effectiveness of BCG vaccine, ketoconazole
Drug/Food
Do not give with high-tyramine foods

NURSING CONSIDERATIONS

Assess:
• Hepatic studies qwk: ALT, AST, bilirubin; increased test results may indicate hepatitis
• Mental status often: affect, mood, behavioral changes; psychosis may occur
• Hepatic status: decreased appetite, jaundice, dark urine, fatigue
• For paresthesia in hands, feet
Administer:
• PO with meals to decrease GI symptoms; better to take on empty stomach 1 hr ac or 2 hr pc
• Antiemetic if vomiting occurs
• After C&S is completed; qmo to detect resistance
• IM deep in large muscle mass, massage, rotate inj site, warm inj to room temperature to dissolve crystals
Evaluate:
• Therapeutic response: decreased symptoms of TB
Teach patient/family:
• That compliance with dosage schedule, duration is necessary, not to skip or double dose
• That scheduled appointments must be kept or relapse may occur
🅐 To avoid alcohol while taking drug, may increase risk of hepatic injury

• That if diabetic, use blood glucose monitor to obtain correct result

⚠ To report weakness, fatigue, loss of appetite, nausea, vomiting, jaundice of skin or eyes, tingling/numbness of hands/feet

Treatment of overdose: Pyridoxine

Rarely Used

isoproterenol (R)
(eye-soe-proe-ter′e-nole)
Aerolone, Dispos-a-
Medisoproterenol HCl,
Isoproterenol HCl, Isuprel,
Isuprel Glossets, Isuprel
Mistometer, Medihaler-Iso,
Vapo-Iso
Func. class.: β-Adrenergic agonist

Uses: Bronchospasm, asthma, heart block, ventricular dysrhythmias, shock

DOSAGE AND ROUTES
Asthma, bronchospasm
• *Adult:* **SL** 10-20 mg q6-8h, max 60 mg/day; **INH** 1 puff, may repeat in 2-5 min, maintenance 1-2 puffs 4-6 ×/day; **IV** 10-20 mcg during anesthesia
• *Child:* **SL** 5-10 mg q6-8h; **INH** 1 puff, may repeat in 2-5 min, maintenance 1-2 puffs 4-6 ×/day
Shock
• *Adult:* **IV INF** 0.5-5 mcg/min 1 mg/ 500 ml D₅W, titrate to B/P, CVP, hourly urine output

Contraindications: Hypersensitivity to sympathomimetics, narrow-angle glaucoma, tachydysrhythmias

isosorbide dinitrate (R)
(eye-soe-sor′bide)
Apo-ISDN ♣, Cedocard-SR ♣,
Coronex ♣, Dilatrate-SR,
ISDN, Iso-Bid, Isonate,
Isorbid, Isordil, Isosorbide
dinitrate, Isotrate,
Novasorbide ♣, Sorbitrate
**isosorbide
mononitrate**
(eye-soe-sor′bide) Imdur,
ISMO, Isotrate ER,
Monoket
Func. class.: Antianginal, vasodilator
Chem. class.: Nitrate

Do not confuse:
Monoket/Monopril
Imdur/Imuran/Inderal/K-Dur
Action: Relaxation of vascular smooth muscle which leads to decreases pre-load, after-load, which is responsible for decreasing left ventricular end-diastolic pressure, systemic vascular resistance and reducing cardiac O_2 demand
Uses: Treatment, prevention of chronic stable angina pectoris

DOSAGE AND ROUTES
Dinitrate
• *Adult:* **PO** 5-40 mg qid; **SL,** buccal 2.5-5 mg, may repeat q5-10 min × 3 doses; **CHEW TAB** 5-10 mg prn or q2-3h as prophylaxis; **SUS REL** 40-80 mg q8-12h
Mononitrate
• *Adult:* **PO** ISMO, Monoket: 10-20 mg bid, 7 hr apart; Imdur: initiate at 30-60 mg/day as a single dose, increase q3d as needed, may increase to 120 mg daily, max 240 mg/day
Available forms:
Dinitrate: Caps sus rel (SR) 40 mg; tabs 5, 10, 20, 30, 40 mg; SL tabs 2.5, 5, 10 mg; chew tabs 5, 10 mg
Mononitrate: Tabs 10, 20 mg (ISMO, Monoket); ext rel (Imdur, ER) 30, 60, 120 mg

SIDE EFFECTS

CNS: Vascular headache, flushing, dizziness, weakness, faintness
CV: Postural hypotension, tachycardia, *collapse,* syncope, palpitations
GI: Nausea, vomiting, diarrhea
INTEG: Pallor, sweating, rash
MISC: Twitching, hemolytic anemia, *methemoglobinemia*

Contraindications: Hypersensitivity to this drug or nitrates, severe anemia, increased intracranial pressure, cerebral hemorrhage, acute MI

Precautions: Pregnancy (C), postural hypotension, lactation, children, MI, CHF, severe renal, hepatic disease

PHARMACOKINETICS

Mononitrate
SUS REL: Duration 6-8 hr
Dinitrate
PO: Onset 15-30 min, duration 4-6 hr
SUS REL: Onset up to 4 hr, duration 6-8 hr
SL: Onset 2-5 min, duration 1-4 hr
CHEW TAB: Onset 3 min, duration ½-3 hr
Metabolized by liver, excreted in urine as metabolites (80%-100%)

INTERACTIONS

⚠ Fatal hypotension: sildenafil, tadalafil, vardenafil
Increase: hypotension—β-blockers, diuretics, antihypertensives, alcohol, calcium channel blockers, phenothiazines
Drug/Herb
Decrease: antianginal effect—blue cohosh

NURSING CONSIDERATIONS

Assess:
• Pain: duration, time started, activity being performed, character
• B/P, pulse, respirations during beginning therapy
• Tolerance if taken over long period

• Headache, light-headedness, decreased B/P; may indicate a need for decreased dosage
Administer:
• Do not break, crush, or chew sus rel caps, SL tabs
• After checking expiration date
• PO with 8 oz H_2O on empty stomach
• SL tabs should be placed under the tongue until dissolved
Evaluate:
• Therapeutic response: decrease or prevention of anginal pain
Teach patient/family:
• To leave tabs in original container
• To avoid alcohol products
• That drug may cause headache, but tolerance usually develops; taking with meals may reduce or eliminate headache
• That drug may be taken before stressful activity (exercise, sexual activity)
• That SL may sting when drug comes in contact with mucous membranes
• To avoid hazardous activities if dizziness occurs
• The importance of complying with complete medical regimen
• To make position changes slowly to prevent orthostatic hypotension

Rarely Used

isotretinoin (℞)
(eye-soe-tret′i-noyn)
Func. class.: Antiacne agent

Uses: Severe recalcitrant cystic acne

DOSAGE AND ROUTES

• *Adult:* **PO** 0.5-2 mg/kg/day in 2 divided doses × 15-20 wk; if relapse occurs, repeat after 2 mo off drug
Contraindications: Pregnancy (X), hypersensitivity, inflamed skin

isradipine (℞)

(is-ra'di-peen)

DynaCirc, DynaCirc CR

Func. class.: Antihypertensive, anti-anginal (calcium channel blocker)

Chem. class.: Dihydropyridine

Do not confuse:

DynaCirc/Dynabac/Dynacin

Action: Inhibits calcium ion influx across cell membrane during cardiac depolarization; produces relaxation of coronary vascular smooth muscle, peripheral vascular smooth muscle; dilates coronary vascular arteries

Uses: Essential hypertension, angina pectoris, vasospastic angina

DOSAGE AND ROUTES

• *Adult:* **PO** 2.5 mg bid; increase at 2-4 wk intervals up to 10 mg bid or 5 mg daily; **CONT REL** may be increased q2-4wk, max 20 mg/day

Available forms: Caps 2.5, 5 mg, cont rel tabs (CR) 5, 10 mg

SIDE EFFECTS

CNS: Headache, fatigue, dizziness, fainting, sleep disturbances, weakness, depression, drowsiness

CV: Peripheral edema, tachycardia, hypotension, chest pain, ***dysrhythmias,*** syncope

GI: Nausea, vomiting, diarrhea, gastric upset, constipation, ***hepatitis,*** abdominal pain, distention, dry mouth

GU: Nocturia, urinary frequency

HEMA: ***Leukopenia***

INTEG: Rash, pruritus, urticaria

MISC: Flushing

Contraindications: Sick sinus syndrome, 2nd- or 3rd-degree heart block, hypotension less than 90 mm Hg systolic, hypersensitivity

Precautions: Pregnancy (C), CHF, hypotension, hepatic disease, lactation, children, renal disease, elderly

PHARMACOKINETICS

Metabolized in liver; metabolites excreted in urine, feces; secreted in breast milk, peak plasma levels at 1.5 hr immediate rel, 7-18 hr cont rel

INTERACTIONS

Additive/synergistic effect: β-blockers

Bradycardia, conduction defects: disopyramide

Increase: hypotension—nitrates, fentanyl, other antihypertensives

Increase: serum conc of isradipine—cimetidine, ranitidine

Decrease: serum conc of isradipine—rifampin

Decrease: conc—fluvastatin, lovastatin

Drug/Herb

Increase: toxicity, death—aconite

Increase: antihypertensive effect—barberry, betony, black catechu, black cohosh, bloodroot, broom, burdock, cat's claw, dandelion, goldenseal, Irish moss, Jamaican dogwood, kelp, khella, mistletoe, parsley

Increase or decrease: antihypertensive effect—astragalus, cola tree

Decrease: antihypertensive effect—coltsfoot, guarana, khat, licorice

NURSING CONSIDERATIONS

Assess:

• I&O ratio, daily weight, watch for CHF: edema, dyspnea, weight gain, crackles, jugular vein distention

• Renal, hepatic studies, electrolytes prior to and during treatment

• Cardiac status: B/P, pulse, respiration, ECG; assess anginal pain, precipitating, ameliorating factors

Administer:

• Do not break, crush, or chew cont rel tabs

• Without regard to meals

Evaluate:

• Therapeutic response: decreased anginal pain, decreased B/P

Teach patient/family:

• To avoid hazardous activities until

stabilized on drug, dizziness is no longer a problem
- To limit caffeine consumption
- To avoid OTC drugs unless directed by prescriber
- The importance of compliance in all areas of regimen: diet, exercise, stress reduction, drug therapy
- To notify prescriber of irregular heartbeat, shortness of breath, swelling of feet and hands, pronounced dizziness, constipation, nausea, hypotension

Treatment of overdose: Defibrillation, β-agonists, IV calcium inotropic agents, diuretics, atropine for AV block, vasopressor for hypotension

---

itraconazole (R)
(it-ra-con′a-zol)
Sporanox
Func. class.: Antifungal, systemic
Chem. class.: Triazole derivative

Action: Alters cell membranes and inhibits several fungal enzymes
Uses: Systemic candidiasis, chronic mucocandidiasis, oral thrush, candiduria, histoplasmosis, chromomycosis, para-coccidioidomycosis, blastomycosis (pulmonary and extrapulmonary), aspergillosis onychomycosis
Investigational uses: Dermatomycosis, chromoblastomycosis, coccidioidomycosis, pityriasis versicolor, sebopsoriasis, vaginal candidiasis, cryptococcus, subcutaneous mycoses, dimorphic infections, leishmaniasis, fungal keratitis, alternariosis, zygomycosis

DOSAGE AND ROUTES

Dose varies with type of infection
- *Adult:* **PO** 200 mg daily with food; may increase to 400 mg daily if needed; life-threatening infections may require a loading dose of 200 mg tid × 3 days; **IV** 200 mg bid × 4 doses, then 200 mg daily, give each dose over 1 hr; maintenance **PO** 200-400 mg/day
- *Child:* **PO** 3-5 mg/kg/day

Available forms: Caps 100 mg; oral sol 10 mg/ml; inj 10 mg/ml

SIDE EFFECTS

CNS: Headache, dizziness, insomnia, somnolence, depression
CV: Hypertension
GI: Nausea, vomiting, anorexia, diarrhea, cramps, abdominal pain, flatulence, *GI bleeding, hepatotoxicity*
GU: Gynecomastia, impotence, decreased libido
INTEG: Pruritus, fever, *rash, toxic epidermal necrolysis*
MISC: Edema, fatigue, malaise, hypokalemia, tinnitus, *rhabdomyolysis*
Contraindications: Hypersensitivity, fungal meningitis, onychomycosis or dermatomycosis in cardiac dysfunction
Precautions: Pregnancy (C), hepatic disease, cardiac disease, achlorhydria or hypochlorhydria (drug-induced), children, lactation

PHARMACOKINETICS

PO: Peak 3-5 hr, half-life 21 hr; metabolized in liver; excreted in bile, feces; requires acid pH for absorption; distributed poorly to CSF; highly protein bound; inhibits CYP4503A4

INTERACTIONS

Tinnitus, hearing loss: quinidine
Hepatotoxicity: other hepatotoxic drugs
Edema: calcium channel blockers
Severe hypoglycemia: oral hypoglycemics
⚠ Life-threatening CV reactions: pimozide, quinidine, dofetilide
Increase: sedation—triazolam, oral midazolam
Increase: levels, toxicity—busPIRone, busulfan, clarithromycin, cycloSPORINE, diazepam, digoxin, felodipine, indinavir, isradipine, niCARdipine, niFEDipine, nimodipine, phenytoin, quinidine, ritonavir, saquinavir, tacrolimus, warfarin
Decrease: effect of oral contraceptives

⚠ Safety alert   *"Tall Man" lettering

Decrease: itraconazole action—antacids, H$_2$-receptor antagonists, rifamycins, didanosine

Drug/Herb

Nephrotoxicity: gossypol

Drug/Food

Food increases absorption

NURSING CONSIDERATIONS

Assess:

• For type of infection, may begin treatment prior to obtaining results

• For infection: temp, WBC, sputum, baseline and periodically

• I&O ratio, potassium levels

• Hepatic studies (ALT, AST, bilirubin) if on long-term therapy

• For allergic reaction: rash, photosensitivity, urticaria, dermatitis

⚠ For hepatotoxicity: nausea, vomiting, jaundice, clay-colored stools, fatigue

Administer:

• In the presence of acid products only; do not use alkaline products or antacids within 2 hr of drug; may give coffee, tea, acidic fruit juices

PO route

• Swallow caps whole; do not break, crush, or chew caps

• Do not use oral sol, caps interchangeably

• Oral sol: patient should swish in mouth vigorously, use on empty stomach

• Give caps after full meal to ensure absorption

• Oral sol and caps are not interchangeable on an mg/mg basis

IV route

• After adding full contents 25-50 ml bag of 0.9% NaCl mix, use infusion pump, give at a rate of 1 ml/min, flush line with 0.9% NaCl after infusion; do not use by bolus

Perform/provide:

• Storage in tight container at room temperature, do not freeze

Evaluate:

• Therapeutic response: decreased fever, malaise, rash, negative C&S for infecting organism

Teach patient/family:

• That long-term therapy may be needed to clear infection (1 wk-6 mo depending on infection)

• To avoid hazardous activities if dizziness occurs

• To take 2 hr ac administration of other drugs that increase gastric pH (antacids, H$_2$-blockers, omeprazole, sucralfate, anticholinergics); to notify health care provider of all medications taken; to take after a full meal (caps), on empty stomach (oral sol)

• The importance of compliance with drug regimen, to use alternative method of contraceptive

• To notify prescriber of GI symptoms, signs of hepatic dysfunction (fatigue, nausea, anorexia, vomiting, dark urine, pale stools)

K

Rarely Used

kanamycin (℞)
(kan-a-mye′sin)
kanamycin sulfate, Kantrex
Func. class.: Antiinfective

Uses: Severe systemic infections of CNS; respiratory, GI, urinary tract; bone, skin, soft tissues caused by *Escherichia coli, Acinetobacter, Proteus, Klebsiella pneumoniae, Pseudomonas aeruginosa;* also used as adjunct in hepatic coma, peritonitis, preoperatively to sterilize bowel; decreases ammonia-producing bacteria in bowel and intraperitoneally after fecal spill during surgery

DOSAGE AND ROUTES

Severe systemic infections

• *Adult and child:* **IV INF** 15 mg/kg/day in divided doses q8-12h; diluted 500 mg/200 ml of NS or D$_5$W given over 30-60 min, not to exceed 1.5 g/day; **IM** 15 mg/kg/day in divided doses q8-12h, not to exceed 1.5 g/day, irrigation not to exceed 1.5 g/day; **INH** 250 mg qid

Preoperative bowel sterilization
• *Adult:* **PO** 1 g qh × 4 doses, then q6h × 36-72 hr
Renal dose
• *Adult:* **IM/IV** 7.5 mg/kg, may increase or decrease dose based on renal status
Contraindications: Pregnancy (D), bowel obstruction, severe renal disease, hypersensitivity

---

ketoconazole (℞)
(kee-toe-koe′na-zole)
Nizoral
Func. class.: Antifungal
Chem. class.: Imidazole derivative

Do not confuse:
Nizoral/ Nasarel/Neoral
Action: Alters cell membrane permeability and inhibits several fungal enzymes leading to cell death
Uses: Systemic candidiasis, chronic mucocandidiasis, oral thrush, candiduria, coccidioidomycosis, histoplasmosis, chromomycosis, para-coccidioidomycosis, blastomycosis; tinea cruris, tinea corporis, tinea versicolor, *Pityrosporum ovale*
Investigational uses: Cushing's syndrome, advanced prostatic cancer

DOSAGE AND ROUTES

• *Adult:* **PO** 200-400 mg daily for 1-2 wk (candidiasis), 6 wk (other infections); 400 mg tid (prostate cancer—unlabeled)
• *Child >2 yr:* **PO:** 3.3-6.6 mg/kg/day as single daily dose
Available forms: Tabs 200 mg; oral susp 100 mg/5 ml ✤

SIDE EFFECTS

CNS: Headache, dizziness, somnolence
GI: Nausea, vomiting, anorexia, diarrhea, abdominal pain, ***hepatotoxicity***
GU: Gynecomastia, impotence
HEMA: ***Thrombocytopenia, leukopenia, hemolytic anemia***

INTEG: Pruritus, fever, chills, photophobia, rash, dermatitis, purpura, urticaria
SYST: **Anaphylaxis**
Contraindications: Hypersensitivity, lactation, fungal meningitis; coadministration with terfenadine or drugs that prolong QTc interval
Precautions: Pregnancy (C), renal disease, hepatic disease, achlorhydria (drug-induced), children <2 yr, other hepatotoxic agents including terfenadine, other drugs metabolized by CYP450

PHARMACOKINETICS

PO: Peak 1-2 hr, half-life 2 hr, terminal 8 hr; metabolized in liver; excreted in bile, feces; requires acid pH for absorption; distributed poorly to CSF; highly protein bound

INTERACTIONS

Ketoconazole may decrease theophylline effect
Hepatotoxicity: other hepatotoxic drugs, alcohol
Inhibition of CYP 4503A4 pathway, toxicity: alfentanil, alprazolam, amprenavir, atorvastatin, calcium channel blockers, carbamazepine, cerivastatin, clarithromycin, corticosteroids, cyclophosphamide, cycloSPORINE, donepezil, erythromycin, fentanyl, ifosfamide, indinavir, lovastatin, midazolam, nelfinavir, nisoldipine, quinidine, ritonavir, saquinavir, sildenafil, simvastatin, sufentanil, tamoxifen, triazolam, vinBLAStine, vinca alkaloids, vinCRIStine, zolpidem
Inhibited metabolism: paclitaxel
Increase: anticoagulant effect—warfarin, anticoagulants
Decrease: action of ketoconazole—antacids, H_2-receptor antagonists, anticholinergics, phenytoin, isoniazid, rifampin, ddI, gastric acid pump inhibitors
Decrease: effect of oral contraceptives
Drug/Herb
Nephrotoxicity: gossypol
Decrease: ketoconazole action—yew

NURSING CONSIDERATIONS

Assess:

• For infection symptoms before and after treatment

• Hepatic studies (ALT, AST, bilirubin) if on long-term therapy

• For allergic reaction: rash, photosensitivity, urticaria, dermatitis

⚠ For hepatotoxicity: nausea, vomiting, jaundice, clay-colored stools, fatigue

Administer:

• In the presence of acid products only; do not use alkaline products, proton pump inhibitors, H₂-antagonists, antacids within 2 hr of drug; may give coffee, tea, acidic fruit juices, cola

• With food to decrease GI symptoms

• With HCl if achlorhydria is present; dissolve tab/4 ml of aqueous sol 0.2 N hydrochloric acid, use straw to avoid contact, rinse with water afterward and swallow

Perform/provide:

• Storage in tight container at room temperature

Evaluate:

• Therapeutic response: decreased fever, malaise, rash, negative C&S for infecting organism, absence of scaling

Teach patient/family:

• That long-term therapy may be needed to clear infection (1 wk-6 mo depending on infection)

• To avoid hazardous activities if dizziness occurs

• To take 2 hr ac administration of other drugs that increase gastric pH (antacids, H₂-blockers, omeprazole, sucralfate, anticholinergics)

• The importance of compliance with drug regimen

⚠ To notify prescriber of GI symptoms, signs of hepatic dysfunction (fatigue, nausea, anorexia, vomiting, dark urine, pale stools)

• Use sunglasses to prevent photophobia

• To use alternative method of contraception while taking this drug

---

ketoconazole topical
See Appendix C

---

ketoprofen (otc, ℞)

(ke-toe-proe'fen)

Actron, Apo-Keto ✦, Apo-Keto-E ✦, ketoprofen, Orudis, Orudis-E ✦, Orudis-KT, Orudis-SR ✦, Oruvail, Rhodis ✦

Func. class.: Nonsteroidal antiinflammatory (NSAID), antirheumatic

Chem. class.: Propionic acid derivative

Do not confuse:

Oruvail/Clinoril

Oruvail/Elavil

Action: Inhibits prostaglandin synthesis by decreasing enzyme needed for biosynthesis; analgesic, antiinflammatory, antipyretic

Uses: Mild to moderate pain, osteoarthritis, rheumatoid arthritis, dysmenorrhea

DOSAGE AND ROUTES

Antiinflammatory

• *Adult:* **PO** 150-300 mg in divided doses tid-qid, not to exceed 300 mg/day or **EXT REL** 150-200 mg daily

Analgesic

• *Adult:* **PO** 25-50 mg q6-8h

Available forms: Caps 25, 50, 75 mg; ext rel cap 100, 150, 200 mg; tabs 12.5 mg

SIDE EFFECTS

CNS: Dizziness, drowsiness, fatigue, tremors, confusion, insomnia, anxiety, depression, headache

CV: Tachycardia, peripheral edema, palpitations, dysrhythmias, hypertension

EENT: Tinnitus, hearing loss, blurred vision

GI: Nausea, anorexia, vomiting, diarrhea, jaundice, **hepatitis**, constipation,

---

flatulence, cramps, dry mouth, peptic ulcer, *GI bleeding*
*GU: **Nephrotoxicity: dysuria, hematuria, oliguria, azotemia***
*HEMA: **Blood dyscrasias***
INTEG: Purpura, rash, pruritus, sweating
*SYST: **Anaphylaxis***

Contraindications: Avoid in 2nd/3rd trimester, hypersensitivity, asthma, severe renal disease, severe hepatic disease, ulcer disease

Precautions: Pregnancy (B) 1st trimester, lactation, children, bleeding disorders, GI disorders, cardiac disorders, hypersensitivity to other antiinflammatory agents, elderly

PHARMACOKINETICS

PO: Peak 2 hr, half-life 2-4 hr; metabolized in liver; excreted in urine (metabolites); excreted in breast milk; 99% plasma protein binding

INTERACTIONS

Increase: hypoglycemia—insulin, sulfonylureas
Increase: toxicity—cycloSPORINE, lithium, methotrexate, phenytoin, alcohol
Increase: bleeding risk—cefamandole, cefoperazone, cefotetan, clopidogrel, eptifibatide, plicamycin, thrombolytics, ticlopidine, tirofiban, valproic acid, warfarin
Increase: ketoprofen levels—aspirin, probenecid
Increase: adverse GI reactions—aspirin, corticosteroids, NSAIDs, alcohol
Increase: hematologic toxicity—radiation
Decrease: effect of diuretics, antihypertensives

Drug/Herb
Increase: bleeding risk—anise, arnica, bogbean, chondroitin chamomile, clove, dong quai, feverfew, garlic, ginger, ginkgo, ginseng *(Panax)*
Increase: gastric irritation—arginine, gossypol
Increase: NSAIDs effect—bearberry, bilberry

Drug/Lab Test
Increase: Potassium, BUN, alk phosphatase, AST, ALT, LDH, creatinine, bleeding time
Decrease: Blood glucose, HCT, Hgb, platelets, CCr, leukocyte
Interference: Urine albumin, 17 KS, 17-hydroxycorticosteroid, bilirubin

NURSING CONSIDERATIONS

Assess:
• For pain: type, location, intensity, ROM before and 1-2 hr after treatment
• Renal, hepatic, blood studies: BUN, creatinine, AST, ALT, Hgb, before treatment, periodically thereafter
A For aspirin sensitivity, asthma; these patients may be more likely to develop hypersensitivity to NSAIDs
• Audiometric, ophthalmic exam before, during, after treatment
• For eye, ear problems: blurred vision, tinnitus; may indicate toxicity
• For GI bleeding: blood in sputum, emesis, stools

Administer:
• Do not break, crush, or chew ext rel caps
• With food to decrease GI symptoms; however, taking on empty stomach best facilitates absorption

Perform/provide:
• Storage at room temperature

Evaluate:
• Therapeutic response: decreased pain, stiffness in joints, decreased swelling in joints, ability to move more easily; decreased fever

Teach patient/family:
• To report blurred vision, ringing, roaring in ears; may indicate toxicity
• To avoid driving, other hazardous activities if dizziness, drowsiness occurs, especially elderly
• To report change in urine pattern, increased weight, edema, increased pain in joints, fever, blood in urine; indicate nephrotoxicity; rash, itching, blurred vision, ringing in the ears, flulike symptoms
• That therapeutic effects may take up to

1 mo, to take with 8 oz of water and sit upright for ½ hr after administration to prevent GI irritation
• To avoid aspirin, alcohol, steroids, acetaminophen or other medications, supplements unless approved by prescriber
• To wear sunscreen to prevent photosensitivity

---

ketorolac (R)

(kee-toe'role-ak)

Acular, Toradol

Func. class.: Nonsteroidal antiinflammatory/nonopioid analgesic

Chem. class.: Acetic acid

Do not confuse:

Toradol/Tegretol/Foradil/Toradol/
Inderal

Toradol/Torecan/Toradol/tramadol

Action: Inhibits prostaglandin synthesis by decreasing an enzyme needed for biosynthesis; analgesic, antiinflammatory, antipyretic effects

Uses: Mild to moderate pain; seasonal allergic conjunctivitis (ophth)

DOSAGE AND ROUTES

• *Adult <65 yr:* **PO** 20 mg then 10 mg q4-6h prn, max 40 mg/day
• *Adult >65 yr, renal disease, <50 kg:* **PO** 10 mg q4-6h prn, max 40 mg/day
• *Adult <65 yr:* **IM** (single dose) 60 mg **IV** 30 mg; **IM** (multiple dosing) 15 mg q6h, max 60 mg/day × 5 day combined either **PO/IM/IV**
• *Adult >65 yr, renal disease, <50 kg:* **IM** single dose 30 mg; **IV** 15 mg **IM/IV** (multiple dosing) 15 mg q6h, max 60 mg/day × 5 days combined either **PO/IM/IV**

Available forms: Inj 15, 30 mg/ml (prefilled syringes); ophth 0.5% sol; tab 10 mg

SIDE EFFECTS

CNS: Dizziness, *drowsiness,* tremors
CV: Hypertension, flushing, syncope, pallor, edema, vasodilation

EENT: Tinnitus, hearing loss, blurred vision
GI: Nausea, anorexia, vomiting, diarrhea, constipation, flatulence, cramps, dry mouth, peptic ulcer, ***GI bleeding, perforation,*** taste change
GU: ***Nephrotoxicity: dysuria, hematuria, oliguria, azotemia***
HEMA: ***Blood dyscrasias,*** prolonged bleeding
INTEG: Purpura, rash, pruritus, sweating
Contraindications: Hypersensitivity, asthma, severe renal disease, severe hepatic disease, peptic ulcer disease, L&D, lactation, CV bleeding
Precautions: Pregnancy (C), children, bleeding disorders, GI disorders, cardiac disorders, hypersensitivity to other antiinflammatory agents, elderly, CCr <25 ml/min

PHARMACOKINETICS

PO: Peak 2-3 hr, duration 4-6 hr
IM: Peak 50 min, half-life 6 hr, enters breast milk, <50% metabolized by liver, excreted by kidneys

INTERACTIONS

Increase: toxicity—methotrexate, lithium, cycloSPORINE
Increase: bleeding risk—anticoagulants, cefamandole, cefoperazone, cefotetan, clopidogrel, eptifibatide, plicamycin, salicylates, ticlopidine, tirofiban, thrombolytics, valproic acid
Increase: renal impairment—ACE inhibitors
Increase: ketorolac levels—aspirin, probenecid
Increase: GI effects—steroids, alcohol, aspirin, NSAIDs, potassium products
Decrease: effects—antihypertensives, diuretics
Drug/Herb
Increase: gastric irritation—arginine, gossypol
Increase: NSAIDs effect—bearberry, bilberry
Increase: bleeding risk—anise, arnica, bogbean, chamomile, chondroitin, clove,

K

---

dong quai, feverfew, garlic, ginger, ginkgo, ginseng *(Panax)*

Drug/Lab Test

Increase: Hepatic studies, bleeding time, BUN, creatinine, potassium

NURSING CONSIDERATIONS

Assess:

• Patients with aspirin sensitivity, asthma; may be more likely to develop hypersensitivity to NSAIDs, monitor for hypersensitivity

• For pain: type, location, intensity, ROM before and 1 hr after treatment

• Eyes: redness, swelling, tearing, itching (ophthalmic)

• Renal, hepatic, blood studies: BUN, creatinine, AST, ALT, Hgb before treatment, periodically thereafter; check for dehydration

• Bleeding times; check for bruising, bleeding; test for occult blood in urine

• For eye, ear problems: blurred vision, tinnitus (may indicate toxicity)

⚠ Hepatic dysfunction: jaundice, yellow sclera and skin, clay-colored stools

• Audiometric, ophthalmic exam before, during, after treatment

• GI bleeding: blood in sputum, emesis, stools

Administer:

• IM/IV for 5 days or less; continue therapy with PO

IV route

• Give undiluted over ≥15 sec

Solution compatibility: D_5W, 0.9% NaCl, LR, D_5, plasmalate

Syringe compatibilities: Sufentanil

Y-site compatibilities: Cisatracurium, remifentanil, sufentanil

Perform/provide:

• Storage at room temperature

Evaluate:

• Therapeutic response: decreased pain, stiffness, swelling in joints, ability to move more easily; decreased ocular itching (ophth)

Teach patient/family:

• To report blurred vision or ringing, roaring in ears (may indicate toxicity)

• To avoid driving, other hazardous activities if dizziness or drowsiness occurs

• To report change in urine pattern, weight increase, edema, pain increase in joints, fever, blood in urine (indicates nephrotoxicity)

• To avoid alcohol, salicylates, other NSAIDs, acetaminophen

• This drug may cause redness, burning if soft contact lenses are worn (ophth)

---

ketorolac ophthalmic
See Appendix C

---

ketotifen ophthalmic
See Appendix C

---

labetalol (℞)
(la-bet′a-lole)
Normodyne, Trandate
Func. class.: Antihypertensive, antianginal
Chem. class.: α/β-Blocker

Do not confuse:
Trandate/Tridrate

Action: Produces decreases in B/P without reflex tachycardia or significant reduction in heart rate through mixture of α-blocking, β-blocking effects; elevated plasma renins are reduced

Uses: Mild to moderate hypertension; treatment of severe hypertension (IV)

Investigational uses: Hypertension in patients with pheochromocytoma, hypertension in clonidine withdrawal

DOSAGE AND ROUTES

Hypertension

• *Adult:* **PO** 100 mg bid; may be given with a diuretic; may increase to 200 mg bid after 2 days; may continue to increase q1-3d; max 2400 mg/day in divided doses

---

Hypertensive crisis
• *Adult:* **IV INF** 200 mg/160 ml D$_5$W, run at 2 ml/min; stop inf at desired response, repeat q6-8h as needed; **IV BOL** 20 mg over 2 min, may repeat 40-80 mg q10min, not to exceed 300 mg

Available forms: Tabs 100, 200, 300 mg; inj 5 mg/ml in 20 ml amps

SIDE EFFECTS

CNS: Dizziness, mental changes, drowsiness, fatigue, headache, catatonia, depression, anxiety, nightmares, paresthesias, lethargy

CV: Orthostatic hypotension, bradycardia, CHF, chest pain, *ventricular dysrhythmias,* AV block, scalp tingling

EENT: Tinnitus, visual changes, sore throat, double vision, dry, burning eyes

GI: Nausea, vomiting, diarrhea, dyspepsia, taste distortion

GU: Impotence, dysuria, ejaculatory failure

HEMA: Agranulocytosis, thrombocytopenia, purpura (rare)

INTEG: Rash, alopecia, urticaria, pruritus, fever

RESP: Bronchospasm, dyspnea, wheezing

Contraindications: Hypersensitivity to β-blockers, cardiogenic shock, heart block (2nd or 3rd degree), sinus bradycardia, CHF, bronchial asthma

Precautions: Pregnancy (C), major surgery, lactation, diabetes mellitus, renal disease, thyroid disease, COPD, well-compensated heart failure, CAD, nonallergic bronchospasm, elderly, hepatic disease

PHARMACOKINETICS

PO: Onset ½-2 hr, peak 2-4 hr, duration 8-12 hr

IV: Onset 5 min, peak 15 min, duration 2-4 hr

Half-life 6-8 hr; metabolized by liver (metabolites inactive); excreted in urine; crosses placenta; excreted in breast milk

INTERACTIONS

Do not use within 2 wk of MAOIs

Myocardial depression: hydantoins, general anesthetics, verapamil

Increase: hypotension—diuretics, other antihypertensives, cimetidine, nitroglycerin, alcohol

Decrease: effects—sympathomimetics, lidocaine, indomethacin, theophylline, β-blockers, bronchodilators, xanthines

Decrease: labetolol effect—glutethimide

Drug/Herb

Increase: toxicity, death—aconite

Increase: antihypertensive effect—barberry, betony, black catechu, black cohosh, bloodroot, broom, burdock, cat's claw, dandelion, goldenseal, Irish moss, Jamaican dogwood, kelp, khella, mistletoe, parsley

Increase or decrease: antihypertensive effect—astragalus, cola tree

Decrease: antihypertensive effect—coltsfoot, guarana, khat, licorice

Drug/Lab Test

Increase: ANA titer, blood glucose, alk phosphatase, LDH, AST, ALT, BUN, potassium, triglyceride, uric acid

False increase: Urinary catecholamines

NURSING CONSIDERATIONS

Assess:

⚠ I&O, weight daily; fluid overload: weight gain, jugular venous distention, edema, crackles in lungs

• B/P during beginning treatment, periodically thereafter, pulse q4hr; note rate, rhythm, quality

• Apical/radial pulse before administration; notify prescriber of any significant changes

• Baselines in renal, hepatic studies before therapy begins

• Edema in feet, legs daily

• Skin turgor, dryness of mucous membranes for hydration status

Administer:

• PO ac, at bedtime; tab may be crushed or swallowed whole, give with meals to increase absorption

• Reduced dosage in renal dysfunction
IV route
• Undiluted or diluted in LR, D_5W, D_5 in 0.2%, 0.9%, 0.33% NaCl or Ringer's inj, give undiluted 20 mg or less/2 min; inf is titrated to patient response; 200 mg of drug/160 ml sol = 1 mg/ml; 300 mg of drug/240 ml sol = 1 mg/ml; 200 mg of drug/250 ml sol = 2 mg/3 ml; use infusion pump
• Keeping patient recumbent during and for 3 hr after administration, monitor VS q5-15min
Solution compatibilities: D_5R, D_5LR, $D_{2½}/0.45\%$ NaCl, $D_5/0.2\%$ NaCl, $D_5/0.33\%$ NaCl, $D_50.9\%$ NaCl, D_5W, Ringer's, LR
Y-site compatibilities: Amikacin, aminophylline, amiodarone, ampicillin, butorphanol, calcium gluconate, cefazolin, ceftazidime, ceftizoxime, chloramphenicol, cimetidine, clindamycin, diltiazem, DOBUTamine, DOPamine, enalaprilat, epINEPHrine, erythromycin, esmolol, famotidine, fentanyl, gentamicin, hydromorphone, lidocaine, lorazepam, magnesium sulfate, meperidine, metronidazole, midazolam, milrinone, morphine, niCARdipine, nitroglycerin, norepinephrine, nitroprusside, oxacillin, penicillin G potassium, piperacillin, potassium chloride, potassium phosphate, propofol, ranitidine, sodium acetate, tobramycin, trimethoprim-sulfamethoxazole, vancomycin, vecuronium
Perform/provide:
• Storage in dry area at room temperature; do not freeze
Evaluate:
• Therapeutic response: decreased B/P after 1-2 wk
Teach patient/family:
• Not to discontinue drug abruptly; taper over 2 wk; may cause precipitate angina
• Not to use OTC products containing α-adrenergic stimulants (nasal decongestants, OTC cold preparations) unless directed by prescriber
• To report bradycardia, dizziness, confusion, depression, fever

• To take pulse at home, advise when to notify prescriber
• To avoid alcohol, smoking, sodium intake
• To comply with weight control, dietary adjustments, modified exercise program
• To carry emergency ID to identify drug, allergies
• To avoid hazardous activities if dizziness is present
• To report symptoms of CHF: difficulty breathing, especially on exertion or when lying down, night cough, swelling of extremities
• To take medication at bedtime to prevent effect of orthostatic hypotension, to rise slowly
• To wear support hose to minimize effects of orthostatic hypotension
Treatment of overdose: Lavage, IV atropine for bradycardia, IV theophylline for bronchospasm, digitalis, O_2, diuretic for cardiac failure; hemodialysis is useful for removal, hypotension; administer vasopressor (norepinephrine)

---

lactulose (℞)

(lak′tyoo-lose)
Cephulac, Cholac, Chronulac, Constilac, Constulose, Duphalac, Enulose, Evalose, Heptalac, Kristalose, Lactulax ✦, Lactulose PSE, Portalac
Func. class.: Laxative; ammonia detoxicant (hyperosmotic)
Chem. class.: Lactose synthetic derivative

Action: Prevents absorption of ammonia in colon; increases water in stool
Uses: Chronic constipation, portal-systemic encephalopathy in patients with hepatic disease

DOSAGE AND ROUTES
Constipation
• *Adult:* **PO** 15-60 ml daily or 10-20 g **POWDER** for oral sol daily

---

• *Child* (unlabeled): **PO** 7.5 ml daily
Encephalopathy
• *Adult:* **PO** 30-45 ml tid or qid until
stools are soft; **RETENTION ENEMA**
300 ml diluted
• *Infant:* (unlabeled) **PO** 2.5-10 ml/day
in divided doses
• *Child:* (unlabeled) **PO** 40-90 ml/day
in divided doses given 2-4 ×/day
Available forms: Syr 10 g/15 ml;
single-use packets (Kristalose) 10, 20 g

SIDE EFFECTS

GI: Nausea, vomiting, anorexia, abdominal cramps, diarrhea, flatulence,
distention, belching
Contraindications: Hypersensitivity,
low-galactose diet
Precautions: Pregnancy (B), lactation,
diabetes mellitus, elderly, debilitated
patients

PHARMACOKINETICS

Metabolized in intestine, excreted by
kidneys; onset 1-2 days, peak unknown, duration unknown

INTERACTIONS

Drug/Herb
Do not use with laxatives
Increase: laxative action—flax, senna
Decrease: lactulose effects—neomycin,
other oral antiinfectives

NURSING CONSIDERATIONS

Assess:
• Stool: amount, color, consistency
• Blood ammonia level (30-70 mg/100
ml); may decrease ammonia level by
25%-50%
• Blood, urine electrolytes if drug is
used often; may cause diarrhea, hypokalemia, hyponatremia
• I&O ratio to identify fluid loss
• Cause of constipation; determine
whether fluids, bulk, or exercise is missing from lifestyle, constipating drugs
• Cramping, rectal bleeding, nausea,
vomiting; if these symptoms occur, drug
should be discontinued

• Clearing of confusion, lethargy, restlessness, irritability if portal-systemic
encephalopathy
Administer:
PO route
• With 8 oz fruit juice, water, milk to
increase palatability of oral form
RECT route
• Retention enema by diluting 300 ml
lactose/700 ml of water; administer by
rectal balloon catheter
• Increased fluids to 2 L/day; do not give
with other laxatives; if diarrhea occurs,
reduce dosage
Evaluate:
• Therapeutic response: decreased
constipation, decreased blood ammonia
level, clearing of mental state
Teach patient/family:
• Not to use laxatives long-term
• To dilute with water or fruit juice to
counteract sweet taste
• To store in cool environment; do not
freeze
• To take on an empty stomach for rapid
action
• To report diarrhea; may indicate overdose

---

lamivudine (R)

(lam-i-voo′deen)
Epivir, Epivir-HBV
Func. class.: Antiretroviral
Chem. class.: Nucleoside reverse
transcriptase inhibitor

Do not confuse:
lamivudine/lamotrigine
Action: Inhibits replication of HIV virus
by incorporating into cellular DNA by
viral reverse transcriptase, thereby terminating cellular DNA chain
Uses: HIV-1 infection in combination
with other antiretrovirals; chronic hepatitis B (Epivir-HBV)
Investigational uses: Prophylaxis of
HIV—postexposure with indinavir and
zidovudine

Side effects: *italics* = common; ***bold italics*** = life-threatening

DOSAGE AND ROUTES

HIV

• *Adult and child >16 yr:* **PO** 150 mg bid or 300 mg daily

• *Child 3 mo to 16 yr:* **PO** 4 mg/kg bid, max 150 mg bid

Renal dose

• *Adult:* **PO** CCr 30-49 ml/min 150 mg daily; CCr 15-29 ml/min 150 mg 1st dose, then 100 mg daily; CCr 5-14 ml/min 150 mg daily, then 50 mg daily; CCr <5 ml/min, 50 mg 1st dose, then 25 mg daily

Chronic hepatitis B

• *Adult:* **PO** 100 mg daily

Available forms: Epivir: oral sol 10 mg/ml; tabs 150, 300 mg; Epivir-HBV: oral sol 5 mg/ml; tabs 100 mg

SIDE EFFECTS

*CNS: Fever, headache, malaise, dizziness, insomnia, depression, fatigue, chills, **seizures***

EENT: Taste change, hearing loss, photophobia

GI: Nausea, vomiting, diarrhea, anorexia, cramps, dyspepsia, ***hepatomegaly with steatosis, pancreatitis***

*HEMA: **Neutropenia, anemia, thrombocytopenia***

INTEG: Rash

MS: Myalgia, arthralgia, pain

RESP: Cough

*SYST: **Lactic acidosis, anaphylaxis, Stevens-Johnson syndrome***

Contraindications: Hypersensitivity

Precautions: Pregnancy (C), granulocyte count <1000/mm^3 or Hgb <9.5 g/dl, lactation, children, renal disease, severe hepatic dysfunction, pancreatitis, elderly

PHARMACOKINETICS

Rapidly absorbed, distributed to extravascular space, excreted unchanged in urine, protein binding <36%, terminal half-life 5-7 hr

INTERACTIONS

May decrease both drugs: zalcitabine

Increase: lamivudine level—trimethoprim-sulfamethoxazole

Increase: level—zidovudine

Drug/Lab Test

Increase: ALT, bilirubin

Decrease: Hgb, neutrophil, platelet count

NURSING CONSIDERATIONS

Assess:

• Blood counts q2wk; watch for neutropenia, thrombocytopenia, Hgb, CD4, viral load; if low, therapy may have to be discontinued and restarted after hematologic recovery; blood transfusions may be required

• Hepatic studies: AST, ALT, bilirubin; amylase, lipase, triglycerides, CD4, viral load periodically during treatment

• Children for pancreatitis: abdominal pain, nausea, vomiting

⚠ Lactic acidosis, severe hepatomegaly with steatosis: obtain baseline LFTs, if elevated discontinue treatment; discontinue even if LFTs are normal if lactic acidosis, severe hepatomegaly develop

Administer:

• PO daily or bid, without regard to meals

Perform/provide:

• With other antiretrovirals only

• Storage in cool environment; protect from light

Evaluate:

• Blood dyscrasias: bruising, fatigue, bleeding, poor healing

Teach patient/family:

• That GI complaints, insomnia resolve after 3-4 wk of treatment

• That drug is not a cure for HIV, but will control symptoms

• To notify prescriber of sore throat, swollen lymph nodes, malaise, fever; other infections may occur

• That patient is still infective, may pass HIV virus on to others

• That follow-up visits must be contin-

ued since serious toxicity may occur; blood counts must be done q2wk
• That drug must be taken as prescribed, even if patient feels better
• That other drugs may be necessary to prevent other infections
• That drug may cause fainting or dizziness

lamotrigine (℞)
(la-mot'ri-geen)
Lamictal, Lamictal Chewable Dispersible
Func. class.: Anticonvulsant, misc.
Chem. class.: Phenyltriazine

Do not confuse:
Lamictal/Lomotil/Lamisil
lamotrigine/lamivudine
Action: Unknown, may inhibit voltage-sensitive sodium channels
Uses: Adjunct in the treatment of partial seizures; children with Lennox-Gastaut syndrome, bipolar disorder
Investigational uses: Generalized tonic-clonic, absence, atypical absence and myoclonic seizures

DOSAGE AND ROUTES
Seizures: Monotherapy
• *Adult:* PO 50 mg/day for wk 1-2, then increase to 100 mg divided bid for wk 3-4; maintenance, 300-500 mg/day
• *Child:* 2 mg/kg/day in 2 divided doses × 2 wk, then 10 mg/kg/day, max 15 mg/kg/day or 400 mg/day
Seizures: Multiple therapy
• *Adult:* PO 25 mg every other day wk 1-4, then 150 mg/day in divided doses
• *Child:* 0.1-0.2 mg/kg/day initially, then increase q2wk as needed to 2 mg/kg/day or 150 mg/day
Hepatic Dose (Child-Pugh Grade B)
• *Adult:* PO Reduce by 50%; *(Child-Pugh Grade C)* Reduce by 75%
Bipolar disorder
• *Adult:* PO wk 1-2 25 mg daily; wk 3-4 50 mg daily; wk 5 100 mg daily; wk 6-7 200 mg daily; for patients taking valproic acid: wk 1-2 25 mg every other day, wk

3-4 25 mg daily; wk 5 50 mg daily; wk 6 100 mg daily; wk 7 100 mg daily
Available forms: Tabs 25, 100, 150, 200 mg; chew dispersible tabs 2, 5, 25 mg

SIDE EFFECTS
CNS: Dizziness, ataxia, *headache,* fever, insomnia, tremor, depression, anxiety
EENT: Nystagmus, diplopia, blurred vision
*GI: Nausea, vomiting, anorexia, abdominal pain, **hepatotoxicity***
GU: Dysmenorrhea
*INTEG: **Rash (potentially life-threatening),*** alopecia, photosensitivity
*SYST: **Stevens-Johnson syndrome***
Contraindications: Hypersensitivity
Precautions: Pregnancy (C), lactation, child <16 yr, renal, hepatic disease, elderly, cardiac disease, severe depression, suicidal, blood dyscrasias

PHARMACOKINETICS
Half-life varies depending on dose; rapidly, completely absorbed; metabolized by slucuronic acid conjunction

INTERACTIONS
Decrease: metabolic clearance of lamotrigine—valproic acid
Decrease: lamotrigine serum concentration—carbamazepine, rifamycins, oral contraceptives, acetaminophen, phenytoin, primodone, phenobarbital, oxcarbazepine, succinimides
Drug/Herb
Increase: anticonvulsant effect—ginkgo
Decrease: anticonvulsant effect—ginseng, santonica

NURSING CONSIDERATIONS
Assess:
• For seizure activity: duration, type, intensity, halo before seizure
⚠ For rash (Stevens-Johnson syndrome or toxic epidermal necrolysis) in pediat-

ric patients, drug should be discontinued at first sign of rash

Administer:
• Chewable dispersible tabs; swallow whole, chew, or dispersed in water or diluted fruit juice; if chewed, drink a small amount of water

Evaluate:
• Therapeutic response: decrease in severity of seizures

Teach patient/family:
• To take PO doses divided with or after meals to decrease adverse effects, not to discontinue drug abruptly; seizures may occur
• To avoid hazardous activities until stabilized on drug
• To carry emergency ID, to notify prescriber of skin rash or increased seizure activity, to use sunscreen and protective clothing if photosensitivity occurs
• To notify prescriber if pregnant or intend to become pregnant

---

lansoprazole (R)
(lan-so-prey′zole)
Prevacid
Func. class.: Antiulcer, proton pump inhibitor
Chem. class.: Benzimidazole

Do not confuse:
Prevacid/Pravachol/Prinivil
Action: Suppresses gastric secretion by inhibiting hydrogen/potassium ATPase enzyme system in gastric parietal cell; characterized as gastric acid pump inhibitor, since it blocks final step of acid production
Uses: Gastroesophageal reflux disease (GERD), severe erosive esophagitis, poorly responsive systemic GERD, pathologic hypersecretory conditions (Zollinger-Ellison syndrome, systemic mastocytosis, multiple endocrine adenomas); possibly effective for treatment of duodenal, gastric ulcers, maintenance of healed duodenal ulcers

DOSAGE AND ROUTES
NG tube
• *Adult:* Use intact granules mixed in 40 ml of apple juice and injected through NG tube, then flush with apple juice
Duodenal ulcer
• *Adult:* **PO** 15 mg daily before eating for 4 wk, then 15 mg daily to maintain healing of ulcers; associated with *Helicobacter pylori*—30 mg lansoprazole, 500 mg clarithromycin, 1 g amoxicillin bid × 14 days or 30 mg lansoprazole, 1 g amoxicillin tid × 14 days
Erosive esophagitis
• *Adult:* **PO** 30 mg daily before eating for up to 8 wk, may use another 8-wk course if needed
Pathologic hypersecretory conditions
• *Adult:* **PO** 60 mg daily, may give up to 90 mg bid, administer doses of >120 mg/day in divided doses
GERD/esophagitis
• *Child 1-11 yr: (>30 kg):* **PO** 30 mg daily ≤12 wk
• *Child 1-11 yr (≤30 kg):* **PO** 15 mg daily ≤12 wk
Available forms: Del rel caps 15, 30 mg; granules for oral susp 15, 30 mg/packet

SIDE EFFECTS
CNS: Headache, dizziness, confusion, agitation, amnesia, depression
CV: Chest pain, angina, tachycardia, bradycardia, palpitations, *CVA,* hypertension/hypotension, *MI, shock,* vasodilation
EENT: Tinnitus, taste perversion, deafness, eye pain, otitis media
GI: Diarrhea, abdominal pain, vomiting, nausea, constipation, flatulence, acid regurgitation, anorexia, irritable colon
GU: **Hematuria,** glycosuria, impotence, kidney calculus, breast enlargement
HEMA: **Hemolysis,** anemia
INTEG: Rash, urticaria, pruritus, alopecia
META: Weight gain/loss, gout
RESP: Upper respiratory infections, cough, epistaxis, asthma, bronchitis, dyspnea
Contraindications: Hypersensitivity

Precautions: Pregnancy (B), lactation, children

PHARMACOKINETICS

Absorption after granules leave stomach—rapid; plasma half-life 1½ hr, protein binding 97%, extensively metabolized in liver, excreted in urine, feces; clearance decreased in the elderly, renal and hepatic impairment

INTERACTIONS

Delayed lansoprazole absorption: sucralfate

Decrease: absorption of ketoconazole, itraconazole, ampicillin, iron, digoxin, theophylline

NURSING CONSIDERATIONS

Assess:
• GI system: bowel sounds q8h, abdomen for pain, swelling, anorexia
• Hepatic studies: AST, ALT, alk phosphatase during treatment

Administer:
• Swallow capsule whole before eating; do not crush or chew caps; caps may be opened and contents sprinkled on food

Evaluate:
• Therapeutic response: absence of epigastric pain, swelling, fullness

Teach patient/family:
• To report severe diarrhea; drug may have to be discontinued
• That diabetic patient should know that hypoglycemia may occur
• To avoid hazardous activities; dizziness may occur
• To avoid alcohol, salicylates, ibuprofen; may cause GI irritation

Rarely Used

lanthanum (℞)
(lan′-tha-num)
Fosrenol
Func. class.: Phosphate binder

Uses: End-stage renal disease

DOSAGE AND ROUTES

• *Adult:* **PO** 750-1500 mg daily in divided doses with meals; titrate dose q2-3wk until an acceptable phosphate level is reached; tablets should be chewed completely before swallowing; intact tablets should not be swallowed

Contraindications: Hypophosphatemia, hypersensitivity

Rarely Used

laronidase (℞)
(lah-rah′nih-daze)
Aldurazyme
Func. class.: Miscellaneous drug

Uses: Mucopolysaccharidosis I (MPSI), patients with Hurler and Hurler-Scheie forms of MPSI

DOSAGE AND ROUTES

• *Adult:* **IV INF** 0.58 mg/kg qwk. Pretreat with antipyretic and/or antihistamines 1 hr prior to **IV INF**

Contraindications: Hypersensitivity

latanoprost ophthalmic
See Appendix C

leflunomide (℞)
(leh-floo′noh-mide)
Arava
Func. class.: Antirheumatic (DMARDs)
Chem. class.: Immune modulator, pyrimidine synthesis inhibitor

Action: Inhibits an enzyme involved in pyrimidine synthesis and has antiproliferative, antiinflammatory effect

Uses: Rheumatoid arthritis, to reduce disease process and symptoms

Investigational uses: Juvenile rheumatoid arthritis

Side effects: *italics* = common; ***bold italics*** = life-threatening

DOSAGE AND ROUTES
Rheumatoid arthritis
• *Adult:* **PO** loading dose 100 mg/day × 3 days, maintenance 20 mg/day, may be decreased to 10 mg/day if not well tolerated
Juvenile rheumatoid arthritis (off-label)
• *Adolescents and child:* **PO** 10 mg (10-19.9 kg); 15 mg (20-40 kg); 20 mg (>40 kg)
Available forms: Tabs 10, 20, 100 mg

SIDE EFFECTS
CNS: Headache, dizziness, insomnia, depression, paresthesia, anxiety, migraine, neuralgia
CV: Palpitations, hypertension, chest pain, angina pectoris, peripheral edema
EENT: Pharyngitis, oral candidiasis, stomatitis, dry mouth, blurred vision
*GI: Nausea, anorexia, vomiting, constipation, flatulence, diarrhea, elevated LFTs, **hepatotoxicity***
HEMA: Anemia, ecchymosis, hyperlipidemia
INTEG: Rash, pruritus, alopecia, acne, hematoma, herpes infections
RESP: Pharyngitis, rhinitis, bronchitis, cough, respiratory infection, pneumonia, sinusitis
Contraindications: Pregnancy (X), hypersensitivity, lactation, jaundice, lactase deficiency, hepatic disease
Precautions: Renal disorders, vaccinations, infection, alcoholism, children, immunosuppression

PHARMACOKINETICS
PO: metabolized in liver to active metabolite, excreted in urine

INTERACTIONS
Increase: NSAIDs effect—NSAIDs
Increase: leflunomide side effects—hepatotoxic agents, methotrexate
Increase: rifampin levels—rifampin
Decrease: antibody response—live virus vaccines
Decrease: leflunomide effect—activated charcoal, cholestyramine

NURSING CONSIDERATIONS
Assess:
• Arthritic symptoms: ROM, mobility, swelling of joints baseline and during treatment
• Hepatic studies: if ALT elevations are > twofold ULN, reduce dose to 10 mg/day
Administer:
• With food for GI upset
• To eliminate drug: give cholestyramine 8 g tid × 11 days, check levels
Evaluate:
• Therapeutic response: decreased inflammation, pain in joints
Teach patient/family:
• That drug must be continued for prescribed time to be effective
• To take with food, milk, or antacids to avoid GI upset
• To use caution when driving; drowsiness, dizziness may occur
• To take with a full glass of water to enhance absorption
• To avoid pregnancy while taking this drug; not to breastfeed while taking this drug; men should also discontinue drug and begin leflunomide removal protocol if a pregnancy is planned
• That hair may be lost, review alternatives
• To avoid vaccinations during treatment (live virus)

🅰 High Alert

lepirudin (℞)
(lep-ih-roo′din)
Refludan
Func. class.: Anticoagulant
Chem. class.: Thrombin inhibitor, hirudin

Action: Direct inhibitor of thrombin that is highly specific
Uses: Heparin-induced thrombocytopenia and other thromboembolic conditions

Investigational uses: Adjunct therapy in unstable angina, acute MI without ST elevation, prevention of deep vein thrombosis, percutaneous coronary intervention

DOSAGE AND ROUTES

• *Adult:* IV 0.4 mg/kg over 15-20 sec; then 0.15 mg/kg/hr as a cont inf for 2-10 days or longer

Concomitant use with thrombolytic therapy

• *Adult:* IV BOLUS 0.2 mg/kg initially
• *Adult:* CONT IV INF 0.1 mg/kg/hr

Renal dose

• *Adult:* IV BOLUS 0.2 mg/kg over 15-20 sec, then CCr 45-60 ml/min 0.075 mg/kg/hr, CCr 30-44 ml/min 0.045 mg/kg/hr, CCr 15-29 ml/min 0.0225 mg/kg/hr

Available forms: Powder for inj 50 mg

SIDE EFFECTS

CNS: Fever, **intracranial bleeding**
CV: **Heart failure, pericardial effusion, ventricular fibrillation**
GI: GI bleeding, abnormal LFTs
GU: **Hematuria,** abnormal kidney function, vaginal bleeding
HEMA: **Hemorrhage, thrombocytopenia**
INTEG: Allergic skin reactions
RESP: Pneumonia
SYST: **Multiorgan failure, sepsis, anaphylaxis**

Contraindications: Hypersensitivity to hirudins

Precautions: Pregnancy (B), intracranial bleeding, lactation, children, hepatic disease, recent major surgery, hemorrhagic diathesis bacterial endocarditis, severe uncontrolled hypertension, advanced renal disease, recent active peptic ulcer, recent CVA, stroke, intracerebral surgery, elderly, women

PHARMACOKINETICS

May be metabolized by the release of amino acids during catabolism; 50% unchanged in urine

INTERACTIONS

Increase: bleeding risk—warfarin derivatives, thrombolytics, NSAIDs, plicamycin, cefamandole, cefotetan, cefoperazone, aspirin, clopidogrel, dipyridamole, eptifibatide, ticlopidine, tirofiban, valproic acid

Drug/Herb
Increase: risk of bleeding—agrimony, alfalfa, angelica, anise, basil, bay, bilberry, black haw, bogbean, bromelain, buchu, chondroitin, cinchona bark, dong quai, fenugreek, feverfew, garlic, ginger, ginkgo, ginseng, horse chestnut, Irish moss, kelp, kelpware, khella, lovage, lungwort, meadowsweet, motherwort, mugwort, nettle, papaya, parsley (large amts), pau d'arco, pineapple, poplar, prickly ash, safflower, saw palmetto, tonka bean, turmeric, wintergreen, yarrow
Decrease: anticoagulant effect—chamomile, coenzyme Q10, flax, glucomannan, goldenseal, guar gum

NURSING CONSIDERATIONS

Assess:
• Obtain baseline in APTT before treatment; do not start treatment if APTT ratio ≥2.5, then APTT 4 hr after initiation of treatment and at least daily thereafter; if APTT above target, stop inf for 2 hr, then restart at 50%, take APTT in 4 hr; if below target, increase inf rate by 20%, take APTT in 4 hr, do not exceed inf rate of 0.21 mg/kg/hr without checking for coagulation abnormalities
• APTT, which should be 1.5-2.5 × control
⚠ Bleeding gums, petechiae, ecchymosis, black tarry stools, hematuria/epistaxis, B/P, vaginal bleeding and possible hemorrhage
• Fever, skin rash, urticaria

Administer:
• Avoiding all IM inj
• After reconstitution and further dilution under sterile conditions; use water for inj or 0.9% NaCl; for further dilution 0.9% NaCl or D_5; for rapid and complete

reconstitution, inject 1 ml of diluent into vial and shake gently, use immediately, warm to room temp before use

IV BOL route

• Reconstitute each vial with 1 ml sterile water or 0.9% NaCl, shake gently, transfer content of vial into 10-ml syringe and dilute to a volume of 10 ml with sterile water for inj, D_5W, or 0.9% NaCl, final conc 5 mg/ml

IV INF route

• Reconstitute 2 vials with 1 ml each of sterile water for inj, or 0.9% NaCl, transfer contents into infusion bag containing 250 or 500 ml 0.9% NaCl or D_5W for a conc 0.2 mg/ml or 0.4 mg/ml, infuse at 0.15 mg/kg/hr; use infusion pump

Evaluate:

• Therapeutic response

Teach patient/family:

• To use soft-bristle toothbrush to avoid bleeding gums, avoid contact sports, use electric razor, avoid IM inj

• To report any signs of bleeding: gums, under skin, urine, stools

---

letrozole (℞)

(let′tro-zohl)

Femara

Func. class.: Antineoplastic, nonsteroidal aromatase inhibitor

---

Action: Binds to the heme group of aromatase. Inhibits conversion of androgens to estrogens to reduce plasma estrogen levels. 30% of breast cancers decrease in size when deprived of estrogen

Uses: Metastatic breast cancer in postmenopausal women

DOSAGE AND ROUTES

• *Adult:* **PO** 2.5 mg daily

Available forms: Tabs 2.5 mg

SIDE EFFECTS

CNS: Headache, lethargy, somnolence, dizziness, depression, anxiety

CV: Hypertension

*GI: Nausea, vomiting, anorexia, **hep-**

atotoxicity, constipation, heartburn, diarrhea

INTEG: Rash, pruritus, alopecia, sweating, hot flashes

RESP: Dyspnea, cough

Contraindications: Pregnancy (D), hypersensitivity

Precautions: Hepatic disease, respiratory disease

PHARMACOKINETICS

Metabolized in liver, excreted in urine

INTERACTIONS

None known

NURSING CONSIDERATIONS

Assess:

• Monitor temp q4h; may indicate beginning infection

• Hepatic studies before, during therapy (bilirubin, AST, ALT, LDH) as needed or monthly

• Jaundiced skin, sclera, dark urine, clay-colored stools, itchy skin, abdominal pain, fever, diarrhea

Administer:

• Without regard to meals

Perform/provide:

• Liquid diet, including cola, Jell-O; dry toast or crackers as ordered may be added if patient is not nauseated or vomiting

• Nutritious diet with iron and vitamin supplements as ordered

Evaluate:

• Therapeutic response: decrease in size of tumor

Teach patient/family:

• To report any complaints, side effects to nurse or prescriber

• That drowsiness may occur and to avoid driving or operating heavy machinery

---

leucovorin (R)

(loo-koe-vor'in)
citrovorum factor, folinic
acid, leucovorin calcium,
Wellcovorin
Func. class.: Vitamin, folic acid/
methotrexate antagonist antidote
Chem. class.: Tetrahydrofolic acid
derivative

Do not confuse:
leucovorin/Leukeran
leucovorin/leukine

Action: Needed for normal growth
patterns; prevents toxicity during antineoplastic therapy by protecting normal
cells

Uses: Megaloblastic or macrocytic anemia caused by folic acid deficiency, overdose of folic acid antagonist, methotrexate toxicity, toxicity caused by
pyrimethamine or trimethoprim, pneu-
mocystosis, toxoplasmosis

DOSAGE AND ROUTES
*Megaloblastic anemia caused by
enzyme deficiency*
• *Adult and child:* PO/IV/IM up to 6
mg/day
*Megaloblastic anemia caused by
deficiency of folate*
• *Adult and child:* IM 1 mg or less daily
until adequate response
Methotrexate toxicity
• *Adult and child:* PO/IM/IV normal
elimination given 6 hr after dose of methotrexate (10 mg/m^2) until methotrexate
is $<10^{-8}$ M; CCr is $>50\%$ above prior
level or methotrexate level is 5×10 at 24
hr, or at 48-hr level is $>9 \times 10$ M, give
leucovorin 100 mg/m^2 q3h until level
drops to <10 M
Pyrimethamine toxicity
• *Adult and child:* PO/IM 5-15 mg daily
Trimethoprim toxicity
• *Adult and child:* PO/IM 400 mg daily
Advanced colorectal cancer
• *Adult:* IV 200 mg/m^2, then 5-FU 370
mg/m^2; or leucovorin 20 mg/m^2, then

5-FU 425 mg/m^2; give daily $\times$ 5 days
q4-5wk
Available forms: Tabs 5, 10, 15, 25
mg; inj 3, 5 mg/ml; powder for inj 10
mg/ml

SIDE EFFECTS
HEMA: Thrombocytosis (intraarterial)
INTEG: Rash, pruritus, erythema, urticaria
RESP: Wheezing
Contraindications: Hypersensitivity,
anemias other than megaloblastic not
associated with vit B$_{12}$ deficiency
Precautions: Pregnancy (C)

INTERACTIONS
Increase: metabolism of phenobarbital,
hydantoins
Decrease: folate levels—
chloramphenicol

NURSING CONSIDERATIONS
Assess:
• CCr, creatinine before leucovorin res-
cue and daily to detect nephrotoxicity;
methotrexate level
• I&O; watch for nausea and vomiting
• Other drugs taken: alcohol, hydanto-
ins, trimethoprim may cause increased
folic acid use by body
Administer:
• Within 1 hr of folic acid antagonist
IM route
• No reconstitution needed
• Treatment of megaloblastic anemia
uses IM dosing
IV route
• For IV reconstitute 50 mg/5 ml bacte-
riostatic or sterile H$_2$O for inj (10 mg/
ml) or (100 mg/10 ml); use immediately
if sterile H$_2$O is used
• Give by direct IV over 160 mg/min or
less (16 ml of 10 mg/ml sol/min)
• Give by intermittent inf after diluting in
100-500 ml of 0.9% NaCl, D$_5$W, D$_{10}$W,
LR, Ringer's sol
Additive compatibilities: Cisplatin,
cisplatin/floxuridine, floxuridine
Syringe compatibilities: Bleomycin,
cisplatin, cyclophosphamide, DOXOrubicin, fluorouracil, furosemide, heparin,

L

methotrexate, metoclopramide, mitomycin, vinBLAStine, vinCRIStine

Y-site compatibilities: Amifostine, aztreonam, bleomycin, cefepime, cisplatin, cladribine, cyclophosphamide, DOXOrubicin, DOXOrubicin liposome, filgrastim, fluconazole, fluorouracil, furosemide, granisetron, heparin, methotrexate, metoclopramide, mitomycin, piperacillin/tazobactam, tacrolimus, teniposide, thiotepa, vinBLAStine, vinCRIStine

Perform/provide:
• Increase fluid intake if used to treat folic acid inhibitor overdose
• Protection from light and heat

Evaluate:
• Therapeutic response: increased weight; improved orientation, well-being; absence of fatigue; reversal of toxicity (methotrexate, folic acid antagonist overdose)

Teach patient/family:
• For leucovorin rescue have patient drink 3 L fluid daily of rescue
• For folic acid deficiency eat folic acid rich foods: bran, yeast, dried beans, nuts, fresh, green leafy vegetables
• To take drug exactly as prescribed
• To notify prescriber of side effects
• To report signs of hyposensitivity reaction immediately

⚠ High Alert

leuprolide (℞)
(loo-proe'lide)
Leupron Depo PED, Lupron, Lupron Depot, Lupron Depot-3 month, Viadur
Func. class.: Antineoplastic hormone
Chem. class.: Gonadotropin-releasing hormone

Do not confuse:
Lupron/Nuprin
Lupron/Lopurin

Action: Causes initial increase in circulating levels of LH, FSH; continuous administration results in decreased LH, FSH; in men, testosterone is reduced to castrate levels; in premenopausal women, estrogen is reduced to menopausal levels

Uses: Metastatic prostate cancer, management of endometriosis, central precocious puberty

DOSAGE AND ROUTES

Prostate cancer
• *Adult:* **SUBCUT** 1 mg/day; **IM:**
• 7.5 mg/dose qmo; Viadur implant (72 mg) qyr; or **IM** 22.5 mg q3mo; or **IM** 30 mg q4mo

Endometriosis/fibroids
• *Adult:* **IM** 3.75 mg qmo or 11.25 q3mo or 30 mg q4mo

Central precocious puberty
• *Child:* **SUBCUT** 50 mcg/kg/day; may increase by 10 mcg/kg/day as needed
• *Child >37.5 kg:* **IM** 15 mg q4wk
• *Child 25-37.5 kg:* **IM** 11.25 mg q4wk
• *Child ≤25 kg:* **IM** 7.5 mg q4wk

Available forms: Inj (depot) 3.75 mg, 7.5 mg single dose, multiple-dose vials (5 mg/ml), single-use kit 11.25 mg vial, pediatric depot 7.5, 11.25, 15 mg; 3 mo depot 22.5 mg single use; Viadur once a yr implant

SIDE EFFECTS

CV: **MI, pulmonary emboli, dysrhythmias**
GI: Anorexia, diarrhea, **GI bleeding**
GU: Edema, hot flashes, impotence, decreased libido, amenorrhea, vaginal dryness, gynecomastia

Contraindications: Pregnancy (X), hypersensitivity to GnRH or analogs, thromboembolic disorders, lactation, undiagnosed vaginal bleeding

Precautions: Edema, hepatic disease, CVA, MI, seizures, hypertension, diabetes mellitus

PHARMACOKINETICS

SUBCUT: Onset 1-2 wk, peak 2-4 wk; absorbed rapidly (SUBCUT), slowly (IM depot); half-life 3 hr

---

⚠ Safety alert   *"Tall Man" lettering

INTERACTIONS

Increase: antineoplastic action—flutamide, megestrol

NURSING CONSIDERATIONS

Assess:

• For symptoms of endometriosis (lower abdominal pain)/fibroids (pelvic pain, excessive vaginal bleeding, bloating) before, during, and after treatment

• For central precocious puberty (CPP) if treatment is for this condition; secondary S_4 characteristics to child <9 yr, estradiol/testosterone levels, GnRH test, tomography of head, adrenal steroids, chorionic gonadotropin, wrist x-ray, height, weight

• Hepatic studies before, during therapy (bilirubin, AST, ALT, LDH) as needed or monthly, PSA in prostate cancer

• Pituitary gonadotropic and gonadal function during therapy and 4-8 wk after therapy is decreased

• Worsening of signs and symptoms; normal during beginning therapy

• Fatigue, increased pulse, pallor, lethargy; edema in feet, joints; stomach pain

⚠ Symptoms indicating severe allergic reaction: rash, pruritus, urticaria, purpuric skin lesions, itching, flushing

Administer:

• IM/SUBCUT using syringe and drug packaged together, give deep in large muscle mass, rotate sites

• Use depot IM only

• Monthly: reconstitute single-use vial with 1 ml of diluent, if multiple vials used, withdraw 0.5 ml and inject into each vial (1 ml), withdraw all and inject

• 3-month: reconstitute microspheres using 1.5 ml of diluent, and inject in vial, shake, withdraw, and inject

• 12-month: insert into upper arm; at the end of 12 months, implant must be removed

Perform/provide:

• Nutritious diet with iron, vitamin supplements as ordered

• Storage in tight container at room temperature

Evaluate:

• Therapeutic response: decreased tumor size and spread of malignancy, decrease in lesions, pain in endometriosis, fibroids, correction of CCP

Teach patient/family:

• To notify prescriber if menstruation continues; menstruation should stop

• To use a nonhormonal method of contraception during therapy

• That bone pain will disappear after 1 wk

• To report any complaints, side effects to nurse or prescriber; hot flashes may occur; record weight, report gain of >2 lb/day

• How to prepare, give; to rotate sites for SUBCUT inj

• To keep accurate records of dose

• That tumor flare may occur: increase in size of tumor, increased bone pain, will subside rapidly; may take analgesics for pain; premenopausal women must use mechanical birth control; ovulation may be induced

• Do not breastfeed while taking this drug

• Voiding problems may increase in beginning of therapy, but will decrease in several weeks

---

levalbuterol (℞)

(lev-al-byoo'ter-ole)
Xopenex
Func. class.: Bronchodilator, adrenergic β_2-agonist

Action: Causes bronchodilation by action on β_2 (pulmonary) receptors by increasing levels of cAMP, which relaxes smooth muscle; produces bronchodilation, CNS, cardiac stimulation, as well as increased diuresis and gastric acid secretion

Uses: Treatment or prevention of bronchospasm (reversible obstructive airway disease)

DOSAGE AND ROUTES

• *Adult and child ≥12 yr:* **INH** 0.63 mg tid, q6-8h by nebulization, may increase 1.25 mg q8h

• *Child 6-11 yr:* **INH** 0.31 mg tid by nebulization, max 0.63 mg tid

Available forms: Sol, inh 0.63 mg, 1.25 mg/3 ml

SIDE EFFECTS

CNS: **Tremors, anxiety,** insomnia, headache, dizziness, stimulation, *restlessness,* hallucinations, flushing, irritability

CV: Palpitations, tachycardia, hypertension, angina, hypotension, dysrhythmias

EENT: Dry nose, irritation of nose and throat

GI: Heartburn, nausea, vomiting

META: Hypokalemia, hyperglycemia

MS: Muscle cramps

Contraindications: Hypersensitivity to sympathomimetics, tachydysrhythmias, severe cardiac disease

Precautions: Pregnancy (C), lactation, cardiac disorders, hyperthyroidism, diabetes mellitus, hypertension, prostatic hypertrophy, narrow-angle glaucoma, seizures

PHARMACOKINETICS

Metabolized in the liver and tissues, crosses placenta, breast milk, blood-brain barrier

INH: Onset 5-15 min, peak 1-1½ hr, duration 6-8 hr

INTERACTIONS

Increase: action of aerosol bronchodilators

Increase: levalbuterol action—tricyclics, MAOIs, other adrenergics

Decrease: levalbuterol action—other β-blockers

Drug/Herb

Increase: stimulation—black/green tea, coffee, cola nut, guarana, yerba maté

NURSING CONSIDERATIONS

Assess:

• Respiratory function: vital capacity, forced expiratory volume, ABGs, lung sounds, heart rate and rhythm (baseline); character of sputum: color, consistency, amount

• For evidence of allergic reactions, paradoxical bronchospasm

Administer:

• By nebulization q6-8h; wait at least 1 min between inhalation of aerosols

Evaluate:

• Therapeutic response: absence of dyspnea, wheezing after 1 hr, improved airway exchange, improved ABGs

Teach patient/family:

• Not to use OTC medications; excess stimulation may occur

• To avoid getting aerosol in eyes; blurring may result

• To avoid smoking, smoke-filled rooms, persons with respiratory infections

⚠ That paradoxic bronchospasm may occur and to stop drug immediately, contact prescriber

• To limit caffeine products such as chocolate, coffee, tea, and colas or herbs such as cola nut, guarana, yerba maté

Treatment of overdose: Administer a β₁-adrenergic blocker

---

levetiracetam (Ŗ)
(lev-eh-teer-ass'eh-tam)
Keppra
Func. class.: Anticonvulsant

Action: Unknown, may inhibit nerve impulses by limiting influx of sodium ions across cell membrane in motor cortex

Uses: Adjunctive therapy in partial onset seizures

DOSAGE AND ROUTES

• *Adult:* **PO** 500 mg bid, may increase by 1000 mg/day q2wk max 3000 mg/day

Available forms: Tabs 250, 500, 750 mg; oral sol 100 mg/ml

⚠ Safety alert   *"Tall Man" lettering

SIDE EFFECTS

CNS: Dizziness, somnolence, asthenia
HEMA: Lowered Hct, Hgb, RBC, infection
MISC: Infection, abdominal pain, pharyngitis

Contraindications: Hypersensitivity
Precautions: Pregnancy (C), renal disease, cardiac disease, psychosis, lactation, children, elderly

PHARMACOKINETICS

Rapidly absorbed, not protein bound, excreted via kidneys 66% unchanged; half-life 6-8 hr, longer in elderly

NURSING CONSIDERATIONS

Assess:
• Renal studies: urinalysis, BUN, urine creatinine q3mo
• Blood studies: RBC, Hct, Hgb
• Description of seizures
• Mental status: mood, sensorium, affect, behavioral changes; if mental status changes, notify prescriber

Administer:
• Swallow tab whole; do not break, crush, or chew
• With food, milk to decrease GI symptoms (rare)

Perform/provide:
• Storage at room temperature
• Assistance with ambulation during early part of treatment; dizziness occurs

Evaluate:
• Therapeutic response: decreased seizure activity, document on patient's chart

Teach patient/family:
• To carry emergency ID stating patient's name, drugs taken, condition, prescriber's name, phone number
• Use oral sol; if swallowing is a problem, measure oral sol in medicine cup or dropper, don't use teaspoon
• To notify prescriber if pregnant or intend to become pregnant
• To avoid driving, other activities that require alertness
• Not to discontinue medication quickly

after long-term use, withdrawal seizure may occur

---

levobetaxolol ophthalmic
See Appendix C

---

levobunolol ophthalmic
See Appendix C

Rarely Used

levobupivacaine (R)
(lee-voh-bu-piv′ah-kane)
Chirocaine
Func. class.: Local anesthetic

Uses: Local, regional anesthesia, surgical anesthesia, pain management, continuous epidural analgesia

DOSAGE AND ROUTES

• Varies with route of anesthesia
Contraindications: Hypersensitivity, children <12 yr, elderly, severe hepatic disease

---

levocabastine ophthalmic
See Appendix C

---

levodopa (R)
(lee′voe-doe-pa)
Dopar, Larodopa, L-Dopa
Func. class.: Antiparkinson agent
Chem. class.: Dopamine agonist

Do not confuse:
L-dopa (levodopa)/methyldopa
Action: Decarboxylation to dopamine, which increases dopamine levels in brain
Uses: Parkinson's disease
Research note: Levodopa may be the

---

cause of sleep attacks (daytime) in patients

DOSAGE AND ROUTES

• *Adult:* **PO** 0.5-1 g daily divided bid-qid with meals; may increase by up to 0.75 g q3-7d not to exceed 8 g/day unless closely supervised

Available forms: Caps 100, 250, 500 mg; tabs 100, 250, 500 mg

SIDE EFFECTS

CNS: Involuntary choreiform movements, hand tremors, fatigue, headache, anxiety, twitching, numbness, weakness, confusion, agitation, insomnia, nightmares, psychosis, hallucination, hypomania, severe depression, dizziness

CV: Orthostatic hypotension, tachycardia, hypertension, palpitation

EENT: Blurred vision, diplopia, dilated pupils

GI: Nausea, vomiting, anorexia, abdominal distress, dry mouth, flatulence, dysphagia, bitter taste, diarrhea, constipation

HEMA: **Hemolytic anemia, leukopenia, agranulocytosis**

INTEG: Rash, sweating, alopecia

MISC: Urinary retention, incontinence, weight change, dark urine

Contraindications: Hypersensitivity, narrow-angle glaucoma, undiagnosed skin lesions

Precautions: Pregnancy (C), renal disease, cardiac disease, hepatic disease, respiratory disease, MI with dysrhythmias, convulsions, peptic ulcer, asthma, endocrine disease, affective disorders, psychosis, lactation, children <12 yr, peptic ulcer

PHARMACOKINETICS

PO: Peak 1-3 hr, excreted in urine (metabolites)

INTERACTIONS

⚠ Hypertensive crisis: MAOIs
Increase: levodopa effects—antacids

Decrease: levodopa effects—anticholinergics, hydantoins, papaverine, pyridoxine

Drug/Herb
Increase: parkinsonian symptoms—kava
Decrease: levodopa action, increase EPS—Indian snakeroot

Drug/Food
Decrease: levodopa absorption—high-protein foods

Drug/Lab Test
Decrease: VMA
False positive: Urine ketones, urine glucose, Coombs' test
False negative: Urine glucose (glucose oxidase)
False increase: Uric acid, urine protein

NURSING CONSIDERATIONS

Assess:
• Renal, hepatic studies: AST, ALT, alk phosphatase, LDH, bilirubin, CBC, BUN, protein-bound iodine
• Involuntary movements in parkinsonism: akinesia, tremors, staggering gait, muscle rigidity, drooling
⚠ Levodopa toxicity: mental, personality changes, hallucinations, increased twitching, grimacing, tongue protrusion, GI side effects
• B/P, respiration during initial treatment; hypo/hypertension should be reported
• Mental status: affect, mood, behavioral changes, depression; complete suicide assessment

Administer:
• Drug until NPO before surgery
• Adjust dosage to patient response
• With meals; limit protein taken with drug
• Only after MAOIs have been discontinued for 2 wk

Perform/provide:
• Assistance with ambulation during beginning therapy, orthostatic hypotension may occur

---

⚠ Safety alert   *"Tall Man" lettering

• Testing for diabetes mellitus, acromegaly if on long-term therapy

Evaluate:

• Therapeutic response: decrease in akathisia, increased mood

Teach patient/family:

• That therapeutic effects may take several weeks to a few months

• To change positions slowly to prevent orthostatic hypotension

• To report side effects: twitching, eye spasms; indicate overdose

• To use drug exactly as prescribed; if drug is discontinued abruptly, parkinsonian crisis may occur

• That urine, sweat may darken

• To avoid vit B₆ preparations, vitamin-fortified foods containing B₆; these foods can reverse effects of levodopa

---

levofloxacin (℞)

(lee-voh-floks'a-sin)
Levaquin
Func. class.: Antiinfective
Chem. class.: Fluoroquinolone

Action: Interferes with conversion of intermediate DNA fragments into high-molecular-weight DNA in bacteria; DNA gyrase inhibitor

Uses: Acute sinusitis, acute chronic bronchitis, community-acquired pneumonia, uncomplicated skin infections, complicated UTI, acute pyelonephritis caused by *Streptococcus pneumoniae, Haemophilus influenzae, Haemophilis parainfluenzae, Moraxella catarrhalis, Escherichia coli, Serratia marcescens, Klebsiella pneumoniae, Chlamydia pneumoniae, Legionella pneumophilia, Mycoplasma pneumoniae, Enterococcus faecalis, Staphylococcus epidermidis, Staphylococcus pyogenes*

DOSAGE AND ROUTES

• *Adult:* IV INF 500 mg by slow inf over 1 hr q24h × 7-14 days depending on infection; PO: 500 mg q24h × 7-14 days depending on infection

Renal disease

• *Adult:* **PO/IV** CCr 20-49 ml/min initial 500 mg, then 250 mg, q24h; CCr 10-19 ml/min 250 or 500 mg, depending on condition; then 250 mg q48h

Available forms: Single-use vials 500, 750 mg; premixed flexible containers 250 mg/50 ml D₅W, 500 mg/100 ml D₅W, 750 mg/150 ml D₅W; tabs 250, 500, 750 mg

SIDE EFFECTS

CNS: Headache, dizziness, *insomnia,* anxiety, ***seizures,*** encephalopathy, paresthesia

CV: Chest pain, palpitations, vasodilation

EENT: Dry mouth

GI: Nausea, flatulence, *vomiting,* diarrhea, abdominal pain, ***pseudomembranous colitis***

GU: Vaginitis, crystalluria

HEMA: Eosinophilia, ***hemolytic anemia,*** lymphopenia

INTEG: Rash, pruritus, *photosensitivity*

MISC: Hypoglycemia, hypersensitivity

RESP: Pneumonitis

*SYST: **Anaphylaxis, multisystem organ failure, Stevens-Johnson syndrome***

Contraindications: Hypersensitivity to quinolones, photosensitivity

Precautions: Pregnancy (C), lactation, children

PHARMACOKINETICS

Metabolized in liver, excreted in urine unchanged, half-life 6-8 hr

INTERACTIONS

Do not use with magnesium in the same IV line

Increase: CNS stimulation, seizures—NSAIDs, foscarnet

Increase: bleeding risk—warfarin

Decrease: levofloxacin absorption—antacids containing aluminum, magnesium; sucralfate, zinc, iron, calcium

L

Side effects: *italics* = common; ***bold italics*** = life-threatening

Decrease: clearance of—theophylline, toxicity may result

Drug/Herb

Increase: antiinfective effect—cola tree

Drug/Lab Test

Decrease: Glucose, lymphocytes

NURSING CONSIDERATIONS

Assess:

• For previous sensitivity reaction

• For signs and symptoms of infection: characteristics of sputum, WBC >10,000/mm³, fever; obtain baseline information before and during treatment

• C&S before beginning drug therapy to identify if correct treatment has been initiated

⚠ For allergic reactions and anaphylaxis: rash, urticaria, pruritus, chills, fever, joint pain; may occur a few days after therapy begins; epINEPHrine and resuscitation equipment should be available for anaphylactic reaction

• Bowel pattern daily; if severe diarrhea occurs, drug should be discontinued

⚠ For overgrowth of infection: perineal itching, fever, malaise, redness, pain, swelling, drainage, rash, diarrhea, change in cough, sputum

Administer:

• PO 4 hr before or 2 hr after antacids, iron, calcium, zinc

• Not to use theophylline with this product, toxicity may result

IV route

• Only by slow IV infusion over 1 hr

• Discard any unused sol in the single-dose vial

• Using premix, tear outer wrap at notch and remove sol container, check for leaks, close control clamps; remove cover from port at bottom of container, insert pin into port with a twist; suspend container from hanger, squeeze and release drip chamber to proper fluid level, open flow control to expel air, close clamp; regulate rate with flow control clamps

Solution compatibilities: 0.9% NaCl, D₅W, D₅/0.9% NaCl, D₅LR, D₅/0.45% NaCl, sodium lactate

Perform/provide:

• Increase fluid intake to 2 L/day to prevent crystalluria

Evaluate:

• Therapeutic response: absence of signs/symptoms of infection (WBC <10,000/mm³, temp WNL)

Teach patient/family:

• To contact prescriber if vaginal itching, loose, foul-smelling stools, furry tongue occur (may indicate superinfection); report itching, rash, pruritus, urticaria

• To notify prescriber of diarrhea with blood or pus

• To take 4 hr before or 2 hr after antacids, iron, calcium, zinc products

• To complete full course of therapy

• To avoid hazardous activities until response is known

• To use frequent rinsing of mouth, sugarless candy or gum for dry mouth

• To avoid other medication unless approved by prescriber

• To prevent sun exposure or use sunscreen to prevent phototoxicity

---

levofloxacin ophthalmic
See Appendix C

---

levonorgestrel implant (℞)
(lee-voe-nor-jess′trel)
Norplant, Mirena
Func. class.: Contraceptive system
Chem. class.: Synthetic progestin

Action: As a progestin, transforms proliferative endometrium into secretory endometrium; inhibits secretion of pituitary gonadotropins, which prevents follicular maturation and ovulation

Uses: Prevention of pregnancy for 5 yr

DOSAGE AND ROUTES

• *Adult:* 6 caps subdermally implanted in the upper arm during first 7 days after onset of menses, replace q5yr

---

Available forms: Kit of 6 caps, 36 mg/cap

SIDE EFFECTS

CNS: Dizziness, headache, nervousness
CV: ***Cerebral hemorrhage, coronary thrombosis, pulmonary embolism, cerebral thrombosis***
GI: Nausea, abdominal discomfort
GU: Amenorrhea, cervical erosion, breakthrough bleeding, dysmenorrhea, vaginal candidiasis, breast changes, vaginitis
INTEG: Alopecia, dermatitis, hirsutism, acne, hypertrichosis, infection at site, pain/itching at site
OTHER: Change in appetite, weight gain
Contraindications: Pregnancy (X), hypersensitivity, thrombophlebitis, undiagnosed genital bleeding, liver tumors, breast carcinoma, liver disease
Precautions: Depression, psychosis, lactation, fluid retention, contact lens wearers, family history of breast cancer

PHARMACOKINETICS

Onset 1 mo, peak 1 mo, duration 5 yr

INTERACTIONS

Decrease: contraception—phenytoin, carbamazepine, penicillins, chloramphenicol, dihydroergotamine, mineral oil, corticosteroids, phenylbutazone, primidone, protease inhibitors, antiretrovirals, tetracyclines
Drug/Herb
Possible toxicity: β-blockers, benzodiazepines, cycloSPORINE, corticosteroids, tricyclics, theophylline
Decrease: contraception—St. John's wort

NURSING CONSIDERATIONS

Assess:
• Blood studies: cholesterol, triglycerides; may be increased or decreased; sex hormone—binding globulin, thyroxine, T₃ uptake, LDL, HDL
• Menstrual irregularities: spotting,

prolonged bleeding, amenorrhea; usually diminish
• For jaundice, thrombophlebitis; implants should be removed, hepatic studies
• For acne, dermatitis, hirsutism, alopecia
Administer:
• 8 cm (3 in) above the crease of the elbow; implantation should be during first 7 days after onset of menses; implantation should be fanlike, 15 degrees apart
Evaluate:
• Therapeutic response: absence of pregnancy
Teach patient/family:
• To notify prescriber if pregnancy is suspected
• To use
• That this product only prevents pregnancy, does not protect against HIV or other STDs
• That if vision problems occur, an ophthalmologist should be seen
• That physical examinations are necessary
⚠ To report fluid retention: weight gain, edema; hepatic symptoms: yellowing skin or eyes, clay-colored stools, dark urine; thrombosis: blurred vision, headache, tenderness in extremities

---

levothyroxine (T₄) (℞)

(lee-voe-thye-rox′een)
Eltroxin ✦, Levo-T, Levothroid, levothyroxine sodium, Levoxyl, PMS-Levothyroxine Sodium ✦, Synthroid, T₄
Func. class.: Thyroid hormone
Chem. class.: Levoisomer of thyroxine

Do not confuse:
Synthroid/Symmetrel
Action: Increases metabolic rate, controls protein synthesis, increases cardiac output, renal blood flow, O₂ consumption, body temp, blood volume, growth,

---

development at cellular level, exact mechanism unknown
Uses: Hypothyroidism, myxedema coma, thyroid hormone replacement, congenital hypothyroidism, thyrotoxicosis, congenital hypothyroidism, some types of thyroid cancer

DOSAGE AND ROUTES
Severe hypothyroidism
• *Adult:* **PO** 50 mcg/day, increase by 25 mcg/day every 2-3 wk, average dose 100-200 mcg/day; max 200 mcg/day
IM/IV 50-100 mcg/day as a single dose or 50% of usual oral dosage
• *Child >12 yr:* **PO** 2-3 mcg/kg/day as a single dose AM
• *Child 6-12 yr:* **PO** 4-5 mcg/kg/day as a single dose AM
• *Child 1-5 yr:* **PO** 5-6 mcg/kg/day as a single dose AM
• *Child 6-12 mo:* **PO** 6-8 mcg/kg/day as a single dose AM
• *Child to 6 mo:* **PO** 8-10 mcg/kg/day as a single dose AM
Myxedema coma
• *Adult:* **IV** 200-500 mcg, may increase by 100-300 mcg after 24 hr; place on oral medication as soon as possible
Available forms: Powder for inj 200, 500 mcg/vial; tabs 0.025, 0.05, 0.075, 0.088, 0.1, 0.112, 0.125, 0.137, 0.15, 0.175, 0.2, 0.3 mg

SIDE EFFECTS
CNS: Anxiety, insomnia, tremors, headache, ***thyroid storm***
CV: Tachycardia, palpitations, angina, dysrhythmias, hypertension, ***cardiac arrest***
GI: Nausea, diarrhea, increased or decreased appetite, cramps
MISC: Menstrual irregularities, weight loss, sweating, heat intolerance, fever, alopecia
Contraindications: Adrenal insufficiency, recent MI, thyrotoxicosis, hypersensitivity to beef, alcohol intolerance (inj only)
Precautions: Pregnancy (A), elderly,

angina pectoris, hypertension, ischemia, cardiac disease, lactation, diabetes

PHARMACOKINETICS
PO: Onset 3-5 days, peak 2-4 wk, duration 1-3 wk
IV: Onset 6-8 hr, peak 24 hr, duration unknown
Half-life euthyroid 6-7 days; hypothyroid 9-10 days; hyperthyroid 3-4 days; distributed throughout body tissues

INTERACTIONS
Increase: cardiac insufficiency risk—epINEPHrine products
Increase: effects of anticoagulants, sympathomimetics, tricyclics
Decrease: levothyroxine absorption—cholestyramine, colestipol, ferrous sulfate
Decrease: effects of digitalis drugs, insulin, hypoglycemics
Decrease: levothyroxine effects—estrogens, SSRIs
Drug/Herb
Decrease: thyroid hormone effect—agar, bugleweed carnitine, kelpware, soy, spirulina
Drug/Lab Test
Increase: CPK, LDH, AST, PBI, blood glucose
Decrease: Thyroid function tests

NURSING CONSIDERATIONS
Assess:
• B/P, pulse periodically during treatment
• Weight daily in same clothing, using same scale, at same time of day
• Height, growth rate of a child
• T$_3$, T$_4$, FTIs, which are decreased; radioimmunoassay of TSH, which is increased; radio uptake, which is increased if patient is on too low a dose of medication
• PT may require decreased anticoagulant; check for bleeding, bruising
• Increased nervousness, excitability, irritability, which may indicate too high

dose of medication, usually after 1-3 wk of treatment

• Cardiac status: angina, palpitation, chest pain, change in VS

Administer:

• IV after diluting with provided diluent 0.5 mg/5 ml; shake; give through Y-tube or 3-way stopcock; give 0.1 mg or less over 1 min; do not add to IV inf; 0.1 mg = 1 ml

• Considered to be incompatible in syringe with all other drugs

• In AM if possible as a single dose to decrease sleeplessness, at same time each day to maintain drug level, take on empty stomach

• Only for hormone imbalances; not to be used for obesity, male infertility, menstrual conditions, lethargy

• Lowest dose that relieves symptoms; lower dose to the elderly and in cardiac diseases

• Crushed and mixed with water, nonsoy formula, or breast milk for infants/ children

Perform/provide:

• Storage in tight, light-resistant container; sol should be discarded if not used immediately

• Withdrawal of medication 4 wk before RAIU test

Evaluate:

• Therapeutic response: absence of depression; increased weight loss, diuresis, pulse, appetite; absence of constipation, peripheral edema, cold intolerance; pale, cool, dry skin; brittle nails, alopecia, coarse hair, menorrhagia, night blindness, paresthesias, syncope, stupor, coma, rosy cheeks

Teach patient/family:

• That hair loss will occur in child, is temporary

• To report excitability, irritability, anxiety, which indicate overdose

• Not to switch brands unless approved by prescriber

• That drug may be discontinued after giving birth, thyroid panel evaluated after 1-2 mo

• That hypothyroid child will show al-

most immediate behavior/personality change

• That drug is not to be taken to reduce weight

• To avoid OTC preparations with iodine; read labels

• To avoid iodine food, iodized salt, soybeans, tofu, turnips, high-iodine seafood, some bread

• That drug is not a cure but controls symptoms and treatment is lifelong

---

⚠ High Alert

lidocaine (parenteral) (℞)
(lye'doe-kane)
LidoPen Auto-Injector,
Xylocaine, Xylocard ✦
Func. class.: Antidysrhythmic (Class Ib)
Chem. class.: Aminoacyl amide

L

Action: Increases electrical stimulation threshold of ventricle, His-Purkinje system, which stabilizes cardiac membrane, decreases automaticity

Uses: Ventricular tachycardia, ventricular dysrhythmias during cardiac surgery, myocardial infarction, digitalis toxicity, cardiac catheterization

DOSAGE AND ROUTES

• *Adult:* **IV BOL** 50-100 mg (1 mg/kg) over 2-3 min, repeat q3-5min, not to exceed 300 mg in 1 hr; begin **IV INF; IV INF** 20-50 mcg/kg/min; **IM** 200-300 mg (4.3 mg/kg) in deltoid muscle, may repeat in 1-1½ hr if needed

• *Elderly, CHF, reduced hepatic function:* **IV BOL** give ½ adult dose

• *Child:* **IV BOL** 1 mg/kg, then **IV INF** 30 mcg/kg/min

Available forms: IV INF 0.2% (2 mg/ ml), 0.4% (4 mg/ml), 0.8% (8 mg/ml); IV ad 4% (40 mg/ml), 10% (100 mg/ ml), 20% (200 mg/ml); IV dir 1% (10 mg/ml), 2% (20 mg/ml); IM 10% 300 mg/ml

---

Side effects: *italics* = common; ***bold italics*** = life-threatening

SIDE EFFECTS

CNS: Headache, dizziness, involuntary movement, confusion, tremor, drowsiness, euphoria, *convulsions*
CV: Hypotension, bradycardia, heart block, cardiovascular collapse, arrest
EENT: Tinnitus, blurred vision
GI: Nausea, vomiting, anorexia
INTEG: Rash, urticaria, edema, swelling
MISC: Febrile response, phlebitis at inj site
RESP: Dyspnea, *respiratory depression*

Contraindications: Hypersensitivity to amides, severe heart block, supraventricular dysrhythmias, Adams-Stokes syndrome, Wolff-Parkinson-White syndrome

Precautions: Pregnancy (B), lactation, children, renal disease, hepatic disease, CHF, respiratory depression, malignant hyperthermia, elderly, myasthenia gravis, weight <50 kg

PHARMACOKINETICS

IV: Onset 2 min, duration 20 min
IM: Onset 5-15 min, duration 1½ hr; half-life 8 min, 1-2 hr (terminal); metabolized in liver; excreted in urine; crosses placenta

INTERACTIONS

Increase: neuromuscular blockade—neuromuscular blockers, tubocurarine
Increase: lidocaine effects—cimetidine, phenytoin, propranolol, metoprolol
Decrease: lidocaine effects—barbiturates

Drug/Herb
Increase: lidocaine action—aloe, buckthorn, cascara sagrada, senna
Increase: toxicity, death—aconite
Increase: effect—aloe, broom, chronic buckthorn use, cascara sagrada (chronic use), Chinese rhubarb, figwort, fumitory, goldenseal, kudzu, licorice
Increase: serotonin effect—horehound
Decrease: effect—coltsfoot

Drug/Lab Test
Increase: CPK

NURSING CONSIDERATIONS

Assess:
⚠ ECG continuously to determine increased PR or QRS segments; if these develop, discontinue or reduce rate; watch for increased ventricular ectopic beats; may have to rebolus, B/P
• IV infusion rate using infusion pump; run at less than 4 mg/min
• Blood levels (therapeutic level: 1.5-5 mcg/ml)
• I&O ratio, electrolytes (K, Na, Cl)
⚠ Malignant hyperthermia: tachypnea, tachycardia, changes in B/P, increased temp
• Respiratory status: rate, rhythm, lung fields for crackles, watch for respiratory depression; lung fields, bilateral crackles may occur in CHF patient; increased respiration, increased pulse; drug should be discontinued
• CNS effects: dizziness, confusion, psychosis, paresthesias, convulsions; drug should be discontinued

Administer:
• IM inj in deltoid; aspirate to avoid intravascular administration; check site daily for infiltration or extravasation
IV route
• Bolus undiluted (1%, 2% only) give 50 mg or less over 1 min or dilute 1 g/250-500 ml of D₅W; titrate to patient response; use infusion pump; pediatric inf is 120 mg of lidocaine/100 ml D₅W; 1-2.5 ml/kg/hr = 20-50 mcg/kg/min; use only 1%, 2% sol for IV bol

Additive compatibilities: Alteplase, aminophylline, amiodarone, atracurium, bretylium, calcium chloride, calcium gluceptate, calcium gluconate, chloramphenicol, chlorothiazide, cimetidine, dexamethasone, digoxin, diphenhydrAMINE, DOBUTamine, DOPamine, epHEDrine, erythromycin lactobionate, floxacillin, flumazenil, furosemide, heparin, hydrocortisone, hydrOXYzine, insulin (regular), mephentermine, metaraminol, nafcillin, nitroglycerin, penicillin G potassium, pentobarbital, phenylephrine, potassium chloride, procainamide, prochlorperazine, promazine, ranitidine, sodium bicarbonate, sodium lactate, theophylline, verapamil, vit B/C

Solution compatibilities: D₅W, D₅/0.9% NaCl, D₅/0.45% NaCl, D₅/LR, LR, 0.9% NaCl, 0.45% NaCl

Syringe compatibilities: Cloxacillin, glycopyrrolate, heparin, hydrOXYzine, methicillin, metoclopramide, milrinone, moxalactam, nalbuphine

Y-site compatibilities: Alteplase, amiodarone, amrinone, cefazolin, ciprofloxacin, cisatracurium, diltiazem, DOBUTamine, DOPamine, enalaprilat, etomidate, famotidine, haloperidol, heparin, heparin/hydrocortisone, labetalol, meperidine, morphine, nitroglycerin, nitroprusside, potassium chloride, propofol, remifentanil, streptokinase, theophylline, vit B/C, warfarin

Evaluate:

• Therapeutic response: decreased dysrhythmias

Teach patient/family:

• The use of automatic lidocaine injection device if ordered for personal use

Treatment of overdose: O₂, artificial ventilation, ECG; administer DOPamine for circulatory depression, diazepam or thiopental for convulsions; decrease drug if needed

---

lidocaine topical
See Appendix C

---

lindane (℞)

(lin′dane)
GBH ✤, G-Well, Hexit ✤, Kwell, lindane, PMS-Lindane ✤, Scabene

Func. class.: Scabicide, pediculicide
Chem. class.: Chlorinated hydrocarbon (synthetic)

Action: Stimulates nervous system of arthropods, resulting in seizures, death of organism

Uses: Scabies, lice (head/pubic/body), nits

DOSAGE AND ROUTES

Lice

• *Adult and child:* **CREAM/LOTION** wash area with soap, water; remove visible crusts; apply to skin surfaces; remove with soap, water in 8-12 hr; may reapply in 1 wk if needed; shampoo using 30 ml: work into lather, rub for 5 min, rinse, dry with towel; comb with fine-toothed comb to remove nits

Scabies

• *Adult and child:* **TOP** apply 1% cream/lotion to skin, neck to bottom of feet, toes; repeat in 1 wk prn

Available forms: Lotion, shampoo, cream (1%)

SIDE EFFECTS

CNS: Tremors, ***seizures, CNS toxicity,*** stimulation, dizziness (chronic inhalation of vapors)

CV: ***Ventricular fibrillation*** (chronic inhalation of vapors)

GI: *Nausea, vomiting, diarrhea,* liver damage (inhalation of vapors)

GU: ***Kidney damage*** (chronic inhalation of vapors)

HEMA: ***Aplastic anemia*** (chronic inhalation of vapors)

INTEG: *Pruritus, rash, irritation, contact dermatitis*

Contraindications: Hypersensitivity; premature neonate; patients with known

seizure disorders; inflammation of skin, abrasions, or skin breaks
Precautions: Pregnancy (B), avoid contact with eyes, children <10 yr, infants, lactation

INTERACTIONS

Oils may increase absorption; if an oil-based hair dressing is used, shampoo, rinse, dry hair before applying lindane shampoo

NURSING CONSIDERATIONS

Assess:
• Head, hair for lice and nits before and after treatment; if scabies are present check all skin surfaces
• Identify source of infection: school, family, sexual contacts

Administer:
• To body areas, scalp only; do not apply to face, lips, mouth, eyes, any mucous membrane, anus, or meatus
• Topical corticosteroids as ordered to decrease contact dermatitis
• Antihistamines
• Lotions of menthol or phenol to control itching
• Topical antibiotics for infection

Perform/provide:
• Isolation until areas on skin, scalp have cleared and treatment is completed
• Removal of nits by using a fine-toothed comb rinsed in vinegar after treatment; use gloves

Evaluate:
• Therapeutic response: decreased crusts, nits, brownish trails on skin, itching papules in skin folds, decreased itching after several weeks

Teach patient/family:
• To wash all inhabitants' clothing, using insecticide; preventive treatment may be required of all persons living in same house, using lotion or shampoo to decrease spread of infection; use rubber gloves when applying drug
• That itching may continue for 4-6 wk
• That drug must be reapplied if accidentally washed off, or treatment will be ineffective

• Not to apply to face; if accidental contact with eyes occurs, flush with water
• Instruct patient to remove after specified time to prevent toxicity
• To treat sexual contacts simultaneously
• To check for CNS toxicity: dizziness, cramps, anxiety, nausea, vomiting, seizures

Treatment of ingestion: Gastric lavage, saline laxatives, IV diazepam (Valium) for convulsions

---

linezolid (℞)
(line-zoe′lide)
Zyvox
Func. class.: Broad-spectrum antiinfective
Chem. class.: Oxazolidinone

Action: Binds to bacterial 23S ribosomal RNA of the 50S subunit preventing formation of the bacterial translation process
Uses: Vancomycin-resistant *Enterococcus faecium* infections, nosocomial pneumonia, uncomplicated or complicated skin and skin structure infections, community-acquired pneumonia

DOSAGE AND ROUTES

Vancomycin-resistant Enterococcus faecium *infections*
• *Adult:* **IV/PO** 600 mg q12h × 14-28 days
Nosocomial pneumonia/complicated skin infections/community-acquired pneumonia/concurrent bacterial infection
• *Adult:* **IV/PO** 600 mg q12h × 10-14 days
Uncomplicated skin infections
• *Adult:* **PO** 400 mg q12h ×10-14 days
• *Adolescents:* **PO** 600 mg q12h × 10-14 days
Available forms: Tab 400, 600 mg; oral sus 100 mg/5 ml; inj 2 mg/ml

SIDE EFFECTS

CNS: Headache, dizziness
GI: Nausea, diarrhea, increased ALT,

⚠ Safety alert   *‶Tall Man" lettering

AST, *vomiting*, taste change, tongue color change

*HEMA: **Myelosuppression***

MISC: Vaginal moniliasis, fungal infection, oral moniliasis

Contraindications: Hypersensitivity

Precautions: Pregnancy (C), lactation, children, thrombocytopenia

PHARMACOKINETICS

Rapidly and extensively absorbed, protein binding 31%, metabolized by oxidation of the morpholine ring

INTERACTIONS

Increase: effects of adrenergic agents, serotonergic agents

NURSING CONSIDERATIONS

Assess:

• CBC weekly, assess for myelosuppression (anemias, leukopenia, pancytopenia, thrombocytopenia)

• CNS symptoms: headache, dizziness

• Hepatic studies: AST, ALT

• Allergic reactions: fever, flushing, rash, urticaria, pruritus

🅐 For pseudomembranous colitis

Administer:

PO route

• With or without food

• Store reconstituted oral suspension at room temperature, use within 3 wk

IV route

• 30-120 min; do not use IV infusion bag in series connections, do not use with additives in sol, do not use with another drug, administer separately

Y-site compatibilities: acyclovir, alfentanil, amikacin, aminophylline, ampicillin, aztreonam, bretylium, buprenorphine, butorphanol, calcium gluconate, carboplatin, cefazolin, cefoperazone, cefotetan, cefoxitin, ceftazidine, ceftizoxime, ceftriaxone, cefuroxime, cimetidine, ciprofloxacin, cisatracurium, cisplatin, clindamycin, cyclophosphamide, cycloSPORINE, cytarabine, hydromorphone, ifosfamide, labetalol, leucovorin, levofloxacin, lidocaine, lorazepam, magnesium sulfate, mannitol, meperidine, meropenem, mesna, methotrexate, methylPREDNISolone, metoclopramide, metronidazole, midazolam, minocycline, mitoxantrone, morphine, nalbuphine, naloxone, nitroglycerin, ofloxacin, ondansetron, paclitaxel, pentobarbital, phenobarbital, piperacillin, potassium chloride, prochlorperazine, promethazine, propranolol, ranitidine, remifentanil, sufentanil, theophylline, ticarcillin, tobramycin, vancomycin, vecuronium, verapamil, vinCRIStine, zidovudine

Solution compatibilities: D₅, 0.9% NaCl, LR

Evaluate:

• Therapeutic response: decreased symptoms of infection, blood cultures negative

Teach patient/family:

• If dizziness occurs, to ambulate, perform activities with assistance

• To complete full course of drug therapy

• To contact prescriber if adverse reaction occurs

• To inform prescriber if SSRIs or cold products, decongestants are being used

• To inform prescriber if there is a history of hypertension

• To avoid large amounts of high-tyramine foods, drinks (provide list)

L

liothyronine (T₃) (℞)

(lye-oh-thye′roe-neen)
Cytomel, ✦triiodothyronine, T₃, liothyronine sodium, Triostat

Func. class.: Thyroid hormone
Chem. class.: Synthetic T₃

Action: Increases metabolic rates, cardiac output, O₂ consumption, body temp, blood volume, growth, development at cellular level; exact mechanism unknown

Uses: Hypothyroidism, myxedema coma, thyroid hormone replacement, congenital hypothyroidism, nontoxic goiter, T₃ suppression test

DOSAGE AND ROUTES

• *Adult:* PO 25 mcg daily, increased by 12.5-25 mcg q1-2wk until desired response, maintenance dose 25-75 mcg daily, max 100 mcg/day
• *Geriatric:* PO 5 mcg/day, increase by 5 mcg/day q1-2wk, maintenance 25-75 mcg/day

Congenital hypothyroidism

• *Child >3 yr:* PO 50-100 mcg daily
• *Child <3 yr:* PO 5 mcg daily, increased by 5 mcg q3-4d titrated to response, maintenance 20 mcg/day

Myxedema, severe hypothyroidism

• *Adult:* PO 25-50 mcg then may increase by 5-10 mcg q1-2wk; maintenance dose 50-100 mcg daily

Myxedema coma/precoma

• *Adult:* IV 25-50 mcg initially, 5 mcg in elderly, 10-20 mcg in cardiac disease; give doses q4-12h

Nontoxic goiter

• *Adult:* PO 5 mcg daily, increased by 12.5-25 mcg q1-2wk; maintenance dose 75 mcg daily

Suppression test

• *Adult:* PO 75-100 mcg daily × 1 wk; radioactive ^{131}I is given before and after 1-wk dose

Available forms: Tabs 5, 25, 50 mcg; inj 10 mcg/ml

SIDE EFFECTS

CNS: Insomnia, tremors, headache, **thyroid storm**
CV: Tachycardia, palpitations, angina, dysrhythmias, hypertension, **cardiac arrest**
GI: Nausea, diarrhea, increased or decreased appetite, cramps
MISC: Menstrual irregularities, weight loss, sweating, heat intolerance, fever, alopecia

Contraindications: Adrenal insufficiency, myocardial infarction, thyrotoxicosis

Precautions: Pregnancy (A), elderly, angina pectoris, hypertension, ischemia, cardiac disease, lactation, diabetes

PHARMACOKINETICS

PO/IV: Peak 12-48 hr, duration 72 hr, half-life 1-2 days

INTERACTIONS

Increase: effects of anticoagulants, sympathomimetics, tricyclics, amphetamines, decongestants, vasopressors
Decrease: absorption of liothyronine—cholestyramine, colestipol
Decrease: effects of digoxin, insulin, hypoglycemics
Decrease: effects of liothyronine—estrogens
Drug/Herb
Decrease: thyroid hormone effect—agar, bugleweed, carnitine, kelpware, soy, spirulina
Drug/Lab Test
Increase: CPK, LDH, AST, PBI, blood glucose
Decrease: Thyroid function tests

NURSING CONSIDERATIONS

Assess:

• B/P, pulse, periodically during treatment
• Weight daily in same clothing, using same scale, at same time of day
• Height, growth rate of child
• T$_3$, T$_4$, which are decreased; radioimmunoassay of TSH, which is increased; radio uptake, which is increased if patient is on too low a dose of medication
• PT may require decreased anticoagulant; check for bleeding, bruising
• Increased nervousness, excitability, irritability, which may indicate too high dose of medication, usually after 1-3 wk of treatment
• Cardiac status: angina, palpitation, chest pain, change in VS

Administer:

• In AM if possible as a single dose to decrease sleeplessness
• At same time each day to maintain drug level
• Only for hormone imbalances; not to

be used for obesity, male infertility, menstrual conditions, lethargy
• Lowest dose that relieves symptoms
• Liothyronine after discontinuing other thyroid preparation

Perform/provide:
• Removal of medication 4 wk before RAIU test

Evaluate:
• Therapeutic response: absence of depression; increased weight loss, diuresis, pulse, appetite; absence of constipation, peripheral edema, cold intolerance; pale, cool, dry skin; brittle nails, alopecia, coarse hair, menorrhagia, night blindness, paresthesia, syncope, stupor, coma, rosy cheeks

Teach patient/family:
• That hair loss will occur in child but is temporary
• To report excitability, irritability, anxiety, which indicates overdose
• Not to switch brands unless approved by prescriber
• That hypothyroid child will show almost immediate behavior/personality change
• That drug is not to be taken to reduce weight
• To avoid OTC preparations with iodine; read labels
• To avoid iodine food, iodized salt, soybeans, tofu, turnips, high iodine seafood, some bread
• That drug controls symptoms but does not cure; treatment is lifelong

liotrix (R)
(lye′oh-trix)
Thyrolar, T₃/T₄
Func. class.: Thyroid hormone
Chem. class.: Levothyroxine/liothyronine (synthetic T₄, T₃)

Do not confuse:
Thyrolar/Thyrar
Action: Increases metabolic rates, cardiac output, O_2 consumption, body temp, blood volume, growth, development at cellular level, exact mechanism unknown

Uses: Hypothyroidism, thyroid hormone replacement

DOSAGE AND ROUTES
• *Adult:* PO a single dose of Thyrolar ¼ or ½, adjust as needed at 2-wk intervals
• *Geriatric:* PO ¼ tab, initially, adjust q6-8 wks

Available forms: Tabs: Levothyoxine 12.5 mcg/liothyronine 3.1 mcg; levothyroxine 25 mcg/liothyronine 6.25 mcg (Tyrolar-½); levothyroxine 50 mcg/liothyronine 12.5 mcg (Thyrolar-1); levothyroxine 100 mcg/liothyronine 25 mcg (Thyrolar-2); levothyroxine 150 mcg/liothyronine 37.5 mcg (Thyrolar-3)

SIDE EFFECTS
CNS: Insomnia, tremors, headache, ***thyroid storm***
CV: Tachycardia, palpitations, angina, dysrhythmias, hypertension, ***cardiac arrest***
GI: Nausea, diarrhea, increased or decreased appetite, cramps
MISC: Menstrual irregularities, weight loss, sweating, heat intolerance, fever
Contraindications: Adrenal insufficiency, myocardial infarction, thyrotoxicosis
Precautions: Pregnancy (A), elderly, angina pectoris, hypertension, ischemia, cardiac disease, lactation, diabetes

PHARMACOKINETICS
PO (T_4): Onset unknown, peak 1-3 wk, duration 1-3 wk
PO (T_3): Onset unknown, peak 24-72 hr, duration 72 hr, half-life 1 wk

INTERACTIONS
Increase: effects of amphetamines, decongestants, vasopressors, anticoagulants, sympathomimetics, tricyclics, catecholamines
Decrease: absorption of liotrix—cholestyramine, colestipol
Decrease: effects of digoxin, insulin, hypoglycemics
Decrease: effects of liotrix—estrogens

L

Side effects: *italics* = common; ***bold italics*** = life-threatening

Drug/Herb
Decrease: thyroid hormone effect—agar, bugleweed, carnitine, kelpware, soy, spirulina

Drug/Lab Test
Increase: CPK, LDH, AST, PBI, blood glucose
Decrease: Thyroid function tests

NURSING CONSIDERATIONS

Assess:
• B/P, pulse periodically during treatment
• Weight daily in same clothing, using same scale, at same time of day
• Height, growth rate of child
• T_3, T_4, FTIs, which are decreased; radioimmunoassay of TSH, which is increased; radio uptake, which is increased if patient is on too low a dose of medication
• PT may require decreased anticoagulant; check for bleeding, bruising
• Increased nervousness, excitability, irritability, which may indicate too high dose of medication, usually after 1-3 wk of treatment
• Cardiac status: angina, palpitation, chest pain, change in VS

Administer:
• In AM if possible as a single dose to decrease sleeplessness
• At same time each day to maintain drug level
• Only for hormone imbalances; not to be used for obesity, male infertility, menstrual conditions, lethargy
• Lowest dose that relieves symptoms

Perform/provide:
• Withdrawal of medication 4 wk before RAIU test
• Storage in airtight, light-resistant container

Evaluate:
• Therapeutic response: absence of depression; increased weight loss, diuresis, pulse, appetite; absence of constipation, peripheral edema, cold intolerance; pale, cool, dry skin; brittle nails, coarse hair, menorrhagia, night blindness, par-

esthesias, syncope, stupor, coma, rosy cheeks

Teach patient/family:
• That hair loss will occur in child, is temporary
• To report excitability, irritability, chest pain, increased pulse rate, palpitations, excessive sweating, heat intolerance, nervousness, anxiety, which indicate overdose
• Not to switch brands unless approved by prescriber
• That hypothyroid child will show almost immediate behavior/personality change
• That drug is not to be taken to reduce weight
• To avoid OTC preparations with iodine; read labels
• To avoid iodine food, iodized salt, soybeans, tofu, turnips, high iodine seafood, some bread
• That drug does not cure, but controls symptoms, treatment is lifelong

---

lisinopril (℞)
(lyse-in'oh-pril)
Prinivil, Zestril
Func. class.: Antihypertensive, angiotensin converting enzyme inhibitor (ACE)
Chem. class.: Enalaprilat lysine analog

Do not confuse:
lisinopril/Risperdal
Prinivil/Plendil/Proventil
Prinivil/Prilosec

Action: Selectively suppresses renin-angiotensin-aldosterone system; inhibits ACE, preventing conversion of angiotensin I to angiotensin II
Uses: Mild to moderate hypertension, adjunctive therapy of systolic CHF, acute MI

DOSAGE AND ROUTES

Hypertension
• *Adult:* PO 10-40 mg daily; may increase to 80 mg daily if required

---

• *Geriatric:* **PO** 2.5-5 mg/day, increase q7d

CHF

• *Adult:* **PO** 5 mg initially with diuretics/digitalis, range 5-20 mg

Available forms: Tabs 2.5, 5, 10, 20, 30, 40 mg

SIDE EFFECTS

CNS: Vertigo, depression, **stroke,** insomnia, paresthesias, headache, *fatigue,* asthenia, dizziness
CV: Chest pain, hypotension
EENT: Blurred vision, nasal congestion
GI: Nausea, vomiting, anorexia, constipation, flatulence, GI irritation, diarrhea
*GU: **Proteinuria, renal insufficiency,*** sexual dysfunction, impotence
INTEG: Rash, pruritus
MISC: Muscle cramps
RESP: Dry cough, dyspnea
*SYST: **Angioedema***

Contraindications: Pregnancy (D) 2nd/3rd trimesters, hypersensitivity
Precautions: Pregnancy (C) 1st trimester, lactation, renal disease, hyperkalemia, renal artery stenosis

PHARMACOKINETICS

Onset 1 hr, peak 6-8 hr, duration 24 hr; excreted unchanged in urine

INTERACTIONS

Hyperkalemia: potassium salt substitutes, potassium-sparing diuretics, potassium supplements, cycloSPORINE
Possible toxicity: lithium, digoxin
Increase: hypotensive effect—diuretics, other hypertensives, probenecid, phenothiazines, nitrates, acute alcohol ingestion
Increase: hypersensitivity—allopurinol
Decrease: lisinopril effects—aspirin, indomethacin, NSAIDs

Drug/Herb

Increase: toxicity, death—aconite
Increase: antihypertensive effect—barberry, betony, black catechu, black cohosh, bloodroot, broom, burdock, cat's claw, dandelion, goldenseal, Irish moss, Jamaican dogwood, kelp, khella, mistletoe, parsley

Increase or decrease: antihypertensive effect—astragalus, cola tree
Decrease: antihypertensive effect—coltsfoot, guarana, khat, licorice

Drug/Food

High-potassium diet (bananas, orange juice, avocados, nuts, spinach) should be avoided; hyperkalemia may occur

Drug/Lab Test

Interference: Glucose/insulin tolerance tests, ANA titer

NURSING CONSIDERATIONS

Assess:

⚠ Blood studies, platelets; WBC with diff baseline and periodically q3mo; if neutrophils <1000/mm^3, discontinue treatment (recommended in collagen-vascular disease)
• B/P, pulse q4h; note rate, rhythm, quality
• Electrolytes: K, Na, Cl
• Apical/pedal pulse before administration; notify prescriber of any significant changes
• Baselines in renal, hepatic studies before therapy begins and periodically LFTs, uric acid and glucose may be increased
• Edema in feet, legs daily, weight daily in CHF
• Skin turgor, dryness of mucous membranes for hydration status
• Symptoms of CHF: edema, dyspnea, wet crackles

Administer:

• Severe hypotension may occur after 1st dose of this medication; may be prevented by reducing or discontinuing diuretic therapy 3 days before beginning lisinopril therapy

Evaluate:

• Therapeutic response: decreased B/P, CHF symptoms

Teach patient/family:

• Not to discontinue drug abruptly
• To rise slowly to sitting or standing position to minimize orthostatic hypotension
• To avoid increasing potassium in the diet

Treatment of overdose: Lavage, IV atropine for bradycardia, IV theophylline for bronchospasm, digitalis, O_2, diuretic for cardiac failure

---

lithium (℞)

(li'thee-um)
Carbolith ✿, Duralith ✿,
Eskalith, Eskalith-CR, lithium
carbonate, Lithizine ✿,
Lithonate, Lithotabs
Func. class.: Antimanic, antipsychotic
Chem. class.: Alkali metal ion salt

Action: May alter sodium, potassium ion transport across cell membrane in nerve, muscle cells; may balance biogenic amines of norepinephrine, serotonin in CNS areas involved in emotional responses

Uses: Bipolar disorders (manic phase), prevention of bipolar manic-depressive psychosis

DOSAGE AND ROUTES

• *Adult:* **PO** 300-600 mg tid, maintenance 300 mg tid or qid; **SLOW REL TABS** 300 mg bid; dose should be individualized to maintain blood levels at 0.5-1.5 mEq/L
• *Geriatric:* **PO** 300 mg bid, increase q7 days by 300 mg to desired dose
• *Child:* **PO** 15-20 mg (0.4-0.5 mEq/kg/day in 2-3 divided doses, increase as needed, do not exceed adult doses)
Renal dose
• **PO** CCr 10-50 ml/min 50%-75% of dose; CCr <10 ml/min 25%-50% of dose
Available forms: Caps 150, 300, 600 mg; tabs 300 mg; tabs ext rel 300, 450 mg; syr 300 mg/5 ml (8 mEq/5 ml); cap slow rel 150, 300 mg ✿

SIDE EFFECTS

CNS: Headache, drowsiness, dizziness, tremors, twitching, ataxia, *seizure,* slurred speech, restlessness, confusion, stupor, memory loss, clonic movements, fatigue

CV: Hypotension, ECG changes, ***dysrhythmias, circulatory collapse,*** edema

EENT: Tinnitus, blurred vision

ENDO: Hyponatremia, hypothyroidism, goiter, hyperglycemia, hyperthyroidism

GI: Dry mouth, anorexia, nausea, vomiting, diarrhea, incontinence, abdominal pain, metallic taste

*GU: **Polyuria, glycosuria, proteinuria, albuminuria,*** urinary incontinence, polydipsia

*HEMA: **Leukocytosis***

INTEG: Drying of hair, alopecia, rash, pruritus, hyperkeratosis, acneiform lesions, folliculitis

MS: Muscle weakness

Contraindications: Pregnancy (D), hepatic disease, brain trauma, OBS, lactation, children <12 yr, schizophrenia, severe cardiac disease, severe renal disease, severe dehydration

Precautions: Elderly, thyroid disease, seizure disorders, diabetes mellitus, systemic infection, urinary retention

PHARMACOKINETICS

PO: Onset rapid, peak ½-4 hr, half-life 18-36 hr depending on age; crosses blood-brain barrier; 80% of filtered lithium is reabsorbed by the renal tubules, excreted in urine; crosses placenta; enters breast milk; well absorbed by oral method

INTERACTIONS

Neurotoxicity: haloperidol, thioridazine

Increase: hypothyroid effects—antithyroid agents, calcium iodide, potassium iodide, iodinated glycerol

Increase: effects of neuromuscular blocking agents, phenothiazines

Increase: renal clearance—sodium bicarbonate, acetaZOLAMIDE, mannitol, aminophylline

Increase: toxicity—indomethacin, diuretics, nonsteroidal antiinflammatories, losartan

---

Increase: lithium effect/toxicity—carbamazepine, fluoxetine, methyldopa, NSAIDs, thiazide diuretics, probenecid
Decrease: lithium effects—theophyllines, urea, urinary alkalinizers

Drug/Herb
Increase: lithium effects, increase toxicity—broom, buchu, dandelion, goldenrod, horsetail, juniper, nettle, parsley
Decrease: lithium levels—black/green tea, coffee, cola nut, guarana, plantain, yerba maté

Drug/Food
Significant changes in sodium intake will alter lithium excretion

Drug/Lab Test
Increase: Potassium excretion, urine glucose, blood glucose, protein, BUN
Decrease: VMA, T_3, T_4, PBI, ^{131}I

NURSING CONSIDERATIONS
Assess:
• Weight daily; check for and report edema in legs, ankles, wrists
• Sodium intake; decreased sodium intake with decreased fluid intake may lead to lithium retention; increased sodium and fluids may decrease lithium retention
• Skin turgor at least daily
• Urine for albuminuria, glycosuria, uric acid during beginning treatment, q2mo thereafter
• Neurologic status: LOC, gait, motor reflexes, hand tremors
• Serum lithium levels qwk initially, then q2mo (therapeutic level: 0.5-1.5 mEq/L)

Administer:
• Do not break, crush, or chew caps, ext rel tabs
• Reduced dose to elderly
• With meals to avoid GI upset
• Adequate fluids (2-3 L/day) to prevent dehydration during initial treatment, 1-2 L/day during maintenance

Evaluate:
• Therapeutic response: decrease in excitement, manic phase

Teach patient/family:
• The symptoms of minor toxicity: vomiting, diarrhea, poor coordination, fine motor tremors, weakness, lassitude; major toxicity: coarse tremors, severe thirst, tinnitus, diluted urine
• To monitor urine specific gravity, emphasize need for follow-up care to determine lithium levels; monitor lithium levels to ensure effective levels and treatment
• That contraception is necessary, since lithium may harm fetus
• Not to operate machinery until lithium levels are stable
• That beneficial effects may take 1-3 wk
• About drugs that interact with lithium (provide list) and discuss need for adequate stable intake of salt and fluids

Treatment of overdose: Induce emesis or lavage, maintain airway, respiratory function; dialysis for severe intoxication

---

Iodoxamide ophthalmic
See Appendix C

L

---

lomefloxacin (℞)
(lo-meh-flox′a-sin)
Maxaquin
Func. class.: Antiinfective
Chem. class.: Fluoroquinolone

Action: Interferes with conversion of intermediate DNA fragments into high-molecular-weight DNA in bacteria; DNA gyrase inhibitor

Uses: Treatment of lower respiratory tract infections (pneumonia, bronchitis), genitourinary infections (prostatitis, UTIs), preoperatively to reduce UTIs in transurethral surgical procedures; gram-negative bacteria: *Aeromonas, Citrobacter, Enterobacter, Escherichia coli, Haemophilus influenzae, Klebsiella, Legionella, Moraxella catarrhalis, Morganella morganii, Proteus vulgaris, Proteus mirabilis, Providencia alcalifaciens, Providencia rettgeri, Pseudomonas aeruginosa, Serratia;* gram-positive bacteria: *Staphylococcus*

Side effects: *italics* = common; ***bold italics*** = life-threatening

aureus, Staphylococcus epidermidis,
Staphylococcus saprophyticus

DOSAGE AND ROUTES

Lower respiratory tract infection/
uncomplicated cystitis
• *Adult:* **PO** 400 mg daily × 10 day
Complicated UTI
• *Adult:* **PO** 400 mg daily × 14 days
depending on type of infection
Surgical prophylaxis
• *Adult:* **PO** 400 mg 2-6 hr before sur-
gery
Renal dose
• *Adult:* **PO** CCr ≤40 ml/min 400 mg,
then 200 mg/day
Available forms: Tabs 400 mg

SIDE EFFECTS

CNS: Dizziness, headache, somnolence,
depression, insomnia, nervousness,
confusion, agitation, ***seizures***
EENT: Visual disturbances
GI: Diarrhea, *nausea,* vomiting, anorexia, flatulence, heartburn, dry mouth;
increased AST, ALT; constipation, abdominal pain, oral thrush, glossitis, stomatitis, ***pseudomembranous colitis***
INTEG: Rash, pruritus, urticaria, *photo-*
sensitivity
*SYST: **Anaphylaxis, Stevens-Johnson***
syndrome
Contraindications: Hypersensitivity
to quinolones
Precautions: Pregnancy (C), lactation,
children, elderly, renal disease, seizure
disorders, excessive exposure to sunlight, psychosis, increased intracranial
pressure

PHARMACOKINETICS

PO: Peak 1-2 hr, half-life 6-8 hr; excreted in urine as active drug, metabolites

INTERACTIONS

Increase: CNS stimulation, seizures—
NSAIDs
Increase: lomefloxacin toxicity—
cimetidine, probenecid

Increase: levels—cycloSPORINE, warfarin, watch for toxicity
Decrease: absorption—antacids containing aluminum, magnesium, sucralfate, zinc, iron
Drug/Herb
Increase: antiinfective effect—cola tree

NURSING CONSIDERATIONS
Assess:
• Renal, hepatic studies: BUN, creatinine, AST, ALT
• I&O ratio; urine pH, <5.5 is ideal
• CNS symptoms: insomnia, vertigo,
headache, agitation, confusion
⚠ Allergic reactions and anaphylaxis:
rash, flushing, urticaria, pruritus, chills,
fever, joint pain; may occur a few days
after therapy begins; epINEPHrine and
resuscitation equipment should be available for anaphylactic reaction
• Bowel pattern daily, if severe diarrhea
occurs, drug should be discontinued
• For overgrowth of infection: perineal
itching, fever, malaise, redness, pain,
swelling, drainage, rash, diarrhea,
change in cough, sputum
Administer:
• After clean-catch urine for C&S
• 4 hr before or 2 hr after antacids, iron,
calcium, zinc products
Evaluate:
• Therapeutic response: negative C&S,
absence of signs/symptoms of infection
Teach patient/family:
• That fluids must be increased to 2
L/day to avoid crystallization in kidneys
• That if dizziness or light-headedness
occurs, to ambulate, perform activities
with assistance
• To complete full course of drug ther-
apy
• To contact prescriber if adverse reac-
tions occur
• To avoid iron- or mineral-containing
supplements or antacids within 4 hr
before and after dosing
• That photosensitivity may occur and
sunscreen should be used
• To use frequent rinsing of mouth,
sugarless candy or gum for dry mouth

⚠ Safety alert   *"Tall Man" lettering

• To avoid other medication unless approved by prescriber

lomustine (R)

(loe-mus′teen)

CCNU, CeeNU

Func. class.: Antineoplastic alkylating agent

Chem. class.: Nitrosourea

Action: Responsible for crosslinking DNA strands, which leads to cell death; activity is not cell cycle phase specific

Uses: Hodgkin's disease, lymphomas, melanomas, multiple myeloma; brain, lung, bladder, kidney, colon cancer

Investigational uses: Brain, breast, renal, GI tract, bronchogenic carcinoma; melanomas

DOSAGE AND ROUTES

• *Adult:* **PO** 130 mg/m^2 as a single dose q6wk; titrate dose to WBC; do not give repeat dose unless WBC >4000/mm^3, platelet count >100,000/mm^3

Available forms: Caps 10, 40, 100 mg

SIDE EFFECTS

*GI: Nausea, vomiting, anorexia, stomatitis, **hepatotoxicity***

GU: Azotemia, renal failure

*HEMA: **Thrombocytopenia, leukopenia, myelosuppression, anemia***

*RESP: **Fibrosis, pulmonary infiltrate***

Contraindications: Pregnancy (D), hypersensitivity, leukopenia, thrombocytopenia, lactation, "blastic" phase of CML

Precautions: Radiation therapy

PHARMACOKINETICS

Metabolized in liver, excreted in urine; half-life 16-48 hr; 50% protein bound; crosses blood-brain barrier; appears in breast milk

INTERACTIONS

Lomustine potentiation: succinylcholine

Increase: bleeding—aspirin, anticoagulants

Increase: toxicity—barbiturates, phenytoin, chloral hydrate

Increase: lomustine metabolism—phenobarbital

Increase: bone marrow depression—allopurinol

Drug/Lab Test

False positive: Cytology tests for breast, bladder, cervix, lung

NURSING CONSIDERATIONS

Assess:

• CBC, differential, platelet count qwk; withhold drug if WBC <4000/mm^3 or platelet count <100,000/mm^3; notify prescriber

• Pulmonary function tests, chest x-ray films before, during therapy; chest film should be obtained q2wk during treatment

• Renal studies: BUN, serum uric acid, urine CCr before, during therapy

• I&O ratio; report fall in urine output of 30 ml/hr

• Monitor temp q4h (may indicate beginning infection); no rectal temps

• Hepatic studies before, during therapy (bilirubin, AST, ALT, LDH) as needed or monthly

• Bleeding: hematuria, guaiac, bruising or petechiae, mucosa or orifices q8h

• Dyspnea, crackles, unproductive cough, chest pain, tachypnea

• Food preferences; list likes, dislikes

• Jaundiced skin and sclera, dark urine, clay-colored stools, itchy skin, abdominal pain, fever, diarrhea

• Inflammation of mucosa, breaks in skin

• Buccal cavity q8h for dryness, sores or ulceration, white patches, oral pain, bleeding, dysphagia

• Local irritation, pain, burning, discoloration at inj site

⚠ Symptoms indicating severe allergic

reaction: rash, pruritus, urticaria, purpuric skin lesions, itching, flushing

Administer:
• Antiemetic 30-60 min before giving drug to prevent vomiting
• Antibiotics for prophylaxis of infection

Perform/provide:
• Storage in tight container at room temperature
• Strict medical asepsis, protective isolation if WBC levels are low
• Deep-breathing exercises with patient tid-qid; place in semi-Fowler's position
• Rinsing of mouth tid-qid with water, club soda; brushing of teeth bid-tid with soft brush or cotton-tipped applicators for stomatitis; use unwaxed dental floss

Evaluate:
• Therapeutic response: decreased tumor size, spread of malignancy

Teach patient/family:
• About protective isolation
• To report any changes in breathing or coughing
• To avoid foods with citric acid, hot or rough texture if buccal inflammation is present
• To report any bleeding, white spots, or ulcerations in mouth to prescriber; tell patient to examine mouth daily
• To report signs of infection: fever, sore throat, flulike symptoms
• To use essective contraception, aviod breast feeding
• To report signs of anemia: fatigue, headache, faintness, shortness of breath, irritability
• To avoid use of razors, commercial mouthwash
• To avoid use of all OTC meds
• To take entire dose at one time

---

loperamide (otc, ℞)
(loe-per′a-mide)
loperamide solution, Imodium, Imodium A-D, Imodium A-D Caplet, loperamide, Kaopectate II Caplets, Maalox Antidiarrheal Caplets, Neo-Diaral, Pepto Diarrhea Control
Func. class.: Antidiarrheal
Chem. class.: Piperidine derivative

Action: Direct action on intestinal muscles to decrease GI peristalsis; reduces volume, increases bulk, electrolytes not lost

Uses: Diarrhea (cause undetermined), travelers diarrhea, chronic diarrhea, to decrease amount of ileostomy discharge

DOSAGE AND ROUTES
• *Adult:* **PO** 4 mg, then 2 mg after each loose stool, max 16 mg/day
• *Child 9-11 yr:* **PO** 2 mg, then 1 mg after each loose stool, max 6 mg/24 hr
• *Child 2-5 yr:* **PO** 1 mg then 0.1 mg/kg after each loose stool, max 4 mg/24 hr
Available forms: Caps 2 mg; liq 1 mg/5 ml; tabs 2 mg

SIDE EFFECTS
CNS: Dizziness, drowsiness, fatigue, fever
GI: Nausea, dry mouth, vomiting, constipation, abdominal pain, anorexia, *toxic megacolon*
INTEG: Rash

Contraindications: Hypersensitivity, severe ulcerative colitis, pseudomembranous colitis, acute diarrhea associated with *Escherichia coli*

Precautions: Pregnancy (B), lactation, children <2 yr, hepatic disease, dehydration, bacterial disease

PHARMACOKINETICS
PO: Onset ½-1 hr, duration 4-5 hr, half-life 7-14 hr; metabolized in liver; excreted in feces as unchanged drug; small amount in urine

---

INTERACTIONS

Increase: CNS depression—alcohol, antihistamines, analgesics, opioids, sedative/hypnotics

Drug/Herb

Increase: CNS depression—chamomile, hops, kava, skullcap, valerian

Increase: antidiarrheal effect—nutmeg

NURSING CONSIDERATIONS

Assess:

• Stools: volume, color, characteristics
• Electrolytes (K, Na, Cl) if on long-term therapy
• Skin turgor q8h if dehydration is suspected
• Bowel pattern before; for rebound constipation
• Response after 48 hr; if no response, drug should be discontinued
• Dehydration, CNS problems in children
• Abdominal distention, toxic megacolon; may occur in ulcerative colitis

Administer:

• Do not break, crush, or chew caps
• For 48 hr only
• Do not mix oral sol with other sols

Perform/provide:

• Storage in tight container

Evaluate:

• Therapeutic response: decreased diarrhea

Teach patient/family:

• To avoid OTC products unless directed by prescriber
• That ileostomy patient may take this drug for extended time
• That if drowsiness occurs, not to operate machinery
• To use hard candy, sips of water for dry mouth

loracarbef
See cephalosporins—2nd generation

loratadine (OTC, ℞)
(lor-a'ti-deen)
Alavert, Claritin, Claritin Non-Drowsy Allergy, Claritin Reditabs, Tavist ND
Func. class.: Antihistamine, 2nd generation
Chem. class.: Selective histamine (H_1)-receptor antagonist

Action: Binds to peripheral histamine receptors, providing antihistamine action without sedation
Uses: Seasonal rhinitis, chronic idiopathic urticaria for those ≥2 yr

DOSAGE AND ROUTES

• *Adult and child ≥6 yr:* **PO** 10 mg daily
• *Child 2-5 yr:* **PO** 5 mg daily

Renal dose

• *Adult:* 10 mg every other day (CCr <30 ml/min)

Hepatic dose

• *Adult:* **PO** 10 mg every other day

Available forms: Tabs 10 mg; tabs rapid-disintegrating 10 mg; tabs, orally disintegrating 10 mg; syr 1 mg/ml; susp 5 mg/ml

SIDE EFFECTS

CNS: Sedation (more common with increased doses), headache
Contraindications: Hypersensitivity, acute asthma attacks, lower respiratory tract disease
Precautions: Pregnancy (B), increased intraocular pressure, bronchial asthma

PHARMACOKINETICS

Onset 1-3 hr, peak 8-12 hr, duration <24 hr, elimination half-life; metabolized in liver to active metabolites, excreted in urine; active metabolite desloratadine half-life 17-28 hr

INTERACTIONS

Increase: antihistamine effects—MAOIs
Increase: CNS depressant effects—

Side effects: *italics* = common; ***bold italics*** = life-threatening

alcohol, antidepressants, other antihistamines, sedative/hypnotics

Increase: loratadine level—cimetidine, ketoconazole, macrolides (clarithromycin, erythromycin)

Drug/Herb

Increase: CNS depression—chamomile, hops, Jamaican dogwood, kava, khat, senega, skullcap, valerian

Increase: anticholinergic effect—corkwood, henbane leaf

Drug/Lab Test

False negative: Skin allergy tests (discontinue antihistamine 3 days before testing)

NURSING CONSIDERATIONS

Assess:

• Allergy: hives, rash, rhinitis; monitor respiratory status

Administer:

• Rapid-disintegrating tabs by placing on tongue, then swallow after disintegrated with or without water

• Use within 6 mo of opening pouch, immediately after opening blister pack

• On empty stomach daily

Perform/provide:

• Storage in tight container at room temperature

Evaluate:

• Therapeutic response: absence of running or congested nose, other allergy symptoms

Teach patient/family:

• To avoid driving, other hazardous activities if drowsiness occurs

• To use sunscreen or stay out of the sun to prevent photosensitivity

• To avoid use of other CNS depressants

---

lorazepam (℞)

(lor-a′ze-pam)
Apo-Lorazepam ✦, Ativan, lorazepam, Novo-Lorazem ✦, Nu-Loraz ✦
Func. class.: Sedative, hypnotic; antianxiety
Chem. class.: Benzodiazepine

Controlled Substance Schedule IV

Do not confuse:
lorazepam/alprazolam/clonazepam

Action: Potentiates the actions of GABA, especially in system and reticular formation

Uses: Anxiety, irritability in psychiatric or organic disorders, preoperatively, insomnia, adjunct in endoscopic procedures

Investigational uses: Antiemetic prior to chemotherapy, status epilepticus, rectal use

DOSAGE AND ROUTES

Anxiety

• *Adult:* **PO** 2-6 mg/day in divided doses, max 10 mg/day

• *Geriatric:* **PO** 0.5-1 mg/day in divided doses; or 0.5-1 mg at bedtime

• *Child:* **PO** 0.05 mg/kg/dose, q4-8h

Insomnia

• *Adult:* **PO** 2-4 mg at bedtime; only minimally effective after 2 wk continuous therapy

• *Geriatric:* **PO** 1-2 mg initially

Preoperatively

• *Adult:* **IM** 50 mcg/kg 2 hr prior to surgery; **IV** 44 mcg/kg 15-20 min prior to surgery, max 2 mg 15-20 min prior to surgery

• *Child:* **IV** 0.05 mg/kg

Status epilepticus

• *Neonate:* **IV** 0.05 mg/kg

• *Child:* **IV** 0.1 mg/kg up to 4 mg/dose; rectal (off label) 0.05-0.1 mg ×2; wait 7 min before giving 2nd dose

Available forms: Tabs 0.5, 1, 2 mg; inj 2, 4 mg/ml; conc oral sol 2 mg/ml

---

SIDE EFFECTS

CNS: Dizziness, drowsiness, confusion, headache, anxiety, tremors, stimulation, fatigue, depression, insomnia, hallucinations, weakness, unsteadiness

*CV: Orthostatic hypotension, **ECG changes, tachycardia,** hypotension; **apnea, cardiac arrest (IV, rapid)***

EENT: Blurred vision, tinnitus, mydriasis

GI: Constipation, dry mouth, nausea, vomiting, anorexia, diarrhea

INTEG: Rash, dermatitis, itching

Contraindications: Pregnancy (D), hypersensitivity to benzodiazepines, narrow-angle glaucoma, psychosis, lactation, history of drug abuse, COPD

Precautions: Elderly, debilitated, hepatic disease, renal disease, child <12 yr

PHARMACOKINETICS

PO: Onset ½ hr, peak 1-6 hr, duration 24-48 hr

IM: Onset 15-30 min, peak 1-1½ hr, duration 24-48 hr

IV: Onset 5-15 min, peak unknown, duration 24-48 hr

Metabolized by liver; excreted by kidneys; crosses placenta, breast milk; half-life 14 hr

INTERACTIONS

Increase: lorazepam effects—CNS depressants, alcohol, disulfiram, oral contraceptives

Decrease: lorazepam effects—valproic acid

Drug/Herb

Increase: hypotension—black cohosh

Increase: CNS depression—catnip, chamomile, clary, cowslip, hops, kava, lavender, mistletoe, nettle, pokeweed, poppy, Queen Anne's lace, senega, skullcap, valerian

Drug/Lab Test

Increase: AST, ALT, serum bilirubin

Decrease: RAIU

False increase: 17-OHCS

NURSING CONSIDERATIONS

Assess:

• B/P (lying, standing), pulse; if systolic B/P drops 20 mm Hg, hold drug, notify prescriber; respirations q5-15min if given IV

• Blood studies: CBC during long-term therapy; blood dyscrasias have occurred rarely

• Hepatic studies: AST, ALT, bilirubin, creatinine, LDH, alk phosphatase

• Mental status: mood, sensorium, affect, sleeping pattern, drowsiness, dizziness

• Physical dependency, withdrawal symptoms: headache, nausea, vomiting, muscle pain, weakness, tremors, convulsions, after long-term, excessive use

⚠ Suicidal tendencies

Administer:

• With food or milk for GI symptoms

• Crushed if patient is unable to swallow medication whole

• Sugarless gum, hard candy, frequent sips of water for dry mouth

• Deep into large muscle mass (IM inj)

IV route

• Prepare immediately before use, short stability time

• IV after diluting in equal vol sterile H_2O, 5% dextrose or 0.9% NaCl for inj; give through Y-tube or 3-way stopcock; give at 2 mg or less over 1 min

Syringe compatibilities: Cimetidine, hydromorphone

Y-site compatibilities: Acyclovir, albumin, allopurinol, amifostine, amikacin, amoxicillin, amoxicillin/clavulanate, amphotericin B cholesteryl, amsacrine, atracurium, bumetanide, cefepime, cefmetazole, cefotaxime, ciprofloxacin, cisatracurium, cisplatin, cladribine, clonidine, cyclophosphamide, cytarabine, dexamethasone, diltiazem, DOBUTamine, DOPamine, DOXOrubicin, DOXOrubicin liposome, epINEPHrine, erythromycin, etomidate, famotidine, fentanyl, filgrastim, fluconazole, fludarabine, furosemide, gentamicin, granisetron, haloperidol, heparin, hydrocortisone, hydromorphone, ketanserin, labetalol, melphalan, methotrexate, metronidazole, midazolam, milrinone, morphine, niCARdipine, nitroglycerin, norepinephrine, paclitaxel, pancuronium, piperacillin, piperacillin/tazobactam, potassium chloride, propofol, ranitidine, remifentanil, tacrolimus, teniposide, thiotepa, trimethoprim-sulfamethoxazole, vancomycin, vecuronium, vinorelbine, zidovudine

Perform/provide:

• Assistance with ambulation during beginning therapy, since drowsiness/dizziness occurs

• Check to see if PO medication has been swallowed

• Refrigerate parenteral form

Evaluate:

• Therapeutic response: decreased anxiety, restlessness, insomnia

Teach patient/family:

• That drug may be taken with food

• Not to use drug for everyday stress or used longer than 4 mo unless directed by prescriber

• Not to take more than prescribed amount; may be habit forming

• To avoid OTC preparations (cough, cold, hay fever) unless approved by prescriber

• To avoid driving, activities that require alertness, since drowsiness may occur

• To avoid alcohol ingestion, other psychotropic medications, unless directed by prescriber

• Not to discontinue medication abruptly after long-term use

• To rise slowly or fainting may occur, especially elderly

• That drowsiness may worsen at beginning of treatment

• To use birth control if child-bearing age

Treatment of overdose: Lavage, VS, supportive care, flumazenil

---

losartan (Rx)

(lo-zar'tan)

Cozaar

Func. class.: Antihypertensive

Chem. class.: Angiotensin II receptor (type AT_1)

Do not confuse:

Cozaar/Zocor

losartan/valsartan

Action: Blocks the vasoconstrictor and aldosterone-secreting effects of angiotensin II; selectively blocks the binding of angiotensin II to the AT_1 receptor found in tissues

Uses: Hypertension, alone or in combination, nephropathy in type 2 diabetes, hypertension with left ventricular hypertrophy

DOSAGE AND ROUTES

Hypertension

• *Adult:* **PO** 50 mg daily alone or 25 mg daily when used in combination with diuretic

Hepatic dose

• *Adult:* **PO** 25 mg daily as starting dose

Hypertension with left ventricular hypertrophy

• *Adult:* **PO** 50 mg daily, add hydrochlorothiazide 12.5 mg/day and/or increase losartan to 100 mg daily, then increase hydrochlorothiazide to 25 mg daily

Nephropathy in type 2 diabetic patients

• *Adult:* **PO** 50 mg daily, may increase to 100 mg daily

Available forms: Tabs 25, 50, 100 mg

SIDE EFFECTS

CNS: Dizziness, insomnia, anxiety, confusion, abnormal dreams, migraine, tremor, vertigo, headache

CV: Angina pectoris, 2nd-degree AV block, ***cerebrovascular accident,*** hypotension, ***myocardial infarction,*** dysrhythmias

---

EENT: Blurred vision, burning eyes, conjunctivitis

GI: Diarrhea, dyspepsia, anorexia, constipation, dry mouth, flatulence, gastritis, vomiting

GU: Impotence, nocturia, urinary frequency, UTI, ***renal failure***

HEMA: Anemia

INTEG: Alopecia, dermatitis, dry skin, flushing, photosensitivity, rash, pruritus, sweating, ***angioedema***

META: Gout

MS: Cramps, myalgia, pain, stiffness

RESP: Cough, upper respiratory infection, congestion, dyspnea, bronchitis

Contraindications: Pregnancy (D) 2nd/3rd trimesters, hypersensitivity

Precautions: Pregnancy (C) 1st trimester; hypersensitivity to ACE inhibitors; lactation, children, elderly

PHARMACOKINETICS

Extensively metabolized, half-life 2 hr, metabolite 6-9 hr, highly bound to plasma proteins, excreted in urine and feces

INTERACTIONS

Increase: lithium toxicity—lithium

Increase: antihypertensive effect—fluconazole

Decrease: antihypertensive effect—phenobarbital, rifamycin

Drug/Herb

Increase: toxicity, death—aconite

Increase: antihypertensive effect—barberry, betony, black catechu, black cohosh, bloodroot, broom, burdock, cat's claw, dandelion, goldenseal, Irish moss, Jamaican dogwood, kelp, khella, mistletoe, parsley

Increase or decrease: antihypertensive effect—astragalus, cola tree

Decrease: antihypertensive effect—coltsfoot, guarana, khat, licorice

NURSING CONSIDERATIONS

Assess:

• B/P with position changes, pulse q4h; note rate, rhythm, quality

• Electrolytes: K, Na, Cl

• Baselines in renal, hepatic studies before therapy begins

• Edema in feet, legs daily

• Skin turgor, dryness of mucous membranes for hydration status

Administer:

• Without regard to meals

Evaluate:

• Therapeutic response: decreased B/P

Teach patient/family:

• To avoid sunlight or wear sunscreen if in sunlight; photosensitivity may occur

• To comply with dosage schedule, even if feeling better

• To notify prescriber of mouth sores, fever, swelling of hands or feet, irregular heartbeat, chest pain

• That excessive perspiration, dehydration, vomiting, diarrhea may lead to fall in blood pressure; consult prescriber if these occur

• That drug may cause dizziness, fainting; light-headedness may occur

• To rise slowly to sitting or standing position to minimize orthostatic hypotension

• To use contraception while taking this product

---

loteprednol ophthalmic
See Appendix C

---

lovastatin (℞)

(loh-vah-stat′in)

Altocor, Mevacor

Func. class.: Antilipemic

Chem. class.: HMG-CoA reductase inhibitor

Do not confuse:

lovastatin/Lotensin

Action: Inhibits HMG-CoA reductase enzyme, which reduces cholesterol synthesis

Uses: As an adjunct in primary hypercholesterolemia (types IIa, IIb), atherosclerosis, primary and secondary prevention of coronary events

DOSAGE AND ROUTES

• *Adult:* PO 20 mg daily with evening meal; may increase to 20-80 mg/day in single or divided doses, not to exceed 80 mg/day; dosage adjustments should be made qmo, reduce dose in renal disease; **EXT REL** 20-60 mg daily at bedtime

Available forms: Tabs 10, 20, 40 mg; ext rel tab (Altocor) 10, 20, 40, 60 mg

SIDE EFFECTS

CNS: Dizziness, headache, tremor, insomnia, paresthesia

EENT: Blurred vision, lens opacities

GI: Flatus, nausea, constipation, diarrhea, dyspepsia, abdominal pain, heartburn, hepatic dysfunction, vomiting, acid regurgitation, dry mouth, dysgeusia

HEMA: **Thrombocytopenia, hemolytic anemia, leukopenia**

INTEG: Rash, pruritus, photosensitivity

MS: Muscle cramps, myalgia, myositis, rhabdomyolysis, leg, shoulder or localized pain

Contraindications: Pregnancy (X), hypersensitivity, lactation, active liver disease

Precautions: Past hepatic disease, alcoholism, severe acute infections, trauma, hypotension, uncontrolled seizure disorders, severe metabolic disorders, electrolyte imbalances, visual disorder, children

PHARMACOKINETICS

PO: Peak 2-4 hr, metabolized in liver (metabolites), highly protein bound; excreted in urine 10%, feces 83%; crosses placenta, excreted in breast milk; half-life 3-4 hr

INTERACTIONS

Possible toxicity: grapefruit juice

Increase: myalgia, myositis—cycloSPOR-INE, gemfibrozil, niacin, erythromycin, clofibrate, azole antifungals

Increase: bleeding—warfarin

Increase: effects of digoxin

Decrease: effects of lovastatin—bile acid sequestrants

Drug/Herb

Increase: effect—glucomannan

Decrease: effect—gotu kola

Drug/Food

Increase: levels of lovastatin with food, must be taken with food

Drug/Lab Test

Increase: CPK, LFTs

NURSING CONSIDERATIONS

Assess:

• Diet, obtain diet history including fat, cholesterol in diet

• Fasting cholesterol, LDL, HDL, triglycerides periodically during treatment

• Hepatic studies q1-2mo during the first 1½ yr of treatment; AST, ALT, LFTs may increase

• Renal function in patients with compromised renal system: BUN, creatinine, I&O ratio

⚠ For muscle pain, tenderness, obtain CPK baseline and if these occur, drug may need to be discontinued

Administer:

• In evening with meal; if dose is increased, take with breakfast and evening meal

Perform/provide:

• Storage in cool environment in air-tight, light-resistant container

Evaluate:

• Therapeutic response: cholesterol at desired level after 8 wk

Teach patient/family:

• To report suspected pregnancy

• That blood work and ophthalmic exam will be necessary during treatment

• To report blurred vision, severe GI symptoms, dizziness, headache, muscle pain, weakness

• To use sunscreen or stay out of the sun to prevent photosensitivity

• That previously prescribed regimen will continue: low-cholesterol diet, exercise program, smoking cessation

• That drug should be taken with food

loxapine (R)

(lox'a-peen)

Loxapac ✤, loxapine succinate ✤, Loxitane, Loxitane IM, Loxitane-C
Func. class.: Antipsychotic, neuroleptic
Chem. class.: Dibenzoxazepine

Do not confuse:

Loxitane/Soriatane

Action: Depresses cerebral cortex, hypothalamus, limbic system, which control activity and aggression; blocks neurotransmission produced by dopamine at synapse; exhibits strong α-adrenergic, anticholinergic blocking action; mechanism for antipsychotic effects is unclear

Uses: Psychotic disorders, nonpsychotic symptoms associated with dementia
Investigational uses: Depression, anxiety

DOSAGE AND ROUTES

• *Adult:* **PO** 10 mg bid-qid initially, may be rapidly increased depending on severity of condition, maintenance 60-100 mg/day; **IM** 12.5-50 mg q4-6h or more until desired response, then start **PO** form
• *Geriatric:* **PO** 5-10 mg daily-bid, increase q4-7d by 5-10 mg, max 125 mg
Available forms: Caps 5, 10, 25, 50 mg; tabs 5, 10, 25, 50 mg; conc 25 mg/ml; inj 50 mg/ml

SIDE EFFECTS

CNS: EPS: pseudoparkinsonism, akathisia, dystonia, tardive dyskinesia, drowsiness, headache, seizures, confusion, ***neuroleptic malignant syndrome***
*CV: Orthostatic hypotension, **cardiac arrest**,* ECG changes, tachycardia
EENT: Blurred vision, glaucoma
GI: Dry mouth, nausea, vomiting, anorexia, constipation, diarrhea, jaundice, weight gain

GU: Urinary retention, urinary frequency, enuresis, impotence, amenorrhea, gynecomastia
*HEMA: **Anemia, leukopenia, leukocytosis, agranulocytosis***
INTEG: Rash, photosensitivity, dermatitis
*RESP: **Laryngospasm**, dyspnea, **respiratory depression***
Contraindications: Hypersensitivity, blood dyscrasias, coma, brain damage, bone marrow depression, alcohol and barbiturate withdrawal states, severe CNS depression, narrow-angle glaucoma
Precautions: Pregnancy (C), lactation, seizure disorders, hepatic disease, cardiac disease, prostatic hypertrophy, cardiac conditions, child <16 yr, elderly

PHARMACOKINETICS

PO: Onset 20-30 min, peak 2-4 hr, duration 12 hr
IM: Onset 15-30 min, peak 15-20 min, duration 12 hr
Metabolized by liver; excreted in urine; crosses placenta; enters breast milk; initial half-life 5 hr; terminal half-life 19 hr

INTERACTIONS

Toxicity: epINEPHrine
Increase: EPS—other antipsychotics
Increase: CNS depression—MAOIs, antidepressants, alcohol
Decrease: effects—guanadrel, guanethidine
Drug/Herb
Increase: CNS depression—chamomile, cola tree, hops, kava, nettle, nutmeg, skullcap, valerian
Increase: EPS—betel palm, kava

NURSING CONSIDERATIONS

Assess:

• Mental status before initial administration
• Swallowing of PO medication; check for hoarding or giving of medication to other patients
• I&O ratio; palpate bladder if low uri-

L

nary output occurs, urinary retention may be the cause

• Bilirubin, CBC, LFTs qmo

• Urinalysis is recommended before and during prolonged therapy

• Affect, orientation, LOC, reflexes, gait, coordination, sleep pattern disturbances

• B/P standing and lying; take pulse and respirations q4h during initial treatment; establish baseline before starting treatment; report drops of 30 mm Hg

• Dizziness, faintness, palpitations, tachycardia on rising

• EPS including akathisia (inability to sit still, no pattern to movements), tardive dyskinesia (bizarre movements of the jaw, mouth, tongue, extremities), pseudoparkinsonism (rigidity, tremors, pill rolling, shuffling gait)

A For neuroleptic malignant syndrome: muscle rigidity, increased CPK, altered mental status, hyperthermia

• Constipation, urinary retention daily; if these occur, increase bulk, water in diet

Administer:

• Reduced dose to elderly

• Antiparkinsonian agent if EPS symptoms occur

IM route

• IM inj into large muscle mass

PO route

• Concentrate mixed in orange or grapefruit juice

Perform/provide:

• Decreased sensory input by dimming lights, avoiding loud noises

• Supervised ambulation until stabilized on medication; do not involve in strenuous exercise program because fainting is possible; patient should not stand still for long periods

• Increased fluids to prevent constipation

• Sips of water, candy, gum for dry mouth

• Storage in airtight, light-resistant container

Evaluate:

• Therapeutic response: decrease in emotional excitement, hallucinations, delusions, paranoia; reorganization of patterns of thought, speech

Teach patient/family:

• That orthostatic hypotension may occur and to rise from sitting or lying position gradually

• To remain lying down after IM injection for at least 30 min

• To avoid hot tubs, hot showers, tub baths, as hypotension may occur; that in hot weather heat stroke may occur; take extra precautions to stay cool

• To avoid abrupt withdrawal of this drug, or EPS may result; drug should be withdrawn slowly

• To avoid OTC preparations (cough, hay fever, cold) unless approved by prescriber; serious drug interactions may occur; avoid use with alcohol, CNS depressants; increased drowsiness may occur

• To avoid hazardous activities until stabilized on medication

• To use sunscreen during sun exposure to prevent burns

• About necessity for meticulous oral hygiene, since oral candidiasis may occur

• To report impaired vision, jaundice, tremors, muscle twitching

Treatment of overdose: Lavage if orally ingested; provide an airway

lymphocyte immune globulin (antithymocyte) (℞)

Atgam
Func. class.: Immune globulins—immunosuppressant

Action: Produces immunosuppression by inhibiting the function of lymphocytes (T)

Uses: Organ transplants to prevent rejection, aplastic anemia

Investigational uses: Multiple sclerosis; myasthenia gravis; immunosuppressant in liver, bone marrow, heart, and other organ transplants; pure red-cell aplasia; scleroderma

DOSAGE AND ROUTES

Renal allograft
• *Adult:* **IV** 10-30 mg/kg/day
• *Child:* **IV** 5-25 mg/kg/day

Delay of renal allograft rejection
• *Adult:* **IV** 15 mg/kg/day × 14 days, then every other day × 14 days for a total of 21 doses in 28 days

Aplastic anemia
• *Adult:* **IV** 10-20 mg/kg/day × 8-14 days

Available forms: Inj 50 mg horse gamma globulin/ml

SIDE EFFECTS

Renal transplant
CNS: Fever, chills, headache, dizziness, weakness, faintness, *seizures*
CV: Chest pain, hypertension, tachycardia
GI: Diarrhea, nausea, vomiting, epigastric pain
INTEG: Rash, pruritus, urticaria, wheal
SYST: ***Anaphylaxis***

Aplastic anemia
CNS: Fever, chills, headache, *seizures,* lightheadedness, encephalitis, postviral encephalopathy
CV: Bradycardia, myocarditis, irregularity
GI: Nausea, LFTs abnormality

Contraindications: Hypersensitivity
Precautions: Pregnancy (C), severe renal disease, severe hepatic disease, lactation, children

PHARMACOKINETICS

Onset rapid, half-life 5-7 days

INTERACTIONS

None known

NURSING CONSIDERATIONS

Assess:
• For infection; if infection occurs, evaluation will be needed to continue therapy
• Renal studies: BUN, creatinine at least monthly during treatment, 3 mo after treatment

• Hepatic studies: alk phosphatase, AST, ALT, bilirubin

Administer:
• Do not infuse <4 hr

Aplastic anemia
• Skin testing must be completed prior to treatment; use intradermal inj of 0.1 ml of a 1:1000 dilution (5 mcg horse IgG) in 0.9% NaCl, if a wheal or rash >10 mm or both, use caution during inf
• Dilute in saline sol before inf, invert IV bag, so undiluted drug does not contact the air inside, concentration should not be >1 mg/ml
• Keep emergency equipment nearby for severe allergic reaction

Evaluate:
• Therapeutic response: absence of rejection; hematologic recovery (aplastic anemia)

Teach patient/family:
• To report fever, chills, sore throat, fatigue, since serious infections may occur
• To use contraceptive measures during treatment, for 12 wk after ending therapy

M

mafenide topical
See Appendix C

magaldrate (OTC)
(mag'al-drate)
Losapan ✦, Lowsium, Riopan, Riopan Extra Strength ✦
Func. class.: Antacid
Chem. class.: Aluminum/magnesium hydroxide

Action: Neutralizes gastric acidity; drug is dissolved in gastric contents; combination of aluminum, magnesium
Uses: Antacid, peptic ulcer disease (adjunct), duodenal, gastric ulcers, reflux esophagitis, hyperacidity, indigestion, heartburn

---

DOSAGE AND ROUTES

• *Adult:* **SUSP** 5-10 ml (400-800 mg) with H_2O between meals, at bedtime, not to exceed 100 ml/day

Available forms: Susp 540 mg/5 ml, liquid 540 mg/5 ml

SIDE EFFECTS

GI: Constipation, diarrhea

META: Hypermagnesemia, hypophosphatemia

Contraindications: Hypersensitivity to this drug or aluminum

Precautions: Pregnancy (C), elderly, fluid restriction, decreased GI motility, GI obstruction, dehydration, renal disease, sodium-restricted diets

PHARMACOKINETICS

PO: Duration 60 min

INTERACTIONS

Increase: action when taken in large amounts—quinidine, flecainide, amphetamines

Decrease: absorption of anticholinergics, chlordiazepoxide, cimetidine, corticosteroids, fluoroquinolones, iron salts, isoniazid, ketoconazole, phenothiazines, phenytoin, salicylates, tetracyclines

Decrease: action when taken in large amounts—salicylates

NURSING CONSIDERATIONS

Assess:

• GI status: location of pain, intensity, characteristics, heartburn, hematemesis

• Serum magnesium levels with impaired renal function; calcium, phosphate, potassium if using long term; may increase calcium, decrease phosphate

• Constipation: increase bulk in diet if needed

Administer:

• Laxatives or stool softeners if constipation occurs

• After shaking; give between meals and bedtime

Evaluate:

• Therapeutic response: absence of pain, decreased acidity

Teach patient/family:

• To separate enteric-coated drugs and antacid by 2 hr

• To notify prescriber immediately of coffee-ground emesis, emesis with frank blood, black tarry stools

Rarely Used

magnesium salicylate (OTC, R)

Doan's Pills, Magan, Mobidin

Func. class.: Nonopioid analgesic, nonsteroidal antiinflammatory

Uses: Mild to moderate pain or fever including arthritis, juvenile rheumatoid arthritis

DOSAGE AND ROUTES

Arthritis

• *Adult:* **PO** not to exceed 4.8 g/day in divided doses

Pain/fever

• *Adult:* **PO** 600 mg qid or 1160 mg tid

Contraindications: Pregnancy (D) 1st trimester, hypersensitivity to salicylates, GI bleeding, bleeding disorders, children <12 yr, vit K deficiency

magnesium salts
(mag-nee'zee-um)

magnesium chloride (℞)
Chloromag, Slo-Mag

magnesium citrate (OTC)
Citrate of Magnesia, Citroma, CitroMag ✦

magnesium gluconate (OTC)
Almoate, Magonate, magtrate OTC

magnesium oxide (OTC)
Mag-Ox 400, Maox, Uro-Mag

magnesium hydroxide (OTC)
Phillips' Magnesia Tablets, Phillips' Milk of Magnesia, MOM

magnesium sulfate (OTC, ℞)
epsom salts; magnesium sulfate (IV)—**HIGH ALERT**

Func. class.: Electrolyte; anticonvulsant; saline laxative, antacid

Action: Increases osmotic pressure, draws fluid into colon, neutralizes HCl
Uses: Constipation, bowel preparation before surgery or exam, anticonvulsant in preeclampsia, eclampsia (magnesium sulfate), electrolyte

DOSAGE AND ROUTES

Laxative
• *Adult:* **PO** 30-60 ml at bedtime (Milk of Magnesia), 300 mg
• *Adult and child >6 yr:* **PO** 15 g in 8 oz H_2O (magnesium sulfate); **PO** 10-20 ml (Concentrated Milk of Magnesia); **PO** 5-10 oz at bedtime (magnesium citrate)
• *Child 2-6 yr:* 5-15 ml/day (Milk of Magnesia)
Prevention of magnesium deficiency
• *Adult and child ≥10 yr:* **PO** male:
350-400 mg/day; female: 280-300 mg/day; lactation: 335-350 mg/day; pregnancy 320 mg/day
• *Child 8-10 yr:* **PO** 170 mg/day
• *Child 4-7 yr:* **PO** 120 mg/day
• *Child infant to 4 yr:* 40-80 mg/day
Magnesium sulfate
Deficiency
• *Adult:* **PO** 200-400 mg in divided doses tid-qid; **IM** 1 g q6h × 4 doses; **IV** 5 g (severe)
• *Child 6-12 yr:* 3-6 mg/kg/day in divided doses tid-qid
Pre-eclampsia/eclampsia magnesium sulfate
• *Adult:* **IM/IV** 4-5 g **IV inf;** with 5 g **IM** in each gluteus, then 5 g q4h or 4 g **IV INF,** then 1-2 g/hr **CONT INF,** max 40 g/day or 20 g/48 hr in severe renal disease

Available forms:
• Chloride: sus rel tabs 535 mg (64 mg Mg) enteric tabs 833 mg (100 mg Mg)
• Citrate: oral sol 240, 296, 300 ml bottles (77 mEq/100 ml)
• Hydroxide: Liq 400 mg/5 ml; conc liq 800 mg/5 ml; chew tabs 300, 600 mg
• Oxide: Tabs 400 mg; caps 140 mg
• Sulfate: Powder for oral; bulk packages; epsom salts, bulk packages; inj 10%, 12.5%, 25%, 50%

SIDE EFFECTS

CNS: Muscle weakness, flushing, sweating, confusion, sedation, depressed reflexes, ***flaccid paralysis,*** hypothermia
CV: Hypotension, heart block, ***circulatory collapse***
GI: Nausea, vomiting, anorexia, cramps
META: Electrolyte, fluid imbalances
RESP: Respiratory depression
Contraindications: Hypersensitivity, abdominal pain, nausea/vomiting, obstruction, acute surgical abdomen, rectal bleeding
Precautions: Pregnancy (A); (B) magnesium sulfate, renal disease, cardiac disease

M

PHARMACOKINETICS

PO: Onset 3-6 hr
IM: Onset 1 hr, duration 4 hr
IV: Duration ½ hr
Excreted by kidney, effective anticonvulsant serum levels 2.5-7.5 mEq/L

INTERACTIONS

Increase: effect of neuromuscular blockers
Decrease: absorption of tetracyclines, aminoquinolones, nitrofurantoin

NURSING CONSIDERATIONS

Assess:
• I&O ratio; check for decrease in urinary output
• Cause of constipation; lack of fluids, bulk, exercise
• Cramping, rectal bleeding, nausea, vomiting; drug should be discontinued
⚠ Magnesium toxicity: thirst, confusion, decrease in reflexes

Administer:
PO route
• With 8 oz H_2O
• Refrigerate magnesium citrate before giving
• Shake susp before using as antacid at least 2 hr pc

IM route (magnesium sulfate)
• Give deeply in gluteal site

IV route (magnesium sulfate)
• Only when calcium gluconate available for magnesium toxicity

IV, direct route
• IV undiluted 1.5 ml of 10% sol over 1 min
• May dilute to 20% sol, infuse over 3 hr
• IV at less than 150 mg/min; circulatory collapse may occur
• Use infusion pump

Additive compatibilities: Cephalothin, chloramphenicol, cisplatin, heparin, hydrocortisone, isoproterenol, meropenem, methyldopate, norepinephrine, penicillin G potassium, potassium phosphate, verapamil

Y-site compatibilities: Acyclovir, aldesleukin, amifostine, amikacin, ampicillin, aztreonam, cefamandole, cefazolin, cefmetazole, cefoperazone, cefotaxime, cefoxitin, cephalothin, cephapirin, chloramphenicol, cisatracurium, DOBUTamine, doxycycline, DOXOrubicin liposome, enalaprilat, erythromycin, esmolol, famotidine, fludarabine, gallium, gentamicin, granisetron, heparin, hydromorphone, idarubicin, insulin, kanamycin, labetalol, meperidine, metronidazole, minocycline, morphine, moxalactam, nafcillin, ondansetron, oxacillin, paclitaxel, penicillin G potassium, piperacillin, piperacillin/tazobactam, potassium chloride, propofol, remifentanil, sargramostim, thiotepa, ticarcillin, tobramycin, trimethoprim-sulfamethoxazole, vancomycin, vit B complex/C

Evaluate:
• Therapeutic response: decreased constipation

Teach patient/family:
• Not to use laxatives for long-term therapy; bowel tone will be lost
• That chilling helps the taste of magnesium citrate
• To shake suspension well
• To not give at bedtime as a laxative; may interfere with sleep
• To give citrus fruit after administering to counteract unpleasant taste

---

mannitol (℞)
(man′i-tole)
mannitol, Osmitrol, Resectisol
Func. class.: Diuretic, osmotic
Chem. class.: Hexahydric alcohol

Action: Acts by increasing osmolarity of glomerular filtrate, which raises osmotic pressure of fluid in renal tubules; decrease in reabsorption of water, electrolytes; increase in urinary output, sodium, chloride excretion
Uses: Edema, promote systemic diuresis in cerebral edema, decrease intraocular pressure, improve renal function in acute renal failure, chemical poisoning

---

⚠ Safety alert   *"Tall Man" lettering

DOSAGE AND ROUTES

Oliguria, prevention
• *Adult:* IV 50-100 g 5%-25% sol, may use test dose 0.2 g/kg over 3-5 min

Oliguria, treatment
• *Adult:* IV 300-400 mg/kg 20%-25% sol up to 100 g 15%-20% sol, run over 30-60 min
• *Child:* IV 0.25-2 g/kg as 15%-20% sol run over 2-6 hr

Intraocular pressure/intracranial pressure
• *Adult:* IV 1½-2 g/kg 15%-25% sol over ½-1 hr
• *Child:* IV 1-2 g/kg (30-60 g/m^2) as 15%-20% sol run over ½-1 hr

Renal failure
• *Adult:* IV 50-200 g/24 hr, adjusted to maintain output of 30-50 mg/hr

Diuresis in drug intoxication
• *Adult and child >12 yr:* 5%-10% sol continuously up to 200 g IV, while maintaining 100-500 ml urine output/hr

Available forms: Inj 5%, 10%, 15%, 20%, 25%; GU irrigation: 5%

SIDE EFFECTS

CNS: Dizziness, headache, ***convulsions, rebound increased ICP,*** confusion
CV: Edema, thrombophlebitis, hypotension, hypertension, ***tachycardia,*** angina-like chest pains, fever, chills, ***CHF***
EENT: Loss of hearing, blurred vision, nasal congestion, decreased intraocular pressure
ELECT: Fluid, electrolyte imbalances, *acidosis,* electrolyte loss, dehydration
GI: *Nausea, vomiting,* dry mouth, diarrhea
GU: Marked diuresis, urinary retention, thirst
RESP: Pulmonary congestion

Contraindications: Active intracranial bleeding, hypersensitivity, anuria, severe pulmonary congestion, edema, severe dehydration, progressive heart, renal failure
Precautions: Pregnancy (C), dehydration, severe renal disease, CHF, lactation

PHARMACOKINETICS

IV: Onset 30-60 min for diuresis, ½-1 hr for intraocular pressure, 25 min for cerebrospinal fluid; duration 4-6 hr for intraocular pressure, 3-8 hr for cerebrospinal fluid; excreted in urine, half-life 100 min

INTERACTIONS

Decrease: effect—lithium
Drug/Food
Potassium foods: increased hyperkalemia
Drug/Lab Test
Interference: Inorganic phosphorus, ethylene glycol

NURSING CONSIDERATIONS

Assess:
• Weight, I&O daily to determine fluid loss; effect of drug may be decreased if used daily; output qh prn
• Rate, depth, rhythm of respiration, effect of exertion
• B/P lying, standing; postural hypotension may occur
• Electrolytes: K, Na, Cl; include BUN, CBC, serum creatinine, blood pH, ABGs, CVP, PAP
• Signs of metabolic acidosis: drowsiness, restlessness
• Signs of hypokalemia: postural hypotension, malaise, fatigue, tachycardia, leg cramps, weakness
• Rashes, temp daily
• Confusion, especially in elderly; take safety precautions if needed
• Hydration including skin turgor, thirst, dry mucous membranes
• For blurred vision, pain in eyes, before and during treatment (increased intraocular pressure); neurologic checks, intracranial pressure during treatment (increased intracranial pressure)

Administer:
IV route
• In 15%-25% sol with filter; give over ½-1½ hr; rapid infusion may worsen CHF; warm in hot water and shake to dissolve crystals

M

• Test dose in severe oliguria, 0.2 g/kg over 3-5 min; if no urine increase, give second test dose; if no response, reassess patient

Irrigation
• 100 ml of 25%/900 ml of sterile water for inj (2.5% sol)

Additive compatibilities: Amikacin, bretylium, cefamandole, cefoxitin, cimetidine, cisplatin, DOPamine, fosphenytoin, furosemide, gentamicin, metoclopramide, netilmicin, nizatidine, ofloxacin, ondansetron, sodium bicarbonate, tobramycin, verapamil

Y-site compatibilities: Allopurinol, amifostine, amphotericin B cholesteryl, aztreonam, cisatracurium, cladribine, fludarabine, fluorouracil, gallium, idarubicin, melphalan, ondansetron, paclitaxel, piperacillin, propofol, remifentanil, sargramostim, teniposide, thiotepa, vinorelbine

Evaluate:
• Therapeutic response: improvement in edema of feet, legs, sacral area daily if medication is being used in CHF; decreased intraocular pressure, prevention of hypokalemia, increased excretion of toxic substances; decreased ICP

Teach patient/family:
• To rise slowly from lying or sitting position
• The reason for and method of treatment
• To report signs of electrolyte imbalance; confusion

Treatment of overdose: Discontinue infusion; correct fluid, electrolyte imbalances; hemodialysis; monitor hydration, CV, renal function

---

mebendazole (℞)
(me-ben′da-zole)
Vermox
Func. class.: Anthelmintic
Chem. class.: Carbamate

Action: Inhibits glucose uptake, degeneration of cytoplasmic microtubules in the cell; interferes with absorption, secretory function

Uses: Pinworms, roundworms, hookworms, whipworms, thread-worms, pork tapeworms, dwarf tapeworms, beef tapeworms, hydatid cyst

DOSAGE AND ROUTES
• *Adult and child >2 yr:* **PO** 100 mg as a single dose (pinworms) or bid × 3 days (whipworms, roundworms, or hookworms); course may be repeated in 3 wk if needed

Available forms: Tabs, chew 100 mg

SIDE EFFECTS
CNS: Dizziness, fever, headache
GI: Transient diarrhea, abdominal pain, nausea, vomiting
Contraindications: Hypersensitivity
Precautions: Pregnancy (C) (1st trimester), child <2 yr, lactation, Crohn's disease, hepatic disease, IBD, ulcerative colitis

PHARMACOKINETICS
PO: Peak ½-7 hr; excreted in feces primarily (metabolites), small amount in urine (unchanged); highly bound to plasma proteins 95%

INTERACTIONS
Decrease: mebendazole effect—carbamazepine, hydantoins
Drug/Food
Increase: absorption—high-fat meal

NURSING CONSIDERATIONS
Assess:
• Stools during entire treatment; specimens must be sent to lab while still warm, also 1-3 wk after treatment is completed
• For allergic reaction: rash (rare)
• For diarrhea during expulsion of worms; avoid self-contamination with patient's feces
• For infection in other family members, since infection from person to person is common

---

• Blood studies: AST, ALT, alk phosphatase, BUN, CBC during treatment
Administer:
• May be crushed, chewed, swallowed whole, mixed with food
• PO after meals to avoid GI symptoms, since absorption is not altered by food
• Second course after 3 wk if needed; usually recommended
Perform/provide:
• Storage in tight container
Evaluate:
• Therapeutic response: expulsion of worms and 3 negative stool cultures after completion of treatment
Teach patient/family:
• Proper hygiene after BM, including hand-washing technique; tell patient to avoid putting fingers in mouth; clean fingernails
• That infected person should sleep alone; do not shake bed linen, change bed linen daily, wash in hot water, change and wash undergarments daily
• To clean toilet daily with disinfectant (green soap solution)
• The need for compliance with dosage schedule, duration of treatment
• To wear shoes, wash all fruits and vegetables well before eating; use commercial fruit/vegetable cleaner
• That all members of the family should be treated (pinworms)

---

mecasermin
See Appendix A—Selected New Drugs

---

mechlorethamine (R)
(me-klor-eth'a-meen)
Mustargen, nitrogen mustard
Func. class.: Antineoplastic alkylating agent
Chem. class.: Nitrogen mustard

Action: Responsible for cross-linking DNA strands leading to cell death; rapidly

degraded, a vesicant; activity is not cell cycle phase-specific
Uses: Hodgkin's disease, leukemias, lymphomas, lymphosarcoma; ovarian, breast, lung carcinoma; neoplastic effusions

DOSAGE AND ROUTES
• *Adult:* IV 0.4 mg/kg or 10 mg/m^2 as 1 dose or 2-4 divided doses over 2-4 days; second course after 3 wk depending on blood cell count
Neoplastic effusions
• *Adult:* INTRACAVITARY 0.4 mg/kg, may be 200-400 mcg/kg
Available forms: Inj 10 mg

SIDE EFFECTS
CNS: Headache, dizziness, drowsiness, paresthesia, peripheral neuropathy, ***coma***
EENT: Tinnitus, hearing loss
GI: Nausea, vomiting, diarrhea, stomatitis, weight loss, colitis, ***hepatotoxicity***
*HEMA: **Thrombocytopenia, leukopenia, agranulocytosis,*** anemia
INTEG: Alopecia, pruritus, herpes zoster, extravasation
Contraindications: Pregnancy (D), lactation, myelosuppression, acute herpes zoster
Precautions: Radiation therapy, chronic lymphocytic leukopenia

PHARMACOKINETICS
Metabolized in liver, excreted in urine

INTERACTIONS
Blood dyscrasias: amphotericin B
Increase: bleeding—aspirin, anticoagulants
Increase: toxicity—antineoplastics, radiation
Decrease: antibody reaction—live virus vaccines

NURSING CONSIDERATIONS
Assess:
• CBC, differential, platelet count qwk; withhold drug if WBC is <1000/mm^3 or

M

platelet count is <75,000/mm³; notify prescriber, recovery of WBCs, platelets within 20 days

• Renal function tests: BUN, serum uric acid, urine CCr before, during therapy

• I&O ratio; report fall in urine output of 30 ml/hr

• Monitor temp q4h (may indicate beginning infection); no rectal temps

• Hepatic studies before, during therapy (bilirubin, AST, ALT, LDH) as needed or monthly

• Bleeding: hematuria, guaiac, bruising or petechiae, mucosa or orifices q8h

• Jaundiced skin and sclera, dark urine, clay-colored stools, itchy skin, abdominal pain, fever, diarrhea

• Effects of alopecia on body image; discuss feelings about body changes

• Buccal cavity q8h for dryness, sores, ulceration, white patches, oral pain, bleeding, dysphagia

• Local irritation, pain, burning, discoloration at inj site

A Symptoms indicating severe allergic reaction: rash, pruritus, urticaria, purpuric skin lesions, itching, flushing

Administer:

• After using guidelines for preparation of cytotoxic drugs

• Antiemetic 30-60 min before giving drug and prn

• IV after diluting 10 mg/10 ml sterile H₂O or NaCl; leave needle in vial, shake, withdraw dose, give through Y-tube or 3-way stopcock or directly over 3-5 min

• Watch for infiltration; infiltrate area with isotonic sodium thiosulfate or 1% lidocaine; apply ice for 6-12 hr

• Topical or systemic analgesics for pain

• Local or systemic drugs for infection

Y-site compatibilities: Amifostine, aztreonam, filgrastim, fludarabine, granisetron, melphalan, ondansetron, sargramostim, teniposide, vinorelbine

Perform/provide:

• Storage at room temperature in dry form

• Increase fluid intake to 2-3 L/day to prevent urate deposits, calculi formation

• Diet low in purines: organ meats (kidney, liver), dried beans, peas to maintain alkaline urine

• Preparation under hood using gloves and mask

• Rinsing of mouth tid-qid with water, club soda; brushing of teeth bid-tid with soft brush or cotton-tipped applicators for stomatitis; use unwaxed dental floss

• Warm compresses at inj site for inflammation

Evaluate:

• Therapeutic response: decreased tumor size, spread of malignancy

Teach patient/family:

• The rationale for and techniques of protective isolation

• That sterility, amenorrhea can occur; reversible after discontinuing treatment

• That hair may be lost during treatment; a wig or hairpiece may make patient feel better; new hair may be different in color, texture

• To avoid foods with citric acid, hot or rough texture

• To report any bleeding, white spots, or ulcerations in mouth to prescriber; tell patient to examine mouth daily

• To report signs of infection: fever, sore throat, flulike symptoms

• To report signs of anemia: fatigue, headache, faintness, shortness of breath, irritability

• To avoid use of razors, commercial mouthwash

• To avoid use of aspirin products, NSAIDs

• To notify prescriber if pregnancy is suspected; to use contraception during treatment

---

meclizine (OTC, ℞)

(mek'li-zeen)
Antivert, Antrizine, Bonamine ♣, Bonine, Dramamine Less Drowsy Formula, meclizine HCl, Meni-D, Vergan

Func. class.: Antiemetic, antihistamine, anticholinergic

Chem. class.: H_1-receptor antagonist, piperazine derivative

Action: Acts centrally by blocking chemoreceptor trigger zone, which in turn acts on vomiting center

Uses: Vertigo, motion sickness

DOSAGE AND ROUTES

Vertigo
• *Adult:* **PO** 25-100 mg daily in divided doses

Motion sickness
• *Adult:* **PO** 12.5-25 mg 1 hr before traveling, repeat dose q12-24h prn

Available forms: Tabs 12.5, 25, 50 mg; chew tabs 25 mg; caps 25, 30 mg

SIDE EFFECTS

CNS: Drowsiness, fatigue, restlessness, headache, insomnia
CV: Hypotension
EENT: Dry mouth, blurred vision
GI: Nausea, anorexia, constipation, increased appetite
GU: Urinary retention

Contraindications: Hypersensitivity to cyclizines, shock

Precautions: Pregnancy (B), children, narrow-angle glaucoma, glaucoma, urinary retention, lactation, prostatic hypertrophy, elderly, CV disease, hypertension, seizure disease

PHARMACOKINETICS

PO: Onset 1 hr, duration 8-24 hr, half-life 6 hr

INTERACTIONS

Increase: effect of alcohol, opioids, other CNS depressants

Drug/Herb
Increase: anticholinergic effect—corkwood, henbane leaf
Increase: sedative effect—hops, Jamaican dogwood, khat, senega

Drug/Lab Test
False negative: Allergy skin testing

NURSING CONSIDERATIONS

Assess:
• VS, B/P
⚠ Signs of toxicity of other drugs or masking of symptoms of disease: brain tumor, intestinal obstruction
• Observe for drowsiness, dizziness, level of consciousness

Administer:
PO route
• Tablets may be swallowed whole, chewed, or allowed to dissolve; give with food to decrease GI upset
• Lowest possible dose in elderly, anticholinergic effects

Evaluate:
• Therapeutic response: absence of dizziness, vomiting

Teach patient/family:
• That a false-negative result may occur with skin testing for allergies; these procedures should not be scheduled for 4 days after discontinuing use
• To avoid hazardous activities, activities requiring alertness; dizziness may occur; instruct patient to request assistance with ambulation
• To avoid alcohol, other depressants

M

*medroxyPROGES-TERone (R)

(me-drox′ee-proe-jess′te-rone)
Amen, Curretab, Cycrin, Depo-Provera, medroxyPRO-GESTERone, Provera
Func. class.: Antineoplastic, hormone, contraceptive
Chem. class.: Progesterone derivative

Do not confuse:

Amen/Ambien
medroxyPROGESTERone/
methylPREDNISolone
Provera/Premarin
Action: Inhibits secretion of pituitary gonadotropins, which prevents follicular maturation and ovulation; stimulates growth of mammary tissue; antineoplastic action against endometrial cancer
Uses: Uterine bleeding (abnormal), secondary amenorrhea, prevent endometrial changes associated with estrogen replacement therapy (ERT)

DOSAGE AND ROUTES

Secondary amenorrhea
• *Adult:* **PO** 5-10 mg daily × 5-10 days
Uterine bleeding
• *Adult:* **PO** 5-10 mg daily × 5-10 days starting on 16th or 21st day of menstrual cycle
With ERT
• *Adult:* **PO** monophasic 2.5 mg daily; Biphasic 5 mg days 15-28 of cycle
Available forms: Tabs 2.5, 5, 10 mg; inj susp 50, 100, 150, 400 mg/ml

SIDE EFFECTS

CNS: Dizziness, headache, migraines, depression, fatigue
CV: Hypotension, thrombophlebitis, edema, ***thromboembolism, stroke, pulmonary embolism, MI***
EENT: Diplopia
GI: Nausea, vomiting, anorexia, cramps, increased weight, ***cholestatic jaundice***

GU: Amenorrhea, cervical erosion, breakthrough bleeding, dysmenorrhea, vaginal candidiasis, breast changes, *gynecomastia, testicular atrophy, impotence,* endometriosis, ***spontaneous abortion***
INTEG: Rash, urticaria, acne, hirsutism, alopecia, oily skin, seborrhea, purpura, melasma, photosensitivity
META: Hyperglycemia
*SYST: **Angioedema, anaphylaxis***
Contraindications: Pregnancy (X), breast cancer, hypersensitivity, thromboembolic disorders, reproductive cancer, genital bleeding (abnormal, undiagnosed)
Precautions: Lactation, hypertension, asthma, blood dyscrasias, gallbladder disease, CHF, diabetes mellitus, bone disease, depression, migraine headache, convulsive disorders, hepatic disease, renal disease, family history of cancer of breast or reproductive tract

PHARMACOKINETICS

PO: Duration 24 hr, excreted in urine and feces, metabolized in liver

INTERACTIONS

Decrease: medroxyPROGESTERone action—aminoglutethimide
Drug/Lab Test
Increase: Alk phosphatase, sodium (urine), pregnanediol, amino acids
Decrease: GTT, HDL

NURSING CONSIDERATIONS

Assess:
⚠ Symptoms indicating severe allergic reaction, angioedema, have epINEPHrine and rescusitative equipment available
• Weight daily; notify prescriber of weekly weight gain >5 lb
• B/P at beginning of treatment and periodically
• I&O ratio; be alert for decreasing urinary output, increasing edema
• Hepatic studies: ALT, AST, bilirubin, periodically during long-term therapy

---

⚠ Safety alert   *"Tall Man" lettering

- Edema, hypertension, cardiac symptoms, jaundice
- Mental status: affect, mood, behavioral changes, depression

Administer:
- Titrated dose; use lowest effective dose
- Oil solution deep in large muscle mass (IM), rotate sites
- With food or milk to decrease GI symptoms (PO)

Perform/provide:
- Storage in dark area

Evaluate:
- Therapeutic response: decreased abnormal uterine bleeding, absence of amenorrhea

Teach patient/family:
- To avoid sunlight or use sunscreen; photosensitivity can occur
- Cushingoid symptoms: weight gain, moon face, buffalo hump, acne
⚠ To report breast lumps, vaginal bleeding, edema, jaundice, dark urine, clay-colored stools, dyspnea, headache, blurred vision, abdominal pain, numbness or stiffness in legs, chest pain; male to report impotence or gynecomastia
- To report suspected pregnancy

medrysone ophthalmic
See Appendix C

megestrol (℞)
(me-jess'trole)
Megace, megestrol
Func. class.: Antineoplastic hormone
Chem. class.: Progestin

Do not confuse:
Megace/Reglan

Action: Affects endometrium by antiluteinizing effect; this is thought to bring about cell death

Uses: Breast, endometrial cancer, renal cell cancer; cachexia anorexia weight loss in AIDs

Investigational uses:
Hot flashes

DOSAGE AND ROUTES
Endometrial/ovarian carcinoma
- *Adult:* PO 40-320 mg/day in divided doses

Breast carcinoma
- *Adult:* PO 40 mg qid or 160 mg daily

Anorexia (AIDS)
- *Adult:* PO 800 mg daily (oral susp)

Hot flashes (off-label)
- *Adult:* PO 20 mg daily

Available forms: Tabs 20, 40 mg; oral susp 40 mg/ml

SIDE EFFECTS
CNS: Mood swings
CV: ***Thrombophlebitis, thromboembolism***
GI: Nausea, vomiting, diarrhea, abdominal cramps, weight gain
GU: Gynecomastia, fluid retention, hypercalcemia, vaginal bleeding, discharge, impotence, decreased libido
INTEG: Alopecia, rash, pruritus, purpura, itching

Contraindications: Pregnancy D (tabs); X (susp), hypersensitivity

PHARMACOKINETICS
PO: Duration 1-3 days, half-life 60 min; metabolized in liver; excreted in feces, breast milk

Drug/Lab Test
Increase: Alk phosphatase, urinary sodium, urinary pregnanediol, plasma amino acids
Decrease: HDL, glucose tolerance test
False positive: Urine glucose

NURSING CONSIDERATIONS
Assess:
- I&O ratio; weights
- Effects of alopecia on body image; discuss feelings about body changes
⚠ Symptoms indicating severe allergic reaction: rash, pruritus, urticaria, purpuric skin lesions, itching, flushing
- Frequency of stools, characteristics:

M

cramping, acidosis, signs of dehydration (rapid respirations, poor skin turgor, decreased urine output, dry skin, restlessness, weakness)

• Anorexia, nausea, vomiting, constipation, weakness, loss of muscle tone

⚠ Thrombophlebitis: Homans' sign, edema, pain in calf, thigh, notify prescriber immediately

Administer:

• Oral susp for AIDS patients; shake well

• Tablets for carcinoma

Perform/provide:

• Nutritious diet with iron, vitamin supplements as ordered

• Storage in tight container at room temperature

Evaluate:

• Therapeutic response: decreased tumor size, spread of malignancy; weight gain in AIDS patients

Teach patient/family:

• To report vaginal bleeding

• That nonhormonal contraception should be used during and 4 mo after treatment

• That gynecomastia can occur; reversible after discontinuing treatment

⚠ To recognize signs of fluid retention, thromboemboli and to report immediately

---

meloxicam (℞)

(mel-ox′i-kam)
Mobic
Func. class.: Nonsteroidal antiinflammatory/nonopioid analgesic (NSAIDs)
Chem. class.: Oxicam

Action: Inhibits prostaglandin synthesis by decreasing an enzyme needed for biosynthesis; analgesic, antiinflammatory, antipyretic effects

Uses: Osteoarthritis, rheumatoid arthritis, juvenile arthritis

DOSAGE AND ROUTES

• *Adult:* **PO** 7.5 mg daily, may increase to 15 mg daily

Available forms: Tabs 7.5 mg; susp 7.5 mg/ml

SIDE EFFECTS

CNS: Dizziness, drowsiness, tremors, headache, nervousness, malaise, fatigue, insomnia, depression, *seizures*
CV: Hypertension, angina, *cardiac failure, MI,* hypotension, palpitations, *dysrhythmias,* tachycardia
EENT: Tinnitus, hearing loss
GI: Pancreatitis, nausea, colitis, GERD, vomiting, diarrhea, constipation, flatulence, cramps, dry mouth, peptic ulcer, *GI bleeding, perforation*
GU: Nephrotoxicity: dysuria, hematuria, oliguria, azotemia
HEMA: Blood dyscrasias, anemia, prolonged bleeding
INTEG: Rash, urticaria, photosensitivity
SYST: Angioedema, anaphylaxis
Contraindications: Pregnancy (D) 2nd/3rd trimester; hypersensitivity, asthma, severe renal disease, severe hepatic disease, peptic ulcer disease, L&D, lactation, CV bleeding
Precautions: Pregnancy (C), children, bleeding disorders, GI disorders, cardiac disorders, hypersensitivity to other antiinflammatory agents, elderly, CCr <25 ml/min

PHARMACOKINETICS

PO: Peak 4-5 hr
IM: Peak 50 min, half-life 6 hr, enters breast milk, <50% metabolized by liver, excreted by kidneys

INTERACTIONS

Nephrotoxicity: cycloSPORINE
Increase: meloxicam action—phenytoin, sulfonamides, salicylates
Increase: action of aminoglycosides, hydantoins, diuretics, anticoagulants
Decrease: meloxicam action—cholestyramine
Decrease: action of β-blockers
Drug/Herb
Increase: gastric irritation—arginine, gossypol

Increase: NSAIDs effect—bearberry, bilberry

Increase: bleeding risk—bogbean, chondroitin

NURSING CONSIDERATIONS

Assess:

• Renal, hepatic, blood studies: BUN, creatinine, AST, ALT, Hgb before treatment, periodically thereafter

• Bleeding times; check for bruising, bleeding; test for occult blood in urine

⚠ For anaphylaxis and angioedema; emergency equipment should be nearby

⚠ Hepatic dysfunction: jaundice, yellow sclera and skin, clay-colored stools

• Audiometric, ophthalmic exam before, during, after treatment

• GI condition, hypertension, cardiac conditions

Administer:

• May take without regard to meals, to take with food for GI upset

• Take with full glass of water and sit upright for ½ hr

Perform/provide:

• Storage at room temperature

Evaluate:

• Therapeutic response: decreased pain, stiffness, swelling in joints, ability to move more easily

Teach patient/family:

• To report blurred vision or ringing, roaring in ears (may indicate toxicity)

• To avoid driving, other hazardous activities if dizziness or drowsiness occurs

• To report change in urine pattern, weight increase, edema, pain increase in joints, fever, blood in urine (indicates nephrotoxicity); to report rash, black stools, or continuing headache

• To avoid alcohol, aspirin, acetaminophen without consulting prescriber

---

⚠ High Alert

melphalan (℞)

(mel′fa-lan)

Alkeran, L-PAM, phenylalanine mustard

Func. class.: Antineoplastic, alkylating agent

Chem. class.: Nitrogen mustard

Do not confuse:

melphalan/Myleran

Action: Responsible for cross-linking DNA strands leading to cell death; activity is not cell cycle phase specific

Uses: Multiple myeloma, malignant melanoma, advanced ovarian cancer

Investigational uses: Breast, testicular, prostate carcinoma; osteogenic sarcoma, chronic myelogenous leukemia

DOSAGE AND ROUTES

Multiple myeloma

• *Adult:* **PO** 150 mcg/kg/day × 1 wk, then 21 days after, then 50 mcg/kg/day or 100-150 mcg/kg/day or 250 mcg/kg/day × 4 days for 2-3 wk, then 2-4 wk after, then 2-4 mg/day or 7 mg/m² × 5 day q5-6wk

• *Adult:* **IV INF** 16 mg/m², reduce in renal insufficiency, give over 15-20 min, give at 2-wk intervals × 4 doses, then at 4-wk intervals

Ovarian carcinoma

• *Adult:* **PO** 200 mcg/kg/day for 5 days q4-5wk

Available forms: Tabs 2 mg, powder for inj 50 mg

SIDE EFFECTS

GI: Nausea, vomiting, stomatitis, diarrhea

GU: Amenorrhea, hyperuricemia, gonadal suppression

*HEMA: **Thrombocytopenia, neutropenia, leukopenia,** anemia*

INTEG: Rash, urticaria, alopecia, pruritus

*RESP: **Fibrosis, dysplasia***

*SYST: **Anaphylaxis,** allergic reactions*

Contraindications: Pregnancy (D),

M

---

lactation, hypersensitivity to this drug or other nitrogen mustards

Precautions: Radiation therapy, bone marrow depression, infections, renal disease, children

PHARMACOKINETICS

Metabolized in liver, excreted in urine, half-life 1½ hr

INTERACTIONS

Increase: toxicity—antineoplastics, radiation

Increase: pulmonary toxicity—carmustine

Increase: renal failure risk—cycloSPORINE

Increase: enterocolitis risk—nalidixic acid

Decrease: antibody response—live virus vaccines

NURSING CONSIDERATIONS

Assess:

• CBC, differential, platelet count qwk; withhold drug if WBC is <3000/mm³ or platelet count is <100,000/mm³; notify prescriber; recovery usually occurs in 6 wk

• Renal studies: BUN, serum uric acid, urine CCr before, during therapy

• I&O ratio; report fall in urine output to 30 ml/hr

• For infection: fever, cough, temp, sore throat, notify prescriber

• For bleeding: bruising, blood in urine, stools, emesis

• Hepatic studies before, during therapy (bilirubin, AST, ALT, LDH) as needed or monthly

• Bleeding: hematuria, guaiac, bruising or petechiae, mucosa or orifices q8h

• Jaundiced skin and sclera, dark urine, clay-colored stools, itchy skin, abdominal pain, fever, diarrhea

• Buccal cavity q8h for dryness, sores, ulceration, white patches, oral pain, bleeding, dysphagia

• Local irritation, pain, burning, discoloration at inj site

⚠ Symptoms indicating severe allergic reaction: rash, pruritus, urticaria, purpuric skin lesions, itching, flushing; assess allergy to chlorambucil, cross-sensitivity may occur

Administer:

• Antiemetic 30-60 min before giving drug to prevent vomiting

IV route

• Give by intermittent inf after reconstituting with 10 ml diluent provided (5 mg/ml), shake, dilute dose with 0.9% NaCl (≤0.45 mg/ml), give within 1 hr, run over ≥15 min

Y-site compatibilities: Acyclovir, amikacin, aminophylline, ampicillin, aztreonam, bleomycin, bumetanide, buprenorphine, butorphanol, calcium gluconate, carboplatin, carmustine, cefazolin, cefepime, cefoperazone, cefotaxime, cefotetan, ceftazidime, ceftizoxime, ceftriaxone, cefuroxime, cimetidine, cisplatin, clindamycin, cyclophosphamide, cytarabine, dacarbazine, dactinomycin, DAUNOrubicin, dexamethasone, diphenhydrAMINE, DOXOrubicin, doxycycline, droperidol, enalaprilat, etoposide, famotidine, floxuridine, fluconazole, fludarabine, fluorouracil, furosemide, gallium, ganciclovir, gentamicin, granisetron, haloperidol, heparin, hydrocortisone, hydrocortisone sodium phosphate, hydromorphone, hydrOXYzine, idarubicin, ifosfamide, imipenem-cilastatin, lorazepam, mannitol, mechlorethamine, meperidine, mesna, methotrexate, methylPREDNISolone, metoclopramide, metronidazole, miconazole, minocycline, mitomycin, mitoxantrone, morphine, nalbuphine, netilmicin, ondansetron, pentostatin, piperacillin, plicamycin, potassium chloride, prochlorperazine, promethazine, ranitidine, sodium bicarbonate, streptozocin, teniposide, thiotepa, ticarcillin, ticarcillin/clavulanate, tobramycin, trimethoprim-sulfamethoxazole, vancomycin, vinBLAStine, vinCRIStine, vinorelbine, zidovudine

---

⚠ Safety alert   *"Tall Man" lettering

Perform/provide:
• Storage in airtight, light-resistant container
• Strict medical asepsis, protective isolation if WBC levels are low
• Increase fluid intake to 2-3 L/day to prevent urate deposits, calculi formation
• Diet low in purines: organ meats (kidney, liver), dried beans, peas to maintain alkaline urine
• Rinsing of mouth tid-qid with water, club soda; brushing of teeth bid-tid with soft brush or cotton-tipped applicators for stomatitis; use unwaxed dental floss
• Warm compresses at inj site for inflammation

Evaluate:
• Therapeutic response: decreased tumor size, spread of malignancy

Teach patient/family:
• That sterility, amenorrhea can occur; reversible after discontinuing treatment
• To avoid foods with citric acid, hot or rough texture
• To report any bleeding, white spots, or ulcerations in mouth to prescriber; tell patient to examine mouth daily
• To report signs of infection: fever, sore throat, flulike symptoms
• To report suspected pregnancy; to use contraception during treatment
• To report signs of anemia: fatigue, headache, faintness, shortness of breath, irritability
• To avoid use of razors, commercial mouthwash
• To avoid use of aspirin products, NSAIDs, alcohol

---

memantine (Ŗ)

(me-man′teen)
Namenda
Func. class.: Anti-Alzheimer agent
Chem. class.: NMDA receptor antagonist

Action: Antagonist action of CNS NMDA receptors that may contribute to the symptoms of Alzheimer's disease

Uses: Treatment of moderate to severe dementia in Alzheimer's disease
Investigational uses: Vascular dementia

DOSAGE AND ROUTES

• *Adult:* **PO** 5 mg daily, may increase dose in 5 mg increments ≥1 wk intervals; recommended target dose 20 mg/day
Available forms: Tabs 5, 10 mg

SIDE EFFECTS

CNS: Dizziness, confusion, somnolence, headache, hallucinations
CV: Hypertension
GI: Vomiting, constipation
INTEG: Rash
MISC: Back pain, fatigue, pain
RESP: Coughing, dyspnea
Contraindications: Hypersensitivity
Precautions: Pregnancy (B), renal disease, GU conditions that raise urine pH, lactation, children

PHARMACOKINETICS

Rapidly absorbed PO, 44% protein binding, very little metabolism, 57%-82% excreted unchanged in urine, terminal elimination half-life 60-80 hr

INTERACTIONS

May alter levels of both drugs: hydrochlorothiazide, triamterene, cimetidine, quinidine, ranitidine, nicotine
Decrease: clearance of memantine—drugs which makes the urine alkaline (sodium bicarbonate, carbonic anhydrase inhibitors)

NURSING CONSIDERATIONS

Assess:
• B/P: hypertension
• Mental status: affect, mood, behavioral changes; hallucinations, confusion
• GI status: vomiting, constipation, add bulk, increase fluids for constipation
• GU status: urinary frequency

Administer:
• Can be taken without regard to meals
• Twice a day if dose >5 mg

M

• Dosage adjusted to response no more than q1wk

Perform/provide:

• Assistance with ambulation during beginning therapy; dizziness may occur

Evaluate:

• Therapeutic response: decrease in confusion, improved mood

Teach patient/family:

• To report side effects: restlessness, psychosis, visual hallucinations, stupor, loss of consciousness; indicate overdose

• To use drug exactly as prescribed; drug is not a cure

---

menotropins (R)

(men-oh-troe′pins)
Humegon, Pergonal, Repronex
Func. class.: Gonadotropin
Chem. class.: Exogenous gonadotropin

Action: In women, increases follicular growth, maturation; in men, when given with hCG, stimulates spermatogenesis

Uses: Infertility, anovulation in women, stimulates spermatogenesis in men

DOSAGE AND ROUTES

Infertility

• *Men:* **IM** 1 ampule 3 × wk with hCG 2000 units 2 × wk × 4 mo

• *Women:* **IM** 75 international units FSH, LH daily × 9-12 days, then 10,000 units hCG 1 day after these drugs; repeat × 2 menstrual cycles, then increase to 150 international units FSH, LH daily × 9-12 days, then 10,000 units hCG 1 day after these drugs × 2 menstrual cycles

Anovulation

• *Women:* **IM** 75 international units FSH, LH daily × 9-12 days, then 10,000 units hCG 1 day after last dose of these drugs; repeat × 1-3 menstrual cycles

Available forms: Powder for inj lyophilized 75 international units FSH, LH activity 150 international units FSH, LH activity

SIDE EFFECTS

CNS: Fever

*CV: **Hypovolemia***

GI: Nausea, vomiting, diarrhea, anorexia

GU: Ovarian enlargement, abdominal distention/pain, multiple births, ovarian hyperstimulation: sudden ovarian enlargement, ascites with or without pain; gynecomastia in men

*HEMA: **Hemoperitoneum, arterial thromboembolism***

*RESP: **ARDS, pulmonary embolism, pulmonary infarction, pleural effusion***

*SYST: **Anaphylaxis***

Contraindications: Pregnancy (X), primary ovarian failure, abnormal bleeding, thyroid/adrenal dysfunction, organic intracranial lesion, ovarian cysts, primary testicular failure

NURSING CONSIDERATIONS

Assess:

• Weight daily; notify prescriber if weight increases rapidly

• Estrogen excretion level; if >100 mcg/24 hr, drug is withheld; hyperstimulation syndrome may occur

• I&O ratio; be alert for decreasing urinary output

• Ovarian enlargement, abdominal distention/pain; report symptoms immediately

Administer:

IM route

• After reconstituting with 1-2 ml sterile saline inj; use immediately

Evaluate:

• Therapeutic response: ovulation, pregnancy

Teach patient/family:

• That multiple births are possible; if pregnancy occurs, usually 4-6 wk after start of treatment

• To keep appointment during treatment daily × 2 wk

A High Alert

meperidine (℞)
(me-per'i-deen)
Demerol, meperidine,
Pethidine
Func. class.: Opioid analgesic
Chem. class.: Phenylpiperidine derivative

Controlled Substance Schedule II
Do not confuse:
Demerol/Dilaudid
meperidine/hydromorphone/
meprobamate/morphine
Action: Depresses pain impulse transmission at the spinal cord level by interacting with opioid receptors
Uses: Moderate to severe pain, preoperatively, postoperatively
Investigational uses: Rigors

DOSAGE AND ROUTES

Pain
• *Adult:* **PO/SUBCUT/IM** 50-150 mg q3-4h prn; **IV** 15-35 mg/hr as a **CONT INF**; PCA 10 mg, then 1-5 mg incremental dose; lockout interval 6-10 min
• *Child:* **PO/SUBCUT/IM** 1 mg/kg q3-4h prn, not to exceed 100 mg q4h
Labor analgesia
• *Adult:* **SUBCUT/IM** 50-100 mg given when contractions are regularly spaced, repeat q1-3h prn
Preoperatively
• *Adult:* **IM/SUBCUT** 50-100 mg q30-90 min before surgery; dose should be reduced if given **IV**
• *Child:* **IM/SUBCUT** 1-2.2 mg/kg 30-90 min before surgery
Renal disease
• CCr 10-50 ml/min 75% of dose; CCr <10 ml/min 50% of dose
Available forms include:
Inj 10, 25, 50, 75, 100 mg/ml; tabs 50, 100 mg; syr 50 mg/5 ml

SIDE EFFECTS

CNS: Drowsiness, dizziness, confusion, headache, sedation, euphoria, **in-**creased intracranial pressure, **seizures**
CV: Palpitations, bradycardia, change in B/P, tachycardia (IV)
EENT: Tinnitus, blurred vision, miosis, diplopia, depressed corneal reflex
GI: Nausea, vomiting, anorexia, constipation, cramps
GU: Urinary retention, dysuria
INTEG: Rash, urticaria, bruising, flushing, diaphoresis, pruritus
RESP: **Respiratory depression**
Contraindications: Hypersensitivity, addiction (opioid)
Precautions: Pregnancy (B), addictive personality, lactation, increased intracranial pressure, MI (acute), severe heart disease, respiratory depression, hepatic disease, renal disease, child <18 yr, elderly

PHARMACOKINETICS

Absorption 50% (PO), well absorbed IM, SUBCUT
PO: Onset 15 min, peak ½-1 hr, duration 2-4 hr
SUBCUT/IM: Onset 10 min, peak ½-1 hr, duration 2-4 hr
IV: Onset 5 min, duration 2 hr
Metabolized by liver (to active/inactive metabolites), excreted by kidneys; crosses placenta, excreted in breast milk; half-life 3-4 hr; toxic by-product can result from regular use

INTERACTIONS

⚠ May cause fatal reaction: MAOIs, procarbazine
Increase: effects with other CNS depressants, alcohol, opioids, sedative/hypnotics, antipsychotics, skeletal muscle relaxants
Increase: adverse reactions—protease inhibitor antiretrovirals
Decrease: meperidine effect—phenytoin
Drug/Herb
Increase: CNS depression—chamomile, hops, Jamaican dogwood, kava, lavender,

Side effects: *italics* = common; **bold italics** = life-threatening

mistletoe, nettle, pokeweed, poppy, senega, skullcap, valerian

Increase: Parsley may promote serotonin syndrome; avoid concurrent medicinal use

Drug/Lab Test

Increase: Amylase, lipase

NURSING CONSIDERATIONS

Assess:

• Pain: location, type, character; give before pain becomes extreme; reassess after 60 min (IM, SUBCUT, PO) and 5-10 min (IV)

• Renal function prior to initiating therapy; poor renal function can lead to accumulation of toxic metabolite and seizures

• I&O ratio; check for decreasing output; may indicate urinary retention

• For constipation; increase fluids, bulk in diet; give laxatives if needed

• CNS changes: dizziness, drowsiness, hallucinations, euphoria, LOC, pupil reactions; at chronic or high-dose use

• Allergic reactions: rash, urticaria

• Respiratory dysfunction: depression, character, rate, rhythm; notify prescriber if respirations are <12/min

• CNS stimulation: occurs with chronic or high doses

Administer:

• Patient should remain recumbent for 1 hr after IM/SUBCUT route

• With antiemetic for nausea, vomiting

• When pain is beginning to return; determine dosage interval by patient response

• In gradually decreasing dose after long-term use; withdrawal symptoms may occur

IV route

• After diluting with 5 ml or more sterile H$_2$O or NS; give directly over 4-5 min; may be further diluted in sol to 1 mg/ml during anesthesia in D$_5$W or NS; if diluted in NS, may be given through patient-controlled inf device

Additive compatibilities: Cefazolin, DOBUTamine, ondansetron, scopol-amine, succinylcholine, trifluoperazine, verapamil

Syringe compatibilities: Atropine, benzquinamide, butorphanol, chlor-proMAZINE, cimetidine, dimenhyDRINATE, diphenhydrAMINE, droperidol, fentanyl, glycopyrrolate, hydrOXYzine, ketamine, metoclopramide, midazolam, pentazocine, perphenazine, prochlorper-azine, promazine, promethazine, raniti-dine, scopolamine

Y-site compatibilities: Amifostine, amikacin, ampicillin, atenolol, aztre-onam, bumetanide, cefamandole, cefazo-lin, cefmetazole, cefotaxime, cefotetan, cefoxitin, ceftazidime, ceftizoxime, ceftri-axone, cefuroxime, cephalothin, cepha-pirin, chloramphenicol, cisatracurium, cladribine, clindamycin, dexamethasone, diltiazem, diphenhydrAMINE, DOB-UTamine, DOPamine, DOXOrubicin lipo-some, doxycycline, droperidol, erythro-mycin, famotidine, filgrastim, fluconazole, fludarabine, gallium, genta-micin, granisetron, heparin, hydrocorti-sone, insulin (regular), kanamycin, labetalol, lidocaine, methyldopate, mag-nesium sulfate, melphalan, methylPRED-NISolone, metoclopramide, metoprolol, metronidazole, moxalactam, on-dansetron, oxacillin, oxytocin, paclitaxel, penicillin G potassium, piperacillin, potassium chloride, propofol, propranolol, ranitidine, remifentanil, sargramostim, teniposide, thiotepa, ticar-cillin, ticarcillin/clavulanate, tobramycin, trimethoprim-sulfamethoxazole, vanco-mycin, verapamil, vinorelbine

Perform/provide:

• Storage in light-resistant container at room temperature

• Assistance with ambulation

• Safety measures: night-light, call bell within easy reach

Evaluate:

• Therapeutic response: decrease in pain

Teach patient/family:

• To report any symptoms of CNS changes, allergic reactions

• That physical dependency may result from extended use

• That drowsiness, dizziness may occur; to call for assistance

• That withdrawal symptoms may occur: nausea, vomiting, cramps, fever, faintness, anorexia

• To make position changes slowly; orthostatic hypotension can occur

• To avoid OTC medications, alcohol unless directed by prescriber

Treatment of overdose: Naloxone (Narcan) 0.2-0.8 mg IV, O_2, IV fluids, vasopressors

---

mercaptopurine (℞)

(mer-kap-toe-pyoor′een)
Purinethol, 6-MP
Func. class.: Antineoplastic-antimetabolite
Chem. class.: Purine analog

Action: Inhibits purine metabolism at multiple sites, which inhibits DNA and RNA synthesis, S phase of cell cycle specific

Uses: Chronic myelocytic or acute lymphoblastic leukemia in children, acute myelogenous leukemia

Investigational uses: Polycythemia vera, psoriatic arthritis, colitis, lymphoma

DOSAGE AND ROUTES

• *Adult:* PO 80-100 mg/m^2 daily max 5 mg/kg/day; maintenance 1.5-2.5 mg/kg/day

• *Child:* PO 75 mg/m^2/day; maintenance 1.5-2.5 mg/kg/day

Available forms: Tabs 50 mg

SIDE EFFECTS

CNS: Fever, headache, weakness
GI: Nausea, vomiting, anorexia, diarrhea, stomatitis, **hepatotoxicity** (high doses), jaundice, gastritis
*GU: **Renal failure**, hyperuricemia, **oliguria**, crystalluria, **hematuria**
*HEMA: **Thrombocytopenia, leukopenia, myelosuppression, anemia***
INTEG: Rash, dry skin, urticaria

Contraindications: Pregnancy (D), patients with prior drug resistance, leukopenia (<2500/mm^3), thrombocytopenia (<100,000/mm^3), anemia, lactation

Precautions: Renal disease

PHARMACOKINETICS

Incompletely absorbed when taken orally; metabolized in liver, excreted in urine

INTERACTIONS

Reversal of neuromuscular blockade: nondepolarizing muscle relaxants
Increase: toxicity—radiation or other antineoplastics
Increase: bone marrow depression—allopurinol, co-trimoxazole
Increase or decrease: anticoagulant action—warfarin
Decrease: antibodies—live virus vaccines

NURSING CONSIDERATIONS
Assess:

• CBC, differential, platelet count qwk; withhold drug if WBC is <3500 or platelet count is <100,000; notify prescriber; drug should be discontinued

• Renal studies: BUN, serum uric acid, urine CCr, electrolytes before, during therapy

• I&O ratio; report fall in urine output to <30 ml/hr

• Monitor temp q4h; fever may indicate beginning infection; no rectal temps

• Hepatic studies before, during therapy: bilirubin, alk phosphatase, AST, ALT, qwk during beginning therapy

• Bleeding: hematuria, guaiac, bruising, petechiae; mucosa or orifices q8h

• Buccal cavity q8h for dryness, sores, ulceration, white patches, oral pain, bleeding, dysphagia

⚠ Symptoms indicating severe allergic reaction: rash, urticaria, itching, flushing

Administer:

• Antacid before oral agent; give drug after evening meal before bedtime

• Allopurinol or sodium bicarbonate to

M

maintain uric acid levels, alkalinization of urine

Perform/provide:

• Strict medical asepsis, protective isolation if WBC levels are low

• Increase fluid intake to 2-3 L/day to prevent urate deposits, calculi formation, unless contraindicated

• Diet low in purines: absence of organ meats (kidney, liver), dried beans, peas to maintain alkaline urine

• Rinsing of mouth tid-qid with water, club soda; brushing of teeth bid-tid with soft brush or cotton-tipped applicators for stomatitis; use unwaxed dental floss

• Nutritious diet with iron, vitamin supplements as ordered

• Storage in tightly closed container in cool environment

Evaluate:

• Therapeutic response: decreased size of tumor, spread of malignancy

Teach patient/family:

• To avoid foods with citric acid, hot or rough texture for stomatitis

• To report stomatitis: any bleeding, white spots, ulcerations in mouth; tell patient to examine mouth daily, report symptoms

• That contraceptive measures are recommended during therapy; to avoid breastfeeding

• To drink 10-12 (8 oz) glasses of fluid/day

• To notify prescriber of fever, chills, sore throat, nausea, vomiting, anorexia, diarrhea, bleeding, bruising, which may indicate blood dyscrasias

• To report signs of infection: fever, sore throat, flulike symptoms

• To report signs of anemia: fatigue, headache, faintness, shortness of breath, irritability

• To report bleeding: avoid use of razors, commercial mouthwash

• To avoid use of aspirin products, NSAIDs

• To take entire dose at one time

---

meropenem (Ƀ)
(mer-oh-pen'em)
Merrem IV
Func. class.: Antiinfective, miscellaneous
Chem. class.: Carbapenem

Action: Interferes with cell wall replication of susceptible organisms; osmotically unstable cell wall swells, bursts from osmotic pressure

Uses: Serious infections caused by gram-positive bacteria: *Streptococcus pneumoniae*, group A β-hemolytic streptococci, enterococcus; gram-negative: *Klebsiella, Proteus, Escherichia coli, Pseudomonas aeruginosa;* appendicitis, peritonitis caused by *viridans* group streptococci; *Bacteroides fragilis, Bacteroides thetaiotaomicron,* bacterial meningitis (≥3 mo)

DOSAGE AND ROUTES

• *Adult:* **IV** 1 g q8h, given over 15-30 min or as an **IV BOL** 5-20 ml given over 3-5 min

• *Child ≥3 mo:* **IV** 20-40 mg/kg q8h (max 2g q8h meningitis)

• *Child >50 kg:* **IV** 1 g q8h (intraabdominal infection) or 2 g q8h (meningitis) given over 15-30 min or as an **IV BOL** 5-20 ml over 3-5 min

Renal disease

• *Adult:* **IV** CCr 26-50 ml/min 1 g q12h; CCr 10-25 ml/min 500 mg q12h; CCr <10 ml/min 500 mg q24h

Available forms: Inj 500 mg, 1 g

SIDE EFFECTS

CNS: Fever, somnolence, *seizures,* dizziness, weakness, myoclonia, *headache*
CV: Hypotension, palpitations
GI: Diarrhea, nausea, vomiting, *pseudomembranous colitis, hepatitis,* glossitis
HEMA: Eosinophilia, neutropenia, decreased Hgb, Hct
INTEG: Rash, urticaria, *pruritus,* pain at inj site, phlebitis, erythema at inj site

---

RESP: Chest discomfort, dyspnea, hyperventilation
SYST: ***Anaphylaxis***
Contraindications: Hypersensitivity to meropenem or imipenem
Precautions: Pregnancy (B), lactation, elderly, renal disease

PHARMACOKINETICS

IV: Onset immediate, peak dose dependent, half-life 1 hr, hepatic metabolism

INTERACTIONS

Increase: meropenem plasma levels—probenecid
Drug/Lab Test
Increase: AST, ALT, LDH, BUN, alk phosphatase, bilirubin, creatinine
False positive: Direct Coombs' test

NURSING CONSIDERATIONS

Assess:
• Sensitivity to carbapenem antibiotics, penicillins
• Renal disease: lower dose may be required
• Bowel pattern daily; if severe diarrhea occurs, drug should be discontinued; may indicate pseudomembranous colitis
• For infection: temp, sputum, characteristics of wound, before, during, and after treatment
🅰 Allergic reactions, anaphylaxis: rash, urticaria, pruritus; may occur few days after therapy begins
• Overgrowth of infection: perineal itching, fever, malaise, redness, pain, swelling, drainage, rash, diarrhea, change in cough, sputum
Administer:
• By IV inf or IV bol
• After C&S is taken
• Reconstitute with 0.9% NaCl, D₅W, LR, dilute in 5-20 ml comp sol, give by direct IV over 3-5 min; give by intermittent inf, dilute in 5-20 ml of comp sol, give over 15-30 min
Additive compatibilities: Aminophylline, atropine, cimetidine, dexamethasone, DOBUTamine, DOPamine, enalaprilat, fluconazole, furosemide, gentamicin, heparin, insulin (regular), magnesium sulfate, metoclopramide, morphine, norepinephrine, phenobarbital, ranitidine, vancomycin
Y-site compatibilities: Aminophylline, atenolol, atropine, cimetidine, dexamethasone, digoxin, diphenhydrAMINE, enalaprilat, fluconazole, furosemide, gentamicin, heparin, insulin (regular), metoclopramide, morphine, norepinephrine, phenobarbital, vancomycin
Evaluate:
• Therapeutic response: negative C&S; absence of symptoms and signs of infection
Teach patient/family:
• To report severe diarrhea; may indicate pseudomembranous colitis
• To report sore throat, bruising, bleeding, joint pain; may indicate blood dyscrasias (rare)
• To report overgrowth of infection: black, furry tongue; vaginal itching; foul-smelling stools
• To avoid breastfeeding; drug is excreted in breast milk
Treatment of overdose: EpINEPHrine, antihistamines; resuscitate if needed (anaphylaxis)

M

---

mesalamine (Ⓡ)
(mez-al′a-meen)
Asacol, Canasa, Mesasal, Pentasa, Rowasa Salofalk ✦
Func. class.: GI antiinflammatory
Chem. class.: 5-Aminosalicylic acid

Do not confuse:
Asacol/Ansaid
Action: May diminish inflammation by blocking cyclooxygenase, inhibiting prostaglandin production in colon; local action only
Uses: Mild to moderate active distal ulcerative colitis, proctosigmoiditis, proctitis
Investigational uses: Crohn's disease

Side effects: *italics* = common; ***bold italics*** = life-threatening

DOSAGE AND ROUTES

• *Adult:* **RECT** 60 ml (4 g) at bedtime, retained for 8 hr × 3-6 wk; **PO** 800 mg tid × 6 wk; **SUPP** 500 mg bid × 3-6 wk, retain 1-3 hr

Available forms: Rect susp 4 g/60 ml; supp 500 mg; tab del rel 400 mg; con rel cap 250 mg (Pentasa)

SIDE EFFECTS

CNS: Headache, fever, dizziness, insomnia, asthenia, weakness, fatigue
CV: Pericarditis, myocarditis
EENT: Sore throat, cough, pharyngitis, rhinitis
GI: Cramps, gas, nausea, diarrhea, rectal pain, constipation
INTEG: Rash, itching, acne
SYST: Flulike symptoms, malaise, back pain, peripheral edema, leg and joint pain, arthralgia, dysmenorrhea, *anaphylaxis,* acute intolerance syndrome
Contraindications: Hypersensitivity to this drug or salicylates
Precautions: Pregnancy (B), renal disease, lactation, children, sulfite sensitivity, elderly, pyloric stenosis

PHARMACOKINETICS

RECT: Primarily excreted in feces but some in urine as metabolite; half-life 1 hr, metabolite half-life 5-10 hr

INTERACTIONS

Increase: mesalamine absorption—omeprazole
Increase: action of—azathioprine
Decrease: digoxin level—digoxin
Decrease: mesalamine absorption—lactulose
Drug/Lab Test
Increase: AST, ALT, alk phosphatase, LDH, GGTP, amylase, lipase

NURSING CONSIDERATIONS

Assess:
• For allergy to salicylates, sulfonamides, if allergic reactions occur, discontinue drug

• Renal studies: BUN, creatinine before and during treatment
• GI symptoms: cramps, gas, nausea, diarrhea, rectal pain; if severe, drug should be discontinued
• I&O ratios, increase fluids to 1500 ml daily to prevent crystalluria

Administer:
PO route
• Swallow tabs whole; do not break, crush, or chew tabs
Rectal route
• Drug should be given at bedtime, retained until morning; empty bowel before insertion

Perform/provide:
• Storage at room temperature

Evaluate:
• Therapeutic response: absence of pain, bleeding from GI tract, decrease in number of diarrhea stools

Teach patient/family:
• That usual course of therapy is 3-6 wk
• To shake bottle well (rectal susp)
• Method of rectal administration
• To inform prescriber of GI symptoms
• To report abdominal cramping, pain, diarrhea with blood, headache, fever, rash, chest pain; drug should be discontinued

---

metaproterenol (℞)

(met-a-proe-ter′e-nole)
Alupent, Arm-a-Med, Dey-Lute
Func. class.: Bronchodilator-selective β₂-agonist

Do not confuse:
Alupent/Atrovent
Action: Relaxes bronchial smooth muscle by direct action on β₂-adrenergic receptors with increased levels of cAMP with increased bronchodilation, diuresis, cardiac CNS stimulation
Uses: Bronchial asthma, bronchospasm

DOSAGE AND ROUTES

• *Adult and child >12 yr:* **INH** 2-3 inhalations; may repeat q3-4h, not to

---

exceed 12 inhalations/day; **IPPB** or **NEB** 0.2-0.3 ml of 5% sol diluted in 2.5 ml of ½NS or NS; or 2.5 ml of 0.4, 0.6% sol q4h prn

• *Adult:* **PO** 20 mg q6-8h
• *Geriatric:* **PO** 10 mg tid-qid, initially
• *Child 6-12 yr:* **IPPB/NEB** 0.1-0.2 ml of a 5% sol diluted in NS to a final volume of 3 ml q4h prn
• *Child >9 yr or >27 kg:* **PO** 20 mg q6-8h or 0.4-0.9 mg/kg tid
• *Child 6-9 yr or <27 kg:* **PO** 10 mg q6-8h or 0.4-0.9 mg/kg tid
• *Child 2-6 yr:* **PO** 1.3-2.6 mg/kg divided q6-8h

Available forms: Tabs 10, 20 mg; aerosol inhaler 0.65 mg/dose; syr 10 mg/5 ml; Neb inhaler 0.4%, 0.6%, 5%

SIDE EFFECTS

CNS: Tremors, anxiety, insomnia, headache, dizziness, stimulation
CV: Palpitations, tachycardia, hypertension, dysrhythmias, ***cardiac arrest*** (high dose)
GI: Nausea, vomiting, dry mouth
RESP: ***Paradoxical bronchospasm***
Contraindications: Hypersensitivity to sympathomimetics, narrow-angle glaucoma, cardiac dysrhythmias with tachycardia
Precautions: Pregnancy (C), cardiac disorders, hyperthyroidism, diabetes mellitus, prostatic hypertrophy, seizure disorder, elderly, child <6 yr (PO)

PHARMACOKINETICS

PO: Onset 15 min, peak 1 hr, duration 1-4 hr, excreted in urine as metabolites
INH: Onset 1 min, peak 1 hr, duration 1-2½ hr
NEB: Onset 5-30 min, peak 1 hr, duration 1-2½ hr

INTERACTIONS

⚠ Hypertensive crisis: MAOIs
Increase: effects of both drugs—other sympathomimetics, bronchodilators
Decrease: β-blockers action

Drug/Herb
Increase: effect—black/green tea, coffee, cola nut, guarana, yerba maté
Drug/Lab Test
Decrease: Potassium

NURSING CONSIDERATIONS

Assess:
• Respiratory function: vital capacity, forced expiratory volume, ABGs; also B/P; lung sounds, secretions before and after treatment
• Tolerance over long-term therapy; dose may have to be changed; check for rebound bronchospasm
Administer:
• 2 hr before bedtime to avoid sleeplessness
• PO with food for GI upset
Perform/provide:
• Storage at room temperature; do not use discolored sol
• Spacer device for elderly
Evaluate:
• Therapeutic response: absence of dyspnea, wheezing; improved ABGs
Teach patient/family:
• To increase fluid intake (2-3 L/day) to liquefy secretions unless contraindicated
• Not to use OTC medications; excess stimulation may occur
• To notify prescriber of headaches, chest pain, weakness, dizziness, anxiety
• Use of inhaler; review package insert with patient
• To avoid getting aerosol in eyes
• To wash inhaler in warm water and dry daily
• All aspects of drug; avoid smoking, smoke-filled rooms, persons with respiratory infections

M

metformin (℞)

(met-for′min)
Fortamet, Glucophage,
Glucophage XR,
Novo-Metformin ✲, Riomet
Func. class.: Antidiabetic, oral
Chem. class.: Biguanide

Action: Inhibits hepatic glucose production and increases sensitivity of peripheral tissue to insulin
Uses: Type 2 diabetes mellitus

DOSAGE AND ROUTES

• *Adult:* **PO** 500 mg bid initially, then increase to desired response 1-2 g; dosage adjustment q2-3wk or 850 mg daily with morning meal with dosage increased every other wk, max 2500 mg/day, **EXT REL** max 2000 mg/day
• *Geriatric:* **PO,** use lowest effective dose
Available forms: Tabs 500, 850, 1000 mg; ext rel tab 500 mg; oral sol (Riomet) 500 mg/5 ml

SIDE EFFECTS

CNS: Headache, weakness, dizziness, drowsiness, tinnitus, fatigue, vertigo, *agitation*
*ENDO: **Lactic acidosis,*** hypoglycemia
GI: Nausea, vomiting, diarrhea, heartburn, anorexia, metallic taste
*HEMA: **Thrombocytopenia,*** decreased vit B_{12} levels
INTEG: Rash
Contraindications: Hypersensitivity, hepatic, creatinine >1.5 mg/ml (males) ≥1.4 (females), CHF, alcoholism, cardiopulmonary disease, history of lactic acidosis
Precautions: Pregnancy (B), previous hypersensitivity, elderly, thyroid disease

PHARMACOKINETICS

Excreted by the kidneys unchanged 35%-50%, half-life 1½-5 hr, terminal 6-20 hr, peak 1-3 hr

INTERACTIONS

Do not give with radiologic contrast media; may cause renal failure
Increase: metformin level—cimetidine, digoxin, morphine, procainamide, quinidine, ranitidine, triamterene, vancomycin
Increase: hypoglycemia—cimetidine, calcium channel blockers, corticosteroids, estrogens, oral contraceptives, phenothiazines, sympathomimetics, diuretics, phenytoin
Drug/Herb
Hyperglycemia: glucosamine
Hypoglycemia: chromium, coenzyme Q-10, fenugreek
Increase: metformin level—quinine
Increase: antidiabetic effect—alfalfa, aloe, basil, bay, bilberry, bitter melon, black catechu, buchu, burdock, coriander, dandelion, eyebright (po), fenugreek, garlic, ginseng, glucomannan, glucosamine, goat's rue, gymnema, horehound, horse chestnut, jambul, myrrh, myrtle
Decrease: antidiabetic effect—bee pollen, blue cohosh, broom, chromium, elecampane, eucalyptus, gotu kola

NURSING CONSIDERATIONS

Assess:
• For hypoglycemic reactions (sweating, weakness, dizziness, anxiety, tremors, hunger), hyperglycemic reactions soon after meals
• CBC (baseline, q3mo) during treatment; check LFTs periodically AST, LDH, renal studies: BUN, creatinine during treatment; glucose, A1c
⚠ For lactic acidosis: malaise, myalgia, abdominal distress; risk increases with age, poor renal function; monitor electrolytes, lactate, pyruvate, blood pH, ketones, glucose
Administer:
PO route
• Do not break, crush, chew ext rel tab
• Twice a day given with meals to decrease GI upset and provide best absorption, may also be taken as a single dose
• Tabs crushed and mixed with meal or

fluids for patients with difficulty swallowing

Perform/provide:
• Conversion from other oral hypoglycemic agents; change may be made without gradual dosage change; monitor serum or urine glucose and ketones tid during conversion
• Storage in tight container in cool environment

Evaluate:
• Therapeutic response: decrease in polyuria, polydipsia, polyphagia; clear sensorium; absence of dizziness; stable gait, blood glucose at normal level

Teach patient/family:
⚠ Lactic acidosis symptoms: hyperventilation, fatigue, malaise, chills, myalgia, somnolence; to notify prescriber immediately
• To use regular self-monitoring of blood glucose using blood glucose meter
• The symptoms of hypo/hyperglycemia, what to do about each
• That drug must be continued on daily basis; explain consequence of discontinuing drug abruptly
• To avoid OTC medications unless approved by prescriber
• That diabetes is a lifelong illness; that this drug is not a cure; only controls symptoms
• That all food included in diet plan must be eaten to prevent hypoglycemia
• To carry emergency ID and glucagon emergency kit for emergencies
• That Glucophage XR tab may appear in stool

Treatment of overdose: Glucose 25 g IV via dextrose 50% sol, 50 ml or 1 mg glucagon

---

⚠ High Alert

methadone (℞)
(meth'a-done)
Dolophine, methadone, Methadose
Func. class.: Opioid analgesic
Chem. class.: Synthetic diphenylheptane derivative

Controlled Substance Schedule II
Do not confuse:
methadone/methylphenidate
Action: Depresses pain impulse transmission at the spinal cord level by interacting with opioid receptors, produce CNS depression
Uses: Severe pain, opioid withdrawal

DOSAGE AND ROUTES
Severe pain
• *Adult:* **PO/SUBCUT/IM** 2.5-10 mg q3-4h prn
Opioid withdrawal
• *Adult:* **PO** 15-40 mg/day individualized initially, then 20-120 mg/day titrated to patient response
• *Child:* 0.05-0.1 mg/kg/dose q6-12h
Renal disease
• *Adult:* CCr 10-50 ml/min dose q8h; CCr <10 ml/min dose q8-12h
Available forms: Inj 10 mg/ml; tabs 5, 10 mg; oral sol 5, 10 mg/5 ml; dispersible tabs 40 mg; oral conc 10 mg/ml; oral sol 5 mg/5 ml, 10 mg/5 ml, 10 mg/10 ml

SIDE EFFECTS
CNS: Drowsiness, dizziness, confusion, headache, sedation, euphoria, ***seizures***
CV: Palpitations, bradycardia, change in B/P, ***cardiac arrest, shock***
EENT: Tinnitus, blurred vision, miosis, diplopia
GI: Nausea, vomiting, anorexia, constipation, cramps, biliary tract spasm
GU: Increased urinary output, dysuria, urinary retention
INTEG: Rash, urticaria, bruising, flushing, diaphoresis, pruritus

M

Side effects: *italics* = common; ***bold italics*** = life-threatening

RESP: **Respiratory depression, respiratory arrest**

Contraindications: Hypersensitivity to this drug or chlorobutanol (inj), addiction (opiate)

Precautions: Pregnancy (C), addictive personality, lactation, increased intracranial pressure, MI (acute), severe heart disease, respiratory depression, hepatic disease, renal disease, children <18 yr, elderly

PHARMACOKINETICS

PO: Onset 30-60 min, peak 1½-2 hr, duration 6-8 hr, cumulative 22-48 hr; PO half as active as INJ

SUBCUT/IM: Onset 10-20 min, peak 1½-2 hr, duration 4-6 hr, cumulative 22-48 hr

Metabolized by liver; excreted by kidneys; crosses placenta; excreted in breast milk; half-life 15-30 hr, extended interval with continued dosing; 90% bound to plasma proteins

INTERACTIONS

⚠ Unpredictable reactions: MAOIs, do not use together

Increase: effects with other CNS depressants—alcohol, opiates, sedative/hypnotics, antipsychotics, skeletal muscle relaxants

Decrease: analgesia—rifampin, phenytoin, nalbuphine, pentazine

Drug/Herb

Increase: CNS depression—chamomile, hops, Jamaican dogwood, kava, lavender, mistletoe, nettle, pokeweed, poppy, senega, skullcap, valerian

Increase: anticholinergic effect—corkwood

Drug/Lab Test

Increase: Amylase, lipase

NURSING CONSIDERATIONS

Assess:

• For pain: type, location, intensity, grimacing before and 1½-2 hr after administration; use pain scoring

• I&O ratio; check for decreasing output; may indicate urinary retention

• CNS changes: dizziness, drowsiness, hallucinations, euphoria, LOC, pupil reaction

• Allergic reactions: rash, urticaria

• Respiratory dysfunction: respiratory depression, character, rate, rhythm; notify prescriber if respirations are <10/min

• For opioid detoxification: no analgesia occurs, only prevention of withdrawal symptoms

• B/P, pulse

• Bowel changes, bulk, fluids, laxatives should be used for constipation

Administer:

• With antiemetic if nausea/vomiting occurs

• When pain is beginning to return; determine dosage interval by patient response

• Rotating inj sites, give deep in large muscle mass (IM)

Perform/provide:

• Storage in light-resistant container at room temperature

• Assistance with ambulation

• Safety measures: night-light, call bell within easy reach

Evaluate:

• Therapeutic response: decrease in pain, successful opioid withdrawal

Teach patient/family:

• To report any symptoms of CNS changes, allergic reactions

• That physical dependency may result from extended use

⚠ Withdrawal symptoms may occur: nausea, vomiting, cramps, fever, faintness, anorexia

Treatment of overdose: Naloxone (Narcan) 0.2-0.8 mg IV, O_2, IV fluids, vasopressors

methimazole (Ŗ)

(meth-im´a-zole)
Tapazole
Func. class.: Thyroid hormone antagonist (antithyroid)
Chem. class.: Thioamide

Action: Inhibits synthesis of thyroid hormones by decreasing iodine use in manufacture of thyroglobin and iodothyronine; does not affect circulatory T_4, T_3

Uses: Hyperthyroidism, preparation for thyroidectomy, thyrotoxic crisis, thyroid storm

DOSAGE AND ROUTES

Hyperthyroidism
• *Adult:* **PO** 15 mg/day (mild hyperthyroidism); 30-40 mg/day (moderate-severe); 60 mg/day (severe); maintenance 5-15 mg/day

• *Child:* **PO** 0.4 mg/kg/day in divided doses q8h; continue until euthyroid; maintenance dose 0.2 mg/kg/day in divided doses q8h, max 30 mg/24 hr

Preparation and thyroidectomy
• *Adult and child:* **PO** same as above; iodine may be added × 10 days before surgery

Thyrotoxic crisis
• *Adult and child:* **PO** same as hyperthyroidism with iodine and propranolol

Available forms: Tabs 5, 10 mg

SIDE EFFECTS

CNS: Drowsiness, headache, vertigo, fever, paresthesias, neuritis
ENDO: Enlarged thyroid
*GI: Nausea, diarrhea, vomiting, **jaundice**, **hepatitis**,* loss of taste
*GU: **Nephritis***
*HEMA: **Agranulocytosis, leukopenia, thrombocytopenia, hypothrombinemia, lymphadenopathy,*** bleeding, vasculitis
INTEG: Rash, urticaria, pruritus, alopecia, hyperpigmentation, lupus-like syndrome

MS: Myalgia, arthralgia, nocturnal muscle cramps

Contraindications: Pregnancy (D), hypersensitivity, lactation

Precautions: Infection, bone marrow depression, hepatic disease

PHARMACOKINETICS

PO: Onset 12-18 hr, duration 36-72 hr, half-life 4-12 hr; excreted in urine, breast milk; crosses placenta

INTERACTIONS

Agranulocytosis: phenothiazines
Increase: bone marrow depression—radiation, antineoplastic agents
Increase: response to digitalis, warfarin
Decrease: effectiveness—amiodarone, potassium iodide

Drug/Lab Test
Increase: PT, AST, ALT, alk phosphatase

NURSING CONSIDERATIONS

Assess:
• Pulse, B/P, temp
• I&O ratio; check for edema: puffy hands, feet, periorbits; indicate hypothyroidism
• Weight daily; same clothing, scale, time of day
• T_3, T_4, which are increased; serum TSH, which is decreased; free thyroxine index, which is increased if dosage is too low; discontinue drug 3-4 wk before RAIU

⚠ Blood work: CBC for blood dyscrasias: leukopenia, thrombocytopenia, agranulocytosis, if these occur, drug should be discontinued and other treatment initiated; LFTs

• Hypersensitivity: rash, enlarged cervical lymph nodes; drug may have to be discontinued
• Hypoprothrombinemia: bleeding, petechiae, ecchymosis
• Clinical response: after 3 wk should include increased weight, pulse; decreased T_4

⚠ Bone marrow depression: sore throat, fever, fatigue

M

Administer:
- With meals to decrease GI upset
- At same time each day to maintain drug level
- Lowest dose that relieves symptoms; discontinue before RAIU

Perform/provide:
- Storage in light-resistant container
- Fluids to 3-4 L/day, unless contraindicated

Evaluate:
- Therapeutic response: weight gain, decreased pulse, decreased T_4, B/P

Teach patient/family:
- Not to breastfeed
- To take pulse daily
- To report redness, swelling, sore throat, mouth lesions, fever, which indicate blood dyscrasias
- To keep graph of weight, pulse, mood
- To avoid OTC products that contain iodine
- That seafood, other iodine products may be restricted
- Not to discontinue this medication abruptly; thyroid crisis may occur; stress patient response
- That response may take several mo if thyroid is large
- The symptoms and signs of overdose: periorbital edema, cold intolerance, mental depression
- The symptoms of inadequate dose: tachycardia, diarrhea, fever, irritability
- To take medication as prescribed; do not skip or double dose

---

methocarbamol (℞)
(meth-oh-kar′ba-mole)
Carbacot, methocarbamol, Robaxin
Func. class.: Skeletal muscle relaxant, central acting
Chem. class.: Carbamate derivative

Action: Depresses multisynaptic pathways in the spinal cord, causing skeletal muscle relaxation
Uses: Adjunct for relief of spasm and pain in musculoskeletal conditions

DOSAGE AND ROUTES
MS pain
- *Adult:* **PO** 1.5 g qid × 2-3 days, then 1 g qid; **IM** 500 mg in each gluteal region, may repeat q8h; **IV BOL** 1-3 g/day at max 3 ml/min; **IV INF** 1 g/250 ml D_5W or NS, not to exceed 3 g/day
- *Geriatric:* **PO** 500 mg qid, titrate to needed dose

Tetanus management
- *Adult:* **IV Direct** 1-2 g or **IV INF** 1-3 g q6h
- *Child:* **IV** 15 mg/kg q6h prn

Available forms: Tabs 500, 750 mg; inj 100 mg/ml

SIDE EFFECTS
CNS: Dizziness, weakness, drowsiness, headache, tremor, depression, insomnia; *seizures* (IV, IM use)
CV: Postural hypotension, *bradycardia*
EENT: Diplopia, temporary loss of vision, blurred vision, nystagmus
GI: Nausea, vomiting, hiccups, anorexia, metallic taste
GU: Brown, black, green urine
HEMA: Hemolysis, increased hemoglobin (IV only)
INTEG: Rash, pruritus, fever, facial flushing, urticaria, phlebitis
SYST: Anaphylaxis (IM, IV)
Contraindications: Hypersensitivity, child <12 yr, intermittent porphyria
Precautions: Pregnancy (C), renal disease, hepatic disease, addictive personalities, myasthenia gravis, epilepsy

PHARMACOKINETICS
IM/IV: Onset rapid
PO: Onset ½ hr, peak 1-2 hr, half-life 1-2 hr
Metabolized in liver, excreted in urine unchanged, crosses placenta

INTERACTIONS
Increase: CNS depression—alcohol, tricyclics, opioids, barbiturates, sedatives, hypnotics

---

⚠ Safety alert   *"Tall Man" lettering

Drug/Herb
Increase: CNS depression—chamomile, hops, kava, skullcap, valerian
Drug/Lab Test
False increase: VMA, urinary 5-HIAA

NURSING CONSIDERATIONS
Assess:
• Blood studies: CBC, WBC, differential; blood dyscrasias may occur
• During and after inj: CNS effects, rash, conjunctivitis, nasal congestion may occur
• Hepatic studies: AST, ALT, alk phosphatase; hepatitis may occur
• ECG in epileptic patients; poor seizure control has occurred
• Allergic reactions: rash, fever, respiratory distress
• Severe weakness, numbness in extremities
• Tolerance: increased need for medication, more frequent requests for medication, increased pain
• CNS depression: dizziness, drowsiness, psychiatric symptoms
Administer:
PO route
• With meals for GI symptoms
IM route
• IM deep in large muscle mass; rotate sites
• Do not give SUBCUT
• Considered incompatible with any drug in sol or syringe
IV route
• IV undiluted over 1 min or more, give 300 mg or less/1 min or longer; may be diluted in 250 ml or less D₅ or isotonic NaCl sol for slow IV infusion
• By slow IV to prevent phlebitis; keep recumbent for 15 min to prevent orthostatic hypotension; check for extravasation
• Considered incompatible with any drug in sol or syringe
Perform/provide:
• Storage in tight container at room temperature
• Assistance with ambulation if dizziness/drowsiness occurs
• Recumbent position during and 10-15 min after IV administration
Evaluate:
• Therapeutic response: decreased pain, spasticity
Teach patient/family:
• Not to discontinue medication quickly; insomnia, nausea, headache, spasticity, tachycardia will occur; drug should be tapered off over 1-2 wk
• That urine may turn green, black, or brown
• Not to take with alcohol, other CNS depressants
• To avoid altering activities while taking this drug
• To avoid hazardous activities if drowsiness, dizziness occurs
• To avoid using OTC medication: cough preparations, antihistamines, unless directed by prescriber
Treatment of overdose: Induce emesis of conscious patient, lavage, dialysis; have epINEPHrine, antihistamines, and corticosteroids available, enhance elimination with osmotic diuresis, IV fluids for hypotension

⚠ High Alert

methotrexate (amethopterin, MTX) (℞)
(meth-oh-trex′ate)
methotrexate, Rheumatrex Dose Pack, Trexall
Func. class.: Antineoplastic-antimetabolite
Chem. class.: Folic acid antagonist

Do not confuse:
methotrexate/metolazone
Action: Inhibits an enzyme that reduces folic acid, which is needed for nucleic acid synthesis in all cells; S phase of cell cycle specific; immunosuppressive
Uses: Acute lymphocytic leukemia, in combination for breast, lung, head, neck carcinoma; lymphosarcoma, gestational choriocarcinoma, hydatidiform mole,

psoriasis, rheumatoid arthritis, mycosis fungoides

Investigational uses: Used investigationally to produce abortion

DOSAGE AND ROUTES

Acute lymphocytic leukemia
- *Adult and child:* **PO/IM/IV** 3.3 mg/m^2/day × 4-6 wk until remission, then 20-30 mg/m^2 **PO/IM** qwk in 2 divided doses or 2.5 mg/kg **IV** × 2 wk

Choriocarcinoma
- *Adult and child:* **PO/IM** 15-30 mg/m^2 daily × 5 days, then off 1 wk; may repeat

Meningeal leukemia
- *Adult and child:* 12 mg/m^2 **INTRATHECALLY** q2-5d until CSF is normal, then 1 additional dose, max 15 mg

Burkitt's lymphoma (stages I, II, III)
- *Adult:* **PO** 10-25 mg daily × 4-8 days with 7-day rest period

Lymphosarcoma (stage III)
- *Adult:* **PO/IM/IV** 0.625-2.5 mg/kg/day

Osteosarcoma
- *Adult and child:* **IV** 12 g/m^2 given over 4 hr, then leucovorin rescue

Mycosis fungoides
- *Adult:* **PO** 2.5-10 mg/day until cleared (may be many months); **IM** 50 mg qwk or 25 mg 2 ×/wk

Psoriasis
- *Adult:* **PO/IM/IV** 10-25 mg qwk or 2.5 mg **PO** q12h × 3 doses, may increase to 25 mg qwk

Breast cancer
- *Adult:* **IV** 40 mg/m^2 on days 1 and 8 with other antineoplastics

Rheumatoid arthritis
- *Adults:* **PO** 7.5 mg/wk or divided doses of 2.5 mg q12h × 3 given qwk; max 20 mg/wk

Polyarticular-course-juvenile RA
- *Child:* **PO** 10 mg/m^2 qwk

Available forms: Tabs 2.5, 5, 7.5, 10, 15 mg; inj 25 mg/ml; powder for inj 20, mg, 1 g

SIDE EFFECTS

CNS: Dizziness, *seizures, leukencephalopathy,* headache, confusion, hemiparesis, malaise, fatigue, chills, fever; *arachnoiditis* (intrathecal)

GI: Nausea, vomiting, anorexia, diarrhea, ulcerative stomatitis, *hepatotoxicity,* cramps, ulcer, gastritis, *GI hemorrhage,* abdominal pain, hematemesis, *hepatic fibrosis, acute toxicity*

GU: Urinary retention, *renal failure,* menstrual irregularities, defective spermatogenesis, *hematuria, azotemia, uric acid nephropathy*

HEMA: Leukopenia, thrombocytopenia, myelosuppression, anemia

INTEG: Rash, alopecia, dry skin, urticaria, photosensitivity, folliculitis, vasculitis, petechiae, ecchymosis, acne, alopecia, *severe fatal skin reaction*

RESP: Methotrexate-induced lung disease

SYST: Sudden death, pneumocystis carinii

Contraindications: Pregnancy (X), hypersensitivity, leukopenia (<3500/mm^3), thrombocytopenia (<100,000/mm^3), anemia, psoriatic patients with severe renal/hepatic disease, alcoholism, HIV

Precautions: Renal disease, lactation, children

PHARMACOKINETICS

PO: Readily absorbed
PO/IM/IV: Onset unknown; duration unknown
IT: Onset, peak, duration unknown
Not metabolized; excreted in urine (unchanged); crosses placenta, blood-brain barrier; 50% plasma protein bound

INTERACTIONS

Increase: toxicity—salicylates, sulfa drugs, other antineoplastics, radiation, alcohol, probenecid, NSAIDs, phenylbutazone, theophylline, penicillins
Increase: hypoprothrombinemia—oral anticoagulants
Decrease: effect of oral digoxin, vaccines, phenytoin, fosphenytoin

Decrease: effect of methotrexate—folic acid supplements

NURSING CONSIDERATIONS

Assess:

PO

• Make sure that drug is taken weekly in RA, JRA

⚠ CBC, differential, platelet count weekly; withhold drug if WBC is <3500/mm³ or platelet count is <100,000/mm³; notify prescriber; drug should be discontinued; WBC, platelet nadirs occur on day 7

• Renal studies: BUN, serum uric acid, urine CCr, electrolytes before, during therapy

• I&O ratio; report fall in urine output to <30 ml/hr

• Monitor temp q4h; fever may indicate beginning infection; no rectal temps

• Hepatic studies before and during therapy: bilirubin, alk phosphatase, AST, ALT; liver biopsy should be done before start of therapy (psoriasis patients)

• Bleeding time, coagulation time during treatment; bleeding: hematuria, guaiac, bruising or petechiae, mucosa or orifices q8h

• Effects of alopecia on body image; discuss feelings about body changes

⚠ Hepatotoxicity: jaundiced skin and sclera, dark urine, clay-colored stools, pruritus, abdominal pain, fever, diarrhea

• Monitor methotrexate levels, adjust leucovorin dose based on the level

• Buccal cavity q8h for dryness, sores, ulceration, white patches, oral pain, bleeding, dysphagia

⚠ Symptoms indicating severe allergic reaction: rash, urticaria, itching, flushing

Administer:

• Antacid before oral agent; give drug after evening meal before bedtime

• Antiemetic 30-60 min before giving drug

• Allopurinol or sodium bicarbonate to maintain uric acid levels, alkalinization of urine (pH >6.5), adequate fluids

IV route

• After diluting 5 mg/2 ml of sterile H_2O for inj; give through Y-tube or 3-way stopcock at 10 mg or less/min

⚠ Leucovorin calcium within 24 hr of this drug to prevent tissue damage; check agency policy, continue until methotrexate level <10^{-8}m

⚠ Give sodium bicarbonate tabs or IV fluids to prevent precipitation of drug at high doses; urine pH should be >7; may need to reduce dosage if BUN 20-30 mg/dl or creatinine is 1.2-2 mg/dl; stop drug if BUN >30 mg/dl or creatinine is >2 mg/dl

Additive compatibilities: Cephalothin, cyclophosphamide, cytarabine, fluorouracil, hydrOXYzine, mercaptopurine, ondansetron, sodium bicarbonate, vinCRIStine

Solution compatibilities: Amino acids, 4.25%/D$_{25}$, D$_5$W, sodium bicarbonate 0.05 mol/L, sodium chloride 0.9%

Syringe compatibilities: Bleomycin, cisplatin, cyclophosphamide, doxapram, DOXOrubicin, fluorouracil, furosemide, heparin, leucovorin, mitomycin, vinBLAStine, vinCRIStine

Y-site compatibilities: Allopurinol, amifostine, amphotericin B cholesteryl, asparaginase, aztreonam, bleomycin, cefepime, ceftriaxone, cimetidine, cisplatin, cyclophosphamide, cytarabine, DAUNOrubicin, dexchlorpheniramine, diphenhydrAMINE, DOXOrubicin, DOXOrubicin liposome, etoposide, famotidine, filgrastim, fludarabine, fluorouracil, furosemide, gallium, ganciclovir, granisetron, heparin, hydromorphone, imipenem/cilastatin, leucovorin, lorazepam, melphalan, mesna, methylPREDNISolone, metoclopramide, mitomycin, morphine, ondansetron, oxacillin, paclitaxel, piperacillin/tazobactam, prochlorperazine, ranitidine, sargramostim, teniposide, thiotepa, vinBLAStine, vinCRIStine, vinorelbine

Perform/provide:

• Strict medical asepsis and protective isolation if WBC levels are low

M

• Liquid diet: carbonated beverage, Jell-O; dry toast, crackers may be added when patient is not nauseated or vomiting

• Increased fluid intake to 2-3 L/day to prevent urate deposits, calculi formation, unless contraindicated

• Diet low in purines: absence of organ meats (kidney, liver), dried beans, peas to maintain alkaline urine

• Rinsing of mouth tid-qid with water, club soda; brushing of teeth bid-tid with soft brush or cotton-tipped applicators for stomatitis; use unwaxed dental floss

• Nutritious diet with iron, vitamin supplements

• Storage in tightly closed container in cool environment; store injection, powder for inj in dark, dry area

Evaluate:

• Therapeutic response: decreased tumor size, spread of malignancy

Teach patient/family:

• To report any complaints, side effects to nurse or prescriber: black tarry stools, chills, fever, sore throat, bleeding, bruising, cough, shortness of breath, dark or bloody urine

• That hair may be lost during treatment; wig or hairpiece may make patient feel better; tell patient that new hair may be different in color, texture (alopecia is rare)

• To avoid foods with citric acid, hot or rough texture if stomatitis is present

• To report stomatitis: any bleeding, white spots, ulcerations in mouth to prescriber; tell patient to examine mouth daily, report symptoms to nurse, use good oral hygiene

• That contraceptive measures are recommended during therapy and for at least 8 wk following cessation of therapy, to discontinue breastfeeding; toxicity to infant may occur

• To drink 10-12 glasses of fluid/day

• To avoid alcohol, salicylates, live vaccines

• To avoid use of razors, commercial mouthwash

• To use sunblock to prevent burns

methylcellulose (otc)

(meth-ill-sell'yoo-lose)
Citrucel
Func. class.: Laxative, bulk
Chem. class.: Hydrophilic semisynthetic cellulose derivative

Do not confuse:

Citrucel/Citracal

Action: Attracts water, expands in intestine to increase peristalsis; also absorbs excess water in stool; decreases diarrhea

Uses: Chronic constipation

DOSAGE AND ROUTES

• *Adult:* **PO** up to 6 g daily in divided doses

• *Child 6-12 yr:* **PO** 3 g daily in divided doses

Available forms: Powder 105 mg/g, 196 mg/g

SIDE EFFECTS

GI: **Obstruction,** abdominal distention

Contraindications: Hypersensitivity, GI obstruction, hepatitis

PHARMACOKINETICS

PO: Onset 12-24 hr, peak 1-3 days

INTERACTIONS

Decrease: absorption—antibiotics, digitalis, nitrofurantoin, salicylates, tetracyclines, oral anticoagulants

Drug/Herb

Increase: laxative action—flax senna

NURSING CONSIDERATIONS

Assess:

• Blood, urine electrolytes if used often

• I&O ratio to identify fluid loss

• Cause of constipation; lack of fluids, bulk, exercise, constipating drugs

• Cramping, rectal bleeding, nausea, vomiting; drug should be discontinued

Administer:

PO route

• Alone for better absorption; do not take within 1 hr of other drugs

• In morning or evening (oral dose)

⚠ Safety alert   *"Tall Man" lettering

Evaluate:
• Therapeutic response: decrease in constipation

Teach patient/family:
• To mix powder in water
• To increase fluid intake
• That normal bowel movements do not always occur daily
• Not to use in presence of abdominal pain, nausea, vomiting
• To notify prescriber if constipation unrelieved or if symptoms of electrolyte imbalance occur: muscle cramps, pain, weakness, dizziness, excessive thirst

---

methyldopa/methyl-dopate (℞)

(meth-ill-doe′pa)

Aldomet, Apo-Methyldopa ✦, Dopamet ✦, methyldopa/methyldopate, Novamedopa ✦, Nu-Medopa ✦

Func. class.: Antihypertensive
Chem. class.: Centrally acting α-adrenergic inhibitor

Do not confuse:
methyldopa/ʟ-dopa (levodopa)

Action: Stimulates central inhibitory α-adrenergic receptors or acts as false transmitter, resulting in reduction of arterial pressure

Uses: Hypertension, hypertensive crisis

DOSAGE AND ROUTES

• *Adult:* **PO** 250-500 mg bid or tid, then adjusted q2d as needed, 0.5-2 g daily in 2-4 divided doses (maintenance), not to exceed 3 g/day; **IV** 250-500 mg in 100 ml D_5W q6h, run over 30-60 min, not to exceed 1 g q6h, switch to oral as soon as possible
• *Geriatric:* **PO** 125 mg bid-tid, increase q2d as needed, max 3 g/day
• *Child:* **PO** 10 mg/kg/day in 2-4 divided doses, not to exceed 65 mg/kg or 3 g/day, whichever is less; **IV** 20-40 mg/kg/day in 4 divided doses, not to exceed 65 mg/kg or 3 g, whichever is less

Available forms: Methyldopa: tabs 125, 250, 500 mg; oral susp 50 mg/ml; methyldopate: inj 50 mg/ml

SIDE EFFECTS

CNS: Drowsiness, weakness, dizziness, sedation, headache, depression, psychosis paresthesias, parkinsonism, Bell's palsy, nightmares
CV: Bradycardia, ***myocarditis,*** orthostatic hypotension, angina, edema, weight gain, ***CHF,*** paradoxical pressor response (IV use)
EENT: Nasal congestion
ENDO: Breast enlargement, gynecomastia, lactation, amenorrhea
GI: Nausea, vomiting, diarrhea, constipation, ***hepatic dysfunction,*** sore or "black" tongue, ***pancreatitis,*** colitis, flatulence
GU: Impotence, failure to ejaculate
HEMA: ***Leukopenia, thrombocytopenia, hemolytic anemia, granulocytopenia,*** positive Coombs' test
INTEG: Rash, ***toxic epidermal necrolysis,*** lupuslike syndrome
Contraindications: Active hepatic disease, hypersensitivity
Precautions: Pregnancy (B) (PO); (C) (IV), hepatic disease, eclampsia, severe cardiac disease, renal disease

PHARMACOKINETICS

PO: Peak 2-4 hr, duration 12-24 hr
IV: Peak 2 hr, duration 10-16 hr
Metabolized by liver, excreted in urine

INTERACTIONS

Lithium toxicity: lithium
Increase: pressor effect—sympathomimetic amines, MAOIs
Increase: hypotension, CNS toxicity—levodopa
Increase: hypotension—diuretics, other antihypertensives
Increase: psychosis—haloperidol
Increase: CNS depression—alcohol, antihistamines, antidepressants, analgesics, sedative/hypnotics
Increase: B/P—phenothiazines,

M

β-blockers, amphetamines, NSAIDs, tricyclics, barbiturates
Increase: hypoglycemia—TOLBUTamide
Drug/Herb
Increase: toxicity, death—aconite
Increase: antihypertensive effect—barberry, betony, black catechu, black cohosh, bloodroot, broom, burdock, cat's claw, dandelion, goldenseal, Irish moss, Jamaican dogwood, kelp, khella, mistletoe, parsley
Increase or decrease: antihypertensive effect—astragalus, cola tree
Decrease: effect—capsicum, Indian snakeroot
Decrease: antihypertensive effect—coltsfoot, guarana, khat, licorice
Drug/Lab Test
Interference: Urinary uric acid, serum creatinine, AST
False increase: Urinary catecholamines

NURSING CONSIDERATIONS

Assess:
• Blood studies: neutrophils, decreased platelets
• Direct Coombs' test before/after 6, 12 mo of therapy
• Baselines in renal, hepatic studies, before therapy begins
• B/P when beginning treatment, periodically thereafter, report significant changes
• Allergic reaction: rash, fever, pruritus, urticaria; drug should be discontinued if antihistamines fail to help
• CNS symptoms, especially in the elderly, depression, change in mental status
• Symptoms of CHF: edema, dyspnea, wet crackles, B/P
• Renal symptoms: polyuria, oliguria, urinary frequency; I&O ratio, weight, report weight gain >5 lb
Administer:
PO route
• Shake susp before use
IV route
• After diluting with 100 ml D_5W; run over ½-1 hr

Additive compatibilities: Aminophylline, ascorbic acid, chloramphenicol, diphenhydrAMINE, heparin, magnesium sulfate, multivitamins, netilmicin, potassium chloride, promazine, sodium bicarbonate, succinylcholine, verapamil, vit B/C
Solution compatibilities: D_5W, D_5/0.9% NaCl, Ringer's, sodium bicarbonate 5%, 0.9% NaCl, amino acids 4.25%/D_{25}, Dextran$_6$/0.9% NaCl, Normosol R, Normosol M/D_5W
Y-site compatibilities: Esmolol, heparin, meperidine, morphine, theophylline
Perform/provide:
• Storage of tabs in tight container
Evaluate:
• Therapeutic response: decrease in B/P in hypertension
Teach patient/family:
• To avoid hazardous activities
• Not to discontinue drug abruptly, or withdrawal symptoms may occur: anxiety, increased B/P, headache, insomnia, increased pulse, tremors, nausea, sweating
• Not to use OTC (cough, cold, allergy) products unless directed by prescriber
• To comply with dosage schedule even if feeling better
• To rise slowly to sitting or standing position to minimize orthostatic hypotension
• To notify prescriber of mouth sores, sore throat, fever, swelling of hands or feet, irregular heartbeat, chest pain, signs of angioedema
• That excessive perspiration, dehydration, vomiting, diarrhea may lead to fall in blood pressure; consult prescriber
• That dizziness, fainting, light-headedness may occur during first few days of therapy
• That compliance is necessary; not to skip or stop drug unless directed by prescriber
• That drug may cause skin rash or impaired perspiration
Treatment of overdose: Gastric evacuation, sympathomimetics may be indicated; if severe, hemodialysis

---

methylergonovine (℞)

(meth-ill-er-goe-noe'veen)
Methergine,
methylergonovine
Func. class.: Oxytocic
Chem. class.: Ergot alkaloid

Action: Stimulates uterine, vascular, smooth muscle, causing contractions; decreases bleeding

Uses: Treatment of hemorrhage postpartum or postabortion, uterine contractions

DOSAGE AND ROUTES

• *Adult:* **PO** 200-400 mcg q6-12h × 2-7 days **IM/IV** 200 mcg q2-4h for 1-5 doses

Available forms: Inj 200 mcg/ml; tabs 200 mcg

SIDE EFFECTS

CNS: *Headache, dizziness,* **seizures**
CV: **Hypotension,** chest pain, palpitation, *hypertension,* **dysrhythmias;** **CVA (IV)**
EENT: Tinnitus
GI: *Nausea, vomiting*
GU: Cramping
INTEG: Sweating, rash, allergic reactions
RESP: Dyspnea

Contraindications: Hypersensitivity to ergot preparations, indication of labor, before delivery of placenta, hypertension, pelvic inflammatory disease, respiratory disease, cardiac disease, peripheral vascular disease

Precautions: Pregnancy (C), severe hepatic disease, severe renal disease, jaundice, diabetes mellitus, convulsive disorders, sepsis

PHARMACOKINETICS

PO: Onset 5-25 min, duration 3 hr
IM: Onset 2-5 min, duration 3 hr
IV: Onset immediate, duration 45 min
Metabolized in liver, excreted in urine

INTERACTIONS

Increase: vasoconstriction—vasopressors, nicotine

NURSING CONSIDERATIONS

Assess:
• B/P, pulse, character and amount of vaginal bleeding; watch for indications of hemorrhage
• Respiratory rate, rhythm, depth; notify prescriber of abnormalities
• For uterine relaxation; observe for severe cramping
⚠ Ergot toxicity: tinnitus, hypertension, palpitations, chest pain, nausea, vomiting, weakness; cold, numb extremities

Administer:
• Only during fourth stage of labor; not to be used to augment labor
• IM in deep muscle mass; rotate injection sites of additional doses

IV route
• Undiluted through Y-tube or 3-way stopcock; give 0.2 mg or less/min or diluted in 5 ml 0.9% NaCl given through Y-site
• With crash cart available on unit; IV route used only in emergencies

Y-site compatibilities: Heparin, hydrocortisone sodium succinate, potassium chloride, vit B/C

Evaluate:
• Therapeutic response: absence of hemorrhage

Teach patient/family:
• To report increased blood loss, severe abdominal cramps, fever or foul-smelling lochia
• To avoid smoking
• Not to breastfeed while taking this drug

M

methylphenidate (R)

(meth-ill-fen'i-date)
Concerta, Metadate CD,
Metadate ER, Methylin,
Methylin ER, PMS-
methylphenidate, Methidate,
PMS-Methylphenidate ✦,
Riphenidate ✦, Ritalin, Ritalin
LA, Ritalin SR
Func. class.: Cerebral stimulant
Chem. class.: Piperidine derivative

Controlled Substance Schedule II
Do not confuse:
methylphenidate/methadone

Action: Increases release of norepinephrine, dopamine in cerebral cortex to reticular activating system; exact action not known

Uses: Attention deficit disorder (ADD), attention deficit hyperactivity disorder (ADHD); narcolepsy (except Concerta, Metadate, CD, Ritalin LA)

Investigational uses: Depression in the elderly, cancer, post-stroke patients, HIV, brain injury, improvement in pain control, sedation in patients receiving opiates

DOSAGE AND ROUTES

Attention deficit hyperactivity disorder
• *Child >6 yr:* **PO** (immediate release tabs, chew tabs, oral sol) 5 mg before breakfast and lunch, increasing by 5-10 mg/wk, not to exceed 60 mg/day; **EXT REL** 20 mg daily-tid

Narcolepsy
• *Adult:* **PO** 10 mg bid-tid, 30-45 min before meals, may increase up to 40-60 mg/day

Depression (elderly)
• *Geriatric:* **PO** 2.5 mg q$_{AM}$, increase q3d by 2.5 mg to desired dose, max 20 mg/day

Available forms: Tabs 5, 10, 20 mg; tabs ext rel 10, 20, mg; tabs, ext rel (Concerta): 18, 27, 36, 54 mg; cap, ext rel 10, 20, 30, 40 mg; oral sol 5 mg, 10 mg/ml; tabs, chew (methylin) 2.5, 5, 10 mg

SIDE EFFECTS

CNS: **Hyperactivity, insomnia, restlessness, talkativeness,** dizziness, drowsiness, toxic psychosis, headache, akathisia, dyskinesia, masking or worsening of Gilles de la Tourette's syndrome, **seizures**
CV: **Palpitations, tachycardia,** B/P changes, angina, **dysrhythmias**
ENDO: Growth retardation
GI: Nausea, anorexia, dry mouth, weight loss, abdominal pain
HEMA: **Leukopenia, anemia, thrombocytopenic purpura**
INTEG: **Exfoliative dermatitis,** urticaria, rash, erythema multiforme
MISC: Fever, arthralgia, scalp hair loss

Contraindications: Hypersensitivity, anxiety, history of Gilles de la Tourette's syndrome; children <6 yr, glaucoma, anorexia nervosa, tartrazine dye hypersensitivity

Precautions: Pregnancy (C), hypertension, depression, seizures, lactation, drug abuse

PHARMACOKINETICS

PO: Onset ½-1 hr, duration 4-6 hr, metabolized by liver, excreted by kidneys

INTERACTIONS

Hypertensive crisis: MAOIs or within 14 days of MAOIs, vasopressors
Increase: effects of tricyclics, anticonvulsants, SSRIs
Decrease: effect of guanethidine
Drug/Herb
Synergistic effect: melatonin
Increase: CNS stimulation—cola nut, guarana, horsetail, yerba maté, yohimbe
Drug/Food
Increase: stimulation—caffeine

NURSING CONSIDERATIONS

Assess:
• VS, B/P; may reverse antihypertensives; check patients with cardiac disease more often for increased B/P

• CBC, urinalysis, in diabetes: blood glucose, urine glucose; insulin changes may have to be made, since eating will decrease

• Height, growth rate q3mo in children; growth rate may be decreased

• Mental status: mood, sensorium, affect, stimulation, insomnia, aggressiveness

A Withdrawal symptoms: headache, nausea, vomiting, muscle pain, weakness

• Appetite, sleep, speech patterns

• For attention span, decreased hyperactivity in ADHD persons

Administer:

• Do not crush or chew time-released medication; caps may be opened and beads sprinkled over spoonful of applesauce

• At least 6 hr before bedtime to avoid sleeplessness (regular release); at least 10 hr (ext rel)

• Gum, hard candy, frequent sips of water for dry mouth

• Chew tab with adequate water to prevent choking; contains phenylalanine

Evaluate:

• Therapeutic response: decreased hyperactivity (ADHD) or ability to stay awake (narcolepsy)

Teach patient/family:

• To decrease caffeine consumption (coffee, tea, cola, chocolate); may increase irritability, stimulation; not to use guarana, yerba maté, cola nut

• To avoid OTC preparations unless approved by prescriber

• To taper off drug over several weeks, or depression, increased sleeping, lethargy will occur

• To avoid driving, hazardous activities if dizziness, blurred vision occur

• To avoid alcohol ingestion

• To avoid hazardous activities until stabilized on medication

• To get needed rest; patients will feel more tired at end of day

• That shell of Concerta tab may appear in stools

Treatment of overdose: Administer fluids; hemodialysis or peritoneal dialysis; antihypertensive for increased B/P; administer short-acting barbiturate before lavage

---

*methylPRED-NISolone (R)

(meth-il-pred-niss'oh-lone)
A-Methapred, depMedalone, Depoject, Depo-Medrol, Depopred, Depo-Predate, Medrol, Duralone, Medralone, Rep-Pred, Solu-Medrol

Func. class.: Corticosteroid, synthetic

Chem. class.: Glucocorticoid, immediate acting

Do not confuse:

methylPREDNISolone/ predniSONE
methylPREDNISolone/ medroxyPROGESTERone
methylPREDNISolone/ methylTESTOSTERone

Action: Decreases inflammation by suppression of migration of polymorphonuclear leukocytes, fibroblasts; reversal of increased capillary permeability and lysosomal stabilization

Uses: Severe inflammation, shock, adrenal insufficiency, collagen disorders, management of acute spinal cord injury, multiple sclerosis

DOSAGE AND ROUTES

Adrenal insufficiency/inflammation

• *Adult:* **PO** 2-60 mg in 4 divided doses; **IM** 10-80 mg (acetate); **IM/IV** 10-250 mg (succinate); intraarticular 4-30 mg (acetate); **RECT** 40 mg 3-7 × wk for ≥2 wk

• *Child:* **IV** 117 mcg-1.66 mg/kg in 3-4 divided doses (succinate); **RECT** 0.5-1 mg/kg (15-30 mg/m^2) daily or every other day × 1 wk or more

Shock

• *Adult:* **IV** 100-250 mg q2-6h or 30 mg/kg, then q4-6h prn, for 2-3 days (succinate)

M

Multiple sclerosis
• *Adult:* **PO** 160 mg/day × 1 wk, then 64 mg every other day × 30 days
Available forms: Tabs 2, 4, 6, 8, 16, 24, 32 mg; inj 20, 40, 80 mg/ml acetate; inj 40, 125, 500, 1000, 2000 mg/vial succinate; susp for inj 20, 40, 80 mg/ml; dose pack 4 mg tabs; enema 40 mg

SIDE EFFECTS

CNS: Depression, flushing, sweating, headache, mood changes
CV: Hypertension, ***circulatory collapse, thrombophlebitis, embolism,*** tachycardia
EENT: Fungal infections, increased intraocular pressure, blurred vision, cataracts
GI: Diarrhea, nausea, abdominal distention, ***GI hemorrhage,*** increased appetite, pancreatitis
HEMA: ***Thrombocytopenia***
INTEG: Acne, poor wound healing, ecchymosis, petechiae
MS: Fractures, osteoporosis, weakness
Contraindications: Psychosis, hypersensitivity, idiopathic thrombocytopenia, acute glomerulonephritis, amebiasis, fungal infections, non-asthmatic bronchial disease, child <2 yr, AIDS, TB
Precautions: Pregnancy (C), lactation, diabetes mellitus, glaucoma, osteoporosis, seizure disorders, ulcerative colitis, CHF, myasthenia gravis, renal disease, esophagitis, peptic ulcer

PHARMACOKINETICS

Well absorbed PO, IM
PO: Peak 1-2 hr, duration 1½ days
IM: Peak 4-8 days, duration 1-4 wk
Intraarticular: Peak 1 wk
Half-life >3½ hr (plasma), 18-36 hr (tissue); crosses placenta, enters breast milk in small amounts; metabolized in liver, excreted by kidneys (unchanged)

INTERACTIONS

Increase: side effects—amphotericin B, diuretics

Increase: methylPREDNISolone action—oral contraceptives
Decrease: methylPREDNISolone action—rifampin, phenytoin, theophylline
Decrease: effects of antidiabetics, vaccines, somatrem
Drug/Herb
Increase: hypokalemia—aloe, buckthorn, cascara sagrada, Chinese rhubarb, senna
Increase: corticosteroid effect—aloe, licorice, perilla
Drug/Food
Do not use with grapefruit juice, level of methylPREDNISolone will be increased
Drug/Lab Test
Increase: Cholesterol, sodium, blood glucose, uric acid, calcium, urine glucose
Decrease: Ca, K, T_4, T_3, thyroid ^{131}I uptake test, urine 17-OHCS, 17-KS
False negative: Skin allergy tests

NURSING CONSIDERATIONS

Assess:
• Potassium depletion: parethesias, fatigue, nausea, vomiting, depression, polyuria, dysrhythmias, weakness
• Edema, hypertension, cardiac symptoms
• Mental status: affect, mood, behavioral changes, aggression
• Potassium, blood glucose, urine glucose while on long-term therapy; hypokalemia and hyperglycemia
• Joint mobility, pain, edema if given intraarticularly
• B/P q4h, pulse; notify prescriber of chest pain, crackles
• I&O ratio; be alert for decreasing urinary output, increasing edema; weight daily; notify prescriber of weekly gain >5 lb
• Adrenal insufficiency: weight loss, nausea, vomiting, confusion, anxiety, hypotension, weakness
• Plasma cortisol levels during long-term therapy (normal level: 138-635 nmol/L SI units when drawn at 8 AM)

• Growth in children on long-term treatment

Administer:
• Titrated dose; use lowest effective dose
• IM inj deep in large muscle mass; rotate sites; avoid deltoid; use 21G needle; after shaking suspension (parenteral)
• In one dose in AM to prevent adrenal suppression; avoid SUBCUT administration; may damage tissue
• With food or milk to decrease GI symptoms (PO)
⚠ Do not give Solu-Medrol intrathecally

IV route
• After diluting with diluent provided; agitate slowly; give 500 mg or less/1 min or longer; may be given as IV infusion in its own diluent over 10-20 min

Additive compatibilities: Chloramphenicol, cimetidine, clindamycin, DOPamine, granisetron, heparin, norepinephrine, penicillin G potassium, ranitidine, theophylline, verapamil

Syringe compatibilities: Granisetron, metoclopramide

Y-site compatibilities: Acyclovir, amifostine, amphotericin B cholesteryl, amrinone, aztreonam, cefepime, cisplatin, cladribine, cyclophosphamide, cytarabine, DOPamine, DOXOrubicin, enalaprilat, famotidine, fludarabine, granisetron, heparin, melphalan, meperidine, methotrexate, metronidazole, midazolam, morphine, piperacillin/tazobactam, remifentanil, sodium bicarbonate, tacrolimus, teniposide, theophylline, thiotepa

Perform/provide:
• Assistance with ambulation in patient with bone tissue disease to prevent fractures

Evaluate:
• Therapeutic response: ease of respirations, decreased inflammation; decreased symptoms of adrenal insufficiency
• Infection: increased temp, WBC, even after withdrawal of medication; drug masks infection

Teach patient/family:
• To increase intake of potassium, calcium, protein
• To carry emergency ID (steroid user)
• To notify prescriber if therapeutic response decreases; dosage adjustment may be needed
• Not to discontinue abruptly, or adrenal crisis can result
• To avoid OTC products: salicylates, alcohol in cough products, cold preparations unless directed by prescriber; to avoid vaccinations, since immunosuppression occurs
• About cushingoid symptoms
• To recognize the symptoms of adrenal insufficiency: nausea, anorexia, fatigue, dizziness, dyspnea, weakness, joint pain

methylPREDNISolone topical
See Appendix C

metipranolol ophthalmic
See Appendix C

metoclopramide (℞)
(met-oh-kloe-pra′mide)
Apo-Metoclop ✦, Emex ✦, Maxeran ✦, metoclopramide, Octamide, Reglan, Sensamide IV
Func. class.: Cholinergic, antiemetic
Chem. class.: Central dopamine receptor antagonist

Do not confuse:
metoclopramide/metolazone
Reglan/Megace

Action: Enhances response to acetylcholine of tissue in upper GI tract, which causes contraction of gastric muscle; relaxes pyloric, duodenal segments; increases peristalsis without stimulating secretions, blocks dopamine in chemoreceptor trigger zone of CNS

Uses: Prevention of nausea, vomiting induced by chemotherapy, radiation, delayed gastric emptying, gastroesophageal reflux

Investigational uses: Hiccups, migraines, lactation induction, lung cancer

DOSAGE AND ROUTES

Renal dose
- *Adult:* CCr <40 ml/min 50% of dose

Nausea/vomiting
- *Adult:* **IV** 1-2 mg/kg 30 min before administration of chemotherapy, then q2h × 2 doses, then q3h × 3 doses
- *Child:* **IV** 0.1-0.2 mg/kg/dose

Facilitate small bowel intubation, in radiologic exams
- *Adult and child >14 yr:* **IV** 10 mg over 1-2 min
- *Child <6 yr:* **IV** 0.1 mg/kg
- *Child 6-14 yr:* **IV** 2.5-5 mg

Diabetic gastroparesis
- *Adult:* **PO** 10 mg 30 min ac, at bedtime × 2-8 wk
- *Geriatric:* **PO** 5 mg ½ hr ac, at bedtime, increase to 10 mg if needed

Hiccups (off-label)
- *Adult:* **PO/IM/IV** 10 mg q6h

Gastroesophageal reflux
- *Adult:* **PO** 10-15 mg qid 30 min ac
- *Child:* **PO** 0.4-0.8 mg/kg/day in 4 divided doses

Lactation induction (off-label)
- *Adult:* **PO** 10 mg bid-tid, may increase to 20-45 mg/day in divided doses

Non–small cell lung cancer (NSCLC) radiation sensitizer (off-label)
(Sensamide IV)
- *Adult:* **IV** 2 mg/kg given 1 hr prior to radiation therapy 3 ×/wk

Available forms: Tabs 5, 10 mg; syr 5 mg/5 ml; inj 5 mg/ml; conc sol 10 mg/ml

SIDE EFFECTS

CNS: Sedation, fatigue, restlessness, headache, sleeplessness, dystonia, dizziness, drowsiness, ***suicide ideation, seizures,*** EPS

CV: Hypotension, supraventricular tachycardia

GI: Dry mouth, constipation, nausea, anorexia, vomiting, diarrhea

GU: Decreased libido, prolactin secretion, amenorrhea, galactorrhea

HEMA: ***Neutropenia, leukopenia, agranulocytosis***

INTEG: Urticaria, rash

Contraindications: Hypersensitivity to this drug or procaine or procainamide, seizure disorder, pheochromocytoma, breast cancer (prolactin dependent), GI obstruction

Precautions: Pregnancy (B), lactation, GI hemorrhage, CHF, Parkinson's disease, tardive dyskinesia

PHARMACOKINETICS

IV: Onset 1-3 min, duration 1-2 hr
PO: Onset ½-1 hr, duration 1-2 hr
IM: Onset 10-15 min, duration 1-2 hr
Metabolized by liver, excreted in urine, half-life 4 hr

INTERACTIONS

Avoid use with MAOIs
Increase: sedation—alcohol, other CNS depressants
Increase: risk of EPS—haloperidol, phenothiazines
Decrease: action of metoclopramide—anticholinergics, opiates
Drug/Lab Test
Increase: Prolactin, aldosterone, thyrotropin

NURSING CONSIDERATIONS

Assess:
- For EPS and tardive dyskinesia, more likely to occur in elderly patient
- Mental status: depression, anxiety, irritability
- GI complaints: nausea, vomiting, anorexia, constipation
Administer:
PO route
- ½-1 hr before meals for better absorption

⚠ Safety alert   *"Tall Man" lettering

• Gum, hard candy, frequent rinsing of mouth for dry oral cavity

IV route

• DiphenhydrAMINE IV for EPS

• Undiluted if dose is ≤10 mg; give over 2 min; more than 10 mg may be diluted in 50 ml or more D₅W, NaCl, Ringer's, LR and given over 15 min or more

Syringe compatibilities: Aminophylline, ascorbic acid, atropine, benztropine, bleomycin, butorphanol, chlorproMAZINE, cisplatin, cyclophosphamide, cytarabine, dexamethasone, dimenhyDRINATE, diphenhydrAMINE, DOXOrubicin, droperidol, fentanyl, fluorouracil, heparin, hydrocortisone, hydrOXYzine, insulin (regular), leucovorin, lidocaine, magnesium sulfate, meperidine, methotrimeprazine, methylPREDNISolone, midazolam, mitomycin, morphine, pentazocine, perphenazine, prochlorperazine, promazine, promethazine, ranitidine, scopolamine, sufentanil, vinBLAStine, vinCRIStine, vit B/C

Y-site compatibilities: Acyclovir, aldesleukin, amifostine, aztreonam, bleomycin, ciprofloxacin, cisatracurium, cisplatin, cladribine, cyclophosphamide, cytarabine, diltiazem, DOXOrubicin, droperidol, famotidine, filgrastim, fluconazole, fludarabine, fluorouracil, foscarnet, gallium, granisetron, heparin, idarubicin, leucovorin, melphalan, meperidine, meropenem, methotrexate, mitomycin, morphine, ondansetron, paclitaxel, piperacillin/tazobactam, propofol, remifentanil, sargramostim, sufentanil, tacrolimus, teniposide, thiotepa, vinBLAStine, vinCRIStine, vinorelbine, zidovudine

Perform/provide:

• Protect from light with aluminum foil during infusion

• Discard open ampules

Evaluate:

• Therapeutic response: absence of nausea, vomiting, anorexia, fullness

Teach patient/family:

• To avoid driving, other hazardous activities until patient is stabilized on this medication

• To avoid alcohol, other CNS depressants that will enhance sedating properties of this drug

---

metolazone (R)

(me-tole′a-zone)
Mykrox, Zaroxolyn
Func. class.: Diuretic, antihypertensive
Chem. class.: Thiazide-like quinazoline derivative

Do not confuse:
metolazone/methotrexate
metolazone/metoclopramide

Action: Acts on distal tubule and cortical thick ascending limb of the loop of Henle by increasing excretion of water, sodium, chloride, potassium, magnesium, bicarbonate

Uses: Edema, hypertension, CHF, nephrotic syndrome

DOSAGE AND ROUTES

Edema

• *Adult:* **PO** 5-20 mg/day

Hypertension

• *Adult:* **PO** 2.5-5 mg/day (Zaroxolyn)

• *Child:* **PO** 0.2-0.4 mg/kg/day divided q12-24h

• *Adult:* **PO** 0.5 mg (Mykrox) daily in AM, may increase to 1 mg

Available forms: Tabs 0.5 (Mykrox), 2.5, 5, 10 mg (Zaroxolyn)

SIDE EFFECTS

CNS: Drowsiness, paresthesia, anxiety, depression, headache, *dizziness, fatigue, weakness*

CV: Irregular pulse, orthostatic hypotension, palpitations, volume depletion

EENT: Blurred vision

ELECT: Hypokalemia, hypomagnesemia, hypercalcemia, hyponatremia, hypochloremia, hypophosphatemia

GI: Nausea, vomiting, anorexia, constipation, diarrhea, cramps, pancreatitis, GI irritation, ***hepatitis***

M

GU: Urinary frequency, polyuria, ***uremia, glucosuria***
*HEMA: **Aplastic anemia, hemolytic anemia, leukopenia, agranulocytosis, neutropenia***
INTEG: Rash, urticaria, purpura, photosensitivity, fever
META: Hyperglycemia, increased creatinine, BUN

Contraindications: Hypersensitivity to thiazides or sulfonamides, anuria, lactation

Precautions: Pregnancy (B), hypokalemia, renal disease, hepatic disease, gout, COPD, lupus erythematosus, diabetes mellitus, elderly

PHARMACOKINETICS

PO: Onset 1 hr, peak 2 hr, duration 12-24 hr; excreted unchanged by kidneys; crosses placenta; enters breast milk; half-life 8 hr

INTERACTIONS

Increase: hypokalemia—mezlocillin, piperacillin, amphotericin B, glucocorticoids, digoxin, stimulant laxatives
Increase: hypotension—alcohol (large amounts), nitrates, antihypertensives, barbiturates, opioids
Increase: toxicity—lithium
Decrease: action of metolazone—NSAIDs, salicylates

Drug/Herb
Increase: hypokalemia—aloe, buckthorn, cascara sagrada, rhubarb, senna
Increase: toxicity, death—aconite
Increase: antihypertensive effect—barberry, betony, black catechu, black cohosh, bloodroot, broom, burdock, cat's claw, dandelion, goldenseal, Irish moss, Jamaican dogwood, kelp, khella, mistletoe, parsley
Increase or decrease: antihypertensive effect—astragalus, cola tree
Decrease: antihypertensive effect—coltsfoot, guarana, khat, licorice

Drug/Lab Test
Increase: BSP retention, calcium, amylase, parathyroid test
Decrease: PBI, PSP

NURSING CONSIDERATIONS

Assess:
• Weight, I&O daily to determine fluid loss; effect of drug may be decreased if used daily
• Rate, depth, rhythm of respiration, effect of exertion
• B/P lying, standing; postural hypotension may occur
• Electrolytes: K, Mg, Na, Cl; include BUN, blood glucose, CBC, serum creatinine, blood pH, ABGs, uric acid, calcium
• Improvement in edema of feet, legs, sacral area daily if medication is being used in CHF
• Improvement in CVP q8h
• Signs of metabolic alkalosis: drowsiness, restlessness
• Signs of hypokalemia: postural hypotension, malaise, fatigue, tachycardia, leg cramps, weakness
• Rashes, fever daily
• Confusion, especially in elderly; take safety precautions if needed

Administer:
• In AM to avoid interference with sleep if using drug as a diuretic
• Potassium replacement if potassium <3 mg/dl
• With food, if nausea occurs; absorption may be decreased slightly
• Extended product is Zaroxolyn; prompt product is Mykrox, they are not interchangeable

Evaluate:
• Therapeutic response: decreased edema, B/P

Teach patient/family:
• To increase fluid intake to 2-3 L/day unless contraindicated, to rise slowly from lying or sitting position
• To notify prescriber of muscle weakness, cramps, nausea, dizziness
• That drug may be taken with food or milk
• To use sunscreen for photosensitivity
• That blood glucose may be increased in diabetics
• To take early in day to avoid nocturia
• To avoid alcohol

 Safety alert   *"Tall Man" lettering

• To avoid sodium food, increase potassium foods in diet
Treatment of overdose: Lavage if taken orally; monitor electrolytes; administer dextrose in saline; monitor hydration, CV, renal status

metoprolol (℞)

(meh-toe′proe-lole)
Betaloc ♣, Betaloc Durules ♣, Lopresor ♣, Lopressor, Lopressor SR ♣, Nu-Metop ♣, Novometoprol ♣, Toprol-XL
Func. class.: Antihypertensive, antianginal
Chem. class.: β₁-Blocker

Do not confuse:
metoprolol/misoprostol
Action: Lowers B/P by β-blocking effects; reduces elevated renin plasma levels; blocks β₂-adrenergic receptors in bronchial, vascular smooth muscle only at high doses
Uses: Mild to moderate hypertension, acute MI to reduce cardiovascular mortality, angina pectoris, NYHA class II, III heart failure
Investigational uses: Atrial ectopy, antipsychotic induced akathisia, rapid heart rate control, unstable angina, variceal bleeding in portal hypotension, migraine prevention

DOSAGE AND ROUTES
Hypertension
• *Adult:* PO 50 mg bid, or 100 mg daily; may give up to 200-450 mg in divided doses; **EXT REL** give daily
• *Geriatric:* PO 25 mg/day initially, increase weekly as needed
Myocardial infarction
• *Adult:* (early treatment) **IV BOL** 5 mg q2min × 3, then 50 mg **PO** 15 min after last dose and q6h × 48 hr; (late treatment) **PO** maintenance 100 mg bid for 3 mo
Angina
• *Adult:* PO 100 mg daily as a single

dose or in two divided doses, increase qwk prn or 100 mg **EXT REL** daily
Migraine prevention (off-label)
• *Adult:* **PO** 50-100 mg bid-qid
Available forms: Tabs 50, 100 mg; inj 1 mg/ml; ext rel tab (succinate) (XL) 25, 50, 100, 200 mg; ext rel tabs, tartrate: 100 mg

SIDE EFFECTS
CNS: Insomnia, dizziness, mental changes, hallucinations, ***depression,*** anxiety, headaches, nightmares, confusion, fatigue
CV: Hypotension, ***bradycardia, CHF, palpitations,*** dysrhythmias, ***cardiac arrest, AV block, pulmonary edema, chest pain***
EENT: Sore throat; dry, burning eyes
GI: Nausea, vomiting, colitis, cramps, ***diarrhea,*** constipation, flatulence, dry mouth, *hiccups*
GU: Impotence
*HEMA: **Agranulocytosis, eosinophilia, thrombocytopenia, purpura***
INTEG: Rash, purpura, alopecia, dry skin, urticaria, pruritus
*RESP: **Bronchospasm,*** dyspnea, wheezing
Contraindications: Hypersensitivity to β-blockers, cardiogenic shock, heart block (2nd, 3rd degree), sinus bradycardia, bronchial asthma
Precautions: Pregnancy (C), major surgery, lactation, diabetes mellitus, renal disease, thyroid disease, COPD, CAD, nonallergic bronchospasm, hepatic disease, CHF, elderly

PHARMACOKINETICS
PO: Peak 2-4 hr, duration 13-19 hr
PO-ER: Peak 6-12 hr, duration 24 hr
IV: Onset immediate, peak 20 min, duration 6-8 hr
Half-life 3-4 hr; metabolized in liver (metabolites); excreted in urine; crosses placenta; enters breast milk

INTERACTIONS

Do not use with MAOIs

Increase: hypotension, bradycardia—reserpine, hydrALAZINE, methyldopa, prazosin, amphetamines, epINEPHrine, H₂-antagonists, calcium channel blockers

Increase: hypoglycemic effects—insulin, oral antidiabetics

Increase: metoprolol effect—cimetidine

Increase: effects of benzodiazepines

Decrease: antihypertensive effect—salicylates, NSAIDs

Decrease: metoprolol level—barbiturates

Decrease: effects of DOPamine, DOBUTamine, xanthines

Drug/Herb

Increase: toxicity, death—aconite

Increase: antihypertensive effect—barberry, betony, black catechu, black cohosh, bloodroot, broom, burdock, cat's claw, dandelion, goldenseal, Irish moss, Jamaican dogwood, kelp, khella, mistletoe, parsley

Increase or decrease: antihypertensive effect—astragalus, cola tree

Decrease: antihypertensive effect—coltsfoot, guarana, khat, licorice

Drug/Food

Increase: absorption with food

Drug/Lab Test

Increase: BUN, potassium, ANA titer, serum lipoprotein, triglycerides, uric acid, alk phosphatase, LDH, AST, ALT

NURSING CONSIDERATIONS

Assess:

• ECG directly when giving IV during initial treatment

• I&O, weight daily

• B/P during initial treatment, periodically thereafter; pulse q4h; note rate, rhythm, quality

• Apical/radial pulse before administration; notify prescriber of any significant changes or pulse <50 bpm

• Baselines in renal, hepatic studies before therapy begins

• Edema in feet, legs daily

• Skin turgor, dryness of mucous membranes for hydration status

Administer:

PO route

• Do not break, crush, or chew ext rel tabs

• After meals, at bedtime; tab may be crushed or swallowed whole; take at same time each day

Ext rel tab

IV route

• IV, undiluted, give over 1 min, × 3 doses at 2-5 min intervals; start **PO** 15 min after last IV dose

Y-site compatibilities: Alteplase, meperidine, morphine

Perform/provide:

• Storage in dry area at room temperature, do not freeze

Evaluate:

• Therapeutic response: decreased B/P after 1-2 wk

Teach patient/family:

• To take immediately after meals

• Not to discontinue drug abruptly; taper over 2 wk; may cause precipitate angina

• Not to use OTC products containing α-adrenergic stimulants (nasal decongestants, OTC cold preparations) unless directed by prescriber

• To report bradycardia, dizziness, confusion, depression, fever, sore throat, shortness of breath to prescriber

• To take pulse at home; advise when to notify prescriber

• To avoid alcohol, smoking, sodium intake

• To comply with weight control, dietary adjustments, modified exercise program

• To carry emergency ID to identify drug, allergies

• To avoid hazardous activities if dizziness is present

• To report symptoms of CHF: difficult breathing, especially on exertion or when lying down, night cough, swelling of extremities

• To take medication at bedtime to prevent effect of orthostatic hypotension

---

⚠ Safety alert   *"Tall Man" lettering

• To wear support hose to minimize effects of orthostatic hypotension
Treatment of overdose: Lavage, IV atropine for bradycardia, IV theophylline for bronchospasm, digitalis, O_2, diuretic for cardiac failure, hemodialysis, hypotension administer vasopressor (norepinephrine)

---

metronidazole (R)

(me-troe-ni′da-zole)
Apo-Metronidazole ✦, Flagyl, Flagyl ER, Flagyl IV, Flagyl IV RTU, metronidazole, Novonidazole ✦, Protostat, Trikacide ✦
Func. class.: Antiinfective, miscellaneous
Chem. class.: Nitroimidazole derivative

Action: Direct-acting amebicide/trichomonacide binds, degrades DNA in organism
Uses: Intestinal amebiasis, amebic abscess, trichomoniasis, refractory trichomoniasis, bacterial anaerobic infections, giardiasis, septicemia, endocarditis, bone, joint infections, lower respiratory tract infections

DOSAGE AND ROUTES
Trichomoniasis
• *Adult:* **PO** 250 mg tid × 7 days or 2 g in single dose; do not repeat treatment for 4-6 wk
• *Child:* **PO** 5 mg/kg tid × 7 days
Refractory trichomoniasis
• *Adult:* **PO** 250 mg bid × 10 days
Amebic hepatic abscess
• *Adult:* **PO** 500-750 mg tid × 5-10 days
• *Child:* **PO** 35-50 mg/kg/day in 3 divided doses × 10 days
Intestinal amebiasis
• *Adult:* **PO** 750 mg tid × 5-10 days
• *Child:* **PO** 35-50 mg/kg/day in 3 divided doses × 10 days; then oral iodoquinol

Anaerobic bacterial infections
• *Adult:* **IV INF** 15 mg/kg over 1 hr, then 7.5 mg/kg **IV** or **PO** q6h, not to exceed 4 g/day; first maintenance dose should be administered 6 hr following loading dose
Giardiasis
• *Adult:* **PO** 250 mg tid × 5 days
• *Child:* **PO** 5 mg/kg tid × 5 days
Antibiotic-associated pseudomembranous colitis
• *Adult:* **PO** 250-500 mg 3-4 ×/day × 10-14 days
• *Child:* **PO** 20 mg/kg/day (max 2 g) divided q6h
Available forms: Tabs 250, 375, 500 mg; tab, ext rel (ER) 750 mg; inj 500 mg/100 ml; powder for inj 500 mg single dose

SIDE EFFECTS
CNS: Headache, dizziness, confusion, irritability, restlessness, ataxia, depression, fatigue, drowsiness, insomnia, paresthesia, peripheral neuropathy, *seizures,* incoordination, depression
CV: Flattening of T waves
EENT: Blurred vision, sore throat, retinal edema, dry mouth, metallic taste, furry tongue, glossitis, stomatitis
GI: Nausea, vomiting, diarrhea, epigastric distress, *anorexia,* constipation, *abdominal cramps,* metallic taste, *pseudomembranous colitis*
GU: Darkened urine, vaginal dryness, polyuria, *albuminuria,* dysuria, cystitis, decreased libido, *neurotoxicity,* incontinence, dyspareunia
HEMA: Leukopenia, bone marrow, depression, aplasia
INTEG: Rash, pruritus, urticaria, flushing
Contraindications: Pregnancy, 1st trimester, hypersensitivity to this drug, renal disease, hepatic disease, contracted visual or color fields, blood dyscrasias, lactation, CNS disorders
Precautions: Pregnancy (B) 2nd/3rd trimesters, *Candida* infections

M

PHARMACOKINETICS

IV: Onset immediate, peak end of inf
PO: Peak 1-2 hr, half-life 6-11 hr
Crosses placenta, enters breast milk,
excreted in feces; absorbed PO (80%-85%)

INTERACTIONS

Disulfiram reaction: alcohol
Increase: action of warfarin
Increase: Leukopenia—azathioprine,
fluorouracil
Decrease: metronidazole action—
phenobarbital, phenytoin, cimetidine
Drug/Lab Test
Altered: AST, ALT, LDH

NURSING CONSIDERATIONS

Assess:
• For infection: WBC, wound symptoms,
fever, skin or vaginal secretions; start
treatment after C&S
• Stools during entire treatment; should
be clear at end of therapy; stools should
be free of parasites for 1 yr before patient
is considered cured (amebiasis)
• Vision by ophthalmic exam during,
after therapy; vision problems often occur
• I&O; weight daily; stools for number,
frequency, character
⚠ Neurotoxicity: peripheral neuropathy,
seizures, dizziness, uncoordination,
pruritus, joint pains; drug may be discontinued
• Allergic reaction: fever, rash, itching,
chills; drug should be discontinued if
these symptoms occur
• Superinfection: fever, monilial growth,
fatigue, malaise
• Renal and reproductive dysfunction:
dysuria, polyuria, impotence, dyspareunia, decreased libido
Administer:
PO route
• PO with or after meals to avoid GI
symptoms, metallic taste; crush tabs if
needed
IV route
• Prediluted; metronidazole IV, dilute

with 4.4 ml sterile H_2O or 0.9% NaCl;
must be diluted further with 8 mg/ml or
more 0.9% NaCl, D_5W, or LR; must neutralize with 5 mEq $NaCO_3$/500 mg; CO_2
gas will be generated and may require
venting; run over 1 hr or more; primary
IV must be discontinued; may be given as
continuous infusion; do not use aluminum products; IV may require venting
Additive compatibilities: Amikacin,
aminophylline, cefazolin, cefotaxime,
ceftazidime, ceftizoxime, ceftriaxone,
cefuroxime, chloramphenicol, ciprofloxacin, clindamycin, disopyramide,
floxacillin, fluconazole, gentamicin,
heparin, moxalactam, multielectrolyte
concentrate, multivitamins, netilmicin,
penicillin G potassium, tobramycin
Y-site compatibilities: Acyclovir,
allopurinol, amifostine, amiodarone,
cefepime, cisatracurium, cyclophosphamide, diltiazem, DOPamine, DOXOrubicin liposome, enalaprilat, esmolol, fluconazole, foscarnet, granisetron,
heparin, hydromorphone, labetalol,
lorazepam, magnesium sulfate, melphalan, meperidine, methylPREDNISolone,
midazolam, morphine, perphenazine,
piperacillin/tazobactam, remifentanil,
sargramostim, tacrolimus, teniposide,
theophylline, thiotepa, vinorelbine
Perform/provide:
• Storage in light-resistant container; do
not refrigerate
Evaluate:
• Therapeutic response: decreased
symptoms of infection
Teach patient/family:
• That urine may turn dark-reddish
brown, drug may cause metallic taste
• Proper hygiene after BM; handwashing technique
• To notify physician for numbness or
tingling of extremities
• To avoid hazardous activities, since
dizziness can occur
• Need for compliance with dosage
schedule, duration of treatment
• To use condoms if treatment for
trichomoniasis, or cross-contamination
may occur

• To use frequent sips of water, sugarless gum, candy for dry mouth
• That treatment of both partners is necessary in trichomoniasis
• Not to drink alcohol or use preparations containing alcohol during use or for 48 hr after use of drug; disulfiram-like reaction can occur

---

metronidazole topical
See Appendix C

---

mexiletine (℞)
(mex-il'e-teen)
Mexitil
Func. class.: Antidysrhythmic (Class IB)
Chem. class.: Lidocaine analog

Action: Increases electrical stimulation threshold of ventricle, His-Purkinje system, which stabilizes cardiac membrane
Uses: Life-threatening ventricular tachycardia; because of proarrhythmic effects, use with lesser dysrhythmias not recommended
Investigational uses: Diabetic neuropathy, ventricular tachycardia, other ventricular dysrhythmias in acute phase of MI

DOSAGE AND ROUTES
• *Adult:* **PO** 200-400 mg (loading dose), then 200 mg q8h, then 200-400 mg q8h
Diabetic neuropathy (off-label)
• *Adult:* **PO** 150 mg/day for 3 days, then 300 mg/day for 3 days, followed by 10 mg/kg/day
Available forms: Caps 150, 200, 250 mg

SIDE EFFECTS
CNS: Headache, dizziness, confusion, *seizures,* tremors, psychosis, nervousness, paresthesias, weakness, fatigue, coordination difficulties, change in sleep habits

CV: Hypotension, bradycardia, angina, PVCs, *heart block, cardiovascular collapse or arrest,* sinus node slowing, *left ventricular failure,* syncope, *cardiogenic shock, AV conduction disturbances, CHF, atrial dysrhythmias, palpitations, ventricular dysrhythmias, ventricular tachycardia, other ventricular arrhythmias in acute phase of MI*
EENT: Blurred vision, tinnitus
GI: Nausea, vomiting, anorexia, diarrhea, abdominal pain, *hepatitis,* dry mouth, peptic ulcer, altered taste, *GI bleeding,* constipation
GU: Urinary hesitancy, decreased libido
HEMA: *Thrombocytopenia, leukopenia, agranulocytosis*
INTEG: Rash, alopecia, dry skin
MISC: Edema, arthralgia, fever, systemic lupus erythematosus syndrome
RESP: Dyspnea
Contraindications: Hypersensitivity, cardiogenic shock, severe heart block (if no pacemaker)
Precautions: Pregnancy (C), lactation, children, hepatic disease, CHF, seizure disorder, hypotension

PHARMACOKINETICS
PO: Peak 2-3 hr; half-life 12 hr, metabolized by liver, excreted unchanged by kidneys (10%), excreted in breast milk

INTERACTIONS
Smoking: decrease drug effect
Increase: mexiletine effects—metoclopramide, urinary alkalinizers
Increase: levels of caffeine, theophylline
Decrease or increase: mexiletine effects—cimetidine
Decrease: mexiletine levels—phenytoin, phenobarbital, rifampin, urinary acidifiers, aluminum/magnesium hydroxide, atropine, opiates
Drug/Herb
Increase: hypokalemia, increase antidysrhythmic action—aloe, buckthorn, cascara sagrada, rhubarb, senna

---

M

Increase: toxicity, death—aconite
Increase: effect—aloe, broom, chronic buckthorn use, cascara sagrada (chronic use), Chinese rhubarb, figwort, fumitory, goldenseal, kudzu, licorice
Increase: serotonin effect—horehound
Decrease: effect—coltsfoot
Drug/Lab Test
Increase: CPK

NURSING CONSIDERATIONS

Assess:
• ECG continuously for increased PR or QRS segments; discontinue or reduce rate; watch for increased ventricular ectopic beats; may have to rebolus
• Blood levels (therapeutic level 0.5-2 mcg/ml)
• B/P continuously for fluctuations in cardiac rate
• I&O ratio, electrolytes (K, Na, Cl), liver enzymes
⚠ Malignant hyperthermia: tachypnea, tachycardia, changes in B/P, fever
• Respiratory status: rate, rhythm, lung fields for crackles, watch for respiratory depression
• CNS effects: dizziness, confusion, psychosis, paresthesias, convulsions; drug should be discontinued
• Lung fields, bilateral crackles may occur in CHF patient
• Increased respiration, increased pulse; drug should be discontinued
Administer:
• With food for GI upset
Evaluate:
• Therapeutic response: decreased dysrhythmias
Teach patient/family:
• To take with food or antacid
• Avoid changes in diet that could drastically acidify or alkalinize urine
• Notify prescriber of side effects
Treatment of overdose: O₂, artificial ventilation, ECG; administer DOPamine for circulatory depression, diazepam or thiopental for convulsions, to acidify urine

---

miconazole topical
See Appendix C

---

miconazole vaginal antifungal
See Appendix C

---

midazolam (℞)
(mid'ay-zoe-lam)
Versed
Func. class.: Sedative, hypnotic, antianxiety
Chem. class.: Benzodiazepine, short-acting

Controlled Substance Schedule IV
Do not confuse:
Versed/Vepesid
Versed/Vistaril
Action: Depresses subcortical levels in CNS; may act on limbic system, reticular formation; may potentiate γ-aminobutyric acid (GABA) by binding to specific benzodiazepine receptors
Uses: Preoperative sedation, general anesthesia induction, sedation for diagnostic endoscopic procedures, intubation
Investigational uses: Epileptic seizures, refractory status epilepticus

DOSAGE AND ROUTES

Preoperative sedation
• *Adult and child ≥12 yr:* **IM** 0.07-0.08 mg/kg ½-1 hr before general anesthesia
• *Child 1-6 mo:* **IM** 0.1-0.15 mg/kg, may give up to 0.5 mg/kg if needed
• *Child 6 mo-5 yr:* **PO** 0.25-1 mg/kg, max 20 mg as a single dose
• *Child 6 yr-11 yr:* 0.25-0.5 mg/kg, max 20 mg as a single dose
Induction of general anesthesia
• *Adult and child 12-16 yr:* **IV** (unpremedicated patients) 0.3-0.35 mg/kg over 30 sec, wait 2 min, follow with 25% of initial dose if needed; (premedicated

patients) 0.15-0.35 mg/kg over 20-30
sec, allow 2 min for effect
• *Child 6-12 yr:* **IV** 0.025-0.05 mg/kg,
total dose up to 0.4 mg/kg may be
needed
• *Child 6 mo-5 yr:* **IV** 0.05-0.1 mg/kg,
total dose up to 0.6 mg/kg may be
needed
• *Child <6 mo:* Titrate with small increments, adjust as needed
**Continuous infusion for intubation
(critical care)**
• *Adult:* **IV** 0.01-0.05 mg/kg over several min; repeat at 10-15 min intervals,
until adequate sedation; then 0.02-0.10
mg/kg/hr maintenance, adjust as needed
• *Child:* **IV** 0.05-0.2 mg/kg over 2-3
min, then 0.06-0.12 mg/kg/hr by cont
inf; adjust as needed
• *Neonates:* **IV** 0.03-0.06 mg/kg/hr,
titrate using lowest dose
Available forms: Inj 1, 5 mg/ml, syr 2
mg/ml

SIDE EFFECTS

CNS: Retrograde amnesia, euphoria,
confusion, headache, anxiety, insomnia,
slurred speech, paresthesia, tremors,
weakness, chills
CV: Hypotension, PVCs, tachycardia,
bigeminy, nodal rhythm, ***cardiac arrest***
EENT: Blurred vision, nystagmus, diplopia, loss of balance
GI: Nausea, vomiting, increased salivation, hiccups
INTEG: Urticaria, pain at injection site,
swelling at inj site, rash, pruritus at injection site
RESP: Coughing, ***apnea, bronchospasm, laryngospasm,*** dyspnea,
respiratory depression
Contraindications: Pregnancy (D),
hypersensitivity to benzodiazepines,
shock, coma, alcohol intoxication, acute
narrow-angle glaucoma
Precautions: COPD, CHF, chronic renal
failure, chills, elderly, debilitated, children, lactation, neonates (contains benzyl alcohol)

PHARMACOKINETICS

IM: Onset 15 min, peak ½-1 hr, duration 2-3 hr
IV: Onset 3-5 min, onset of anesthesia 1½-2½ min, duration 2 hr
Protein binding 97%; half-life 1.2-
12.3 hr
Metabolized in liver; metabolites excreted in urine; crosses placenta,
blood-brain barrier

INTERACTIONS

Extended half-life: oral contraceptives
Increase: respiratory depression—
other CNS depressants, alcohol, barbiturates, opiate analgesics, verapamil,
ritonavir, indinavir, fluvoxamine
Decrease: midazolam metabolism—
azole antifungals, cimetidine, erythromycin, ranitidine, theophylline
Drug/Herb
Increase: hypotension—black cohosh
Increase: CNS depression—catnip,
chamomile, clary, cowslip, hops, kava,
lavender, mistletoe, nettle, pokeweed,
poppy, Queen Anne's lace, senega, skullcap, valerian
Drug/Food
Increase: (PO) midazolam effect—
grapefruit juice

NURSING CONSIDERATIONS
Assess:
• Injection site for redness, pain, swelling
• Degree of amnesia in elderly; may be
increased
• Anterograde amnesia
• Vital signs for recovery period in obese
patient, since half-life may be extended
• Apnea, respiratory depression that
may be increased in the elderly
Administer:
PO route
• Remove cap of press-in bottle adaptor
and push adaptor into neck of bottle,
close with cap, remove cap and insert tip
of dispenser and insert into adaptor; turn
upside-down and withdraw correct dose;
place in mouth

M

IM route
• IM deep into large muscle mass
IV route
• May be given diluted or undiluted
• After diluting with D_5W or 0.9% NaCl to 0.25 mg/ml; give over 2 min (conscious sedation) or over 30 sec (anesthesia induction)
Additive compatibility: Hydromorphone
Syringe compatibilities: Alfentanil, atracurium, atropine, benzquinamide, buprenorphine, butorphanol, chlorproMAZINE, cimetidine, cisatracurium, diphenhydrAMINE, droperidol, fentanyl, glycopyrrolate, hydromorphone, hydrOXYzine, ketamine, meperidine, metoclopramide, morphine, nalbuphine, promazine, promethazine, remifentanil, scopolamine, sufentanil, thiethylperazine, trimethobenzamide
Y-site compatibilities: Abciximab, alfentamil, amikacin, amiodarone, argatroban, atracurium, atropine, aztreonam, benzotropine, calcium gluconate, cefazolin, cefotaxime, cefoxitine, ceftriaxone, cimetidine, ciprofloxacin, cisplatin, clindamycin, clonidine, cyanocobalamin, cyclosporine, dactinomycin, digoxin, diltiazem, diphenhydramine, docetaxal, DOPamine, doxycyclin, enalaprilate, epINEPHrine, erythromycin, esmolol, etomidate, etoposide, famotidine, fentanyl, fluconazole, folic acid, gatifloxacin, gemcitabine, gentamicin, glycopyrrolate, granisetron, heparin, hetastarch, hydromorphone, hydroxyzine, inamrinone, isoproterenol, labetalol, lactated ringer's, levofloxacin, lidocaine, linezolid, lorazepam, magnesium, mannitol, meperdine, methadone, methyldopa, methylPREDNISolone, metoclopromide, metomolol, metronidazole, milrinone, morphine, nalbuphine, naloxone, niCARdipine, nitroglycerin, nitroprusside, norepinephrine, ondansetron, oxacillin, oxytocin, paclitaxel, palonasetron, pancuronium, papaverin, phentolamine, phytonadione, piperacillin, potassium chloride, propanolol, protamine, pyridoxine, ranitidine, remifentanil, sodium nitroprusside, streptokinase, succinylcholine, sufentanil, teniposide, theophylline, thiotepa, ticarcillin, tobramycin, vancomycin, vasopressin, vecuronium, verapamil, voriconazole
Perform/provide:
• Assistance with ambulation until drowsy period relieved
• Storage at room temperature, protect from light
• Immediate availability of resuscitation equipment, O_2 to support airway; do not give by rapid bolus
Evaluate:
• Therapeutic response: induction of sedation, general anesthesia
Teach patient/family:
• That amnesia occurs; events may not be remembered
Treatment of overdose: Flumazenil, O_2

---

midodrine (R)
(mye′doh-dreen)
ProAmatine
Func. class.: Vasopressor

Do not confuse:
ProAmatine/Protamine
Action: Activates α-adrenergic receptors of arteriolar, venous vasculature by increasing vascular tone
Uses: Orthostatic hypotension

DOSAGE AND ROUTES
• *Adult:* **PO** 10 mg tid
Renal dose
• *Adult:* **PO** 2.5 mg tid
Available forms: Tabs 2.5, 5 mg

SIDE EFFECTS
CNS: Drowsiness, restlessness, headache, *paresthesia, pain,* chills, confusion
CV: **Supine hypertension,** vasodilation, flushing face
EENT: Dry mouth, blurred vision
GI: Nausea, anorexia
GU: Dysuria
INTEG: Pruritus, piloerection, rash
Contraindications: Hypersensitivity,

---

severe organic heart disease, acute renal disease, urinary retention, pheochromocytoma, thyrotoxicosis, thyroid disease, visual disturbance dialysis, urinary retention, persistent/excessive supine hypertension, thyroid disease, visual disturbance, dialysis, urinary retention
Precautions: Pregnancy (C), children, lactation, prostatic hypertrophy, hepatic function impairment, orthostatic diabetic patients

PHARMACOKINETICS

PO: Peak 1-2 hr, half-life 3-4 hr, bioavailability 90%

INTERACTIONS

Increase: bradycardia—β-blockers, psychotropics, cardiac glycosides, tricyclics
Increase: pressor effects—α-agonist
Increase: supine hypertension—fludrocortisone
Increase: lactic acidosis—metformin

NURSING CONSIDERATIONS
Assess:
• VS, B/P (standing, supine); notify prescriber if B/P supine is increased
• Observe for drowsiness, dizziness, LOC
Administer:
• Tablets may be swallowed whole, chewed, or allowed to dissolve
• Upon arising, midday, and late afternoon (no later than 6 PM)
• Avoid administering if patient is to be supine during day
Evaluate:
• Therapeutic response: decreased orthostatic hypotension
Teach patient/family:
• To avoid hazardous activities, activities requiring alertness; dizziness may occur; instruct patient to request assistance with ambulation
• To avoid alcohol, other depressants

---

mifepristone (R)
(mif-ee-press'tone)
Mifeprex
Func. class.: Abortifacient
Chem. class.: Antiprogestational

Action: Stimulates uterine contractions, causing complete abortion
Uses: Abortion through 49 days' gestation
Investigational uses: Postcoital contraception/contragestation, intrauterine fetal death, endometriosis, Cushing's syndrome, unresectable meningioma

DOSAGE AND ROUTES
• *Adult:* **PO** 600 mg day 1, 400 mcg misoprostol day 3
Available forms: Tabs 200 mg

SIDE EFFECTS

CNS: Dizziness, insomnia, anxiety, syncope, fainting, headache
GI: Nausea, vomiting, diarrhea, dyspepsia
GU: Uterine cramping, uterine hemorrhage, vaginitis, pelvic pain
MISC: Fatigue, back pain, fever, viral infections, chills, sinusitis
Contraindications: Hypersensitivity, severe hepatic disease, severe renal disease, IUD, ectopic pregnancy, chronic adrenal failure, bleeding disorder, inherited porphyrias, PID, respiratory disease, cardiac disease
Precautions: Pregnancy (C), asthma, anemia, jaundice, diabetes mellitus, convulsive disorders, women >35 yr/ smoke ≥10 cigarettes/day, past uterine surgery

PHARMACOKINETICS

Rapidly absorbed, peak 90 min, 98% bound to plasma proteins, albumin, glycoprotein, excretion via feces, urine

INTERACTIONS

Decrease: metabolism of erythromycin, ketoconazole, itraconazole

M

Side effects: *italics* = common; ***bold italics*** = life-threatening

Drug/Herb
Decrease: by—St. John's wort
Drug/Food
Decrease: metabolism of mifepristone: grapefruit juice

NURSING CONSIDERATIONS

Assess:
• B/P, pulse; watch for change that may indicate hemorrhage
• Respiratory rate, rhythm, depth; notify prescriber of abnormalities
• For length, duration of contraction; notify prescriber of contractions lasting over 1 min or absence of contractions
• For incomplete abortion, pregnancy must be terminated by another method; drug is teratogenic

Perform/provide:
• Emotional support before and after abortion

Evaluate:
• Therapeutic response: expulsion of fetus

Teach patient/family:
• To report increased blood loss, abdominal cramps, increased temp, foul-smelling lochia
• Some methods of comfort control and pain control
• Must continue with follow-up
• That cramping and vaginal bleeding will occur

---

miglitol (℞)
(mig'lih-tol)
Glyset
Func. class.: Oral hypoglycemic
Chem. class.: α-Glucosidase inhibitor

Action: Delays digestion of ingested carbohydrates, results in smaller rise in blood glucose after meals; does not increase insulin production
Uses: Type 2 diabetes mellitus

DOSAGE AND ROUTES

• *Adult:* **PO** 25 mg tid initially, with first bite of meal; maintenance dose may be increased to 50 mg tid; may be increased to 100 mg tid if needed (only in patients >60 kg) with dosage adjustment at 4-8 wk intervals
Available forms: Tabs 25, 50, 100 mg

SIDE EFFECTS

GI: Abdominal pain, diarrhea, flatulence, ***hepatotoxicity***
HEMA: Low iron
INTEG: Rash

Contraindications: Hypersensitivity, diabetic ketoacidosis, cirrhosis, inflammatory bowel disease, colonic ulceration, partial intestinal obstruction, chronic intestinal disease
Precautions: Pregnancy (B), renal disease, lactation, children, hepatic disease

PHARMACOKINETICS

Peak 2-3 hr, not metabolized, excreted in urine as unchanged drug, half-life 2 hr

INTERACTIONS

Decrease: levels of digoxin, propranolol, ranitidine
Decrease: miglitol levels—digestive enzymes, intestinal adsorbents; do not use together
Drug/Herb
Improved glucose tolerance: karela
Decrease: hypoglycemic effect—broom, buchu, dandelion, juniper
Increase or decrease: hypoglycemic effect—chromium, fenugreek, ginseng
Drug/Food
Increase: diarrhea; carbohydrates

NURSING CONSIDERATIONS

Assess:
• Hypoglycemia, hyperglycemia; even though drug does not cause hypoglycemia, if patient is on sulfonylureas or insulin, hypoglycemia may be additive
• Blood glucose levels, hemoglobin, A1c

⚠ Safety alert   *"Tall Man" lettering

LFTs; if hypoglycemia occers with monotherapy, treat with glucose

Administer:

• Tid with first bite of each meal

Perform/provide:

• Storage in tight container in cool environment

Evaluate:

• Therapeutic response: decreased signs/symptoms of diabetes mellitus (polyuria, polydipsia, polyphagia, clear sensorium, absence of dizziness, stable gait)

Teach patient/family:

• The symptoms of hypo/hyperglycemia, what to do about each, that during periods of stress, infection, surgery, insulin may be required

• That medication must be taken as prescribed; explain consequences of discontinuing medication abruptly

• To avoid OTC medications unless approved by health care provider

• That diabetes is lifelong illness; that this drug is not a cure

• To carry ID for emergency purposes

• That diet and exercise regimen must be followed

Rarely Used

miglustat (℞)

(mih′glue-stat)

Zavesca

Func. class.: Miscellaneous agent

Uses: Adults with mild to moderate type 1 Gaucher disease

DOSAGE AND ROUTES

• *Adult:* **PO** 100 mg tid, without regard to food

Contraindications: Pregnancy (X), hypersensitivity

⚠ High Alert

milrinone (℞)

(mill′rih-nohn)

Primacor

Func. class.: Inotropic/vasodilator agent with phosphodiesterase activity

Chem. class.: Bipyridine derivative

Action: Positive inotropic agent, increases contractility of cardiac muscle with vasodilator properties; reduces preload and afterload by direct relaxation on vascular smooth muscle

Uses: Short-term management of advanced CHF that has not responded to other medication; can be used with digitalis

DOSAGE AND ROUTES

• *Adult:* **IV BOL** 50 mcg/kg given over 10 min; start inf of 0.375-0.75 mcg/kg/min; reduce dose in renal impairment

Available forms: Inj 1 mg/ml; premixed inj 200 mcg/ml in D_5W

SIDE EFFECTS

CV: **Dysrhythmias,** hypotension, chest pain

GI: Nausea, vomiting, anorexia, abdominal pain, **hepatotoxicity, jaundice**

HEMA: **Thrombocytopenia**

MISC: Headache, hypokalemia, tremor

Contraindications: Hypersensitivity to this drug, severe aortic disease, severe pulmonic valvular disease, acute myocardial infarction

Precautions: Pregnancy (C), lactation, children, renal disease, hepatic disease, atrial flutter/fibrillation, elderly

PHARMACOKINETICS

IV: Onset 2-5 min, peak 10 min, duration variable; half-life 2.4 hr; metabolized in liver; excreted in urine as drug (83%) and metabolites (12%)

M

Side effects: *italics* = common; ***bold italics*** = life-threatening

NURSING CONSIDERATIONS
Assess:
⚠️ ECG continuously during IV, ventricular dysrhythmia can occur

• B/P and pulse q5min during infusion; if B/P drops 30 mm Hg, stop infusion and call prescriber

• Electrolytes: K, Na, Cl, Ca; renal studies: BUN, creatinine; blood studies: platelet count

• ALT, AST, bilirubin daily

• I&O ratio and weight daily; diuresis should increase with continuing therapy

• If platelets are <150,000/mm^3, drug is usually discontinued and another drug started

• Extravasation; change site q48h

Administer:
• Potassium supplements if ordered for potassium levels <3 mg/dl

IV route
• Give IV loading dose undiluted over 10 min

• Into running dextrose infusion through Y-connector or directly into tubing; dilute with 0.9% NaCl to 1-3 mg/ml; do not mix with glucose for long-term infusion

• By inf pump for doses other than bolus

Additive compatibilities: Quinidine

Syringe compatibilities: Atropine, calcium chloride, digoxin, epINEPHrine, lidocaine, morphine, propranolol, sodium bicarbonate, verapamil

Y-site compatibilities: Digoxin, diltiazem, DOBUTamine, DOPamine, epINEPHrine, fentanyl, heparin, hydromorphone, labetalol, lorazepam, midazolam, morphine, niCARdipine, nitroglycerin, norepinephrine, propranolol, quinidine, ranitidine, thiopental, vecuronium

Evaluate:
• Therapeutic response: increased cardiac output, decreased PCWP, adequate CVP, decreased dyspnea, fatigue, edema, ECG

Teach patient/family:
• To report angina immediately during infusion

• To report headache, which can be treated with analgesics

Treatment of overdose: Discontinue drug, support circulation

---

minocycline (℞)
(min-oh-sye′kleen)
Arestin, Dynacin, Minocin, Vectrin
Func. class.: Broad-spectrum antiinfective
Chem. class.: Tetracycline

Action: Inhibits protein synthesis, phosphorylation in microorganisms by binding to 30S ribosomal subunits, reversibly binding to 50S ribosomal subunits; bacteriostatic

Uses: Syphilis, *Chlamydia trachomatis,* gonorrhea, lymphogranuloma venereum, rickettsial infections, inflammatory acne, *Neisseria meningitidis, Neisseria gonorrhoeae, Treponema pallidum, Chlamydia trachomatis, Ureaplasma urealyticum, Mycoplasma pneumoniae, Nocardia,* periodontitis

Investigational uses: Rheumatoid arthritis

DOSAGE AND ROUTES
• *Adult:* **PO/IV** 200 mg, then 100 mg q12h or 50 mg q6h, not to exceed 400 mg/24 hr **IV; SUBGINGIVAL** inserted into periodontal pocket

• *Child >8 yr:* **PO/IV** 4 mg/kg then 4 mg/kg/day **PO** in divided doses q12h

Gonorrhea
• *Adult:* **PO** 200 mg, then 100 mg q12h × 4 days

Chlamydia trachomatis
• *Adult:* **PO** 100 mg bid × 7 days

Syphilis
• *Adult:* **PO** 200 mg, then 100 mg q12h × 10-15 days

Uncomplicated gonococcal urethritis in men
• *Adult:* **PO** 100 mg q12h × 5 days

Rheumatoid arthritis (off-label)
• *Adult:* **PO** 100 mg bid for ≤48 wk

Available forms: Caps 50, 75, 100

---

mg; oral susp 50 mg/5 ml; powder for inj 100 mg; caps, pellet filled 50, 100 mg; tabs 50, 75, 100 mg

SIDE EFFECTS

CNS: Dizziness, fever, light-headedness, vertigo
CV: Pericarditis
EENT: Dysphagia, glossitis, decreased calcification of deciduous teeth, permanent discoloration of teeth, oral candidiasis
GI: Nausea, abdominal pain, *vomiting, diarrhea,* anorexia, enterocolitis, **hepatotoxicity,** flatulence, abdominal cramps, epigastric burning, stomatitis
GU: Increased BUN, polyuria, polydipsia, **renal failure, nephrotoxicity**
HEMA: **Eosinophilia, neutropenia, thrombocytopenia, hemolytic anemia**
*INTEG: Rash, urticaria, photosensitivity, increased pigmentation, **exfoliative dermatitis,*** pruritus, blue-gray color of skin, mucous membranes
*SYST: **Angioedema***
Contraindications: Pregnancy (D), hypersensitivity to tetracyclines, children <8 yr
Precautions: Hepatic disease, lactation

PHARMACOKINETICS

PO: Peak 2-3 hr, half-life 11-17 hr; excreted in urine, feces, breast milk; crosses placenta; 70%-75% protein bound

INTERACTIONS

Increase: effect of warfarin, digoxin, insulin, oral anticoagulants, theophylline
Decrease: effect of minocycline—antacids, sodium bicarbonate, alkali products, iron, kaolin/pectin, cimetidine
Decrease: effect of barbiturates, carbamazepine, phenytoin, penicillins, oral contraceptives, calcium
Drug/Lab Test
False negative: Urine glucose with Clinistix or Tes-Tape

NURSING CONSIDERATIONS

Assess:
• I&O ratio
• Blood tests: PT, CBC, AST, ALT, BUN, creatinine
• Signs of anemia: Hct, Hgb, fatigue
• Allergic reactions: rash, itching, pruritus, angioedema
• Nausea, vomiting, diarrhea; administer antiemetic, antacids as ordered
• Overgrowth of infection: fever, malaise, redness, pain, swelling, drainage, perineal itching, diarrhea, changes in cough or sputum, black, furry tongue
Administer:
• After C&S obtained
• With a full glass of water; with food for GI symptoms
PO route
• 2 hr before or after laxative or ferrous products; 3 hr after antacid
IV route
• After diluting 100 mg/5 ml sterile H_2O for inj; further dilute in 500-1000 ml of NaCl, dextrose sol, LR, Ringer's sol; run 100 mg/6 hr
Y-site compatibilities: Aztreonam, cisatracurium, cyclophosphamide, filgrastim, fludarabine, granisetron, heparin, hydrocortisone, magnesium sulfate, melphalan, perphenazine, potassium chloride, remifentanil, sargramostim, teniposide, vinorelbine, vit B/C
Perform/provide:
• Storage in airtight, light-resistant container at room temperature
Evaluate:
• Therapeutic response: decreased temp, absence of lesions, negative C&S
Teach patient/family:
• To avoid sunlight; sunscreen does not seem to decrease photosensitivity
• That all prescribed medication must be taken to prevent superinfection; not to use outdated product, Fanconi's syndrome may occur

M

minoxidil (R, otc)
(mi-nox′i-dill)
Loniten, minoxidil, Rogaine (top)
Func. class.: Antihypertensive
Chem. class.: Vasodilator, peripheral

Do not confuse:
Loniten/Lotensin
minoxidil/Monopril
Action: Directly relaxes arteriolar smooth muscle, causing vasodilation
Uses: Severe hypertension unresponsive to other therapy (use with diuretic); topically to treat alopecia

DOSAGE AND ROUTES
Severe hypertension
• *Adult:* **PO** 2.5-5 mg/day not to exceed 100 mg daily, usual range 10-40 mg/day in single doses
• *Geriatric:* **PO** 2.5 mg daily, may be increased gradually
• *Child <12 yr:* **PO** (initial) 0.2 mg/kg/day; (effective range) 0.25-1 mg/kg/day; (max) 50 mg/day
Alopecia
• *Adult:* **TOP** 1 ml bid, rub into scalp daily, max 2 ml/day
Available forms: Tabs 2.5, 10 mg; top 2% sol

SIDE EFFECTS
Systemic
CNS: Headache, fatigue
CV: Severe rebound hypertension on withdrawal in children, tachycardia, angina, increased T wave, *CHF, pulmonary edema, pericardial effusion,* edema, sodium, water retention
GI: Nausea, vomiting
GU: Breast tenderness
HEMA: Hct, Hgb, erythrocyte count may decrease initially
INTEG: Pruritus, *Stevens-Johnson syndrome,* rash, hirsutism
Contraindications: Acute MI, dissecting aortic aneurysm, hypersensitivity, pheochromocytoma

Precautions: Pregnancy (C), lactation, children, renal disease, CAD, CHF, elderly

PHARMACOKINETICS
PO: Onset 30 min, peak 2-3 hr, duration 75 hr; half-life 4.2 hr; metabolized in liver; metabolites excreted in urine, feces

INTERACTIONS
Orthostatic hypotension: antihypertensives
Drug/Lab Test
Increase: Renal studies
Decrease: Hgb/Hct/RBC

NURSING CONSIDERATIONS
Assess:
⚠ Monitor closely, usually given with β-blocker to prevent tachycardia and increased myocardial workload, usually given with diuretic to prevent serious fluid accumulation, patient should be hospitalized during beginning treatment
• Nausea, edema in feet, legs daily
• Skin turgor, dryness of mucous membranes for hydration status
• Crackles, dyspnea, orthopnea
• Electrolytes: K, Na, Cl, CO_2
• Renal studies: catecholamines, BUN, creatinine
• Hepatic studies: AST, ALT, alk phosphatase
• B/P, pulse
• Weight daily, I&O
Administer:
PO route
• With meals for better absorption, to decrease GI symptoms
• With β-blocker and/or diuretic for hypertension
TOP route
• 1 ml no matter how much balding has occurred; increasing dosage does not speed growth
Perform/provide:
• Storage protected from light and heat
Evaluate:
• Therapeutic response: decreased B/P or increased hair growth

---

⚠ Safety alert   *"Tall Man" lettering

Teach patient/family:

• That body hair will increase but is reversible after discontinuing treatment

• Not to discontinue drug abruptly

• To report pitting edema, dizziness, weight gain >5 lb, shortness of breath, bruising or bleeding, heart rate >20 beats/min over normal, severe indigestion, dizziness, light-headedness, panting, new or aggravated symptoms of angina

• To take drug exactly as prescribed, or serious side effects may occur

Topical

• That for topical use, treatment must continue long-term or new hair will be lost

• Not to use except on scalp

Treatment of overdose: Administer normal saline IV, vasopressors

---

mirtazapine (R)
(mer-ta′za-peen)
Remeron, Remeron Soltab
Func. class.: Antidepressant
Chem. class.: Tetracyclic

Action: Blocks reuptake of norepinephrine, serotonin into nerve endings, increasing action of norepinephrine, serotonin in nerve cells

Uses: Depression, dysthymic disorder, bipolar disorder—depressed, agitated depression

DOSAGE AND ROUTES

• *Adult:* **PO** 15 mg/day at bedtime, maintenance to continue for 6 mo, titrate up to 45 mg/day; orally disintegrating tabs: open blister pack, place tab on tongue, allow to disintegrate, swallow

• *Geriatric:* **PO** 7.5 mg at bedtime, increase by 7.5 mg q1-2wk to desired dose, max 45 mg/day

Available forms: Tabs 15, 30 mg; orally disintegrating tab (soltab) 15, 30, 45 mg

SIDE EFFECTS

CNS: Dizziness, drowsiness, confusion, headache, anxiety, tremors, stimulation, weakness, insomnia, nightmares, EPS (elderly), increased psychiatric symptoms, *seizures*

CV: Orthostatic hypotension, ECG changes, tachycardia, hypertension, palpitations

EENT: Blurred vision, tinnitus, mydriasis

GI: Diarrhea, dry mouth, nausea, vomiting, *paralytic ileus,* increased appetite, cramps, epigastric distress, constipation, *jaundice, hepatitis,* stomatitis

GU: Urinary retention, acute renal failure

HEMA: Agranulocytosis, thrombocytopenia, eosinophilia, leukopenia

INTEG: Rash, urticaria, sweating, pruritus, photosensitivity

SYST: Flulike symptoms

Contraindications: Hypersensitivity to tricyclics, recovery phase of MI, convulsive disorders, prostatic hypertrophy

Precautions: Pregnancy (C), suicidal patients, severe depression, increased intraocular pressure, narrow-angle glaucoma, urinary retention, cardiac disease, renal disease, hepatic disease, hypothyroidism, hyperthyroidism, electroshock therapy, elective surgery, elderly

PHARMACOKINETICS

PO: Peak 12 hr, metabolized by liver; excreted in urine, feces; crosses placenta; half-life 20-40 hr

INTERACTIONS

⚠ Hyperpyretic crisis, seizures, hypertensive episode: MAOIs

Increase: CNS depression, alcohol, barbiturates, benzodiazepines, other CNS depressants

Decrease: effects of clonidine, indirect-acting sympathomimetics (epHEDrine)

Drug/Herb

Serotonin syndrome: SAM-e, St. John's wort

Increase: anticholinergic effect—belladonna, henbane

Increase: antidepressant action—scopolia

Side effects: *italics* = common; ***bold italics*** = life-threatening

Increase: CNS depression—chamomile, hops, kava, skullcap, valerian
Drug/Lab Test
Increase: Serum bilirubin, blood glucose, alk phosphatase
Decrease: VMA, 5-HIAA
False increase: Urinary catecholamines

NURSING CONSIDERATIONS

Assess:
• B/P (lying, standing), pulse q4h; if systolic B/P drops 20 mm Hg, hold drug, notify prescriber; take vital signs q4h in patients with cardiovascular disease
• Blood studies: CBC, leukocytes, differential, cardiac enzymes if patient is receiving long-term therapy
• Hepatic studies: AST, ALT, bilirubin, creatinine
• Weight qwk; appetite may increase with drug
• ECG for flattening of T wave, bundle branch block, AV block, dysrhythmias in cardiac patients
• EPS primarily in elderly: rigidity, dystonia, akathisia
• Mental status: mood, sensorium, affect, suicidal tendencies, increase in psychiatric symptoms: depression, panic
• Alcohol consumption; if alcohol is consumed, hold dose until morning
Administer:
• Increased fluids, bulk in diet for constipation, especially elderly
• With food, milk for GI symptoms
• Dosage at bedtime if oversedation occurs during day; may take entire dose at bedtime; elderly may not tolerate once/day dosing
• Gum, hard candy, or frequent sips of water for dry mouth
• Orally disintegrating tab: no water needed; allow to dissolve on tongue
Perform/provide:
• Storage in tight container at room temperature; do not freeze
• Assistance with ambulation during beginning therapy, since drowsiness/dizziness occurs
• Safety measures, including side rails, primarily in elderly

• Checking to see PO medication swallowed
Evaluate:
• Therapeutic response: decreased depression
Teach patient/family:
• That therapeutic effects may take 2-3 wk
• To use caution in driving, other activities requiring alertness, because of drowsiness, dizziness, blurred vision
• To report immediately urinary retention
• To avoid alcohol ingestion, other CNS depressants
Treatment of overdose: ECG monitoring, induce emesis; lavage, activated charcoal; administer anticonvulsant

---

misoprostol (℞)
(mye-soe-prost′ole)
Cytotec
Func. class.: Gastric mucosa protectant, antiulcer
Chem. class.: Prostaglandin E$_1$-analog

Do not confuse:
cytotec/Cytoxan
misoprostol/metoprolol
Action: Inhibits gastric acid secretion; may protect gastric mucosa; can increase bicarbonate, mucus production
Uses: Prevention of nonsteroidal antiinflammatory drug-induced gastric ulcers
Investigational uses: Used investigationally with methotrexate to produce abortion, chronic idiopathic constipation, postpartum hemorrhage; cervical ripening/labor induction (vaginal)

DOSAGE AND ROUTES

• *Adult:* **PO** 200 mcg qid with food for duration of nonsteroidal antiinflammatory therapy with last dose at bedtime; if 200 mcg is not tolerated, 100 mcg may be given
Available forms: Tabs 100, 200 mcg

⚠ Safety alert　　*"Tall Man" lettering

SIDE EFFECTS

GI: Diarrhea, nausea, vomiting, flatulence, constipation, dyspepsia, abdominal pain

GU: Spotting, cramps, hypermenorrhea, menstrual disorders

Contraindications: Pregnancy (X), hypersensitivity to this drug or prostaglandins

Precautions: Lactation, children, elderly, renal disease, CV disease

PHARMACOKINETICS

PO: Peak 12 min, plasma steady state achieved within 2 days, excreted in urine

INTERACTIONS

Drug/Food
Decrease: maximum concentrations when taken with food

NURSING CONSIDERATIONS

Assess:
• GI symptoms: hematemesis, occult or frank blood in stools, gastric aspirate, cramping, severe diarrhea
• Obtain a negative pregnancy test; miscarriages are common
• Gastric pH (>5 should be maintained)

Administer:
• PO with meals for prolonged drug effect; avoid use of magnesium antacids

Perform/provide:
• Storage at room temperature

Evaluate:
• Therapeutic response: absence of pain or GI complaints; prevention of ulcers

Teach patient/family:
• To take only as directed, read patient information leaflet
• Not to take if pregnant (can cause miscarriage) and not to become pregnant while taking this medication; if pregnancy occurs during therapy, discontinue drug, notify prescriber; not to administer to nursing mothers
• Not to give drug to anyone else or take for more than 4 wk unless directed by prescriber

• To avoid OTC preparations: aspirin, cough, cold products; condition may worsen

⚠ High Alert

mitomycin (℞)
(mye-toe-mye'sin)
mitomycin, Mutamycin
Func. class.: Antineoplastic, antibiotic

Action: Inhibits DNA synthesis, primarily; derived from *Streptomyces caespitosus;* appears to cause crosslinking of DNA, a vesicant

Uses: Pancreas, stomach cancer, head and neck or breast cancer

Investigational uses: Palliative treatment of head, neck, colon, breast, biliary, cervical, lung malignancies

DOSAGE AND ROUTES

• *Adult:* **IV** 10-20 mg/m^2 q6-8wk

Available forms: Inj 5, 20, 40 mg/vial

SIDE EFFECTS

CNS: Fever, headache, confusion, drowsiness, syncope, fatigue

EENT: Blurred vision

GI: Nausea, vomiting, anorexia, stomatitis, **bepatotoxicity,** diarrhea

GU: Urinary retention, **renal failure,** edema

HEMA: **Thrombocytopenia, leukopenia, anemia**

INTEG: Rash, alopecia, **extravasation**

MISC: **Hemolytic uremic syndrome**

RESP: **Fibrosis, pulmonary infiltrate,** dyspnea

Contraindications: Pregnancy (D) 1st trimester, hypersensitivity, as a single agent, thrombocytopenia, coagulation disorders, lactation

Precautions: Renal disease, bone marrow depression

PHARMACOKINETICS

Half-life 1 hr, metabolized in liver, 10% excreted in urine (unchanged)

INTERACTIONS

Increase: toxicity—other antineoplastics, radiation

NURSING CONSIDERATIONS

Assess:

• CBC, differential, platelet count weekly; withhold drug if WBC is <2000/mm³, granulocyte count <1000/mm³, or platelet count is <100,000/mm³; notify prescriber

• Pulmonary function tests, chest x-ray before, during therapy; chest x-ray should be obtained q2wk during treatment

⚠ Fatal hemolytic uremic syndrome: hypertension, thrombocytopenia, microangiopathic hemolytic anemia, occurs in those on long-term therapy

• Renal studies: BUN, serum uric acid, urine CCr, electrolytes before, during therapy

• I&O ratio; report fall in urine output to <30 ml/hr

• Monitor temp q4h; fever may indicate beginning infection

• Hepatic studies before, during therapy: bilirubin, AST, ALT, alk phosphatase as needed or monthly; check for jaundiced skin and sclera, dark urine, clay-colored stools, itchy skin, abdominal pain, fever, diarrhea

• Bleeding: hematuria, guaiac, bruising, petechiae, mucosa or orifices q8h

⚠ Pulmonary fibrosis: bronchospasm

• Dyspnea, crackles, unproductive cough; chest pain, tachypnea, fatigue, increased pulse, pallor, lethargy

• Effects of alopecia on body image; discuss feelings about body changes

• Inflammation of mucosa, breaks in skin

• Buccal cavity q8h for dryness, sores, ulceration, white patches, oral pain, bleeding, dysphagia

• Local irritation, pain, burning at inj site

• GI symptoms: frequency of stools, cramping

• Acidosis, signs of dehydration: rapid respirations, poor skin turgor, decreased urine output, dry skin, restlessness, weakness

Administer:

• Apply ice compress for extravasation; stop infusion

• Antiemetic 30-60 min before giving drug to prevent vomiting

• IV after diluting 5 mg/10 ml or 10 mg/40 ml sterile H_2O for inj; shake, allow to stand, give through Y-tube or 3-way stopcock; give over 5-10 min, color of reconstituted sol is gray

Additive compatibilities: Dexamethasone, hydrocortisone

Solution compatibilities: LR, 0.3% NaCl, 0.5% NaCl

Syringe compatibilities: Bleomycin, cisplatin, cyclophosphamide, DOXOrubicin, droperidol, fluorouracil, furosemide, heparin, leucovorin, methotrexate, metoclopramide, vinBLAStine, vinCRIStine

Y-site compatibilities: Allopurinol, amifostine, bleomycin, cisplatin, cyclophosphamide, DOXOrubicin, droperidol, fluorouracil, furosemide, granisetron, heparin, leucovorin, melphalan, methotrexate, metoclopramide, ondansetron, teniposide, thiotepa, vinBLAStine, vinCRIStine

Perform/provide:

• Rinsing of mouth tid-qid with water; brushing of teeth with baking soda bid-tid with soft brush or cotton-tipped applicators for stomatitis; use unwaxed dental floss

• Storage at room temperature 1 wk after reconstituting or 2 wk refrigerated

Evaluate:

• Therapeutic response: decreased tumor size, spread of malignancy

Teach patient/family:

• To report any complaints, side effects to nurse or prescriber

• That hair may be lost during treatment and wig or hairpiece may make the patient feel better; tell patient that new hair may be different in color, texture

• To avoid foods with citric acid, hot or rough texture

⚠ Safety alert   *"Tall Man" lettering

• To report any bleeding, white spots, ulcerations in mouth; tell patient to examine mouth daily

• To avoid crowds, persons with infections if granulocyte count is low

Rarely Used

mitotane (℞)
(mye′toe-tane)
Lysodren, p′-DDD
Func. class.: Antineoplastic

Uses: Adrenocortical carcinoma

DOSAGE AND ROUTES

• *Adult:* PO 9-10 g/day in divided doses tid or qid; may have to decrease dose for severe reaction

Contraindications: Hypersensitivity

⚠ High Alert

mitoxantrone (℞)
(mye-toe-zan′trone)
Novantrone
Func. class.: Antineoplastic, antiinfective, immunomodulator
Chem. class.: Synthetic anthraquinone

Action: DNA reactive agent, cytocidal effect on both proliferating and nonproliferating cells, suggesting lack of cell cycle phase specificity (vesicant)
Uses: Acute nonlymphocytic leukemia (adult), relapsed leukemia, breast cancer; used with steroids to treat bone pain (advanced prostate cancer), multiple sclerosis (MS)
Investigational uses: Liver malignancies, non-Hodgkin's lymphoma

DOSAGE AND ROUTES
Induction
• *Adult:* IV INF 12 mg/m^2/day on days 1-3, and 100 mg/m^2 cytosine arabinoside × 7 days as a continuous 24-hr inf

Consolidation
• *Adult:* IV 12 mg/m^2 given as a short 5-15 min inf
Multiple sclerosis
• *Adult:* IV INF 12 mg/m^2 as a 5-15 min inf q3mo
Available forms: Inj 2 mg/ml

SIDE EFFECTS

CNS: Headache, *seizures*
CV: **CHF, cardiopathy, dysrhythmias**
EENT: Conjunctivitis, blue/green sclera
GI: Nausea, vomiting, diarrhea, anorexia, mucositis, **hepatotoxicity**
HEMA: **Thrombocytopenia, leukopenia, myelosuppression, anemia**
INTEG: Rash, necrosis at inj site, dermatitis, thrombophlebitis at injection site, alopecia
MISC: Fever
RESP: Cough, dyspnea
Contraindications: Pregnancy (D), hypersensitivity
Precautions: Myelosuppression, lactation, cardiac disease, children; renal, hepatic disease; gout

PHARMACOKINETICS

Highly bound to plasma proteins, metabolized in liver, excreted via renal, hepatobiliary systems; half-life 24-72 hr

INTERACTIONS

Do not mix with heparin; precipitate will form
Do not mix with any other drug
Increase: bone marrow depression toxicity—radiation, other antineoplastics
Increase: adverse reactions—live virus vaccines

NURSING CONSIDERATIONS
Assess:
• CBC, differential, platelet count qwk; withhold drug if WBC is <4000/mm^3 or platelet count is <75,000/mm^3; notify prescriber of these results
• Hepatic studies before, during therapy:

M

Side effects: *italics* = common; **bold italics** = life-threatening

bilirubin, AST, ALT, alk phosphatase prn or qmo

• Renal studies: BUN, serum uric acid, urine CCr, electrolytes before, during therapy

• Bleeding, hematuria, guaiac, bruising or petechiae, mucosa or orifices q8h

• Jaundiced skin and sclera, dark urine, clay-colored stools, itchy skin, abdominal pain, fever, diarrhea

⚠ ECG, ECHO, chest x-ray RAI angiography to assess ejection fraction before and during treatment, cardiotoxic, may develop during treatment or months to years after treatment

• Acidosis, signs of dehydration: rapid respirations, poor skin turgor, decreased urine output, dry skin, restlessness, weakness

⚠ For secondary acute myelogenous leukemia (AML) that can develop after taking this drug

⚠ For MS: obtain MUGA, LVEF baselines; repeat LVEF if symptoms of CHF occur or if cumulative dose is >100 mg/m²; do not administer to patients who have received a lifetime dose of ≥140 mg/m² or if LVEF <50% or significant LVEF

• Do not administer to patients with MS if neutrophils <1500 cells/mm³

• Obtain pregnancy test in all women of childbearing age, even if birth control is used

Administer:

• Medications by oral route if possible; avoid IM, SUBCUT, IV routes to prevent infections

• Antiemetic 30-60 min before giving drug to prevent vomiting

IV route

• IV after diluting with 50 ml or more NS or D_5W; give over 3-5 min, running IV of D_5W or NS; may be diluted further in D_5W, NS and run over 15-30 min; check for extravasation

Additive compatibilities: Cyclophosphamide, cytarabine, fluorouracil, hydrocortisone, potassium chloride

Solution compatibilities: D_5/0.9 NaCl, D_5W, 0.9% NaCl

Y-site compatibilities: Allopurinol, amifostine, cladribine, filgrastim, fludarabine, granisetron, melphalan, ondansetron, sargramostim, teniposide, thiotepa, vinorelbine

Perform/provide:

• Liquid diet: carbonated beverages, Jell-O; dry toast, crackers may be added if patient is not nauseated or vomiting

• Rinsing of mouth tid-qid with water, club soda; brushing of teeth bid-qid with soft brush or cotton-tipped applicators for stomatitis; use unwaxed dental floss

• Increase fluids to 2-3 L/day unless contraindicated

Evaluate:

• Therapeutic response: decreased tumor size, spread of malignancy

Teach patient/family:

• To report side effects to nurse or physician

• To avoid foods with citric acid, rough texture, or hot

• To report any bleeding, white spots, ulcerations in mouth; tell patient to examine mouth daily

• To avoid crowds, persons with infections

• That sclera, urine may turn blue or green, hair loss may occur

• To notify prescriber if pregnancy is suspected or planned, use effective contraception

---

⚠ High Alert

mivacurium (℞)
(miv-a-kure′ee-um)
Mivacron
Func. class.: Neuromuscular blocker—nondepolarizing

Do not confuse:
Mivacron/Mazicon
Action: Inhibits transmission of nerve impulses by binding competitively with cholinergic receptor sites, antagonizing action of acetylcholine
Uses: Facilitation of endotracheal intubation, skeletal muscle relaxation during

---

mechanical ventilation, surgery, or general anesthesia

DOSAGE AND ROUTES
• *Adult:* **IV** 0.15 mg/kg; maintenance 0.10/mg/Kg q15min
• *Child 2-12 yr:* **IV** 0.2 mg/kg for a 10 min block
Available forms: 5, 10 ml single-use vial (2 mg/ml); premixed infusion in D₅W 50-ml flex container

SIDE EFFECTS
CV: Decreased B/P, bradycardia, tachycardia
EENT: Diplopia
INTEG: Rash, urticaria
MS: Weakness, prolonged skeletal muscle relaxation, *paralysis*
RESP: ***Prolonged apnea, bronchospasm, wheezing, respiratory depression***
Contraindications: Hypersensitivity
Precautions: Pregnancy (C), renal or hepatic disease, lactation, children <3 mo, fluid and electrolyte imbalances, neuromuscular disease, respiratory disease, obesity, elderly

PHARMACOKINETICS
Rapidly hydrolyzed by plasma cholinesterases, peak 2-3 min, reversal within 15-30 min

INTERACTIONS
Increase: neuromuscular blockade—aminoglycosides, amphotericin B, bacitracin, carbamazepine, clindamycin, colistin, diuretics, enflurane, halothane, isoflurane, lincomycin, lithium, local anesthetics, magnesium, phenytoin, polymyxin antibiotics, procainamide, quinidine, tetracyclines

NURSING CONSIDERATIONS
Assess:
• For electrolyte imbalances (K, Mg); may lead to increased action of this drug
• VS (B/P, pulse, respirations, airway)

until fully recovered; rate, depth, pattern of respirations, strength of hand grip
• I&O ratio; check for urinary retention, frequency, hesitancy
• Recovery: decreased paralysis of face, diaphragm, leg, arm, rest of body
• Allergic reactions: rash, fever, respiratory distress, pruritus; drug should be discontinued
Administer:
• Using nerve stimulator by anesthesiologist to determine neuromuscular blockade
• Anticholinesterase to reverse neuromuscular blockade
• By slow IV over 1-2 min (only by qualified persons, usually an anesthesiologist)
• Only fresh sol
Y-site compatibilities: Etomidate, thiopental
Perform/provide:
• Storage at room temperature; do not freeze
• Reassurance if communication is difficult during recovery from neuromuscular blockade
• Frequent (q2h) instillation of artificial tears and covering eyes to prevent drying of cornea
Evaluate:
• Therapeutic response: paralysis of jaw, eyelid, head, neck, rest of body
Treatment of overdose: Neostigmine, monitor VS; may require mechanical ventilation

Rarely Used
modafinil (℞)
(moh-daf'ih-nil)
Provigil
Func. class.: Cerebral stimulant

Controlled Substance Schedule IV
Uses: Narcolepsy, sleep apnea
Investigational use: Fatigue

DOSAGE AND ROUTES
• *Adult:* **PO** 200 mg daily in the AM, may increase to 400 mg daily if needed

Hepatic dose
• Reduce dose by 50%

Contraindications: Hypersensitivity, hyperthyroidism, hypertension, glaucoma, severe arteriosclerosis, drug abuse, cardiovascular disease, anxiety

---

moexipril (℞)
(moe-ex'ih-prill)
Univasc
Func. class.: Antihypertensive
Chem. class.: Angiotensin-converting enzyme inhibitor

Action: Selectively suppresses renin-angiotensin-aldosterone system; inhibits ACE; prevents conversion of angiotensin I to angiotensin II; results in dilation of arterial, venous vessels

Uses: Hypertension, alone or in combination with thiazide diuretics

DOSAGE AND ROUTES

• *Adult:* PO 7.5 mg 1 hr ac initially, may be increased or divided depending on B/P response; maintenance dosage 7.5-30 mg daily in 1-2 divided doses 1 hr ac
Renal dose
• *Adult:* PO CCr <40 ml/min 3.75 mg/day titrate to desired dose
Available forms: Tabs 7.5, 15 mg

SIDE EFFECTS

CNS: Fever, chills
CV: Hypotension, postural hypotension
GI: Loss of taste
GU: Impotence, dysuria, nocturia, proteinuria, nephrotic syndrome, acute reversible renal failure, polyuria, oliguria, frequency
HEMA: **Neutropenia**
INTEG: Rash
META: Hypokalemia
RESP: **Bronchospasm,** dyspnea, dry cough
SYST: **Angioedema, anaphylaxis**
Contraindications: Pregnancy (D) 2nd/3rd trimesters, hypersensitivity, children, lactation, heart block, bilateral renal stenosis, history of angioedema
Precautions: Pregnancy (C) 1st trimester, dialysis patients, hypovolemia, leukemia, scleroderma, lupus erythematosus, blood dyscrasias, CHF, diabetes mellitus, renal disease, thyroid disease, COPD, asthma, potassium-sparing diuretics

PHARMACOKINETICS

Metabolized by liver (metabolites), excreted in urine; crosses placenta; excreted in breast milk

INTERACTIONS

Do not use with potassium-sparing diuretics, sympathomimetics, potassium supplements
Increase: hypotension—diuretics, other antihypertensives, ganglionic blockers, adrenergic blockers, phenothiazines
Increase: toxicity—digoxin, lithium
Increase: hyperkalemia—cyclo-SPORINE, potassium-sparing diuretics
Decrease: antihypertensive effect—NSAIDs
Drug/Lab Test
False positive: Urine acetone

NURSING CONSIDERATIONS

Assess:
• Blood tests: neutrophils, decreased platelets
• B/P
• Renal studies: protein, BUN, creatinine; watch for increased levels that may indicate nephrotic syndrome
• Baselines in renal, hepatic studies before therapy begins
• Potassium levels, although hyperkalemia rarely occurs
• Edema in feet, legs daily
• Allergic reaction: rash, fever, pruritus, urticaria; drug should be discontinued if antihistamines fail to help
• Symptoms of CHF; edema, dyspnea, wet crackles, B/P
• Renal symptoms: polyuria, oliguria, frequency

Administer:
• PO 1 hr before meals
• Do not use with potassium-sparing diuretics, sympathomimetics, potassium supplements

Perform/provide:
• Storage in tight container at 86° F (30° C) or less

Evaluate:
• Therapeutic response: decrease in B/P in hypertension

Teach patient/family:
• To take 1 hr ac
• Not to discontinue drug abruptly
• Not to use OTC (cough, cold, or allergy) products unless directed by prescriber
• To comply with dosage schedule, even if feeling better
• To rise slowly to sitting or standing position to minimize orthostatic hypotension
• To notify prescriber of mouth sores, sore throat, fever, swelling of hands or feet, irregular heartbeat, chest pain, signs of angioedema
• That excessive perspiration, dehydration, vomiting, diarrhea may lead to fall in blood pressure; consult prescriber if these occur
• That dizziness, fainting, lightheadedness may occur during first few days of therapy
• That skin rash or impaired perspiration may occur
• How to take B/P

Treatment of overdose: 0.9% NaCl IV inf, hemodialysis

mometasone nasal agent
See Appendix C

mometasone topical
See Appendix C

montelukast (℞)
(mon-teh-loo'kast)
Singulair
Func. class.: Bronchodilator
Chem. class.: Leukotriene antagonist, cysteinyl

Action: Inhibits leukotriene (LTD$_4$) formation; leukotrienes exert their effects by increasing neutrophil, eosinophil migration; aggregation of neutrophils, monocytes; smooth muscle contraction, capillary permeability; these actions further lead to bronchoconstriction, inflammation, edema

Uses: Chronic asthma in adults and children, seasonal allergic rhinitis
Investigational uses: Chronic urticaria

DOSAGE AND ROUTES

• *Adult and child ≥15 yr:* **PO** 10 mg daily PM
• *Child 6-14 yr:* **PO** 5 mg chew tab daily PM
• *Child 2-5 yr:* **PO** chew tab 4 mg daily
Asthma
• *Child 12-23 mo:* **PO** 1 packet (4 mg) of granules taken PM
Available forms: Tabs 10 mg; chew tabs 4, 5 mg; oral granules 4 mg/packet

SIDE EFFECTS

CNS: Dizziness, fatigue, headache
GI: Abdominal pain, dyspepsia
INTEG: Rash
MS: Asthenia
RESP: Influenza, cough, nasal congestion
Contraindications: Hypersensitivity
Precautions: Pregnancy (B), acute attacks of asthma, alcohol consumption, lactation, child <6 yr, aspirin sensitivity

PHARMACOKINETICS

Rapidly absorbed, peak 3-4 hr, half-life 2.7-5.5 hr; protein binding 99%; metabolized by liver, excreted via bile

M

INTERACTIONS

Decrease: montelukast levels—phenobarbital, rifampin

Drug/Herb

Increase: stimulation—black, green tea, guarana

Drug/Lab Test

Increase: ALT, AST

NURSING CONSIDERATIONS

Assess:

A Adult patients carefully for symptoms of Churg-Strauss syndrome (rare), including eosinophilia, vasculitic rash, worsening pulmonary symptoms, cardiac complications, and/or neuropathy

• CBC, blood chemistry, during treatment

• Respiratory rate, rhythm, depth; auscultate lung fields bilaterally; notify prescriber of abnormalities

• Allergic reactions: rash, urticaria; drug should be discontinued

Administer:

PO route

• In PM daily

Granules

• May give directly in the mouth or mixed with a spoonful of soft food (carrots, applesauce, ice cream, rice)

• Do not open packet until ready to use, mix whole dose, give within 15 min

Evaluate:

• Therapeutic response: ability to breathe more easily

Teach patient/family:

• To check OTC medications, current prescription medications for epHEDrine, which will increase stimulation; to avoid alcohol

• To avoid hazardous activities; dizziness may occur

• That drug is not to be used for acute asthma attacks

• If aspirin sensitivity is known, do not take NSAIDs while taking this product

• To continue to use inhaled beta-agonists if exercise-induced asthma occurs

---

moricizine (Ŗ)
(more-i'siz-een)
Ethmozine
Func. class.: Antidysrhythmic, group 1A
Chem. class.: Phenothiazine

Action: Decreased rate of rise of action potential, prolonging refractory period and shortening the action potential duration; depression of inward influx if sodium mediates the effects; drug may slow atrial and AV nodal conduction

Uses: Life-threatening ventricular dysrhythmias

DOSAGE AND ROUTES

Hospitalization is required when initiating therapy

• *Adult:* PO 10-15 mg/kg/day or 600-900 mg/day in 2-3 divided doses

Hepatic dose

• *Adult:* PO 600 mg or less daily

Available forms: Film-coated tabs 200, 250, 300 mg

SIDE EFFECTS

CNS: Dizziness, headache, fatigue, perioral numbness, euphoria, nervousness, sleep disorders, depression, tinnitus, fatigue, anxiety

CV: Palpitations, chest pain, **CHF,** hypertension, syncope, dysrhythmias, bradycardia, **MI, thrombophlebitis,** ECG abnormalities, **cardiac arrest**

GI: Nausea, abdominal pain, vomiting, diarrhea

GU: Sexual dysfunction, difficult urination, dysuria, incontinence, urinary retention

MISC: Sweating, musculoskeletal pain, drug fever, blurred vision, dry mouth

RESP: Dyspnea, hyperventilation, **apnea,** asthma, pharyngitis, cough

Contraindications: 2nd-/3rd-degree AV block, right bundle branch block, cardiogenic shock, hypersensitivity

Precautions: Pregnancy (B), CHF, hypokalemia, hyperkalemia, sick sinus

---

A Safety alert   *"Tall Man" lettering

syndrome, lactation, children, impaired hepatic and renal function, cardiac dysfunction

PHARMACOKINETICS

Half-life 1.5-3.5 hr; peak 0.5-2.2 hr; metabolized by the liver; metabolites excreted in feces and urine, protein binding >90%

INTERACTIONS

Digoxin or propranolol may enhance some cardiac effects of moricizine; moricizine may decrease effects of theophylline

Increase: plasma levels of moricizine—cimetidine
Decrease: effects of theophylline
Drug/Herb
Increase: anticholinergic effect—henbane
Increase: hypokalemia, increase antidysrhythmic action—aloe, buckthorn, cascara sagrada, rhubarb, senna
Increase: toxicity, death—aconite
Increase: effect—aloe, broom, chronic buckthorn use, cascara sagrada (chronic use), Chinese rhubarb, figwort, fumitory, goldenseal, kudzu, licorice
Increase: serotonin effect—horehound
Decrease: effect—coltsfoot
Drug/Lab Test
Increase: CPK

NURSING CONSIDERATIONS
Assess:
• GI status: bowel pattern, number of stools
• Cardiac status: rate, rhythm, quality
• Chest x-ray, pulmonary function test during treatment
• I&O ratio; check for decreasing output
• B/P for fluctuations
• Lung fields: bilateral crackles may occur in CHF patient
• Increased respirations, increased pulse; drug should be discontinued
⚠ Toxicity: fine tremors, dizziness, emesis, lethargy, coma, syncope, hypotension, conduction disturbances

• Cardiac status: respiration, rate, rhythm, character continuously
Administer:
• Initiate therapy in hospital
• Dosage adjustment should be ≥3 days
Evaluate:
• Therapeutic response: absence of dysrhythmias
Teach patient/family:
• To report side effects to prescriber
• To take exactly as prescribed, take consistently with respect to meals
Treatment of overdose: O_2 artificial ventilation, ECG; administer DOPamine for circulatory depression, diazepam or thiopental for convulsions

---

⚠ High Alert

morphine (℞)
(mor'feen)
Astramorph, Astramorph PF, Avinza, Duramorph, Epimorph ✤, Infumorph, Kadian, morphine sulfate, Morphitec ✤, M.O.S. ✤, M.O.S.-S.R. ✤, MS Contin, MSIR, OMS Concentrate, Oramorph SR, RMS, Roxanol, Roxanol Rescudose, Roxanol-T, Statex
Func. class.: Opioid analgesic

Controlled Substance Schedule II
Do not confuse:
morphine/hydromorphone
Roxanol/Roxicet
Action: Depresses pain impulse transmission at the spinal cord level by interacting with opioid receptors
Uses: Severe pain

DOSAGE AND ROUTES
• *Adult:* **SUBCUT/IM** 5-20 mg q4h prn; **PO** 10-30 mg q4h prn; **EXT REL** 70-kg patient q8-12h; **RECT** 10-30 mg q4h prn; **IV** 4-10 mg diluted in 4-5 ml H_2O for inj, over 5 min; **SUS REL** cap pellets (Kadian); Kadian is not bioequivalent to

other controlled release forms. Caps may be opened and sprinkled on applesauce immediately before use. The pellets in the cap should not be chewed, crushed, or dissolved, which may lead to overdose. Adjustments may need to be made when converting from another form of morphine. Avinza, for those with no tolerance to opioids, 30 mg daily; may adjust by no more than 30 mg q4d.

• *Child:* **SUBCUT/IV** 0.1-0.2 mg/kg, not to exceed 15 mg; **PO** 0.2-0.5 mg/kg q4-6h (reg rel), q12h (sus rel)

Available forms: Inj 0.5, 1, 2, 3, 4, 5, 8, 10, 15, 25, 50 mg/ml; sol tabs 10, 15, 30 mg; oral sol 10, 20 mg/5 ml, 20 mg/10 ml, 20 mg/ml; oral tabs 15, 30 mg; rect supp 5, 10, 20, 30 mg; ext rel tabs 15, 30, 60, 100, 200 mg; caps 15, 30 mg; syr 1, 5 mg/ml; cont rel cap pellets (Kadian) 20, 30, 50, 60, 100 mg; ext rel caps (Avinza) 30, 60, 90, 120 mg

SIDE EFFECTS

CNS: Drowsiness, dizziness, confusion, headache, sedation, euphoria

CV: Palpitations, ***bradycardia,*** change in B/P, ***shock, cardiac arrest***

EENT: Tinnitus, blurred vision, miosis, diplopia

GI: Nausea, vomiting, anorexia, constipation, cramps, biliary tract pressure

GU: Urinary retention

HEMA: ***Thrombocytopenia***

INTEG: Rash, urticaria, bruising, flushing, diaphoresis, pruritus

RESP: ***Respiratory depression, respiratory arrest, apnea***

Contraindications: Hypersensitivity, addiction (opioid), hemorrhage, bronchial asthma, increased intracranial pressure

Precautions: Pregnancy (C), addictive personality, lactation, acute MI, severe heart disease, elderly, respiratory depression, hepatic disease, renal disease, child <18 yr

PHARMACOKINETICS

PO: Onset variable, peak variable, duration variable

IM: Onset ½ hr, peak ½-1 hr, duration 3-7 hr

SUBCUT: Onset 15-20 min, peak 50-90 min, duration 3-5 hr

IV: Peak 20 min

RECT: Peak ½-1 hr, duration 4-5 hr

Intrathecal: Onset rapid, duration up to 24 hr

Metabolized by liver, crosses placenta; excreted in urine, breast milk; half-life 1½-2 hr

INTERACTIONS

Unpredictable reaction, avoid use: MAOIs

Increase: effects with other CNS depressants—alcohol, opiates, sedative/hypnotics, antipsychotics, skeletal muscle relaxants

Decrease: morphine action—rifampin

Drug/Herb

Increase: anticholinergic effect—corkwood

Increase: CNS depression—chamomile, hops, Jamaican dogwood, kava, lavender, mistletoe, nettle, pokeweed, poppy, senega, skullcap, valerian

Decrease: morphine effect—cranberry juice (excessive amounts), oats

Drug/Lab Test

Increase: Amylase

NURSING CONSIDERATIONS

Assess:

• Pain: location, type, character; give dose before pain becomes severe

• Bowel status; constipation common

• I&O ratio; check for decreasing output; may indicate urinary retention

• B/P, pulse, respirations (character, depth, rate)

• CNS changes: dizziness, drowsiness, hallucinations, euphoria, LOC, pupil reaction

• Allergic reactions: rash, urticaria

• Respiratory dysfunction: depression,

character, rate, rhythm; notify prescriber
if respirations are <12/min
Administer:
• Do not break, crush, or chew controlled or sustained release products
• With antiemetic for nausea, vomiting
• When pain is beginning to return; determine dosage interval by response; continuous dosing is more effective than prn
• May be given by patient: controlled analgesia
• Epidural cautiously in the elderly
IV route
• After diluting with 5 ml or more sterile H_2O or NS; give 15 mg or less over 4-5 min; give through Y- tube or 3-way stopcock; may be added to IV sol, each 0.1-1 mg diluted in 1 ml D_5W, $D_{10}W$, 0.9% NaCl, 0.45% NaCl, Ringer's sol, LR, given with inf pump titrated to patient response

Additive compatibilities: Alteplase, atracurium, baclofen, bupivacaine, DOBUTamine, fluconazole, furosemide, meropenem, metoclopramide, succinylcholine, verapamil

Syringe compatibilities: Atropine, benzquinamide, bupivacaine, butorphanol, cimetidine, dimenhyDRINATE, diphenhydrAMINE, droperidol, fentanyl, glycopyrrolate, hydrOXYzine, ketamine, metoclopramide, midazolam, milrinone, pentazocine, perphenazine, promazine, ranitidine, scopolamine

Y-site compatibilities: Allopurinol, amifostine, amikacin, aminophylline, amiodarone, ampicillin, ampicillin/sulbactam, amsacrine, atenolol, atracurium, aztreonam, bumetanide, calcium chloride, cefamandole, cefazolin, cefmetazole, cefo perazone, cefotaxime, cefotetan, cefoxitin, ceftazidime, ceftizoxime, ceftriaxone, cefuroxime, cephalothin, cephapirin, chloramphenicol, cisatracurium, cisplatin, cladribine, clindamycin, cyclophosphamide, cytarabine, dexamethasone, digoxin, diltiazem, DOBUTamine, DOPamine, doxycycline, enalaprilat, epINEPHrine, erythromycin, esmolol, etomidate, famotidine, fentanyl,

filgrastim, fluconazole, fludarabine, foscarnet, gentamicin, granisetron, heparin, hydrocortisone, hydromorphone, IL-2, insulin (regular), kanamycin, labetalol, lidocaine, lorazepam, magnesium sulfate, melphalan, meropenem, methotrexate, methyldopate, methylPREDNISolone, metoclopramide, metoprolol, metronidazole, mezlocillin, midazolam, milrinone, moxalactam, nafcillin, niCARdipine, nitroglycerin, norepinephrine, ondansetron, oxacillin, oxytocin, paclitaxel, pancuronium, penicillin G potassium, piperacillin, piperacillin/tazobactam, potassium chloride, propofol, propranolol, ranitidine, remifentanil, sodium bicarbonate, sodium nitroprusside, teniposide, thiotepa, ticarcillin, ticarcillin/clavulanate, tobramycin, trimethoprim-sulfamethoxazole, vancomycin, vecuronium, vinorelbine, vit B/C, warfarin, zidovudine

Perform/provide:
• Storage in light-resistant container at room temperature
• Assistance with ambulation
• Safety measures: side rails, night-light, call bell within easy reach
• Gradual withdrawal after long-term use

Evaluate:
• Therapeutic response; decrease in pain intensity

Teach patient/family:
• To change position slowly; orthostatic hypotension may occur
• To report any symptoms of CNS changes, allergic reactions
• That physical dependency may result from long-term use
• To avoid use of alcohol, CNS depressants
• That withdrawal symptoms may occur: nausea, vomiting, cramps, fever, faintness, anorexia

Treatment of overdose: Naloxone (Narcan) 0.2-0.8 mg IV, O_2, IV fluids, vasopressors

M

Side effects: *italics* = common; ***bold italics*** = life-threatening

moxifloxacin
Avelox, Avelox IV
Func. class.: Antiinfective
Chem. class.: Fluoroquinolone

Action: Interferes with conversion of intermediate DNA fragments into high-molecular-weight DNA in bacteria; DNA gyrase inhibitor

Uses: Acute bacterial sinusitis: *Streptococcus pneumoniae, Haemophilus influenzae, Moraxella catarrhalis;* acute bacterial exacerbation of chronic bronchitis: *S. pneumoniae, H. influenzae, Haemophilus parainfluenzae, Klebsiella pneumoniae, Staphylococcus aureus, M. catarrhalis;* community-acquired pneumonia: *S. pneumoniae, H. influenzae, Mycoplasma pneumoniae, Chlamydia pneumoniae, M. catarrhalis;* uncomplicated skin/skin structure infections: *S. aureus, Streptococcus pyogenes*

DOSAGE AND ROUTES
Acute bacterial sinusitis
• *Adult:* **PO/IV** 400 mg q24h × 10 days
Acute bacterial exacerbation of chronic bronchitis
• *Adult:* **PO/IV** 400 mg q24h × 5 days
Community acquired pneumonia
• *Adult:* **PO/IV** 400 mg q24h × 7-14 days
Uncomplicated skin/skin structure infections
• *Adult:* **PO/IV** 400 mg q24h × 7 days
Available forms: Tabs 400 mg; inj premix 400 mg

SIDE EFFECTS
CNS: Headache, dizziness, fatigue, insomnia, depression, *restlessness, seizures,* confusion
CV: Prolonged QT interval, *dysrhythmias*
EENT: Blurred vision, tinnitus
GI: Nausea, diarrhea, increased ALT, AST, flatulence, heartburn, *vomiting,* oral candidiasis, dysphagia, *pseudomembranous colitis*
INTEG: Rash, pruritus, urticaria, photosensitivity, flushing, fever, chills
MS: Tremor, arthralgia, tendon rupture
*SYST: **Anaphylaxis, Stevens-Johnson syndrome***

Contraindications: Hypersensitivity to quinolones

Precautions: Pregnancy (C), lactation, children, renal disease, epilepsy, uncorrected hypokalemia, prolonged QT interval, patients receiving class IA, III antidysrhythmics

PHARMACOKINETICS
Excreted in urine as active drug, metabolites

INTERACTIONS
Prolonged QT: antidysrhythmics class IA, III
Increase: moxifloxacin serum levels—probenecid
Increase: warfarin, cycloSPORINE effect
Decrease: moxifloxacin absorption—magnesium antacids, aluminum hydroxide, zinc, iron, sucralfate, calcium, enteral feeding, didanosine
Drug/Herb
Increase: antiinfective effect—cola tree

NURSING CONSIDERATIONS
Assess:
• CNS symptoms: headache, dizziness, fatigue, insomnia, depression, *seizures*
• Renal, hepatic studies: BUN, creatinine, AST, ALT
• I&O ratio, urine pH <5.5 is ideal
A Allergic reactions and anaphylaxis: fever, flushing, rash, urticaria, pruritus; keep epINEPHrine, emergency equipment nearby for anaphylaxis
Administer:
PO route
• 4 hr before or 8 hr after antacids, zinc, iron, calcium
IV route
• Discontinue primary IV while administering moxifloxacin

A Safety alert   *"Tall Man" lettering

• Do not give SUBCUT, IM
Solution compatibilities: 0.9% NaCl, D_5, D_{10}, LR, sterile water for inj
Perform/provide:
• Limited intake of alkaline foods, drugs: milk, dairy products, alkaline antacids, sodium bicarbonate
• That fluids must be increased to 3 L/day to avoid crystallization in kidneys
Evaluate:
• Therapeutic response: decreased pain, C&S; absence of infection
Teach patient/family:
• Not to take any products containing magnesium or calcium (such as antacids), iron, or aluminum with this drug or within 8 hr of drug
• That photosensitivity may occur; patient should avoid sunlight or use sunscreen to prevent burns
• To use frequent rinsing of mouth, sugarless candy or gum for dry mouth
• To take as prescribed, not to double or miss doses
• If dizziness occurs, to ambulate, perform activities with assistance
• To complete full course of drug therapy
• To contact prescriber if adverse reaction occurs or if inflammation or pain in tendon occurs

---

moxifloxacin ophthalmic
See Appendix C

---

multivitamins (otc, ℞)
Adavite, Dayalets, LKV Drops, Multi-75, Multiday, One-A-Day, Optilets, Poly-Visol, Quin tabs, Ru-Lets, Sesame Street Vitamins, Tab-A-Vite, Therabid, Theragram, Unicaps, Vita-Bob, Vita-Kid, many other brands
Func. class.: Vitamins, multiple

Do not confuse:
Theragran/Phenergan
Action: Needed for adequate metabolism
Uses: Prevention and treatment of vitamin deficiencies

DOSAGE AND ROUTES
• *Adult and child:* **PO/IV**—depends on brand
Available forms: Many

SIDE EFFECTS
None known at recommended dosage
Precautions: Pregnancy (A)

NURSING CONSIDERATIONS
Assess:
• Vitamin deficiency: usually more than one vitamin is deficient
Administer:
• Liquid multivitamins diluted or dropped into patient's mouth using dropper provided with some brands
• Chew tabs should be chewed, not swallowed whole
• Give by cont IV inf only after diluting 5-10 ml multivitamins/500-1000 ml of D_5W, $D_{10}W$, $D_{20}W$, LR, D_5/LR, $D_5/0.9\%$ NaCl, 0.9% NaCl, 3% NaCl
• Do not use sol with crystals, precipitate, or color other than bright yellow
Additive compatibilities: Cefoxitin, isoproterenol, methyldopa, metoclopramide, metronidazole, netilmicin, norepinephrine, sodium bicarbonate, verapamil
Y-site compatibilities: Acyclovir,

M

ampicillin, cefazolin, cephalothin, cephapirin, diltiazem, erythromycin, fludarabine, gentamicin, tacrolimus

Evaluate:

• Therapeutic response: check each individual vitamin for guidelines

Teach patient/family:

• That adequate nutrition must be maintained to prevent further deficiencies

• To comply with regimen

• To avoid presenting flavored multivitamins as candy; child may overdose

• To store out of children's reach

---

mupirocin topical
See Appendix C

---

muromonab-CD3 (℞)
(mur-oo-mone'ab)
Orthoclone OKT3
Func. class.: Immunosuppressant
Chem. class.: Murine monoclonal antibody

Action: Reverses graft rejection by blocking T-cell function

Uses: Acute allograft rejection in renal, cardiac/hepatic transplant patients

DOSAGE AND ROUTES

• *Adult:* **IV BOL** 5 mg/day × 10-14 days
• *Child:* **IV** 100 mcg/kg/day × 10-14 days

Cardiac/hepatic allograft rejection, steroid resistant

• *Adult:* **IV BOL** 5 mg/day × 10-14 days; begin when it is known that rejection has not been reversed by steroids

Available forms: Inj 5 mg/5 ml

SIDE EFFECTS

*CNS: Pyrexia, chills, tremors, **aseptic meningitis***
CV: Chest pain
GI: Vomiting, nausea, diarrhea
*MISC: **Infection, cytokine release syndrome, anaphylaxis***

*RESP: Dyspnea, wheezing, **pulmonary edema***

Contraindications: Hypersensitivity to murine origin, fluid overload

Precautions: Pregnancy (C), child <2 yr, fever

PHARMACOKINETICS

Trough level steady state 3-14 days

INTERACTIONS

Increase: immunosuppression—immunosuppressants
Increase: infection risk—cycloSPORINE, corticosteroids, azathioprine
Increase: CNS symptoms—indomethacin
Decrease: immune response—vaccines

Drug/Herb

Interference with immunosuppression: astragalus, echinacea, melatonin
Decrease: effect—ginseng, maitake, mistletoe, schisandra, St. John's wort, turmeric

NURSING CONSIDERATIONS

Assess:

⚠ For cytokine release syndrome (CRS): nausea, vomiting, chills, fever, joint pain, weakness, dizziness, diarrhea, tremors, abdominal pain

⚠ For hypersensitivity, *anaphylaxis:* dyspnea, bronchospasm, urticaria, tachycardia, angioedema; emergency equipment must be available

• Blood studies: Hgb, WBC, platelets during treatment qmo; if leukocytes are <3000/mm^3, drug should be discontinued; CD3, CD4, CD8, CD3 ≤25 cells/mm^3

• Hepatic studies: alk phosphatase, AST, ALT, bilirubin

⚠ Hepatotoxicity: dark urine, jaundice, itching, light-colored stools; drug should be discontinued

• For infection: sore throat, fever, chills, temp, notify prescriber immediately

⚠ For aseptic meningitis: fever, headache, photophobia

⚠ For fluid overload: increased weight, I&O, edema, crackles

Administer:

• For several days before transplant surgery

• All medications PO if possible; avoid IM injection, since infection may occur

IV route

• IV undiluted; withdraw with a 0.2-0.22 low protein-binding μm filter, discard and use new needle for administration; give over 1 min

• Incompatible with any drug in syringe or sol

Evaluate:

• Therapeutic response: absence of graft rejection

Teach patient/family:

• To report fever, chills, sore throat, fatigue, since serious infection may occur; rash, dyspnea, fast heartbeat

• To use contraceptive measures during treatment

• To report cytokine release syndrome, give symptoms

• To avoid vaccinations during treatment

• To avoid persons with infections, crowds; infections may occur

---

mycophenolate (℞)

(mye-koe-phen'oh-late)

CellCept, Myfortic

Func. class.: Immunosuppressant

Action: Inhibits inflammatory responses that are mediated by the immune system; prolongs the survival of allogenic transplants

Uses: Organ transplants (to prevent rejection); prophylaxis of organ rejection in allogenic cardiac, hepatic, renal transplants

Investigational uses: Refractory uveitis, second-line therapy for Churg-Strauss syndrome, diffuse proliferative lupus nephritis (in combination), rheumatoid arthritis, psoriasis

DOSAGE AND ROUTES

Renal transplant

• *Adult:* **PO/IV** give initial dose 72 hr prior to transplantation; 1 g bid given to renal transplant patients in combination with corticosteroids, cycloSPORINE; **TAB ER** 720 mg bid on empty stomach

• *Child:* **PO-ER** 400 mg/m² bid, max 720 mg bid

Renal dose

• *Adult:* **PO/IV** GFR <25 ml/min, max 2 g/day

Cardiac transplant

• *Adult:* **PO/IV** 1.5 g bid, IV can be started ≤24 hr after transplant, switch to **PO** when able

Hepatic transplant

• *Adult:* **PO/IV** 1.5 g bid; give IV over ≥2 hr

Available forms: Caps 250 mg; tabs 500 mg; inj (powder) 500 mg/20-ml vial; powder for oral susp 200 mg/ml; tab, ext rel (Myfortic) 180, 360 mg

SIDE EFFECTS

M

CNS: Tremor, dizziness, insomnia, headache, fever

CV: Hypertension, chest pain

GI: Diarrhea, constipation, nausea, vomiting, stomatitis, **GI bleeding**

GU: UTI, hematuria, **renal tubular necrosis**

HEMA: **Leukopenia, thrombocytopenia, anemia, pancytopenia**

INTEG: Rash

META: Peripheral edema, hypercholesterolemia, hypophosphatemia, edema, hyperkalemia, hypokalemia, hyperglycemia

MS: Arthralgia, muscle wasting

RESP: Dyspnea, respiratory infection, increased cough, pharyngitis, bronchitis, pneumonia

SYST: **Lymphoma,** *nonmelanoma skin carcinoma,* **sepsis**

Contraindications: Hypersensitivity to this drug or mycophenolic acid

Precautions: Pregnancy (C), lymphomas, malignancies, neutropenia, renal disease, lactation

---

PHARMACOKINETICS

Rapidly and completely absorbed, metabolized to active metabolite (MPA), excreted in urine, feces, protein binding (MPA) 97%, half-life (MPA) 17.9 hr

INTERACTIONS

Avoid administration with azathioprine

Increase: effects of phenytoin, theophylline

Increase: concentration of both drugs—acyclovir, ganciclovir

Increase: mycophenolate levels—probenecid, salicylates

Decrease: mycophenolate levels—antacids, cholestyramine

Decrease: protein binding of phenytoin, theophylline

Decrease: effect of live attenuated vaccines, oral contraceptives

Drug/Herb

Interference with immunosuppressant astragalus, echinacea, melatonin

Drug/Food

Decrease: absorption if taken with food

NURSING CONSIDERATIONS

Assess:

• Blood studies: CBC during treatment monthly

• Hepatic studies: alk phosphatase, AST, ALT, bilirubin

Administer:

• 72 hr prior to transplantation; may be given in combination with corticosteroids, cycloSPORINE

PO route

• Do not break, crush, or chew tabs; do not open caps

• Avoid inhalation or direct contact with skin, mucous membranes, teratogenic in animals

• Oral susp: tap the closed bottle several times to loosen powder, use 94 ml of water in graduated cylinder, add ½ the total amount of water for constitution and shake the closed bottle, add remaining water and shake, again remove child

resistant cap and push adapter into neck of the bottle, close tightly

• Give alone for better absorption

IV route

• Do not give by rapid or bolus inj; reconstitute and dilute to 6 mg/ml with D₅W, give over ≥2 hr

• Do not admix with mycophenolate IV in infusion catheter or with other IV drugs or infusion admixtures

Evaluate:

• Therapeutic response: absence of graft rejection

Teach patient/family:

• To report fever, rash, severe diarrhea, chills, sore throat, fatigue, since serious infections may occur

• To reduce risk of infection by avoiding crowds

• The need for repeated lab tests

• To limit exposure to sunlight/UV light

• To use contraception before, during, and 6 wk after therapy

---

nabumetone (Ⓡ)

(na-byoo'me-tone)

Relafen

Func. class.: Nonsteroidal antiinflammatory

Chem. class.: Acetic acid derivative

Action: Inhibits prostaglandin synthesis by decreasing enzyme needed for biosynthesis; analgesic, antiinflammatory

Uses: Osteoarthritis, rheumatoid arthritis, acute or chronic treatment

DOSAGE AND ROUTES

• *Adult:* **PO** 1 g as a single dose; may increase to 2 g/day if needed; may give daily or bid as a divided dose

Available forms: Tabs 500, 750 mg

SIDE EFFECTS

CNS: Dizziness, headache, drowsiness, fatigue, tremors, confusion, insomnia, anxiety, depression, nervousness

CV: Tachycardia, peripheral edema, palpitations, dysrhythmias, *CHF*

⚠ Safety alert *"Tall Man" lettering

EENT: Tinnitus, hearing loss, blurred vision

GI: Nausea, anorexia, vomiting, diarrhea, jaundice, ***cholestatic hepatitis***, constipation, flatulence, cramps, dry mouth, peptic ulcer, gastritis, ***ulceration, perforation***

GU: ***Nephrotoxicity, dysuria, hematuria, oliguria, azotemia***, cystitis

HEMA: ***Blood dyscrasias***

INTEG: Purpura, rash, pruritus, sweating, photosensitivity

RESP: Dyspnea, pharyngitis, ***bronchospasm***

SYST: ***Anaphylaxis, angioneurotic edema***

Contraindications: Hypersensitivity to this drug or aspirin, iodides, NSAIDs, asthma, severe renal disease, severe hepatic disease, avoid in late pregnancy

Precautions: Pregnancy (C); lactation, children, bleeding disorders, GI disorders, cardiac disorders, renal disorders, hepatic dysfunction, elderly

PHARMACOKINETICS

PO: Peak 2½-4 hr, plasma protein binding >90%, half-life 22-30 hr; metabolized in liver to active metabolite; excreted in urine (metabolites), breast milk

INTERACTIONS

Increase: bleeding risk—anticoagulants, thrombolytics, valproic acid, cefamandole, cefotetan, cefoperazone, plicamycin, clopidogrel, eptifibatide, ticlopidine

Increase: hematologic reactions risk—antineoplastics, radiation

Increase: GI reactions—salicylates, NSAIDs, alcohol, potassium, corticosteroids

Decrease: effect of—diuretics, antihypertensives

Drug/Herb

Increase: gastric irritation—arginine, gossypol

Increase: NSAIDs effect—bearberry, bilberry

Increase: bleeding risk—bogbean, chondroitin

NURSING CONSIDERATIONS

Assess:
• Pain: frequency, intensity, characteristics; relief of pain after med
• Asthma, aspirin sensitivity or nasal polyps; increased hypersensitivity reactions
• Renal, hepatic studies: BUN, creatinine, AST, ALT, Hgb, LDH, blood glucose, WBC, platelets, CCr before treatment, periodically thereafter
• Audiometric, ophthalmic exam before, during, after treatment
• For eye, ear problems: blurred vision, tinnitus; may indicate toxicity

Administer:
• With food for GI symptoms

Perform/provide:
• Storage at room temperature

Evaluate:
• Therapeutic response: decreased pain and stiffness in joints

Teach patient/family:
• To avoid alcoholic beverages and aspirin
• To report blurred vision, ringing, roaring in ears; may indicate toxicity
• To avoid driving, other hazardous activities if dizziness, drowsiness occur
• To report change in urine pattern, increased weight, edema, increased pain in joints, fever, blood in urine; indicates nephrotoxicity
• That therapeutic effects may take up to 1 mo
• To take with a full glass of water to enhance absorption and sit upright
• To report dark stools; may indicate GI bleeding

N

Side effects: *italics* = common; ***bold italics*** = life-threatening

nadolol (R)

(nay-doe'lole)

Corgard, Syn-Nadolol ✢

Func. class.: Antihypertensive, antianginal

Chem. class.: β-Adrenergic receptor blocker

Do not confuse:

Corgard/Cognex

Action: Long-acting, nonselective β-adrenergic receptor blocking agent; mechanism is similar to that of propranolol

Uses: Chronic stable angina pectoris, mild to moderate hypertension

Investigational uses: Tachydysrhythmias, aggression, anxiety, tremors, esophageal varices (rebleeding only), hyperthyroidism adjunctive therapy, prophylaxis of migraine headaches

DOSAGE AND ROUTES

• *Adult:* **PO** 40 mg daily, increase by 40-80 mg q3-7d; maintenance 40-240 mg/day for angina, 40-320 mg/day for hypertension

• *Geriatric:* **PO** 20 mg/day, may increase by 20 mg until desired dose

Renal dose

• *Adult:* **PO** CCr 31-50 ml/min give q24-36h; CCr 10-30 ml/min give q24-48h; CCr <10 ml/min give q40-60h

Available forms: Tabs 20, 40, 80, 120, 160 mg

SIDE EFFECTS

CNS: Depression, dizziness, *fatigue,* lethargy, paresthesias, headache, *weakness,* insomnia, memory loss, nightmares

CV: **Bradycardia,** *hypotension,* **CHF,** palpitations, **AV block,** chest pain, peripheral ischemia, flushing, edema, vasodilation, conduction disturbances

EENT: Blurred vision, dry eyes, nasal congestion

ENDO: Hyperglycemia, hypoglycemia

GI: Nausea, vomiting, diarrhea, colitis, constipation, cramps, dry mouth, flatulence, hepatomegaly, **pancreatitis,** taste distortion

GU: Impotence, decreased libido

HEMA: **Agranulocytosis, thrombocytopenia**

INTEG: Rash, pruritus, fever, alopecia

RESP: Dyspnea, respiratory dysfunction, **bronchospasm,** cough, wheezing, **pulmonary edema,** pharyngitis, **laryngospasm**

Contraindications: Hypersensitivity to this drug, cardiac failure, cardiogenic shock, 2nd, 3rd degree heart block, bronchospastic disease, sinus bradycardia, CHF, COPD

Precautions: Pregnancy (C), diabetes mellitus, renal disease, lactation, hyperthyroidism, peripheral vascular disease, myasthenia gravis, major surgery, nonallergic bronchospasm

PHARMACOKINETICS

PO: Onset variable, peak 3-4 hr, duration 17-24 hr; half-life 20-24 hr; not metabolized; excreted in urine (unchanged), bile, breast milk; protein binding 30%

INTERACTIONS

Do not use with MAOIs, bradycardia may occur

Peripheral ischemia: ergots

Increase: bradycardia—digoxin

Increase: hypotension, bradycardia—clonidine, epINEPHrine

Increase: hypotensive effects—other hypotensive agents, phenothiazines

Decrease: β-blocking effect—thyroid hormones

Decrease: antihypertensive effect—NSAIDs

Drug/Herb

Increase: toxicity, death—aconite

Increase: antihypertensive effect—barberry, betony, black catechu, black cohosh, bloodroot, broom, burdock, cat's claw, dandelion, goldenseal, Irish moss, Jamaican dogwood, kelp, khella, mistletoe, parsley

Increase or decrease: antihypertensive effect—astragalus, cola tree
Decrease: antihypertensive effect—coltsfoot, guarana, khat, licorice
Drug/Lab Test
Increase: Serum potassium, serum uric acid, ALT, AST, alk phosphatase, LDH, blood glucose, cholesterol

NURSING CONSIDERATIONS

Assess:
• B/P, pulse, respirations during beginning therapy, orthostatic hypotension
• Weight daily; report gain of 5 lb
• I&O ratio, CCr if kidney damage is diagnosed
• Pain: duration, time started, activity being performed, character
• Headache, light-headedness, decreased B/P; may indicate a need for decreased dosage
Administer:
• With 8 oz water
Evaluate:
• Therapeutic response: decreased B/P, symptoms of angina
Teach patient/family:
• That drug may mask signs of hypoglycemia or alter blood glucose in diabetics
⚠ Not to discontinue abruptly, serious dysrhythmias may occur
• To avoid OTC drugs unless prescriber approves
• To avoid hazardous activities if dizziness occurs
• To comply with complete medical regimen
• To rise slowly to prevent orthostatic hypotension
• How and when to check B/P and pulse; to hold dose if pulse ≤50 bpm

nafarelin (℞)
(naf-ah-rell'in)
Synarel
Func. class.: Gonadotropin
Chem. class.: Analog of gonadotropin-releasing hormone

Action: Stimulates the release of LH and FSH, which increases ovarian steroid production; repeated dosing prevents stimulation of the pituitary gland
Uses: Endometriosis, gonadotropin-dependent precocious puberty

DOSAGE AND ROUTES

• *Adult:* **NASAL** 400 mcg/day as one spray (200 mcg) into one nostril in morning and one spray into other nostril in evening; start treatment between days 2 and 4 of menstrual cycle; may increase to 800 mcg/day (one spray into each nostril twice a day); recommended duration of treatment is 6 mo
• *Child:* **NASAL** 2 sprays in each nostril AM and PM, may increase to 3 sprays alternating nostril tid
Available forms: Nasal spray 2 mg/ml (200 mcg/spray)

SIDE EFFECTS

CNS: Headache, flushing, depression, insomnia, emotional lability, hot flashes
GU: Decreased libido, vaginal dryness, breast tenderness, increased pubic hair
INTEG: Nasal irritation, acne
MISC: Body odor, seborrhea, rhinitis
SENSITIVITY: Shortness of breath, chest pain, urticaria, pruritus
Contraindications: Pregnancy (X), hypersensitivity, lactation, undiagnosed abnormal vaginal bleeding
Precautions: Children

PHARMACOKINETICS

Rapidly absorbed, peak 10-40 min, half-life 3 hr; 80% bound to plasma proteins

INTERACTIONS

Decrease: nafarelin absorption—nasal decongestants (nasal sprays)

NURSING CONSIDERATIONS

Assess:
- Pain in endometriosis during treatment
- Endocrine studies, bone age, sex steroids, RHCG, GnRH, baseline q8wk
- For precocious puberty including secondary sex characteristics
- Test results: pituitary/hypothalamus dysfunction (decreased LH); postmenopausal (increased LH)

Administer:
- Repeated doses may be necessary to elevate pituitary gonadotropin reserve

Perform/provide:
- Storage at room temperature; protect from light

Evaluate:
- Therapeutic response: decreased symptoms of endometriosis; adequate resolution of central precocious puberty

Teach patient/family:
- To use nonhormonal contraception
- About correct nasal use, one spray in right nostril AM, one in left nostril PM
- That medication may cause hot flashes, decreased libido, vaginal dryness

---

nafcillin (R)

(naf-sill'in)
nafcillin sodium, Nallpen, Unipen
Func. class.: Antiinfective, broad-spectrum
Chem. class.: Penicillinase-resistant penicillin

Action: Interferes with cell wall replication of susceptible organisms; osmotically unstable cell wall swells, bursts from osmotic pressure
Uses: Effective for gram-positive cocci *(Staphylococcus aureus, Streptococcus viridans, Streptococcus pneumoniae),* infections caused by penicillinase-producing *Staphylococcus*

DOSAGE AND ROUTES

- *Adult:* **IV** 500-1000 mg q4h
- *Child and infant >1 mo:* **IV** 50-200 mg/kg/day in divided doses q4-6h
- *Neonates >7 days (weight >2 kg):* **IV** 25 mg/kg q8h
- *Neonates ≤7 days (weight <2 kg):* **IV** 25 mg/kg q12h

Meningitis
- *Adult:* **IV** 100-200 mg/kg/day divided q4-6h
- *Neonates >7 days (weight >2 kg):* **IV** 50 mg/kg q6h
- *Neonates ≤7 days (weight <2 kg):* **IV** 50 mg/kg q12h

Available forms: Powder for inj 1, 2 g

SIDE EFFECTS

CNS: Lethargy, hallucinations, anxiety, depression, twitching, ***coma, seizures***
GI: Nausea, vomiting, diarrhea, increased AST, ALT, abdominal pain, glossitis, ***pseudomembranous colitis***
GU: Oliguria, ***proteinuria, hematuria,*** vaginitis, moniliasis, ***glomerulonephritis,*** interstitial nephritis
HEMA: Anemia, increased bleeding time, ***bone marrow depression, granulocytopenia***
SYST: ***Anaphylaxis, serum sickness***
Contraindications: Hypersensitivity to penicillins
Precautions: Pregnancy (B), hypersensitivity to cephalosporins, neonates

PHARMACOKINETICS

Half-life 1 hr, metabolized by liver, excreted in bile, urine

INTERACTIONS

Increase: nafcillin concentrations—probenecid
Decrease: effect—oral contraceptives, heparin

Drug/Herb

Do not use with antiinfectives: acidophilus

Decrease: absorption—khat

Drug/Food

Decrease: absorption—food, carbonated drinks, citrus fruit juices

Drug/Lab Test

False-positive: Urine glucose, urine protein

NURSING CONSIDERATIONS

Assess:

• I&O ratio; report hematuria, oliguria, since penicillin in high doses is nephrotoxic

A Any patient with compromised renal system, since drug is excreted slowly in poor renal system function; toxicity may occur rapidly

• Hepatic studies: AST, ALT

• Blood studies: WBC, RBC, H&H, bleeding time

• Renal studies: urinalysis, protein, blood, BUN, creatinine

• C&S before drug therapy; drug may be given as soon as culture is taken

• Bowel pattern before and during treatment

• Respiratory status: rate, character, wheezing, and tightness in chest

A Allergies before initiation of treatment; monitor for anaphylaxis, dyspnea, rash, laryngeal edema; stop drug; keep emergency equipment nearby; skin eruptions after administration of penicillin to 1 wk after discontinuing drug

• Differential WBC in patients on long-term therapy

Administer:

• Drug after C&S has been completed

IV route

• After diluting 1 g/3.4 ml or 2 g/6.8 ml to 250 mg/ml sterile H_2O for inj; further dilute 15-30 ml sterile H_2O or NS sol; give through Y-tube or 3-way stopcock; 500 mg or less/5-10 min; may be further diluted and run over 24 hr

Additive compatibilities: Chloramphenicol, chlorothiazide, dexamethasone, diphenhydrAMINE, epHEDrine, heparin, hydrOXYzine, lidocaine, potassium chloride, prochlorperazine, sodium bicarbonate, sodium lactate

Syringe compatibilities: Cimetidine, heparin

Y-site compatibilities: Acyclovir, atropine, cyclophosphamide, diazepam, enalaprilat, esmolol, famotidine, fentanyl, fluconazole, foscarnet, hydromorphone, magnesium sulfate, morphine, perphenazine, propofol, theophylline, zidovudine

Perform/provide:

• Adrenalin, suction, tracheostomy set, endotracheal intubation equipment

• Adequate fluid intake (2 L) during diarrhea episodes

• Scratch test to assess allergy after securing order from prescriber; usually done when penicillin is only drug of choice

• Storage in tight container; refrigerate reconstituted sol

Evaluate:

• Therapeutic response: absence of fever, draining wounds

Teach patient/family:

• To report sore throat, fever, fatigue (may indicate superinfection)

• To wear or carry emergency ID if allergic to penicillins

• To notify nurse of diarrhea

Treatment of anaphylaxis: Withdraw drug; maintain airway; administer epINEPHrine, aminophylline, O_2, IV corticosteroids

---

naftifine topical
See Appendix C

Side effects: *italics* = common; ***bold italics*** = life-threatening

⚠ High Alert

nalbuphine (℞)
(nal′byoo-feen)
Nubain, nalbuphine HCl
Func. class.: Opioid analgesic
Chem. class.: Synthetic opioid agonist, antagonist

Action: Depresses pain impulse transmission at the spinal cord level by interacting with opioid receptors
Uses: Moderate to severe pain

DOSAGE AND ROUTES

Analgesic
• *Adult:* **SUBCUT/IM/IV** 10-20 mg q3-6h prn, not to exceed 160 mg/day
Balanced anesthesia supplement
• *Adult:* **IV** 0.3-3 mg/kg given over 10-15 min, may give 0.25-0.5 mg/kg as needed for maintenance
Available forms: Inj 10, 20 mg/ml

SIDE EFFECTS

CNS: Drowsiness, dizziness, confusion, headache, sedation, euphoria, dysphoria (high doses), hallucinations, dreaming, tolerance, physical, psychological dependency
CV: Palpitations, bradycardia, change in B/P, orthostatic hypotension
EENT: Tinnitus, blurred vision, miosis, diplopia
GI: Nausea, vomiting, anorexia, constipation, cramps
GU: Increased urinary output, dysuria, urinary retention, urgency
INTEG: Rash, urticaria, bruising, flushing, diaphoresis, pruritus
RESP: Respiratory depression, pulmonary edema
Contraindications: Hypersensitivity, addiction (opiate)
Precautions: Pregnancy (C), addictive personality, lactation, increased intracranial pressure, MI (acute), severe heart disease, respiratory depression, hepatic disease, renal disease

PHARMACOKINETICS

SUBCUT/IM/IV: Duration 3-6 hr; metabolized by liver, excreted by kidneys, half-life 5 hr

INTERACTIONS

⚠ Avoid use with MAOIs, unpredictable reactions may occur
Increase: effects with other CNS depressants—alcohol, opiates, sedative/hypnotics, antipsychotics, skeletal muscle relaxants
Drug/Herb
Increase: CNS depression—chamomile, hops, Jamaican dogwood, kava, lavender, mistletoe, nettle, pokeweed, poppy, senega, skullcap, valerian
Increase: anticholinergic effect—corkwood
Drug/Lab Test
Increase: Amylase

NURSING CONSIDERATIONS

Assess:
• I&O ratio; check for decreasing output; may indicate urinary retention
⚠ For withdrawal reactions in opiate-dependent individuals: pulmonary embolus, vascular occlusion; abscesses, ulcerations, nausea, vomiting, seizures; however, there is a low potential for dependence
• CNS changes: dizziness, drowsiness, hallucinations, euphoria, LOC, pupil reaction
• Allergic reactions: rash, urticaria
• Respiratory dysfunction: respiratory depression, character, rate, rhythm; notify prescriber if respirations are <10/min
• Need for pain medication by pain sedation scoring, physical dependency
Administer:
• With antiemetic if nausea, vomiting occur
• When pain is beginning to return; determine dosage interval by response
IM route
• IM deep in large muscle mass, rotate inj sites

IV route
• Undiluted 10 mg or less over 3-5 min

Syringe compatibilities: Atropine, cimetidine, diphenhydrAMINE, droperidol, glycopyrrolate, hydrOXYzine, lidocaine, midazolam, prochlorperazine, ranitidine, scopolamine, trimethobenzamide

Y-site compatibilities: Amifostine, aztreonam, cefmetazole, cisatracurium, cladribine, filgrastim, fludarabine, granisetron, melphalan, paclitaxel, propofol, remifentanil, teniposide, thiotepa, vinorelbine

Perform/provide:
• Storage in light-resistant area at room temperature
• Assistance with ambulation
• Safety measures: night-light, call bell within easy reach

Evaluate:
• Therapeutic response: decrease in pain

Teach patient/family:
• To report any symptoms of CNS changes, allergic reactions
• That physical dependency may result from long-term use
• That withdrawal symptoms may occur: nausea, vomiting, cramps, fever, faintness, anorexia

Treatment of overdose: Naloxone (Narcan) 0.2-0.8 mg IV, O_2, IV fluids, vasopressors

---

naloxone (℞)
(nal-oks'one)
naloxone HCl, Narcan
Func. class.: Opioid antagonist, antidote
Chem. class.: Thebaine derivative

Do not confuse:
Narcan/Norcuron

Action: Competes with opioids at opiate receptor sites

Uses: Respiratory depression induced by opioids, pentazocine, propoxyphene; refractory circulatory shock, asphyxia neonatorum, coma, hypotension

Investigational uses: IBS, opiate agonist dependence, opiate agonist-induced constipation, pruritus

DOSAGE AND ROUTES
Opioid-induced respiratory depression
• *Adult:* **IV/SUBCUT/IM** 0.4-2 mg; repeat q2-3min if needed
• *Child:* **IV/SUBCUT/IM** 0.01 mg/kg slowly or as **INF** titrated to response

Postoperative opioid-induced respiratory depression
• *Adult:* **IV** 0.1-0.2 mg q2-3min prn
• *Child:* **IV/SUBCUT/IM** 0.01 mg/kg q2-3min prn

Opioid overdose
• *Adult:* **IV/SUBCUT/IM** 0.4 mg (10 mcg/kg) (not opioid dependent) may repeat q2-3min; 0.1-0.2 mg q2-3min (opioid dependent)
• *Child:* **IV/SUBCUT/IM** 10 mcg (0.01 mg/kg) q2-3min

Available forms: Inj 0.02, 0.4 mg/ml

SIDE EFFECTS
CNS: Drowsiness, nervousness
CV: Rapid pulse, increased systolic B/P (high doses), ***ventricular tachycardia, fibrillation***
GI: Nausea, vomiting
RESP: Hyperpnea

Contraindications: Hypersensitivity
Precautions: Pregnancy (B), children, cardiovascular disease, opioid dependency, lactation, seizure disorder

PHARMACOKINETICS
Well absorbed IM, SUBCUT; metabolized by liver, crosses placenta; excreted in urine, breast milk; half-life 1 hr
IV: Onset 1 min, duration 45 min
IM/SUBCUT: Onset 2-5 min, duration 45-60 min

INTERACTIONS
Decrease: effect of opioid analgesics

N

Side effects: *italics* = common; ***bold italics*** = life-threatening

Drug/Lab Test
Interference: Urine VMA, 5-HIAA, urine glucose

NURSING CONSIDERATIONS

Assess:
- Withdrawal: cramping, hypertension, anxiety, vomiting, signs of withdrawal in drug-dependent individuals may occur up to 2 hr after administration
- VS q3-5min
- ABGs including Po_2, Pco_2
- Cardiac status: tachycardia, hypertension; monitor ECG
- Respiratory dysfunction: respiratory depression, character, rate, rhythm; if respirations are <10/min, administer naloxone; probably due to opioid overdose; monitor LOC
- For pain: duration, intensity, location, before and after administration; may be used for respiratory depression

Administer:
- Only with resuscitative equipment, O_2 nearby
- Only sol prepared within 24 hr

IV route
- Undiluted with sterile H_2O for inj; may be further diluted with NS or D_5 and given as an inf; give 0.4 mg or less over 15 sec or titrate inf to response

Additive compatibilities: Verapamil
Syringe compatibilities: Benzquinamide, heparin
Y-site compatibilities: Propofol

Perform/provide:
- Dark storage at room temperature

Evaluate:
- Therapeutic response: reversal of respiratory depression; LOC-alert

---

naltrexone (℞)
(nal-trex'one)
ReVia, Trexan
Func. class.: Opioid antagonist
Chem. class.: Thebaine derivative

Action: Competes with opioids at opioid receptor sites
Uses: Blockage of opioid analgesics,
used in treatment of opiate addiction, alcoholism
Investigational uses: Nicotine withdrawal

DOSAGE AND ROUTES

- *Adult:* **PO** 25 mg, may give 25 mg after 1 hr if no withdrawal symptoms; 50-150 mg may be given daily depending on need, maintenance 50 mg q24h; 100-150 mg may be given on alternate days or 3 days per wk

Pruritus (off-label)
- *Adult:* **PO** 50 mg daily

Available forms: Tabs 50 mg

SIDE EFFECTS

*CNS: Stimulation, drowsiness, dizziness, confusion, **seizures,** headache, flushing, hallucinations, nervousness, irritability, **suicidal ideation***
*CV: Rapid pulse, **pulmonary edema,** hypertension*
EENT: Tinnitus, hearing loss, blurred vision
*GI: Nausea, vomiting, diarrhea, heartburn, anorexia, **hepatitis,** constipation*
GU: Delayed ejaculation, decreased potency
INTEG: Rash, urticaria, bruising, oily skin, acne, pruritus
MISC: Increased thirst, chills, fever
MS: Joint and muscle pain
RESP: Wheezing, hyperpnea, nasal congestion, rhinorrhea, sneezing, sore throat

Contraindications: Hypersensitivity, opioid dependence, hepatic failure, hepatitis
Precautions: Pregnancy (C), hepatic disease, lactation, children

PHARMACOKINETICS

PO: Onset 15-30 min, peak 1-2 hr, duration is dose dependent
Metabolized by liver, excreted by kidneys; crosses placenta, excreted in breast milk; half-life 4 hr; extensive first-pass metabolism

---

⚠ Safety alert   *"Tall Man" lettering

INTERACTIONS

Increase: lethargy—phenothiazines
Increase: hepatotoxicity—disulfiram
Decrease: effect of analgesics, antidiarrheals, cough preparations

NURSING CONSIDERATIONS

Assess:
- VS q3-5min
- ABGs including Po_2, Pco_2
- Signs of withdrawal in drug-dependent individuals
- Cardiac status: tachycardia, hypertension
- Respiratory dysfunction: respiratory depression, character, rate, rhythm; if respirations are <10/min, respiratory stimulant should be administered

Administer:
- Only if resuscitative equipment is nearby

Perform/provide:
- Storage in tight container

Evaluate:
- Therapeutic response: blocking opiate ingestion

Teach patient/family:
- That they must be drug-free to start treatment
- That using opioid while taking this drug could prove fatal because high dose is needed to overcome this antagonist
- To carry emergency ID stating med used
- If surgery is needed, all involved should be aware of this drug

---

nandrolone (℞)
(nan′droe-lone)
Deca-Durabolin, Hybolin Decanoate, Kabolin
Func. class.: Androgenic anabolic steroid, antianemic
Chem. class.: Halogenated testosterone derivative

Controlled Substance Schedule III
Action: May stimulate bone marrow

development, stimulates erythropoietin production
Uses: Anemia associated with renal disease

DOSAGE AND ROUTES

- *Adult and child ≥14 yr:* **IM** women 50-100 mg qwk; men 100-200 mg qwk
- *Child 2-13 yr:* **IM** 25-50 mg q3-4wk

SIDE EFFECTS

CNS: Dizziness, headache, fatigue, tremors, paresthesias, flushing, sweating, anxiety, lability, insomnia, carpal tunnel syndrome, chills
CV: Increased B/P
EENT: Conjunctival edema, nasal congestion
ENDO: Abnormal GTT
GI: Nausea, vomiting, constipation, weight gain, ***cholestatic jaundice***
GU: ***Hematuria,*** amenorrhea, vaginitis, decreased libido, decreased breast size, clitoral hypertrophy, testicular atrophy, priapism
INTEG: Rash, acneiform lesions, oily hair/skin, flushing, sweating, acne vulgaris, alopecia, hirsutism
MS: Cramps, spasms
Contraindications: Pregnancy (X), severe renal, severe cardiac, severe hepatic disease, hypersensitivity, lactation, abnormal genital bleeding, males with cancer of breast, prostate
Precautions: Diabetes mellitus, CV disease, MI

PHARMACOKINETICS

Well absorbed, peak up to 6 days

INTERACTIONS

Increase: bleeding—anticoagulants, NSAIDs, salicylates
Increase: hepatotoxicity—hepatotoxics
Drug/Lab Test
Increase: Serum cholesterol, blood glucose, urine glucose
Decrease: Serum calcium, serum potassium, T_4, T_3, thyroid ^{131}I uptake test, urine 17-OHCS, 17-KS, PBI, BSP

N

Side effects: *italics* = common; ***bold italics*** = life-threatening

NURSING CONSIDERATIONS

Assess:

- Anemia symptoms: dyspnea, fatigue, weakness, pallor
- Weight daily; notify prescriber if weekly weight gain is >5 lb
- B/P q4h
- I&O ratio; be alert for decreasing urinary output, increasing edema
- Growth rate in children, since growth rate may be uneven (linear/bone growth) with extended use
- Electrolytes: K, Na, Cl, Ca; cholesterol
- Hepatic studies: ALT, AST, bilirubin
- Edema, hypertension, cardiac symptoms, jaundice
- Mental status: affect, mood, behavioral changes, aggression
- Signs of masculinization in female: increased libido, deepening of voice, decreased breast tissue, enlarged clitoris, menstrual irregularities; male: gynecomastia, impotence, testicular atrophy
- Hypercalcemia: lethargy, polyuria, polydipsia, nausea, vomiting, constipation, drug may have to be decreased
- Hypoglycemia in diabetics, since oral antidiabetic action is increased

Administer:

- Titrated dose; use lowest effective dose
- Inject deeply, use large muscle mass

Perform/provide:

- Diet with increased calories, protein; decrease sodium if edema occurs

Evaluate:

- Therapeutic response: increased appetite, increased stamina

Teach patient/family:

- That drug must be combined with complete health plan: diet, rest, exercise
- To notify prescriber if therapeutic response decreases
- Not to discontinue abruptly
- About changes in sex characteristics
- That females should report menstrual irregularities

---

naphazoline nasal agent
See Appendix C

---

naphazoline ophthalmic
See Appendix C

---

naproxen (OTC, ℞)
(na-prox'en)
Apo-Naproxen ✦, EC-Naprosyn, Naprelan, Napron X, Naprosyn, Naprosyn-E ✦, Naprosyn-SR ✦, Naxen ✦, Novo-Naprox ✦, Nu-Naprox ✦

naproxen sodium
Aleve, Anaprox, Anaprox DS, Apo-Napro-Na ✦, Apo-Napro-Na DS, Naprelan, Novo-Naprox Sodium ✦, Novo-Naprox Sodium DS ✦, Synflex ✦, Synflex DS ✦

Func. class.: Nonsteroidal antiinflammatory, nonopioid analgesic
Chem. class.: Propionic acid derivative

Action: Inhibits prostaglandin synthesis by decreasing an enzyme needed for biosynthesis; analgesic, antiinflammatory, antipyretic
Uses: Mild to moderate pain, osteoarthritis, rheumatoid, gouty arthritis, juvenile arthritis, primary dysmenorrhea

DOSAGE AND ROUTES

Anti-Inflammatory/analgesic/antidysmenorrheal
- *Adult:* PO 250-500 mg bid, max 1.5 g/day; **DEL REL** 375-500 mg bid
- *Child ≥2 yr:* PO 5 mg/kg/day bid

Antigout
- *Adult:* PO 750 mg, then 250 mg q8h

OTC Use
- *Adult:* PO 200 mg q8-12h or 400 mg, then 200 mg q12h, max 600 mg/24hr

---

• *Geriatric >65 yr:* **PO** max 200 mg q12h

Available forms: Tabs, naproxen: 250, 375, 500 mg; cont rel tabs (Naprelan) 375, 500 mg; tabs, del rel (EC-Naprosyn, Naprosyn-E) 250 ✤, 375, 500 mg; tabs, oral susp 125 mg/5 ml; ext rel tabs (SR) 750 mg ✤naproxen sodium tabs, cont rel 421.5, 550 mg; tabs 275, 550 mg; supp (Naprosyn, Naxen) 500 mg ✤

SIDE EFFECTS

CNS: Dizziness, drowsiness, fatigue, tremors, confusion, insomnia, anxiety, depression
CV: Tachycardia, peripheral edema, palpitations, dysrhythmias
EENT: Tinnitus, hearing loss, blurred vision
GI: Nausea, anorexia, vomiting, diarrhea, jaundice, ***cholestatic hepatitis,*** constipation, flatulence, cramps, dry mouth, peptic ulcer, ***GI ulceration, bleeding, perforation***
GU: ***Nephrotoxicity: dysuria, hematuria, oliguria, azotemia***
HEMA: ***Blood dyscrasias***
INTEG: Purpura, rash, pruritus, sweating
SYST: ***Anaphylaxis***

Contraindications: Pregnancy (D) 2nd/3rd trimester, hypersensitivity, asthma, severe renal disease, severe hepatic disease, ulcer disease
Precautions: Pregnancy (B) 1st trimester, lactation, children <2 yr, bleeding disorders, GI disorders, cardiac disorders, hypersensitivity to other antiinflammatory agents, elderly, CCr <25 ml/min

PHARMACOKINETICS

PO: Peak 2-4 hr, half-life 3-3½ hr; metabolized in liver; excreted in urine (metabolites), breast milk; 99% protein binding

INTERACTIONS

Possible renal impairment: ACE inhibitors

Toxicity risk: methotrexate, lithium, antineoplastics, radiation treatment
Increase: bleeding risk—oral anticoagulants, thrombolytic agents, eptifibatide, tirofiban, cefamandole, cefotetan, cefoperazone, clopidogrel, ticlopidine, plicamycin, valproic acid
Increase: GI side effects risk—aspirin, corticosteroids, alcohol, NSAIDs
Decrease: effect of antihypertensives, diuretics

Drug/Herb
Bleeding risk: anise, arnica, bogbean, chamomile, chondroitin, clove, dong quai, fenugreek, feverfew, garlic, ginger, ginkgo, ginseng *(Panax),* licorice
Increase: gastric irritation—arginine, gossypol
Increase: NSAIDs effect—bearberry, bilberry
Drug/Lab Test
Increase: BUN, alk phosphatase
False increase: 5-HIAA, 17KS

NURSING CONSIDERATIONS
Assess:
• Pain: frequency, characteristics, intensity; relief prior to and 1-2 hr after med
⚠ Asthma, aspirin hypersensitivity or nasal polyps, increased risk of hypersensitivity
• Renal, hepatic, blood studies: BUN, creatinine, AST, ALT, Hgb, LDH, blood glucose, Hct, WBC, platelets CCr before treatment, periodically thereafter
• Audiometric, ophthalmic exam before, during, after treatment
• For eye, ear problems: blurred vision, tinnitus (may indicate toxicity)
Administer:
• With food to decrease GI symptoms; take on empty stomach to facilitate absorption
Perform/provide:
• Storage at room temperature
Evaluate:
• Therapeutic response: decreased pain, stiffness, swelling in joints, ability to move more easily

N

Teach patient/family:

• To use sunscreen to prevent photosensitivity

• To report blurred vision, ringing, roaring in ears (may indicate toxicity)

• To avoid driving, other hazardous activities if dizziness or drowsiness occurs

• To report change in urine pattern, weight increase, edema (face, lower extremities), pain increase in joints, fever, blood in urine (indicates nephrotoxicity); black stools, flulike symptoms

• That therapeutic effects may take up to 1 mo

• To avoid ASA, alcohol, steroids

---

naratriptan (℞)

(nair'ah-trip-tan)
Amerge
Func. class.: Antimigraine agent
Chem. class.: 5-HT₁ receptor agonist

Action: Binds selectively to the vascular 5-HT₁ receptor subtype, exerts antimigraine effect; causes vasoconstriction in cranial arteries

Uses: Acute treatment of migraine with or without aura

DOSAGE AND ROUTES

• *Adult:* **PO** 1 or 2.5 mg with fluids, if headache returns, repeat once after 4 hr, max 5 mg/24 hr
Hepatic/renal dose
• Max 2.5 mg/24 hr
Available forms: Tabs 1, 2.5 mg

SIDE EFFECTS

CNS: Dizziness, sedation, fatigue
CV: Increased B/P, palpitations, ***tachydysrhythmias, PR, QTc prolongation, ST/T wave changes, PVCs, atrial flutter/fibrillation, coronary vasospasm***
EENT: EENT infections, photophobia
GI: Nausea, vomiting

MISC: Temperature change sensations; tightness, pressure sensations
MS: Weakness, neck stiffness, myalgia
Contraindications: Hypersensitivity, angina pectoris, history of MI, documented silent ischemia, ischemic heart disease, concurrent ergotamine-containing preparations, uncontrolled hypertension, CV syndromes, hemiplegic or basilar migraines, severe renal disease (CCr <15 ml/min); severe hepatic disease (Child-Pugh grade C)
Precautions: Pregnancy (C), postmenopausal women, men >40 yr, risk factors for CAD, hypercholesterolemia, obesity, diabetes, impaired hepatic or renal function, lactation, children, elderly, peripheral vascular disease

PHARMACOKINETICS

Onset ½ hr, peak 2-3 hr, 28%-31% protein binding, half-life 6 hr, metabolized in the liver (metabolite), excreted in urine, feces; may be excreted in breast milk

INTERACTIONS

Weakness, hyperreflexia, incoordination: SSRIs (fluoxetine, fluvoxamine, paroxetine, sertraline)
Increase: vasospastic effects—ergot, ergot derivatives, other 5-HT₁ agonists
Increase: adverse reactions risk—MAOIs, do not use together
Drug/Herb
Serotonin syndrome: SAM-e, St. John's wort
Increase: effect—butterbur

NURSING CONSIDERATIONS
Assess:

• For stress level, activity, recreation, coping mechanisms

• Neurologic status: LOC blurred vision, nausea, vomiting, tingling in extremities preceding headache

---

🅐 Safety alert   *"Tall Man" lettering

Administer:
• With fluids as soon as symptoms appear, may take another dose after 4 hr; do not take >5 mg in any 24-hr period
Perform/provide:
• Quiet, calm environment with decreased stimulation for noise, bright light, excessive talking
Evaluate:
• Therapeutic response: decrease in frequency, severity of headache
Teach patient/family:
• To report pain, tightness in chest, neck, throat, or jaw; notify prescriber immediately if sudden, severe abdominal pain occurs
• Not to use if another 5-HT$_1$ agonist or an ergot preparation has been used in the past 24 hr
• Advise patient to notify prescriber if pregnancy is planned or suspected, avoid breastfeeding

---

natamycin ophthalmic
See Appendix C

---

nedocromil (℞)
(ned-o-kroe'mill)
Tilade
Func. class.: Antiasthmatic
Chem. class.: Mast cell stabilizer

Action: Stabilizes the membrane of the sensitized mast cell, preventing release of chemical mediators after an antigen-IgE interaction
Uses: Severe perennial bronchial asthma, exercise-induced bronchospasm (prevention), prevention of acute bronchospasm induced by environmental pollutants; *not* for treatment of acute asthma attacks

DOSAGE AND ROUTES
• *Adult and child >12 yr:* **INH** 2 inhalations 2-4 ×/day at regular intervals to provide 14 g/day

Available forms: 1.75 mg nedocromil sodium per activation in 16.2 g canisters providing at least 112 metered inhalations

SIDE EFFECTS
CNS: Headache, dizziness, neuritis, dysphonia
EENT: Throat irritation, cough, nasal congestion, burning eyes, rhinitis
GI: Nausea, vomiting, anorexia, dry mouth, bitter taste
MISC: **Anaphylaxis**
Contraindications: Hypersensitivity to this drug or lactose, status asthmaticus
Precautions: Pregnancy (B), lactation, children

PHARMACOKINETICS
INH: Peak 15 min, duration 4-6 hr; excreted unchanged in urine; half-life 80 min

NURSING CONSIDERATIONS
Assess:
• Pulmonary function testing baseline (asthma)
• Respiratory status: rate, rhythm, characteristics, cough, wheezing, dyspnea
Administer:
• By inhalation only, with spacer device if needed
• Gargle, sip of water to decrease irritation in throat
Evaluate:
• Therapeutic response: decrease in asthmatic symptoms, congested, runny nose
Teach patient/family:
• To clear mucus before using
• The proper technique: exhale; using inhaler, inhale deeply with head tipped back to open airway; remove, hold breath, exhale; use Halermatic or Spinhaler with Intal caps
• That therapeutic effect may take up to 4 wk

N

• That drug is preventive only, not restorative

nelarabine
See Appendix A—Selected New Drugs

nelfinavir (R)
(nell-fin'a-ver)
Viracept
Func. class.: Antiretroviral
Chem. class.: HIV protease inhibitor

Action: Inhibits human immunodeficiency virus (HIV-1) protease, which prevents maturation of the infectious virus

Uses: HIV-1 in combination with other antiretrovirals

DOSAGE AND ROUTES
HIV infection
• *Adult and child >13 yr:* **PO** 750 mg tid or 1250 mg bid
• *Child 2-13 yr:* **PO** 20-30 mg/kg tid, max 750 mg tid
Prevention of HIV infection after exposure
• *Adult:* **PO** 750 mg tid with two other antiretroviral agents × 4 wks
Available forms: Tabs 250, 625 mg; powder, oral 50 mg/g

SIDE EFFECTS

CNS: Headache, asthenia, poor concentration, *seizures, suicidal ideation*
CV: Bleeding
ENDO: Hypoglycemia, hyperlipidemia
GI: *Diarrhea,* anorexia, dyspepsia, *nausea, flatulence, hepatitis, pancreatitis*
HEMA: Anemia, leukopenia, thrombocytopenia, Hgb abnormalities
INTEG: *Rash,* dermatitis
MS: Pain, arthralgia, myalgia, myopathy
OTHER: *Hypoglycemia,* redistribution/accumulation of body fat

Contraindications: Hypersensitivity to protease inhibitors
Precautions: Pregnancy (B), hepatic disease, lactation, renal disease, hemophilia, PKU, pancreatitis

PHARMACOKINETICS
Half-life 3½-5 hr, excreted urine/feces, peak 2-4 hr, 98% protein binding

INTERACTIONS
Drug/Herb
⚠ Serious dysrhythmias: amiodarone, ergots, lovastatin, midazolam, pimozide, quinidine, simvastatin, triazolam
Increase: effect—atorvastatin, azithromycin, rifabutin
Increase: nelfinavir levels—ketoconazole, indinavir, ritonavir
Increase: protease inhibitor levels—delavirdine, HIV protease inhibitors
Decrease: nelfinavir levels—rifamycins, nevirapine, phenobarbital, phenytoin, carbamazepine
Decrease: effect of didanosine, methadone, oral contraceptives, phenytoin
Drug/Herb
Decrease: antiretroviral effect—St. John's wort
Drug/Food
Increase: absorption with food

NURSING CONSIDERATIONS
Assess:
• Signs of infection, anemia
• Hepatic studies: ALT, AST
• C&S before drug therapy; drug may be taken as soon as culture is taken; repeat C&S after treatment; determine the presence of other sexually transmitted diseases
• Bowel pattern before, during treatment; if severe abdominal pain with bleeding occurs, drug should be discontinued; monitor hydration
• Skin eruptions, rash, urticaria, itching

⚠ Safety alert   *"Tall Man" lettering

• Allergies before treatment, reaction of each medication; place allergies on chart
• Viral load, CD4 cell counts baseline and throughout treatment

Administer:
• With food
• Oral powder mixed with fluids if desired, do not mix with juice or acidic fluids, stable mixed for 6 hr

Teach patient/family:
• To avoid taking with other medications unless directed by prescriber
• That drug does not cure, but does manage symptoms; does not prevent transmission of HIV to others
• To use a nonhormonal form of birth control while taking this drug
• If dose is missed, to take as soon as remembered up to 1 hr before next dose; do not double dose
• To take with food

Rarely Used

neomycin (R)
(nee-oh-mye'sin)
Mycifradin, Myciguent
Func. class.: Antiinfective

Uses: Severe systemic infections of CNS, respiratory, GI, urinary tract, eye, bone, skin, soft tissues caused by *Pseudomonas aeruginosa, Escherichia coli, Enterobacter, Klebsiella pneumoniae, Proteus vulgaris;* also used for hepatic coma, preoperatively to sterilize bowel, infectious diarrhea caused by enteropathogenic *E. coli*

DOSAGE AND ROUTES

Hepatic encephalopathy
• *Adult:* PO 4-12 g/day in divided doses × 5-6 days
• *Child:* PO 50-100 mg/kg/day in divided doses

Preoperative intestinal antisepsis
• *Adult:* PO on 3rd day of a 3-day regimen, give 1 g early PM, repeat in 1 hr, repeat at bedtime (given with

erythromycin); give saline cathartic before giving this drug
• *Child:* PO 14.7 mg/kg or 4.7 mg/m² q4h × 3 days

Contraindications: Bowel obstruction (oral use), severe renal disease, hypersensitivity, infants, children

---

neomycin topical
See Appendix C

---

neostigmine (R)
(nee-oh-stig'meen)
neostigmine, Prostigmin
Func. class.: Cholinergic stimulant; anticholinesterase
Chem. class.: Quaternary compound

Action: Inhibits destruction of acetylcholine, which increases concentration at sites where acetylcholine is released; this facilitates transmission of impulses across myoneural junction
Uses: Myasthenia gravis, nondepolarizing neuromuscular blocker antagonist, urinary retention, postoperative ileus

DOSAGE AND ROUTES

Myasthenia gravis
• *Adult:* PO 15 mg q3-4h, may increase to 375 mg/day; IM/IV 0.5-2 mg q1-3h
• *Child:* PO 2 mg/kg/day q3-4h

Nondepolarizing neuromuscular blocker antagonist
• *Adult:* IV 0.5-2 mg slowly, may repeat if needed (give 0.6-1.2 mg atropine before this drug)
• *Infant/child:* IV 0.025-0.1 mg/kg/dose

Abdominal distention/postoperative ileus
• *Adult:* IM/SUBCUT 0.25-1 mg (1:4000) q4-6h depending on condition × 2-3 days

N

Renal dose
• CCr 10-50 ml/min 50% of dose; CCr
<10 ml/min 25% of dose
Available forms: Tabs 15 mg; inj
1:1000, 1:2000, 1:4000

SIDE EFFECTS

CNS: Dizziness, headache, sweating,
weakness, ***convulsions,*** incoordination, ***paralysis,*** drowsiness, loss of
consciousness
CV: Tachycardia, dysrhythmias, bradycardia, hypotension, AV block, ECG changes,
cardiac arrest, syncope
EENT: Miosis, blurred vision, lacrimation,
visual changes
*GI: Nausea, diarrhea, vomiting,
cramps,* increased peristalsis, salivary
and gastric secretions
GU: Urinary frequency, incontinence,
urgency
INTEG: Rash, urticaria, flushing
RESP: ***Respiratory depression,
bronchospasm, constriction, laryngospasm, respiratory arrest,*** dyspnea
Contraindications: Obstruction of
intestine, renal system, bromide sensitivity, peritonitis, urinary tract obstruction,
ileus
Precautions: Pregnancy (C), bradycardia, hypotension, seizure disorders,
bronchial asthma, coronary occlusion,
hyperthyroidism, dysrhythmias, peptic
ulcer, megacolon, poor GI motility, lactation, children

PHARMACOKINETICS

PO: Onset 45-75 min, duration 2½-4
hr
IM/SUBCUT: Onset 10-30 min,
duration 2½-4 hr
IV: Onset 4-8 min; duration 2-4 hr;
metabolized in liver, excreted in
urine

INTERACTIONS

Increase: action of decamethonium,
succinylcholine
Decrease: neostigmine action—
aminoglycosides, antihistamines, antidepressants, atropine, anticholinergics,
local/general anesthetics, corticosteroids, haloperidol, phenothiazines, quinidine, disopyramide
Drug/Herb
Increase: effect: pill—bearing spurge

NURSING CONSIDERATIONS

Assess:
• VS, respiration q8h
• I&O ratio; check for urinary retention
or incontinence
🅰 For bradycardia, hypotension, bron-
chospasm, headache, dizziness, convul-
sions, respiratory depression; drug
should be discontinued if toxicity occurs
Administer:
• Only with atropine sulfate available for
cholinergic crisis
• Only after all other cholinergics have
been discontinued
• Increased doses, as ordered if toler-
ance occurs
• Larger doses after exercise or fatigue,
as ordered
PO route
• On empty stomach for better absorp-
tion
IV route
• Undiluted, give through Y-tube or
3-way stopcock; give 0.5 mg or less over
1 min
Additive compatibilities: Netilmicin
Syringe compatibilities: Glycopyr-
rolate, heparin, pentobarbital, thiopental
Y-site compatibilities: Heparin, hy-
drocortisone, potassium chloride, vit B/C
Perform/provide:
• Storage at room temperature
Evaluate:
• Therapeutic response: increased mus-
cle strength, hand grasp, improved gait,
absence of labored breathing (if severe)
Teach patient/family:
• That drug is not a cure; it only relieves
symptoms
• To wear emergency ID specifying my-
asthenia gravis, drugs taken
Treatment of overdose: Respiratory
support, atropine 1-4 mg (IV)

🅰 Safety alert   *"Tall Man" lettering

⚠ High Alert

nesiritide (℞)
(neh-seer'ih-tide)
Natrecor
Func. class.: Vasodilator
Chem. class.: Human B-type natri-
uretic peptide

Action: Uses DNA technology; human
B-type natriuretic peptide binds to the
receptor in vascular smooth muscle and
endothelial cells, leading to smooth muscle relaxation
Uses: Acutely decompensated CHF

DOSAGE AND ROUTES

• *Adult:* **IV BOL** 2 mcg/kg, then **IV INF**
0.01 mcg/kg/min
Available forms: Powder for inj, 1.5
mg single-use vial

SIDE EFFECTS

CNS: Headache, insomnia, dizziness,
anxiety, confusion, paresthesia, tremor
CV: Hypotension, **tachycardia**, dysrhythmias, bradycardia, ventricular
tachycardia, ventricular extrasystoles,
atrial fibrillation
GI: Vomiting, nausea
INTEG: Rash, sweating, pruritus, inj site
reaction
MISC: Abdominal pain, back pain
RESP: Increased cough, hemoptysis, **apnea**
Contraindications: Hypersensitivity,
cardiogenic shock or B/P <90 mm Hg as
primary therapy
Precautions: Pregnancy (C); mitral
stenosis; significant valvular stenosis,
restriction, or obstructive cardiomyopathy, or any condition that is dependent
upon venous return; renal disease, lactation, children

PHARMACOKINETICS

Half-life 18 min

INTERACTIONS

Increase: symptomatic hypotension with
ACE inhibitors

NURSING CONSIDERATIONS

Assess:
• PCWP, RAP, cardiac index, MPAP
• B/P, pulse during treatment until stable
Administer:
IV route
• Do not administer nesiritide through a
central catheter containing other drugs;
administer other drugs through a separate catheter
• Prime IV fluid with infusion of 25 ml
before connecting to patient's vascular
access port and before bolus dose or IV
infusion
• Reconstitute one 1.5 mg vial/5 ml of
diluent from prefilled 250-ml plastic IV
bag with diluent of choice (D_5, 0.9%
NaCl, D_5/½ NaCl, D_5/0.2% NaCl); do not
shake vial, roll gently; use only clear sol
• Withdraw all contents of reconstituted
vial and add to the 250-ml plastic IV bag
(6 mcg/ml), invert bag several times
• Use within 24 hr of reconstituting
Evaluate:
• Therapeutic response: improvement in
CHF with improved PCWP, RAP, MPAP
Teach patient/family:
• To explain purpose of medication and
expected results

---

nevirapine
(ne-veer'a-peen)
Viramune
Func. class.: Antiretroviral
Chem. class.: Nonnucleoside reverse
transcriptase inhibitor (NNRTI)

Do not confuse
nevirapine/nelfinavir
viramune/viracept
Action: Binds directly to reverse transcriptase and blocks RNA, DNA, causing a
disruption of the enzyme's site
Uses: HIV-1 in combination with other

N

highly active antiretroviral treatments (HAART)

DOSAGE AND ROUTES

• *Adult:* **PO** 200 mg daily × 2 wk, then 200 mg bid in combination
• *Child ≥8 yr:* **PO** 4 mg/kg/daily × 2 wk, then 4 mg/kg/bid, max 200 mg bid
• *Child 2 mo-8 yr:* **PO** 4 mg/kg daily × 2 wk, then 7 mg/kg bid
Available forms: Tabs 200 mg; oral susp 50 mg/5 ml

SIDE EFFECTS

CNS: Paresthesia, headache, fever, peripheral neuropathy
GI: Diarrhea, abdominal pain, *nausea, stomatitis,* **hepatotoxicity**
HEMA: **Neutropenia, anemia, thrombocytopenia**
INTEG: Rash, toxic epidermal necrolysis
MISC: **Stevens-Johnson syndrome**
MS: Pain, myalgia

Contraindications: Hypersensitivity
Precautions: Pregnancy (C), hepatic disease, lactation, children, renal disease

PHARMACOKINETICS

Rapidly absorbed, peak 4 hr, 60% bound to plasma proteins, metabolized by liver; metabolized by hepatic P450 enzyme system, excreted 91% in urine, terminal half-life 2.5-3 hr

INTERACTIONS

Increase: nevirapine levels—cimetidine, macrolide antiinfectives
Decrease: effects of protease inhibitors, oral contraceptives, ketoconazole, methadone
Decrease: nevirapine levels—rifamycins, anticonvulsants, clonazepam, diazepam, warfarin
Drug/Herb
Decrease: action of antiretroviral—St. John's wort, do not use concurrently
Drug/Lab Test
Increase: ALT, AST, GGT, bilirubin, Hgb
Decrease: Neutrophil count

NURSING CONSIDERATIONS

Assess:
• Signs of infection, anemia
• Hepatic, blood studies during treatment: ALT, AST, viral load, CD4; renal studies; if LFTs are elevated significantly, drug should be withheld
• C&S before drug therapy; drug may be taken as soon as culture is taken; repeat C&S after treatment; determine the presence of other sexually transmitted disease
• Bowel pattern before, during treatment; if severe abdominal pain with bleeding occurs, drug should be discontinued; monitor hydration
🅰 Allergies before treatment, reaction to each medication; skin eruptions; rash, urticaria, itching; if rash is severe or systemic symptoms occur, discontinue immediately
Administer:
• Without regard to meals
Teach patient/family:
🅰 To report any right quadrant pain, jaundice, rash immediately
• That drug may be taken with food, antacids, didanosine
• To take as prescribed; if dose is missed, take as soon as remembered up to 1 hr before next dose; do not double dose
• That drug is not a cure, controls symptoms of HIV
• To avoid OTC agents unless approved by prescriber
• To use a nonhormonal form of contraception during treatment
• That drug must be taken in equal intervals around the clock to maintain blood levels for duration of therapy

---

🅰 Safety alert   *"Tall Man" lettering

niacin (otc, R)
(nye'a-sin)
Edur-Acin, Nia-Bid, Niac, Ni-acels, Niacor, Niaspan, Nico-bid, Nico-400, Nicolar, Nic-otinex
nicotinic acid (otc, R)
Novo-Niacin ✦, Slo-Niacin, vitamin B
niacinamide (otc, R)
nicotinamide (otc, R)
Func. class.: Vit B_3, antihyperlipid-emic
Chem. class.: Water-soluble vitamin

Do not confuse:
Nicobid/Nitro-Bid
Action: Needed for conversion of fats, protein, carbohydrates, by oxidation reduction; acts directly on vascular smooth muscle, causing vasodilation, reduces LDL, HDL, triglycerides, and lipoprotein A
Uses: Pellagra, hyperlipidemias (types 4, 5), peripheral vascular disease that presents a risk for pancreatitis

DOSAGE AND ROUTES
Niacin deficiency
• *Adult:* PO 100-500 mg/day in divided doses; **IM/SUBCUT** 5-100 mg 5 or more ×/day; **IV** 25-100 mg bid or tid
• *Child:* PO up to 300 mg/day in divided doses
Adjunct in hyperlipidemia
• *Adult:* PO 250 mg after evening meal; may increase dose at 1-4 wk intervals to 1-2 g tid, max 6 g/day; ext rel 500 mg at bedtime, × 4 wk, then 1000 mg at bed-time for wk 5-8, do not increase by more than 500 mg q4wk, max 2000 mg/day
Pellagra
• *Adult:* PO 300-500 mg daily in divided doses
• *Child:* PO 100-300 mg daily in divided doses
Peripheral vascular disease
• *Adult:* PO 250-800 mg daily in divided doses

Available forms: Niacin tabs 25, 50, 100, 250, 500, 1000 mg; caps, time rel 250, 500 mg; tabs, timed rel 250, 500 mg; cap, ext rel 250, 400 mg; sus rel tabs 500 mg; cont rel tabs 250, 500, 750 mg; sus rel cap 125, 500 mg; elix 50 mg/5 ml; nicotinamide—tabs 100, 250, 500 mg

SIDE EFFECTS
CNS: Paresthesias, headache, dizziness, anxiety
CV: Postural hypotension, vasovagal at-tacks, dysrhythmias, vasodilation
EENT: Blurred vision, ptosis
GI: Nausea, vomiting, anorexia, ***jaun-dice, hepatotoxicity,*** diarrhea, peptic ulcer, dyspepsia
GU: Hyperuricemia, ***glycosuria, hypo-albuminemia***
INTEG: Flushing, dry skin, rash, pruritus, itching, tingling
Contraindications: Hypersensitivity, peptic ulcer, hepatic disease, lactation, hemorrhage, severe hypotension
Precautions: Pregnancy (C), glau-coma, cardiovascular disease, CAD, dia-betes mellitus, gout, schizophrenia, lac-tation

N

PHARMACOKINETICS
PO: Peak 30-70 min (depends on formulatiton) half-life 45 min; metabo-lized in liver; 30% excreted unchanged in urine

INTERACTIONS
Myopathy, rhabdomyolysis: HMG-CoA reductase inhibitors
Postural hypotension: ganglionic block-ers
Increase: flushing, pruritus—alcohol, avoid use
Drug/Lab Test
Increase: Bilirubin, alk phosphatase, hepatic enzymes, LDH, uric acid, glucose
Decrease: Cholesterol
False increase: Urinary catecholamines
False-positive: Urine glucose

✦ Canada only   Side effects: *italics* = common; ***bold italics*** = life-threatening

NURSING CONSIDERATIONS

Assess:
- Hepatic studies: AST, ALT, bilirubin, uric acid, alk phosphatase; blood glucose before and during treatment
- Cardiac status: rate, rhythm, quality; postural hypotension, dysrhythmias
- Nutritional status: liver, yeast, legumes, organ meat, lean poultry; fat in diet
- Hepatic dysfunction: clay-colored stools, itching, dark urine, jaundice
- CNS symptoms: headache, paresthesias, blurred vision
- For symptoms of niacin deficiency: nausea, vomiting, anemia, poor memory, confusion, dermatitis
- For lipid, triglyceride, cholesterol level, if using for hyperlipidemia

Administer:
- Do not break, crush, or chew ext rel tabs, caps
- With meals for GI symptoms, and 81-325 mg aspirin or NSAIDs ½ hr before dose to decrease flushing

Evaluate:
- Therapeutic response: decreased lipids, warm extremities, absence of numbness in extremities

Teach patient/family:
- That flushing and increase in feelings of warmth will occur several hr after taking drug (PO); after 2 wk of therapy, these side effects diminish
- To remain recumbent if postural hypotension occurs; to rise slowly to prevent orthostatic hypotension
- To abstain from alcohol if drug is prescribed for hyperlipidemia
- To avoid sunlight if skin lesions are present

⚠ To report clay-colored stools, anorexia, jaundiced sclera, skin; dark urine, hepatotoxicity may occur

*niCARdipine (℞)

(nye-card′i-peen)
Cardene, Cardene IV,
Cardene SR

Func. class.: Calcium channel blocker, antianginal, antihypertensive

Chem. class.: Dihydropyridine

Do not confuse:
niCARdipine/NIFEdipine
Cardene/Cardizem
Cardene SR/Cardizem SR

Action: Inhibits calcium ion influx across cell membrane during cardiac depolarization; produces relaxation of coronary vascular smooth muscle, peripheral vascular smooth muscle; dilates coronary vascular arteries; increases myocardial oxygen delivery in patients with vasospastic angina

Uses: Chronic stable angina pectoris, hypertension

DOSAGE AND ROUTES

Hypertension
- *Adult:* **PO** 20 mg tid initially, may increase after 3 days (range 20-40 mg tid) or 30 mg bid sus rel, may increase to 60 mg bid or **IV** 5 mg/hr, may increase by 2.5 mg/hr q15min, max 15 mg/hr

Angina
- *Adult:* **PO** 20 mg tid, may be adjusted q3d, may use 20-40 mg tid

Renal dose
- *Adult:* **PO** 20 mg tid; or 30 mg bid (sus rel)

Hepatic dose
- *Adult:* **PO** 20 mg bid

Available forms: Caps 20, 30 mg; caps sus rel 30, 45, 60 mg; inj 2.5 mg/ml

SIDE EFFECTS

CNS: Headache, dizziness, anxiety, depression, confusion, paresthesia, somnolence
CV: Edema, bradycardia, hypotension, palpitations, ***pulmonary edema***, chest pain, tachycardia, increased angina, ***arrhythmias***, ***CHT***

GI: Nausea, vomiting, gastric upset, constipation, ***hepatitis,*** abdominal cramps, dry mouth, sore throat
GU: Nocturia, polyuria, ***acute renal failure***
INTEG: Rash, infusion site discomfort
Stevens-Johnson syndrome
OTHER: Blurred vision, flushing, sweating, shortness of breath, impotence
Contraindications: Sick sinus syndrome, 2nd-/3rd-degree heart block, hypersensitivity
Precautions: Pregnancy (C), CHF, hypotension, hepatic injury, lactation, children, renal disease, elderly

PHARMACOKINETICS

PO: Onset 30 min, peak 1-2 hr, duration 8 hr
PO-SR: Onset unknown, peak 2-6 hr, duration 10-12 hr, half-life 2-5 hr
Metabolized by liver, excreted in urine 60%, 35% feces

INTERACTIONS

Increase: effects of digitalis, neuromuscular blocking agents, theophylline, other antihypertensives, nitrates, alcohol, quinidine
Increase: niCARdipine effects—cimetidine
Increase: toxicity risk—cycloSPORINE, prazosin, carbamazepine, quinidine, propranolol
Decrease: antihypertensive effect—NSAIDs, rifampin

Drug/Herb
Increase: effect—barberry, betel palm, burdock, goldenseal, khat, khella, lily of the valley, plantain
Decrease: effect—yohimbe

Drug/Food
Increase: hypotensive effect—grapefruit juice

NURSING CONSIDERATIONS
Assess:
⚠ Cardiac status: B/P, pulse, respiration, ECG during long-term treatment

• Anginal pain: intensity, location, duration, alleviating factors
• Potassium, renal, hepatic studies, periodically
⚠ CHF: weight gain, crackles, jugular venous distention, dyspnea, I&O

Administer:
PO route
• Do not break, crush, chew, or open sus rel cap
• Without regard to meals

IV route
• Dilute each 25 mg/240 ml of compatible sol (0.1 mg/ml), give slowly
• Stable at room temperature 24 hr

Solution compatibilities: D₅W, D₅/0.45% NaCl, D₅/0.9% NaCl
Y-site compatibilities: Diltiazem, DOBUTamine, DOPamine, epINEPHrine, fentanyl, hydromorphone, labetalol, lorazepam, midazolam, milrinone, morphine, nitroglycerin, norepinephrine, ranitidine, vecuronium

Evaluate:
• Therapeutic response: decreased anginal pain, decreased B/P

Teach patient/family:
• To avoid hazardous activities until stabilized on drug, dizziness is no longer a problem
• To limit caffeine consumption, take no alcohol products
• To avoid OTC drugs unless directed by prescriber
• To comply in all areas of medical regimen: diet, exercise, stress reduction, drug therapy
⚠ To notify prescriber of irregular heartbeat, shortness of breath, swelling of feet and hands, pronounced dizziness, constipation, nausea, hypotension
Treatment of overdose: Defibrillation, β-agonists, IV calcium, diuretics, atropine for AV block, vasopressor for hypotension

N

nicotine (otc, ℞)
(nik'o-teen)
nicotine chewing gum (otc, ℞)
Nicorette
nicotine inhaler (otc, ℞)
Nicotrol Inhaler
nicotine nasal spray (℞)
Nicotrol NS
nicotine transdermal (℞)
Clear Nicoderm CQ, Habitrol, Nicoderm CQ, Nicotrol
Func. class.: Smoking deterrent
Chem. class.: Ganglionic cholinergic agonist

Action: Agonist at nicotinic receptors in peripheral, central nervous systems; acts at sympathetic ganglia, on chemoreceptors of aorta, carotid bodies; also affects adrenalin-releasing catecholamines
Uses: Deter cigarette smoking
Investigational uses: Gilles de la Tourette's syndrome

DOSAGE AND ROUTES

Nicotine chewing gum
• *Adult:* Gum 1 piece chewed × ½ hr as needed to abstain from smoking, not to exceed 30/day
Nicotine inhaler
• *Adult:* INH 6 cartridges/day for first 3-6 wk, max 16/day × 12 wk
Nicotine nasal spray
• *Adults:* 1 spray in each nostril 1-2 ×/hr, max 5 ×/hr or 40 ×/day, max 3 mo
Nicotine transdermal/inhaler system
• *Habitrol, Nicoderm:* 21 mg/day × 4-8 wk; 14 mg/day × 2-4 wk; 7 mg/day × 2-4 wk
• *Nicotrol:* 15 mg/day × 12 wk; 10 mg/day × 2 wk; 5 mg/day × 2 wk
• *Nicotrol Inhaler:* delivers 30% of what

a smoker receives from an actual cigarette
Gilles de la Tourette's syndrome (off-label)
• *Adult/child:* Chewing gum: 2 mg chewed × ½ hr bid for 1-6 mo; TD: 7- or 10-mg patch daily × 2 days
Available forms: Transdermal patch delivering 7, 14, 21 mg/day (Habitrol, Nicoderm, nicotine transdermal system); 5, 10, 15 mg/day (Nicoderm); nicotine inhaler: 4 mg delivered; nasal spray: 0.5 mg nicotine/actuation; gum: 2 mg/piece

SIDE EFFECTS

CNS: Dizziness, vertigo, insomnia, headache, confusion, convulsions, depression, euphoria, numbness, tinnitus, strange dreams
CV: Dysrhythmias, tachycardia, palpitations, edema, flushing, hypertension
EENT: Jaw ache, irritation in buccal cavity
GI: Nausea, vomiting, anorexia, indigestion, diarrhea, abdominal pain, constipation, eructation
RESP: Breathing difficulty, cough, hoarseness, sneezing, wheezing
Contraindications: Pregnancy (X), gum; (D), transdermal; hypersensitivity, immediate post MI recovery period, severe angina pectoris
Precautions: Vasospastic disease, dysrhythmias, diabetes mellitus, hyperthyroidism, pheochromocytoma, coronary disease, esophagitis, peptic ulcer, lactation, hepatic/renal disease

PHARMACOKINETICS

Onset 15-30 min, metabolized in liver, excreted in urine, half-life 2-3 hr, 30-120 hr (terminal)

INTERACTIONS

Smoking cessation increases diuretic effects of furosemide
Increase: absorption—SUBCUT insulin
Increase: blood levels with cessation of smoking—caffeine, theophylline, pentazocine, imipramine, oxazepam, propranolol, acetaminophen

⚠ Safety alert   *"Tall Man" lettering

Decrease: absorption—glutethimide
Decrease: metabolism of propoxyphene
Drug/Herb
Increase: effect—blue cohosh, lobelia
Decrease: effect—oats

NURSING CONSIDERATIONS

Assess:
• Adverse reaction: irritation of buccal cavity, dislike of taste, jaw ache

Administer:
Gum
• Chew gum slowly for 30 min to promote buccal absorption of the drug; do not chew over 45 min
• Begin drug withdrawal after 3 mo use; do not exceed 6 mo

Transdermal patch
• Once a day to a nonhairy, clean, dry area of skin on upper body or upper outer arm; rotate sites to prevent skin irritation

Inhaler
• Puffing on mouthpiece delivers nicotine through the mouth

Evaluate:
• Therapeutic response: decrease in urge to smoke, decreased need for gum after 3-6 mo

Teach patient/family:
Gum
• All aspects of drug use; give package insert to patient and explain
• That gum will not stick to dentures, dental appliances
• That gum is as toxic as cigarettes; to be used only to deter smoking
• Not to use during pregnancy; birth defects may occur

Transdermal patch
• That patch is as toxic as cigarettes; to be used only to deter smoking
• Not to use during pregnancy; birth defects may occur
• To keep used and unused system out of reach of children and pets
• To stop smoking immediately when beginning patch treatment
• To apply promptly after removing from protective patch; system may lose strength

---

*NIFEdipine (℞)

(nye-fed′i-peen)
Adalat, Adalat CC,
Apo-Nifed ✿, NIFEdipine,
Novo-Nifedin ✿, Nu-Nifedin ✿,
Procardia, Procardia XL
Func. class.: Calcium-channel blocker, antianginal, antihypertensive
Chem. class.: Dihydropyridine

Do not confuse:
NIFEdipine/niCARdipine
Action: Inhibits calcium ion influx across cell membrane during cardiac depolarization; relaxes coronary vascular smooth muscle; dilates coronary arteries; increases myocardial oxygen delivery in patients with vasospastic angina; dilates peripheral arteries
Uses: Chronic stable angina pectoris, vasospastic angina, hypertension
Investigational uses: Migraines, CHF, Raynaud's disease, anal fissures, preterm labor

DOSAGE AND ROUTES

• *Adult:* **PO** immediate release 10 mg tid, increase in 10 mg increments q7-14d, not to exceed 180 mg/24 hr or single dose of 30 mg; **SUS REL** 30-60 mg daily, may increase q7-14d, doses >120 mg not recommended
• *Child:* **PO** 0.25-0.5 mg/kg/dose q4-6h, max 1-2 mg/kg/day
Available forms: Caps 5, 10, 20 mg; tabs, ext rel (CC, XL) 10 ✿, 20 ✿, 30, 60, 90 mg; tabs 10 mg

SIDE EFFECTS

CNS: Headache, fatigue, drowsiness, dizziness, anxiety, depression, weakness, insomnia, light-headedness, paresthesia, tinnitus, blurred vision, nervousness, tremor
CV: **Dysrhythmias,** edema, hypotension, palpitations, tachycardia
GI: Nausea, vomiting, diarrhea, gastric

---

upset, constipation, increased LFTs, dry mouth, flatulence, gingival hyperplasia, *hepatotoxicity*
GU: Nocturia, polyuria
INTEG: Rash, pruritus, flushing, hair loss
MISC: Sexual difficulties, cough, fever, chills
SYST: Stevens-Johnson syndrome
Contraindications: Hypersensitivity
Precautions: Pregnancy (C), CHF, hypotension, sick sinus syndrome, 2nd-, 3rd-degree heart block, hypotension less than 90 mm Hg systolic, hepatic injury, lactation, children, renal disease

PHARMACOKINETICS

Well-absorbed PO
PO-ER: Duration 24 hr
PO: Onset 20 min, peak 0.5-6 hr, duration 6-8 hr, half-life 2-5 hr
Metabolized by liver, excreted in urine 60-80% (metabolites); feces 15%

INTERACTIONS

Increase: level of—digoxin, phenytoin, cyclosporine, prazosin, carbamazepine
Increase: NIFEdipine, toxicity—cimetidine, ranitidine
Increase: effects of β-blockers, antihypertensives
Decrease: antihypertensive effect—NSAIDs
Decrease: effects of quinidine
Decrease: NIFEdipine level—smoking
Drug/Herb
Increase: effect—barberry, betel palm, burdock, goldenseal, khat, khella, lily of the valley, plantain
Decrease: effect—yohimbe
Food/Drug
Increase: NIFEdipine level—grapefruit juice
Drug/Lab Test
Increase: CPK, LDH, AST
Positive: ANA, direct Coombs' test

NURSING CONSIDERATIONS

Assess:
• Anginal pain: location, intensity, duration, character, alleviating, aggravating factors

• Cardiac status: B/P, pulse, respiration, ECG
• Potassium, renal/hepatic studies periodically during treatment
Administer:
• Do not break, crush, or chew ext rel tabs
• Without regard to meals
• SL: may puncture liquid-filled cap and squeeze drug into buccal pouch
Evaluate:
• Therapeutic response: decreased anginal pain, B/P, activity tolerance
Teach patient/family:
• To avoid hazardous activities until stabilized on drug, dizziness is no longer a problem
• To limit caffeine consumption; take no alcohol products
• To avoid OTC drugs unless directed by a prescriber
• That ext rel nonabsorbable shell may appear in stools
• To comply with all areas of medical regimen: diet, exercise, stress reduction, drug therapy
• To change position slowly; orthostatic hypotension is common
⚠ To notify prescriber of dyspnea, edema of extremities, nausea, vomiting, severe ataxia, severe rash
• To increase fluid intake to prevent constipation
• To check for gingival hyperplasia and report promptly
Treatment of overdose: Defibrillation, atropine for AV block, vasopressor for hypotension

---

nilutamide
(nye-loo'ta-mide)
Anandron ✦, Nilandron
Func. class.: Antineoplastic-hormone
Chem. class.: Antiandrogen

Action: Interferes with testosterone uptake in the nucleus or testosterone activity in target tissues; arrests tumor growth in androgen-sensitive tissue (e.g., prostate gland); prostatic carcinoma is androgen-sensitive, so tumor growth is arrested

Uses: Metastatic prostatic carcinoma, stage D2 in combination with surgical castration

DOSAGE AND ROUTES

• *Adult:* **PO** 300 mg daily × 30 days, then 150 mg daily

Available forms: Tabs 100 ♣, 150 mg

SIDE EFFECTS

CNS: Hot flashes, drowsiness, insomnia, dizziness, hyperthesia, depression
EENT: Delay in adaptation to dark
GI: Diarrhea, nausea, vomiting, increased liver function studies, constipation, dyspepsia, ***hepatotoxicity***
GU: Decreased libido, impotence, testicular atrophy, UTI, hematuria, nocturia, gynecomastia
HEMA: Anemia
INTEG: Rash, sweating, alopecia, dry skin
MISC: Edema
RESP: Dyspnea, URI, pneumonia, ***interstitial pneumonitis***

Contraindications: Hypersensitivity, severe hepatic impairment, severe respiratory disease, women

Precautions: Pregnancy (C)

PHARMACOKINETICS

Rapidly and completely absorbed; excreted in urine and feces as metabolites

INTERACTIONS

Increase: toxicity of vit K, phenytoin, theophylline

NURSING CONSIDERATIONS
Assess:

⚠ Hepatic studies: AST, ALT, alk phosphatase, which may be elevated; if elevated 3× normal, discontinue drug
• For CNS symptoms: drowsiness, insomnia, dizziness
• Chest x-rays, routinely, baseline pulmonary function studies, dyspnea,

cough, which may indicate interstitial pneumonitis; discontinue treatment if this condition is suspected
• For hyperglycemia, increased BUN, creatinine, alk phosphatase leukopenia

Administer:
• Without regard to meals

Perform/provide:
• Storage at room temperature

Evaluate:
• Therapeutic response: decrease in prostatic tumor size, decrease in spread of cancer

Teach patient/family:
⚠ To report side effects: decreased libido, impotence, breast enlargement, hot flashes, diarrhea, dyspnea, cough, shortness of breath; if SOB occurs notify prescriber immediately
⚠ To report signs of hepatotoxicity: dark urine, abdominal pain, clay-colored stools, jaundice eyes, skin
• To wear tinted lens to alleviate delay in adapting to the dark
• That drug is started on day of or day after surgical castration
• To avoid alcohol consumption

Treatment of overdose: Induce vomiting, provide supportive care

nisoldipine
(nye-sole'dih-peen)
Sular
Func. class.: Calcium channel blocker, antihypertensive
Chem. class.: Dihydropyridine

Action: Inhibits calcium ion influx across cell membrane, resulting in dilation of peripheral arteries
Uses: Essential hypertension, alone or with other antihypertensives

DOSAGE AND ROUTES

• *Adult:* **PO** 20 mg daily initially, may increase by 10 mg/wk, usual dose 20-40 mg daily, max 60 mg/day

• *Geriatric/hepatic dose:* **PO** 10 mg/day, increase by 10 mg/wk

Available forms: Tabs, ext rel 10, 20, 30, 40 mg

SIDE EFFECTS

CNS: Headache, fatigue, drowsiness, dizziness, anxiety, depression, nervousness, insomnia, light-headedness, paresthesia, tinnitus, psychosis, somnolence, ataxia, confusion, malaise, migraine
CV: Dysrhythmia, edema, CHF, hypotension, palpitations, *MI, pulmonary edema,* tachycardia, syncope, AV block, angina, chest pain, ECG abnormalities
GI: Nausea, vomiting, diarrhea, gastric upset, constipation, increased LFTs, dry mouth, dyspepsia, dysphagia, flatulence
GU: Nocturia, hematuria, dysuria
HEMA: Anemia, leukopenia, petechia
INTEG: Rash, pruritus
MISC: Sexual difficulties, cough, nasal congestion, SOB, wheezing, epistaxis, dyspnea, gingival hyperplasia, chills, fever, gout, sweating

Contraindications: Hypersensitivity, sick sinus syndrome, 2nd-, 3rd-degree heart block

Precautions: Pregnancy (C), CHF, hypotension <90 mm Hg systolic, hepatic injury, lactation, children, renal disease, elderly, acute MI, unstable angina

PHARMACOKINETICS

Metabolized by liver, excreted in urine, peak 6-12 hr, highly protein bound

INTERACTIONS

Increase: effects of β-blockers, antihypertensives, digitalis
Increase: nisoldipine level—cimetidine, ranitidine, azole antifungals
Decrease: nisoldipine effect—hydantoins

Drug/Herb
Increase: effect—barberry, betel palm, burdock, goldenseal, khat, khella, lily of the valley, plantain
Decrease: effect—yohimbe

Drug/Food
Increase: nisoldipine level—high-fat foods; increased hypotensive effect: grapefruit juice

NURSING CONSIDERATIONS

Assess:
• Cardiac status: B/P, pulse, respiration, ECG
• I&O ratios, weight daily
• For CHF: weight gain, jugular vein distention, edema, crackles

Administer:
• Swallow whole; do not break, crush, or chew
• Once daily as whole tablet; avoid high-fat foods, grapefruit juice

Evaluate:
• Therapeutic response: decreased B/P

Teach patient/family:
• To avoid hazardous activities until stabilized on drug, dizziness is no longer a problem
• To report nausea, dizziness, edema, shortness of breath, palpitations
• To limit caffeine consumption
• To avoid OTC drugs unless directed by a prescriber
• The importance of complying with all areas of medical regimen: diet, exercise, stress reduction, drug therapy
• To rise slowly to prevent orthostatic hypotension

Treatment of overdose: Defibrillation, atropine for AV block, vasopressor for hypotension

---

nitazoxanide (Ŗ)
(nye-taz-ox′a-nide)
Alinia
Func. class.: Antiprotozoal

Action: Interferes with DNA/RNA synthesis in protozoa
Uses: Diarrhea caused by *Cryptosporidium parvum* or *Giardia lamblia*

DOSAGE AND ROUTES

• *Child 4-11 yr:* **PO** 10 ml (200 mg) q12h × 3 days

• *Child 12-47 mos:* **PO** 5 ml (100 mg) q12h × 3 days
Available forms: Powder for oral susp 100 mg/5 ml

SIDE EFFECTS

CNS: Dizziness, fever, headache
CV: Hypotension
GI: Nausea, anorexia, flatulence, increased appetite, enlarged salivary glands, abdominal pain, diarrhea, vomiting
HEMA: Anemia, ***leukopenia,*** neutropenia
INTEG: Pruritus, sweating
MISC: Increased creatinine, pale yellow eye discoloration, rhinitis, discolored urine, infection, malaise
Contraindications: Hypersensitivity
Precautions: Pregnancy (B), renal, hepatic disease, lactation, child <1 yr or >11 yr, diabetes mellitus (contains sucrose)

PHARMACOKINETICS

Excreted in urine, bile, feces; hydrolyzed to active metabolite, which undergoes conjugation; metabolite protein binding >99%

INTERACTIONS

• Competes for binding sites: other highly protein-bound drugs

NURSING CONSIDERATIONS

Assess:
• Signs of infection
• Bowel pattern before, during treatment
Administer:
PO route
• With food
Evaluate:
• Therapeutic response: C&S negative for organism
Teach patient/family:
• To take with food; shake susp well before each dose

---

nitrofurantoin (℞)

(nye-troe-fyoor'an-toyn)
Apo-Nitrofurantoin ✦, Furadantin, Macrobid, Macrodantin, nitrofurantoin
Func. class.: Urinary tract antiinfective
Chem. class.: Synthetic nitrofuran derivative

Action: Appears to inhibit bacterial enzymes

Uses: Urinary tract infections caused by *Escherichia coli, Klebsiella, Pseudomonas, Proteus vulgaris, Proteus morganii, Serratia, Citrobacter, Staphylococcus aureus, Staphylococcus epidermidis, Enterococcus, Salmonella, Shigella*

DOSAGE AND ROUTES

Active infections
• *Adult and child >12 yr:* **PO** 50-100 mg qid pc or 50-100 mg at bedtime for long-term treatment
• *Child 1 mo-3 yr:* **PO** 5-7 mg/kg/day in 4 divided doses; 1-3 mg/kg/day for long-term treatment
Chronic suppression
• *Adult:* **PO** 50-100 mg qPM
• *Child:* **PO** 1 mg/kg/day qPM
Available forms: Caps 25, 50, 100 mg; tabs 50, 100 mg; susp 25 mg/5 ml; macrocrystal caps (Macrodantin) 25, 50, 100 mg; Macrobid cap 100 mg (25 macrocrystals, 75 monohydrate)

SIDE EFFECTS

CNS: Dizziness, headache, drowsiness, peripheral neuropathy, chills
GI: Nausea, vomiting, abdominal pain, diarrhea, ***cholestatic jaundice,*** loss of appetite, ***pseudomembranous colitis***
INTEG: Pruritus, rash, urticaria, angioedema, alopecia, tooth staining
Contraindications: Hypersensitivity, anuria, severe renal disease, infants <1 mo

N

Side effects: *italics* = common; ***bold italics*** = life-threatening

Precautions: Pregnancy (B), lactation, G6PD deficiency, elderly, CCr <60

PHARMACOKINETICS

PO: Half-life 20-60 min; crosses blood-brain barrier, placenta; enters breast milk; excreted as inactive metabolites in liver, unchanged in urine

INTERACTIONS

Antagonistic effect: norfloxacin
Increase: levels of nitrofurantoin—probenecid
Decrease: absorption of magnesium trisilicate antacid

NURSING CONSIDERATIONS

Assess:
• Blood count during chronic therapy
• I&O ratio: C&S before treatment, after completion; symptoms of UTI
• CNS symptoms: insomnia, vertigo, headache, drowsiness, convulsions
• Allergy: fever, flushing, rash, urticaria, pruritus
Administer:
PO route
• Do not break, crush, chew, or open tabs, caps
• After clean-catch urine for C&S
• Two daily doses if urine output is high or if patient has diabetes
Evaluate:
• Therapeutic response: decreased dysuria, fever; neg C&S
Teach patient/family:
• To take with food or milk; avoid alcohol
• To protect susp from freezing and shake well before taking
• That drug may cause drowsiness; instruct client to seek aid in walking and other activities; advise client not to drive or operate machinery while on medication
• That diabetics should monitor blood glucose level
• That drug may turn urine rust-yellow to brown

🅐 To notify prescriber of symptoms of pseudomembranous colitis: fever, diarrhea with mucous, pus, or blood

---

nitrofurazone topical
See Appendix C

---

nitroglycerin (℞)
(nye-troe-gli'ser-in)
transmucosal tablets (℞)
Nitrogard, Nitrogard SR
extended release (℞)
Nitrocot, Nitroglyn E-R, Nitropar, Nitro-Time, Nitrong
extended-release buccal tabs (℞)
Nitrogard, Nitrogard SR ✦
IV (℞)
Nitro-Bid I.V., Tridil
ointment (℞)
Nitro-Bid, Nitrol
SL (℞)
Nitrostat, NitroQuick
spray (℞)
Nitrolingual Translingual Spray
transdermal (℞)
Deponit, Minitran, Nitrek, Nitrocine, Nitrodisc, Nitro-Dur, Transderm-Nitro
Func. class.: Coronary vasodilator, antianginal
Chem. class.: Nitrate

Do not confuse:
Nitro-Bid/Nicobid
Action: Decreases preload, afterload, which is responsible for decreasing left ventricular end-diastolic pressure, systemic vascular resistance; dilates coronary arteries, improves blood flow through coronary vasculature, dilates arterial, venous beds systemically
Uses: Chronic stable angina pectoris, prophylaxis of angina pain, CHF associ-

---

🅐 Safety alert   *"Tall Man" lettering

ated with acute MI, controlled hypotension in surgical procedures

DOSAGE AND ROUTES

• *Adult:* **SL** dissolve tab under tongue when pain begins; may repeat q5min until relief occurs; take no more than 3 tabs/15 min; use 1 tab prophylactically 5-10 min before activities; **SUS CAP** q6-12h on empty stomach; **TOP** 1-2 in q8h, increase to 4 in q4h as needed; **IV** 5 mcg/min, then increase by 5 mcg/min q3-5min; if no response after 20 mcg/min, increase by 10-20 mcg/min until desired response; **TRANS** apply a pad daily to a site free of hair; remove patch at bedtime to provide 10-12h nitrate-free interval to avoid tolerance

• *Child:* **IV** initial: 0.25-0.5 mcg/kg/min, titrate to patient response, usual dose 1-3 mcg/kg/min transmucosal

Available forms: Buccal tabs 1, 2, 3 mg; translingual aero 0.4 mg/metered spray; sus rel caps 2.5, 6.5, 9, 13 mg; tabs, sus rel 2.6, 6.5, 9 mg; SL tabs 0.3, 0.4, 0.6 mg; oint 2%; trans syst 0.1, 0.2, 0.3, 0.4, 0.6, 0.8 mg/hr; inj sol 25 mg/250 ml, 50 mg/250 ml, 50 mg/500 ml, 100 mg/250 ml, 200 mg/500 ml

SIDE EFFECTS

CNS: Headache, flushing, dizziness
*CV: Postural hypotension, tachycardia, **collapse**, syncope, palpitations*
GI: Nausea, vomiting
INTEG: Pallor, sweating, rash
Contraindications: Hypersensitivity to this drug or nitrites, severe anemia, increased intracranial pressure, cerebral hemorrhage, closed-angle glaucoma
Precautions: Pregnancy (C), postural hypotension, lactation, children, severe hepatic/renal disease

PHARMACOKINETICS

SUS REL: Onset 20-45 min, duration 3-8 hr
SL: Onset 1-3 min, duration 30 min
TRANSDERMAL: Onset ½-1 hr, duration 12-24 hr

IV: Onset 1-2 min, duration 3-5 min
TRANSMUC: Onset 1-2 min, duration 3-5 hr
AEROSOL: Onset 2 min, duration 30-60 min
TOP OINT: Onset 30-60 min, duration 2-12 hr
Metabolized by liver, excreted in urine, half-life 1-4 min

INTERACTIONS

Severe hypotension, CV collapse: alcohol
Increase: effects of β-blockers, diuretics, antihypertensives, calcium channel blockers
Increase: hypotension—sildenafil, tadalafil, vardenafil
Increase: nitrate level—aspirin
Decrease: heparin—IV nitroglycerin

NURSING CONSIDERATIONS

Assess:
• Orthostatic B/P, pulse
• Pain: duration, time started, activity being performed, character
• Tolerance if taken over long period
• Headache, light-headedness, decreased B/P; may indicate a need for decreased dosage

Administer:
PO route
• Swallow sus rel whole; do not break, crush, or chew
• With 8 oz H_2O on empty stomach (oral tablet) 1 hr before or 2 hr after meals
• SL should be dissolved under tongue, not swallowed
• Aerosol sprayed under tongue, not inhaled

Transdermal route
• Transmucosal tab should be placed between cheek and gum line
• Topical ointment should be measured on papers supplied
• Apply a new TD patch daily and remove after 12-14 hr to prevent tolerance

IV route
• Diluted in amount specified D_5, D_5W, 0.9% NaCl for infusion; use glass infusion

N

bottles, non–polyvinyl chloride infusion tubing; titrate to patient response; do not use filters

Y-site compatibilities: Amiodarone, amphotericin B cholesteryl, amrinone, atracurium, cefmetazole, cisatracurium, diltiazem, DOBUTamine, DOPamine, epINEPHrine, esmolol, famotidine, fentanyl, fluconazole, furosemide, haloperidol, heparin, hydromorphone, insulin (regular), labetalol, lidocaine, lorazepam, midazolam, milrinone, morphine, niCARdipine, norepinephrine, pancuronium, propofol, ranitidine, remifentanil, sodium nitroprusside, streptokinase, tacrolimus, theophylline, thiopental, vecuronium, warfarin

Evaluate:

• Therapeutic response: decrease, prevention of anginal pain

Teach patient/family:

• To place buccal tab between lip and gum above incisors or between cheek and gum

• To keep tabs in original container

• If 3 SL tabs in 15 min do not relieve pain, to seek immediate medical attention

• To avoid alcohol

• That drug may cause headache; tolerance usually develops; use nonopioid analgesic

• That drug may be taken before stressful activity: exercise, sexual activity

• That SL may sting when drug comes in contact with mucous membranes

• To avoid hazardous activities if dizziness occurs

• To comply with complete medical regimen

• To make position changes slowly to prevent fainting

> ### ⚠ High Alert
>
> **nitroprusside (℞)**
> (nye-troe-pruss'ide)
> Nitropress, sodium nitroprusside
> *Func. class.:* Antihypertensive, vasodilator

Action: Directly relaxes arteriolar, venous smooth muscle, resulting in reduction in cardiac preload, afterload

Uses: Hypertensive crisis, to decrease bleeding by creating hypotension during surgery, acute CHF

DOSAGE AND ROUTES

• *Adult:* IV INF dissolve 50 mg in 2-3 ml of D_5W, then dilute in 250-1000 ml of D_5W; run at 0.5-8 mcg/kg/min

• *Child:* IV 0.3-0.5 mcg/kg/min, titrate to response

Available forms: Inj 50 mg

SIDE EFFECTS

CNS: Dizziness, headache, agitation, twitching, decreased reflexes, restlessness

CV: Bradycardia, ECG changes, tachycardia

GI: Nausea, vomiting, abdominal pain

INTEG: Pain, irritation at inj site, sweating

MISC: Cyanide, thiocyanate toxicity, flushing, hypothyroidism

Contraindications: Hypersensitivity, hypertension (compensatory) due to aortic coarctation or AV shunting, acute CHF associated with reduced peripheral vascular resistance

Precautions: Pregnancy (C), lactation, children, fluid, electrolyte imbalances, hepatic disease, renal disease, hypothyroidism, elderly

PHARMACOKINETICS

IV: Onset 1-2 min, duration 1-10 min, half-life 3 days in patients with abnormal renal function, circulating half-life 2 min; metabolized in liver, excreted in urine

---

⚠ Safety alert   *"Tall Man" lettering

INTERACTIONS

Severe hypotension: ganglionic blockers, volatile liquid anesthetics, halothane, enflurane, circulatory depressants

Drug/Herb

Increase: toxicity, death—aconite
Increase: antihypertensive effect—barberry, betony, black catechu, black cohosh, bloodroot, broom, burdock, cat's claw, dandelion, goldenseal, Irish moss, Jamaican dogwood, kelp, khella, mistletoe, parsley
Increase or decrease: antihypertensive effect—astragalus, cola tree
Decrease: antihypertensive effect—coltsfoot, guarana, khat, licorice

NURSING CONSIDERATIONS

Assess:

• Electrolytes: K, Na, Cl, CO_2, CBC, serum glucose, serum methemoglobin if pulmonary O_2 levels are decreased
• Renal studies: catecholamines, BUN, creatinine
• Hepatic studies: AST, ALT, alk phosphatase
• B/P by direct means if possible; check ECG continuously; pulse, jugular vein distention; PCWP; rebound hypertension may occur after nitroprusside is discontinued
• Weight daily, I&O
⚠ Thiocyanate, lactate, cyanide levels if on long-term treatment, thiocyanate level should be ≤1 mmol/L
• Nausea, vomiting, diarrhea
• Edema in feet, legs daily; skin turgor, dryness of mucous membranes for hydration status
• Crackles, dyspnea, orthopnea q30min
• For decrease in bicarbonate, P_{CO_2} blood pH, acidosis

Administer:

IV route

• Depending on B/P reading q15min
• IV after diluting 50 mg/2-3 ml of D_5W, further dilute in 250 ml of D_5W; use an infusion pump only; wrap bottle with aluminum foil to protect from light; observe for color change in the infusion;

discard if highly discolored (blue, green, dark red); titrate to patient response
Syringe compatibilities: Heparin
Y-site compatibilities: Amrinone, atracurium, diltiazem, DOBUTamine, DOPamine, enalaprilat, famotidine, lidocaine, nitroglycerin, pancuronium, tacrolimus, theophylline, vecuronium

Evaluate:

• Therapeutic response: decreased B/P, absence of bleeding

Teach patient/family:

• To report headache, dizziness, loss of hearing, blurred vision, dyspnea, faintness, dizziness

---

nizatidine (otc, ℞)

(ni-za′ti-deen)
Axid, Axid AR
Func. class.: H_2-receptor antagonist
Chem. class.: Substituted thiazole

Action: Blocks H_2-receptors, thereby reducing gastric acid output
Uses: Benign gastric and duodenal ulceration, prevention of duodenal ulcer recurrence, symptomatic relief of gastroesophageal reflux, heartburn prevention

DOSAGE AND ROUTES

Gastric and duodenal ulcer

• *Adult:* **PO** 300 mg at night or 150 mg bid for 4-8 wk; maintenance 150 mg at night

Prophylaxis of duodenal ulcer

• *Adult:* **PO** 150 mg daily at bedtime

Gastroesophageal reflux

• *Adult:* **PO** 150 mg bid

Heartburn prevention

• *Adult:* **PO** 75 mg before eating

Renal dose

• *Adult:* **PO** CCr 20-50 ml/min give 150 mg/day; CCr <20 ml/min give 150 mg every other day

Available forms: Caps 150, 300 mg; tabs 75 mg

SIDE EFFECTS

CNS: Headache, somnolence, confusion, abnormal dreams, dizziness

---

CV: **Cardiac dysrhythmias, cardiac arrest**
ENDO: Gynecomastia
GI: Elevated hepatic enzymes, **hepatitis,** jaundice, nausea
HEMA: **Thrombocytopenia, agranulocytosis, aplastic anemia**
INTEG: Pruritus, sweating, urticaria, **exfoliative dermatitis**
METAB: Hyperuricemia
MS: Myalgia
RESP: **Bronchospasm, laryngeal edema**
Contraindications: Hypersensitivity
Precautions: Pregnancy (B), renal or hepatic impairment (reduce dose in renal impairment), lactation

PHARMACOKINETICS

Partially metabolized by liver, excreted by kidneys, plasma half-life 1½ hr, 70% absorbed orally, small amount (0.1% of plasma concentration) enters breast milk, 35% bound to plasma proteins

NURSING CONSIDERATIONS

Assess:
⚠ CBC with differential if on long-term therapy, agranulocytosis may occur
• Gastric pH (>5 should be maintained)
• Fluid balance, I&O
Administer:
• With meals for prolonged drug effect; antacids 1 hr before or 1 hr after drug
Evaluate:
• Mental status, confusion, dizziness, depression, anxiety, weakness, tremors, psychosis, diarrhea, jaundice, report immediately
• For GI symptoms: nausea, vomiting, diarrhea, cramps
Teach patient/family:
• That gynecomastia, impotence may occur, are reversible
• To avoid driving or other hazardous activities until patient is stabilized on this medication; dizziness may occur
• To avoid black pepper, caffeine, alcohol, harsh spices, extremes in temp of food
• To avoid OTC preparations: aspirin, cough, cold preparations
Treatment of overdose: Symptomatic and supportive therapy is recommended; activated charcoal, emesis, or lavage may reduce absorption

---

⚠ High Alert

norepinephrine (℞)
(nor-ep-i-nef′rin)
Levophed
Func. class.: Adrenergic
Chem. class.: Catecholamine

Do not confuse:
norepinephrine/epINEPHrine
Action: Causes increased contractility and heart rate by acting on β-receptors in heart; also acts on α-receptors, causing vasoconstriction in blood vessels; B/P is elevated, coronary blood flow improves, cardiac output increases
Uses: Acute hypotension, shock

DOSAGE AND ROUTES

• *Adult:* **IV INF** 8-12 mcg/min titrated to B/P
• *Child:* **IV INF** 0.05-0.1 mcg/kg/min titrated to B/P
Available forms: Inj 1 mg/ml

SIDE EFFECTS

CNS: **Headache,** anxiety, dizziness, insomnia, restlessness, tremor
CV: **Palpitations, tachycardia, hypertension, ectopic beats, angina**
GI: **Nausea,** vomiting
GU: Decreased urine output
INTEG: Necrosis, tissue sloughing with extravasation, **gangrene**
RESP: Dyspnea
SYST: **Anaphylaxis**
Contraindications: Hypersensitivity, ventricular fibrillation, tachydysrhythmias, pheochromocytoma
Precautions: Pregnancy (C), lactation, arterial embolism, peripheral vascular

disease, hypertension, hyperthyroidism, elderly, heart disease

PHARMACOKINETICS

IV: Onset 1-2 min; metabolized in liver; excreted in urine (inactive metabolites); crosses placenta

INTERACTIONS

Dysrhythmias: general anesthetics, bretylium

Incompatible with alkaline solutions: sodium, HCO_3^-

Severe hypertension—guanethidine

⚠ Do not use within 2 wk of MAOIs, antihistamines, ergots, methyldopa, oxytocics, tricyclics, guanethidine, or hypertensive crisis may result

Increase: B/P—oxytocics

Increase: pressor effect—tricyclics, MAOIs

Decrease: norepinephrine action—α-blockers

NURSING CONSIDERATIONS

Assess:
• I&O ratio; notify prescriber if output <30 ml/hr
• ECG during administration continuously; if B/P increases, drug is decreased
• B/P and pulse q2-3min after parenteral route
• CVP or PWP during infusion if possible
• For paresthesias and coldness of extremities; peripheral blood flow may decrease
• Inj site: tissue sloughing; administer phentolamine mixed with 0.9% NaCl
• Sulfite sensitivity, which may be life-threatening

Administer:
• Plasma expanders for hypovolemia
• IV after diluting with 500-1000 ml D_5W or D_5/0.9% NaCl; average dilution is 4 mg/1000 ml diluent (4 mcg base/ml); give as infusion 2-3 ml/min; titrate to response
• Using 2-bottle setup so drug may be

discontinued while IV is still running; use infusion pump

Additive compatibilities: Amikacin, calcium chloride, calcium gluconate, cimetidine, corticotropin, dimenhyDRINATE, DOBUTamine, heparin, hydrocortisone, magnesium sulfate, meropenem, methylPREDNISolone, multivitamins, netilmicin, potassium chloride, succinylcholine, verapamil, vit B/C

Syringe compatibilities: Heparin

Y-site compatibilities: Amiodarone, amrinone, cisatracurium, diltiazem, DOBUTamine, DOPamine, epINEPHrine, esmolol, famotidine, fentanyl, furosemide, haloperidol, heparin, hydrocortisone, hydromorphone, labetalol, lorazepam, meropenem, midazolam, milrinone, morphine, niCARdipine, nitroglycerin, potassium chloride, propofol, ranitidine, remifentanil, vecuronium, vit B/C

Perform/provide:
• Storage of reconstituted sol in refrigerator no longer than 24 hr
• Do not use discolored sol

Evaluate:
• Therapeutic response: increased B/P with stabilization

Teach patient/family:
• The reason for drug administration and to report dyspnea, dizziness, chest pain

Treatment of overdose: Administer fluids, electrolyte replacement

---

norethindrone (℞)
(nor-eth-in'drone)
Aygestin, Camila, Errin, Micronor, Nora-BE, Nor-QD
Func. class.: Progestogen
Chem. class.: Progesterone derivative

Action: Inhibits secretion of pituitary gonadotropins, which prevents follicular maturation, ovulation; stimulates growth of mammary tissue; antineoplastic action against endometrial cancer
Uses: Uterine bleeding (abnormal),

Side effects: *italics* = common; ***bold italics*** = life-threatening

amenorrhea, endometriosis, contraception

DOSAGE AND ROUTES

Amenorrhea, abnormal uterine bleeding (Aygestin)
• *Adult:* PO 2.5-10 mg daily days 5-25 of menstrual cycle

Endometriosis (Aygestin)
• *Adult:* PO 5 mg daily × 2 wk, then increased by 2.5 mg daily × 2 wk, up to 15 mg daily

Contraception
• *Adult:* PO 0.35 mg on 1st day of menses, then 0.35 mg daily

Available forms: Tabs 5 mg (Aygestin); tabs 0.35 mg

SIDE EFFECTS

CNS: Dizziness, headache, migraines, depression, fatigue

CV: Hypotension, ***thrombophlebitis***, edema, ***thromboembolism, CVA, stroke, pulmonary embolism, MI***

EENT: Diplopia

GI: Nausea, vomiting, anorexia, cramps, increased weight, ***cholestatic jaundice***

GU: Amenorrhea, cervical erosion, breakthrough bleeding, dysmenorrhea, vaginal candidiasis, breast changes, (gynecomastia, testicular atrophy, impotence), endometriosis, ***spontaneous abortion***

INTEG: Rash, urticaria, acne, hirsutism, alopecia, oily skin, seborrhea, purpura, melasma

META: Hyperglycemia

Contraindications: Pregnancy (X), breast cancer, hypersensitivity, thromboembolic disorders, reproductive cancer, genital bleeding (abnormal, undiagnosed)

Precautions: Lactation, hypertension, asthma, blood dyscrasias, gallbladder disease, CHF, diabetes mellitus, bone disease, depression, migraine headache, convulsive disorders, hepatic disease, renal disease, family history of breast or reproductive tract cancer

PHARMACOKINETICS

PO: Duration 24 hr, excreted in urine, feces, metabolized in liver

INTERACTIONS

Decrease: progestin effect—barbiturates, carbamazepine, fosphenytoin, phenytoin, rifampin

Drug/Herb
Increase: stimulation—black/green tea, coffee, cola nut, guarana, yerba maté
Decrease: contraception—St. John's wort

Drug/Food
Caffeine: increase caffeine level

Drug/Lab Test
Increase: Alk phosphatase, nitrogen (urine), pregnanediol, amino acids, factors VII, VIII, IX, X
Decrease: GTT, HDL

NURSING CONSIDERATIONS

Assess:
• Weight daily: notify prescriber of weekly weight gain >5 lb
• B/P at beginning of treatment and periodically
• I&O ratio; be alert for decreasing urinary output, increasing edema
• Hepatic studies: ALT, AST, bilirubin, periodically during long-term therapy
• Edema, hypertension, cardiac symptoms, jaundice, thromboembolism
• Mental status: affect, mood, behavioral changes, depression
• Hypercalcemia

Administer:
• Titrated dose; use lowest effective dose
• In one dose in AM
• With food or milk to decrease GI symptoms

Perform/provide:
• Storage in dark area

Evaluate:
• Therapeutic response: decreased abnormal uterine bleeding, absence of amenorrhea

Teach patient/family:
• About cushingoid symptoms
• To report breast lumps, vaginal bleed-

ing, amenorrhea, edema, jaundice, dark urine, clay-colored stools, dyspnea, headache, blurred vision, abdominal pain, numbness or stiffness in legs, chest pain; male to report impotence or gynecomastia

• To report suspected pregnancy immediately, to wait ≥3 mo after stopping medication to become pregnant

• To avoid smoking; CV reactions may occur

norfloxacin (℞)
(nor-flox-a-sin)
Noroxin
Func. class.: Urinary antiinfective
Chem. class.: Fluoroquinolone

Action: Interferes with conversion of intermediate DNA fragments into high-molecular-weight DNA in bacteria, inhibits DNA gyrase

Uses: Adult urinary tract infections (including complicated) caused by *Escherichia coli, Enterobacter cloacae, Proteus mirabilis, Klebsiella pneumoniae,* group D strep, indole-positive *Proteus, Citrobacter freundii, Staphylococcus aureus;* uncomplicated gonorrhea

DOSAGE AND ROUTES
Uncomplicated infections
• *Adult:* **PO** 400 mg bid × 3-10 days 1 hr before or 2 hr after meals
Complicated infections
• *Adult:* **PO** 400 mg bid × 10-21 days; 400 mg daily × 7-10 days in impaired renal function
Uncomplicated gonorrhea
• *Adult:* **PO** 800 mg as a single dose
Prostatitis
• *Adult:* **PO** 400 mg bid × 4 wk
Renal dose
• *Adult:* **PO** CCr ≤30 ml/min 400 mg **PO** daily
Available forms: Tabs 400 mg

SIDE EFFECTS
CNS: Headache, dizziness, fatigue, somnolence, depression, insomnia
EENT: Visual disturbances
GI: Nausea, constipation, increased ALT, AST, flatulence, heartburn, vomiting, diarrhea, dry mouth
INTEG: Rash

Contraindications: Hypersensitivity to quinolones
Precautions: Pregnancy (C), lactation, children, renal disease, seizure disorders

PHARMACOKINETICS
Peak 1 hr, half-life 3-4 hr; steady state 2 days; excreted in urine as active drug, metabolites

INTERACTIONS
Antagonizes effects of norfloxacin: nitrofurantoin, monitor closely
Possible increase levels, toxicity: theophylline, caffeine, do not use together
Increase: serum concentrations of cycloSPORINE
Increase: norfloxacin level—probenecid
Increase: anticoagulation—warfarin
Decrease: norfloxacin effect—antacids, iron products, sucralfate; give 2 hr apart
Drug/Lab Test
Increase: AST, ALT, BUN, creatinine, alk phosphatase

NURSING CONSIDERATIONS
Assess:
• Renal, hepatic studies: BUN, creatinine, AST, ALT
• I&O ratio
• CNS symptoms: insomnia, vertigo, headache, agitation, confusion
• Allergic reactions: fever, flushing, rash, urticaria, pruritus
Administer:
• After clean-catch urine for C&S
• Two daily doses if urine output is high or if patient has diabetes
Evaluate:
• Therapeutic response: decreased pain,

N

frequency, urgency, C&S, absence of infection

Teach patient/family:

• That if dizziness occurs, to walk, perform activities with assistance

• To complete full course of drug therapy, to take at same time of day

• To contact prescriber if adverse reaction occurs

• To take 1 hr before or 2 hr after meals; not to take antacids with or within 2 hr of this drug; to sip water or use hard candy for dry mouth

---

norfloxacin ophthalmic
See Appendix C

---

norgestrel (R)
(nor-jess'trel)
Ovrette
Func. class.: Progestogen
Chem. class.: Progesterone derivative

Action: Inhibits secretion of pituitary gonadotropins, which prevents follicular maturation, ovulation, stimulates growth of mammary tissue, antineoplastic action against endometrial cancer

Uses: Female contraception

DOSAGE AND ROUTES

• *Adult:* PO 1 tab daily
Available forms: Tabs 0.075 mg

SIDE EFFECTS

CNS: Dizziness, headache, migraines, depression, fatigue

CV: Hypotension, *thrombophlebitis,* edema, *thromboembolism, stroke, pulmonary embolism, myocardial infarction*

EENT: Diplopia

GI: Nausea, vomiting, anorexia, cramps, increased weight, *cholestatic jaundice*

GU: Amenorrhea, cervical erosion, breakthrough bleeding, dysmenorrhea,

vaginal candidiasis, breast changes, *gynecomastia, testicular atrophy, impotence,* endometriosis, ***spontaneous abortion***

INTEG: Rash, urticaria, acne, hirsutism, alopecia, oily skin, seborrhea, purpura, melasma

META: Hyperglycemia

Contraindications: Pregnancy (X), lactation, breast cancer, hypersensitivity, thromboembolic disorders, reproductive cancer, genital bleeding (abnormal, undiagnosed), cerebral hemorrhage

Precautions: Hypertension, asthma, blood dyscrasias, gallbladder disease, CHF, diabetes mellitus, bone disease, depression, migraine headache, convulsive disorders, hepatic disease, renal disease, family history of breast or reproductive tract cancer

PHARMACOKINETICS

PO: Duration 24 hr; excreted in urine, feces; metabolized in liver

Drug/Lab Test
Increase: Alk phosphatase, nitrogen (urine), pregnanediol, amino acids, factors VII, VIII, IX, X
Decrease: GTT, HDL

NURSING CONSIDERATIONS

Assess:

• Weight daily; notify prescriber of weekly weight gain >5 lb

• B/P at beginning of treatment and periodically

• I&O ratio; be alert for decreasing urinary output, increasing edema

• Hepatic studies: ALT, AST, bilirubin, periodically during long-term therapy

• Edema, hypertension, cardiac symptoms, jaundice

• Mental status: affect, mood, behavioral changes, depression

• Hypercalcemia

Administer:

• Titrated dose; use lowest effective dose

• In one dose in AM

A Safety alert   *"Tall Man" lettering

- With food or milk to decrease GI symptoms
- After warming to dissolve crystals

Perform/provide:
- Storage in dark area

Evaluate:
- Therapeutic response: absence of pregnancy

Teach patient/family:
- About cushingoid symptoms
- To report breast lumps, vaginal bleeding, edema, jaundice, dark urine, clay-colored stools, dyspnea, headache, blurred vision, abdominal pain, numbness or stiffness in legs, chest pain
- To report suspected pregnancy, to wait ≥3 mo after stopping medication to get pregnant
- To monitor blood glucose if diabetic

---

nortriptyline (℞)

(nor-trip'ti-leen)
Aventyl, Pamelor
Func. class.: Antidepressant, tricyclic
Chem. class.: Dibenzocycloheptene—secondary amine

Do not confuse:
nortriptyline/amitriptyline
Action: Blocks reuptake of norepinephrine, serotonin into nerve endings, increasing action of norepinephrine, serotonin in nerve cells
Uses: Major depression
Investigational uses: Chronic pain management

DOSAGE AND ROUTES

- *Adult:* **PO** 25 mg tid or qid; may increase to 150 mg/day; may give daily dose at bedtime
- *Geriatric:* **PO** 10-25 mg at bedtime, increase by 10-25 mg at weekly intervals to desired dose; usual maintenance 75 mg
Available forms: Caps 10, 25, 50, 75 mg; sol 10 mg/5 ml

SIDE EFFECTS

CNS: Dizziness, drowsiness, confusion, headache, anxiety, tremors, stimulation, weakness, insomnia, nightmares, EPS (elderly), increased psychiatric symptoms
*CV: Orthostatic hypotension, ECG changes, tachycardia, **hypertension,*** palpitations
EENT: Blurred vision, tinnitus, mydriasis
GI: Constipation, dry mouth, nausea, vomiting, ***paralytic ileus,*** increased appetite, cramps, epigastric distress, jaundice, ***hepatitis,*** stomatitis
*GU: Urinary retention, **acute renal failure***
*HEMA: **Agranulocytosis, thrombocytopenia, eosinophilia, leukopenia***
INTEG: Rash, urticaria, sweating, pruritus, photosensitivity
Contraindications: Hypersensitivity to tricyclics, recovery phase of MI, convulsive disorders, prostatic hypertrophy
Precautions: Pregnancy (C), suicidal patients, severe depression, increased intraocular pressure, narrow-angle glaucoma, urinary retention, cardiac disease, hepatic disease, hyperthyroidism, electroshock therapy, elective surgery, lactation, children

PHARMACOKINETICS

PO: Steady state 4-19 days; metabolized by liver; excreted by kidneys; crosses placenta; excreted in breast milk; half-life 18-28 hr

INTERACTIONS

Heavy smoking: decreased drug effect
⚠ Hyperpyretic crisis, convulsions, hypertensive episode: MAOI
Increase: effects of direct-acting sympathomimetics (epINEPHrine), alcohol, barbiturates, benzodiazepines, CNS depressants
Decrease: effects of guanethidine, clonidine, indirect-acting sympathomimetics (epHEDrine)

N

Drug/Herb

Serotonin syndrome: SAM-e, St. John's wort

Increase: anticholinergic effect—belladonna, corkwood, henbane, jimsonweed

Increase: antidepressant action—scopolia

Increase: CNS effect—hops, lavender

Drug/Lab Test

Increase: Serum bilirubin, blood glucose, alk phosphatase

Decrease: VMA, 5-HIAA

False increase: Urinary catecholamines

NURSING CONSIDERATIONS

Assess:

• B/P (lying, standing), pulse q4h; if systolic B/P drops 20 mm Hg, hold drug, notify prescriber; take vital signs q4h in patients with cardiovascular disease

• Blood studies: CBC, leukocytes, differential, cardiac enzymes if patient is receiving long-term therapy

• Hepatic studies: AST, ALT, bilirubin

• Weight qwk; appetite may increase with drug

• ECG for flattening of T wave, bundle branch block, AV block, dysrhythmias in cardiac patients

• EPS primarily in elderly: rigidity, dystonia, akathisia

• Mental status changes: mood, sensorium, affect, suicidal tendencies, increase in psychiatric symptoms, depression, panic

• Urinary retention, constipation; constipation is more likely to occur in children

⚠ Withdrawal symptoms: headache, nausea, vomiting, muscle pain, weakness; do not usually occur unless drug was discontinued abruptly

• Alcohol intake; if alcohol is consumed, hold dose until AM

Administer:

• Increased fluids, bulk in diet if constipation occurs

• With food, milk for GI symptoms

• Dosage at bedtime for oversedation during day; may take entire dose at bedtime; elderly may not tolerate once/day dosing

• Gum, hard candy, frequent sips of water for dry mouth

• Concentrate with fruit juice, water, or milk to disguise taste

Perform/provide:

• Storage in tight, light-resistant container at room temperature

• Assistance with ambulation during beginning therapy, since drowsiness/dizziness occurs

• Safety measures including side rails, primarily for elderly

• Checking to see if PO medication swallowed

Evaluate:

• Therapeutic response: decreased depression

Teach patient/family:

• That therapeutic effects may take 2-3 wk

• To use caution in driving, other activities requiring alertness because of drowsiness, dizziness, blurred vision

• To avoid alcohol ingestion, other CNS depressants

• Not to discontinue medication quickly after long-term use; may cause nausea, headache, malaise

• To wear sunscreen or large hat, since photosensitivity occurs

• To report immediately urinary retention

Treatment of overdose: ECG monitoring; induce emesis; lavage, activated charcoal; administer anticonvulsant

---

nystatin (R)

(nye-stat′in)

Mycostatin, Nadostine ✦, Nilstat, Nystex, PMS-Nystatin ✦, Pastilles, nystatin

Func. class.: Antifungal

Chem. class.: Amphoteric polyene

Action: Interferes with fungal DNA replication; binds sterols in fungal cell membrane, which increases permeability, leaking of cell nutrients

---

Uses: Lozenges, oral: *Candida* species causing oral, intestinal infections

DOSAGE AND ROUTES

Oral infection
• *Adult:* **SUSP** 400,000-600,000 units qid, use ½ dose in each side of mouth, swish and swallow
• *Infants:* 200,000 units qid (100,000 units in each side of mouth)
• *Newborn and premature infant:* **SUSP** 100,000 units qid
• *Adult and child:* Troches 200,000-400,000 units qid × up to 2 wk

GI infection
• *Adult:* **PO** 500,000-1,000,000 units tid

Available forms: Tabs 500,000 units; powder 50 million, 150 million, 500 million, 1 billion, 2 billion, 5 billion units; susp 100,000 units per ml; troches 200,000 units

Side effects/adverse reactions:
GI: Nausea, vomiting, anorexia, diarrhea, cramps
INTEG: Rash, urticaria (rare)

Contraindications: Hypersensitivity
Precautions: Pregnancy (B)

PHARMACOKINETICS

PO: Little absorption, excreted in feces

NURSING CONSIDERATIONS

Assess:
• For allergic reaction: rash, urticaria; drug may have to be discontinued
• For predisposing factors: antibiotic therapy, pregnancy, diabetes mellitus, sexual partner infection (vaginal infections)

Administer:
• Oral susp dose by placing ½ in each cheek, then swallow
• Topical dose after cleansing area; mouth may be swabbed

Perform/provide:
• Storage in refrigerator for oral susp; tabs in tight, light-resistant containers at room temperature

Evaluate:
• Therapeutic response: culture negative for *Candida*

Teach patient/family:
• That long-term therapy may be needed to clear infection; to complete entire course of medication
• Using no commercial mouthwashes for mouth infection
• Shake susp before measuring each dose
• To notify prescriber of irritation; drug may have to be discontinued

---

nystatin topical
See Appendix C

---

nystatin vaginal antifungal
See Appendix C

---

octreotide (℞)
(ok-tree′oh-tide)
Sandostatin, Sandostatin LAR Depot
Func. class.: Hormone, antidiarrheal
Chem. class.: Octapeptide

Action: A potent growth hormone similar to somatostatin

Uses: Sandostatin: acromegaly, improves symptoms in carcinoid tumors, vasoactive intestinal peptide tumors (VIPomas); LAR Depot: long-term maintenance of acromegaly, carcinoid tumors, VIPomas

Investigational uses: GI fistula, variceal bleeding, diarrheal conditions, pancreatic fistula, irritable bowel syndrome, dumping syndrome

DOSAGE AND ROUTES

Acromegaly
• *Adult:* **SUBCUT/IV** 50-100 mcg tid, adjust q2wk based on growth hormone

---

levels (Sandostatin), or **IM** 20 mg q4wk × 3 mo, adjust by growth hormone levels (Sandostatin LAR)

VIPomas
• *Adult:* **SUBCUT/IV** 0.2-0.3 mg daily in 2-4 doses for 2 wk, not to exceed 0.45 mg daily (Sandostatin), or **IM** 20 mg q2wk × 2 mo, adjust dose (Sandostatin LAR)

Carcinoid tumors
• *Adult:* **SUBCUT/IV** 0.1-0.6 mg daily in 2-4 doses for 2 wk, titrated to patient response (Sandostatin), or **IM** 20 mg q4wk × 2 mo, adjust dose (Sandostatin LAR)

GI fistula
• *Adult:* **SUBCUT** 50-200 mcg q8h

Antidiarrheal in AIDS patients
• *Adult:* **SUBCUT/IV** 100-1800 mcg/day

Irritable bowel syndrome
• *Adult:* **SUBCUT** 100 mcg single dose to 125 mcg bid

Dumping syndrome
• *Adult:* **SUBCUT** 50-150 mcg/day

Variceal bleeding
• *Adult:* **IV** 25-50 mcg/hr CONT **IV** INF for 18 hr-5 days

Available forms: Sandostatin: inj 0.05, 0.1, 0.2, 0.5, 1 mg/ml; LAR depot: inj 10, 20, 30 mg/5 ml

SIDE EFFECTS

CNS: Headache, dizziness, fatigue, weakness, depression, anxiety, tremors, *seizure,* paranoia

CV: Sinus bradycardia, conduction abnormalities, dysrhythmias, chest pain, SOB, thrombophlebitis, ischemia, *CHF,* hypertension, palpitations

ENDO: Hyperglycemia, ketosis, hypothyroidism, hypoglycemia, galactorrhea, diabetes insipidus

GI: Diarrhea, nausea, abdominal pain, vomiting, flatulence, distention, constipation, hepatitis, increased LFTs, *GI bleeding, pancreatitis*

GU: UTI, pollakiuria

HEMA: Hematoma of inj site, bruise

INTEG: Rash, urticaria, pain; inflammation at inj site

MS: Joint and muscle pain

Contraindications: Hypersensitivity

Precautions: Pregnancy (B), diabetes mellitus, hypothyroidism, elderly, lactation, children, renal disease

PHARMACOKINETICS

Absorbed rapidly, completely, peak ½ hr, half-life 1.7 hr, duration 12 hr, excreted unchanged in urine

INTERACTIONS

CycloSPORINE: Possible increase rejection

Drug/Food

Decreased: absorption of dietary fat, decreased vit B_{12} levels

NURSING CONSIDERATIONS

Assess:

• Growth hormone antibodies, IGF-1, 1-4 hr intervals for 8-12 hr post dose in acromegaly; 5-HIAA, plasma serotonin, plasma substance P in carcinoid; VIP in VIPomas

• Thyroid function tests: T_3, T_4, T_7, TSH to identify hypothyroidism

• Fecal fat, serum carotene

• Allergic reaction: rash, itching, fever, nausea, wheezing

• For cardiac status: bradycardia, conduction abnormalities, dysrhythmias; monitor ECG for QT prolongation, low voltage, axis shifts, early repolarization, R/S transition, early wave progression

Administer:

SUBCUT route

• Rotate inj site, use hip, thigh, abdomen

• Avoid using medication that is cold; allow to reach room temperature

IM route

• Reconstitute with diluent provided; give into gluteal

IV route

• May use IV bolus if required; give over 3 min

• To use by intermittent infusion, dilute in 50-200 ml D_5W, 0.9% NaCl; give 15-30 min

Perform/provide:

• Storage in refrigerator for unopened amps, vials; or room temperature for 2 wk, protect from light; do not use discolored or cloudy sol

Evaluate:

• Therapeutic response: relief of diarrhea in AIDS, improves symptoms in carcinoid or VIP tumors, data is insufficient if drugs decrease size/rate of tumor growth, decreasing symptoms of acromegaly

Teach patient/family:

• Regular assessments are required
• Regarding SUBCUT inj if patient or other persons will be giving inj
• To change position slowly to prevent orthostatic hypotension

---

ofloxacin (℞)

(o-flox′a-sin)

Floxin

Func. class.: Antiinfective

Chem. class.: Fluoroquinolone

Action: Interferes with conversion of intermediate DNA fragments into high-molecular-weight DNA in bacteria, inhibits DNA gyrase

Uses: Treatment of lower respiratory tract infections (pneumonia, bronchitis), genitourinary infections (prostatitis, UTIs) caused by *Escherichia coli, Klebsiella pneumoniae, Chlamydia trachomatis, Neisseria gonorrhoeae;* skin and skin structure infections; conjunctivitis (ophthalmic) (refer to appendix C)

DOSAGE AND ROUTES

Lower respiratory tract infections/ skin and skin structure infections
• *Adult:* **PO, IV** 400 mg q12h × 10 days

Cervicitis, urethritis
• *Adult:* **PO, IV** 300 mg q12h × 7 days

Prostatitis
• *Adult:* **PO, IV** 300 mg q12h × 6 wk

Acute, uncomplicated gonorrhea
• *Adult:* **PO, IV** 400 mg as a single dose

Urinary tract infection
• *Adult:* **PO, IV** 200-400 mg q12h × 3-10 days

Renal dose
• *Adult:* **PO** CCr 20-50 ml/min give

q24h; CCr <20 ml/min give ½ of dose q24h

Available forms: Tabs 200, 300, 400 mg; inj 20, 40 mg/ml; 200 mg/50 ml; 400 mg/100 ml

SIDE EFFECTS

CNS: Dizziness, headache, fatigue, somnolence, depression, insomnia, lethargy, malaise, *seizures*

EENT: Visual disturbances

GI: Diarrhea, nausea, vomiting, anorexia, flatulence, heartburn, dry mouth, increased AST, ALT, abdominal pain, constipation, *pseudomembranous colitis*

INTEG: Rash, pruritus

SYST: Anaphylaxis, Stevens-Johnson syndrome

Contraindications: Hypersensitivity to quinolones

Precautions: Pregnancy (C), lactation, children, elderly, renal disease, seizure disorders, excessive sunlight

PHARMACOKINETICS

PO: Peak 1-2 hr, half-life 9 hr, steady state 2 days; excreted in urine as active drug, metabolites; 90%-95% bioavailability

INTERACTIONS

May alter blood glucose levels: antidiabetics

Possible theophylline toxicity: theophylline, do not use together

Increase: CNS stimulation, seizures—NSAIDs

Increase: anticoagulation—warfarin

Decrease: absorption—antacids with aluminum, magnesium, iron products, sucralfate, zinc products; separate by 2 hr

Drug/Herb

Increase: effect—cola nut

NURSING CONSIDERATIONS

Assess:

• Renal, hepatic studies: BUN, creatinine, AST, ALT

- CNS symptoms: insomnia, vertigo, headache, agitation, confusion
- Allergic reactions: rash, flushing, urticaria, pruritus

Administer:

PO route

- 2 hr before or 2 hr after antacids, calcium, iron, zinc products
- After clean-catch urine for C&S

IV route

- Dilute to 4 mg/ml with 0.9% NaCl, D_5W, D_5/LR, $D_5/0.9\%$ NaCl, 5% NaCO$_3$, D_5 plasmalyte 56, sodium lactate; give over 1 hr or more

Y-site compatibilities: Ampicillin, cisatracurium, docetaxel, etoposide, gemcitabine, granisetron, linezolid, propofol, remifentanil, thiotepa

Perform/provide:

- Storage for 2 wk refrigerated or 6 mo frozen after reconstitution

Evaluate:

- Therapeutic response: urine culture, absence of symptoms of infection

Teach patient/family:

- That if dizziness or light-headedness occurs, ambulate, perform activities with assistance
- To complete full course of therapy
- To avoid iron- or mineral-containing supplements within 2 hr before or after dose
- To avoid sun exposure, photosensitivity can occur

---

ofloxacin ophthalmic
See Appendix C

---

olanzapine
(oh-lanz'a-peen)
Zyprexa, Zyprexa
IntraMuscular, Zydis
Func. class.: Antipsychotic, neuroleptic
Chem. class.: Thienbenzodiazepine

Action: Unknown; may mediate antipsychotic activity by both dopamine and serotonin type 2 (5-HT2) antagonist; also, may antagonize muscarinic receptors, histaminic (H_1)- and α-adrenergic receptors

Uses: Schizophrenia, acute manic episodes in bipolar disorder

Investigational uses: Dementia related to Alzheimer's disease, OCD

DOSAGE AND ROUTES

Schizophrenia

- *Adult:* **PO** 5-10 mg initially daily, may increase dosage by 5 mg at 1 wk or more intervals; orally disintegrating tabs: open blister pack, place tab on tongue, let disintegrate, swallow
- *Elderly:* **PO** 5 mg, may increase cautiously at 1-wk intervals

Bipolar mania

- *Adult:* **PO** 10-15 mg daily, may increase dose >24 hr, by 5 mg

Agitation associated with schizophrenia, bipolar I mania

- *Adult:* **IM** 10 mg

Available forms: Tab 2.5, 5, 7.5, 10, 15 mg; orally disintegrating tabs 5, 10, 15, 20 mg; powder for inj 10 mg

SIDE EFFECTS

CNS: EPS: pseudoparkinsonism, akathisia, dystonia, tardive dyskinesia, ***seizures,*** headache, ***neuroleptic malignant syndrome (rare),*** somnolence, agitation, nervousness, hostility, *dizziness,* hypertonia, *tremor,* euphoria, confusion, *drowsiness,* fatigue, *abnormal gait, insomnia, fever*

CV: Hypotension, tachycardia, chest pain

ENDO: Increased prolactin levels

GI: Dry mouth, nausea, vomiting, appetite, dyspepsia, anorexia, *constipation,* abdominal pain, *weight gain*
GU: Urinary retention, urinary frequency, enuresis, impotence, amenorrhea, gynecomastia, breast engorgement, premenstrual syndrome
INTEG: Rash
MISC: Peripheral edema, accidental injury, hypertonia
MS: Joint pain, twitching
RESP: Cough, pharyngitis
Contraindications: Hypersensitivity
Precautions: Pregnancy (C), lactation, hypertension, hepatic disease, cardiac disease, elderly

PHARMACOKINETICS

Well absorbed (60%), peak 6 hr, metabolized by liver, glucuronidation/oxidation by CYP1A2 and CYP2D6, excreted in urine (57%), feces (30%), 93% bound to plasma proteins, half-life 21-54 hr, extended in elderly; clearance decreased in women, increased in smokers

INTERACTIONS

Oversedation: other CNS depressants, alcohol, barbiturate anesthetics, antihistamines, sedatives/hypnotics, antidepressants
Increase: olanzapine levels—CYP1A2 inhibitors (fluvoxamine)
Increase: hypotension—antihypertensives, alcohol, diazepam
Increase: anticholinergic effects—anticholinergics
Decrease: olanzapine levels—CYP1A2 inducers: carbamazepine, omeprazole, rifampin
Decrease: antiparkinson activity—levodopa, bromocriptine, other DOPamine agonists

Drug/Herb
Increase: EPS—betel palm, kava
Increase: effect—cola tree, hops, nettle, nutmeg

Drug/Lab Test
Increase: LFTs, prolactin, CPK

NURSING CONSIDERATIONS
Assess:
• Mental status: orientation, mood, behavior, presence of hallucinations and type before initial administration and monthly
• Swallowing of PO medication: check for hoarding or giving of medication to other patients
• I&O ratio; palpate bladder if low urinary output occurs, urinary retention may be the cause especially in elderly
• Bilirubin, CBC
• Urinalysis recommended before, during prolonged therapy
• Affect, orientation, LOC, reflexes, gait, coordination, sleep pattern disturbances
• B/P sitting, standing, lying: take pulse and respirations q4h during initial treatment; establish baseline before starting treatment; report drops of 30 mm Hg; obtain baseline ECG
• Dizziness, faintness, palpitations, tachycardia on rising
⚠ For neuroleptic malignant syndrome: hyperpyrexia, muscle rigidity, increased CPK, altered mental status, for acute dystonia (check chewing, swallowing, eyes, pill rolling)
• EPS, including akathisia (inability to sit still, no pattern to movements), tardive dyskinesia (bizarre movements of the jaw, mouth, tongue, extremities), pseudoparkinsonism (rigidity, tremors, pill rolling, shuffling gait)
• Skin turgor daily
• Constipation, urinary retention daily; increase bulk, H_2O in diet
Administer:
• Antiparkinsonian agent for EPS
• Decreased dose in elderly
PO route
• PO with full glass of water, milk; or with food to decrease GI upset
• Orally disintegrating tabs: open blister pack, place tab on tongue until dissolved, swallow; no water needed
IM route
• Dissolve contents of vials with 2.1 ml

sterile water for injection (5 mg/ml), use immediately

• Do not use IV or SUBCUT

• Inject slowly, deep into muscle mass

Perform/provide:

• Decreased stimuli by dimming light, avoiding loud noises

• Supervised ambulation until stabilized on medication; do not involve in strenuous exercise program because fainting is possible; patient should not stand still for long periods

• Increased fluids, bulk in diet to prevent constipation

• Sips of water, candy, gum for dry mouth

• Storage in tight, light-resistant container

Evaluate:

• Therapeutic response: decrease in emotional excitement, hallucinations, delusion, paranoia, reorganization of patterns of thought, speech

Teach patient/family:

• To use good oral hygiene; frequent rinsing of mouth, sugarless gum, candy, ice chips for dry mouth

• To avoid hazardous activities until drug response is determined

• That orthostatic hypotension occurs often and to rise from sitting or lying position gradually

• To avoid hot tubs, hot showers, tub baths, since hypotension may occur

• To avoid abrupt withdrawal of this drug, or EPS may result; drug should be withdrawn slowly

• To avoid OTC preparations (cough, hay fever, cold) unless approved by prescriber, since serious drug interactions may occur; avoid use with alcohol, CNS depressants; increased drowsiness may occur

• That in hot weather, heat stroke may occur; take extra precautions to stay cool

Treatment of overdose: Lavage if orally ingested; provide airway; do not induce vomiting or use epINEPHrine

olmesartan medoxomil (℞)

(ol-meh-sar'tan)

Benicar

Func. class.: Antihypertensive

Chem. class.: Angiotensin II receptor (type AT$_1$) antagonist

Action: Blocks the vasoconstrictor and aldosterone-secreting effects of angiotensin II; selectively blocks the binding of angiotensin II to the AT$_1$ receptor found in tissues

Uses: Hypertension, alone or in combination with other antihypertensives

DOSAGE AND ROUTES

• *Adult:* **PO,** single agent 20 mg daily initially in patients who are not volume depleted, may be increased to 40 mg daily if needed after 2 wk

Available forms: Tabs 5, 20, 40 mg

SIDE EFFECTS

CNS: Dizziness, fatigue, headache, insomnia

CV: Chest pain, peripheral edema, tachycardia

EENT: Sinusitis, rhinitis, pharyngitis

GI: Diarrhea, abdominal pain

MS: Arthralgia, pain

RESP: Upper respiratory infection, bronchitis

*SYST: **Angioedema***

Contraindications: Pregnancy (D) 2nd/3rd trimesters, hypersensitivity

Precautions: Pregnancy (C) 1st trimester, hypersensitivity to ACE inhibitors; lactation; children; elderly; hepatic disease

PHARMACOKINETICS

Excreted in urine and feces

INTERACTIONS

Drug/Herb

Increase: toxicity, death—aconite

Increase: antihypertensive effect—barberry, betony, black catechu, black cohosh, bloodroot, broom, burdock, cat's claw, dandelion, goldenseal, Irish moss, Jamaican dogwood, kelp, khella, mistletoe, parsley

Increase or decrease: antihypertensive effect—astragalus, cola tree

Decrease: antihypertensive effect—coltsfoot, guarana, khat, licorice

NURSING CONSIDERATIONS

Assess:

• For pregnancy, this drug can cause fetal death when given in pregnancy

• Response and adverse reactions especially in renal disease

• B/P, pulse q4h; note rate, rhythm, quality; electrolytes: K, Na, Cl; baselines in renal, hepatic studies before therapy begins

• Skin turgor, dryness of mucous membranes for hydration status; for angioedema: facial swelling, dyspnea

Administer:

• Without regard to meals

Evaluate:

• Therapeutic response: decreased B/P

Teach patient/family:

• To comply with dosage schedule, even if feeling better

• To notify prescriber of mouth sores, fever, swelling of hands or feet, irregular heartbeat, chest pain

• That excessive perspiration, dehydration, vomiting, diarrhea may lead to fall in blood pressure; to consult prescriber if these occur

• That drug may cause dizziness, fainting; light-headedness may occur

• To rise slowly to sitting or standing position to minimize orthostatic hypotension

• To notify prescriber immediately if pregnant; not to use during lactation

• To avoid all OTC medications, unless approved by prescriber

• To inform all health care providers of medication use

• To use proper technique for obtaining B/P and acceptable parameters

---

olopatadine ophthalmic

See Appendix C

---

olsalazine (℞)

(ohl-sal'ah-zeen)

Dipentum ✦

Func. class.: Antiinflammatory

Chem. class.: Salicylate derivative

Action: Bioconverted to 5-amino-salicylic acid, which decreases inflammation

Uses: Maintenance of remission of ulcerative colitis in patients intolerant to sulfasalazine

DOSAGE AND ROUTES

• *Adult:* **PO** 500 mg bid

Available forms: Caps 250 mg

SIDE EFFECTS

CNS: Headache, hallucinations, depression, vertigo, fatigue, dizziness

GI: Nausea, vomiting, abdominal pain, ***hepatitis,*** diarrhea, bloating

HEMA: ***Leukopenia, neutropenia, thrombocytopenia, agranulocytosis, anemia***

INTEG: Rash, dermatitis, urticaria

Contraindications: Hypersensitivity to salicylates

Precautions: Pregnancy (C), child <14 yr, lactation; impaired hepatic, renal function; severe allergy; bronchial asthma

PHARMACOKINETICS

PO: Partially absorbed, peak 1½ hr, half-life 5-10 hr, excreted in urine as 5-aminosalicylic acid and metabolites, crosses placenta

Drug/Lab Test

False positive: Urinary glucose test

O

NURSING CONSIDERATIONS
Assess:
⚠ Blood dyscrasias: skin rash, fever, sore throat, bruising, bleeding, fatigue, joint pain (rare)

• Allergic reaction: rash, dermatitis, urticaria, pruritus, dyspnea, bronchospasm

Administer:
• Medication after C&S; repeat C&S after full course of medication

• Total daily dose evenly spaced to minimize GI intolerance, with food

Perform/provide:
• Storage in tight, light-resistant container at room temperature

Evaluate:
• Therapeutic response: absence of fever, mucus in stools

---

omalizumab (℞)
(oh-mah-lye-zoo'mab)
Xolair
Func. class.: Monoclonal antibody

Action: Recombinant DNA-derived humanized IgG murine monoclonal antibody that selectively binds to IgE to limit the release of mediators in the allergic response
Uses: Moderate to severe persistent asthma
Investigational uses: Seasonal allergic rhinitis, food allergy

DOSAGE AND ROUTES
• *Adult:* **SUBCUT** 150-375 mg × 2-4 wk, divide inj into 2 sites, if dose is >150 mg; dose is adjusted based on IgE levels, and significant changes in body weight
Available forms: Powder for inj, lyophilized 202.5 mg (150 mg/1.2 ml after reconstitution)

SIDE EFFECTS
INTEG: Pruritus, dermatitis, inj site reactions, rash
MISC: Earache, dizziness, fatigue, pain, ***malignancies***, viral infections, ***anaphylaxis***
MS: Arthralgia, fracture, leg, arm pain
RESP: Sinusitis, upper respiratory infections, pharyngitis
Contraindications: Hypersensitivity to this drug or hamster protein
Precautions: Pregnancy (B), acute attacks of asthma, lactation, children <12 yr, lymphoma, nephrotic disease

PHARMACOKINETICS
Slowly absorbed, peak 7-8 days, half-life 26 days, degradation by liver, excretion in bile

---

INTERACTIONS
None known

NURSING CONSIDERATIONS
Assess:
• Respiratory rate, rhythm, depth; auscultate lung fields bilaterally; notify prescriber of abnormalities

• Allergic reactions: rash, urticaria; drug should be discontinued

Administer:
SUBCUT route
• Given q2-4 wk, product is viscous, if >150 mg is given divide into two sites, the inj may take 5-10 seconds to administer

Evaluate:
• Therapeutic response: ability to breathe more easily

Teach patient/family:
• That improvement will not be immediate

• Not to stop taking or decrease current asthma medications unless instructed by prescriber

• Avoid live virus vaccines while taking this product

---

omeprazole (R)

(oh-mep'ray-zole)

Losec ✤, Prilosec

Func. class.: Antiulcer, proton pump inhibitor

Chem. class.: Benzimidazole

Do not confuse:

Prilosec/Prinivil

Prilosec/Prozac

Prilosec/predniSONE

Action: Suppresses gastric secretion by inhibiting hydrogen/potassium ATPase enzyme system in gastric parietal cell; characterized as gastric acid pump inhibitor, since it blocks final step of acid production

Uses: Gastroesophageal reflux disease (GERD), severe erosive esophagitis, poorly responsive systemic GERD, pathologic hypersecretory conditions (Zollinger-Ellison syndrome, systemic mastocytosis, multiple endocrine adenomas); treatment of active duodenal ulcers with or without antiinfectives for *Helicobacter pylori*

Investigational uses: Posterior laryngitis, enhancing pancreatin

DOSAGE AND ROUTES

Active duodenal ulcers

• *Adult:* **PO** 20 mg daily × 4-8 wk; associated with *H. pylori* 40 mg q AM and clarithromycin 500 mg tid on day 1-14, then 20 mg daily on day 15-28

Severe erosive esophagitis/poorly responsive GERD

• *Adult:* **PO** 20 mg daily × 4-8 wk

Pathologic hypersecretory conditions

• *Adult:* **PO** 60 mg/day; may increase to 120 mg tid; daily doses >80 mg should be divided

Gastric ulcer

• *Adult:* **PO** 40 mg daily 4-8 wk

• *Elderly:* ≤20 mg/day

Laryngitis (unlabeled)

• *Adult:* **PO** 20-40 mg at bedtime × 6-24 wk or 20 mg bid × 4-12 wk

Available forms: Caps, delayed rel 10, 20, 40 mg

SIDE EFFECTS

CNS: Headache, dizziness, asthenia

CV: Chest pain, angina, tachycardia, bradycardia, palpitations, peripheral edema

EENT: Tinnitus, taste perversion

GI: Diarrhea, abdominal pain, vomiting, nausea, constipation, flatulence, acid regurgitation, abdominal swelling, anorexia, irritable colon, esophageal candidiasis, dry mouth

GU: UTI, urinary frequency, increased creatinine, *proteinuria, hematuria,* testicular pain, glycosuria

*HEMA: **Pancytopenia, thrombocytopenia, neutropenia, leukocytosis,*** anemia

INTEG: Rash, dry skin, urticaria, pruritus, alopecia

META: Hypoglycemia, increased hepatic enzymes, weight gain

MISC: Back pain, fever, fatigue, malaise

RESP: Upper respiratory infections, cough, epistaxis

Contraindications: Hypersensitivity

Precautions: Pregnancy (C), lactation, children

PHARMACOKINETICS

Peak ½-3½ hr, half-life ½-1 hr, protein binding 95%, eliminated in urine as metabolites and feces; in elderly elimination rate decreased, bioavailability increased; metabolized by CYP450 enzyme system

INTERACTIONS

Delayed absorption of ampicillin, iron salts, digoxin, ketoconazole, cyanocobalamin

Possible increased bleeding: warfarin

Increase: serum levels of diazepam, phenytoin, flurazepam, triazolam, cycloSPORINE, disulfiram, digoxin

O

✤ Canada only   Side effects: *italics* = common; ***bold italics*** = life-threatening

NURSING CONSIDERATIONS
Assess:

- GI system: bowel sounds q8h, abdomen for pain, swelling, anorexia
- Hepatic enzymes: AST, ALT, alk phosphatase during treatment

Administer:

- Swallow capsule whole; do not break, crush, or chew
- Capsules may be sprinkled over applesauce
- Before eating

Evaluate:

- Therapeutic response: absence of epigastric pain, swelling, fullness

Teach patient/family:

- To report severe diarrhea; drug may have to be discontinued
- That diabetic patient should know hypoglycemia may occur
- To avoid hazardous activities; dizziness may occur
- To avoid alcohol, salicylates, ibuprofen; may cause GI irritation

---

ondansetron (℞)

(on-dan-seh'tron)
Zofran
Func. class.: Antiemetic
Chem. class.: 5-HT$_3$ receptor antagonist

Do not confuse:

Zofran/Zantac

Action: Prevents nausea, vomiting by blocking serotonin peripherally, centrally, and in the small intestine

Uses: Prevention of nausea, vomiting associated with cancer chemotherapy, radiotherapy, and prevention of postoperative nausea, vomiting

Investigational uses: Bulimia; pruritus (rectal use), alcoholism, hyperemesis gravidarum

DOSAGE AND ROUTES

Hepatic dose

- *Adult:* **PO/IM/IV** Max dose 8 mg daily

Prevention of nausea/vomiting of cancer chemotherapy

- *Adult and child 4-18 yr:* **IV** 0.15 mg/kg infused over 15 min, 30 min before start of cancer chemotherapy; 0.15 mg/kg given 4 hr and 8 hr after first dose or 32 mg as a single dose; dilute in 50 ml of D$_5$ or 0.9% NaCl before giving; rectal use (off-label) 16 mg daily 2 hr prior to chemotherapy
- *Adult:* **IV** 0.15 mg/kg 15-30 min prior to chemotherapy, repeat 4, 8 hr later or 32 mg single dose ½ hr prior to chemotherapy; **PO** 8 mg ½ hr prior to chemotherapy, repeat 8 hr later
- *Child 4-18 yr:* **IV** 0.15 mg/kg ½ hr prior to chemotherapy, repeat 4, 8 hr later

Prevention of nausea/vomiting of radiotherapy

- *Adult:* **PO** 8 mg tid, may repeat q8hr

Prevention of postoperative nausea/vomiting

- *Adult:* **IV/IM** 4 mg undiluted over >30 sec prior to induction of anesthesia
- *Child 2-12 yr:* **IV** 0.1 mg/kg (≤40 kg); **IV** 4 mg (≥40 kg) give ≥30 sec

Bulimia (unlabeled)

- *Adult:* **PO** 4 mg tid (base dose); prn during bingeing/purging

Pruritus (unlabeled)

- *Adult:* **PO** 4 mg bid

Alcoholism (off-label)

Adult: **PO** 4 mcg/kg bid

Available forms: Inj 2 mg/ml, 32 mg/50 ml (premixed); tabs 4, 8 mg; oral sol 4 mg/5 ml; oral disintegrating tabs 4, 8 mg

SIDE EFFECTS

CNS: Headache, dizziness, drowsiness, fatigue, EPS
GI: Diarrhea, constipation, abdominal pain
*MISC: Rash, **bronchospasm** (rare), musculoskeletal pain, wound problems, shivering, fever, hypoxia, urinary retention*

Contraindications: Hypersensitivity
Precautions: Pregnancy (B), lactation,

---

children, elderly, granisetron hypersensitivity

PHARMACOKINETICS

IV: Mean elimination half-life 3.5-4.7 hr, plasma protein binding 70%-76%; extensively metabolized in the liver

NURSING CONSIDERATIONS

Assess:

- For absence of nausea, vomiting during chemotherapy
- Hypersensitivity reaction: rash, bronchospasm
- For EPS: shuffling gait, tremors, grimacing, rigidity

Administer:

IV route

- After diluting a single dose in 50 ml NS or D₅W, 0.45% NaCl or NS; give over 15 min

Additive compatibilities: Cisplatin, cyclophosphamide, cytarabine, dacarbazine, dexamethasone, DOXOrubicin, etoposide, fluconazole, hydromorphone, meperidine, methotrexate, morphine

Solution compatibilities: May also be diluted with D₅W, lactated Ringer's, D₅/0.9% NaCl, D₅/0.45% NaCl

Y-site compatibilities: Aldesleukin, amifostine, amikacin, aztreonam, bleomycin, carboplatin, carmustine, cefazolin, cefmetazole, cefotaxime, cefoxitin, ceftazidime, ceftizoxime, cefuroxime, chlorproMAZINE, cimetidine, cisatracurium, cisplatin, cladribine, clindamycin, cyclophosphamide, cytarabine, dacarbazine, dactinomycin, DAUNOrubicin, dexamethasone, diphenhydrAMINE, DOPamine, DOXOrubicin, DOXOrubicin liposome, doxycycline, droperidol, etoposide, famotidine, filgrastim, floxuridine, fluconazole, fludarabine, gallium, gentamicin, haloperidol, heparin, hydrocortisone, hydromorphone, hydrOXYzine, ifosfamide, imipenem/cilastatin, magnesium sulfate, mannitol, mechlorethamine, melphalan, meperidine, mesna, methotrexate, metoclopramide, miconazole, mitomycin, mitoxantrone, morphine, paclitaxel, pentostatin, piperacillin/tazobactam, potassium chloride, prochlorperazine, promethazine, ranitidine, remifentanil, streptozocin, teniposide, thiotepa, ticarcillin, ticarcillin/clavulanate, vancomycin, vinBLAStine, vinCRIStine, vinorelbine, zidovudine

Perform/provide:

- Storage at room temperature 48 hr after dilution

Evaluate:

- Therapeutic response: absence of nausea, vomiting during cancer chemotherapy

Teach patient/family:

- To report diarrhea, constipation, rash, or changes in respirations or discomfort at insertion site

---

orlistat (℞)

(or′lih-stat)
Xenical
Func. class.: Weight control agent
Chem. class.: Lipase inhibitor

Action: Inhibits the absorption of dietary fats

Uses: Obesity management

DOSAGE AND ROUTES

- *Adult:* **PO** 120 mg tid with each main meal containing fat

Available forms: Caps 120 mg

SIDE EFFECTS

CNS: Insomnia, depression, anxiety, dizziness, headache, fatigue
GI: Oily spotting, flatus with discharge, fecal urgency, fatty/oily stool, oily evacuation, fecal incontinence, nausea, vomiting, abdominal pain, infectious diarrhea, rectal pain, tooth disorder, hypovitaminosis
GU: UTI, vaginitis, menstrual irregularity
INTEG: Dry skin, rash
MS: Back pain, arthritis, myalgia, tendinitis
RESP: Influenza, URI, LRI, EENT symptoms

Contraindications: Hypersensitivity,

malabsorption syndrome, cholestasis, lactation

Precautions: Pregnancy (B), hypothyroidism, other organic causes of obesity, children, anorexia nervosa, bulimia, nephrolithiasis

PHARMACOKINETICS

Minimal absorption, peak 8 hr, 99% protein binding, excretion in feces, half-life 1-2 hr

INTERACTIONS

Increase: lipid-lowering effect—pravastatin

Decrease: absorption—fat-soluble vitamins (A, D, E, K), cycloSPORINE

NURSING CONSIDERATIONS

Assess:
• Weight weekly, diabetic patients may need reduction in oral hypoglycemics
• For misuse in certain populations (anorexia nervosa, bulimia)

Administer:
• For obesity only if patient is on weight-reduction program that includes dietary changes, exercise; patient should be on a diet with 30% of calories from fat, omit dose of orlistat if a meal contains no fat

Evaluate:
• Therapeutic response: decrease in weight

Teach patient/family:
• Safety and effectiveness beyond 2 yr have not been determined
• By instructing patient to read patient's information sheet, discuss unpleasant GI side effects
• To take a multivitamin containing fat-soluble vitamins 2 hr before or after orlistat; phyllium taken with each dose or at bedtime may decrease GI symptoms
• To avoid hazardous activities until stabilized on medication, discuss unpleasant side effects
• To notify prescriber if pregnancy is planned or suspected

oseltamivir (Ŗ)

(oss-el-tam′ih-veer)
Tamiflu
Func. class.: Antiviral
Chem. class.: Neuramidase inhibitor

Action: Inhibits influenza virus neuraminidase with possible alteration of virus particle aggregation and release

Uses: Prevention/treatment of influenza type A or B

Investigational uses: Possibly effective for Arian flu (H5N1)

DOSAGE AND ROUTES

Treatment
• *Adult/child >40 kg:* **PO** 75 mg bid × 5 days, begin treatment within 2 days of onset of symptoms
• *Child 23-40 kg and ≥1 yr:* **PO** 60 mg bid
• *Child 15-23 kg and ≥1 yr:* **PO** 45 mg bid
• *Child ≤15 kg and ≥1 yr:* **PO** 30 mg bid

Renal dose
• *Adult:* **PO** CCr <10-30 ml/min 75 mg daily × 5 days

Prevention
• *Adult/child ≥13 yr:* **PO** 75 mg daily × ≥7 days; begin treatment within 2 days of contact, max use 6 wk
• *Adult/child ≥13 yr renal dose:* **PO** CCr 10-30 ml/min 75 mg every other day

Available forms: Caps 75 mg; powder for oral susp 12 mg/ml after reconstitution

SIDE EFFECTS

CNS: Headache, dizziness, fatigue, *insomnia*
GI: Nausea, vomiting, diarrhea, abdominal pain
RESP: Cough

Contraindications: Hypersensitivity
Precautions: Pregnancy (C), hepatic disease, renal disease, elderly

---

PHARMACOKINETICS

Rapidly absorbed, protein binding low, converted to oseltamivir carboxylate, half-life 1-3 hr

NURSING CONSIDERATIONS

Assess:
• Bowel pattern before, during treatment
• Signs of infection: fever, fatigue, sore throat, headache, muscle soreness, aches

Administer:
• Within 2 days of symptoms of influenza; continue for 5 days
• At least 4 hr before bedtime to prevent insomnia

Perform/provide:
• Storage in tight, dry container

Evaluate:
• Therapeutic response: absence of fever, malaise, cough, dyspnea in infection

Teach patient/family:
• About aspects of drug therapy
• To avoid hazardous activities if dizziness occurs
• To take missed dose as soon as remembered within 2 hr of next dose

---

oxacillin (℞)
(ox-a-sill'in)
Bactocill, oxacillin sodium
Func. class.: Broad-spectrum antiinfective
Chem. class.: Penicillinase-resistant penicillin

Do not confuse:
Bactocil/Pathocil
Action: Interferes with cell wall replication of susceptible organisms; osmotically unstable cell wall swells, bursts from osmotic pressure
Uses: Effective for gram-positive cocci *(Staphylococcus aureus, Streptococcus pneumoniae)*, infections caused by penicillinase-producing *Staphylococcus*

DOSAGE AND ROUTES

• *Adult:* **PO** 2-6 g/day in divided doses q4-6h; **IM/IV** 2-12 g/day in divided doses q4-6h
• *Child:* **PO** 50-100 mg/kg/day in divided doses q6h; **IM/IV** 50-100 mg/kg/day in divided doses q4-6h
Available forms: Caps 250, 500 mg; powder for oral susp 250 mg/5 ml; powder for inj 250, 500 mg, 1, 2, 4, 10 g

SIDE EFFECTS

CNS: Lethargy, hallucinations, anxiety, depression, twitching, ***coma, seizures***
GI: Nausea, vomiting, diarrhea, increased AST, ALT, abdominal pain, glossitis, colitis, ***pseudomembranous colitis***
GU: ***Oliguria, proteinuria, hematuria,*** *vaginitis, moniliasis,* ***glomerulonephritis***
HEMA: Anemia, increased bleeding time, ***bone marrow depression, granulocytopenia***
SYST: ***Anaphylaxis, serum sickness***
Contraindications: Hypersensitivity to penicillins
Precautions: Pregnancy (B), hypersensitivity to cephalosporins, neonates

PHARMACOKINETICS

PO/IM: Peak 30-60 min, duration 4-6 hr
IV: Peak 5 min, duration 4-6 hr, half-life 30-60 min
Metabolized in the liver; excreted in urine, bile, breast milk; crosses placenta

INTERACTIONS

Increase: oxacillin concentrations—probenecid
Decrease: oxacillin antimicrobial effectiveness—tetracyclines, rifampin, erythromycins, chloramphenicol, cholestyramine, colestipol
Decrease: oral contraceptives effect
Drug/Herb
Do not use acidophilus with antiinfectives

Decrease: absorption—khat, separate by ≥2 hr

Drug/Lab Test
False positive: Urine glucose, urine protein

NURSING CONSIDERATIONS

Assess:

• I&O ratio; report hematuria, oliguria, since penicillin in high doses is nephrotoxic

⚠ Any patient with compromised renal system, since drug is excreted slowly in poor renal system function; toxicity may occur rapidly

• Hepatic studies: AST, ALT

• Blood studies: WBC, RBC, Hct/Hgb, bleeding time

• Renal studies: urinalysis, protein

• C&S before therapy; drug may be given as soon as culture is taken

• Bowel pattern before and during treatment

• Skin eruptions after administration of penicillin to 1 wk after discontinuing drug

• Respiratory status: rate, character, wheezing, tightness in chest

• Allergies before initiation of treatment, and reaction of each medication

Administer:

• Drug after C&S completed

• PO on empty stomach with full glass of water 1 hr before or 2 hr after meals

• IM inj deep in gluteal muscle

IV route

• After diluting 500 mg or less/5 ml sterile H$_2$O or NaCl for inj; may dilute further in D$_5$W, NS, LR and give 1 g over 10 min; may be given as infusion over 6 hr

Additive compatibilities: Cephapirin, chloramphenicol, DOPamine, potassium chloride, sodium bicarbonate

Y-site compatibilities: Acyclovir, cyclophosphamide, diltiazem, famotidine, fluconazole, foscarnet, heparin, hydrocortisone, hydromorphone, labetalol, magnesium sulfate, meperidine, methotrexate, morphine, perphenazine, potassium chloride, tacrolimus, vit B/C, zidovudine

Perform/provide:

• Adrenalin, suction, tracheostomy set, endotracheal intubation equipment

• Scratch test to assess allergy, after securing order from prescriber; usually done when penicillin is only drug of choice

• Storage in airtight container; refrigerate reconstituted sol up to 2 wk

Evaluate:

• Therapeutic response: absence of fever, draining wounds

Teach patient/family:

• All aspects of drug therapy, including need to complete course of medication to ensure organism death (10-14 days); culture may be taken after completed course

• To report sore throat, fever, fatigue (may indicate superinfection); persistent diarrhea

• To wear or carry emergency ID if allergic to penicillins

Treatment of anaphylaxis: Withdraw drug, maintain airway, administer epINEPHrine, aminophylline, O$_2$, IV corticosteroids

---

oxaliplatin (℞)

(ox-al-i′plat-in)
Eloxitan
Func. class.: Antineoplastic
Chem. class.: Platinum coordination complex

Action: Forms crosslinks, inhibiting DNA replication and transcription, cell-cycle nonspecific

Uses: Metastatic carcinoma of the colon or rectum in combination with 5-FU/leucovorin

DOSAGE AND ROUTES

Dosage protocols may vary

• *Adult:* **IV INF** *Day 1:* oxaliplatin 85 mg/m^2 in 250-500 ml D$_5$W and leucovorin 200 mg/m^2 in D$_5$W, give both over 2

---

hr at the same time in separate bags using a Y-line, followed by 5-FU 400 mg/m^2 **IV BOL** over 2-4 min, then 5-FU 600 mg/m^2 **IV INF** in 500 ml D$_5$W as a 22-hr **CONT INF**; *Day 2:* leucovorin 200 mg/m^2 **IV INF** over 2 hr, then 5-FU 400 mg/m^2 **IV BOL** over 2-4 min, then 5-FU 600 mg/m^2 **IV INF** in 500 D$_5$W as a 22-hr **CONT INF**; repeat cycle q2wk
Available forms: Powder for inj 50, 100 mg single-use vials

SIDE EFFECTS

CNS: Peripheral neuropathy, fatigue, headache, dizziness, insomnia
CV: Cardiac abnormalities
EENT: Decreased visual acuity, tinnitus, hearing loss
GI: Severe nausea, vomiting, diarrhea, weight loss, stomatitis, anorexia, gastro-esophageal reflux, constipation, dyspepsia, mucositis, flatulence
GU: Hematuria, dysuria, creatinine
*HEMA: **Thrombocytopenia, leukopenia, pancytopenia, neutropenia, anemia, hemolytic uremic syndrome***
INTEG: Alopecia, rash, flushing, extravasation, redness, swelling, pain at inj site
META: Hypokalemia
*RESP: **Fibrosis,*** dyspnea, cough, rhinitis, URI, pharyngitis
*SYST: **Anaphylaxis, angioedema***
Contraindications: Pregnancy (D), hypersensitivity to this drug or other platinum products, radiation therapy or chemotherapy within 1 mo, thrombocytopenia, smallpox vaccination
Precautions: Pneumococcus vaccination, lactation, children, elderly

PHARMACOKINETICS

Metabolized in liver, excreted in urine; after administration, 15% of platinum is in systemic circulation, 85% is either in tissues or being eliminated in urine

INTERACTIONS

Risk of bleeding—aspirin, NSAIDs, alcohol

Increase: myelosuppression—myelosuppressive agents, radiation
Increase: nephrotoxicity—aminoglycosides, loop diuretics
Decrease: antibody response—live virus vaccines

NURSING CONSIDERATIONS
Assess:
For bone marrow depression
• CBC, differential, platelet count weekly; withhold drug if WBC is <4000 or platelet count is <100,000; notify prescriber of results
• Renal studies: BUN, creatinine, serum uric acid, urine CCr before, electrolytes during therapy; dose should not be given if BUN <25 mg/dl; creatinine <1.5 mg/dl; I&O ratio; report fall in urine output of <30 ml/hr
⚠ For anaphylaxis: wheezing, tachycardia, facial swelling, fainting; discontinue drug and report to prescriber; resuscitation equipment should be nearby
• Monitor temp q4h (may indicate beginning infection)
• Hepatic studies before, during therapy (bilirubin, AST, ALT, LDH) as needed or monthly
• Bleeding: hematuria, guaiac, bruising or petechiae, mucosa or orifices q8h; obtain prescription for viscous lidocaine (Xylocaine)
• Effects of alopecia on body image; discuss feelings about body changes
• Jaundice of skin, sclera; dark urine; clay-colored stools; itchy skin; abdominal pain; fever; diarrhea
• Edema in feet, joint pain, stomach pain, shaking
Administer:
IV route
• Do not reconstitute or dilute with sodium chloride or any chloride-containing solutions
• Do not use aluminum equipment during any preparation or administration, will degrade platinum; do not refrigerate unopened powder or solution
• Prepare in biologic cabinet using gown, gloves, mask, do not allow drug to

come in contact with skin, use soap and water if contact occurs

• Hydrate patient with 0.9% NaCl over 8-12 hr before treatment

• EpINEPHrine, antihistamines, corticosteroids for hypersensitivity reaction

• Antiemetic 30-60 min before giving drug and prn

• Allopurinol to maintain uric acid levels, alkalinization of urine

• Diuretic (furosemide 40 mg IV) or mannitol after infusion

Perform/provide:

• Comprehensive oral hygiene

• All medications PO, if possible, avoid IM inj when platelets <100,000/mm³

• Increase fluid intake to 2-3 L/day to prevent urate deposits, calculi formation; elimination of drug

Evaluate:

• Therapeutic response: decreased tumor size, spread of malignancy

Teach patient/family:

• To report signs of infection: increased temp, sore throat, flulike symptoms

• To report signs of anemia: fatigue, headache, faintness, shortness of breath, irritability

• To report bleeding: avoid use of razors, commercial mouthwash

• To avoid aspirin, ibuprofen, NSAIDs, alcohol; may cause GI bleeding

• To report any complaints or side effects to nurse or prescriber

• To report any changes in breathing, coughing

• That hair may be lost during treatment; a wig or hairpiece may make patient feel better; new hair may be different in color, texture

• To report numbness, tingling in face or extremities, poor hearing or joint pain, swelling

• Not to receive vaccines during treatment

• To use contraception during treatment and 4 mo after; this drug may cause infertility

oxaprozin (℞)

(ox-a-proe′zin)

Daypro

Func. class.: Nonsteroidal antiinflammatory, antirheumatics

Chem. class.: Propionic acid derivative

Do not confuse:

Daypro/Diupres

Action: May inhibit prostaglandin synthesis by decreasing enzyme needed for biosynthesis; analgesic, antiinflammatory

Uses: Acute and long-term management of osteoarthritis, rheumatoid arthritis, juvenile rheumatoid arthritis

DOSAGE AND ROUTES

• *Adult:* **PO** 600-1200 mg daily; maximum dose 1800 mg/day or 26 mg/kg, whichever is lower

• *Adult <50 kg:* **PO** 600 mg daily

Available forms: Tabs 600 mg

SIDE EFFECTS

CNS: Dizziness, headache, drowsiness, fatigue, tremors, confusion, insomnia, anxiety, depression

CV: Tachycardia, peripheral edema, palpitations, dysrhythmias, CV disease

EENT: Tinnitus, hearing loss, blurred vision

GI: Nausea, anorexia, vomiting, diarrhea, jaundice, ***cholestatic hepatitis,*** constipation, flatulence, cramps, dry mouth, peptic ulcer, ***GI bleeding***

GU: ***Nephrotoxicity: dysuria, hematuria, oliguria, azotemia***

HEMA: ***Increased bleeding time***

INTEG: Purpura, rash, pruritus, sweating

MISC: ***Anaphylaxis, angioneurotic edema***

Contraindications: Hypersensitivity, asthma, patients in whom aspirin and iodides have induced symptoms of allergic reactions or asthma

Precautions: Pregnancy (C), avoid in late pregnancy, lactation, children, bleeding disorders, GI disorders, cardiac

---

disorders, hypersensitivity to other anti-inflammatory agents, severe renal and hepatic disease, elderly, CHF

PHARMACOKINETICS

PO: Onset 1 wk, peak unknown, duration unknown, half-life 40-50 hr; metabolized in liver; excreted in urine (metabolites), breast milk; 99% plasma protein binding

INTERACTIONS

Increase: toxicity—aspirin, cycloSPORINE, methotrexate

Increase: bleeding risk—oral anticoagulants, thrombolytics, cefamandole, cefotetan, cefoperazone, clopidogrel, eptifibatide, plicamycin, ticlopidine, tirofiban

Increase: levels of phenytoin, lithium, avoid concomitant use

Increase: GI side effects—aspirin, corticosteroids, NSAIDs, alcohol, potassium supplements

Decrease: effect—antihypertensives, diuretics

Drug/Herb

NSAIDs effect: bearberry, bilberry

Increase: bleeding risk—anise, arnica, chamomile, clove, dong quai, fenugreek, feverfew, garlic, ginger, ginkgo, ginseng *(Panax)*, licorice, bogbean, chondroitin

Increase: gastric irritation—arginine, gossypol

NURSING CONSIDERATIONS

Assess:

• Pain: frequency, intensity, characteristics; relief of pain after med

⚠ Asthma, aspirin hypersensitivity, oronasal polyps; increased hypersensitivity reactions

• Renal, hepatic, blood studies: BUN, creatinine, AST, ALT, Hgb, before treatment, periodically thereafter

• Audiometric, ophthalmic exam before, during, after treatment

• For eye, ear problems: blurred vision, tinnitus; may indicate toxicity

Administer:

• With food, antacids to decrease GI symptoms

Perform/provide:

• Storage at room temperature

Evaluate:

• Therapeutic response: decreased pain, stiffness in joints, decreased swelling in joints, ability to move more easily

Teach patient/family:

⚠ To report blurred vision, ringing, roaring in ears; may indicate toxicity

• To avoid driving, other hazardous activities if dizziness/drowsiness occurs

⚠ To report change in urine pattern, increased weight, edema, increased pain in joints, fever, blood in urine; indicates nephrotoxicity

• That therapeutic effects may take up to 1 mo

• To take with a full glass of water to enhance absorption, sit upright for ½ hr after dose

---

oxazepam (Ⓡ)

(ox-ay′ze-pam)
Apo-Oxazepam ✦, Novoxapam ✦, oxazepam
Func. class.: Sedative/hypnotic; antianxiety
Chem. class.: Benzodiazepine

O

Controlled Substance Schedule IV
Action: Potentiates the actions of GABA, especially in limbic system and reticular formation
Uses: Anxiety, alcohol withdrawal

DOSAGE AND ROUTES

Anxiety

• *Adult:* **PO** 10-30 mg tid-qid
• *Geriatric:* **PO** 5 mg daily-bid initially, may increase

Alcohol withdrawal

• *Adult:* **PO** 15-30 mg tid-qid
Available forms: Caps 10, 15, 30 mg

SIDE EFFECTS

CNS: Dizziness, drowsiness, confusion, headache, anxiety, tremors, fatigue, de-

pression, insomnia, hallucinations, paradoxical excitement, transient amnesia
*CV: Orthostatic hypotension, **ECG changes, tachycardia,** hypotension*
EENT: Blurred vision, tinnitus, mydriasis
GI: Nausea, vomiting, anorexia
HEMA: Leukopenia
INTEG: Rash, dermatitis, itching
Contraindications: Pregnancy (D), hypersensitivity to benzodiazepines, narrow-angle glaucoma, psychosis, lactation, child <12 yr
Precautions: Elderly, debilitated, hepatic disease, renal disease

PHARMACOKINETICS

PO: Peak 2-4 hr, metabolized by liver, excreted by kidneys, half-life 5-15 hr

INTERACTIONS

Increase: oxazepam effects—CNS depressants, alcohol, disulfiram, oral contraceptives
Decrease: oxazepam effects—oral contraceptives, valproic acid
Drug/Herb
Increase: CNS depression—catnip, chamomile, clary, cowslip, hops, kava, lavender, mistletoe, nettle, pokeweed, poppy, Queen Anne's lace, senega, skullcap, valerian
Increase: hypotension—black cohosh
Drug/Lab Test
Increase: AST, ALT, serum bilirubin
Decrease: RAIU
False increase: 17-OHCS

NURSING CONSIDERATIONS

Assess:
• B/P (lying, standing), pulse; if systolic B/P drops 20 mm Hg, hold drug, notify prescriber
• Blood studies: CBC during long-term therapy; blood dyscrasias have occurred rarely
• Hepatic studies: AST, ALT, bilirubin, creatinine, LDH, alk phosphatase if taking long term
• Mental status: mood, sensorium, affect, sleeping pattern, drowsiness, dizziness
🅰 Physical dependency, withdrawal symptoms: headache, nausea, vomiting, muscle pain, weakness, tremors, convulsions (long-term use)
• Suicidal tendencies
Administer:
• With food, milk for GI symptoms
• Sugarless gum, hard candy, frequent sips of water for dry mouth
Perform/provide:
• Assistance with ambulation during beginning therapy; drowsiness/dizziness occurs
• Safety measures, including side rails
• Check to see if PO medication has been swallowed
Evaluate:
• Therapeutic response: decreased anxiety, restlessness, insomnia
Teach patient/family:
• That drug may be taken with food
• That medication is not to be used for everyday stress or used longer than 4 mo unless directed by prescriber; not to take more than prescribed dose; may be habit forming
• To avoid OTC preparations (cough, cold, hay fever) unless approved by prescriber
• To avoid driving, activities that require alertness, since drowsiness may occur
• To avoid alcohol ingestion, other psychotropic medications unless directed by prescriber
• Not to discontinue medication abruptly after long-term use
• To rise slowly, or fainting may occur, especially elderly
• That drowsiness may worsen at beginning of treatment
Treatment of overdose: Lavage, VS, supportive care, flumazenil

oxcarbazepine (℞)
(ox'kar-baz'uh-peen)
Trileptal
Func. class.: Anticonvulsant

Action: May inhibit nerve impulses by limiting influx of sodium ions across cell membrane in motor cortex

Uses: Partial seizures

Investigational uses: Trigeminal neuralgia, atypical panic disorder, bipolar disorder

DOSAGE AND ROUTES
Seizures, adjunctive therapy
• *Adult:* **PO** 300 mg bid, may be increased to 600 mg/day in divided doses bid; maintenance 1200 mg/day

• *Child 4-16 yr:* **PO** 8-10 mg/kg/day divided bid, max 600 mg/day; dose is determined by weight

Conversion to monotherapy in partial seizures
• *Adult:* **PO** 300 mg bid with reduction in other anticonvulsants, increase oxcarbazepine to max 600 mg/day q1wk over 2-4 wk; withdraw other anticonvulsants over 3-6 wk

Initiation of monotherapy in partial seizures
• *Adult:* **PO** 300 mg bid, increase by 300 mg/day q3d to 1200 mg divided bid

Renal dose
• *Adult:* **PO** CCr <30 ml/min 150 mg bid and increase slowly

Available forms: Tabs, film-coated, 150, 300, 600 mg; oral susp 300 mg/5 ml

SIDE EFFECTS
CNS: Headache, dizziness, confusion, fatigue, feeling abnormal, ataxia, abnormal gait, tremors, anxiety, agitation, ***worsening of seizures***

CV: Hypotension, chest pain, edema

EENT: Blurred vision, diplopia, nystagmus, rhinitis, sinusitis

GI: Nausea, constipation, diarrhea, anorexia, vomiting, abdominal pain, gastritis, dry mouth, thirst, ***rectal hemorrhage***

GU: Frequency, UTI, vaginitis

INTEG: Purpura, rash, acne

Contraindications: Hypersensitivity

Precautions: Pregnancy (C), hypersensitivity to carbamazepine, lactation, child <4 yr, renal disease, fluid restriction

PHARMACOKINETICS
PO: Onset unknown, peak unknown, metabolized by liver to active metabolite; terminal half-life 9 hr metabolite; inhibits P450 CYP2C19, induces CYP3A4/5

INTERACTIONS
Increase: CNS depression—alcohol

Decrease: effects—felodipine, oral contraceptive, carbamazepine

Decrease: oxcarbazepine levels—phenobarbital, phenytoin, valproic acid, verapamil

Drug/Herb
Increase: anticonvulsant effect—ginkgo

Decrease: anticonvulsant effect—ginseng, santonica

NURSING CONSIDERATIONS
Assess:
• Description of seizures: frequency, duration, aura

• Mental status: mood, sensorium, affect, behavioral changes; if mental status changes, notify prescriber

• Eye problems: need for ophthalmic exams before, during, after treatment (slit lamp, funduscopy, tonometry)

Administer:
PO route
• With food, milk to decrease GI symptoms

Perform/provide:
• Storage at room temperature

• Hard candy, gum, frequent rinsing for dry mouth

• Assistance with ambulation during early part of treatment; dizziness occurs

     Side effects: *italics* = common; ***bold italics*** = life-threatening

Evaluate:

• Therapeutic response: decreased seizure activity

Teach patient/family:

• To carry emergency ID stating patient's name, drugs taken, condition, prescriber's name and phone number

• To avoid driving, other activities that require alertness

• Not to discontinue medication quickly after long-term use

• To inform prescriber if hypersensitive to carbamazepine

• To avoid use of alcohol while taking this medication

• To use alternative contraception if using hormonal method

---

oxiconazole topical
See Appendix C

---

oxybutynin (Ɍ)
(ox-i-byoo'ti-nin)
Ditropan, Ditropan XL, oxybutynin, Oxytrol Transdermal
Func. class.: Anticholinergic
Chem. class.: Synthetic tertiary amine

Do not confuse:
Ditropan/diazepam
Action: Relaxes smooth muscles in urinary tract by inhibiting acetylcholine at postganglionic sites
Uses: Antispasmodic for neurogenic bladder, overactive bladder

DOSAGE AND ROUTES

• *Adult:* **PO** 5 mg bid-tid, not to exceed 5 mg qid; **ER** 5 mg daily, may increase by 5 mg, max 30 mg/day; **TD** apply one patch to abdomen, hip, buttock 2 ×/wk (q3-4days)

• *Geriatric:* **PO** 2.5-5 mg tid, increase by 2.5 mg q several days

• *Child >5 yr:* **PO** 5 mg bid, not to exceed 5 mg tid

• *Child 1-5 yr:* **PO** 0.2 mg/kg/dose 2-4 ×/day

Available forms: Syr 5 mg/5 ml; tabs 5 mg; tabs, ext rel 5, 10, 15 mg; TD 3.9 mg/day

SIDE EFFECTS

*CNS: Anxiety, restlessness, dizziness, **convulsions,** headache, drowsiness, confusion*
CV: Palpitations, sinus tachycardia, hypotension
EENT: Blurred vision, increased intraocular tension, dry mouth, throat
GI: Nausea, vomiting, anorexia, abdominal pain, constipation
GU: Dysuria, urinary retention, hesitancy
Contraindications: Hypersensitivity, GI obstruction, GI hemorrhage, GU obstruction, glaucoma, severe colitis, myasthenia gravis, unstable CV status in acute hemorrhage
Precautions: Pregnancy (B), lactation, suspected glaucoma, children <12 yr, elderly

PHARMACOKINETICS

Onset ½-1 hr, peak 3-4 hr, duration 6-10 hr; metabolized by liver, excreted in urine

INTERACTIONS

Increase: levels of atenolol, digoxin, nitrofurantoin
Increase or decrease: levels of phenothiazines
Decrease: levels of acetaminophen, haloperidol, levodopa
Drug/Herb
Increase: constipation—black catechu
Increase: anticholinergic action—butterbur, jimsonweed, scopolia
Decrease: anticholinergic effect—jaborandi tree, pill-bearing spurge

NURSING CONSIDERATIONS
Assess:

• Urinary patterns: distention, nocturia, frequency, urgency, incontinence

---

- Allergic reactions: rash, urticaria; if these occur, drug should be discontinued
- CNS effects: confusion, anxiety; anticholinergic effects in the elderly

Administer:
- Without regard to meals

Evaluate:
- Urinary status: dysuria, frequency, nocturia, incontinence

Teach patient/family:
- To avoid hazardous activities; dizziness, blurred vision may occur
- To avoid OTC medications with alcohol, other CNS depressants
- To prevent photophobia by wearing sunglasses
- Avoid hot weather, strenuous activity, drug decreases perspiration

---

⚠ High Alert

oxycodone (℞)

(ox-i-koe′done)
Endocodone, M-oxy, Oxy Contin, OxyFAST, OxyLR, Roxicodone, Roxicodone Supeudol ✦

oxycodone/aspirin
Endodan ✦, Oxycodan ✦, Percodan, Percodan-Demi, Roxiprin

oxycodone/ acetaminophen
Endocet ✦, Oxycocet ✦, Percocet, Roxicet, Roxilox, Tylox
Func. class.: Opiate analgesic
Chem. class.: Semisynthetic derivative

Controlled Substance Schedule II
Do not confuse:
Percodan/Decadron
Roxicet/Roxanol
Tylox/Xanax
Tylox/Trimox
Tylox/Wymox
Action: Inhibits ascending pain pathways in CNS, increases pain threshold, alters pain perception
Uses: Moderate to severe pain

Investigational uses: Postherpetic neuralgic (cont rel)

DOSAGE AND ROUTES
- *Adult:* PO 10-30 mg q4hr (5 mg q6h for OxyIR, OxyFast) **OxyFast Conc Sol is extremely concentrated; do not use interchangeably**
- *Child:* PO 0.05-0.15 mg/kg/dose up to 5 mg/dose q4-6h; not recommended in children

Available forms: Oxycodone: tabs, cont rel (Oxy Contin) 10, 20, 40, 80, 160 mg; tabs, immediate rel 15, 30 mg; tabs 5 mg; caps, immediate rel 5 mg; oral sol 5 mg/5 ml, 20 mg/ml; oxycodone with acetaminophen: tabs 5 mg/325 mg; cap 5 mg/500 mg; oral sol 5 mg/325 mg/5 ml; oxycodone with aspirin: 2.44 mg/325 mg, 4.88/325 mg

SIDE EFFECTS
CNS: Drowsiness, dizziness, confusion, headache, sedation, euphoria
CV: Palpitations, bradycardia, change in B/P
EENT: Tinnitus, blurred vision, miosis, diplopia
GI: Nausea, vomiting, anorexia, constipation, cramps
GU: Increased urinary output, dysuria, urinary retention
INTEG: Rash, urticaria, bruising, flushing, diaphoresis, pruritus
RESP: ***Respiratory depression***
Contraindications: Hypersensitivity, addiction (opiate)
Precautions: Pregnancy (B), addictive personality, lactation, increased intracranial pressure, MI (acute), severe heart disease, respiratory depression, hepatic disease, renal disease, child <18 yr

PHARMACOKINETICS
PO: Onset 15-30 min, peak 1 hr, duration 4-6 hr; detoxified by liver, excreted in urine, crosses placenta, excreted in breast milk

O

✦ Canada only   Side effects: *italics* = common; ***bold italics*** = life-threatening

INTERACTIONS

Increase: effects with other CNS depressants—alcohol, opioids, sedative/hypnotics, antipsychotics, skeletal muscle relaxants

Drug/Herb

Increase: anticholinergic effect—corkwood

Increase: sedative effect—Jamaican dogwood, lavender, mistletoe, nettle, pokeweed, poppy, senega, valerian

Drug/Lab Test

Increase: Amylase

NURSING CONSIDERATIONS

Assess:

• I&O ratio; check for decreasing output; may indicate urinary retention
• CNS changes: dizziness, drowsiness, hallucinations, euphoria, LOC, pupil reaction
• Allergic reactions: rash, urticaria
• Respiratory dysfunction: respiratory depression, character, rate, rhythm; notify prescriber if respirations are <10/min
• Need for pain medication by pain, sedation scoring; physical dependence

Administer:

• Do not break, crush, or chew controlled release tabs
• 80, 160 mg cont rel tabs only in opioid-tolerant patients
• With antiemetic if nausea, vomiting occur
• When pain is beginning to return; determine dosage interval by response

Perform/provide:

• Storage in light-resistant area at room temperature
• Assistance with ambulation
• Safety measures: night-light, call bell within easy reach

Evaluate:

• Therapeutic response: decrease in pain

Teach patient/family:

• To report any symptoms of CNS changes, allergic reactions

• That physical dependency may result from extended use
• That withdrawal symptoms may occur: nausea, vomiting, cramps, fever, faintness, anorexia

Treatment of overdose: Naloxone (Narcan) 0.2-0.8 mg IV, O₂, IV fluids, vasopressors

---

oxymetazoline nasal agent

See Appendix C

---

oxymetazoline ophthalmic

See Appendix C

⚠ High Alert

oxymorphone (℞)

(ox-i-mor′fone)

Numorphan

Func. class.: Opiate analgesic
Chem. class.: Semisynthetic phenanthrene derivative

Controlled Substance Schedule II

Action: Inhibits ascending pain pathways in CNS, increases pain threshold, alters pain perception

Uses: Moderate to severe pain

DOSAGE AND ROUTES

• *Adult:* **IM/SUBCUT** 1-1.5 mg q4-6h prn; **IV** 0.5 mg q4-6h prn; **RECT** 5 mg q4-6h prn

Labor analgesia

• *Adult:* **IM:** 0.5-1 mg

Available forms: Inj 1, 1.5 mg/ml; supp 5 mg

SIDE EFFECTS

*CNS: Drowsiness, dizziness, confusion, headache, sedation, **seizures,** euphoria (elderly)*

CV: Palpitations, **bradycardia,** change in B/P

⚠ Safety alert   *"Tall Man" lettering

EENT: Tinnitus, blurred vision, miosis, diplopia
GI: Nausea, vomiting, anorexia, constipation, cramps
GU: Increased urinary output, dysuria, urinary retention
INTEG: Rash, urticaria, bruising, flushing, diaphoresis, pruritus
*RESP: **Respiratory depression***
Contraindications: Hypersensitivity, addiction (opiate)
Precautions: Pregnancy (B) (short-term), addictive personality, lactation, increased intracranial pressure, MI (acute), severe heart disease, respiratory depression, hepatic disease, renal disease, child <18 yr

PHARMACOKINETICS

SUBCUT/IM: Onset 10-15 min, peak 1½ hr, duration, 3-6 hr
IV: Onset 5-10 min, peak 15-30 min, duration 3-6 hr
RECT: Onset 15-30 min, duration 3-6 hr
Metabolized by liver, excreted in urine, crosses placenta

INTERACTIONS

Increase: effects with other CNS depressants—alcohol, opiates, sedative/hypnotics, antipsychotics, skeletal muscle relaxants
Drug/Herb
Increase: anticholinergic effect—corkwood
Increase: sedative effect—Jamaican dogwood, lavender, mistletoe, nettle, pokeweed, poppy, senega, valerian
Drug/Lab Test
Increase: Amylase

NURSING CONSIDERATIONS

Assess:
• I&O ratio for decreasing output; may indicate urinary retention
• CNS changes: dizziness, drowsiness, hallucinations, euphoria, LOC, pupil reaction
• Allergic reactions: rash, urticaria

• Respiratory dysfunction: respiratory depression, character, rate, rhythm; notify prescriber if respirations are <10/min
• Need for pain medication, physical dependence
Administer:
• With antiemetic for nausea, vomiting
• When pain is beginning to return; determine interval by response
IV route
• After diluting with 5 ml sterile H_2O or NS for inj; give over 2-5 min through Y-tube or 3-way stopcock
Syringe compatibilities: Glycopyrrolate, hydrOXYzine, ranitidine
Perform/provide:
• Storage in light-resistant area at room temperature
• Assistance with ambulation
• Safety measures: night-light, call bell within easy reach
Evaluate:
• Therapeutic response: decrease in pain
Teach patient/family:
• To report any symptoms of CNS changes, allergic reactions
• That physical dependency may result from extended use
• That withdrawal symptoms may occur: nausea, vomiting, cramps, fever, faintness, anorexia
Treatment of overdose: Naloxone (Narcan) 0.2-0.8 mg IV, O_2, IV fluids, vasopressors

O

> ### ⚠ High Alert
>
> ## oxytocin (℞)
> (ox-i-toe′sin)
> Pitocin
> *Func. class.:* Oxytocic, uterine-active agent
> *Chem. class.:* Hormone

Action: Acts directly on myofibrils, producing uterine contraction; stimulates milk ejection by the breast

---

Uses: Stimulation, induction of labor; missed or incomplete abortion; postpartum bleeding

DOSAGE AND ROUTES
Postpartum hemorrhage
• *Adult:* **IV** 10-40 units in 1000 ml non-hydrating diluent infused at 20-40 mU/min
• *Adult:* **IM** 10 units after delivery of placenta
Fetal stress test
• *Adult:* **IV** 0.5 mU/min, increase q20min until 3 contractions within 10 min
Stimulation of labor
• *Adult:* **IV** 1-2 mU/min, increase by 1-2 mU q15-60min until contractions occur; then decrease dose
Incomplete abortion
• *Adult:* **IV INF** 10 units/500 ml D_5W or 0.9% NaCl at 10-20 mU/min, max 30 units/12 hr
Available forms: Inj 10 units/ml

SIDE EFFECTS
CNS: **Convulsions, tetanic contractions**
CV: Hypotension, hypertension, dysrhythmias, increased pulse, bradycardia, tachycardia, PVC
FETUS: Dysrhythmias, jaundice, hypoxia, **intracranial hemorrhage**
GI: Anorexia, nausea, vomiting, constipation
GU: **Abruptio placentae, decreased uterine blood flow**
HEMA: Increased hyperbilirubinemia
INTEG: Rash
RESP: **Asphyxia**
SYST: Water intoxication of mother
Contraindications: Hypersensitivity, serum toxemia, cephalopelvic disproportion, fetal distress, hypertonic uterus
Precautions: Cervical/uterine surgery, uterine sepsis, primipara >35 yr, 1st, 2nd stage of labor

PHARMACOKINETICS
IM: Onset 3-7 min, duration 1 hr, half-life 12-17 min

IV: Onset 1 min, duration 30 min, half-life 12-17 min

INTERACTIONS
Hypertension: vasopressors
Drug/Herb
Hypertension: ephedra

NURSING CONSIDERATIONS
Assess:
• I&O ratio
• Respiration
• B/P, pulse; watch for changes that may indicate hemorrhage
• Respiratory rate, rhythm, depth; notify prescriber of abnormalities
• Length, intensity, duration of contraction; notify prescriber of contractions lasting over 1 min or absence of contractions; turn patient on her side
• FHTs, fetal distress; watch for acceleration, deceleration; notify prescriber if problems occur; fetal presentation, pelvic dimensions; turn patient on left side if FHT change in rate
⚠ For signs and symptoms of water intoxication; confusion, anuria, drowsiness, headache
Administer:
Labor induction
• After diluting 10 units/L of 0.9% NS or D_5 NS run at 1-2 mU/min at 15-30 min intervals to begin normal labor; dilute 10-40 mU/min, titrate to control postpartum bleeding; dilute 10 units/500 ml sol; run 10 units-20 mU/ml; administer by only 1 route at a time; use inf pump; rotate inf to provide mixing; do not shake
Control of postpartum bleeding
• Dilute 10-40 units/1 L of sol, run at 10-20 mU/min; adjust rate as needed
• With crash cart available on unit (magnesium sulfate at bedside)
Additive compatibilities: Chloramphenicol, metaraminol, netilmicin, sodium bicarbonate, thiopental, verapamil
Y-site compatibilities: Heparin, hydrocortisone, insulin (regular), meperidine, morphine, potassium chloride, vit B/C, warfarin

Evaluate:
• Therapeutic response: stimulation of labor, control of postpartum bleeding

Teach patient/family:
• To report increased blood loss, abdominal cramps, fever, foul-smelling lochia

• That contractions will be similar to menstrual cramps, gradually increasing in intensity

paclitaxel (℞)
(pa-kli-tax'el)
Abraxane, Onxol, Taxol
Func. class.: Antineoplastic—miscellaneous
Chem. class.: Antimicrotubule, natural diterpene

Do not confuse:
paclitaxel/paroxetine
paclitaxel/Paxil
Taxol/Paxil
Taxol/Taxotera

Action: Inhibits reorganization of microtubule network needed for interphase and mitotic cellular functions; also causes abnormal bundles of microtubules during cell cycle and multiple esters of microtubules during mitosis

Uses: Taxol: metastatic carcinoma of the ovary, breast; AIDS-related Kaposi's sarcoma (2nd-line), non–small cell lung cancer (1st-line), adjuvant treatment for node-positive breast cancer; Onxol: failure of other treatment in breast cancer, advanced carcinoma in ovarian cancer

Investigational uses: Advanced head, neck, small cell lung cancer; non–Hodgkin's lymphoma, adenocarcinoma of the upper GI tract, hormone-refractory prostate cancer

DOSAGE AND ROUTES
Ovarian carcinoma
• *Adult:* IV INF 135 mg/m^2 given over 24 hr q3wk then cisplatin 75 mg/m^2; or 175 mg/m^2 over 3 hr q3wk; or 175 mg/m^2 over 3 hr

Advanced ovarian carcinoma
• *Adult:* **IV/INF** 175 mg/m^2 with cisplatin 75 mg/m^2 using a 3-hr regimen q3wk

Breast carcinoma
• *Adult:* **IV INF** 175 mg/m^2 over 3 hr q3wk × 4 courses

AIDS-related Kaposi's sarcoma
• *Adult:* **IV INF** 135 mg/m^2 over 3 hr q3wk or 100 mg/m^2 over 3 hr q2wk

1st-line non–small cell lung cancer
• *Adult:* **IV INF** 135 mg/m^2/24 hr inf with cisplatin 75 mg/m^2 × 3 wk

Available forms: Inj 30 mg/5 ml vial (6 mg/ml); powder for inj, lyophilized 100 mg in single-use vials

SIDE EFFECTS
CV: Bradycardia, *hypotension*, abnormal ECG
GI: *Nausea, vomiting, diarrhea, mucositis, increased bilirubin, alk phosphatase, AST*
HEMA: **Neutropenia, leukopenia, thrombocytopenia, anemia,** bleeding, infections
INTEG: *Alopecia*
MS: Arthralgia, myalgia
NEURO: Peripheral neuropathy
SYST: Hypersensitivity reactions, **anaphylaxis**

Contraindications: Pregnancy (D), hypersensitivity to paclitaxel or other drugs with polyoxyethylated castor oil, neutropenia of <1500/mm^3

Precautions: Children, lactation; hepatic, cardiovascular disease; CNS disorder

PHARMACOKINETICS
89%-98% of drug is serum protein bound, metabolized in liver, excreted in bile and urine; terminal half-life 5.3-17.4 hr

INTERACTIONS
Increase: myelosuppression—other antineoplastics, radiation
Increase: DOXOrubicin levels—DOXOrubicin

Decrease: paclitaxel metabolism—ketoconazole, verapamil, diazepam, cycloSPORINE, teniposide, etoposide, quinidine, dexamethasone, vinCRIStine, testosterone

Decrease: immune response—live virus vaccines

NURSING CONSIDERATIONS
Assess:
• CBC, differential, platelet count prior to and qwk; withhold drug if WBC is <1500/mm^3 or platelet count is <100,000/mm^3, notify prescriber
• Monitor temp q4h (may indicate beginning infection)
• Hepatic studies before, during therapy (bilirubin, AST, ALT, LDH) prn or qmo, check for jaundiced skin and sclera, dark urine, clay-colored stool, itchy skin, abdominal pain, fever, diarrhea
• VS during 1st hr of infusion, check IV site for signs of infiltration
⚠ Hypersensitive reactions, anaphylaxis including hypotension, dyspnea, angioedema, generalized urticaria; discontinue infusion immediately
• Bleeding: hematuria, guaiac, bruising or petechiae, mucosa or orifices q8h; obtain prescription for viscous lidocaine (Xylocaine)
• Effects of alopecia on body image; discuss feelings about body changes
Administer:
• Antiemetic 30-60 min before giving drug and prn
IV route
• After diluting in 0.9% NaCl, D$_5$, D$_5$ and 0.9% NaCl, D$_5$LR to a concentration of 0.3-1.2 mg/ml
• Using an in-line filter ≤0.22 µm
• After premedicating with dexamethasone 20 mg PO 12 hr and 6 hr before paclitaxel, diphenhydrAMINE 50 mg IV ½-1 hr before paclitaxel and cimetidine 300 mg or ranitidine 50 mg IV ½-1 hr before paclitaxel
• Using only glass bottles, polypropylene, polyolefin bags and administration sets; do not use PVC infusion bags or sets

• Using gloves and cytotoxic handling precautions
Abraxane
• Reconstitute vial by injecting 20 ml of 0.9% NaCl
• Slowly inject the 20 ml of 0.9% NaCl over at least 1 min to direct the sol flow on wall of vial
• Do not inject 0.9% NaCl directly onto lyophilized cake (foaming will occur)
• Allow vial to sit for at least 5 min to ensure proper wetting of lyophilized cake
• Gently swirl or invert vial slowly for at least 2 min until completely dissolved
• Calculate dosing by dosing vol/ml = total dose (mg) ÷ 5 (mg/ml)
Y-site compatibilities:
Acyclovir, amikacin, aminophylline, ampicillin/sulbactam, bleomycin, butorphanol, calcium chloride, carboplatin, cefepime, cefotetan, ceftazidime, ceftriaxone, cimetidine, cisplatin, cladribine, cyclophosphamide, cytarabine, dacarbazine, dexamethasone, diphenhydrAMINE, DOXOrubicin, droperidol, etoposide, famotidine, floxuridine, fluconazole, fluorouracil, furosemide, ganciclovir, gentamicin, granisetron, haloperidol, heparin, hydrocortisone, hydromorphone, ifosfamide, lorazepam, magnesium sulfate, mannitol, meperidine, mesna, methotrexate, metoclopramide, morphine, nalbuphine, ondansetron, pentostatin, potassium chloride, prochlorperazine, propofol, ranitidine, sodium bicarbonate, thiotepa, vancomycin, vinBLAStine, vinCRIStine, zidovudine
Perform/provide:
• Confirmation that dexamethasone was given 12 hr and 6 hr before infusion begins
• Storage of prepared sol up to 27 hr in refrigerator
Evaluate:
• Therapeutic response: decreased tumor size, spread of malignancy
Teach patient/family:
• To report signs of infection: fever, sore throat, flulike symptoms
• To report signs of anemia: fatigue,

---

headache, faintness, shortness of breath, irritability

• To report bleeding; avoid use of razors, commercial mouthwash

• To avoid use of aspirin, ibuprofen

• To report any complaints or side effects to nurse or prescriber

• That hair may be lost during treatment; a wig or hairpiece may make patient feel better; new hair may be different in color, texture

• That pain in muscles and joints 2-5 days after infusion is common

• To use nonhormonal type of contraception

• To avoid receiving vaccinations while on this drug

palivizumab (℞)
(pal-ih-viz′uh-mab)
Synagis
Func. class.: Monoclonal antibody

Action: A humanized monoclonal antibody that exhibits neutralizing and fusion-inhibitory activity against respiratory syncytial virus (RSV)

Uses: Prevention of serious lower respiratory tract disease caused by RSV in pediatric patients

DOSAGE AND ROUTES

• *Child:* **IM** 15 mg/kg, those patients who develop RSV should receive monthly doses during RSV season (November-April)

Available forms: Powder for reconstitution: 50, 100 mg; solution 50 mg/0.5 ml, 100 mg/1 ml

SIDE EFFECTS

CNS: Fever
EENT: Otitis media, rhinitis, pharyngitis
GI: Nausea, vomiting, diarrhea, increased AST
INTEG: Rash, inj site reaction
RESP: URI, **apnea,** cough
SYST: **Anaphylaxis**

Contraindications: Hypersensitivity, adults, cyanotic congenital heart disease

Precautions: Pregnancy (C), thrombocytopenia, coagulation disorders, established RSV, congenital heart disease, chronic lung disease, systemic allergic reactions

PHARMACOKINETICS

Mean half-life 20 days

NURSING CONSIDERATIONS
Assess:

• For presence of RSV infection, drug is given to prevent infection. For side effects; report if allergic reaction is evident

⚠ For anaphylaxis: difficulty breathing; drug should be discontinued and have emergency equipment nearby

Administer:

• IM only

• After adding 1 ml of sterile water for inj per 100-mg vial, add 0.6 ml sterile water for inj for 50-mg vial; gently swirl for 30 sec to avoid foaming; do not shake; let stand at room temperature for 20 min until sol clarifies; given within 6 hr of reconstitution

Teach patient/family:

• To report upper respiratory infections, earaches, rash, sore throat

palonosetron (℞)
(pa-lone-o′se-tron)
Aloxi
Func. class.: Antiemetic
Chem. class.: 5-HT₃ receptor antagonist

Action: Prevents nausea, vomiting by blocking serotonin peripherally, centrally, and in the small intestine at the 5-HT₃ receptor

Uses: Prevention of nausea, vomiting associated with cancer chemotherapy

DOSAGE AND ROUTES

• *Adult:* **IV** 0.25 mg as a single dose over 30 secs, ½ hr prior to chemotherapy, max 25 mg IV over q7d

Available forms: Inj 0.25 mg/5 ml

P

SIDE EFFECTS

CNS: Headache, dizziness, drowsiness, fatigue, insomnia
GI: Diarrhea, constipation, abdominal pain
MISC: Weakness, hyperkalemia, anxiety, rash, **bronchospasm** (rare), arthralgia, *fever, urinary retention*

Contraindications: Hypersensitivity

Precautions: Pregnancy (B), lactation, children, elderly, prolongation of QT interval or other cardiac conduction intervals (patients with hypokalemia, hypomagnesium, taking diuretics, congenital QT syndrome and those taking antidysrhythmics or other drugs which many prolong QT interval and cumulative high-dose antithramycline therapy)

PHARMACOKINETICS

62% protein bound; metabolized by liver; unchanged drug and metabolites excreted by kidney; terminal elimination half-life: 40 hr

NURSING CONSIDERATIONS

Assess:
• For absence of nausea, vomiting during chemotherapy
• Hypersensitivity reaction: rash, bronchospasm

Administer:
• Give as a single dose over 30 sec
• Do not mix with other drugs, flush IV line before and after administration

Perform/provide:
• Storage at room temperature

Evaluate:
• Therapeutic response: absence of nausea, vomiting during cancer chemotherapy

Teach patient/family:
• To report diarrhea, constipation, rash, or changes in respirations or discomfort at insertion site

---

pamidronate (℞)
(pam-i-drone′ate)
Aredia
Func. class.: Bone-resorption inhibitor, electrolyte modifier
Chem. class.: Bisphosphonate

Do not confuse:
Aredia/Adriamycin

Action: Inhibits bone resorption, apparently without inhibiting bone formation and mineralization; absorbs calcium phosphate crystals in bone and may directly block dissolution of hydroxyapatite crystals of bone

Uses: Moderate to severe Paget's disease, mild to moderate hypercalcemia associated with malignancy with or without bone metastases, osteolytic bone metastases in breast cancer, multiple myeloma patients

Investigational uses: Postmenopausal osteoporosis, hyperparathyroidism, reduction of bone pain in prostatic carcinoma, immobilization-related hypercalcemia

DOSAGE AND ROUTES

Hypercalcemia of malignancy
• *Adult:* IV INF 60-90 mg as a single dose in moderate hypercalcemia, 90 mg in severe hypercalcemia over 24 hr; dose should be dluted in 1000 ml 0.45% NaCl, 0.9% NaCl or D_5W, wait 7 days before 2nd course

Osteolytic lesions from multiple myeloma
• *Adult:* IV 90 mg/500 ml of D_5W, 0.45% NaCl, or 0.9% NaCl given over 4 hr on a monthly basis

Paget's disease
• *Adult:* IV 90-180 mg/treatment, may use 30 mg daily × 3 days

Available forms: Powder for inj 30, 90 mg/vial; inj 3, 6, 9 mg/ml

SIDE EFFECTS

CNS: Fever, fatigue, psychosis
CV: Hypertension

GI: Abdominal pain, anorexia, constipation, nausea, vomiting, diarrhea, dyspepsia

GU: UTI, fluid overload

INTEG: Redness, swelling, induration, pain on palpation at site of catheter insertion

META: Anemia, hypokalemia, hypomagnesemia, hypophosphatemia, hypocalcemia, hypothyroidism

MS: Bone pain, myalgia

RESP: Coughing, dyspnea, URI

Contraindications: Pregnancy (D), hypersensitivity to bisphosphonates

Precautions: Children, nursing mothers, renal dysfunction

PHARMACOKINETICS

Rapidly cleared from circulation and taken up mainly by bones, primarily in areas of high bone turnover, eliminated primarily by kidneys

INTERACTIONS

Hypomagnesemia, hypokalemia: digoxin

Decrease: pamidronate effect—calcium, vit D

NURSING CONSIDERATIONS

Assess:
• Renal studies, Ca, P, Mg, K
• For hypercalcemia: paresthesia, twitching, laryngospasm, Chvostek's, Trousseau's signs

Administer:

IV route
• After reconstituting by adding 10 ml of sterile water for inj to each vial (30 mg/10 ml, or 60 mg/10 ml, or 90 mg/10 ml depending on vial used), then add to 1000 ml of sterile 0.45%, 0.9% NaCl, D₅W, run over 24 hr for hypercalcemia or 60 mg ≥4 hr, 90 mg over 24 hr; dilute reconstituted sol in 500 ml of 0.9% NaCl, 0.45% NaCl, or D₅W, give over 4 hr (multiple myeloma, Paget's disease)
• Do not mix with calcium-containing infusion sol such as Ringer's sol

Perform/provide:
• Storage of infusion sol up to 24 hr at room temperature
• Reconstituted sol with sterile water may be stored under refrigeration for up to 24 hr

Evaluate:
• Therapeutic response: decreased calcium levels

Teach patient/family
• To report hypercalcemic relapse: nausea, vomiting, bone pain, thirst; unusual muscle twitching, muscle spasms, severe diarrhea, constipation
• To continue with dietary recommendations including calcium and vit D
• To obtain an analgesic from provider for bone pain
• That if nausea/vomiting occur, small, frequent meals may help

---

pancreatin (℞)

(pan'kree-a-tin)

Creon, Donnazyme, Hi-Vegi-Lip, 4× Pancreatin 600 mg, 8× Pancreatin 900 mg, Pancrezyme 4×

Func. class.: Digestant

Chem. class.: Pancreatic enzyme concentrate—bovine/porcine

P

Action: Pancreatic enzyme needed for breakdown of substances released from the pancreas

Uses: Exocrine pancreatic secretion insufficiency, cystic fibrosis (digestive aid)

Dosage and routes:
• *Adult:* **PO** 8000-24,000 USP units with meals

Available forms: Tabs 650, 2000, 12,000 units, others in combination

SIDE EFFECTS

EENT: Buccal soreness

GI: Anorexia, nausea, vomiting, diarrhea, glossitis, anal soreness

GU: Hyperuricuria, hyperuricemia

INTEG: Rash, hypersensitivity

Contraindications: Hypersensitivity to pork, chronic pancreatic disease
Precautions: Pregnancy (C), lactation, ileus, esophageal stricture, Crohn's disease

INTERACTIONS

Decrease: absorption—cimetidine, antacids, oral iron
Decrease: effect of acarbose, miglitol

NURSING CONSIDERATIONS

Assess:
• I&O ratio; watch for increasing urinary output
• Fecal fat, nitrogen, PT, calcium during treatment
• For polyuria, polydipsia, polyphagia (may indicate diabetes mellitus)
• For allergy to pork
Administer:
PO route
• Swallow tabs whole; do not break, crush, or chew enteric coated tabs
• After antacid or H₂-blockers; decreased pH inactivates drug
• Low-fat diet for GI symptoms
Perform/provide:
• Storage in tight container at room temperature
Evaluate:
• Therapeutic response: relief of GI symptoms

---

pancrelipase (℞)
(pan-kre-li′pase)
Cotazym, Cotazym-65B ✦,
Cotazym E.C.S. 8, Cotazym
E.C.S. 20, Cotazym Capsules,
Cotazym-S, Creon, Ilozyme,
Ku-Zyme HP, Lipram-PN16,
Lipram-CR20, Lipram-UL12,
Lipram-PN10, Pancrease
Capsules, Pancrease MT 4,
Pancrease MT 10, Pancrease
MT 16, Protilase, Ultrase MT
12, Ultrase MT 20, Viokase,
Zymase
Func. class.: Digestant
Chem. class.: Pancreatic enzyme—
bovine/porcine

Action: Pancreatic enzyme needed for breakdown of substances released from the pancreas
Uses: Exocrine pancreatic secretion insufficiency, cystic fibrosis (digestive aid), steatorrhea, pancreatic enzyme deficiency

DOSAGE AND ROUTES

Many products listed above are not interchangeable
• *Adult and child:* **PO** 1-3 caps/tabs ac or with meals, or 1 cap/tab with snack or 1-2 powder pkt ac
Available forms: Powder: 16,800 units lipase/70,000 units protease and amylase; caps: 8000 units lipase/30,000 units protease and amylase; cap, delayed rel 4000 units lipase/12,000 units protease and amylase, 4000 units lipase/25,000 units protease/20,000 units amylase, 5000 units lipase/20,000 units protease and amylase, 10,000 units lipase/30,000 units protease and amylase, 12,000 units lipase/24,000 units protease and amylase, 12,000 units lipase/39,000 units protease and amylase, 16,000 units lipase/48,000 units protease and amylase, 20,000 units lipase/65,000 units protease and amy-

lase, 24,000 units lipase/78,000 units protease and amylase

Side effects/adverse reactions:
GI: Anorexia, nausea, vomiting, diarrhea
GU: Hyperuricuria, hyperuricemia
Contraindications: Allergy to pork
Precautions: Pregnancy (C), ileus, pancreatitis, Crohn's disease

INTERACTIONS

Decrease: absorption—cimetidine, antacids, oral iron
Decrease: effect of acarbose, miglitol

NURSING CONSIDERATIONS

Assess:
• For appropriate height, weight development; may be delayed
• I&O ratio; watch for increasing urinary output
• Fecal fat, nitrogen, PT during treatment
• For polyuria, polydipsia, polyphagia (may indicate diabetes mellitus)
• For pork sensitivity, cross-sensitivity may occur

Administer:
• After antacid or cimetidine; decreased pH inactivates drug
• Powder mixed in prepared fruit juice for infants, children
• Low-fat diet for GI symptoms
• With 8 oz water or more, do not allow to sit in mouth, have patient sit up during administration

Perform/provide:
• Storage in tight container at room temperature

Evaluate:
• Therapeutic response: improved digestion of carbohydrates, protein, fat; absence of steatorrhea

Teach patient/family:
• Not to inhale powder; may be very irritating to mucous membranes; some powder may irritate skin
• To notify prescriber of allergic reactions, abdominal pain, cramping, or blood in the urine

---

⚠ High Alert

pancuronium (℞)
(pan-kyoo-roe′nee-um)
pancuronium bromide,
Pavulon
Func. class.: Neuromuscular blocker (nondepolarizing)
Chem. class.: Synthetic curariform

Action: Inhibits transmission of nerve impulses by binding with cholinergic receptor sites, antagonizing action of acetylcholine
Uses: Facilitation of endotracheal intubation, skeletal muscle relaxation during mechanical ventilation, surgery, or general anesthesia

DOSAGE AND ROUTES

• *Adult and child >1 mo:* **IV** 0.04-0.1 mg/kg, then 0.01 mg/kg q½-1h
Available forms: Inj 1, 2 mg/ml

SIDE EFFECTS

CV: Bradycardia; tachycardia; increased, decreased B/P; ventricular extrasystoles, edema
EENT: Increased secretions
INTEG: Rash, flushing, pruritus, urticaria, sweating, salivation
MS: Weakness to prolonged skeletal muscle relaxation
RESP: ***Prolonged apnea, bronchospasm, cyanosis, respiratory depression, wheezing***
SYST: ***Anaphylaxis***
Contraindications: Hypersensitivity to bromide ion
Precautions: Pregnancy (C), renal disease, cardiac disease, hepatic disease, lactation, children <2 yr, electrolyte imbalances, dehydration, neuromuscular disease, respiratory disease

PHARMACOKINETICS

IV: Onset 3-5 min, dose dependent, peak 3-5 min; metabolized (small amounts), excreted in urine (unchanged), crosses placenta

P

INTERACTIONS

Dysrhythmias: theophylline
Increase: neuromuscular blockade—aminoglycosides, clindamycin, enflurane, isoflurane, lincomycin, lithium, local anesthetics, opioid analgesics, polymyxin antiinfectives, quinidine, thiazides

Drug/Lab Test
Decrease: Cholinesterase

NURSING CONSIDERATIONS

Assess:
• For electrolyte imbalances (K, Mg); may lead to increased action of this drug
• VS (B/P, pulse, respirations, airway) until fully recovered; rate, depth, pattern of respirations, strength of hand grip
• I&O ratio; check for urinary retention, frequency, hesitancy
• Recovery: decreased paralysis of face, diaphragm, leg, arm, rest of body; allow to recover fully before neuro assessment
A Allergic reactions, anaphylaxis: rash, fever, respiratory distress, pruritus; drug should be discontinued

Administer:
IV, direct route
• With diazepam or morphine when used for therapeutic paralysis; this drug provides no sedation
• Using nerve stimulator by anesthesiologist to determine neuromuscular blockade
• Atropine to counteract muscarinic effects
• After succinylcholine effects subside
• Anticholinesterase to reverse neuromuscular blockade
• IV undiluted, give over 1-2 min (only by qualified persons)

Additive compatibilities: Verapamil
Syringe compatibilities: Heparin
Y-site compatibilities: Aminophylline, cefazolin, cefuroxime, cimetidine, DOBUTamine, DOPamine, epINEPHrine, esmolol, fentanyl, fluconazole, gentamicin, heparin, hydrocortisone, isoproterenol, lorazepam, midazolam, morphine, nitroglycerin, nitroprusside, ranitidine,

trimethoprim-sulfamethoxazole, vancomycin

Perform/provide:
• Storage in refrigerator; do not store in plastic; use only fresh sol
• Reassurance if communication is difficult during recovery from neuromuscular blockade
• Frequent (q2h) instillation of artificial tears and covering eyes to prevent drying of cornea

Evaluate:
• Therapeutic response: paralysis of jaw, eyelid, head, neck, rest of body

Treatment of overdose: Edrophonium or neostigmine, atropine, monitor VS; may require mechanical ventilation

---

pantoprazole (℞)
(pan-toe-pray'zole)
Protonix, Prontonix IV
Func. class.: Proton pump inhibitor
Chem. class.: Benzimidazole

Action: Suppresses gastric secretion by inhibiting hydrogen/potassium ATPase enzyme system in gastric parietal cell; characterized as gastric acid pump inhibitor, since it blocks final step of acid production
Uses: Gastroesophageal reflux disease (GERD), severe erosive esophagitis, maintenance, long-term pathologic hypersecretory conditions including Zollinger-Ellison syndrome

DOSAGE AND ROUTES

GERD
• *Adult:* **PO** 40 mg daily × 8 wk, may repeat course
Erosive esophagitis
• *Adult:* **IV** 40 mg daily × 7-10 day **PO** 40 mg daily × 8 wk; may repeat **PO** course
Pathological hypersecretory conditions
• *Adult:* **IV** 80 mg q12h; max 240 mg/day

A Safety alert   *"Tall Man" lettering

Available forms: Tabs, delayed rel 20, 40 mg; powder for inj, freeze-dried 40 mg/vial

SIDE EFFECTS

CNS: Headache, insomnia
GI: Diarrhea, abdominal pain, flatulence
INTEG: Rash
META: Hyperglycemia
Contraindications: Hypersensitivity
Precautions: Pregnancy (C), lactation, children

PHARMACOKINETICS

Peak 2.4 hr, duration >24 hr, half-life 1.5 hr, protein binding 97%, eliminated in urine as metabolites and in feces; in elderly elimination rate decreased

INTERACTIONS

May decrease absorption: sucralfate
Increase: pantoprazole serum levels—diazepam, phenytoin, flurazepam, triazolam, clarithromycin
Increase: bleeding—warfarin

NURSING CONSIDERATIONS

Assess:
• GI system: bowel sounds q8h, abdomen for pain, swelling, anorexia
• Hepatic studies: AST, ALT, alk phosphatase during treatment
Administer:
PO route
• Swallow del rel tabs whole: do not break crush, or chew
• Take del rel tabs at same time of day
• May take with or without food
IV route
• Reconstitute with 10 ml 0.9% NaCl, further dilute with 80 ml LR, D₅, 0.9% NaCl (0.8 mg/ml), give over 15 min (≤6 mg/min) using in-line filter provided
Evaluate:
• Therapeutic response: absence of epigastric pain, swelling, fullness

Teach patient/family:
• To report severe diarrhea; drug may have to be discontinued
• That diabetic patient should know hypoglycemia may occur
• To avoid hazardous activities; dizziness may occur
• To avoid alcohol, salicylates, ibuprofen; may cause GI irritation
• To notify prescriber if pregnant or plan to become pregnant, do not breastfeed

Rarely Used

papaverine (℞)
(pa-pav′er-een)
Func. class.: Peripheral vasodilator

Uses: Arterial spasm resulting in cerebral and peripheral ischemia; myocardial ischemia associated with vascular spasm or dysrhythmias; angina pectoris; peripheral pulmonary embolism; visceral spasm as in ureteral, biliary, GI colic, peripheral vascular disease

DOSAGE AND ROUTES

• *Adult:* **SUS REL** 150-300 mg q8-12h; **IM/IV** 30-120 mg
Contraindications: Hypersensitivity, complete AV heart block

Rarely Used

paraldehyde (℞)
(par-al′de-hyde)
Func. class.: Anticonvulsant

Uses: Refractory seizures, status epilepticus, sedation, insomnia, alcohol withdrawal, tetanus, eclampsia

DOSAGE AND ROUTES

Seizures
• *Adult:* **IM** 5-10 ml; divide 10 ml into 2 inj; **IV** 0.2-0.4 ml/kg in **NS** inj
• *Child:* **IM** 0.15 ml/kg; **RECT** 0.3 ml/kg q4-6h or 1 ml/yr of age, not to

P

exceed 5 ml; may repeat in 1 hr prn; **IV** 5 ml/90 ml **NS** inj; begin infusion at 5 ml/hr; titrate to patient response

Alcohol withdrawal
• *Adult:* **PO/RECT** 5-10 ml, not to exceed 60 ml; **IM** 5 ml q4-6h × 24 hr, then q6h on following days, not to exceed 30 ml

Sedation
• *Adult:* **PO/REC** 4-10 ml; **IM** 5 ml; **IV** 3-5 ml in emergency only; Child: **PO/REC/IM** 0.15 ml/kg

Tetanus
• *Adult:* **IV** 4-5 ml or 12 ml by gastric tube q4h diluted with water; **IM** 5-10 ml prn

Contraindications: Hypersensitivity, gastroenteritis with ulceration

---

paricalcitol (R)
(par-ih-cal′sih-tol)
Zemplar
Func. class.: Vit D analong
Chem. class.: Fat-soluble vitamin

Action: Reduces parathyroid hormone (PTH) levels; suppresses PTH levels in patients with chronic renal failure with absence of hypercalcemia/hyperphosphatemia. Serum PO_4, calcium, CaXP may increase

Uses: Hyperparathyroidism in chronic renal failure

DOSAGE AND ROUTES

• *Adult:* **IV BOL** 0.04-0.1 mcg/kg (2.8-7 mcg) no more than every other day during dialysis; may increase by 2-4 mcg q2-4wk until target serum intact Pth $(1.5 - 3 \times$ nonuremic upper limit of normal) is achieved

Available forms: Inj 5 mcg/ml

SIDE EFFECTS

CNS: Lightheadedness
CV: Palpitations
GI: Nausea, vomiting, anorexia, dry mouth
OTHER: Pneumonia, edema, chills, fever, flu, *sepsis*

Contraindications: Hypersensitivity, hypercalcemia

Precautions: Pregnancy (C), cardiovascular disease, renal calculi, elderly, lactation, children

INTERACTIONS

Digitalis toxicity: digitalis

NURSING CONSIDERATIONS

Assess:
• Ca, PO_4, q2 ×/wk during initial therapy; after dose is established take calcium and phosphorus qmo

Administer:
• By IV bolus only

Evaluate:
• Decreased hypoparathyroidism in chronic renal disease

Teach patient/family:
• To report weakness, lethargy, headache, anorexia, loss of weight
• To report nausea, vomiting, palpitations

Rarely Used

paromomycin (R)
(par-oh-moe-mye′sin)
Func. class.: Amebicide

Uses: Intestinal amebiasis, adjunct in hepatic coma

DOSAGE AND ROUTES

Intestinal amebiasis
• *Adult and child:* **PO** 25-35 mg/kg/day in 3 divided doses × 5-10 day pc

Hepatic coma
• *Adult:* **PO** 4 g daily in divided doses × 5-6 day

Contraindications: Hypersensitivity, renal disease, GI obstruction

---

paroxetine (℞)

(par-ox'e-teen)

Paxil, Paxil CR

Func. class.: Antidepressant, SSRI

Chem. class.: Phenylpiperidine derivative

Do not confuse:

paroxetine/paclitaxel

Paxil/paclitaxel

Paxil/Taxol

Action: Inhibits CNS neuron uptake of serotonin but not of norepinephrine or dopamine

Uses: Major depressive disorder, obsessive-compulsive disorder, panic disorder, generalized anxiety disorder, posttraumatic stress disorder, premenstrual disorders, social anxiety disorder

Investigational uses: Diabetic neuropathy, headaches, premature ejaculation, bipolar depression with lithium, fibromyalgia

DOSAGE AND ROUTES

Generalized anxiety disorder

• *Adult:* **PO** 20 mg/day AM range 20-50 mg/day

Posttraumatic stress disorder

• *Adult:* **PO** 20 mg/day range 20-50 mg/day

Depression

• *Adult:* **PO** 20 mg daily in AM; after 4 wk if no clinical improvement is noted, dose may be increased by 10 mg/day qwk to desired response, not to exceed 60 mg/day or **CONTROLLED REL** 25 mg/day, may increase by 12.5 mg/day weekly up to 62.5 mg/day

• *Geriatric:* **PO** 10 mg daily, increase by 10 mg to desired dose, max 40 mg/day

Obsessive-compulsive disorder

• *Adult:* **PO** 20 mg/day in AM, start with 20 mg/day, increase 10 mg/day increments, max 60 mg/day

Panic disorder

• *Adult:* **PO** 40 mg/day, start with 10 mg/day and increase in 10 mg/day increments, max 60 mg/day or

CONTROLLED REL 12.5 mg/day, max 75 mg/day

Premenstrual disorders

• *Adult:* **CONT REL** 12.5 mg/day in AM

Renal dose

• *Adult:* **PO** 10 mg daily in AM, may increase by 10 mg/day qwk, max 50 mg daily or **CONTROLLED REL** 12.5 mg/day, max 50 mg/day

Available forms: Tabs 10, 20, 30, 40 mg; oral susp 10 mg/5 ml; controlled rel 12.5, 25, 37.5 mg

SIDE EFFECTS

CNS: Headache, nervousness, insomnia, drowsiness, anxiety, tremor, dizziness, fatigue, sedation, abnormal dreams, agitation, apathy, euphoria, hallucinations, delusions, psychosis

CV: Vasodilation, postural hypotension, palpitations

EENT: Visual changes

GI: Nausea, diarrhea, dry mouth, anorexia, dyspepsia, constipation, cramps, vomiting, taste changes, flatulence, decreased appetite

GU: Dysmenorrhea, decreased libido, urinary frequency, UTI, amenorrhea, cystitis, impotence, abnormal ejaculation (male)

INTEG: Sweating, rash

MS: Pain, arthritis, myalgia, myopathy, myosthenia

RESP: Infection, pharyngitis, nasal congestion, sinus headache, sinusitis, cough, dyspnea

SYST: Asthenia, fever

Contraindications: Hypersensitivity, patients taking MAOIs, alcohol use

Precautions: Pregnancy (D), lactation, children, elderly, seizure history, patients with history of mania, renal and hepatic disease

PHARMACOKINETICS

PO: Peak 5.2 hr; metabolized in liver by CPY50 enzyme system, unchanged drugs and metabolites excreted in feces and urine; half-life 21 hr; protein binding 95%

P

INTERACTIONS

Paroxetine may decrease digoxin levels
⚠ Do not use with MAOIs, thioridazine potentially fatal reactions can occur
Increase: bleeding—warfarin
Increase: paroxetine plasma levels—cimetidine
Increase: agitation—L-tryptophan
Increase: side effects—highly protein-bound drugs
Increase: theophylline levels—theophylline
Decrease: paroxetine levels—phenobarbital and phenytoin

Drug/Herb
Possible serotonin syndrome: SAM-e, St. John's wort
Hypertensive crisis: ephedra
Increase: anticholinergic effect—corkwood, jimsonweed
Increase: sedative—hops, lavender
Increase: CNS stimulation—yohimbe

Drug/Lab Test
Increase: Serum bilirubin, blood glucose, alk phosphatase
Decrease: VMA, 5-HIAA
False increase: Urinary catecholamines

NURSING CONSIDERATIONS

Assess:
• Mental status: mood, sensorium, affect, suicidal tendencies, increase in psychiatric symptoms, depression, panic
• B/P (lying/standing), pulse q4h; if systolic B/P drops 20 mm Hg, hold drug, notify prescriber; take vital signs q4h in patients with cardiovascular disease
• Blood studies: CBC, leukocytes, differential, cardiac enzymes if patient is receiving long-term therapy
• Hepatic studies: AST, ALT, bilirubin, creatinine
• Weight qwk; appetite may decrease with drug
• ECG for flattening of T wave, bundle branch, AV block, dysrhythmias in cardiac patients
• EPS primarily in elderly: rigidity, dystonia, akathisia
• Urinary retention, constipation

• Withdrawal symptoms: headache, nausea, vomiting, muscle pain, weakness; not usual unless drug discontinued abruptly
• Alcohol intake; if alcohol is consumed, hold dose until morning

Administer:
• Increased fluids, bulk in diet for constipation, urinary retention
• With food, milk for GI symptoms
• Crushed if patient is unable to swallow medication whole
• Dosage at bedtime for oversedation during day; may take entire dose at bedtime; elderly may not tolerate once/day dosing
• Gum, hard candy, frequent sips of water for dry mouth
• Avoid use with other CNS depressants

Perform/provide:
• Storage at room temperature; do not freeze
• Assistance with ambulation during therapy, since drowsiness, dizziness occur
• Safety measures primarily in elderly
• Checking to see if PO medication swallowed

Evaluate:
• Therapeutic response: decreased depression

Teach patient/family:
• That therapeutic effect may take 1-4 wk
• To use caution in driving, other activities requiring alertness because of drowsiness, dizziness, blurred vision
• Not to discontinue medication quickly after long-term use; may cause nausea, headache, malaise
• To avoid alcohol ingestion
Treatment of overdose: Airway, for seizures give diazepam, symptomatic treatment

pegaptanib (℞)
(peg-ap′-ta-nib)
Macugen
Func. class.: Ophthalmic agent—miscellaneous

Action: Binds to vascular endothelial growth factor (VEGF), thereby inhibiting angiogenesis
Uses: Treatment of neovascular (wet) age-related macular degeneration; may be used alone or with photodynamic therapy

DOSAGE AND ROUTES
• *Adult:* **Intravitreal INJ** 0.3 mg injected q6wk
Available forms: Inj 0.3 mg, single glass syringes

SIDE EFFECTS
EENT: Anterior chamber inflammation, blurred vision, conjunctival hemorrhage, corneal edema, cataract, eye discharge, eye pain, increased intraocular pressure, punctuate keratitis, reduced visual acuity, vitreous floaters, vitreous opacities, blepharitis, conjunctivitis, photophobia, retinal detachment, iatrogenic traumatic cataract
Contraindications: Hypersensitivity, ocular or periocular infections
Precautions: Pregnancy (B), inflammatory eye disease, ocular hypertension

PHARMACOKINETICS:
Half-life 87-100 hr in vitreous humor of the monkey, may remain fully active in the eye for 7-28 days

INTERACTIONS
None known

NURSING CONSIDERATIONS
Assess:
• Visual acuity periodically
• Treated eye for increased intraocular pressure, infection, endophthalmitis

• Perfusion of the optic nerve head immediately after inj, tonometry ½ hr after inj, biomicroscopy 2-7 days after inj
Administer:
• Anesthesia and a broad-spectrum antiinfective agent before injection
• The inj should be done under aseptic conditions
Perform/provide:
• Storage at 36°-46° F, do not freeze or shake vigorously
Evaluate:
• Therapeutic response: macular degeneration stabilized
Teach patient/family:
• To report any inflammation, bleeding, eye discharge, opacities to prescriber
• To continue with follow-up care during treatment

⚠ High Alert

pegaspargase (℞)
(peg-as′per-gase)
Oncaspar, PEG-L-asparaginase
Func. class.: Antineoplastic
Chem. class.: Escherichia coli enzyme

Action: Indirectly inhibits protein synthesis in tumor cells; without amino acid, DNA, RNA synthesis is halted; asparagine, protein synthesis is halted; G_1 phase; cell-cycle specific; a nonvesicant; a modified version of L-asparaginase
Uses: Acute lymphocytic leukemia in combination with other antineoplastics

DOSAGE AND ROUTES
In combination
• *Adult and child with BSA ≥0.6 m²:* **IV/IM** 2500 international units/m² q14d, run **IV** over 1-2 hr in 100 ml of NaCl or D_5 through a running **IV**; **IM** should be no more than 2 ml in one inj site
• *Child with BSA <0.6 m²:* **IV/IM** 82.5 international units/kg q14d

Sole induction
• *Adult:* IV 2500 international units/m^2 q14d

Available forms: Inj 750 international units/ml in a phosphate buffered saline sol

SIDE EFFECTS

CNS: Neuritis, dizziness, headache, *coma,* depression, fatigue, confusion, hallucinations, *seizures*
CV: Chest pain, *hypertension*
ENDO: Hyperglycemia
GI: Nausea, vomiting, anorexia, cramps, stomatitis, hepatotoxicity, pancreatitis, diarrhea
GU: Urinary retention, *renal failure,* glycosuria, polyuria, azotemia, uric acid neuropathy
HEMA: Thrombocytopenia, leukopenia, myelosuppression, anemia, decreased clotting factors, pancytopenia
INTEG: Rash, urticaria, chills, fever
RESP: Fibrosis, pulmonary infiltrate, severe bronchospasm
SYST: Anaphylaxis, hypersensitivity
Contraindications: Hypersensitivity, infant, lactation, pancreatitis
Precautions: Pregnancy (C), renal disease, hepatic disease, CNS disease

PHARMACOKINETICS

Half-life 5½ days, onset rapid, duration 2 wk, metabolized in reticuloendothelial system

INTERACTIONS

Do not use with radiation
Coagulation factor imbalances: heparin, warfarin, aspirin, NSAIDs
Decrease: action of methotrexate

NURSING CONSIDERATIONS
Assess:
⚠ For signs and symptoms of pancreatitis (nausea, vomiting, severe abdominal pain), anaphylaxis (bronchospasm, dyspnea), cyanosis
• CBC, differential, platelet count qwk; withhold drug if WBC count is <4000 or platelet count is <75,000; notify prescriber of results
• Pulmonary function tests, chest x-ray studies before and during therapy; chest x-ray film should be obtained q2wk during treatment, watch for severe bronchospasm, fibrosis, pulmonary infiltrate
• Renal studies: BUN, serum uric acid, ammonia, urine CCr, electrolytes before and during therapy
• I&O ratio; report fall in urine output to ≤30 ml/hr, may indicate renal failure
• Temp q4h (may indicate beginning infection)
• Hepatic studies before and during therapy (bilirubin, AST, ALT, LDH) as needed or monthly, hepatotoxicity can occur; check for jaundiced skin, sclera; dark urine, clay-colored stools, itchy skin, abdominal pain, fever, diarrhea
• RBC, Hct, Hgb; may be decreased
• Serum, urine glucose levels, glycosuria can occur
• Bleeding: hematuria, stool guaiac, bruising or petechiae, mucosa or orifices q8h
• Dyspnea, crackles, nonproductive cough, chest pain, tachypnea, fatigue, increased pulse, pallor, lethargy, swelling around eyes or lips; anaphylaxis may occur
• B/P, since hypertension can occur
• Local irritation, pain, burning, discoloration at inj site
⚠ Symptoms of severe allergic reaction: rash, pruritus, urticaria, purpuric skin lesions, itching, flushing, dyspnea
• Frequency of stools, characteristics; cramping, acidosis; signs of dehydration: rapid respirations, poor skin turgor, decreased urine output, dry skin, restlessness, weakness
Administer:
• Antispasmodic if GI symptoms occur
• Allopurinol or sodium bicarbonate to reduce uric acid levels, alkalinization of urine
IV INF route
• Using 21, 23, 25G needle; administer by slow IV infusion via Y-tube or 3-way

stopcock of flowing D_5W or NS infusion over 2 hr after diluting
• Considered incompatible with other drugs in syringe or sol

Perform/provide:
• Deep-breathing exercises with patient tid-qid; place in semi-Fowler's position
• Increase fluid intake to 2-3 L/day to prevent urate deposits, calculi formation
• Diet low in purines: no organ meats (kidney, liver); dried beans, peas to maintain alkaline urine
• Rinsing of mouth tid-qid with water, club soda; brushing of teeth bid-tid with soft brush or cotton-tipped applicator for stomatitis; use unwaxed dental floss
• Warm compresses at inj site for inflammation
• Nutritious diet with iron, vitamin supplements
• HOB raised to facilitate breathing

Evaluate:
• Therapeutic response: decreased exacerbations in acute lymphocytic leukemia

Teach patient/family:
• To report nausea, vomiting, bruising, bleeding, stomatitis, severe diarrhea, jaundice, chest pain, abdominal pain, trouble breathing, rash
• To avoid vaccinations without advice of prescriber
• Not to use hard-bristled toothbrush, razors
• To avoid OTC medications, alcohol

Treatment of anaphylaxis: Administer epINEPHrine, diphenhydrAMINE, IV corticosteroids

---

pegfilgrastim (℞)
(peg-fill-grass'stim)
Neulasta
Func. class.: Hematopoietic agent
Chem. class.: Granulocyte colony-stimulating factor

Action: Stimulates proliferation and differentiation of neutrophils
Uses: To decrease infection in patients receiving antineoplastics that are myelosuppressive; to increase WBC in patients with drug-induced neutropenia

DOSAGE AND ROUTES
• *Adult:* **SUBCUT** 6 mg give once per chemotherapy cycle
Available forms: Sol for inj 10 mg/ml

SIDE EFFECTS
CNS: Fever, fatigue, headache, dizziness, insomnia, peripheral edema
GI: Nausea, vomiting, diarrhea, mucositis, anorexia, constipation, dyspepsia, abdominal pain, stomatitis, ***splenic rupture***
*HEMA: **Leukocytosis, granulocytopenia, sickle cell crisis***
INTEG: Alopecia
MISC: Chest pain, hyperuricemia, ***anaphylaxis***
MS: Skeletal pain
*RESP: **Respiratory distress syndrome***
Contraindications: Hypersensitivity to proteins of *Escherichia coli,* filgrastim; ARDS
Precautions: Pregnancy (C), lactation, myeloid malignancies, sickle cell disease, adolescents, child <45 kg

PHARMACOKINETICS
Half-life: 15-80 hr

INTERACTIONS
Do not use this drug concomitantly or 2 wk before or 24 hr after administration of cytotoxic chemotherapy
Increase: release of neutrophils—lithium

Drug/Lab Test
Increase: Uric acid, LDH, alk phosphatase

NURSING CONSIDERATIONS
Assess:
⚠ Allergic reactions, anaphylaxis: rash, urticaria; discontinue this drug, have emergency equipment nearby
• Blood studies: CBC, platelet count before treatment and twice weekly; neu-

trophil counts may be increased for 2 days after therapy
- B/P, respirations, pulse before and during therapy
- Bone pain, give mild analgesics

Administer:
- Using single-use vials; after dose is withdrawn, do not reenter vial
- Do not use 6 mg fixed dose in infants, children, or others <45 kg
- Inspect sol for discoloration, particulates; if present, do not use
- Do not administer in the period 14 days before and 24 hr after cytotoxic chemotherapy

Perform/provide:
- Storage in refrigerator; do not freeze; may store at room temperature up to 6 hr, avoid shaking, protect from light

Evaluate:
- Therapeutic response: absence of infection

Teach patient/family:
- The technique for self-administration: dose, side effects, disposal of containers and needles; provide instruction sheet

---

peginterferon alfa-2a (℞)
(peg-in-ter-feer'on)
Pegasys
Func. class.: Immunomodulator

Action: Stimulates genes to modulate many biologic effects, including inhibition of viral replication; inhibits ion cell proliferation, immunomodulation, stimulates effector proteins, decreases leukocyte, platelet counts
Uses: Chronic hepatitis C infections in adults with compensated liver disease

DOSAGE AND ROUTES
- *Adult:* SUBCUT 180 mcg qwk × 48 wk; if poorly tolerated, reduce dose to 135 mcg qwk; in some cases reduction to 90 mcg may be needed
Available forms: Inj 180 mcg/ml

SIDE EFFECTS
CNS: Headache, insomnia, dizziness, anxiety, hostility, lability, nervousness, depression, fatigue, poor concentration, pyrexia
GI: Abdominal pain, nausea, diarrhea, anorexia, vomiting, dry mouth
HEMA: **Thrombocytopenia,** neutropenia
INTEG: Alopecia, pruritus, rash, dermatitis
MS: Back pain, myalgia, arthralgia
Contraindications: Hypersensitivity to interferons, neonates, infants, autoimmune hepatitis, decompensated hepatic disease prior to use of this drug
Precautions: Pregnancy (C), thyroid disorders, myelosuppression, hepatic, cardiac disease, lactation, children <18 yr, depression/suicide, preexisting ophthalmologic disorders, pancreatitis, renal disease, elderly

PHARMACOKINETICS
Half-life 15-80 hr, large variability in other pharmacokinetics

INTERACTIONS
Use caution when giving with theophylline, myelosuppressive agents

NURSING CONSIDERATIONS
Assess:
- ALT, HCV viral load; patients who show no reduction in ALT, HCV are unlikely to show benefit of treatment after 6 mo
- Platelet counts, heme concentration, ANC, serum creatinine concentration, albumin, bilirubin, TSH, T_4, AFP
- For myelosuppression, hold dose if neutrophil count is <500 × 10^6/L or if platelets are <50 × 10^9/L
- For hypersensitivity: discontinue immediately if hypersensitivity occurs

Administer:
- In evening to reduce discomfort, sleep through some side effects

Evaluate:
- Therapeutic response: decreased

---

chronic hepatitis C signs/symptoms, undetectable viral load
Teach patient/family:
• Provide patient or family member with written, detailed information about drug
• Instructions for home use if appropriate
• Use effective contraception throughout treatment

Rarely Used

pegvisomant (R)
(peg-vi′soe-mant)
Somavert
Func. class.: Miscellaneous agent

Uses: Acromegaly, in those patients who have an inadequate response to other treatment.

DOSAGE AND ROUTES
• *Adult:* SUBCUT Loading dose of 40 mg, under supervision of prescriber, then SUBCUT 10 mg daily, measure IGF-I levels q4-6wk
Contraindications: Hypersensitivity, latex allergy

⚠ High Alert

pemetrexed (R)
(pem-ah-trex′ed)
Alimta
Func. class.: Antineoplastic-antimetabolite
Chem. class.: Folic acid antagonist

Action: Inhibits an enzyme that reduces folic acid, which is needed for cell replication
Uses: Malignant pleural mesothelioma in combination with cisplatin; non–small cell lung cancer as a single agent

DOSAGE AND ROUTES
• *Adult:* IV INF 500 mg/m^2 given over 10 min on day 1 of a 21-day cycle with cisplatin 75 mg/m^2 infused over 2 hr,

beginning ½ hr after end of pemetrexed infusion
• Nadir ANC <500/mm^3 and platelets ≥50,000/mm^3, 75% of previous dose
Available forms: Inj, single-use vials, 500 mg

SIDE EFFECTS
CNS: Fatigue, fever, mood alteration, neuropathy
*CV: **Thrombosis/embolism**, chest pain*
GI: Nausea, vomiting, anorexia, diarrhea, ulcerative stomatitis, constipation, dysphagia, dehydration
*GU: **Renal failure**, creatinine elevation*
*HEMA: **Neutropenia, leukopenia, thrombocytopenia, myelosuppression, anemia***
INTEG: Rash, desquamation
RESP: Dyspnea
*SYST: **Infection with/without neutropenia***

Contraindications: Pregnancy (D), hypersensitivity, ANC <1500 cells/mm^3, CCr <45 ml/min, thrombocytopenia (<100,000/mm^3), anemia
Precautions: Renal disease, lactation, children, hepatic disease

PHARMACOKINETICS
Not metabolized; excreted in urine (unchanged 70%-90%); not known if it is excreted in breast milk; half-life 3.5 hr, 81% protein binding

INTERACTIONS
Decrease: pemetrexed's clearance—nephrotoxic drugs (NSAIDs)

NURSING CONSIDERATIONS
Assess:
⚠ CBC, differential, platelet count, monitor for nadir and recovery; a new cycle should not begin if ANC <1500 cells/mm^3, platelets are <100,000 cells/mm^3, creatinine clearance <45 ml/min
• Renal studies: BUN, serum uric acid,

P

urine CCr, electrolytes before, during therapy

• I&O ratio; report fall in urine output to <30 ml/hr

• Monitor temp q4h; fever may indicate beginning infection; no rectal temps

• Bleeding time, coagulation time during treatment; bleeding: hematuria, guaiac, bruising or petechiae, mucosa or orifices q8h

• Buccal cavity q8h for dryness, sores, ulceration, white patches, oral pain, bleeding, dysphagia

⚠ Symptoms indicating severe allergic reaction: rash, urticaria, itching, flushing

Administer:

• Vit B$_{12}$ and low-dose folic acid as a prophylactic measure to treat related hematologic, GI toxicity; at least 5 daily doses of folic acid must be taken in the 7 days preceding first dose

• Premedicate with a corticosteroid (dexamethasone) given PO bid the day before, day of, and day after administration of pemetrexed

IV route

• Use aseptic technique during reconstitution, dilution

• Reconstitute 500 mg vial/20 ml 0.9% NaCl inj (preservative free) = 25 mg/ml, swirl until dissolved, further dilute with 100 ml 0.9% NaCl inj (preservative free), give as IV infusion over 10 mg

• Use only 0.9% NaCl inj (preservative free) for reconstitution, dilution

Perform/provide:

• Strict medical asepsis and protective isolation if WBC levels are low

• Liquid diet: carbonated beverage, Jell-O; dry toast, crackers may be added when patient is not nauseated or vomiting

• Rinsing of mouth tid-qid with water, club soda; brushing of teeth bid-tid with soft brush or cotton-tipped applicators for stomatitis; use unwaxed dental floss

• Storage at 77° F, excursions permitted 59°-86° F, not light sensitive, discard unused portions

Evaluate:

• Therapeutic response: decreased spread of malignancy

Teach patient/family:

• To report any complaints, side effects to nurse or prescriber: black tarry stools, chills, fever, sore throat, bleeding, bruising, cough, shortness of breath, dark or bloody urine

• To avoid foods with citric acid, hot or rough texture if stomatitis is present

• To report stomatitis: any bleeding, white spots, ulcerations in mouth to prescriber; tell patient to examine mouth daily, report symptoms to nurse, use good oral hygiene

• That contraceptive measures are recommended during therapy and for at least 8 wk after cessation of therapy, to discontinue breastfeeding; toxicity to infant may occur

• To avoid alcohol, salicylates, live vaccines

• To avoid use of razors, commercial mouthwash

---

pemoline (℞)
(pem'oh-leen)
Pem ADD, Pem ADD CT, pemoline
Func. class.: Cerebral stimulant
Chem. class.: Oxazolidinone derivative

Controlled Substance Schedule IV

Action: Exact mechanism unknown; may act through dopaminergic mechanisms; produces CNS stimulation and a paradoxic effect in ADHD

Uses: Attention deficit hyperactivity disorder when other treatment has failed

Investigational uses: Narcolepsy, fatigue, excessive daytime sleepiness

DOSAGE AND ROUTES

• *Child >6 yr:* **PO** 37.5 mg in AM, increasing by 18.75 mg/wk, not to exceed 112.5 mg/day

Available forms: Tabs 18.75, 37.5, 75 mg; chewable tabs 37.5 mg

---

SIDE EFFECTS

CNS: Hyperactivity, insomnia, restlessness, dizziness, depression, headache, stimulation, irritability, aggressiveness, hallucinations, ***seizures, masking or worsening of Gilles de la Tourette's syndrome,*** drowsiness, dyskinetic movements

CV: Tachycardia

GI: Nausea, anorexia, diarrhea, abdominal pain, increased liver enzymes, ***hepatitis,*** jaundice, weight loss, ***life-threatening hepatic failure***

MISC: Rashes, growth suppression in children

Contraindications: Hypersensitivity, hepatic insufficiency

Precautions: Pregnancy (B), renal disease, lactation, drug abuse, child <6 yr, psychosis, tics, seizure disorder

PHARMACOKINETICS

PO: Peak 2-4 hr, duration 8 hr, metabolized (50%) by liver, excreted (40%) by kidneys, half-life 10-30 hr

INTERACTIONS

Increase: CNS stimulation—other CNS stimulants

Decrease: seizure threshold—anticonvulsants

Drug/Herb

Synergistic effect: melatonin

Increase: CNS stimulation—horsetail, yohimbe

NURSING CONSIDERATIONS

Assess:

• For attention span, decreased hyperactivity in ADHD persons

⚠ Hepatic studies: ALT, AST, bilirubin; renal, creatinine, prior to treatment and periodically thereafter; if life-threatening, hepatic failure has occurred; discontinue drug if hepatic symptoms occur

• Height, growth rate q3mo in child; growth rate may be decreased

• Mental status: mood, sensorium, affect, stimulation, insomnia, aggressiveness

Administer:

• In AM

Evaluate:

• Therapeutic response: decreased hyperactivity

Teach patient/family:

• To decrease caffeine consumption (coffee, tea, cola, chocolate); may increase irritability, stimulation

• To avoid OTC preparations unless approved by prescriber

• To withdraw over several weeks

• To avoid alcohol ingestion

• To avoid hazardous activities until patient is stabilized

• That therapeutic effect may take 2-4 wk

• To notify prescriber if tremors, insomnia, palpitations, restlessness, jaundice, bleeding, dark urine occur

• Regarding the possibility of hepatotoxicity and need for blood work

---

penciclovir topical
See Appendix C

P

PENICILLINS

penicillin G benzathine (R)
(pen-i-sill'in)
Bicillin L-A, Megacillin ✿, Permapen

penicillin G (R)
Pfizerpen

penicillin G procaine (R)
Ayercillin ✿, Wycillin

penicillin V (R)
Apo-Pen-VK ✿, Beepen-VK, Nadopen-V ✿, Novopen-VK ✿, Pen-Vee K ✿, PVF K ✿, Veetids

Func. class.: Broad-spectrum antiinfective
Chem. class.: Natural penicillin

Action: Interferes with cell wall replication of susceptible organisms; osmotically unstable cell wall swells, bursts from osmotic pressure, results in cell death

Uses: Respiratory infections, scarlet fever, erysipelas, otitis media, pneumonia, skin and soft tissue infections, gonorrhea; effective for gram-positive cocci *(Staphylococcus, Streptococcus pyogenes, S. viridans, S. faecalis, S. bovis, S. pneumoniae),* gram-negative cocci *(Neisseria gonorrhoeae),* gram-positive bacilli *(Actinomyces, Bacillus anthracis, Clostridium perfringens, C. tetani, Corynebacterium diphtheriae, Listeria monocytogenes),* gram-negative bacilli *(Escherichia coli, Proteus mirabilis, Salmonella, Shigella, Enterobacter, Streptobacillus moniliformis),* spirochetes *(Treponema pallidum)*

DOSAGE AND ROUTES

Penicillin G benzathine
Early syphilis
• *Adult:* **IM** 2.4 million units in single dose

Congenital syphilis
• *Child <2 yr:* **IM** 50,000 units/kg in single dose

Prophylaxis of rheumatic fever, glomerulonephritis
• *Adult and child:* **IM** 1.2 million units in single dose qmo or 600,000 units q2wk

Upper respiratory infections (group A streptococcal)
• *Adult:* **IM** 1.2 million units in single dose
• *Child >27 kg:* **IM** 900,000 units in single dose
• *Child <27 kg:* **IM** 300,000-600,000 units in single dose
Available forms: Inj 300,000, 600,000 units/ml

Penicillin G
• CCr <10 ml/min, give full loading dose, then ½ of loading dose q8-10h

Pneumococcal/streptococcal infections (serious)
• *Adult:* **IM/IV** 5-24 million units in divided doses q4-6h
• *Child <12 yr:* **IV** 150,000 units/kg/day in 4-6 divided doses
Available forms: Powder for inj 1, 5, 20 million units/vial; inj 1, 2, 3 million units/50 ml

Penicillin G procaine
Moderate to severe pneumococcal infections
• *Adult and child:* **IM** 600,000-1.2 million units in 1 or 2 doses/day for 10 days to 2 wk
• *Newborn:*
• Avoid use in newborns

Pneumococcal pneumonia
• *Adult and child >12 yr:* **IM** 600,000-1.2 million units/day × 7-10 days
Available forms: Inj 600,000, 1,200,000 units/unit dose

Penicillin V
• Dosage reduction indicated in renal impairment (CCr <50 ml/min)

Pneumococcal/staphylococcal infections
• *Adult:* **PO** 250-500 mg q6h
• *Child <12 yr:* **PO** 25-50 mg/kg/day in divided doses q6-8h

Streptococcal infections
• *Adult:* **PO** 125-250 mg q6-8h × 10 days

Prevention of recurrence of rheumatic fever/chorea
• *Adult:* **PO** 125-250 mg bid continuously

Vincent's gingivitis/pharyngitis
• *Adult:* **PO** 250-500 mg q6-8h

Available forms: Tabs 250, 500 mg; powder for oral sol 125, 250 mg/5 ml

SIDE EFFECTS

CNS: Lethargy, hallucinations, anxiety, depression, twitching, ***coma, seizures***
GI: Nausea, vomiting, diarrhea, increased AST, ALT, abdominal pain, glossitis, colitis
*GU: **Oliguria, proteinuria, hematuria,** vaginitis, moniliasis, **glomerulonephritis***
HEMA: Anemia; increased bleeding time; ***bone marrow depression, granulocytopenia***
META: Hyperkalemia, hypokalemia, alkalosis, hypernatremia
*MISC: **Anaphylaxis, serum sickness,** local pain,* tenderness and fever with IM inj

Contraindications: Hypersensitivity to penicillins; neonates
Precautions: Pregnancy (B), hypersensitivity to cephalosporins, lactation, severe renal disease

PHARMACOKINETICS

Penicillin G benzathine
IM: Very slow absorption, duration 21-28 days, half-life 30-60 min; excreted in urine, feces, breast milk; crosses placenta
Penicillin G
IV: Peak immediate
IM: Peak ¼-½ hr
PO: Peak 1 hr, duration 6 hr
Excreted in urine unchanged, excreted in breast milk, crosses placenta, half-life 30-60 min

Penicillin G procaine
IM: Peak 1-4 hr, duration 15 hr, excreted in urine
Penicillin V
PO: Peak 30-60 min, duration 6-8 hr, half-life 30 min, excreted in urine, breast milk

INTERACTIONS

Increase: penicillin concentrations—aspirin, probenecid
Increase: effect of heparin
Decrease: effect of oral contraceptives
Decrease: antimicrobial effect of penicillin—tetracyclines
Drug/Herb
Do not use acidophilus with antiinfectives
Decrease: absorption of penicillin—khat
Drug/Lab Test
False positive: Urine glucose, urine protein

NURSING CONSIDERATIONS
Assess:
• For infection: temp, characteristics of sputum, wounds, urine, stools before, during, and after treatment
• I&O ratio; report hematuria, oliguria, since penicillin in high doses is nephrotoxic
⚠ Any patient with compromised renal system, since drug is excreted slowly in poor renal system function; toxicity may occur rapidly
• Hepatic studies: AST, ALT
• Blood studies: WBC, RBC, Hct, Hgb, bleeding time
• Renal tests: urinalysis, protein, blood
• C&S before therapy; drug may be given as soon as culture is taken
• Bowel pattern before and during treatment
• Skin eruptions after administration of penicillin to 1 wk after discontinuing drug
• Respiratory status: rate, character, wheezing, tightness in chest
⚠ Allergies before initiation of treatment, reaction of each medication; be-

Side effects: *italics* = common; ***bold italics*** = life-threatening

cause of prolonged action, allergic reaction may be prolonged and severe; watch for anaphylaxis: rash, dyspnea, pruritus, laryngeal edema

Administer:

Penicillin G benzathine

• Drug after C&S completed

• After shaking well, deep IM inj in large muscle mass; avoid intravascular inj, aspirate

Penicillin G

• Drug after C&S

Y-site compatibilities: Acyclovir, amiodarone, cyclophosphamide, diltiazem, enalaprilat, esmolol, fluconazole, foscarnet, heparin, hydromorphone, labetalol, magnesium sulfate, meperidine, morphine, perphenazine, potassium chloride, tacrolimus, theophylline, verapamil, vit B/C

Penicillin G procaine

• Drug after C&S

• Deep IM inj avoid intravascular inj, aspirate

Penicillin V

• Orally on empty stomach for best absorption

• Drug after C&S

Perform/provide:

• EpINEPHrine, suction, tracheostomy set, endotracheal intubation equipment

• Adequate fluid intake (2 L) during diarrhea episodes

• Scratch test to assess allergy after securing order from prescriber; usually done when penicillin is only drug of choice

• Storage in dry, tight container; oral susp refrigerated 2 wk

Evaluate:

• Therapeutic response: absence of fever, draining wounds

• Allergies before initiation of treatment, reaction of each medication; highlight allergies on chart; hypersensitivity reaction may be delayed

Teach patient/family:

• To report sore throat, fever, fatigue; may indicate superinfection

• To wear or carry emergency ID if allergic to penicillins

• To report diarrhea, prevent dehydration

• To shake susp well before each dose; store in refrigerator for up to 2 wk

• To use all medication prescribed

• To use additional contraception if using any of these drugs

Treatment of anaphylaxis: Withdraw drug; maintain airway; administer epINEPHrine, aminophylline, O_2, IV corticosteroids

---

pentamidine (℞)

(pen-tam'i-deen)

Nebupent, Pentam 300, Pentacarinat ✦, Pneumopent ✦

Func. class.: Antiprotozoal

Chem. class.: Aromatic diamide derivative

Action: Interferes with DNA/RNA synthesis in protozoa

Uses: Treatment/prevention of *Pneumocystis jiroveci* infections

Investigational uses: *Leishmania* infections, *Trypanosoma* infections

DOSAGE AND ROUTES

• *Adult and child:* **IV/IM** 4 mg/kg/day × 2-3 wk; **NEB** 300 mg via specific nebulizer given q4wk for prevention

Available forms: Inj, aerosol 300 mg/vial; sol for aerosol 60 mg/vial ✦

SIDE EFFECTS

CNS: Disorientation, hallucinations, *dizziness,* confusion

CV: Hypotension, ventricular tachycardia, ECG abnormalities, *dysrhythmias*

GI: Nausea, vomiting, anorexia; increased AST, ALT; *acute pancreatitis,* metallic taste

*GU: **Acute renal failure, increased serum creatinine, renal toxicity***

HEMA: Anemia, ***leukopenia, thrombocytopenia***

INTEG: Sterile abscess, pain at injection site, pruritus, urticaria, *rash*

META: Hyperkalemia, hypocalcemia, hypoglycemia

MISC: Fatigue, chills, night sweats, ***anaphylaxis, Stevens-Johnson syndrome***

RESP: Cough, shortness of breath, ***bronchospasm*** (with aerosol)

Precautions: Pregnancy (C), blood dyscrasias, hepatic disease, renal disease, diabetes mellitus, cardiac disease, hypocalcemia, hypertension, hypotension, lactation, children

PHARMACOKINETICS

Excreted unchanged in urine (66%)

INTERACTIONS

Nephrotoxicity: aminoglycosides, amphotericin B, cisplatin, NSAIDs, vancomycin

A Fatal dysrhythmias: erythromycin IV

Increase: QT prolongation—class IA, class III antidysrhythmics, phenothiazines

Increase: myelosuppression—antineoplastics, radiation

NURSING CONSIDERATIONS

Assess:

• Blood tests, blood glucose, CBC, platelets, calcium, magnesium

• I&O ratio; report hematuria, oliguria

• ECG for cardiac dysrhythmias

• Patient should be lying down when receiving drug; severe hypotension may develop; monitor B/P during administration and until B/P stable

A Any patient with compromised renal system; drug is excreted slowly in poor renal system function; toxicity may occur rapidly

• Hepatic studies: AST, ALT

• Renal studies: urinalysis, BUN, creatinine; nephrotoxicity may occur

• Signs of infection, anemia

• Bowel pattern before, during treatment

• Sterile abscess, pain at inj site

• Respiratory status: rate, character, wheezing, dyspnea

• Dizziness, confusion, hallucination

• Allergies before treatment, reaction of each medication; place allergies on chart in bright red letters; notify all people giving drugs

• Diabetic patients, hypoglycemia may occur, then hyperglycemia with prolonged therapy

Administer:

INH route

• Through nebulizer; mix contents in 6 ml of sterile H_2O; do not use low pressure (<20 psi); flow rate should be 5-7 L/min (40-50 psi) air or O_2 source over 30-45 min until chamber is empty

IM route

• 300 mg diluted in 3 ml sterile H_2O; give deep IM by Z-track; painful by this route

IV route

• Reconstitute 300 mg/3-5 ml of sterile water for inj, D_5W, withdraw dose and further dilute in 50-250 ml D_5W, give over 1-2 hr

Y-site compatibilities: Aldesleukin, cefazolin, cefoperazone, cefotaxime, cefoxitin, ceftazidime, ceftriaxone, diltiazem, fluconazole, foscarnet, gatifloxacin, linezolid, zidovudine

Perform/provide:

• Storage in refrigerator protected from light

Evaluate:

• Therapeutic response: decreased temp, increased ability to breathe

Teach patient/family:

• To report sore throat, fever, fatigue (may indicate superinfection)

• To maintain adequate fluid intake

⚠ High Alert

pentazocine (℞)
(pen-taz′oh-seen)
Talwin, Talwin NX
Func. class.: Opiate analgesic, antagonist
Chem. class.: Synthetic benzomorphan

Controlled Substance Schedule IV
Action: Inhibits ascending pain pathways in CNS, increases pain threshold, alters pain perception
Uses: Moderate to severe pain

DOSAGE AND ROUTES

• *Adult:* **PO** 50-100 mg q3-4h prn, not to exceed 600 mg/day; **IV/IM/SUBCUT** 30 mg q3-4h prn, not to exceed 360 mg/day
Labor
• *Adult:* **IM** 60 mg; **IV** 30 mg q2-3h when contractions are regular
Renal dose
• CCr 10-50 ml/min reduce dose by 25%; CCr <10 ml/min reduce dose by 50%
Available forms: Inj 30 mg/ml; tabs 50 mg

SIDE EFFECTS

CNS: Drowsiness, dizziness, confusion, headache, sedation, euphoria, hallucinations, dreaming
CV: Palpitations, bradycardia, change in B/P, tachycardia, increased B/P (high doses)
EENT: Tinnitus, blurred vision, miosis, diplopia
GI: Nausea, vomiting, anorexia, constipation, *cramps,* dry mouth
GU: Increased urinary output, dysuria, urinary retention
INTEG: Rash, urticaria, bruising, flushing, diaphoresis, pruritus, severe irritation at inj sites
RESP: Respiratory depression
Contraindications: Hypersensitivity, addiction (opiate)

Precautions: Pregnancy (C), addictive personality, lactation, increased intracranial pressure, MI (acute), severe heart disease, respiratory depression, hepatic disease, renal disease, seizure disorder, child <18 yr, head trauma

PHARMACOKINETICS

SUBCUT/IM: Onset 15-30 min, peak 1-2 hr, duration 2-4 hr
IV: Onset 2-3 min, duration 4-6 hr; metabolized by liver, excreted by kidneys, crosses placenta, half-life 2-3 hr, extensive first-pass metabolism with less than 20% entering circulation

INTERACTIONS

⚠ Unpredictable reactions: MAOIs
Increase: effects—CNS depressants; alcohol, sedative/hypnotics, antipsychotics, skeletal muscle relaxants
Decrease: effects—opiates
Drug/Lab Test
Increase: Amylase

NURSING CONSIDERATIONS
Assess:
• For pain: intensity, duration, location prior to and 1 hr after dose
• I&O ratio; check for decreasing output; may indicate urinary retention
• For withdrawal symptoms in opiate-dependent patients
• Pulmonary embolism, abscesses, ulcerations, vascular occlusion, WBC
• CNS changes: dizziness, drowsiness, hallucinations, euphoria, LOC, pupil reaction
• Allergic reactions: rash, urticaria
• Respiratory dysfunction: respiratory depression, character, rate, rhythm; notify prescriber if respirations are <10/min
• Need for pain medication, physical dependence
Administer:
• With antiemetic if nausea, vomiting occur
• When pain is beginning to return;

⚠ Safety alert   *"Tall Man" lettering

determine dosage interval by patient response

SUBCUT/IM route

• Give IM deeply into large muscle mass, rotate sites; SUBCUT may cause necrosis with repeated inj

IV route

• Undiluted or diluted 5 mg/ml of sterile H_2O for inj; give 5 mg or less over 1 min

Syringe compatibilities: Atropine, benzquinamide, butorphanol, chlorproMAZINE, cimetidine, dimenhyDRINATE, diphenhydrAMINE, droperidol, fentanyl, hydromorphone, hydrOXYzine, meperidine, metoclopramide, morphine, perphenazine, prochlorperazine, promazine, promethazine, ranitidine, scopolamine

Y-site compatibilities: Heparin, hydrocortisone, potassium chloride, vit B/C

Perform/provide:

• Storage in light-resistant area at room temperature

• Assistance with ambulation

• Safety measures: night-light, call bell within easy reach

Evaluate:

• Therapeutic response: decrease in pain

Teach patient/family:

• To report any symptoms of CNS changes, allergic reactions

• That physical dependency may result from extended use

• That withdrawal symptoms may occur: nausea, vomiting, cramps, fever, faintness, anorexia

Treatment of overdose: Naloxone (Narcan) 0.2-0.8 mg IV, O_2, IV fluids, vasopressors

---

⚠ High Alert

pentobarbital (℞)
(pen-toe-bar'bi-tal)
Nembutal, Novopentobarb ✤,
Nova-Rectal ✤, pentobarbital
sodium
Func. class.: Sedative/hypnotic barbiturate; anticonvulsant
Chem. class.: Barbitone, short acting

Controlled Substance Schedule II (USA), Schedule G (CDSA IV) (Canada)

Do not confuse:
pentobarbital/phenobarbital

Action: Depresses activity in brain cells, primarily in reticular activating system in brain stem; selectively depresses neurons in posterior hypothalamus, limbic structures

Uses: Insomnia, sedation, preoperative medication, increased intracranial pressure, dental anesthetic

DOSAGE AND ROUTES

Insomnia

• *Adult:* **PO** 100-200 mg at bedtime; **IM** 150-200 mg at bedtime; **IV** 100 mg initially, then up to 500 mg; **RECT** 120-200 mg at bedtime

• *Child:* **IM** 2-6 mg/kg, not to exceed 100 mg; **PO** 2-6 mg/kg/day in divided doses; **PO** preoperatively 2-6 mg/kg, max 100 mg/dose; **IV** 100 mg (hypnotic/anticonvulsant)

Available forms: Caps 50, 100 mg; elix 20 mg/5 ml; rect supp 25, 30, 50, 60, 120, 200 mg; inj 50 mg/ml

SIDE EFFECTS

CNS: Lethargy, drowsiness, hangover, dizziness, paradoxical stimulation in elderly and children, light-headedness, dependence, ***CNS depression,*** mental depression, slurred speech
CV: Hypotension, bradycardia
GI: Nausea, vomiting, diarrhea, constipation

P

HEMA: ***Agranulocytosis, thrombocy-***
topenia, megaloblastic anemia
(long-term treatment)
INTEG: *Rash,* urticaria, pain, abscesses at
inj site, angioedema, thrombophlebitis,
Stevens-Johnson syndrome
RESP: ***Respiratory depression, ap-***
nea, laryngospasm, bronchospasm
Contraindications: Pregnancy (D),
hypersensitivity to barbiturates, respiratory depression, addiction to
barbiturates; severe hepatic, renal
impairment; porphyria, uncontrolled
pain
Precautions: Anemia, lactation, hepatic disease, renal disease, hypertension, elderly, acute/chronic pain

PHARMACOKINETICS

PO: Onset 15-30 min, duration 4-6 hr
RECT: Onset slow, duration 4-6 hr
Metabolized by liver, excreted by kid-
neys (metabolites); half-life 15-48 hr

INTERACTIONS

Increase: CNS depression—alcohol,
MAOIs, sedatives, other CNS depressants,
antihistamines, opiates
Increase: half-life of doxycycline
Decrease: effect of oral anticoagulants,
corticosteroids, griseofulvin, quinidine
Drug/Herb
Increase: pentobarbital levels—
eucalyptus, Jamaican dogwood, kava,
lemon balm nettle, pill-bearing spurge,
poppy, quinine, senega, valerian
Drug/Lab Test
False increase: Sulfobromophthalein

NURSING CONSIDERATIONS

Assess:
• VS q30min after parenteral route for 2
hr
• Blood studies: Hct, Hgb, RBCs, serum
folate, vit D (long-term therapy); PT in
patients receiving anticoagulants
• Hepatic studies: AST, ALT, bilirubin; if
increased, drug is usually discontinued
• Mental status: mood, sensorium, affect, memory (long, short)

• Physical dependency: more frequent
requests for medication, shakes, anxiety
⚠ Barbiturate toxicity: hypotension;
pupillary constriction; cold, clammy
skin; cyanosis of lips; insomnia; nausea;
vomiting; hallucinations; delirium;
weakness; coma; mild symptoms may
occur in 8-12 hr without drug
• Respiratory changes: respiratory depression, character, rate, rhythm; hold
drug if respirations are <10/min or if
pupils are dilated
• Blood dyscrasias: fever, sore throat,
bruising, rash, jaundice, epistaxis
Administer:
• For <14 days, since not effective after
that; tolerance develops
• After removal of cigarettes to prevent
fires
• After trying conservative measures for
insomnia
• Avoid use with CNS depressants; seri-
ous CNS depression may result
PO route
• Use elixir alone or diluted in fluids
• ½-1 hr before bedtime for sleepless-
ness
• On empty stomach for best absorption
• Crushed or whole
• Alone; do not mix with other drugs or
inject if there is precipitate
IM route
• Inj deep in large muscle mass to prevent tissue sloughing and abscesses; do
not inject more than 5 ml in one site
IV route
• IV undiluted or dilute in sterile H_2O,
LR, NaCl, give 50 mg or less/min; titrate
to patient response; use only clear sol;
avoid extravasation
• IV only with resuscitative equipment
available; administer at <100 mg/min
(only by qualified personnel)
Additive compatibilities: Amikacin,
aminophylline, calcium chloride, cephapirin, chloramphenicol, dimenhyDRI-
NATE, erythromycin lactobionate, lidocaine, thiopental, verapamil
Syringe compatibilities: Aminophylline, epHEDrine, hydromorphone,

---

neostigmine, scopolamine, sodium bicarbonate, thiopental

Y-site compatibilities: Acyclovir, insulin (regular), propofol

Perform/provide:

• Assistance with ambulation after receiving dose

• Safety measures: night-light, call bell within easy reach

• Checking to see if PO medication has been swallowed

• Storage of suppositories in refrigerator; do not use aqueous solutions that contain precipitate

Evaluate:

• Therapeutic response: ability to sleep at night, less early morning awakening if taking drug for insomnia, or decrease in number, severity of seizures if taking drug for seizure disorder

Teach patient/family:

• That hangover is common

• That drug is indicated only for short-term treatment of insomnia; probably ineffective after 2 wk

• That physical dependency may result from extended use (45-90 days depending on dose)

• To avoid driving, other activities requiring alertness

• To avoid alcohol ingestion

• Not to discontinue medication quickly after long-term use; drug should be tapered over 1-2 wk

• To tell all prescribers that a barbiturate is being taken

• That withdrawal insomnia may occur after short-term use; not to start using drug again; insomnia will improve in 1-3 nights

• That effects may take 2 nights for benefits to be noticed

• Alternative measures to improve sleep (reading, exercise several hr before bedtime, warm bath, warm milk, TV, self-hypnosis, deep breathing)

Treatment of overdose: Lavage, activated charcoal, warming blanket, vital signs, hemodialysis, I&O ratio

⚠ High Alert

pentostatin (℞)
(pen-toh-stat′in)
Nipent
Func. class.: Antineoplastic, enzyme inhibitor
Chem. class.: Streptomyces antibioticus derivative

Action: Inhibits the enzyme adenosine deaminase (ADA), which is able to block DNA synthesis and some RNA synthesis
Uses: α-Interferon-refractory hairy cell leukemia
Investigational uses: Chronic lymphocytic leukemia

DOSAGE AND ROUTES

• *Adult:* **IV** 4 mg/m^2 every other wk; may be given **IV BOL**, or diluted in a larger volume and given over 20-30 min
Available forms: Powder for inj 10 mg/vial

SIDE EFFECTS

CNS: Headache, anxiety, confusion, depression, dizziness, insomnia, nervousness, paresthesia
GI: Nausea, vomiting, anorexia, diarrhea, constipation, flatulence, stomatitis, elevated LFTs
GU: **Hematuria,** dysuria, increased BUN/creatinine
HEMA: **Leukopenia, anemia, thrombocytopenia,** ecchymosis, **lymphadenopathy,** petechiae
INTEG: Rash, eczema, dry skin, pruritus, sweating, herpes simplex/zoster
RESP: Cough, upper respiratory infection, bronchitis, dyspnea, epistaxis, pneumonia, pharyngitis, rhinitis, sinusitis
SYST: Fever, infection, fatigue, pain, allergic reaction, chills, ***death, sepsis,*** chest pain, flulike symptoms
Contraindications: Pregnancy (D), hypersensitivity to this drug or mannitol
Precautions: Renal disease, lactation, children, bone marrow depression

PHARMACOKINETICS

IV: Elimination half-life 5.7 hr, low protein binding, 90% excreted in urine unchanged or as metabolites

INTERACTIONS

⚠ Fatal pulmonary toxicity: fludarabine
Increase: adverse reactions—vidarabine
Drug/Lab Test
Increase: Uric acid

NURSING CONSIDERATIONS

Assess:
• CBC, differential, platelet count qwk; withhold drug if WBC is <2000/mm³ or platelet count is <75,000/mm³; notify prescriber
• Renal studies; BUN, serum uric acid, urine CCr, electrolytes before, during therapy
• I&O ratio; report fall in urine output to <30 ml/hr
• Monitor temp q4h; fever may indicate beginning infection
• Hepatic studies before, during therapy: bilirubin, AST, ALT, alk phosphatase, prn or qmo; check for jaundiced skin and sclera, dark urine, clay-colored stools, itchy skin, abdominal pain, fever, diarrhea
• Bleeding: hematuria, guaiac stools, bruising, petechiae, mucosa or orifices q8h
• Effects of alopecia on body image; discuss feelings about body changes
• Inflammation of mucosa, breaks in skin
• Buccal cavity q8h for dryness, sores, ulceration, white patches, oral pain, bleeding, dysphagia
• Local irritation, pain, burning at inj site
• Symptoms of severe allergic reaction: rash, pruritus, urticaria, purpuric skin lesions, itching, flushing
• GI symptoms: frequency of stools, cramping
• Acidosis, signs of dehydration; rapid respiration, poor skin turgor, decreased urine output, dry skin, restlessness, weakness

Administer:
• Antiemetic 30-60 min before giving drug to prevent vomiting
• Antibiotics as ordered for prophylaxis of infection

IV route
• Hydrate with 500-1000 ml D₅½NS or equivalent before administration; administer another 500 ml D₅ or equivalent after pentostatin
• After diluting, use with 5 ml sterile H₂O for injection and mix thoroughly (2 mg/ml); may be given by bolus or diluted in 25-50 ml 5% dextrose, or 0.9% NaCl (0.33 or 0.18 mg/ml)

Solution compatibilities: D₅W, 0.9% NaCl, LR
Y-site compatibilities: Fludarabine, melphalan, ondansetron, paclitaxel, sargramostim

Perform/provide:
• Hydrocortisone, sodium thiosulfate to infiltration area, and ice compress after stopping infusion
• Strict hand-washing technique, gloves, protective covering
• Liquid diet: carbonated beverages; gelatin may be added if patient is not nauseated or vomiting
• Rinsing of mouth tid-qid with water, club soda; brushing of teeth bid-qid with soft brush or cotton-tipped applicators for stomatitis; use unwaxed dental floss
• Storage in refrigerator; reconstituted or diluted sol may be stored at room temperature up to 8 hr

Evaluate:
• Therapeutic response: decrease in tumor size, spread of malignancy

Teach patient/family:
• To report any complaints, side effects to nurse or prescriber
• That hair may be lost during treatment and wig or hairpiece may make patient feel better; tell patient that new hair may be different in color, texture
• To avoid foods with citric acid, hot or rough texture

- To report any bleeding, white spots, ulcerations in mouth to prescriber; tell patient to examine mouth daily
- To avoid crowds and sources of infection when granulocyte count is low

pentoxifylline (R)

(pen-tox'ih-fill-in)
Trental
Func. class.: Hemorrheologic agent
Chem. class.: Dimethylxanthine derivative

Action: Decreases blood viscosity, stimulates prostacyclin formation, increases blood flow by increasing flexibility of RBCs; decreases RBC hyperaggregation; reduces platelet aggregation, decreases fibrinogen concentration

Uses: Intermittent claudication related to chronic occlusive vascular disease

Investigational uses: Cerebrovascular insufficiency, diabetic neuropathies, TIAs, leg ulcers, strokes, aphthous stomatitis, sickle cell anemia

DOSAGE AND ROUTES

- *Adult:* **PO** 400 mg tid with meals, may decrease to bid if side effects occur; must be taken for ≥8 wk for maximal effect
Stomatitis (off-label)
- *Adult:* **PO** 400 mg tid × 1-6 mo
Available forms: Tabs, cont release 400 mg; tab ext rel 400 mg

SIDE EFFECTS

CNS: Headache, anxiety, *tremors,* confusion, *dizziness*
CV: Angina, dysrhythmias, palpitation, hypotension, chest pain, dyspnea, edema
EENT: Blurred vision, earache, increased salivation, sore throat, conjunctivitis
GI: Dyspepsia, nausea, vomiting, anorexia, bloating, belching, constipation, cholecystitis, dry mouth, thirst, bad taste
INTEG: Rash, pruritus, urticaria, brittle fingernails
MISC: Epistaxis, flulike symptoms, laryngitis, nasal congestion, *leukopenia,* malaise, weight changes

Contraindications: Hypersensitivity to this drug or xanthines, retinal/cerebral hemorrhage

Precautions: Pregnancy (C), angina pectoris, cardiac disease, lactation, children, impaired renal function, recent surgery, peptic ulceration, hepatic disease

PHARMACOKINETICS

PO: Peak 8 wk, half-life ½-1 hr, degradation in liver, excreted in urine

INTERACTIONS

Increase: risk of bleeding—warfarin, salicylates, NSAIDs, thrombolytics, abciximab, eptifibatide, tirofiban, ticlopidine
Increase: theophylline level—theophylline
Increase: hypotension—antihypertensives, nitrates
Increase: pentoxifylline—cimetidine
Drug/Herb
Increase: bleeding potential—anise, arnica, chamomile, clove, dong quai, fenugreek, feverfew, garlic, ginger, ginkgo, ginseng *(Panax),* licorice

NURSING CONSIDERATIONS
Assess:
- B/P, respirations of patient also taking antihypertensives; intermittent claudication baseline and throughout
Administer:
- Do not break, crush, or chew ext rel tabs
- With meals to prevent GI upset
Evaluate:
- Therapeutic response: decreased pain, cramping, increased ambulation
Teach patient/family:
- That therapeutic response may take 2-4 wk, 8-12 wk to reach full benefit
- To observe feet for arterial insufficiency
- To use cotton socks, well-fitted shoes; not to go barefoot

- To watch for bleeding, bruises, petechiae, epistaxis
- To avoid smoking, to prevent blood vessel constriction

pergolide (R)
(per'goe-lide)
Permax
Func. class.: Antiparkinson agent
Chem. class.: Dopamine agonist

Do not confuse:
Permax/ Permitil
Action: Stimulates postsynaptic dopamine receptors, directly. Acts as a dopamine agonist
Uses: Parkinson's disease with carbidopa/levodopa

DOSAGE AND ROUTES
- *Adult:* **PO** 50 mcg/day × 2 days, then increase by 100-150 mcg/day q3d × 12 days, then increase by 250 mcg/day q3d until desired response, max 5 mg/day
Available forms: tab 50 mcg, 250 mcg, 1 mg

SIDE EFFECTS
CNS: Drowsiness, hallucinations, dyskinesia
CV: Orthostatic hypotension, atrial premature contractions, hypertension, palpitations, ***sinus tachycardia, MI***
GI: Nausea, constipation, diarrhea, dry mouth, abdominal pain, dyspepsia
META: Weight gain
MS: Arthralgia, chest, back pain
RESP: Dyspnea
Contraindications: Hypersensitivity to this drug or ergots; lactation
Precautions: Pregnancy (B), psychiatric disorders, children, dysrhythmias

PHARMACOKINETICS

Onset, peak, duration is unknown; well-absorbed, protein binding >90%, metabolized in the liver, excreted by the kidneys

INTERACTIONS
Decrease: action of haloperidol, phenothiazines, reserpine, metoclopramide

NURSING CONSIDERATIONS
Assess:
- For Parkinson's symptoms: tremor, ataxia, muscle weakness and rigidity; baseline and periodically
- Mental status: hallucinations, confusion, notify prescriber
- Monitor cardiac status: B/P, ECG; periodically during beginning treatment
Administer:
- With meals to prevent nausea; continuing therapy usually reduces or eliminates nausea
- Reduced dose of carbidopa/levodopa, cautiously
Evaluate:
- Therapeutic response: Improved symptoms in those with Parkinson's disease
Teach patient/family:
- To change positions slowly to prevent orthostatic hypotension
- To avoid hazardous activities until stabilized; dizziness can occur
- To rinse mouth frequently, use sugarless gum to alleviate dry mouth
- To take as prescribed, not to miss doses or double doses; take missed dose as soon as remembered, if several hours before next dose

perindopril (R)
(per-in'doe-pril)
Aceon
Func. class.: Antihypertensive
Chem. class.: Angiotensin-converting enzyme inhibitor

Action: Selectively suppresses renin-angiotensin-aldosterone system; inhibits ACE; prevents conversion of angiotensin I to angiotensin II, dilation of arterial, venous vessels
Uses: Hypertension

DOSAGE AND ROUTES

Hypertension
• **Adult:** PO 4 mg/day, may increase or decrease to desired response range 4-8 mg/day; may give in 2 divided doses or as a single dose, max 16 mg/day

Patients on diuretics
• Discontinue diuretic 2-3 days prior to perindopril then resume diuretic if needed

Renal impairment
• **Adult:** PO CCr <30 ml/min 2 mg/day, max 8 mg/day

Available forms: Tabs scored 2, 4, 8 mg

SIDE EFFECTS

CNS: Insomnia, dizziness, paresthesias, headache, fatigue, anxiety, depression
CV: Hypotension, chest pain, tachycardia, dysrhythmias, syncope
EENT: Tinnitus, visual changes, sore throat, double vision, dry burning eyes
GI: Nausea, vomiting, colitis, cramps, diarrhea, constipation, flatulence, dry mouth, loss of taste
*GU: **Proteinuria, renal failure,*** increased frequency of polyuria or oliguria
*HEMA: **Agranulocytosis, neutropenia***
INTEG: Rash, purpura, alopecia, hyperhidrosis
META: Hyperkalemia
RESP: Dyspnea, *dry cough,* crackles
*SYST: **Angioedema***

Contraindications: Pregnancy (D) 2nd/3rd trimester, hypersensitivity, history of angioedema
Precautions: Pregnancy (C) 1st trimester, renal disease, hyperkalemia, lactation, hepatic failure, dehydration, bilateral renal artery stenosis

PHARMACOKINETICS

Bioavailability 75%, protein binding 68%, metabolized by liver (active metabolite perindoprilat), half-life 0.8-1 hr, excreted in urine

INTERACTIONS

May increase effects of neuromuscular blocking agents, antihypertensives, lithium
Effects may be increased by diuretics
Hypersensitivity: allopurinol
Severe hypotension: diuretics, other antihypertensives
Hyperkalemia: salt substitutes, potassium-sparing diuretics, potassium supplements
Decrease: effects of NSAIDs
Drug/Herb
Increase: toxicity, death—aconite
Increase: antihypertensive effect—barberry, betony, black catechu, black cohosh, bloodroot, broom, burdock, cat's claw, dandelion, goldenseal, Irish moss, Jamaican dogwood, kelp, khella, mistletoe, parsley
Increase or decrease: antihypertensive effect—astragalus, cola tree
Decrease: antihypertensive effect—coltsfoot, guarana, khat, licorice
Drug/Lab Test
Interference: Glucose/insulin tolerance tests

NURSING CONSIDERATIONS

Assess:
• B/P, pulse q4h; note rate, rhythm, quality
• Electrolytes: K, Na, Cl during 1st 2 wk of therapy
• Baselines in renal, hepatic studies before therapy begins and 1 wk into therapy
• Edema in feet, legs daily
• Skin turgor, dryness of mucous membranes for hydration status, dry mouth
• Symptoms of CHF: edema, dyspnea, wet crackles

Administer:
• As a single dose or in 2 divided doses

Evaluate:
• Therapeutic response: decreased B/P

Teach patient/family:
• Not to use OTC (cough, cold, or allergy) products unless directed by prescriber; to avoid salt substitutes

P

- To avoid sunlight or wear sunscreen for photosensitivity
- To comply with dosage schedule, even if feeling better
- To notify prescriber of mouth sores, sore throat, fever, swelling of hands or feet, irregular heartbeat, chest pains, signs of angioedema
- That excessive perspiration, dehydration, vomiting, diarrhea may lead to fall in blood pressure; consult prescriber if these occur
- That drug may cause dizziness, fainting; light-headedness may occur during 1st few days of therapy
- That drug may cause skin rash or impaired perspiration; angioedema may occur and to discontinue if it occurs
- Not to discontinue drug abruptly
- To rise slowly to sitting or standing position to minimize orthostatic hypotension

Treatment of overdose: Lavage, IV atropine for bradycardia, IV theophylline for bronchospasm, digitalis, O_2, diuretic for cardiac failure

---

Rarely Used

permethrin (OTC, ℞)
(per-meth′rin)
Acticin, Elimite, Nix
Func. class.: Pediculicide

Uses: Lice, nits, ticks, flea nits

DOSAGE AND ROUTES

Lice (head)
- *Adult and child:* Wash hair, towel dry; apply liberally to hair, leave on 10 min, rinse with water

Scabies
- *Adult and child:* **TOP** 5% cream applied and massaged into all skin surfaces; leave cream on 8-14 hr, then wash

Contraindications: Hypersensitivity

---

perphenazine (℞)
(per-fen′a-zeen)
Apo-Perphenazine ✢,
perphenazine, PMS
Perphenazine ✢
Func. class.: Antipsychotic, neuroleptic
Chem. class.: Phenothiazine piperidine

Action: Depresses cerebral cortex, hypothalamus, limbic system, which control activity, aggression; blocks neurotransmission produced by dopamine at synapse; exhibits strong α-adrenergic, anticholinergic blocking action; as antiemetic inhibits medullary chemoreceptor trigger zone; receptor affinity dopamine D_2, histamine H_1, α-adrenergic

Uses: Psychotic disorders, schizophrenia, nausea, vomiting

DOSAGE AND ROUTES

- *Geriatric:* **PO** 2-4 mg daily-bid, increase by 2-4 mg/wk to desired dose

Nausea/vomiting
- *Adult and child >12 yr:* **IM** 5-10 mg prn, max 15 mg in ambulatory patients, 30 mg in hospitalized patients; **PO** 8-16 mg/day in divided doses, up to 24 mg; **IV** not to exceed 5 mg, give diluted or slow **IV** drip

Psychiatric use in hospitalized patients
- *Adult:* **PO** 8-16 mg bid-qid, gradually increased to desired dose, not to exceed 64 mg/day; **IM** 5 mg q6h, not to exceed 30 mg/day
- *Child >12 yr:* **PO** 6-12 mg in divided doses

Nonhospitalized patients
- *Adult:* **PO** 4-8 mg tid

Available forms: Tabs 2, 4, 8, 16 mg; oral conc 16 mg/5 ml; syr 2 mg/5 ml ✢

SIDE EFFECTS

*CNS: EPS: pseudoparkinsonism, akathisia, dystonia, tardive dyskinesia, **sei-***

---

zures, headache, **neuroleptic malignant syndrome,** dizziness

CV: Orthostatic hypotension (elderly), **cardiac arrest,** ECG changes, **tachycardia**

EENT: Blurred vision, glaucoma

GI: Dry mouth, nausea, vomiting, anorexia, constipation, diarrhea, jaundice, weight gain

GU: Urinary retention, urinary frequency, enuresis, impotence, amenorrhea, gynecomastia

HEMA: Anemia, **leukopenia, leukocytosis, agranulocytosis**

INTEG: Rash, photosensitivity, dermatitis

RESP: **Laryngospasm,** dyspnea, **respiratory depression**

Contraindications: Hypersensitivity, blood dyscrasias, coma, child <12 yr, brain damage, bone marrow depression

Precautions: Pregnancy (C), lactation, seizure disorders, hypertension, hepatic disease, cardiac disease, elderly, narrow-angle glaucoma

PHARMACOKINETICS

Bioavailability 20%; metabolized by liver (sulfoxidation, hydroxylation, dealkylation; glucuronidation by CYP2D6); excreted in urine, breast milk; crosses placenta, half-life 9-12 hr

PO: Onset erratic, peak 2-4 hr

IM: Onset 10 min, peak 1-2 hr; duration 6 hr, occasionally 12-24 hr

INTERACTIONS

Oversedation: other CNS depressants, alcohol, barbiturate anesthetics

Toxicity: epINEPHrine

Increase: risk of EPS—lithium

Increase: effects of both drugs—β-adrenergic blockers, alcohol

Increase: anticholinergic effects—anticholinergics

Increase: perphenazine effect—ritonavir

Increase: hypotension—thiazide diuretics, meperidine

Decrease: absorption—aluminum hydroxide or magnesium hydroxide antacids

Decrease: antiparkinson effect—levodopa

Decrease: oral anticoagulant effect—oral anticoagulants

Drug/Herb

Increase: anticholinergic effect—henbane leaf

Increase: EPS—betel palm, kava

Increase: action—cola tree, hops, nettle, nutmeg

Drug/Lab Test

Increase: LFTs, cardiac enzymes, cholesterol, blood glucose, prolactin, bilirubin, PBI, cholinesterase, ^{131}I

Decrease: Hormones (blood, urine)

False positive: Pregnancy tests, PKU

False negative: Urinary steroids, 17-OHCS

NURSING CONSIDERATIONS

Assess:

• Mental status before initial administration

• Swallowing of PO medication; check for hoarding or giving of medication to other patients

• I&O ratio; palpate bladder if urinary output is low, urinary retention may be the cause

• Bilirubin, CBC, LFTs qmo

• Urinalysis is recommended before and during prolonged therapy

• Affect, orientation, LOC, reflexes, gait, coordination, sleep pattern disturbances

• B/P standing and lying; also include pulse, respirations q4h during initial treatment; establish baseline before starting treatment; report drops of 30 mm Hg

• Dizziness, faintness, palpitations, tachycardia on rising

• EPS including akathisia (inability to sit still, no pattern to movements), tardive dyskinesia (bizarre movements of jaw, mouth, tongue, extremities), pseudoparkinsonism (rigidity, tremors, pill rolling, shuffling gait)

• Skin turgor daily

P

⚠ For neuroleptic malignant syndrome: hyperthermia, altered mental status, increased CPK, muscle rigidity

• Constipation, urinary retention daily; increase bulk, water in diet

Administer:

• Antiparkinsonian agent on order from prescriber for EPS
• Avoid use with CNS depressants

PO route

• Concentrate mixed in water, orange, pineapple, apricot, prune, tomato, grapefruit juice; do not mix with caffeine beverages (coffee, cola), tannics (tea), or pectinates (apple juice), since incompatibility may result; use 60 ml diluent for each 5 ml of concentrate

IM route

• IM inj into large muscle mass
• Remain lying down after IM inj for at least 30 min

IV route

• After diluting each 5 mg/9 ml of NaCl, shake, give 0.5 mg or less (1 ml = 0.5 mg) over 1 min; may be further diluted and infused

Additive compatibilities: Ascorbic acid, ethacrynate, netilmicin

Syringe compatibilities: Atropine, benztropine, butorphanol, chlorproMAZINE, cimetidine, dimenhyDRINATE, diphenhydrAMINE, droperidol, fentanyl, hydrOXYzine, meperidine, methotrimeprazine, metoclopramide, morphine, pentazocine, prochlorperazine, promethazine, ranitidine, scopolamine

Y-site compatibilities: Acyclovir, amikacin, ampicillin, azlocillin, cefamandole, cefazolin, cefotaxime, cefoxitin, cefuroxime, cephalothin, cephapirin, chloramphenicol, clindamycin, doxycycline, erythromycin, famotidine, gentamicin, kanamycin, metronidazole, mezlocillin, minocycline, moxalactam, nafcillin, oxacillin, penicillin G potassium, piperacillin, tacrolimus, ticarcillin, ticarcillin/clavulanate, tobramycin, trimethoprimsulfamethoxazole, vancomycin

Perform/provide:

• Supervised ambulation until stabilized on medication; do not involve in strenuous exercise program because fainting is possible; patient should not stand still for long periods
• Increased fluids, bulk in diet to prevent constipation
• Sips of water, sugarless candy, gum, ice chips for dry mouth
• Storage in tight, light-resistant container

Evaluate:

• Therapeutic response: decrease in emotional excitement, hallucinations, delusions, paranoia, reorganization of patterns of thought, speech

Teach patient/family:

• That orthostatic hypotension occurs frequently and to rise from sitting or lying position gradually; to avoid hazardous activities until stabilized on medication
• To avoid hot tubs, hot showers, tub baths, since hypotension may occur; that in hot weather, heat stroke may occur; take extra precautions to stay cool
• To avoid abrupt withdrawal of this drug, or EPS may result; drug should be withdrawn slowly
• To avoid OTC preparations (cough, hay fever, cold) unless approved by prescriber, since serious drug interactions may occur; avoid use with alcohol; increased drowsiness may occur
• To use a sunscreen to prevent burns
• About compliance with drug regimen
• About necessity for meticulous oral hygiene, since oral candidiasis may occur
• To report sore throat, malaise, fever, bleeding, mouth sores; if these occur, CBC should be drawn and drug discontinued
• That urine may turn reddish-brown

Treatment of overdose: Lavage if orally ingested; provide an airway; *do not induce vomiting*

---

phenazopyridine

(R_x, otc)

(fen-az-oh-peer'i-deen)
Azo-Standard, Baridium,
Eridium, Geridium,
Phenazo ❧,
phenazopyridine,
Phenazodine, Prodium,
Pyridiate, Pyridium, Urodine,
Urogesic, Viridium
Func. class.: Nonopioid analgesic
(urinary system)
Chem. class.: Azodye

Action: Exerts analgesic, anesthetic
action on the urinary tract mucosa
Uses: Urinary tract irritation, infection
used with a urinary antiinfective

DOSAGE AND ROUTES

• *Adult:* **PO** 200 mg tid × 2 days or less
when used with antibacterial for UTI
• *Child 6-12 yr:* **PO** 4 mg/kg tid × 2 days
Renal dose
• Do not use in CCr <50 ml/min
Available forms: Tabs 100, 200 mg

SIDE EFFECTS

CNS: Headache
*GI: Nausea, vomiting, diarrhea, heart-
burn,* anorexia, **hepatic toxicity**
GU: Renal toxicity, orange-red urine
*HEMA: Thrombocytopenia, agranu-
locytosis, leukopenia, neutropenia, hemolytic anemia, methemoglobinemia*
INTEG: Rash, skin pigmentation, pruritus
Contraindications: Hypersensitivity,
renal insufficiency
Precautions: Pregnancy (B), lactation,
children <12 yr

PHARMACOKINETICS

Metabolized by liver, excreted by kidneys, crosses placenta, duration 6-8 hr

INTERACTIONS

Drug/Lab Test
Interference: Urinalysis

NURSING CONSIDERATIONS

Assess:

• Urinary status: burning, pain, itching,
urgency, frequency, hematuria, before/
after treatment completed
• Hepatic studies: AST, ALT, bilirubin if
patient is on long-term therapy
🅐 Hepatotoxicity: dark urine, clay-
colored stools, jaundiced skin and
sclera, itching, abdominal pain, fever,
diarrhea if patient is on long-term therapy
• Allergic reactions: rash, urticaria; drug
may have to be discontinued

Administer:

• To patient crushed or whole; chewable
tablets may be chewed
• With food or milk to decrease gastric
symptoms

Evaluate:

• Therapeutic response: decrease in
urinary pain

Teach patient/family:

• Not to exceed recommended dosage
and to take with meals
• To discontinue after pain is relieved
but continue to take concurrent prescribed antiinfective until finished
• That urine may turn red-orange; may
stain clothing or contact lenses
Treatment of overdose: Methylene
blue 1-2 mg/kg IV or 100-200 mg vit C
PO

phenelzine (R_x)

(fen'el-zeen)
Nardil
Func. class.: Antidepressant, MAOI
Chem. class.: Hydrazine

Action: Increases concentrations of
endogenous epinephrine, norepinephrine, serotonin, dopamine in storage
sites in CNS by inhibition of MAO; increased concentration reduces depression
Uses: Depression, when uncontrolled
by other means

P

❧ Canada only
Side effects: *italics* = common; **bold italics** = life-threatening

DOSAGE AND ROUTES

• *Adult:* **PO** 45 mg/day in divided doses; may increase to 60 mg/day; dose should be reduced to 15 mg/day, not to exceed 90 mg/day

• *Geriatric:* **PO** 7.5 mg daily, increase by 7.5-15 mg q3-4d; usual dose 15-60 mg/day in divided doses

Available forms: Tabs 15 mg

SIDE EFFECTS

CNS: Dizziness, drowsiness, confusion, headache, anxiety, tremors, stimulation, weakness, hyperreflexia, mania, insomnia, fatigue, weight gain

CV: Orthostatic hypotension, hypertension, dysrhythmias, **hypertensive crisis,** tachycardia, peripheral edema

EENT: Blurred vision

ENDO: **SIADH-like syndrome**

GI: Constipation, dry mouth, nausea, vomiting, *anorexia,* diarrhea, weight gain

GU: Change in libido, urinary frequency

HEMA: **Anemia**

INTEG: Rash, flushing, increased perspiration

Contraindications: Hypersensitivity to MAOIs, hypertension, CHF, severe hepatic disease, pheochromocytoma, severe renal disease, severe cardiac disease, active alcoholism

Precautions: Pregnancy (C), suicidal patients, convulsive disorders, severe depression, schizophrenia, hyperactivity, diabetes mellitus, child <16 yr

PHARMACOKINETICS

Metabolized by liver, excreted by kidneys

INTERACTIONS

Toxicity: sumatriptan, sulfonamides
Confusion, shivering, hyperreflexia: L-tryptophan

🅐 Hyperpyretic crisis, convulsions, hypertensive episode: tricyclics, SSRIs, meperidine, methylphenidate, amphetamines, nasal decongestants, sinus medications, appetite suppressants, asthma inhalants

Increase: hypotension—thiazide diuretics

Increase: hypoglycemic effect—antidiabetics

Increase: pressor effects—guanethidine, clonidine, indirect-acting or mixed sympathomimetics (epHE-Drine)

Increase: effects of direct-acting sympathomimetics (epINEPHrine)—alcohol, barbiturates, benzodiazepines, CNS depressants, levodopa

Decrease: serotonin, norepinephrine—rauwolfia alkaloids

Drug/Herb

Serotonin syndrome: parsley, St. John's wort

Hypertension: brewer's yeast

Tension headaches, irritability, visual hallucinations, mania: ginseng

Increase: sympathomimetic action—betel palm, butcher's broom, capsicum peppers, galanthamine, green tea (large amounts), guarana (large amounts), night-blooming cereus

Increase: effect—ginkgo, nutmeg, yohimbe

Increase: anticholinergic effect—jimsonweed

Decrease: effect—valerian

Drug/Food

Avoid tyramine foods, caffeine

NURSING CONSIDERATIONS

Assess:

• B/P (lying, standing), pulse; if systolic B/P drops 20 mm Hg, hold drug, notify prescriber

• Blood studies: CBC, leukocytes, cardiac enzymes (long-term therapy)

• Hepatic studies: ALT, AST, bilirubin; hepatotoxicity may occur

🅐 Toxicity: increased headache, palpitation; discontinue drug immediately; prodromal signs of hypertensive crisis

• Mental status changes: mood, sensorium, affect, memory (long, short); increase in psychiatric symptoms

• Urinary retention, constipation, edema; take weight qwk

• Withdrawal symptoms: headache, nausea, vomiting, muscle pain, weakness

Administer:
• Increased fluids, bulk in diet for constipation

• With food, milk for GI symptoms

• Crushed if patient cannot swallow medication whole

• Dosage at bedtime for oversedation during day

• Gum, hard candy, or frequent sips of water for dry mouth

• Phentolamine for severe hypertension

• Avoid use with CNS depressants

Perform/provide:
• Storage in tight container in cool environment

• Ambulation assistance at start of therapy, since drowsiness/dizziness occurs, especially elderly

• Safety measures including side rails

• Checking to see if PO medication swallowed

Evaluate:
• Therapeutic response: decreased depression

Teach patient/family:
• That therapeutic effects may take 1-4 wk

• To avoid driving, other activities requiring alertness

• To avoid alcohol ingestion, OTC medications: cold, weight loss, hay fever, cough syrup

• To rise slowly to prevent orthostatic hypotension

• Not to discontinue medication quickly after long-term use

• To avoid high-tyramine foods: cheese (aged), sour cream, beer, wine, pickled products, liver, raisins, bananas, figs, avocados, meat tenderizers, chocolate, yogurt; provide complete list of tyramine-containing foods; increased caffeine, may cause hypertensive reactions

• To report headache, palpitation, neck stiffness, dizziness, constriction in chest, throat, rash, insomnia, change in strength, changes in urinary patterns, color of urine

Treatment of overdose: Lavage, activated charcoal, monitor electrolytes, vital signs, diazepam IV, $NaHCO_3$

⚠ High Alert

phenobarbital (℞)
(fee-noe-bar′bi-tal)
Ancalixir ✦, Barbita, Luminal, phenobarbital sodium, Solfoton
Func. class.: Anticonvulsant
Chem. class.: Barbiturate

Controlled Substance Schedule IV
Do not confuse:
phenobarbital/pentobarbital
Action: Decreases impulse transmission; increases seizure threshold at cerebral cortex level
Uses: All forms of epilepsy, status epilepticus, febrile seizures in children, sedation, insomnia
Investigational uses: Hyperbilirubinemia, chronic cholestasis

DOSAGE AND ROUTES
Seizures
• *Adult:* **PO** 60-200 mg/day in divided doses tid or total dose at bedtime
• *Child:* **PO** 4-6 mg/kg/day in divided doses q12h; may be given as single dose
Status epilepticus
• *Adult:* **IV INF** 10 mg/kg; run no faster than 50 mg/min; may give up to 20 mg/kg
• *Child:* **IV INF** 5-10 mg/kg; may repeat q10-15min up to 20 mg/kg; run no faster than 50 mg/min
Insomnia
• *Adult:* **PO/IM** 100-320 mg
• *Child:* **PO/IM** 3-5 mg/kg
Sedation
• *Adult:* **PO** 30-120 mg/day in 2-3 divided doses
• *Child:* **PO** 3-5 mg/kg/day in 3 divided doses

Side effects: *italics* = common; ***bold italics*** = life-threatening

Preoperative sedation
- *Adult:* IM 100-200 mg 1-1½ hr before surgery
- *Child:* IM 16-100 mg or **PO/IM/IV** 1-3 mg/kg 1-1½ hr before surgery

Available forms: Caps 15 mg; elix 20 mg/5 ml; tabs 8, 15, 30, 60, 100 mg; inj 30, 60, 65, 130 mg/ml

SIDE EFFECTS

CNS: Paradoxic excitement (elderly), drowsiness, lethargy, hangover headache, flushing, hallucinations, ***coma***
GI: Nausea, vomiting, diarrhea, constipation
INTEG: Rash, urticaria, ***Stevens-Johnson syndrome, angioedema,*** local pain, swelling, necrosis, ***thrombophlebitis***

Contraindications: Pregnancy (D), hypersensitivity to barbiturates, porphyria, hepatic disease, respiratory disease, nephritis, hyperthyroidism, diabetes mellitus, elderly, lactation
Precautions: Anemia

PHARMACOKINETICS

IV: Onset 5 min, peak 30 min, duration 4-6 hr
IM/SUBCUT: Onset 10-30 min, duration 4-6 hr
PO: Onset 20-60 min, peak 8-12 hr, duration 6-10 hr
Metabolized by liver; crosses placenta; excreted in urine, breast milk; half-life 53-118 hr

INTERACTIONS

Increase: effects—CNS depressants, alcohol, chloramphenicol, valproic acid, disulfiram, nondepolarizing skeletal muscle relaxants, sulfonamides
Increase: orthostatic hypotension—furosemide
Decrease: effects—theophylline, oral anticoagulants, corticosteroids, metronidazole, doxycycline, quinidine
Drug/Herb
Increase: phenobarbital levels—quinine

Increase: CNS depression—chamomile, eucalyptus, hops, Jamaican dogwood, kava, lemon balm, nettle, pill-bearing spurge, poppy, senega, skullcap, valerian
Decrease: barbiturate effect—St. John's wort

NURSING CONSIDERATIONS

Assess:
- Mental status: mood, sensorium, affect, memory (long, short)
- For respiratory depression
- Blood dyscrasias: fever, sore throat, bruising, rash, jaundice
- Convulsion activity: type, duration, precipitating factors
- Blood studies, LFTs during long-term treatment
- Therapeutic blood level periodically: 15-40 mcg/ml
- Respiratory status: rate, rhythm, depth

Administer:
- Avoid use with other CNS depressants

IM route
- IM inj deep in large muscle mass to prevent tissue sloughing; use <5 ml in each site

IV route
- Slow IV after dilution with at least 10 ml sterile H_2O for inj regardless of dose; give 65 mg or less/min; titrate to patient response

Additive compatibilities: Amikacin, aminophylline, calcium chloride, calcium gluconate, cephapirin, colistimethate, dimenhyDRINATE, meropenem, polymyxin B, sodium bicarbonate, thiopental, verapamil

Solution compatibilities: D_5W, $D_{10}W$, 0.45% NaCl, 0.9% NaCl, Ringer's, dextrose/saline combinations, dextrose/Ringer's, dextrose/LR combinations, sodium lactate

Syringe compatibilities: Heparin

Y-site compatibilities: Enalaprilat, meropenem, propofol, sufentanil

Perform/provide:
- Supervision of ambulation for dizziness, drowsiness

Evaluate:
• Therapeutic response: decreased seizures, increased sedation

Teach patient/family:
• To use exactly as ordered
• To avoid alcohol use
• To avoid hazardous activities until stabilized on drug; drowsiness may occur
• Never to withdraw drug abruptly; withdrawal symptoms may occur
• That therapeutic effects (PO) may not be seen for 2-3 wk

Treatment of overdose: Lavage, activated charcoal, warming blanket, vital signs, hemodialysis, I&O ratio

---

phentolamine (℞)
(fen-tole′a-meen)
Regitine, Rogitine ✦
Func. class.: Antihypertensive
Chem. class.: α-Adrenergic blocker

Action: α-Adrenergic blocker, binds to α-adrenergic receptors, dilating peripheral blood vessels, lowering peripheral resistances, lowering blood pressure
Uses: Hypertension, pheochromocytoma, prevention, treatment of dermal necrosis following extravasation of norepinephrine or DOPamine
Investigational uses: Impotence, hypertensive crisis due to MAOIs

DOSAGE AND ROUTES
Treatment of hypertensive episodes in pheochromocytoma
• *Adult:* **IV/IM,** 5 mg, repeat if necessary
• *Child:* **IV/IM,** 1 mg, repeat if necessary
Diagnosis of pheochromocytoma
• *Adult:* **IV** 2.5 mg; if negative, repeat with 5 mg IV
• *Child:* **IV** 0.05 mg/kg; if negative, repeat with 0.1 mg/kg IV
Treatment of necrosis
• *Adult:* 5-10 mg/10 ml **NS** injected into area of norepinephrine extravasation within 12 hr
• *Child:* 0.1-0.2 mg/kg, max 10 mg

Prevention of necrosis
• *Adult:* 10 mg/L of norepinephrine-containing sol
• *Child:* **IV** 0.1-0.2 mg/kg, max 10 mg
Available forms: Inj 5 mg/ml

SIDE EFFECTS
CNS: Dizziness, flushing, weakness, ***cerebrovascular spasm***
*CV: Hypotension, tachycardia, angina, dysrhythmias, **MI***
EENT: Nasal congestion
GI: Dry mouth, nausea, vomiting, diarrhea, abdominal pain
Contraindications: Hypersensitivity, MI, coronary insufficiency, angina
Precautions: Pregnancy (C), lactation

PHARMACOKINETICS
IV: Peak 2 min, duration 10-15 min
IM: Peak 15-20 min, duration 3-4 hr
Metabolized in liver, excreted in urine

INTERACTIONS
Increase: effects of epINEPHrine, antihypertensives
Drug/Herb
Increase: toxicity, death—aconite
Increase: antihypertensive effect—barberry, betony, black catechu, black cohosh, bloodroot, broom, burdock, cat's claw, dandelion, goldenseal, Irish moss, Jamaican dogwood, kelp, khella, mistletoe, parsley
Increase or decrease: antihypertensive effect—astragalus, cola tree
Decrease: antihypertensive effect—coltsfoot, guarana, khat, licorice

NURSING CONSIDERATIONS
Assess:
• Weight daily, I&O
• B/P lying, standing before starting treatment, q4h after
• Nausea, vomiting, diarrhea, edema in feet, legs daily; skin turgor, dryness of mucous membranes for hydration status, postural hypotension, cardiac system: pulse, ECG

P

Side effects: *italics* = common; ***bold italics*** = life-threatening

Administer:
• Gum, frequent rinsing of mouth, or hard candy for dry mouth
• With vasopressor available
• After discontinuing all medication for 24 hr
• Treatment during required bed rest, 1 hr after

IV route
• After diluting 5 mg/1 ml sterile H_2O for inj; give 5 mg or less/min; patient to remain recumbent during administration

CONT INF route
• Dilute 5-10 mg/500 ml D_5W, titrate to patient response
• 10 mg/L may be added to norepinephrine in IV sol for prevention of dermal necrosis

Additive compatibilities: DOBUTamine, verapamil
Syringe compatibilities: Papaverine
Y-site compatibilities: Amiodarone
Evaluate:
• Therapeutic response: decreased B/P
Teach patient/family:
• That bed rest is required during treatment, 1 hr after
Treatment of overdose: Administer norepinephrine; discontinue drug

---

phenylephrine (℞)
(fen-ill-ef′rin)
Neo-Synephrine
Func. class.: Adrenergic, direct-acting
Chem. class.: Substituted phenylethylamine

Action: Powerful and selective (α_1) receptor agonist causing contraction of blood vessels
Uses: Hypotension, paroxysmal supraventricular tachycardia, shock, maintain B/P for spinal anesthesia

DOSAGE AND ROUTES
Hypotension
• *Adult:* **SUBCUT/IM** 2-5 mg, may repeat q10-15min if needed, do not exceed initial dose; **IV** 50-100 mcg, may repeat q10-15min if needed, do not exceed initial dose
• *Child:* **IM/SUBCUT** 0.1 mg/kg/dose q1-2h prn

Supraventricular tachycardia
• *Adult:* **IV BOL** 0.5-1 mg given rapidly, not to exceed prior dose by >0.1 mg, total dose ≤1 mg

Shock
• *Adult:* **IV INF** 10 mg/500 ml D_5W given 100-180 mcg/min (if 20 gtt/ml inf device), then maintenance of 40-60 mcg/min. Use infusion device
• *Child:* **IV BOL** 5-20 mcg/kg/dose q10-15min; **IV INF** 0.1-0.5 mcg/kg/min
Available forms: Inj 1% (10 mg/ml)

SIDE EFFECTS
CNS: Headache, anxiety, tremor, insomnia, dizziness
*CV: Palpitations, tachycardia, hypertension, ectopic beats, angina, reflex bradycardia, **dysrhythmias***
GI: Nausea, vomiting
*INTEG: Necrosis, tissue sloughing with extravasation, **gangrene***
*SYST: **Anaphylaxis***
Contraindications: Hypersensitivity, ventricular fibrillation, tachydysrhythmias, pheochromocytoma, narrow-angle glaucoma, severe hypertension
Precautions: Pregnancy (C), lactation, arterial embolism, peripheral vascular disease, elderly, hyperthyroidism, bradycardia, myocardial disease, severe arteriosclerosis, partial heart block

PHARMACOKINETICS
IV: Onset immediate, duration 20-30 min
IM/SUBCUT: Duration 45-60 min

INTERACTIONS
Dysrhythmias: general anesthetics, digoxin, bretylium
⚠ Do not use within 2 wk of MAOIs, or hypertensive crisis may result
Increase: in B/P—oxytocics
Increase: pressor effect—tricyclics, β-blockers, H_1 antihistamines

Decrease: phenylephrine action—α-blockers

NURSING CONSIDERATIONS

Assess:
• I&O ratio; notify prescriber if output <30 ml/hr
• ECG during administration continuously; if B/P increases, drug is decreased
• B/P and pulse q5min after parenteral route
• CVP or PWP during inf if possible
• For paresthesias and coldness of extremities; peripheral blood flow may decrease

Administer:
IV route
• Plasma expanders for hypovolemia
• IV after diluting 1 mg/9 ml sterile H_2O for inj; give dose over ½-1 min; may be diluted 10 mg/500 ml of D_5W or NS; titrate to response (normal B/P); check for extravasation, check site for infiltration, use infusion pump

Additive compatibilities: Chloramphenicol, DOBUTamine, lidocaine, potassium chloride, sodium bicarbonate

Y-site compatibilities: Amiodarone, amrinone, cisatracurium, famotidine, haloperidol, remifentanil, zidovudine

Perform/provide:
• Storage of reconstituted sol if refrigerated for no longer than 24 hr
• Discard discolored sol

Evaluate:
• Therapeutic response: increased B/P with stabilization

Teach patient/family:
• The reason for administration
• To report pain at infusion site or other adverse reactions immediately

Treatment of overdose: Administer an α-blocker

---

phenylephrine nasal agent
See Appendix C

---

phenylephrine ophthalmic
See Appendix C

---

phenytoin (℞)
(fen′i-toh-in)
Dilantin, Dilantin Infatab, Dilantin Kapseals, Dilantin-125, diphenylhydantoin, DPH, Phenytex
Func. class.: Anticonvulsant; antidysrhythmic (IB)
Chem. class.: Hydantoin

Action: Inhibits spread of seizure activity in motor cortex by altering ion transport; increases AV conduction
Uses: Generalized tonic-clonic seizures; status epilepticus; nonepileptic seizures associated with Reye's syndrome or after head trauma; migraines, trigeminal neuralgia, Bell's palsy, ventricular dysrhythmias uncontrolled by antidysrhythmics

DOSAGE AND ROUTES
Seizures
• *Adult:* **PO** 1 g or 20 mg/kg (ext rel) in 3-4 divided doses given q2h, or 400 mg, then 300 mg q2h × 2 doses, maintenance 300-400 mg/day, max 600 mg/day; **IV** 15-20 mg/kg, max 25-50 mg/min, then 100 mg q6-8h
• *Child:* **PO** 5 mg/kg/day in 2-3 divided doses, maintenance 4-8 mg/kg/day in 2-3 divided doses, max 300 mg/day; **IV** 15-20 mg/kg at 1-3 mg/kg/min
Status epilepticus
• *Adult:* **IV** 10-15 mg/kg, max 25-50 mg/min, may give 100 mg q6-8h thereafter
• *Child:* **IV** 15-20 mg/kg, max in divided doses 1-3 mg/kg/min
Neuritic pain
• *Adult:* **PO** 200-600 mg/day in divided doses
Ventricular dysrhythmias
• *Adult:* **PO** loading dose 1 g divided

P

over 24 hr, then 500 mg/day × 2 days; **IV** 250 mg over 5 min until dysrhythmias subside or until 1 g is given, or 100 mg q15min until dysrhythmias subside or until 1 g is given

• *Child*: **PO** 3-8 mg/kg or 250 mg/m²/day as single dose or 2 divided doses; **IV** 3-8 mg/kg over several min, or 250 mg/m²/day as single dose or 2 divided doses

Renal dose

• Do not use loading dose CCr <10 ml/min or hepatic failure

Available forms: Susp 30, 125 mg/5 ml; tabs, chewable 50 mg; inj 50 mg/ml; caps ext rel 30, 100 mg; caps prompt rel 30, 100 mg

SIDE EFFECTS

CNS: Drowsiness, dizziness, insomnia, paresthesias, depression, suicidal tendencies, aggression, headache, confusion, slurred speech

CV: Hypotension, ***ventricular fibrillation***

EENT: Nystagmus, diplopia, blurred vision

ENDO: Diabetes insipidus

GI: Nausea, vomiting, constipation, anorexia, weight loss, ***hepatitis,*** jaundice, gingival hyperplasia

GU: ***Nephritis,*** urine discoloration

HEMA: ***Agranulocytosis, leukopenia, aplastic anemia, thrombocytopenia, megaloblastic anemia***

INTEG: Rash, ***lupus erythematosus, Stevens-Johnson syndrome,*** hirsutism

SYST: Hypocalcemia

Contraindications: Hypersensitivity, psychiatric condition, bradycardia, SA and AV block, Stokes-Adams syndrome, hepatic failure, acute intermittent porphyria

Precautions: Pregnancy (C), allergies, hepatic disease, renal disease, elderly, petit mal seizures, hypotension, myocardial insufficiency

PHARMACOKINETICS

PO-ER: Onset 2-24 hr, peak 4-12 hr, duration 12-36 hr

IV: Onset 1-2 hr, duration 12-24 hr

PO: Onset 2-24 hr, peak 1½-2½ hr, duration 6-12 hr

Metabolized by liver, excreted by kidneys; highly protein-bound, half-life 22 hr, dose dependent

INTERACTIONS

Increase: phenytoin effect—benzodiazepines, cimetidine, tricyclics, salicylates, valproate, cycloSERINE, diazepam, chloramphenicol

Decrease: phenytoin effects—alcohol (chronic use), antacids, barbiturates, carbamazepine, diazoxide, rifampin, folic acid

Drug/Herb

Increase: potassium loss, increase antidysrhythmic action—aloe, buckthorn, cascara sagrada, senna

Increase: action—ginkgo

Decrease: anticonvulsant effect—ginseng, santonica, valerian

Drug/Lab Test

Increase: Glucose, alk phosphatase, BSP

Decrease: Dexamethasone, metyrapone test serum, PBI, urinary steroids

NURSING CONSIDERATIONS

Assess:

A For phenytoin hypersensitivity syndrome 3-12 wk after start of treatment: rash, temp, lymphadenopathy; may cause hepatotoxicity, renal failure, rhabdomyolysis

A For beginning rash that may lead to Stevens-Johnson syndrome or toxic epidermal necrolysis; phenytoin should not be used again

• Drug level: toxic level 30-50 mcg/ml, ther level: 7.5-20 mcg/ml, wait ≥1 wk to draw levels

• For seizures: duration, type, intensity precipitating factors

• Blood studies: CBC, platelets q2wk until stabilized, then qmo × 12, then q3mo; discontinue drug if neutrophils <1600/mm³; renal function: albumin conc

• Mental status: mood, sensorium, affect, memory (long, short)

• Respiratory depression; rate, depth, character
• Blood dyscrasias: fever, sore throat, bruising, rash, jaundice
Administer:
• Do not interchange chewable product with caps, not equivalent; only ext rel caps are to be used for once-a-day dosing
• Shake susp well before each dose G tube/NG tube: dilute susp prior to administration, flush tube with 20 ml H_2O after dose
• Allow 7-10 days between dosage changes
• Divided PO doses with or after meals to decrease adverse effects
• 2 hr before or after antacid or antidiarrheal use
IV route
• After diluting with diluent provided (2.2 ml/100 mg, 5.2 ml/250 mg, 1 ml/50 mg); shake; give through Y-tube or 3-way stopcock; inject slowly <50 mg/min; clear IV tubing first with NS sol; use in-line filter; discard 4 hr after preparation; inject into large veins to prevent purple glove syndrome
Additive compatibilities: Bleomycin, sodium bicarbonate, verapamil
Y-site compatibilities: Esmolol, famotidine, fluconazole, foscarnet, tacrolimus
Evaluate:
• Therapeutic response; decrease in severity of seizures, ventricular dysrhythmias
Teach patient/family:
• That if diabetic, urine glucose should be monitored
• That urine may turn pink
• Not to discontinue drug abruptly; seizures may occur
• Proper brushing of teeth using a soft toothbrush, flossing to prevent gingival hyperplasia; need to see dentist frequently
• To avoid hazardous activities until stabilized on drug
• To carry emergency ID stating drug use

• That heavy use of alcohol may diminish effect of drug; to avoid OTC medications
• Not to change brands or forms once stabilized on therapy; brands may vary

Rarely Used

physostigmine (℞)
(fi-zoe-stig′meen)
Antilirium
Func. class.: Antidote, reversible anticholinesterase

Uses: To reverse CNS effects of anticholinergic

DOSAGE AND ROUTES
Overdose of anticholinergics
• *Adult:* **IM/IV** 2 mg; give no more than 1 mg/min; may repeat
• *Child:* **IM/IV** inj 0.02 mg/kg, not more than 0.5 mg/min; may repeat at 5-10 min intervals until max dose of 2 mg
Postanesthesia
• *Adult:* **IM/IV** 0.5-1 mg; give no more than 1 mg/min **(IV);** can repeat at 10- to 30-min intervals
Contraindications: Hypotension, obstruction of intestine or renal system, asthma, gangrene, CV disease, choline esters, depolarizing neuromuscular blocking agents, diabetes

phytonadione (vit K₁) (℞)
(fye-toe-na-dye′one)
AquaMEPHYTON, Mephyton
Func. class.: Vit K₁, fat-soluble vitamin

Action: Needed for adequate blood clotting (factors II, VII, IX, X)
Uses: Vit K malabsorption, hypoprothrombinemia, prevention of hypoprothrombinemia caused by oral anticoagulants, prevention of hemorrhagic disease of the newborn

DOSAGE AND ROUTES

Hypoprothrombinemia caused by vit K malabsorption

• *Adult:* **PO/IM** 2.5-25 mg, may repeat or increase to 50 mg
• *Child:* **PO/IM** 5-10 mg
• *Infant:* **PO/IM** 2 mg

Prevention of hemorrhagic disease of the newborn

• *Neonate:* **IM** 0.5-1 mg within 1 hr after birth, repeat in 2-3 wk if required

Hypoprothrombinemia caused by oral anticoagulants

• *Adult and child:* **PO/SUBCUT/IM** 1-10 mg, may repeat 12-48 hr after **PO** dose or 6-8 hr after **SUBCUT/IM** dose, based on PT

Available forms: Tabs 5 mg; inj 2 m/10 ml aqueous colloidal; inj aqueous dispersion 10 mg/ml (IM)

SIDE EFFECTS

CNS: Headache, **brain damage** (large doses)
GI: Nausea, decreased LFTs
HEMA: **Hemolytic anemia, hemoglobinuria, hyperbilirubinemia**
INTEG: Rash, urticaria

Contraindications: Hypersensitivity, severe hepatic disease, last few wk of pregnancy
Precautions: Pregnancy (C), neonates

PHARMACOKINETICS

PO/INJ: Metabolized, crosses placenta

INTERACTIONS

Decrease: action of phytonadione—cholestyramine, mineral oil
Decrease: action of oral anticoagulants
Drug/Food
Olestra, decreased vit K levels

NURSING CONSIDERATIONS

Assess:

• For bleeding: emesis, stools, urine
• PT during treatment (2-sec deviation from control time, bleeding time, and clotting time); monitor for bleeding, pulse, and B/P
• Nutritional status: liver (beef), spinach, tomatoes, coffee, asparagus, broccoli, cabbage, lettuce, greens

Administer:

IV route

• After diluting with D₅NS 10 ml or more; give 1 mg/min or more
⚠ IV only when other routes not possible (deaths have occurred)

Additive compatibilities: Amikacin, calcium gluceptate, cephapirin, chloramphenicol, cimetidine, netilmicin, sodium bicarbonate
Syringe compatibilities: Doxapram
Y-site compatibilities: Ampicillin, epINEPHrine, famotidine, heparin, hydrocortisone, potassium chloride, tolazoline, vit B/C

Perform/provide:

• Storage in tight, light-resistant container

Evaluate:

• Therapeutic response: decreased bleeding tendencies, decreased PT, decreased clotting time

Teach patient/family:

• Not to take other supplements unless directed by prescriber
• The necessary foods for diet
• To avoid IM inj site, use soft toothbrush, do not floss, use electric razor until coagulation defect corrected
• To report symptoms of bleeding
• Not to use OTC medications unless approved by prescriber
• The importance of frequent lab tests to monitor coagulation factors

---

pilocarpine ophthalmic
See Appendix C

---

pimecrolimus topical
See Appendix C

---

pindolol (℞)

(pin′doe-lole)
Novo-Pindol ✦, Syn-Pindolol ✦,
Visken

Func. class.: Antihypertensive
Chem. class.: Nonselective β-
blocker

Do not confuse:
pindolol/Parlodel
pindolol/Plendil

Action: Competitively blocks stimulation of β-adrenergic receptor within vascular smooth muscle; decreases rate of SA node discharge, increases recovery time, slows conduction of AV node, decreases heart rate, which decreases O_2 consumption in myocardium; also decreases renin-aldosterone-angiotensin system, at high doses inhibits $β_2$ receptors in bronchial system

Uses: Mild to moderate hypertension

DOSAGE AND ROUTES

• *Adult:* **PO** 5 mg bid, usual dose 15 mg/day (5 mg tid), may increase by 10 mg/day q3-4wk to a max of 60 mg/day
• *Geriatric:* **PO** 5 mg daily, increase by 5 mg q3-4wk

Available forms: Tabs 5, 10 mg

SIDE EFFECTS

CNS: Insomnia, dizziness, hallucinations, anxiety, fatigue, headache, depression
CV: Hypotension, bradycardia, *CHF,* edema, chest pain, palpitation, claudication, tachycardia, *AV block, pulmonary edema, bradycardia, dysrhythmias*
EENT: Visual changes, sore throat, *double vision;* dry, burning eyes, nasal stuffiness
GI: Nausea, vomiting, *ischemic colitis,* diarrhea, *abdominal pain, mesenteric arterial thrombosis,* flatulence, constipation
GU: Impotence, urinary frequency

*HEMA: **Agranulocytosis, thrombocytopenia, purpura***
INTEG: Rash, alopecia, pruritus, fever
MISC: Joint pain, muscle pain
*RESP: **Bronchospasm,** dyspnea,* cough, crackles

Contraindications: Hypersensitivity to β-blockers, cardiogenic shock; 2nd-, 3rd-degree heart block; sinus bradycardia, CHF, cardiac failure, bronchial asthma, severe COPD

Precautions: Pregnancy (B), major surgery, lactation, diabetes mellitus, renal disease, thyroid disease, COPD, well-compensated heart failure, CAD, nonallergic bronchospasm, peripheral vascular disease, hepatic disease

PHARMACOKINETICS

PO: Peak 2-4 hr; half-life 3-4 hr, excreted 30%-45% unchanged; 60%-65% metabolized by liver; excreted in breast milk; protein binding 40%

INTERACTIONS

May alter hypoglycemic effect: insulin, oral hypoglycemics
Increase: hypotension, bradycardia—reserpine, hydrALAZINE, methyldopa, prazosin, anticholinergics
Increase: effects of β-blockers, calcium channel blockers
Decrease: antihypertensive effects—NSAIDs, sympathomimetics, thyroid
Decrease: bronchodilation—theophyllines, $β_2$-agonists
Drug/Herb
Increase: toxicity, death—aconite
Increase: antihypertensive effect—barberry, betony, black catechu, black cohosh, bloodroot, broom, burdock, cat's claw, dandelion, goldenseal, Irish moss, Jamaican dogwood, kelp, khella, mistletoe, parsley
Increase or decrease: antihypertensive effect—astragalus, cola tree
Decrease: antihypertensive effect—coltsfoot, guarana, khat, licorice

P

Drug/Lab Test
Increase: Renal, hepatic studies
Interference: Glucose, insulin tolerance test

NURSING CONSIDERATIONS
Assess:
• I&O, weight daily
• B/P during initial treatment, periodically thereafter; pulse q4h, note rate, rhythm, quality; apical, radial pulse before administration; notify prescriber of any significant changes
• Baselines in renal, hepatic studies before therapy begins
• Skin turgor, dryness of mucous membranes for hydration status; edema in feet, legs daily

Administer:
• PO ac, at bedtime; tablet may be crushed or swallowed whole

Perform/provide:
• Storage in dry area at room temperature; do not freeze

Evaluate:
• Therapeutic response: decreased B/P after 1-2 wk

Teach patient/family:
• To take with or immediately after meals if GI symptoms occur
🅐 Not to discontinue drug abruptly; taper over 2 wk; may cause precipitate angina
• Not to use OTC products containing α-adrenergic stimulants (nasal decongestants, OTC cold preparations) unless directed by prescriber
• To report bradycardia, dizziness, confusion, depression, fever, sore throat, shortness of breath to prescriber
• To take pulse at home; to notify prescriber if pulse <60 bpm
• To avoid alcohol, smoking, sodium
• To comply with weight control, dietary adjustments, modified exercise program
• To carry emergency ID to identify drug, allergies
• To avoid hazardous activities if dizziness is present
• To report symptoms of CHF: difficult breathing, especially on exertion or when

lying down, night cough, swelling of extremities
• To take medication at bedtime to prevent orthostatic hypotension
• To wear support hose to minimize effects of orthostatic hypotension
Treatment of overdose: Lavage, IV atropine for bradycardia, IV theophylline for bronchospasm, digitalis, O_2, diuretic for cardiac failure, hemodialysis, hypotension; give vasopressor (norepinephrine)

---

pioglitazone (℞)
(pie-oh-glye'ta-zone)
Actos
Func. class.: Antidiabetic, oral
Chem. class.: Thiazolidinedione

Action: Specifically targets insulin resistance, an insulin sensitizer; regulates the transcription of a number of insulin responsive genes
Uses: Type 2 diabetes mellitus

DOSAGE AND ROUTES
Monotherapy
• *Adult:* **PO** 15-30 daily, may increase to 45 mg/day
Combination therapy
• *Adult:* **PO** 15-30 mg daily with a sulfonylurea, metformin, or insulin. Decrease sulfonylurea dose if hypoglycemia occurs. Decrease insulin dose by 10%-25% if hypoglycemia occurs or if plasma glucose is <100 mg/dl, max 45 mg/day
Hepatic dose
• Do not use in active hepatic disease or if ALT >2.5 times ULN
Available forms: Tabs 15, 30, 45 mg

SIDE EFFECTS
CNS: Headache
ENDO: Aggravated diabetes mellitus
MISC: Myalgia, sinusitis, URI, pharyngitis
Contraindications: Hypersensitivity to thiazolidinedione, lactation, children, diabetic ketoacidosis

---

🅐 Safety alert   *"Tall Man" lettering

Precautions: Pregnancy (C), elderly, thyroid disease, hepatic, renal disease, edema, CHF

PHARMACOKINETICS

Maximal reduction in FBS after 12 wk; half-life 3-7 hr, terminal 16-24 hr

INTERACTIONS

Decrease: effect of oral contraceptives, use an alternative contraceptive method
Decrease: pioglitazone effect—ketoconazole

Drug/Herb

Poor blood glucose control: glucosamine
Increase: hypoglycemia—chromium, coenzyme Q-10, fenugreek
Increase: antidiabetic effect—alfalfa, aloe, basil, bay, bilberry, bitter melon, black catechu, buchu, burdock, coriander, dandelion, eyebright (po), fenugreek, garlic, ginseng, glucomannan, glucosamine, goat's rue, gymnema, horehound, horse chestnut, jambul, myrrh, myrtle
Decrease: antidiabetic effect—bee pollen, blue cohosh, broom, chromium, elecampane, eucalyptus, gotu kola

NURSING CONSIDERATIONS

Assess:

• For hypoglycemic reactions (sweating, weakness, dizziness, anxiety, tremors, hunger), hyperglycemic reactions soon after meals
• Check LFTs periodically AST, LDH
• FBS, glycosylated Hgb, fasting plasma insulin, plasma lipids/lipoproteins, B/P, body weight during treatment

Administer:

• Once a day; give with meals to decrease GI upset and provide best absorption
• Tabs crushed and mixed with food or fluids for patients with difficulty swallowing

Perform/provide:

• Conversion from other oral hypoglycemic agents; change may be made

with gradual dosage change; monitor serum glucose during conversion
• Storage in tight container in cool environment

Evaluate:

• Therapeutic response: Decrease in polyuria, polydipsia, polyphagia; clear sensorium; absence of dizziness; stable gait, blood glucose at normal level

Teach patient/family:

• To self-monitor using a blood glucose meter
• The symptoms of hypo/hyperglycemia, what to do about each
• That the drug must be continued on daily basis; explain consequence of discontinuing drug abruptly
• To avoid OTC medications or herbal preparations unless approved by prescriber
• That diabetes is lifelong illness; that this drug is not a cure; only controls symptoms
• That all food included in diet plan must be eaten to prevent hypoglycemia
• To carry emergency ID and glucagon emergency kit for emergencies
• To notify prescriber if oral contraceptives are used
• Not to use if breastfeeding
• To report symptoms of hepatic dysfunction (nausea, vomiting, abdominal pain, fatigue, anorexia, dark urine, jaundice)

P

piperacillin (℞)

(pip'er-ah-sill'in)
Pipracil
Func. class.: Broad-spectrum antiinfective
Chem. class.: Extended-spectrum penicillin

Action: Interferes with cell wall replication of susceptible organisms; osmotically unstable cell wall swells and bursts from osmotic pressure
Uses: Respiratory, skin, urinary tract, bone infections; gonorrhea; pneumonia; effective for gram-positive cocci *(Staph-*

ylococcus aureus, Streptococcus pyogenes, Streptococcus viridans, Streptococcus faecalis, Streptococcus bovis, Streptococcus pneumoniae), gram-negative cocci (Neisseria gonorrhoeae, Neisseria meningitidis), gram-positive bacilli (Acinetobacter, Clostridium perfringens, Clostridium tetani), gram-negative bacilli (Bacteroides, Citrobacter, Enterobacter, Escherichia coli, Eubacterium, Fusobacterium nucleatum, Klebsiella, Morganella morganii, Peptococcus, Peptostreptococcus, Proteus mirabilis, Proteus vulgaris, Providencia rettgeri, Pseudomonas aeruginosa, Serratia)

DOSAGE AND ROUTES
Urinary tract infections
• *Adult:* **IV** 8-16 g/day (125-200 mg/kg/day) in divided doses q6-8h
Serious systemic infections
• *Adult and child >12 yr:* **IM/IV** 2-4 g q4-6h (2 g/site **IM**)
• *Child <12 yr:* **IM/IV** 200-300 mg/kg/day in divided doses q4-6h
• *Neonates <36 wk:* **IV** 75 mg/kg q12h in the 1st wk of life, then q8h in 2nd wk
• *Full-term infants:* **IV** 75 mg/kg q8h in 1st wk of life; q6h thereafter
Prophylaxis of surgical infections
• *Adult:* **IV** 2 g ½-1 hr before procedure; may be repeated during surgery or after surgery
Renal dose
• *Adult:* **IV** CCr 20-40 ml/min give q8h; CCr <20 ml/min give q12h
Available forms: Powder for inj 2, 3, 4, 40 g

SIDE EFFECTS
CNS: Lethargy, hallucinations, anxiety, depression, twitching, ***coma, seizures***
GI: Nausea, vomiting, diarrhea; increased AST, ALT; abdominal pain, glossitis, ***pseudomembranous colitis***
GU: **Oliguria, proteinuria, hematuria**, vaginitis, moniliasis, **glomerulonephritis**
HEMA: Anemia, increased bleeding time,

bone marrow depression, thrombocytopenia
META: Hypokalemia, hypernatremia
SYST: **Serum sickness, anaphylaxis**
Contraindications: Hypersensitivity to penicillins, neonates
Precautions: Pregnancy (B), lactation, hypersensitivity to cephalosporins; CHF, renal disease, seizures

PHARMACOKINETICS
IM: Peak 30-50 min
IV: Peak 20-30 min
Half-life 0.7-1.33 hr; excreted in urine, bile, breast milk; crosses placenta

INTERACTIONS
Increase: piperacillin concentrations—aspirin, probenecid
Decrease: antimicrobial effect of piperacillin—tetracyclines (with high concentrations of piperacillin), aminoglycosides
Decrease: effect of oral contraceptives
Drug/Herb
Do not give with antiinfective: acidophilus
Decrease: Absorption—khat
Drug/Lab Test
False positive: Urine glucose, urine protein, Coombs' test

NURSING CONSIDERATIONS
Assess:
• For infection: temp, WBC, sputum, stools, urine, wounds
• I&O ratio; report hematuria, oliguria, since penicillin in high doses is nephrotoxic
⚠ Any patient with compromised renal system, since drug is excreted slowly in poor renal system function; toxicity may occur rapidly
• Hepatic studies: AST, ALT
• Blood studies: WBC, RBC, Hgb, Hct, bleeding time prior to and periodically during treatment
• Renal studies: urinalysis, protein,

blood, BUN, creatinine prior to and periodically during treatment

• C&S before drug therapy; drug may be taken as soon as culture is taken

• Bowel pattern before and during treatment

• Skin eruptions after administration of penicillin to 1 wk after discontinuing drug

• Respiratory status: rate, character, wheezing, tightness in chest

• Allergies before initiation of treatment, reaction of each medication

Administer:

• Drug after C&S completed

IM route

• 2 g/4 ml, 3 g/6 ml, 4 g/8 ml of sterile water, 0.9% NaCl max 2 g/site

IV route

• After diluting 1 g or less/5 ml or more sterile H_2O or 0.9% NaCl; shake; give dose over 3-5 min; may further dilute to 50-100 ml with D_5W, 0.9% NS, and give over ½ hr; discontinue primary IV

Additive compatibilities: Ciprofloxacin, clindamycin, fluconazole, hydrocortisone, ofloxacin, potassium chloride, verapamil

Syringe compatibilities: Heparin

Y-site compatibilities: Acyclovir, allopurinol, amifostine, aztreonam, ciprofloxacin, cyclophosphamide, diltiazem, DOXOrubicin liposome, enalaprilat, esmolol, famotidine, fludarabine, foscarnet, gallium, granisetron, heparin, hydromorphone, IL-2, labetalol, lorazepam, magnesium sulfate, melphalan, meperidine, midazolam, morphine, perphenazine, propofol, ranitidine, remifentanil, tacrolimus, teniposide, theophylline, thiotepa, verapamil, zidovudine

Perform/provide:

• EpINEPHrine, suction, tracheostomy set, endotracheal intubation equipment on unit

• Adequate intake of fluids (2 L) during diarrhea episodes

• Scratch test to assess allergy after securing order from prescriber; usually

done when penicillin is only drug of choice

• Storage of reconstituted sol 24 hr at room temperature or 7 days refrigerated

Evaluate:

• Therapeutic response: absence of fever, purulent drainage, redness, inflammation

Teach patient/family:

• That culture may be taken after completed course of medication

• To report sore throat, fever, fatigue; may indicate superinfection

• To wear or carry emergency ID if allergic to penicillins

• To notify nurse of diarrhea

Treatment of anaphylaxis: Withdraw drug, maintain airway, administer epINEPHrine, aminophylline, O_2, IV corticosteroids

---

piperacillin/tazobactam (℞)
(pip′er-ah-sill′in & ta-zoe-bak′tam)
Zosyn
Func. class.: Antiinfective, broad-spectrum
Chem. class.: Extended-spectrum penicillin, β-lactamase inhibitor

Action: Interferes with cell wall replication of susceptible organisms; osmotically unstable cell wall swells and bursts from osmotic pressure

Uses: Moderate to severe infections: piperacillin-resistant, β-lactamase-producing strains causing infections in respiratory, skin, urinary tract, bone, gonorrhea, pneumonia; effective for resistant *Staphylococcus aureus,* resistant *Escherichia coli, Bacteroides fragilis, Bacteroides ovatus, Bacteroides thetaiotaomicron, Bacteroides vulgatus, Haemophilus influenzae*

DOSAGE AND ROUTES
Nosocomial pneumonia

• *Adult:* **IV** 3.375 g q6-8h with an aminoglycoside × 1-2 wk; continue ami-

---

noglycoside only if *Pseudomonas aeruginosa* is isolated
Other infections
• *Adult:* **IV INF** 6-12 g/day given 2.25 g q8h to 3.375 g q6h over 30 min × 7-10 days
Renal dose
• *Adult:* **IV** CCr 20-40 ml/min give 2.25 g q6h; CCr <20 ml/min give 2.25 g q8h
Available forms: Powder for inj 2 g piperacillin/0.25 tazobactam, 3 g piperacillin/0.375 g tazobactam, 4 g piperacillin/0.5 g tazobactam, 36 g piperacillin/4.5 g tazobactam

SIDE EFFECTS

CNS: Lethargy, hallucinations, anxiety, depression, twitching, insomnia, headache, fever, dizziness
GI: Nausea, vomiting, diarrhea; increased AST, ALT; abdominal pain, glossitis, *pseudomembranous colitis,* constipation
GU: Oliguria, proteinuria, hematuria, vaginitis, moniliasis, glomerulonephritis
HEMA: Anemia, increased bleeding time, *bone marrow depression*
INTEG: Rash, pruritus
META: Hypokalemia, hypernatremia
SYST: Serum sickness, anaphylaxis
Contraindications: Hypersensitivity to penicillins, neonates
Precautions: Pregnancy (B), lactation, hypersensitivity to cephalosporins, CHF, renal insufficiency in children, seizures

PHARMACOKINETICS

IV: Peak completion of IV, duration 6 hr
Half-life 0.7-1.2 hr; excreted in urine, bile, breast milk; crosses placenta; 33% bound to plasma proteins

INTERACTIONS

Increase: effect of neuromuscular blockers, oral anticoagulants
Increase: piperacillin concentrations—aspirin, probenecid
Decrease: antimicrobial effect of

piperacillin—tetracyclines, aminoglycosides IV
Decrease: effect of oral contraceptives
Drug/Herb
Do not use with antiinfectives: acidophilus
Decrease: absorption—khat
Drug/Lab Test
Increase: Platelet count, eosinophilia, neutropenia, leukopenia, serum creatinine, PTT, AST, ALT, alk phosphatase, bilirubin, BUN, electrolytes
Decrease: Hct, Hgb, electrolytes
False positive: Urine glucose, urine protein, Coombs' test

NURSING CONSIDERATIONS
Assess:
• For infection: temp, stools, urine, sputum, wounds
• I&O ratio; report hematuria, oliguria, since penicillin in high doses is nephrotoxic
A Any patient with compromised renal system, since drug is excreted slowly in poor renal system function; toxicity may occur rapidly
• Hepatic studies: AST, ALT prior to and periodically thereafter
• Blood studies: WBC, RBC, Hct, Hgb, bleeding time prior to and periodically thereafter
• Renal studies: urinalysis, protein, blood, BUN, creatinine prior to and periodically thereafter
• C&S before drug therapy; drug may be given as soon as culture is taken
• Bowel pattern before and during treatment
• Skin eruptions after administration of penicillin to 1 wk after discontinuing drug
• Respiratory status: rate, character, wheezing, tightness in chest
• Allergies before initiation of treatment, reaction of each medication
Administer:
• Drug after C&S is complete
IV route
• After diluting 5 ml 0.9% NaCl for injec-

tion or sterile H_2O for inj, dextran 6% in NS, dextrose 5%, KCl 40 mEq, bacteriostatic saline/parabens, bacteriostatic saline/benzyl alcohol, bacteriostatic H_2O/benzyl alcohol per 1 g piperacillin; shake well; further dilute in at least 50 ml compatible IV sol and run as int inf over at least 30 min

Y-site compatibilities: Aminophylline, aztreonam, bleomycin, bumetanide, buprenorphine, butorphanol, calcium gluconate, carboplatin, carmustine, cefepime, cimetidine, clindamycin, cyclophosphamide, cytarabine, dexamethasone, diphenhydrAMINE, DOPamine, enalaprilat, etoposide, floxuridine, fluconazole, fludarabine, fluorouracil, furosemide, gallium, granisetron, heparin, hydrocortisone, hydromorphone, ifosfamide, leucovorin, lorazepam, magnesium sulfate, mannitol, meperidine, mesna, methotrexate, methylPREDNISolone, metoclopramide, metronidazole, morphine, ondansetron, plicamycin, potassium chloride, ranitidine, remifentanil, sargramostim, sodium bicarbonate, thiotepa, trimethoprim-sulfamethoxazole, vinBLAStine, vinCRIStine, zidovudine

Perform/provide:
• EpINEPHrine, suction, tracheostomy set, endotracheal intubation equipment on unit
• Adequate intake of fluids (2 L) during diarrhea episodes
• Scratch test to assess allergy on order from prescriber; usually when penicillin is only drug of choice
• Discard after 24 hr if stored at room temperature or after 48 hr if refrigerated; use single-dose vials immediately after reconstitution; stable in ambulatory IV pump for 12 hr

Evaluate:
• Therapeutic response: absence of fever, purulent drainage, redness, inflammation; culture shows decreased organisms

Teach patient/family:
• That culture may be taken after completed course of medication

• To report sore throat, fever, fatigue (may indicate superinfection)
• To wear or carry emergency ID if allergic to penicillins
• To notify nurse of diarrhea

Treatment of overdose: Withdraw drug, maintain airway, administer epINEPHrine, aminophylline, O_2, IV corticosteroids for anaphylaxis

---

pirbuterol (℞)
(peer-byoo'ter-ole)
Maxair
Func. class.: Bronchodilator
Chem. class.: β-Adrenergic agonist

Action: Causes bronchodilation with little effect on heart rate by action on β-receptors, causing increased cAMP and relaxation of smooth muscle
Uses: Reversible bronchospasm (prevention, treatment) including asthma; may be given with theophylline or steroids

DOSAGE AND ROUTES

• *Adult and child >12 yr:* **INH** 1-2 puffs (0.4 mg) q4-6h; max 12 **INH**/day
Available forms: Aerosol delivery 0.2 mg pirbuterol/actuation

SIDE EFFECTS

CNS: Tremors, anxiety, insomnia, headache, dizziness, stimulation, restlessness, hallucinations, drowsiness, irritability
CV: Palpitations, tachycardia, hypertension, angina, hypotension, dysrhythmias
EENT: Dry nose and mouth, irritation of nose, throat
GI: Gastritis, nausea, vomiting, anorexia
MS: Muscle cramps
RESP: **Paradoxical bronchospasm,** dyspnea, coughing

Contraindications: Hypersensitivity to sympathomimetics, tachycardia
Precautions: Pregnancy (C), lactation, cardiac disorders, hyperthyroidism, diabetes mellitus, prostatic hypertrophy

P

PHARMACOKINETICS

INH: Onset 3 min, peak ½-1 hr, duration 5 hr

INTERACTIONS

⚠ Hypertensive crisis: MAOIs
Increase: action of other aerosol bronchodilators
Increase: pirbuterol action—tricyclics, antihistamines, levothyroxine
Decrease: pirbuterol action—β-blockers
Drug/Herb
Increase: action of both—cola nut, guarana, yerba maté
Increase: effect—green tea (large amounts), guarana

NURSING CONSIDERATIONS

Assess:
• Respiratory function: vital capacity, forced expiratory volume, ABGs, B/P, lung sounds, pulse, characteristics of sputum
⚠ Paradoxical bronchospasm, that can occur rapidly, hold drug, notify prescriber
Administer:
• After shaking; exhale, place mouthpiece in mouth, inhale slowly, hold breath, remove, exhale slowly
• Gum, sips of water for dry mouth
Perform/provide:
• Storage in light-resistant container; do not expose to temperatures over 86° F (30° C)
• Fluid intake >2 L/day to liquefy thick secretions
Evaluate:
• Therapeutic response: absence of dyspnea, wheezing over 1 hr
Teach patient/family:
• Not to use OTC medications; extra stimulation may occur
• Use of inhaler; review package insert with patient
• To avoid getting aerosol in eyes
• Actuator is for Maxair autoinhaler; do not use with other inhaler canister
• About all aspects of drug; avoid smok-

ing, smoke-filled rooms, persons with respiratory infections
• To keep fluid intake >2 L/day to liquefy thick secretions
Treatment of overdose: Administer a β-adrenergic blocker

---

piroxicam (℞)
(peer-ox′i-kam)
Apo-Piroxicam ✦, Feldene, Novopirocam ✦, Nu-Pirox, PMS-Piroxicam ✦
Func. class.: Nonsteroidal antiinflammatory
Chem. class.: Oxicam derivative

Action: Inhibits prostaglandin synthesis by decreasing an enzyme needed for biosynthesis; has analgesic, antiinflammatory, antipyretic properties
Uses: Mild to moderate pain, osteoarthritis, rheumatoid arthritis

DOSAGE AND ROUTES

• *Adult:* **PO** 20 mg daily or 10 mg bid
Available forms: Caps 10, 20 mg

SIDE EFFECTS

CNS: Dizziness, *drowsiness,* fatigue, tremors, confusion, insomnia, anxiety, depression, *headache*
CV: Tachycardia, peripheral edema, palpitations, dysrhythmias, hypertension, *heart failure*
EENT: Tinnitus, hearing loss, blurred vision
GI: Nausea, anorexia, vomiting, diarrhea, jaundice, *cholestatic hepatitis,* constipation, flatulence, cramps, dry mouth, peptic ulcer, *bleeding, ulceration, perforation*
GU: Nephrotoxicity: dysuria, hematuria, oliguria, azotemia
HEMA: Blood dyscrasias
INTEG: Purpura, rash, pruritus, sweating, photosensitivity
SYST: Anaphylaxis
Contraindications: Hypersensitivity, asthma, severe renal disease, severe

hepatic disease, ulcer disease, cardiac disease

Precautions: Pregnancy (B), avoid in late pregnancy, lactation, children, bleeding disorders, GI disorders, cardiac disorders, hypersensitivity to other anti-inflammatory agents, CHF

PHARMACOKINETICS

PO: Peak 2 hr; duration 48-72 hr, half-life 30-80 hr; metabolized in liver; excreted in urine (metabolites), breast milk; 99% protein binding

INTERACTIONS

Hypoglycemia: oral antidiabetics
Increase: toxicity—cycloSPORINE, methotrexate, lithium, alcohol, oral anticoagulants, aspirin, corticosteroids
Decrease: effects of antihypertensives, diuretics

Drug/Herb
Increase: gastric irritation—arginine, gossypol
Increase: NSAIDs effect—bearberry, bilberry
Increase: bleeding risk—bogbean, chondroitin

NURSING CONSIDERATIONS

Assess:
• For pain: location, duration, type, ROM before and 1-2 hr after administration
• Renal, hepatic, blood studies: BUN, creatinine, AST, ALT, Hgb, before treatment, periodically thereafter
• Audiometric, ophthalmic exam before, during, after treatment
• For eye, ear problems: blurred vision, tinnitus (may indicate toxicity)
⚠ Those with aspirin sensitivity, asthma, nasal polyps may develop allergic reactions

Administer:
• Do not break, crush, or chew caps
With food to decrease GI symptoms; take on empty stomach to facilitate absorption; take drug same time daily

Perform/provide:
• Storage at room temperature
• At least 6-8 glasses of water/day
Evaluate:
• Therapeutic response: decreased pain, stiffness, swelling in joints; ability to move more easily

Teach patient/family:
• To report blurred vision or ringing, roaring in ears (may indicate toxicity)
• To avoid driving, other hazardous activities if dizzy or drowsy
• That patient should drink at least 6-8 glasses of water/day
• To report change in urine pattern, weight increase, edema, pain increase in joints, fever, blood in urine (indicates nephrotoxicity)
• That therapeutic effects may take up to 1 mo
• To avoid ASA, other OTC meds, alcohol; advise patient to use sunscreen

---

plasma protein fraction (℞)
Plasmanate, Plasma Plex, Plasmatein, Protenate
Func. class.: Blood derivative
Chem. class.: Human plasma in NaCl

P

Action: Exerts similar oncotic pressure as human plasma, expands blood volume
Uses: Hypovolemic shock, hypoproteinemia, ARDS, preoperative cardiopulmonary bypass, acute hepatic failure, nephrotic syndrome, cardiogenic shock

DOSAGE AND ROUTES

Hypovolemia
• *Adult:* **IV INF** 250-500 ml (12.5-25 g protein), not to exceed 10 ml/min
• *Child:* **IV INF** 22-33 ml/kg at 5-10 ml/min

Hypoproteinemia
• *Adult:* **IV INF** 1000-1500 ml daily, not to exceed 8 ml/min
Available forms: Inj 5%

SIDE EFFECTS

CNS: Fever, chills, headache, paresthesias, flushing

*CV: **Fluid overload**,* hypotension, erratic pulse

GI: Nausea, vomiting, increased salivation

INTEG: Rash, urticaria, cyanosis

RESP: Altered respirations, dyspnea, ***pulmonary edema***

Contraindications: Hypersensitivity, CHF, severe anemia, renal insufficiency

Precautions: Pregnancy (C), decreased salt intake, decreased cardiac reserve, lack of albumin deficiency, hepatic disease

PHARMACOKINETICS

Metabolized as a protein/energy source

INTERACTIONS

Drug/Lab Test
False increase: Alk phosphatase

NURSING CONSIDERATIONS

Assess:

• Blood studies: Hct, Hgb, electrolytes, serum protein; if serum protein declines, dyspnea, hypoxemia can result

• B/P (decreased), pulse (erratic), respiration during infusion

• I&O ratio; urinary output may decrease

• CVP, pulmonary wedge pressure (increases if overload occurs), jugular vein distention

• Allergy: fever, rash, itching, chills, flushing, urticaria, nausea, vomiting, or hypotension requires discontinuation of infusion; use new lot if therapy reinstituted, premedicate with diphenhydrAMINE

⚠ Increased CVP reading: distended neck veins indicate circulatory overload; SOB, anxiety, insomnia, expiratory crackles, frothy blood-tinged cough, cyanosis indicate pulmonary overload

Administer:

• IV access at distant site from infection or trauma; no dilution required; use infusion pump, use large-gauge needle (≥20G), discard unused portion, infuse slowly

• Within 4 hr of opening, discard partially used vials

Additive compatibilities: Carbohydrate and electrolyte sol, whole blood, packed red blood cells, chloramphenicol, tetracycline

Perform/provide:

• Adequate hydration before administration

• Storage—check type of albumin, date; may have to refrigerate

Evaluate:

• Therapeutic response: increased B/P, decreased edema, increased serum albumin

---

⚠ High Alert

plicamycin (Ʀ)
(ply-ka-my′sin)
Mithramycin, Mithracin
Func. class.: Antineoplastic, antibiotic; hypocalcemic
Chem. class.: Crystalline aglycone

Action: Inhibits DNA, RNA, protein synthesis; derived from *Streptomyces plicatus;* replication is decreased by binding to DNA; demonstrates calcium-lowering effect not related to its tumoricidal activity; also acts on osteoclasts and blocks action of parathyroid hormone; a vesicant

Uses: Testicular cancer, hypercalcemia, hypercalciuria, symptomatic treatment of advanced neoplasms

DOSAGE AND ROUTES

Testicular tumors

• *Adult:* **IV** 25-30 mcg/kg/day × 8-10 days, not to exceed 30 mcg/kg/day

Hypercalcemia/hypercalciuria

• *Adult:* **IV** 25 mcg/kg/day × 3-4 days, repeat at intervals of 1 wk

Available forms: Inj 2500 mcg/vial powder

SIDE EFFECTS

CNS: Drowsiness, weakness, lethargy, headache, flushing, fever, depression

---

⚠ Safety alert   *"Tall Man" lettering

GI: *Nausea, vomiting, anorexia, diarrhea, stomatitis,* increased liver enzymes

GU: Increased BUN, creatinine; ***proteinuria***

HEMA: **Hemorrhage, thrombocytopenia,** decreased PT, WBC count

INTEG: *Rash,* cellulitis, ***extravasation,*** facial flushing

META: Decreased serum Ca, P, K

Contraindications: Pregnancy (X), hypersensitivity, thrombocytopenia, bone marrow depression, bleeding disorders, lactation, child <15 yr

Precautions: Renal disease, hepatic disease, electrolyte imbalances

PHARMACOKINETICS

Crosses blood-brain barrier, excreted in urine; little known about pharmacokinetics

INTERACTIONS

Increase: toxicity—other antineoplastics or radiation

Drug/Herb

Increase: bleeding risk—anise, arnica, chamomile, clove, dong quai, fenugreek, garlic, ginger, ginkgo, ginseng *(Panax),* licorice

NURSING CONSIDERATIONS

Assess:

• CBC, differential, platelet count qwk; withhold drug if WBC is <4000/mm³ or platelet count is <50,000/mm³; notify prescriber

• Renal studies: BUN, serum uric acid, urine CCr, electrolytes before, during therapy

• I&O ratio; report urine output <30 ml/hr

• Monitor temp q4h; fever may indicate beginning infection

• Hepatic studies before, during therapy: bilirubin, AST, ALT, alk phosphatase prn or qmo; jaundiced skin, sclera; dark urine, clay-colored stools, itchy skin, abdominal pain, fever, diarrhea

• Alkalosis if severe vomiting is present

⚠ Toxicity: facial flushing, epistaxis, increased PT, thrombocytopenia; drug should be discontinued

⚠ Bleeding: hematuria, guaiac stools, bruising or petechiae, mucosa or orifices q8h; may progress to severe bleeding

• Inflammation of mucosa, breaks in skin

• Buccal cavity q8h for dryness, sores, ulceration, white patches, oral pain, bleeding, dysphagia

• Local irritation, pain, burning at inj site

• Frequency of stools, characteristics, cramping

• Acidosis, signs of dehydration: rapid respirations, poor skin turgor, decreased urine output, dry skin, restlessness, weakness

Administer:

• Antiemetic 30-60 min before giving drug and 4-10 hr after treatment to prevent vomiting

• Transfusion for anemia

• Antispasmodic for diarrhea, phenothiazine for nausea and vomiting

IV route

• Dilute 2.5 mg/4.9 ml of sterile H₂O; (500 mcg/ml) dilute single dose in 1000 ml of D₅W run over 4-6 hr

• EDTA for extravasation, apply ice compress

• Slow IV infusion using 20G, 21G needle

Y-site compatibilities: Allopurinol, amifostine, aztreonam, filgrastim, granisetron, melphalan, piperacillin/tazobactam, teniposide, thiotepa, vinorelbine

Perform/provide:

• Liquid diet: carbonated beverages; gelatin may be added if patient is not nauseated or vomiting

• Rinsing of mouth tid-qid with water; brushing of teeth with baking soda bid-tid with soft brush or cotton-tipped applicator for stomatitis; unwaxed dental floss

• Usage immediately after mixing

Evaluate:

• Therapeutic response: decreased tumor size, spread of malignancy

P

Teach patient/family:
• To report any complaints or side effects to nurse or prescriber
• To avoid foods with citric acid, hot or rough texture
• To use effective contraception, avoid breastfeeding
• To report to prescriber any bleeding, white spots, ulcerations in the mouth; tell patient to examine mouth daily
• To avoid driving, activities requiring alertness; drowsiness may occur
• To report leg cramps, tingling of fingertips, weakness; may indicate hypocalcemia
• To avoid crowds, persons with infections when granulocyte count is low

---

Rarely Used

poly-L-lactic acid (℞)
(pol'-i-el-lak'-tik-as'-id)
Sculptra
Func. class.: Physical adjuncts

Uses: Facial fat loss (lipoatrophy) in those with HIV

DOSAGE AND ROUTES

• *Adult:* INJ injected deep into dermic or subcut layer to avoid superficial inj using a 26G sterile needle; the number of inj depends on quantity of fat loss
Contraindications: Hypersensitivity

---

polymyxin B ophthalmic
See Appendix C

Rarely Used ⚠ High Alert

poractant alfa (℞)
Curosurf
Func. class.: Lung surfactant extract

Uses: Treatment (rescue) of respiratory distress syndrome in premature infants

DOSAGE AND ROUTES

• *Premature infant:* **INTRATRACHEAL INSTILL:** 2.5 ml/kg birth weight up to 2 subsequent doses of 1.25 ml/kg birth weight can be administered at 12-hr intervals, max 5 ml/kg

---

porfimer (℞)
(pour'fih-mur)
Photofrin
Func. class.: Antineoplastic—miscellaneous

Action: Used in photodynamic treatment of tumors (PDT); antitumor and cytotoxic actions are light and O_2 dependent; used with 630 nm laser light
Uses: Esophageal cancer (completely obstructing), endobronchial non–small cell lung cancer, Barrett's esophagus
Investigational uses: AIDs-related cutaneous Kaposi's sarcoma; basal cell, squamous cell carcinoma

DOSAGE AND ROUTES

• Refer to Optiguide for complete instructions
• *Adult:* IV 2 mg/kg, then illumination with laser light 40-50 hr after inj; a second laser light application may be given 96-120 hr after inj; may repeat q30 days × 3
Endobronchial cancer
• *Adult:* 200 joules/cm of tumor length
Available forms: Cake/powder for inj 75 mg

SIDE EFFECTS

CNS: Anxiety, confusion, insomnia
*CV: Hypotension, hypertension, atrial fibrillation, **cardiac failure**, tachycardia*
GI: Abdominal pain, constipation, diarrhea, dyspepsia, dysphagia, eructation, esophageal edema/bleeding, hematemesis, melena, nausea, vomiting, anorexia
MISC: Dehydration, weight decrease,

---

anemia, photosensitivity reaction, UTI, moniliasis

RESP: **Pleural effusion,** pneumonia, dyspnea, respiratory insufficiency, **tracheoesophageal fistula**

Contraindications: Porphyria, porphyrin allergy (porfimer); tracheoesophageal, bronchoesophageal fistula; major blood vessels with eroding tumors (PDT)

Precautions: Pregnancy (C), elderly, lactation, children

PHARMACOKINETICS

Half-life 250 hr, 90% protein bound

INTERACTIONS

Increase: photosensitivity— tetracyclines, sulfonamides, phenothiazines, sulfonylureas, thiazides

NURSING CONSIDERATIONS
Assess:

• Ocular sensitivity: sensitivity to sun, bright lights, car headlights, patients should wear dark sunglasses with an average light transmittance of <4%

• Chest pain: may be so severe as to necessitate opiate analgesics

• For extravasation at inj site: take care to protect from light

Administer:

• As a single slow IV inj over 3-5 min at 2 mg/kg; reconstitute each vial with 31.8 ml D$_5$ or 0.9% NaCl (2.5 mg/ml), shake well; do not mix with other drugs or sol; protect from light and use immediately

• Laser light is initiated 630-nm wave length laser light

Perform/provide:

• Wiping of spills with damp cloth, avoid skin/eye contact, use rubber gloves, eye protection, dispose of material in polyethylene bag according to policy

Teach patient/family:

• To report chest pain, eye sensitivity

• To wear sunglasses; avoid exposure to sunlight or bright light for 30 days

---

potassium acetate

potassium bicarbonate (otc, ℞)

K+ Care ET, K-Electrolyte, K-Ide, Klor-Con EF, K-Lyte, K-Vescent

potassium bicarbonate and potassium chloride (otc, ℞)

Klorvess, Klorvess Effervescent Granules, K-Lyte/Cl, Neo-K ✦

potassium bicarbonate and potassium citrate (otc, ℞)

Effer-K, K-Lyte DS

potassium chloride (otc, ℞)

Apo-K ✦, Cena-K, Gen-K, K+ Care, K+ 10, Kalium Durules ✦, Kaochlor, Kaochlor S-F, Kaon-Cl, Kay Ciel, KCl, K-Dur, K-Lease, K-Long ✦, K-Lor, Klor-Con, Klorvess, Klotrix, K-Lyte/Cl powder, K-med, K-Norm, K-Sol, K-tab, Micro-K, Micro-LS, Potasalan, Roychlor, Rum-K, Slow-K, Ten-K

potassium chloride/ potassium bicarbonate/ potassium citrate (otc, ℞)

Kaochlor Eff

potassium gluconate (otc, ℞)

Kaon, Kaylixir, K-G Elixir, Potassium-Rougier ✦

potassium gluconate/ potassium chloride (otc, ℞)

Kolyum

potassium gluconate/ potassium citrate (otc, ℞)

Twin-K

Func. class.: Electrolyte, mineral replacement

Chem. class.: Potassium

Action: Needed for adequate transmission of nerve impulses and cardiac contraction, renal function, intracellular ion maintenance

Uses: Prevention and treatment of hypokalemia

DOSAGE AND ROUTES

Potassium acetate—hypokalemia
• *Adult and child:* **PO** 40-100 mEq/day in divided doses 2-4 days
Potassium bicarbonate
• *Adult:* **PO** dissolve 25-50 mEq in water daily-qid
Hypokalemia (prevention)
• *Adult and child:* **PO** 20 mEq/day in 2-4 divided doses
Potassium chloride
• *Adult:* **PO** 40-100 mEq in divided doses tid-qid; **IV** 20 mEq/hr when diluted as 40 mEq/1000 ml, not to exceed 150 mEq/day
• *Child:* **PO** 2-4 mEq/kg/day
Potassium gluconate
• *Adult:* **PO** 40-100 mEq in divided doses tid-qid
Potassium phosphate
• *Adult:* **IV** 1 mEq/hr in sol of 60 mEq/L, not to exceed 150 mEq/day; **PO** 40-100 mEq/day in divided doses
• *Child:* **IV** max rate of inf 1 mEq/kg/hr
Available forms: Tabs for sol 6.5, 25 mEq; caps, ext rel 8, 10 mEq; powder for sol 3.3, 5, 6.7, 10, 13.3 mEq/5 ml; tabs 2, 4, 5, 13.4 mEq; tabs, ext rel 6.7, 8, 10 mEq; elix 6.7 mEq/5 ml; oral sol 2.375 mEq/5 ml; inj for prep of IV 1.5, 2, 2.4, 3, 3.2, 4.4, 4.7 mEq/ml

SIDE EFFECTS

CNS: Confusion
CV: Bradycardia, *cardiac depression, dysrhythmias, arrest, peaking T waves, lowered R and depressed RST, prolonged P-R interval, widened QRS complex*
GI: Nausea, vomiting, cramps, pain, *diarrhea,* ulceration of small bowel
GU: Oliguria
INTEG: Cold extremities, rash
Contraindications: Renal disease (severe), severe hemolytic disease, Addi-

son's disease, hyperkalemia, acute dehydration, extensive tissue breakdown
Precautions: Pregnancy (C), cardiac disease, potassium-sparing diuretic therapy, systemic acidosis

PHARMACOKINETICS

PO: Excreted by kidneys and in feces; onset of action ≈30 min
IV: Immediate onset of action

INTERACTIONS

Hyperkalemia: potassium phosphate IV and products containing calcium or magnesium; potassium-sparing diuretic, or other potassium products, ACE inhibitors

NURSING CONSIDERATIONS

Assess:
• ECG for peaking T waves, lowered R, depressed RST, prolonged P-R interval, widening QRS complex, hyperkalemia; drug should be reduced or discontinued
• Potassium level during treatment (3.5-5 mg/dl is normal level)
• I&O ratio; watch for decreased urinary output; notify prescriber immediately
• Cardiac status: rate, rhythm, CVP, PWP, PAWP, if being monitored directly
Administer:
PO route
• Do not crush, break, or chew ext rel tabs/caps or enteric products
• With meal or pc; dissolve effervescent tabs, powder in 8 oz cold water or juice; do not give IM, SUBCUT
• Caps with full glass of liquid
IV route
• Through large-bore needle to decrease vein inflammation; check for extravasation
• In large vein, avoiding scalp vein in child (IV)
• IV after diluting in large volume of IV sol and give as an inf, slowly by IV inf to prevent toxicity; never give IV bolus or IM
Potassium acetate
Additive compatibilities: Metoclopramide

⚠ Safety alert   *"Tall Man" lettering

Y-site compatibilities: Ciprofloxacin

Potassium chloride

Additive compatibilities: Aminophylline, amiodarone, atracurium, bretylium, calcium gluconate, cefepime, cephalothin, cephapirin, chloramphenicol, cimetidine, ciprofloxacin, cisatracurium, clindamycin, cloxacillin, corticotropin, cytarabine, dimenhyDRINATE, DOPamine, DOXOrubicin liposome, enalaprilat, erythromycin, floxacillin, fluconazole, fosphenytoin, furosemide, heparin, hydrocortisone, isoproterenol, lidocaine, metaraminol, methicillin, methyldopate, metoclopramide, mitoxantrone, nafcillin, netilmicin, norepinephrine, oxacillin, penicillin G potassium, phenylephrine, piperacillin, ranitidine, sodium bicarbonate, thiopental, vancomycin, verapamil, vit B/C

Y-site compatibilities: Acyclovir, aldesleukin, allopurinol, amifostine, aminophylline, amiodarone, ampicillin, amrinone, atropine, aztreonam, betamethasone, calcium gluconate, cefmetazole, cephalothin, cephapirin, chlordiazepoxide, chlorproMAZINE, ciprofloxacin, cladribine, cyanocobalamin, dexamethasone, digoxin, diltiazem, diphenhydrAMINE, DOBUTamine, DOPamine, droperidol, edrophonium, enalaprilat, epINEPHrine, esmolol, estrogens, ethacrynate, famotidine, fentanyl, filgrastim, fludarabine, fluorouracil, furosemide, gallium, granisetron, heparin, hydrALAZINE, idarubicin, indomethacin, insulin (regular), isoproterenol, kanamycin, labetalol, lidocaine, lorazepam, magnesium sulfate, melphalan, meperidine, methicillin, methoxamine, methylergonovine, midazolam, minocycline, morphine, neostigmine, norepinephrine, ondansetron, oxacillin, oxytocin, paclitaxel, penicillin G potassium, pentazocine, phytonadione, piperacillin/tazobactam, prednisoLONE, procainamide, prochlorperazine, propofol, propranolol, pyridostigmine, remifentanil, sargramostim, scopolamine, sodium bicarbonate, succinylcholine, tacrolimus, teniposide, theophylline, thiotepa, trimethaphan, trimethoenzamide, vinorelbine, warfarin, zidovudine

Perform/provide:
• Storage at room temperature

Evaluate:
• Therapeutic response: absence of fatigue, muscle weakness; decreased thirst and urinary output; cardiac changes

Teach patient/family:
• To add potassium-rich foods to diet: bananas, orange juice, avocados; whole grains, broccoli, carrots, prunes, cocoa after this medication is discontinued
• To avoid OTC products: antacids, salt substitutes, analgesics, vitamin preparations, unless specifically directed by prescriber
• To report hyperkalemia symptoms (lethargy, confusion, diarrhea, nausea, vomiting, fainting, decreased output) or continued hypokalemia symptoms (fatigue, weakness, polyuria, polydipsia, cardiac changes)
• To dissolve powder or tablet completely in at least 120 ml water or juice
• Importance of regular follow-up visits

---

potassium iodide (℞)

Pima, saturated solution (SSKI), strong iodine solution (Lugol's solution), Thyro-Block

Func. class.: Thyroid hormone antagonist

Chem. class.: Iodine product

Action: Inhibits secretion of thyroid hormone, fosters colloid accumulation in thyroid follicles, decreases vascularity of gland

Uses: Preparation for thyroidectomy, thyrotoxic crisis, neonatal thyrotoxicosis, radiation protectant, thyroid storm

DOSAGE AND ROUTES

Thyrotoxic crisis
• *Adult and child:* **PO** 500 mg q4h (10 gtt SSKI), or 1 ml of strong iodine sol tid; give ≥1 hr after 1st dose of propylthiouracil, or methimazole

---

Side effects: *italics* = common; ***bold italics*** = life-threatening

Preparation for thyroidectomy
• *Adult and child:* **PO** 3-5 gtt strong iodine sol tid, or 1-5 drops SSKI in water tid after meals for 10 days prior to surgery

Available forms: Oral sol (Lugol's solution) iodine 5%/potassium iodide 10%; oral sol (SSKI) 1 g/ml; syrup 325 mg/5 ml; tablets 130 mg

SIDE EFFECTS

CNS: Headache, confusion, paresthesias
EENT: Metallic taste, stomatitis, salivation, periorbital edema, sore teeth and gums, cold symptoms
ENDO: Hypothyroidism, hyperthyroid adenoma
GI: Nausea, diarrhea, vomiting, small-bowel lesions, upper gastric pain
INTEG: Rash, urticaria, **angioneurotic edema,** acne, mucosal hemorrhage, fever
MS: Myalgia, arthralgia, weakness

Contraindications: Pregnancy (D), hypersensitivity to iodine, pulmonary edema, pulmonary TB

Precautions: Lactation, children

PHARMACOKINETICS

PO: Onset 24-48 hr, peak 10-15 days after continuous therapy, uptake by thyroid gland or excreted in urine; crosses placenta

INTERACTIONS

Hypothyroidism: lithium, other antithyroid agents

Drug/Lab Test
Interference: Urinary 17-OHCS

NURSING CONSIDERATIONS

Assess:
• Pulse, B/P, temp
• I&O ratio; check for edema: puffy hands, feet, periorbit; indicate hypothyroidism
• Weight daily; same clothing, scale, time of day
• T_3, T_4, which is increased; serum TSH, which is decreased; free thyroxine index, which is increased if dosage is too low; discontinue drug 3-4 wk before RAIU

⚠ Overdose: peripheral edema, heat intolerance, diaphoresis, palpitations, dysrhythmias, severe tachycardia, fever, delirium, CNS irritability
• Hypersensitivity: rash; enlarged cervical lymph nodes may indicate drug should be discontinued
• Hypoprothrombinemia: bleeding, petechiae, ecchymosis
• Clinical response: after 3 wk should include increased weight, pulse; decreased T_4

Administer:
• Strong iodine solution after diluting with water or juice to improve taste
• Through straw to prevent tooth discoloration
• With meals to decrease GI upset
• At same time each day to maintain drug level
• Lowest dose that relieves symptoms, discontinue before RAIU

Perform/provide:
• Fluids to 3-4 L/day, unless contraindicated

Evaluate:
• Therapeutic response: weight gain, decreased pulse, T_4, size of thyroid gland

Teach patient/family:
• To abstain from breastfeeding after delivery
• To keep graph of weight, pulse, mood
• To avoid OTC products that contain iodine
• That seafood, other iodine products may be restricted
• Not to discontinue this medication abruptly; thyroid crisis may occur; stress response
• That response may take several mo if thyroid is large
• To discontinue drug, notify prescriber of fever, rash, metallic taste, swelling of throat; burning of mouth, throat; sore gums, teeth; severe GI distress, enlargement of thyroid, cold symptoms

pralidoxime (℞)

(pra-li-dox'eem)

Protopam Chloride

Func. class.: Cholinesterase reactivator

Uses: Cholinergic crisis in myasthenia gravis, organophosphate poisoning antidote (early), relief of paralysis of respiratory muscles; used as an adjunct to systemic atropine administration

DOSAGE AND ROUTES

Anticholinesterase overdose
• *Adult:* **IV** 1-2 g, then 250 mg q5min until desired response

Organophosphate poisoning
• *Adult:* **IV INF** 1-2 g/100 ml 0.9% NaCl over 15-30 min; may repeat in 1 hr; **PO** 1-3 g q5h
• *Child:* **IV INF** 20-40 mg/kg/dose diluted in 100 ml 0.9% NaCl over 15-30 min

Contraindications: Hypersensitivity, carbamate insecticide poisoning

pramipexole (℞)

(pra-mi-pex'ol)

Mirapex

Func. class.: Antiparkinson agent

Chem. class.: Dopamine-receptor agonist, non-ergot

Action: Selective agonist for D_2 receptors (presynaptic/postsynaptic sites); binding at D_3 receptor contributes to antiparkinson effects

Uses: Parkinson's disease

Investigational uses: Restless leg syndrome

DOSAGE AND ROUTES

Initial treatment
• *Adult:* **PO** from a starting dose of 0.375 mg/day given in 3 divided doses; increase gradually by 0.125 mg/dose at 5-7 day intervals until total daily dose of 4.5 mg is reached

Maintenance treatment
• *Adult:* **PO** 1.5-4.5 mg daily in 3 divided doses

Restless leg syndrome (off-label)
• *Adult:* **PO** 0.125-0.375 mg 1-2 hr prior to bedtime, increase gradually

Renal dose
• *Adult:* **PO** CCr 35-59 ml/min-0.125 mg bid, may increase q5-7 days to 1.5 mg bid; CCr 15-34 ml/min 0.125 mg daily, increase q5-7 days to 1.5 mg daily

Available forms: Tabs 0.125, 0.25, 1, 1.5 mg

SIDE EFFECTS

CNS: Agitation, insomnia, psychosis, hallucination, depression, dizziness, headache, confusion, ***sleep attacks***
CV: Orthostatic hypotension, edema, syncope, tachycardia
EENT: Blurred vision
GI: Nausea, anorexia, constipation, dysphagia, dry mouth
GU: Impotence, urinary frequency
HEMA: ***Hemolytic anemia, leukopenia, agranulocytosis***

Contraindications: Hypersensitivity
Precautions: Pregnancy (C), renal disease, cardiac disease, MI with dysrhythmias, affective disorders, psychosis, preexisting dyskinesias

PHARMACOKINETICS

Minimally metabolized, peak 2 hr, half-life 8 hr, 12-14 hr in elderly

INTERACTIONS

Increase: pramipexole levels—levodopa, cimetidine, ranitidine, diltiazem, triamterene, verapamil, quinidine
Decrease: pramipexole levels—DOPamine antagonists, phenothiazines, metoclopramide, butyrophenones

Drug/Herb
Decrease: effect of pramipexole—chaste tree fruit, kava

P

Side effects: *italics* = common; ***bold italics*** = life-threatening

NURSING CONSIDERATIONS

Assess:

• Renal studies

• Involuntary movements in parkinsonism: bradykinesia, tremors, staggering gait, muscle rigidity, drooling

• B/P, ECG, respiration during initial treatment; hypo/hypertension should be reported

• Mental status: affect, mood, behavioral changes, depression; complete suicide assessment

A For sleep attacks: may fall asleep during activities without warning; may need to discontinue medication

Administer:

• Adjust dosage to patient response, titrate slowly

• With meals to minimize GI symptoms

Perform/provide:

• Assistance with ambulation during beginning therapy

• Testing for diabetes mellitus, acromegaly if on long-term therapy

Evaluate:

• Therapeutic response: movement disorder improves

Teach patient/family:

• That therapeutic effects may take several weeks to a few months

• To change positions slowly to prevent orthostatic hypotension

• To use drug exactly as prescribed: if drug is discontinued abruptly, parkinsonian crisis may occur, avoid alcohol, OTC sleeping products

• To notify prescriber if pregnancy is planned or suspected

---

pramlintide
See Appendix A—Selected New Drugs

---

pramoxine topical
See Appendix C

---

pravastatin (℞)
(pra'va-sta-tin)
Pravachol
Func. class.: Antilipidemic
Chem. class.: HMG-CoA reductase enzyme

Do not confuse:
Pravachol/Prevacid

Action: Inhibits HMG-CoA reductase enzyme, which reduces cholesterol synthesis

Uses: As an adjunct in primary hypercholesterolemia (types IIa, IIb, III, IV), to reduce the risk of recurrent MI, atherosclerosis, primary/secondary CV events, reduce stroke, TIAs

DOSAGE AND ROUTES

• *Adult:* **PO** 40-80 mg daily at bedtime (range 20-80 mg daily)

• *Adolescent 14-18 yr:* **PO** 40 mg daily

• *Child 8-13 yr:* **PO** 20 mg daily

• *Elderly/renal/hepatic disease:* **PO** 10 mg/day initially

Available forms: Tabs 10, 20, 40, 80 mg

SIDE EFFECTS

CNS: Headache, dizziness, fatigue
EENT: Lens opacities
GI: Nausea, constipation, diarrhea, flatus, abdominal pain, heartburn, ***hepatic dysfunction,*** pancreatitis, ***hepatitis***
INTEG: Rash, pruritus, photosensitivity
MISC: Chest pain, rash, pruritus, photosensitivity
MS: Muscle cramps, myalgia, ***myositis, rhabdomyolysis***
RESP: Common cold, rhinitis, cough

Contraindications: Pregnancy (X), hypersensitivity, lactation, active hepatic disease

Precautions: Past hepatic disease, alcoholism, severe acute infections, trauma, severe metabolic disorders, electrolyte imbalances

---

A Safety alert   *"Tall Man" lettering

PHARMACOKINETICS

Peak 1-1½ hr; metabolized by the liver, protein binding 80%; excreted in urine 20%, feces 70%, breast milk; crosses placenta

INTERACTIONS

Increase: myopathy risk—erythromycin, niacin, cycloSPORINE, gemfibrozil, clofibrate, clarithromycin, itraconazole, protease inhibitors
Increase: effects of warfarin, digoxin
Decrease: bioavailability of pravastatin—bile acid sequestrants
Drug/Herb
Increase: effect—glucomannan
Decrease: effect—gotu kola
Drug/Lab Test
Increase: CPK, LFTs
Altered: thyroid function tests

NURSING CONSIDERATIONS

Assess:
• Fasting lipid profile: LDL, HDL, TG, cholesterol q8wk, then q3-6mo when stable; obtain diet history
• Hepatic studies: baseline, q6wk during the first 3 mo, q8wk for remainder of yr, then q6mo; AST, ALT, LFTs may increase
• Renal studies in patients with compromised renal system: BUN, I&O ratio, creatinine
⚠ For muscle tenderness, pain, obtain CPK baseline and if these occur; rhabdomyolysis may occur, therapy should be discontinued
Administer:
• Without regard to meals, at bedtime
• Give 1 hr ac or 4 hr pc bile acid sequestrants
Perform/provide:
• Storage in cool environment in tight container protected from light
Evaluate:
• Therapeutic response: decrease in cholesterol to desired level after 8 wk
Teach patient/family:
• That blood work will be necessary during treatment
⚠ To report blurred vision, severe GI symptoms, dizziness, headache, muscle pain, weakness, fever
• That regimen will continue: low-cholesterol diet, exercise program
• To report suspected, planned pregnancy, not to use during pregnancy
• To use sunscreen, protective clothing to prevent burns

---

prazosin (℞)
(pray'zoe-sin)
Minipress, prazosin
Func. class.: Antihypertensive
Chem. class.: α₁-Adrenergic blocker

Action: Blocks α-mediated vasoconstriction of adrenergic receptors, inducing peripheral vasodilation
Uses: Hypertension, refractory CHF, Raynaud's vasospasm
Investigational uses: Benign prostatic hypertrophy to decrease urine outflow obstruction

DOSAGE AND ROUTES

Hypertension
• *Adult:* **PO** 1 mg bid or tid, increasing to 20 mg daily in divided doses if required; usual range 6-15 mg/day, not to exceed 1 mg initially; max 20-40 mg/day
• *Child:* **PO** 0.5-7 mg tid
Benign prostatic hyperplasia
• *Adult:* **PO** 1-5 mg bid
Available forms: Caps 1, 2, 5 mg

SIDE EFFECTS

CNS: Dizziness, headache, drowsiness, anxiety, depression, vertigo, weakness, fatigue
CV: Palpitations, orthostatic hypotension, tachycardia, edema, rebound hypertension
EENT: Blurred vision, epistaxis, tinnitus, dry mouth, red sclera
GI: Nausea, vomiting, diarrhea, constipation, abdominal pain
GU: Urinary frequency, incontinence, impotence, priapism, H_2O, sodium retention

P

Side effects: *italics* = common; ***bold italics*** = life-threatening

Contraindications: Hypersensitivity
Precautions: Pregnancy (C), children, lactation

PHARMACOKINETICS

PO: Onset 2 hr, peak 1-3 hr, duration 6-12 hr; half-life 2-3 hr, metabolized in liver, excreted via bile, feces (>90%), in urine (<10%), protein binding 97%

INTERACTIONS

Increase: hypotensive effects—β-blockers, nitroglycerin, alcohol, verapamil
Decrease: antihypertensive effect—NSAIDs, clonidine
Drug/Herb
Increase: toxicity, death—aconite
Increase: antihypertensive effect—barberry, betony, black catechu, black cohosh, bloodroot, broom, burdock, cat's claw, dandelion, goldenseal, Irish moss, Jamaican dogwood, kelp, khella, mistletoe, parsley
Increase or decrease: antihypertensive effect—astragalus, cola tree
Decrease: antihypertensive effect—coltsfoot, guarana, khat, licorice
Drug/Lab Test
Increase: Urinary norepinephrine, VMA

NURSING CONSIDERATIONS

Assess:
• B/P (sitting, standing) during initial treatment, periodically thereafter; pulse, jugular venous distention q4h
• BUN, uric acid if on long-term therapy
• Weight daily, I&O; edema in feet, legs daily
• Skin turgor, dryness of mucous membranes for hydration status
• Crackles, dyspnea, orthopnea q30min
Administer:
• 1st dose at bedtime to avoid fainting
Perform/provide:
• Storage in tight container in cool environment
Evaluate:
• Therapeutic response: decreased B/P

Teach patient/family:
• That fainting occasionally occurs after 1st dose; take 1st dose at bedtime or do not drive or operate machinery for 4 hr after 1st dose
• To change positions slowly, to prevent orthostatic hypotension
• To avoid OTC medications unless approved by prescriber
Treatment of overdose: Administer volume expanders or vasopressors, discontinue drug, place in supine position

---

prednicarbate topical
See Appendix C

---

*prednisoLONE (℞)

(pred-niss'oh-lone)
Articulose-50, Delta-Cortef, Hydeltrasol, Hydeltra-T.B.A., Key-Pred 25, Key-Pred 50, Key-Pred-SP, Orapred, Pediapred, Predaject-50, Predalone 50, Predalone-T.B.A., Predcor-25, Predcor-50, prednisoLONE, PrednisoLONE Acetate, Prednisol TBA, Prelone
Func. class.: Corticosteroid, synthetic
Chem. class.: Glucocorticoid, immediate acting

Do not confuse:
prednisoLONE/predniSONE
Action: Decreases inflammation by suppression of migration of polymorphonuclear leukocytes, fibroblasts; reversal to increase capillary permeability and lysosomal stabilization
Uses: Severe inflammation, immunosuppression, neoplasms

DOSAGE AND ROUTES

• *Adult:* **PO** 2.5-15 mg bid-qid; **IM** 2-30 mg (acetate, phosphate) q12h; **IV** 2-30 mg (phosphate) q12h; 2-30 mg in joint

---

🛑 Safety alert   *"Tall Man" lettering

or soft tissue (phosphate), 4-40 mg in joint of lesion (tebutate)

Asthma/antiinflammatory
• *Child:* **PO/IV** 1 mg/kg q6h × 2 days, then 1-2 mg/kg; max 60 mg/day

Available forms: Tabs 5 mg; syr 5 mg/5 ml, 15 mg/15 ml; acetate: inj 25, 50 mg/ml; tebutate: inj 20 mg/ml; phosphate: inj 20 mg/ml, oral liquid 5 mg/ml, tabs 1, 2.5, 5, 10, 20, 50 mg, oral sol 5 mg/ml, 5 mg/5 ml, syr 5 mg/5 ml

SIDE EFFECTS

CNS: Depression, flushing, sweating, headache, mood changes
CV: Hypertension, ***circulatory collapse, thrombophlebitis, embolism,*** tachycardia
EENT: Fungal infections, increased intraocular pressure, blurred vision
GI: Diarrhea, nausea, abdominal distention, ***GI hemorrhage,*** increased appetite, ***pancreatitis***
HEMA: ***Thrombocytopenia***
INTEG: Acne, poor wound healing, ecchymosis, petechiae
MS: Fractures, osteoporosis, weakness
Contraindications: Psychosis, hypersensitivity, idiopathic thrombocytopenia, acute glomerulonephritis, amebiasis, fungal infections, nonasthmatic bronchial disease, child <2 yr
Precautions: Pregnancy (C), diabetes mellitus, glaucoma, osteoporosis, seizure disorders, ulcerative colitis, CHF, myasthenia gravis

PHARMACOKINETICS

PO: Peak 1-2 hr, duration 2 days
IM: Peak 3-45 hr

INTERACTIONS

Increase: side effects—alcohol, salicylates, indomethacin, amphotericin B, digitalis, cycloSPORINE, diuretics
Increase: prednisoLONE action—salicylates, estrogens, indomethacin, oral contraceptives, ketoconazole, macrolide antibiotics

Decrease: prednisoLONE action—cholestyramine, colestipol, barbiturates, rifampin, epHEDrine, phenytoin, theophylline
Decrease: effects of anticoagulants, anticonvulsants, antidiabetics, ambenonium, neostigmine, isoniazid, toxoids, vaccines, anticholinesterases, salicylates, somatrem

Drug/Herb
Hypokalemia: aloe, buckthorn, cascara sagrada, Chinese rhubarb, senna
Increase: effect—aloe, licorice, perilla

Drug/Lab Test
Increase: Cholesterol, sodium, blood glucose, uric acid, calcium, urine glucose
Decrease: Calcium, potassium, T_4, T_3, thyroid ^{131}I uptake test, urine 17-OHCS, 17-KS, PBI
False negative: Skin allergy tests

NURSING CONSIDERATIONS

Assess:
• Potassium, blood glucose, urine glucose while on long-term therapy; hypokalemia and hyperglycemia
• Weight daily; notify prescriber if weekly gain >5 lb
• B/P q4h, pulse; notify prescriber if chest pain occurs
• I&O ratio; be alert for decreasing urinary output, increasing edema
• Plasma cortisol levels (long-term therapy) (normal level: 138-635 nmol/L SI units when drawn at 8 AM)
• Infection: increased temp, WBC, even after withdrawal of medication; drug masks infection
• Potassium depletion: paresthesias, fatigue, nausea, vomiting, depression, polyuria, dysrhythmias, weakness
• Edema, hypertension, cardiac symptoms
• Mental status: affect, mood, behavioral changes, aggression

Administer:
IM route
• After shaking suspension (parenteral)
• Titrated dose; use lowest effective dose

Side effects: *italics* = common; ***bold italics*** = life-threatening

• IM inj deep in large muscle mass; rotate sites; avoid deltoid; use 21G needle

• In 1 dose in AM to prevent adrenal suppression; avoid SUBCUT administration; may damage tissue

• With food or milk to decrease GI symptoms

IV route

• Undiluted or added to NaCl or D_5 and given by IV inf; give 10 mg or less/1 min; decrease rate if burning occurs

Additive compatibilities: Ascorbic acid, cephalothin, cytarabine, erythromycin, fluorouracil, heparin, methicillin, penicillin G potassium, penicillin G sodium, vit B/C

Y-site compatibilities: Ciprofloxacin, heparin/hydrocortisone, potassium chloride, vit B/C

Perform/provide:

• Assistance with ambulation to patient with bone tissue disease to prevent fractures

Evaluate:

• Therapeutic response: ease of respirations, decreased inflammation

Teach patient/family:

• That emergency ID as steroid user should be carried

• To notify prescriber if therapeutic response decreases; dosage adjustment may be needed

• Not to discontinue abruptly; adrenal crisis can result; take exactly as prescribed

• To avoid OTC products: salicylates, cough products with alcohol, cold preparations unless directed by prescriber

• About cushingoid symptoms

• The symptoms of adrenal insufficiency: nausea, anorexia, fatigue, dizziness, dyspnea, weakness, joint pain

---

**prednisoLONE
ophthalmic**
See Appendix C

---

*predniSONE (℞)
(pred'ni-sone)
Apo-Prednisone ✦,
Deltasone ✦, Liquid Pred,
Meticorten, Orasone,
Panasol-S, Prednicen-M,
PredniSONE, Sterapred,
Winpred
Func. class.: Corticosteroid
Chem. class.: Intermediate-acting glucocorticoid

Do not confuse:
predniSONE/methylPREDNISolone
predniSONE/prednisoLONE
predniSONE/Prilosec

Action: Decreases inflammation by suppression of migration of polymorphonuclear leukocytes, fibroblasts, reversal to increase capillary permeability, and lysosomal stabilization

Uses: Severe inflammation, immunosuppression, neoplasms, multiple sclerosis, collagen disorders, dermatologic disorders

DOSAGE AND ROUTES

• *Adult:* **PO** 5-60 mg daily or divided bid-qid

• *Child:* **PO** 0.05-2 mg/kg/day divided 1-4 ×/day

Nephrosis

• *Child:* **PO** 2 mg/kg/day in divided doses, max 28 days, then 1-1.5 mg/kg/day every other day × 4 wk

Multiple sclerosis

• *Adult:* **PO** 200 mg/day × 1 wk, then 80 mg every other day × 1 mo

Available forms: Tabs 1, 2.5, 5, 10, 20, 50 mg; oral sol 5 mg/5 ml; syr 5 mg/5 ml

SIDE EFFECTS

CNS: Depression, flushing, sweating, headache, mood changes
CV: Hypertension, ***circulatory collapse, thrombophlebitis, embolism,*** tachycardia

---

EENT: Fungal infections, increased intraocular pressure, blurred vision

GI: Diarrhea, nausea, abdominal distention, *GI hemorrhage,* increased appetite, pancreatitis

HEMA: Thrombocytopenia

INTEG: Acne, poor wound healing, ecchymosis, petechiae

META: Hyperglycemia

MS: Fractures, osteoporosis, weakness

Contraindications: Psychosis, hypersensitivity, idiopathic thrombocytopenia, acute glomerulonephritis, amebiasis, fungal infections, nonasthmatic bronchial disease, child <2 yr, AIDS, TB

Precautions: Pregnancy (C), diabetes mellitus, glaucoma, osteoporosis, seizure disorders, ulcerative colitis, CHF, myasthenia gravis, renal disease, esophagitis, peptic ulcer, cataracts, coagulopathy

PHARMACOKINETICS

PO: Well absorbed PO, peak 1-2 hr, duration 1-1½ days, half-life 3½-4 hr
Crosses placenta, enters breast milk, metabolized by liver after conversion, excreted in urine

INTERACTIONS

Increase: side effects—alcohol, salicylates, indomethacin, amphotericin B, digitalis, cycloSPORINE, diuretics

Increase: predniSONE action—salicylates, estrogens, indomethacin, oral contraceptives, ketoconazole, macrolide antiinfectives

Decrease: predniSONE action—cholestyramine, colestipol, barbiturates, rifampin, epHEDrine, phenytoin, theophylline

Decrease: effects of anticoagulants, anticonvulsants, antidiabetics, ambenonium, neostigmine, isoniazid, toxoids, vaccines, anticholinesterases, salicylates, somatrem

Drug/Herb

Hypokalemia: aloe, buckthorn, Chinese rhubarb, senna

Increase: effect—aloe, licorice, perilla

Drug/Lab Test

Increase: Cholesterol, sodium, blood glucose, uric acid, calcium, urine glucose

Decrease: Calcium, potassium, T_4, T_3, thyroid ^{131}I uptake test, urine 17-OHCS, 17-KS, PBI

False negative: Skin allergy tests

NURSING CONSIDERATIONS

Assess:

• Adrenal insufficiency: nausea, vomiting, anorexia, confusion, hypotension

• Potassium, blood glucose, urine glucose while on long-term therapy; hypokalemia and hyperglycemia

• Weight daily; notify prescriber of weekly gain >5 lb

• B/P q4h, pulse; notify prescriber of chest pain; monitor for crackles, dyspnea if edema is present

• I&O ratio; be alert for decreasing urinary output, increasing edema

• Plasma cortisol (long-term therapy) (normal: 138-635 nmol/L SI units drawn at 8 AM)

• Infection: increased temp, WBC, even after withdrawal of medication; drug masks infection

• Potassium depletion: paresthesias, fatigue, nausea, vomiting, depression, polyuria, dysrhythmias, weakness

• Edema, hypertension, cardiac symptoms

• Mental status: affect, mood, behavioral changes, aggression

Administer:

• For long-term use, alternate-day therapy is recommended to decrease adverse reactions

• Titrated dose; use lowest effective dose

• With food or milk to decrease GI symptoms

Perform/provide:

• Assistance with ambulation to patient with bone tissue disease to prevent fractures

Evaluate:

• Therapeutic response: ease of respirations, decreased inflammation

P

Teach patient/family:
• That emergency ID as steroid user should be carried; information on drug being taken and condition
• To notify prescriber if therapeutic response decreases; dosage adjustment may be needed
• To avoid vaccinations
• Not to discontinue abruptly, or adrenal crisis can result
• To avoid OTC products: salicylates, cough products with alcohol, cold preparations unless directed by prescriber
• About cushingoid symptoms: moon face, weight gain
• That drug causes immunosuppression; to report any symptoms of infection (fever, sore throat, cough)
• The symptoms of adrenal insufficiency: nausea, anorexia, fatigue, dizziness, dyspnea, weakness, joint pain

---

primaquine (R)
(prim′a-kween)
Func. class.: Antimalarial
Chem. class.: Synthetic 8-amino-quinolone

Action: Unknown; thought to destroy exoerythrocytic forms by gametocidal action
Uses: Malaria caused by *Plasmodium vivax,* in combination with clindamycin for *Pneumocystis jiroveci* pneumonia

DOSAGE AND ROUTES
• *Adult:* **PO** 15 mg (base) daily × 2 wk; 26.3-mg tab is 15-mg base
• *Child:* **PO** 0.5 mg/kg (0.3 mg/base/day) daily × 2 wk
Available forms: Tabs 26.3 mg, powder

SIDE EFFECTS
CNS: Headache, dizziness
CV: Hypertension
EENT: Blurred vision, difficulty focusing
GI: Nausea, vomiting, anorexia, cramps
HEMA: Agranulocytosis, granulocytopenia, leukopenia, hemolytic

anemia, leukocytosis, mild anemia, *methemoglobinemia*
INTEG: Pruritus, skin eruptions, pallor, weakness
Contraindications: Hypersensitivity, anemia, lupus erythematosus, methemoglobinemia, porphyria, rheumatoid arthritis, methemoglobin reductase deficiency, G6PD deficiency, iodine hypersensitivity
Precautions: Pregnancy (C), bone marrow suppression, lactation, children

PHARMACOKINETICS
PO: Metabolized by liver (metabolites), half-life 3.7-9.6 hr

INTERACTIONS
Toxicity: quinacrine

NURSING CONSIDERATIONS
Assess:
• Ophthalmic test if long-term treatment or drug dosage >150 mg/day
• Hepatic studies qwk: AST, ALT, bilirubin, if on long-term therapy
• Blood studies: CBC; blood dyscrasias occur
• Allergic reactions: pruritus, rash, urticaria
• Blood dyscrasias: malaise, fever, bruising, bleeding (rare)
• For renal status: dark urine, hematuria, decreased output
⚠ For hemolytic reaction: chills, fever, chest pain, cyanosis; drug should be discontinued immediately
Administer:
PO route
• Before or after meals at same time each day to maintain drug level
Evaluate:
• Therapeutic response: decreased symptoms of malaria
Teach patient/family:
• To report visual problems, fever, fatigue, dark urine, bruising, bleeding; may indicate blood dyscrasias
• To complete full course of therapy

⚠ Safety alert   *"Tall Man" lettering

pregabalin
See Appendix A—Selected
New Drugs

---

primidone (R)
(pri'mi-done)
Apo-Primidone ✦, Mysoline,
PMS-Primidone ✦, primidone,
Sertan ✦
Func. class.: Anticonvulsant
Chem. class.: Barbiturate derivative

Action: Raises seizure threshold by
conversion of drug to phenobarbital,
decreases neuron firing
Uses: Generalized tonic-clonic (grand
mal), complex-partial psychomotor
seizures, essential tremors

DOSAGE AND ROUTES
• *Adult and child >8 yr:* **PO** 100-125
mg at bedtime on days 1, 2, 3; then 100-
125 mg bid on days 4, 5, 6; then 100-125
mg tid on days 7, 8, 9; then maintenance
250 mg tid-qid, max 2 g/day in divided
doses
• *Child <8 yr:* **PO** 50 mg at bedtime on
days 1, 2, 3; then 50 mg bid on days 4, 5,
6; then 100 mg bid on days 7, 8, 9; maintenance 125-250 mg tid or 10-25 mg/kg/
day in divided doses
Available forms: Tabs 50, 250
mg;susp 250 mg/5 ml; chew tabs 125
mg ✦

SIDE EFFECTS
CNS: Stimulation, drowsiness, irritability, psychosis, ataxia, vertigo, fatigue,
emotional disturbances, mood changes,
paranoia
EENT: Diplopia, nystagmus, edema of
eyelids
*GI: Nausea, vomiting, anorexia, hepa-
titis*
GU: Impotence
*HEMA: Thrombocytopenia, leukope-
nia, neutropenia, eosinophilia,*
megaloblastic anemia, decreased
serum folate level, lymphadenopathy
INTEG: Rash, edema, alopecia, lupuslike
syndrome
Contraindications: Pregnancy (D),
hypersensitivity, porphyria
Precautions: COPD, hepatic disease,
renal disease, hyperactive children

PHARMACOKINETICS
PO: Peak 4 hr; excreted by kidneys, in
breast milk; half-life 3-12 hr

INTERACTIONS
Primidone levels are decreased by aceta-
ZOLAMIDE, succinimides, carbamaze-
pine
May decrease effect of oral contracep-
tives, acebutolol, metoprolol, proprano-
lol, tricyclics, phenothiazines
Increase: primidone levels—alcohol,
heparin, CNS depressants, hydantoins,
isoniazid, nicotinamide, phenytoin, phe-
nobarbital
Drug/Herb
Increase: effect—ginkgo
Decrease: effect—ginseng, santonica

NURSING CONSIDERATIONS
Assess:
• For seizures: location, duration, type;
folic acid deficiency; fatigue, weakness,
neuropathy, depression
• Drug level: therapeutic level 5-15
mcg/ml; CBC should be done q6mo
• Mental status: mood, sensorium, af-
fect, memory (long, short)
• Respiratory depression, wheezing
• Blood dyscrasias: fever, sore throat,
bruising, rash, jaundice
Administer:
PO route
• After shaking liquid susp well
• With food for GI upset
• Tablets crushed and mixed with food
or fluid for swallowing difficulties
• Avoid use with CNS depressants
Evaluate:
• Therapeutic response: decreased
seizures

P

Side effects: *italics* = common; ***bold italics*** = life-threatening

Teach patient/family:
• Not to withdraw drug quickly; withdrawal symptoms may occur
• To avoid hazardous activities until stabilized on drug; drowsiness, dizziness may occur
• To carry emergency ID with condition and medication
• To recognize the signs of blood dyscrasias; when to notify prescriber
• To avoid alcohol

---

probenecid (℞)
(proe-ben′e-sid)
Benemid, Benuryl ✦, probenecid
Func. class.: Uricosuric, antigout agent
Chem. class.: Sulfonamide derivative

Action: Inhibits tubular reabsorption of urates, with increased excretion of uric acids

Uses: Hyperuricemia in gout, gouty arthritis, adjunct to cephalosporin, cidofovir, or penicillin treatment

DOSAGE AND ROUTES
Gonorrhea
• *Adult:* **PO** 1 g with 3.5 g ampicillin or 1 g ½ hr before 4.8 million units of aqueous penicillin G procaine injected into 2 sites **IM**
Gout/gouty arthritis
• *Adult:* **PO** 250 mg bid for 1 wk, then 500 mg bid, not to exceed 2 g/day; maintenance: 500 mg/day × 6 mo
Adjunct in penicillin/cephalosporin treatment
• *Adult and child >50 kg:* **PO** 500 mg qid
• *Child <50 kg:* **PO** 25 mg/kg, then 40 mg/kg in divided doses qid
Minimize nephrotoxicity in cidofovir therapy
• *Adult:* **PO** 2 g 3 hr prior to cidofovir dose, followed by 1 g at 2 and 8 hr after end of cidofovir infusion

Renal dose
• Avoid use if CCr <50 ml/min
Available forms: Tabs 0.5 g

SIDE EFFECTS
CNS: Drowsiness, headache
CV: Bradycardia
*GI: Gastric irritation, nausea, vomiting, anorexia, **hepatic necrosis***
GU: Glycosuria, thirst, frequency, ***nephrotic syndrome***
INTEG: Rash, dermatitis, pruritus, fever
META: Acidosis, hypokalemia, hyperchloremia, hyperglycemia
*RESP: **Apnea**,* irregular respirations
Contraindications: Hypersensitivity, severe hepatic disease, severe renal disease, CCr <50 mg/min, history of uric acid calculus
Precautions: Pregnancy (B), child <2 yr

PHARMACOKINETICS
PO: Peak 2-4 hr, duration 8 hr, half-life 5-8 hr; metabolized by liver; excreted in urine

INTERACTIONS
Increase: effect of acyclovir, barbiturates, allopurinol, benzodiazepines, dyphylline, zidovudine
Increase: toxicity—sulfa drugs, dapsone, clofibrate, indomethacin, rifampin, naproxen, methotrexate
Decrease: action of probenecid—salicylates
Drug/Lab Test
Increase: BSP/urinary PSP, theophylline levels
False positive: Urine glucose with copper sulfate test (Clinitest)

NURSING CONSIDERATIONS
Assess:
• Uric acid levels (3-7 mg/dl); mobility, joint pain, swelling
• Respiratory rate, rhythm, depth; notify prescriber of abnormalities
• Electrolytes, CO_2 before, during treatment

⚠ Safety alert   *"Tall Man" lettering

• Urine pH, output, glucose during beginning treatment

A For CNS symptoms: confusion, twitching, hyperreflexia, stimulation, headache; may indicate overdose

Administer:
• After meals or with milk if GI symptoms occur
• Increase fluid intake to 2-3 L/day to prevent urinary calculi

Evaluate:
• Therapeutic response: absence of pain, stiffness in joints

Teach patient/family:
• To avoid OTC preparations (aspirin) unless directed by prescriber; increase water intake, avoid alcohol, caffeine

---

procainamide (℞)

(proe-kane-ah′mide)
procainamide, Procanbid,
Promine, Pronestyl,
Pronestyl-SR

Func. class.: Antidysrhythmic (Class IA)

Chem. class.: Procaine HCl amide analog

Action: Depresses excitability of cardiac muscle to electrical stimulation and slows conduction in atrium, bundle of His, and ventricle increases refractory period

Uses: Life-threatening ventricular dysrhythmias

DOSAGE AND ROUTES

Atrial fibrillation/PAT
• *Adult:* **PO** 1-1.25 g; may give another 750 mg if needed; if no response, 500 mg-1 g q2h until desired response; maintenance 50 mg/kg in divided doses q6h

Ventricular tachycardia
• *Adult:* **PO** 1 g; maintenance 50 mg/kg/day given in 3-hr intervals; **SUS REL** 500 mg-1.25 g q6h

Other dysrhythmias
• *Adult:* **IV BOL** 100 mg q5min, given

25-50 mg/min, not to exceed 500 mg; or 17 mg/kg total then **IV INF** 2-6 mg/min

Renal dose
• *Adult:* **IV** CCr 10-50 ml/min give q6-12h; CCr <10 ml/min give q8-24h

Available forms: Caps 250, 375, 500 mg; tabs 250, 375, 500 mg; tabs sus rel 500, 750, 1000 mg; inj 100, 500 mg/ml

SIDE EFFECTS

CNS: Headache, dizziness, confusion, psychosis, restlessness, irritability, weakness

CV: Hypotension, **heart block, cardiovascular collapse, arrest**

GI: Nausea, vomiting, anorexia, diarrhea, hepatomegaly, pain, bitter taste

HEMA: SLE syndrome, **agranulocytosis, thrombocytopenia, neutropenia, hemolytic anemia**

INTEG: Rash, urticaria, edema, swelling (rare), pruritus, flushing

Contraindications: Hypersensitivity, severe heart block, lupus erythematosus, torsades de pointes

Precautions: Pregnancy (C), lactation, children, renal disease, hepatic disease, CHF, respiratory depression, cytopenia, bone marrow failure, dysrhythmia associated with digitalis toxicity, myasthenia gravis, digoxin toxicity

PHARMACOKINETICS

PO: Peak 1-2 hr, duration 3 hr (8 hr extended)
IM: Peak 10-60 min, duration 3 hr; half-life 3 hr
Metabolized in liver to active metabolites, excreted unchanged by kidneys (60%)

INTERACTIONS

Increase: effects of neuromuscular blockers
Increase: procainamide effects—cimetidine, quinidine, trimethoprim, β-blockers, ranitidine
Increase: toxicity—other antidysrhythmics, thioridazine, quinolones

Drug/Herb

Increase: anticholinergic effect—henbane

Increase: toxicity, death—aconite

Increase: effect—aloe, broom, chronic buckthorn use, cascara sagrada (chronic use), Chinese rhubarb, figwort, fumitory, goldenseal, kudzu, licorice

Increase: serotonin effect—horehound

Decrease: effect—coltsfoot

Drug/Lab Test

Increase: ALT, AST, alk phosphatase, LDH, bilirubin

NURSING CONSIDERATIONS

Assess:

⚠ ECG continuously if using IV to determine increased PR or QRS segments; discontinue immediately; watch for increased ventricular ectopic beats, maximum need to rebolus

• Blood levels, 3-10 mcg/ml or NAPA levels 10-20 mcg/ml

⚠ CBC q2wk × 3 mo; leukocyte, neutrophil, platelet counts may be decreased, treatment may need to be discontinued

• I&O ratio; electrolytes (K, Na, Cl), weigh weekly, report gain >2 lb

⚠ Toxicity: confusion, drowsiness, nausea, vomiting, tachydysrhythmias, oliguria

• ANA titer, during long-term treatment, watch for lupuslike symptoms

• Cardiac rate, rhythm, character, B/P continuously for fluctuations

• Respiratory status: rate, rhythm, character, lung fields; bilateral crackles may occur in CHF patient; watch for respiratory depression

⚠ CNS effects: dizziness, confusion, psychosis, paresthesias, seizures; drug should be discontinued

Administer:

PO route

• Do not break, crush, or chew sus rel tabs

IM route

• IM inj in deltoid; aspirate to avoid intravascular administration

IV route

• After diluting 100 mg/ml of D_5W or sterile H_2O for inj; give 20 mg or less/1 min; may dilute 1 g/250-500 ml D_5W, run at 2-6 mg/min

• Check IV site q8h for infiltration or extravasation

Additive compatibilities: Amiodarone, atracurium, DOBUTamine, flumazenil, lidocaine, netilmicin, verapamil

Solution compatibilities: D_5W, D_5/0.9% NaCl, 0.45% NaCl, 0.9% NaCl, water for inj

Y-site compatibilities: Amiodarone, cisatracurium, famotidine, heparin, hydrocortisone, potassium chloride, ranitidine, remifentanil, vit B/C

Evaluate:

• Therapeutic response: decreased dysrhythmias

Teach patient/family:

• That wax matrix may appear in stools

• Not to discontinue without health-care provider's advice

⚠ To notify prescriber immediately if lupuslike symptoms appear (joint pain, butterfly rash, fever, chills, dyspnea)

⚠ To notify prescriber of leukopenia (sore mouth, gums, throat) or thrombocytopenia (bleeding, bruising)

• How to take pulse and when to report to prescriber

Treatment of overdose: O_2 artificial ventilation, ECG, administer DOPamine for circulatory depression, diazepam or thiopental for convulsions, isoproterenol

---

procaine (Rx)

(proe'kane)

Novocain, Unicaine

Func. class.: Local anesthetic

Chem. class.: Ester

Action: Competes with calcium for sites in nerve membrane that control sodium transport across cell membrane; decreases rise of depolarization phase of action potential

Uses: Spinal anesthesia, epidural, peripheral nerve block, perineum, lower extremities, infiltration

---

DOSAGE AND ROUTES

Spinal anesthesia
• *Adult:* 100 mg
Perineum anesthesia
• *Adult:* 50 mg
Available forms: Inj 1%, 2%, 10%

SIDE EFFECTS

CNS: Anxiety, restlessness, **convulsions, loss of consciousness,** drowsiness, disorientation, tremors, shivering
CV: **Myocardial depression, cardiac arrest, dysrhythmias,** bradycardia, hypotension, hypertension, fetal bradycardia
EENT: Blurred vision, tinnitus, pupil constriction
GI: Nausea, vomiting
INTEG: Rash, urticaria, allergic reactions, edema, burning, skin discoloration at inj site, tissue necrosis
RESP: **Status asthmaticus, respiratory arrest, anaphylaxis**
Contraindications: Hypersensitivity, sulfite allergy, myasthenia gravis, child <12 yr, severe hepatic disease
Precautions: Pregnancy (C), elderly, severe drug allergies

PHARMACOKINETICS

Onset 2-5 min, duration 1 hr; metabolized by liver, excreted in urine (metabolites)

INTERACTIONS

Dysrhythmias: epINEPHrine, halothane, enflurane
Hypertension: MAOIs, tricyclics, phenothiazines
Decrease: action of aminosalicylic acid, sulfonamides
Decrease: action of procaine—chloroprocaine

NURSING CONSIDERATIONS

Assess:
• B/P, pulse, respiration during treatment
• Fetal heart tones if drug is used during labor

• Allergic reactions: rash, urticaria, itching
• Cardiac status: ECG for dysrhythmias, pulse, B/P during anesthesia
Administer:
• Only drugs that are not cloudy, do not contain precipitate
• Only with crash cart, resuscitative equipment nearby
• Only drugs without preservatives for epidural or caudal anesthesia
Additive compatibilities: Ascorbic acid, hydrocortisone, penicillin G, penicillin G sodium, vit B/C
Syringe compatibilities: Ampicillin, cloxacillin, glycopyrrolate, hydroxyzine, gentamicin
Solution compatibilities: D_5, D_{10}, NS, LR, Y_2, NS
Perform/provide:
• Use of new sol; discard unused portions, protect from light
Evaluate:
• Therapeutic response: anesthesia necessary for procedure
Treatment of overdose: Airway, O_2, vasopressor, IV fluids, anticonvulsants for seizures

---

procarbazine (℞)
(proe-kar′ba-zeen)
Matulane, Natulan ✦
Func. class.: Antineoplastic, alkylating agent
Chem. class.: Hydrazine derivative

Action: Inhibits DNA, RNA, protein synthesis; has multiple sites of action; a nonvesicant
Uses: Lymphoma, Hodgkin's disease, cancers resistant to other therapy
Investigational uses: Brain, lung malignancies, other lymphomas, multiple myeloma, malignant melanoma, polycythemia vera

DOSAGE AND ROUTES

• *Adult:* **PO** 2-4 mg/kg/day for first wk; maintain dosage of 4-6 mg/kg/day until

platelets and WBC fall; after recovery, 1-2 mg/kg/day
• *Child:* **PO** 50 mg/m^2/day for 7 days, then 100 mg/m^2 until desired response, leukopenia, or thrombocytopenia occurs; 50 mg/day is maintenance after bone marrow recovery
Available forms: Caps 50 mg

SIDE EFFECTS

CNS: Headache, dizziness, insomnia, hallucinations, confusion, ***coma***, pain, chills, fever, sweating, paresthesias, ***seizures***
EENT: Retinal hemorrhage, nystagmus, photophobia, diplopia
GI: Nausea, vomiting, anorexia, diarrhea, constipation, dry mouth, stomatitis
GU: Azoospermia, cessation of menses
HEMA: ***Thrombocytopenia, anemia, leukopenia, myelosuppression, bleeding tendencies,*** purpura, petechiae, epistaxis
INTEG: Rash, pruritus, dermatitis, alopecia, herpes, hyperpigmentation
MS: Arthralgias, myalgias
RESP: Cough, pneumonitis
Contraindications: Pregnancy (D), hypersensitivity, thrombocytopenia, bone marrow depression, lactation
Precautions: Renal disease, hepatic disease, radiation therapy

PHARMACOKINETICS

Half-life 1 hr; concentrates in liver, kidney, skin; metabolized in liver, excreted in urine

INTERACTIONS

Hypotension: meperidine, do not use together
Disulfiram-like reaction: alcohol, MAOIs, tricyclics, tyramine foods, sympathomimetic drugs
Hypertension: guanethidine, levodopa, methyldopa, reserpine, caffeine
Life-threatening hypertension: sympathomimetics
Increase: hypoglycemia—insulin, oral hypoglycemics

Increase: CNS depression—barbiturates, antihistamines, opioids, hypotensive agents, phenothiazines
Drug/Food
Hypertensive crisis: tyramine foods

NURSING CONSIDERATIONS

Assess:
• CBC, differential, platelet count qwk; withhold drug if WBC is <4000/mm^3 or platelet count is <100,000/mm^3; notify prescriber
• Renal studies: BUN, serum uric acid, urine CCr, electrolytes before, during therapy
• I&O ratio, report fall in urine output to <30 ml/hr
• Monitor temp q4h; fever may indicate beginning infection
• Hepatic studies before, during therapy: bilirubin, AST, ALT, alk phosphatase prn or qmo
• CNS changes: confusion, paresthesias, neuropathies, drug should be discontinued
⚠ For tyramine foods in diet, hypertensive crisis can occur
⚠ Toxicity: facial flushing, epistaxis, increased PT, thrombocytopenia; drug should be discontinued
• Bleeding: hematuria, guaiac stools, bruising or petechiae, mucosa or orifices q8h
• Effects of alopecia on body image; discuss feelings about body changes
• Jaundiced skin, sclera; dark urine, clay-colored stools, itchy skin, abdominal pain, fever, diarrhea
• Buccal cavity q8h for dryness, sores or ulceration, white patches, oral pain, bleeding, dysphagia
• Alkalosis if vomiting is severe
• GI symptoms: frequency of stools, cramping
• Acidosis, signs of dehydration: rapid respirations, poor skin turgor, decreased urine output, dry skin, restlessness, weakness
Administer:
• In divided doses and at bedtime to minimize nausea and vomiting

---

⚠ Safety alert   *"Tall Man" lettering

• Nonphenothiazine antiemetic 30-60 min before giving drug and 4-10 hr after treatment to prevent vomiting
• Transfusion for anemia
• Antispasmodic for GI symptoms
Perform/provide:
• Liquid diet: carbonated beverages; gelatin may be added if patient is not nauseated or vomiting
• Storage in tight, light-resistant container in cool environment
Evaluate:
• Therapeutic response: decreased tumor size, spread of malignancy
Teach patient/family:
• To report any complaints, side effects to nurse or prescriber; cough, shortness of breath, fever, chills, sore throat, bleeding, bruising, vomiting blood; black, tarry stools
• That hair may be lost during treatment and wig or hairpiece may make patient feel better; tell patient that new hair may be different in color, texture
• To avoid sunlight or UV exposure, wear sunscreen or protective clothing
• To avoid foods with citric acid, hot, or rough texture
• To report any bleeding, white spots, ulcerations in mouth to prescriber; tell patient to examine mouth daily
• To avoid driving, activities requiring alertness; dizziness may occur
• To use effective contraception, avoid breast-feeding
• To avoid ingestion of alcohol, caffeine, tyramine-containing foods; cold, hay fever, weight-reducing products may cause serious drug interactions
• To avoid crowds, persons with infections if granulocytes are low

prochlorperazine (R)
(proe-klor-pair'a-zeen)
Chlorpazine, Compa-Z, Compazine, Contranzine, Pro-vacin ✤, Stemetil ✤, Ultrazine
Func. class.: Antiemetic, antipsychotic
Chem. class.: Phenothiazine, piperazine derivative

Do not confuse:
Compazine/Coumadin
prochlorperazine/ chlorproMAZINE
Action: Acts centrally by blocking chemoreceptor trigger zone, which in turn acts on vomiting center
Uses: Nausea, vomiting, psychotic disorders

DOSAGE AND ROUTES
Postoperative nausea/vomiting
• *Adult:* **IM** 5-10 mg 1-2 hr before anesthesia; may repeat in 30 min; **IV** 5-10 mg 15-30 min before anesthesia; **IV INF** 20 mg/L D$_5$W or **NS** 15-30 min before anesthesia, not to exceed 40 mg/day
Severe nausea/vomiting
• *Adult:* **PO** 5-10 mg tid-qid; **SUS REL** 15 mg daily in AM or 10 mg q12h; **RECT** 25 mg/bid; **IM** 5-10 mg; may repeat q4h, not to exceed 40 mg/day
• *Child 18-39 kg:* **PO** 2.5 mg tid or 5 mg bid, not to exceed 15 mg/day; **IM** 0.132 mg/kg
• *Child 14-17 kg:* **PO/RECT** 2.5 mg bid-tid, not to exceed 10 mg/day; **IM** 0.132 mg/kg
• *Child 9-13 kg:* **PO/RECT** 2.5 mg daily-bid, not to exceed 7.5 mg/day; **IM** 0.132 mg/kg
Antipsychotic
• *Adult and child ≥12 yr:* **PO** 5-10 mg tid-qid; may increase q2-3d, max 150 mg/day; **IM** 10-20 mg q2-4h up to 4 doses, then 10-20 mg q4-6h, max 200 mg/day; **RECT** 10 mg tid-qid, may increase by 5-10 mg q2-3d as needed

Child 2-12 yr: PO 2.5 mg bid-tid; **IM** 0.132 mg/kg

Antianxiety

• *Adult and child ≥12 yr:* 5 mg tid-qid, max 20 mg/day or >12 wk; **IM** 5-10 mg q3-4h, max 40 mg/day; **IV** 2.5-10 mg; max 40 mg/day

• *Child 2-12 yr:* **IM** 132 mcg/kg

Available forms: Syr 5 mg/ml; inj 5 mg/ml; tabs 5, 10, 25 mg; caps, sus rel 10, 15 mg; supp 2.5, 5, 25 mg

SIDE EFFECTS

CNS: **Neuroleptic malignant syndrome,** *extrapyramidal reactions, tardive dyskinesia, euphoria,* **depression,** drowsiness, restlessness, tremor, dizziness

CV: **Circulatory failure, tachycardia**

EENT: Blurred vision

GI: Nausea, vomiting, anorexia, dry mouth, diarrhea, constipation, weight loss, metallic taste, cramps

HEMA: **Agranulocytosis**

RESP: **Respiratory depression**

Contraindications: Hypersensitivity to phenothiazines, coma, seizure, encephalopathy, bone marrow depression, narrow-angle glaucoma

Precautions: Pregnancy (C), children <2 yr, elderly, lactation

PHARMACOKINETICS

PO: Onset 30-40 min, duration 3-4 hr

SUS REL: Onset 30-40 min, duration 10-12 hr

RECT: Onset 60 min, duration 3-4 hr

IM: Onset 10-20 min, duration 12 hr

Metabolized by liver; excreted in urine, breast milk; crosses placenta

INTERACTIONS

Increase: anticholinergic action—anticholinergics, antiparkinson drugs, antidepressants

Decrease: prochlorperazine effect—barbiturates, antacids

Drug/Herb

Increase: CNS depression—chamomile, cola nut, hops, kava, nettle, nutmeg, skullcap, valerian

Increase: anticholinergic effect—henbane, jimsonweed, scopolia

Increase: EPS—betel palm, kava

Drug/Lab Test

Increase: LFTs, cardiac enzymes, cholesterol, blood glucose, prolactin, bilirubin, PBI, ^{131}I, alk phosphatase, leukocytes, granulocytes, platelets

Decrease: Hormones (blood and urine)

False-positive: Pregnancy tests, urine bilirubin

False-negative: Urinary steroids, 17-OHCS, pregnancy tests

NURSING CONSIDERATIONS

Assess:

• EPS: abnormal movement, tardive dyskinesia, akathisia

• VS, B/P; check patients with cardiac disease more often

⚠ For neuroleptic malignant syndrome: seizures, hyper/hypotension, fever, tachycardia, dyspnea, fatigue, muscle stiffness, loss of bladder control; notify prescriber immediately

⚠ CBC, LFTs during course of treatment, blood dyscrasias, hepatotoxicity may occur

• Respiratory status before, during, after administration of emetic; check rate, rhythm, character; respiratory depression can occur rapidly with elderly or debilitated patients

Administer:

• Avoid other CNS depressants

IM route

• IM inj in large muscle mass; aspirate to avoid IV administration

• Keep patient recumbent for ½ hr

IV route

• IV after diluting 5 mg/9 ml of NaCl for inj (0.5 mg/ml); give 5 mg or less/min; may dilute 10-20 mg/L NaCl and give as infusion; can cause contact dermatitis

Additive compatibilities: Amikacin, ascorbic acid, dexamethasone, dimenhy-DRINATE, erythromycin, ethacrynate, lidocaine, nafcillin, sodium bicarbonate, vit B/C

Syringe compatibilities: Atropine, butorphanol, chlorproMAZINE, cimetidine, diamorphine, diphenhydrAMINE, droperidol, fentanyl, glycopyrrolate, hydrOXYzine, meperidine, metoclopramide, nalbuphine, pentazocine, perphenazine, promazine, promethazine, ranitidine, scopolamine, sufentanil

Y-site compatibilities: Amsacrine, calcium gluconate, cisatracurium, cisplatin, cladribine, cyclophosphamide, cytarabine, DOXOrubicin, DOXOrubicin liposome, fluconazole, granisetron, heparin, hydrocortisone, melphalan, methotrexate, ondansetron, paclitaxel, potassium chloride, propofol, remifentanil, sargramostim, sufentanil, teniposide, thiotepa, vinorelbine, vit B/C

Evaluate:

• Therapeutic response: absence of nausea, vomiting; reduced anxiety, agitation, excitability

Teach patient/family:

• To avoid hazardous activities, activities requiring alertness; dizziness may occur

• To avoid alcohol

• Not to double or skip doses

• That urine may be pink to reddish brown

• To report dark urine, clay-colored stools, bleeding, bruising, rash, blurred vision

• To avoid sun or wear sunscreen, protective clothing

---

progesterone (℞)

(proe-jess′ter-one)

Crinone, progesterone, Prochieve, Prometrium

Func. class.: Progestogen

Chem. class.: Progesterone derivative

Action: Inhibits secretion of pituitary gonadotropins, which prevents follicular maturation, ovulation; stimulates growth of mammary tissue; antineoplastic action against endometrial cancer

Uses: Contraception, amenorrhea, premenstrual syndrome, abnormal uterine bleeding, endometrial hyperplasia prevention, assisted reproductive technology (ART) gel

DOSAGE AND ROUTES

Infertility

• *Adult:* **VAG** 90 mg daily

Amenorrhea/functional uterine bleeding

• *Adult:* **IM** 5-10 mg daily × 6-8 doses

Endometrial hyperplasia prevention

• *Adult:* **PO** 200 mg/day × 12 days

ART

• *Adult:* **GEL** 90 mg (8%) vaginally daily, for supplementation; 90 mg (8%) vaginally bid for replacement; if pregnancy occurs continue × 10-12 wk

Available forms: Inj 50 mg/ml; vag gel 4%, 8%; caps 100, 200 mg

SIDE EFFECTS

CNS: Dizziness, headache, migraines, depression, fatigue

CV: Hypotension, ***thrombophlebitis***, edema, ***thromboembolism, stroke, pulmonary embolism, MI***

EENT: Diplopia, retinal thrombosis

GI: Nausea, vomiting, anorexia, cramps, increased weight, ***cholestatic jaundice***

GU: Amenorrhea, cervical erosion, breakthrough bleeding, dysmenorrhea, vaginal candidiasis, breast changes, *gynecomastia, testicular atrophy, impotence*, endometriosis, ***spontaneous abortion***

INTEG: Rash, urticaria, acne, hirsutism, alopecia, oily skin, seborrhea, purpura, melasma

META: Hyperglycemia

SYST: ***Angioedema, anaphylaxis***

Contraindications: Pregnancy (D), breast cancer, hypersensitivity, thromboembolic disorders, reproductive cancer, genital bleeding (abnormal, undiagnosed), cerebral hemorrhage

Precautions: Lactation, hypertension, asthma, blood dyscrasias, gallbladder disease, CHF, diabetes mellitus, bone

P

Side effects: *italics* = common; ***bold italics*** = life-threatening

disease, depression, migraine headache, convulsive disorders, hepatic disease, renal disease, family history of breast or reproductive tract cancer

PHARMACOKINETICS

IM, RECT, VAG: Duration 24 hr
Excreted in urine, feces; metabolized in liver

Interactions:
Decrease: progesterone effect—barbiturates, phenytoin
Drug/Herb
Increase: hormonal effect—alfalfa
Drug/Lab Test
Increase: Alk phosphatase, nitrogen (urine), pregnanediol, amino acids, factors VII, VIII, IX, X
Decrease: GTT, HDL

NURSING CONSIDERATIONS

Assess:
• Weight daily; notify prescriber of weekly weight gain >5 lb
• B/P at beginning of treatment and periodically
• I&O ratio; be alert for decreasing urinary output, increasing edema
• Hepatic studies: ALT, AST, bilirubin periodically during long-term therapy
• Edema, hypertension, cardiac symptoms, jaundice, thromboembolism
• Mental status: affect, mood, behavioral changes, depression
• Hypercalcemia
Administer:
• Do not break, crush, or chew caps
• Titrated dose; use lowest effective dose
• After warming to dissolve crystals
• In one dose in AM
• With food or milk to decrease GI symptoms
Perform/provide:
• Storage in dark area
Evaluate:
• Therapeutic response: decreased abnormal uterine bleeding, absence of amenorrhea

Teach patient/family:
⚠ To report breast lumps, vaginal bleeding, edema, jaundice, dark urine, clay-colored stools, dyspnea, headache, blurred vision, abdominal pain, numbness or stiffness in legs, chest pain
• To report suspected pregnancy
• To monitor blood glucose if diabetic

---

promethazine (℞)

(proe-meth′a-zeen)
Histanil ✦, Phenadoz, Phenergan, promethazine HCl
Func. class.: Antihistamine, H_1-receptor antagonist
Chem. class.: Phenothiazine derivative

Do not confuse:
Phenergan/Theragran
Action: Acts on blood vessels, GI, respiratory system by competing with histamine for H_1-receptor site; decreases allergic response by blocking histamine
Uses: Motion sickness, rhinitis, allergy symptoms, sedation, nausea, preoperative and postoperative sedation

DOSAGE AND ROUTES

Nausea
• *Adult:* **PO/IM/IV/REC** 12.5-25 mg; q4-6h prn
• *Child >2 yr:* **PO/IM/IV/REC** 0.25-0.5 mg/kg q4-6h prn
Motion sickness
• *Adult:* **PO** 25 mg bid, give ½-1 hr before departure and q8-12h prn
• *Child >2 yr:* **PO/IM/RECT** 12.5-25 mg bid, give ½-1 hr before departure and q8-12h prn
Allergy/rhinitis
• *Adult:* **PO** 12.5 mg qid, or 25 mg at bedtime
• *Child >2 yr:* **PO** 6.25-12.5 mg tid or 25 mg at bedtime
Sedation
• *Adult:* **PO/IM** 25-50 mg at bedtime
• *Child >2 yr:* **PO/IM/RECT** 12.5-25 mg at bedtime

Sedation (preoperative/postoperative)
- *Adult:* **PO/IM/IV** 25-50 mg
- *Child >2 yr:* **PO/IM/IV** 0.5-1.1 mg/kg

Available forms: Tabs 12.5, 25, 50 mg; supp 12.5, 25 mg; inj 25, 50 mg/ml, syr 6.25 mg/5 ml

SIDE EFFECTS

CNS: Dizziness, drowsiness, poor coordination, fatigue, anxiety, euphoria, confusion, paresthesia, neuritis, EPS, *neuroleptic malignant syndrome*
CV: Hypotension, palpitations, tachycardia
EENT: Blurred vision, dilated pupils, tinnitus, nasal stuffiness; dry nose, throat, mouth; photosensitivity
GI: Constipation, dry mouth, nausea, vomiting, anorexia, diarrhea
GU: Urinary retention, dysuria, frequency
HEMA: Thrombocytopenia, agranulocytosis, hemolytic anemia
INTEG: Rash, urticaria, photosensitivity
RESP: Increased thick secretions, wheezing, chest tightness, *apnea in neonates, infants, young children*

Contraindications: Hypersensitivity to H_1-receptor antagonist, acute asthma attack, lower respiratory tract disease; sulfite allergy, child <2 yr
Precautions: Pregnancy (C), increased intraocular pressure, renal disease, cardiac disease, hypertension, bronchial asthma, seizure disorder, stenosed peptic ulcers, hyperthyroidism, prostatic hypertrophy, bladder neck obstruction

PHARMACOKINETICS

PO: Onset 20 min, duration 4-12 hr
IV: Onset 3-5 min
Metabolized in liver; excreted by kidneys, GI tract (inactive metabolites)

INTERACTIONS

Increase: CNS depression—barbiturates, opioids, hypnotics, tricyclics, alcohol
Increase: promethazine effect—MAOIs
Decrease: oral anticoagulants effect—heparin
Drug/Herb
Increase: anticholinergic effect—henbane, jimsonweed, scopolia
Drug/Lab Test
False negative: Skin allergy test
False positive: Urine pregnancy test

NURSING CONSIDERATIONS

Assess:
- I&O ratio; be alert for urinary retention, frequency, dysuria; drug should be discontinued
- **A** CBC during long-term therapy; blood dyscrasias may occur
- Respiratory status: rate, rhythm, increase in bronchial secretions, wheezing, chest tightness
- Cardiac status: palpitations, increased pulse, hypotension

Administer:
- Avoid use with other CNS depressants
PO route
- With meals for GI symptoms; absorption may slightly decrease
- When used for motion sickness, 30 min-1 hr before travel
IM route
- IM inj deep in large muscle; rotate site
IV route
- After diluting each 25-50 mg/9 ml of NaCl for inj; give 25 mg or less/2 min

Additive compatibilities: Amikacin, ascorbic acid, chloroquine, hydromorphone, netilmicin, vit B/C
Syringe compatibilities: Atropine, butorphanol, chlorproMAZINE, cimetidine, dimenhyDRAMINE, droperidol, fentanyl, glycopyrrolate, hydromorphone, hydrOXYzine, meperidine, metoclopramide, midazolam, pentazocine, perphenazine, prochlorperazine, promazine, ranitidine, scopolamine
Y-site compatibilities: Amifostine, amsacrine, aztreonam, ciprofloxacin, cisatracurium, cisplatin, cladribine, cyclophosphamide, cytarabine, DOXOrubicin, filgrastim, fluconazole, fludarabine, granisetron, melphalan, on-

P

---

dansetron, remifentanil, sargramostim, teniposide, thiotepa, vinorelbine

Perform/provide:

- Hard candy, gum, frequent rinsing of mouth for dryness
- Storage in tight, light-resistant container

Evaluate:

- Therapeutic response: absence of running, congested nose, rashes, absence of motion sickness, nausea; sedation

Teach patient/family:

- That drug may cause photosensitivity; to avoid prolonged sunlight
- To notify prescriber of confusion, sedation, hypotension
- To avoid driving, other hazardous activity if drowsy
- To avoid concurrent use of alcohol

---

propafenone (Ŗ)

(pro-paff'e-nown)
Rythmol, Rythmol SR
Func. class.: Antidysrhythmic (Class IC)

Action: Slows conduction velocity; reduces membrane responsiveness; inhibits automaticity; increases ratio of effective refractory period to action potential duration; β-blocking activity

Uses: Life-threatening dysrhythmias, sustained ventricular tachycardia

DOSAGE AND ROUTES

- *Adult:* **PO** 150 mg q8h; allow a 3-4 day interval before increasing dose, max 900 mg/day; **SR** 225 mg q12h, may increase q5d, max 425 mg q12h

Available forms: Tabs 150, 225, 300 mg; caps, sus rel 225, 325, 425 mg

SIDE EFFECTS

CNS: Headache, dizziness, abnormal dreams, syncope, confusion, ***seizures***
CV: ***Supraventricular dysrhythmia, ventricular dysrhythmia, bradycardia,*** prodysrhythmia, palpitations, AV block, intraventricular conduction delay,

AV dissociation, hypotension, chest pain
EENT: Blurred vision, altered taste, tinnitus
GI: Nausea, vomiting, constipation, dyspepsia, cholestasis, ***hepatitis,*** abnormal hepatic studies, dry mouth
HEMA: ***Leukopenia, agranulocytosis, granulocytopenia, thrombocytopenia,*** anemia, bruising
INTEG: Rash
RESP: Dyspnea

Contraindications: 2nd-, 3rd-degree AV block, right bundle branch block, cardiogenic shock, hypersensitivity, bradycardia, uncontrolled CHF, sick-sinus syndrome, marked hypotension, bronchospastic disorders

Precautions: Pregnancy (C), CHF, hypokalemia, hyperkalemia, recent MI, nonallergic bronchospasm, lactation, children, hepatic or renal disease, elderly

PHARMACOKINETICS

Peak 3-5 hr, half-life 2-10 hr; metabolized in liver; excreted in urine (metabolite)

INTERACTIONS

Increase: anticoagulation—warfarin
Increase: CNS effects—local anesthetics
Increase: digoxin level—digoxin
Increase: β-blocker effect—propranolol, metoprolol
Increase: cycloSPORINE levels—cycloSPORINE
Decrease: propafenone effect—rifampin, cimetidine, quinidine
Drug/Herb
Hypokalemia, increased antidysrhythmic action: aloe, buckthorn, cascara sagrada, senna pod/leaf
Increase: toxicity, death—aconite
Increase: effect—aloe, broom, chronic buckthorn use, cascara sagrada (chronic use), Chinese rhubarb, figwort, fumitory, goldenseal, kudzu, licorice
Increase: serotonin effect—horehound
Decrease: effect—coltsfoot

Drug/Lab Test
Increase: CPK

NURSING CONSIDERATIONS

Assess:

• GI status: bowel pattern, number of stools

⚠ Cardiac status: rate, rhythm, quality; ECG or Holter monitor prior to and during therapy; watch for PR, QT prolongation

• Chest x-ray film, pulmonary function test during treatment

• I&O ratio; check for decreasing output; daily weight

• B/P for fluctuations

• Lung fields; bilateral crackles, dyspnea, peripheral edema, weight gain, jugular venous distention may occur in CHF patient

⚠ Toxicity: fine tremors, dizziness, hypotension, drowsiness, abnormal heart rate

• Cardiac function: respiratory rate, rhythm, character continuously

Administer:

• Do not break, crush, chew, or divide contents of SR cap

• SR cap can be taken without regard to food

Evaluate:

• Therapeutic response: absence of dysrhythmias

Teach patient/family:

• To avoid hazardous activities until response is known

• To report fever, chills, sore throat, bleeding, shortness of breath, chest pain, palpitations, blurred vision

• Take reg tab with food, sus rel without regard to food

• To carry emergency ID identifying medication and prescriber

Treatment of overdose: O₂, artificial ventilation, defibrillation ECG; administer DOPamine for circulatory depression, diazepam or thiopental for convulsions, isoproterenol

propantheline (℞)
(proe-pan'the-leen)
Pro-Banthine, Propanthel ✦,
Func. class.: GI anticholinergic, antiulcer agent
Chem. class.: Synthetic quaternary ammonium compound

Action: Inhibits muscarinic actions of acetylcholine at postganglionic parasympathetic neuroeffector sites

Uses: Treatment of urinary incontinence, peptic ulcer disease, irritable bowel syndrome, duodenography

Investigational uses: Antispasmodic uses

DOSAGE AND ROUTES

• *Adult:* **PO** 15 mg tid ac, 30 mg at bedtime

• *Elderly, small patients:* **PO** 7.5 mg tid ac

• *Child:* 0.375 mg/kg (10 mg/m²) qid

Available forms: Tabs 7.5, 15 mg

SIDE EFFECTS

CNS: Confusion, stimulation in elderly, headache, insomnia, dizziness, drowsiness, anxiety, weakness, hallucinations

CV: Palpitations, tachycardia, orthostatic hypotension (elderly)

EENT: Blurred vision, photophobia, mydriasis, cycloplegia, increased ocular tension

*GI: Dry mouth, constipation, **paralytic ileus,*** heartburn, nausea, vomiting, dysphagia, absence of taste

GU: Urinary hesitancy, retention, impotence

INTEG: Urticaria, rash, pruritus, anhidrosis, fever, allergic reactions

Contraindications: Hypersensitivity to anticholinergics, narrow-angle glaucoma, GI obstruction, myasthenia gravis, paralytic ileus, GI atony, toxic megacolon

Precautions: Pregnancy (C), hyperthyroidism, coronary artery disease, dysrhythmias, CHF, ulcerative colitis, hyper-

P

tension, hiatal hernia, hepatic disease, renal disease, urinary retention, prostatic hypertrophy, elderly

PHARMACOKINETICS

PO: Onset 30-45 min, duration 6 hr; metabolized by liver, GI system; excreted in urine, bile

INTERACTIONS

Increase: anticholinergic effect—amantadine, tricyclics, MAOIs, H_1-antihistamines
Decrease: effect of phenothiazines, levodopa, ketoconazole
Drug/Herb
Increase: anticholinergic effect—henbane, jimsonweed, scopolia

NURSING CONSIDERATIONS
Assess:
• VS, cardiac status: checking for dysrhythmias, increased rate, palpitations
• I&O ratio; check for urinary retention or hesitancy
• GI complaints: pain, bleeding (frank or occult), nausea, vomiting, anorexia
Administer:
• ½-1 hr ac for better absorption
• Decreased dose to elderly patients; metabolism may be slowed
• Gum, hard candy, frequent rinsing for dry mouth
• Avoid use with other CNS depressants
Perform/provide:
• Storage in tight container protected from light
• Increased fluids, bulk, exercise to decrease constipation
Evaluate:
• Therapeutic response: absence of epigastric pain, bleeding, nausea, vomiting
Teach patient/family:
• To avoid driving, other hazardous activities until stabilized on medication; may cause blurred vision; to use caution when standing due to orthostatic hypotension

• To avoid alcohol; will enhance sedating properties of this drug
• To drink plenty of fluids
• To report dysphagia

---

proparacaine ophthalmic
See Appendix C

⚠ High Alert

propofol (℞)
(pro'poh-fole)
Diprivan, Disoprofol
Func. class.: General anesthetic

Action: Produces dose-dependent CNS depression; action is unknown
Uses: Induction or maintenance of anesthesia as part of balanced anesthetic technique; sedation in mechanically ventilated patients

DOSAGE AND ROUTES
Induction
• *Adult:* IV 2-2.5 mg/kg, approximately 40 mg q10sec until induction onset
• *Child 3-16 yr:* IV 2.5-3.5 mg/kg over 20-30 sec
• *Elderly:* IV 1-1.5 mg/kg, approximately 20 mg q10sec until induction onset
Maintenance
• *Adult:* IV 0.1-0.2 mg/kg/min (6-12 mg/kg/hr)
• *Child ≥3 yr:* IV 0.125-0.3 mg/kg/min (7.5-18 mg/kg/hr)
• *Elderly:* IV 0.05-0.1 mg/kg/min (3-6 mg/kg/hr)
ICU sedation
• *Adult:* IV 5 mcg/kg/min over 5 min; may give 5-10 mcg/kg/min over 5-10 min until desired response
Available forms: Inj 10 mg/ml in 20 ml ampule, 50 ml and 100 ml vials

SIDE EFFECTS
CNS: Involuntary movement, headache, jerking, fever, dizziness, shivering,

---

⚠ Safety alert   *"Tall Man" lettering

tremor, confusion, somnolence, paresthesia, agitation, abnormal dreams, euphoria, fatigue, ***increased ICP, impaired cerebral flow, seizures***

CV: Bradycardia, hypotension, hypertension, PVC, PAC, tachycardia, abnormal ECG, ST segment depression, ***asystole***

EENT: Blurred vision, tinnitus, eye pain, strange taste, diplopia

GI: Nausea, vomiting, abdominal cramping, dry mouth, swallowing, hypersalivation, ***pancreatitis***

GU: Urine retention, green urine, cloudy urine, oliguria

INTEG: Flushing, phlebitis, hives, burning/stinging at inj site, rash, pain of extremities

MS: Myalgia

*RESP: **Apnea,** cough, hiccups,* dyspnea, hypoventilation, sneezing, wheezing, tachypnea, hypoxia

Contraindications: Hypersensitivity to drug or soybean oil; egg; hyperlipidemia

Precautions: Pregnancy (B), elderly, respiratory depression, severe respiratory disorders, cardiac dysrhythmias, labor and delivery, lactation, children

PHARMACOKINETICS

Onset 15-30 sec, rapid distribution, half-life 1-8 min, terminal elimination half-life 5-10 hr; 70% excreted in urine; metabolized in liver by conjugation to inactive metabolites

INTERACTIONS

Increase: CNS depression—alcohol, opioids, sedative/hypnotics, antipsychotics, skeletal muscle relaxants, inhalational anesthetics

NURSING CONSIDERATIONS

Assess:
• Inj site: phlebitis, burning, stinging
• ECG for changes: PVC, PAC, ST segment changes; monitor VS
• CNS changes: movement, jerking, tremors, dizziness, LOC, pupil reaction
• Allergic reactions: hives

A Respiratory dysfunction: respiratory depression, character, rate, rhythm; notify prescriber if respirations are <10/min

Administer:
• Shake well before use; if diluted, use only D_5W to not less than 2 mg/ml; give over 3-5 min, titrate to needed level of sedation; use only glass containers when mixing, not stable in plastic
• May be given by cont inf; give by inf pump
• Only with resuscitative equipment available
• Only by qualified persons trained in anesthesia

Y-site compatibilities: Acyclovir, alfentanil, aminophylline, ampicillin, aztreonam, bumetanide, buprenorphine, butorphanol, calcium gluconate, carboplatin, cefazolin, cefoperazone, cefotaxime, cefotetan, cefoxitin, ceftizoxime, ceftriaxone, cefuroxime, chlorproMAZINE, cimetidine, cisplatin, clindamycin, cyclophosphamide, cycloSPORINE, cytarabine, dexamethasone, diphenhydrAMINE, DOBUTamine, DOPamine, doxycycline, droperidol, enalaprilat, epHEDrine, epINEPHrine, esmolol, famotidine, fentanyl, fluconazole, fluorouracil, furosemide, ganciclovir, glycopyrrolate, granisetron, haloperidol, heparin, hydrocortisone, hydromorphone, hydrOXYzine, ifosfamide, imipenem/cilastatin, inamrinone, regular insulin, isoproterenol, ketamine, labetalol, levorphanol, lidocaine, lorazepam, magnesium sulfate, mannitol, meperidine, mezlocillin, miconazole, morphine, nafcillin, nalbuphine, naloxone, nitroglycerin, norepinephrine, ofloxacin, paclitaxel, pentobarbital, phenobarbital, piperacillin, potassium chloride, prochlorperazine, propranolol, ranitidine, scopolamine, sodium bicarbonate, sodium nitroprusside, succinylcholine, sufentanil, thiopental ticarcillin, ticarcillin/clavulanate, vecuronium, verapamil

Solution compatibilities: D_5W, D_5LR, LR, $D_5/0.45\%$ NaCl, $D_5/0.2\%$ NaCl

P

Perform/provide:
• Storage in light-resistant area at room temperature, use within 6 hr of opening
• If transferred from original container to another container, complete infusion within 12 hr

Evaluate:
• Therapeutic response: induction of anesthesia

Teach patient/family:
• That this medication will cause dizziness, drowsiness, sedation

Treatment of overdose: Discontinue drug; administer vasopressor agents or anticholinergics, artificial ventilation

---

⚠ High Alert

propoxyphene (℞)
(proe-pox′i-feen)
Darvon, Darvon-N, Dolene,
Novapropoxyn ✦
Func. class.: Opiate analgesic
Chem. class.: Synthetic opiate

Controlled Substance Schedule IV
Action: Depresses pain impulse transmission at the spinal cord level by interacting with opioid receptors
Uses: Mild to moderate pain

DOSAGE AND ROUTES
• *Adult:* **PO** 65 mg q4h prn (HCl)
• *Adult:* **PO** 100 mg q4h prn (napsylate)
Available forms: Propoxyphene HCl Caps 32, 65 mg; propoxyphene napsylate tabs 100 mg; oral susp 50 mg/5 ml

SIDE EFFECTS
CNS: Drowsiness, dizziness, confusion, headache, sedation, euphoria, *seizures, hyperthermia* (elderly)
CV: Palpitations, bradycardia, change in B/P, *dysrhythmias*
EENT: Tinnitus, blurred vision, miosis, diplopia
GI: Nausea, vomiting, anorexia, constipation, cramps
GU: Urinary retention, dysuria

INTEG: Rash, urticaria, bruising, flushing, diaphoresis, pruritus
*RESP: **Respiratory depression***
Contraindications: Hypersensitivity to ASA products (some preparations), addiction (opioid)
Precautions: Pregnancy (C), addictive personality, lactation, increased intracranial pressure, MI (acute), severe heart disease, respiratory depression, hepatic disease, renal disease, child <18 yr, elderly

PHARMACOKINETICS
PO: Onset ½-1 hr, peak 2-2½ hr, duration 4-6 hr
Metabolized by liver, excreted by kidneys (as metabolites), crosses placenta, excreted in breast milk, half-life 6-12 hr (metabolites)

INTERACTIONS
⚠ Possible fatal reactions: MAOIs, alcohol
Increase: effects with other CNS depressants—opioids, sedative/hypnotics, antipsychotics, skeletal muscle relaxants

Drug/Herb
Increase: CNS depression—chamomile, hops, Jamaican dogwood, kava, lavender, mistletoe, nettle, pokeweed, poppy, senega, skullcap, valerian
Increase: anticholinergic effect—corkwood

Drug/Lab Test
Increase: Amylase

NURSING CONSIDERATIONS
Assess:
• For pain: duration, location, type
• I&O ratio; check for decreasing output; may indicate retention
• CNS changes: dizziness, drowsiness, hallucinations, euphoria, loss of consciousness, pupil reaction
• Allergic reactions: rash, urticaria
• Respiratory dysfunction: respiratory depression, character, rate, rhythm;

⚠ Safety alert   *"Tall Man" lettering

notify prescriber if respirations are <10/min
• Need for pain medication; physical dependence

Administer:
• With antiemetic for nausea, vomiting
• When pain is beginning to return; determine dosage interval by response

Perform/provide:
• Storage in light-resistant area at room temperature
• Assistance with ambulation

Evaluate:
• Therapeutic response: decrease in pain

Teach patient/family:
• To report any symptoms of CNS changes, allergic reactions
• That physical dependency may result when used for extended periods; not to exceed dose
• That withdrawal symptoms may occur: nausea, vomiting, cramps, fever, faintness, anorexia

Treatment of overdose: Naloxone (Narcan) 0.2-0.8 mg IV, O₂, IV fluids, vasopressors

---

propranolol (℞)

(proe-pran'oh-lole)
Apo-Propranolol ✦,
Betaclinron E-R ✦,
Detensol ✦, Inderal, Inderal LA, InnoPran XL,
NovoPranol ✦, propranolol HCl, PMS-Propranolol ✦
Func. class.: Antihypertensive, antianginal, antidysrhythmic (class II)
Chem. class.: β-Adrenergic blocker

Do not confuse:
Inderal/Toradol
Inderal/IMDUR
Action: Nonselective β-blocker with negative inotropic, chronotropic, dromotropic properties
Uses: Chronic stable angina pectoris, hypertension, supraventricular dysrhythmias, migraine, prophylaxis, MI, pheochromocytoma, essential tremor, cyanotic spells related to hypertrophic subaortic stenosis

Investigational uses: Anxiety; Parkinson's tremor, prevention of variceal bleeding caused by portal hypertension, akathisia induced by antipsychotics

DOSAGE AND ROUTES

Dysrhythmias
• *Adult:* PO 10-30 mg tid-qid; **IV BOL** 0.5-3 mg give 1 mg/min; may repeat in 2 min, may repeat q4h thereafter
• *Child:* PO 1 mg/kg/day divided in 2 doses; **IV** 0.01-0.1 mg/kg over 5 min

Hypertension
• *Adult:* PO 40 mg bid or 80 mg daily (ext rel) initially; usual dose 120-240 mg/day bid-tid or 120-160 mg daily (ext rel)
• *Child:* PO 0.5-1 mg/kg/day divided q6-12h

Angina
• *Adult:* PO 80-320 mg in divided doses bid-qid or 80 mg daily (ext rel); usual dose 160 mg daily (ext rel)

MI prophylaxis
• *Adult:* PO 180-240 mg/day tid-qid starting 5 days to 2 wk after MI

Pheochromocytoma
• *Adult:* PO 60 mg/day × 3 days preoperatively in divided doses or 30 mg/day in divided doses (inoperable tumor)

Migraine
• *Adult:* PO 80 mg/day (ext rel) or in divided doses; may increase to 160-240 mg/day in divided doses
• *Child:* PO 0.6-1.5 mg/kg/day divided q8h

Essential tremor
• *Adult:* PO 40 mg bid; usual dose 120 mg/day

Available forms: Caps, ext rel 60, 80, 120, 160 mg; tabs 10, 20, 40, 60, 80, 90 mg; inj 1 mg/ml; oral sol 4 mg/ml, 8 mg/ml; conc oral sol 80 mg/ml

SIDE EFFECTS

CNS: Depression, hallucinations, dizziness, fatigue, lethargy, paresthesias, bizarre dreams, disorientation

CV: **Bradycardia**, hypotension, **CHF**, palpitations, AV block, peripheral vascular insufficiency, vasodilation, cold extremities, **pulmonary edema, dysrhythmias**

EENT: Sore throat, **laryngospasm**, blurred vision, dry eyes

GI: Nausea, vomiting, diarrhea, colitis, constipation, cramps, dry mouth, hepatomegaly, gastric pain, acute pancreatitis

GU: Impotence, decreased libido, UTIs

HEMA: **Agranulocytosis, thrombocytopenia**

INTEG: Rash, pruritus, fever

META: Hyperglycemia, hypoglycemia

MISC: Facial swelling, weight change, Raynaud's phenomenon

MS: Joint pain, arthralgia, muscle cramps, pain

RESP: Dyspnea, respiratory dysfunction, **bronchospasm**, cough

Contraindications: Hypersensitivity to this drug; cardiac failure; cardiogenic shock; 2nd-, 3rd-degree heart block; bronchospastic disease; sinus bradycardia; CHF, bronchospasm

Precautions: Pregnancy (C), diabetes mellitus, renal disease, lactation, hyperthyroidism, COPD, hepatic disease, children, myasthenia gravis, peripheral vascular disease, hypotension, CHF

PHARMACOKINETICS

PO: Onset 30 min, peak 1-1½ hr, duration 12 hr
PO-ER: Peak 6 hr, duration 24 hr, half-life 8-11 hr
IV: Onset 2 min, peak 1 min, duration 5 min
Metabolized by liver; crosses placenta, blood-brain barrier; excreted in breast milk, protein binding 90%

INTERACTIONS

Smoking decreases propranolol levels
Increase: effect of calcium channel blockers, neuromuscular blocker
Increase: negative inotropic effects—disopyramide

Increase: β-blocking effect—cimetidine
Increase: hypotension—quinidine, haloperidol, prazosin
Decrease: β-blocking effects—barbiturates

Drug/Herb
Increase: toxicity, death—aconite
Increase: antihypertensive effect—barberry, betony, black catechu, black cohosh, bloodroot, broom, burdock, cat's claw, dandelion, goldenseal, Irish moss, Jamaican dogwood, kelp, khella, mistletoe, parsley
Increase or decrease: antihypertensive effect—astragalus, cola tree
Decrease: antihypertensive effect—coltsfoot, guarana, khat, licorice

Drug/Lab Test
Increase: Serum potassium, serum uric acid, ALT, AST, alk phosphatase, LDH
Decrease: Blood glucose
Interference: Glaucoma testing

NURSING CONSIDERATIONS

Assess:
• B/P, pulse, respirations during beginning therapy; notify prescriber if pulse <50 bpm
• Weight daily; report gain of 5 lb
⚠ I&O ratio, CCr if kidney damage is diagnosed; watch for fluid overload: fatigue, weight gain, jugular distention, dyspnea, peripheral edema, crackles
⚠ ECG continuously if using as antidysrhythmic, IV, PCWP, CVP
• Hepatic enzymes: AST, ALT, bilirubin
• Angina pain: duration, time started, activity being performed, character
• Tolerance (long-term use)
• Headache, light-headedness, decreased B/P; may indicate a need for decreased dosage

Administer:
PO route
• Do not break, crush, chew, or open ext rel cap
• Do not use ext rel cap for essential tremor, MI, cardiac dysrhythmias; do not use InnoPran XL in hypertropic subaortic stenosis, migraine, angina pectoris

- Ext rel caps should be taken daily, InnoPran XL should be taken at bedtime
- May mix oral sol with liquid or semi-solid food, rinse container to get entire dose
- With 8 oz water with food, food enhances bioavailability
- Do not give with aluminum-containing antacid; may decrease GI absorption

IV route
- IV undiluted or diluted 10 ml D_5W for inj; give 1 mg or less/min; may be diluted in 50 ml NaCl and run 1 mg over 10-15 min

Additive compatibilities: DOBU-Tamine, verapamil

Solution compatibilities: 0.9% NaCl, 0.45 NaCl, Ringer's, D_5W, D_5/0.9% NaCl, D_5/0.45% NaCl

Syringe compatibilities: In-amrinone, milrinone

Y-site compatibilities: Alteplase, amrinone, heparin, hydrocortisone, meperidine, milrinone, morphine, potassium chloride, propofol, tacrolimus, vit B/C

Perform/provide:
- Protection from light

Evaluate:
- Therapeutic response: decreased B/P, dysrhythmias

Teach patient/family:
⚠ Not to discontinue abruptly, may precipitate life-threatening dysrhythmias; to take drug at same time each day; to decrease dosage over 2 wk to prevent cardiac damage
- To avoid OTC drugs unless approved by prescriber; avoid alcohol
- To avoid hazardous activities if dizzy
- The importance of compliance with complete medical regimen; monitor blood glucose, may mask symptoms of hypoglycemia
- To make position changes slowly to prevent fainting
- That sensitivity to cold may occur

propylhexadrine nasal agent
See Appendix C

propylthiouracil (℞)
(proe-pill-thye-oh-yoor'a-sill)
propylthiouracil,
Propyl-Thyracil ✦, PTU
Func. class.: Thyroid hormone antagonist (antithyroid)
Chem. class.: Thioamide

Action: Blocks synthesis peripherally of T_3, T_4 (triiodothyronine, thyroxine), inhibits organification of iodine
Uses: Preparation for thyroidectomy, thyrotoxic crisis, hyperthyroidism, thyroid storm

DOSAGE AND ROUTES
Thyrotoxic crisis
- *Adult and child:* PO same as hyperthyroidism with iodine and propranolol
Preparation for thyroidectomy
- *Adult:* 600-1200 mg/day
- *Child:* 10 mg/kg/day in divided doses
Hyperthyroidism
- *Adult:* **PO** 100 mg tid increasing to 300 mg q8h if condition is severe; continue to euthyroid state, then 100 mg daily-tid
- *Child >10 yr:* **PO** 100 mg tid; continue to euthyroid state, then 25 mg tid to 100 mg bid
- *Child 6-10 yr:* **PO** 50-150 mg in divided doses q8h
- *Neonate:* **PO** 10 mg/kg/day in divided doses
Available forms: Tabs 50, 100 mg

SIDE EFFECTS
CNS: Drowsiness, headache, vertigo, fever, paresthesias, neuritis
*GI: Nausea, diarrhea, vomiting, **jaundice, hepatitis,*** loss of taste
*GU: **Nephritis***
*HEMA: **Agranulocytosis, leukope-***

P

---

*nia, **thrombocytopenia, hypothrombinemia, lymphadenopathy,***
bleeding, vasculitis, periarteritis
*INTEG: Rash, urticaria, pruritus, alope-
cia, hyperpigmentation,* lupuslike syndrome
MS: Myalgia, arthralgia, nocturnal muscle
cramps, osteoporosis
Contraindications: Pregnancy (D),
hypersensitivity, lactation
Precautions: Infection, bone marrow
depression, hepatic disease

PHARMACOKINETICS

PO: Onset up to 3 wk, peak 6-10 wk,
duration 1 wk to 1 mo, half-life 1-2 hr;
excreted in urine, bile, breast milk;
crosses placenta; concentration in
thyroid gland

INTERACTIONS

Bone marrow depression: radiation,
antineoplastics
Agranulocytosis: phenothiazines
Increase: anticoagulant effect—
heparin, oral anticoagulants
Increase: effects—potassium/sodium
iodide, lithium
Drug/Lab Test
Increase: PT, AST, ALT, alk phosphatase

NURSING CONSIDERATIONS

Assess:
• Pulse, B/P, temp
• I&O ratio; check for edema: puffy
hands, feet, periorbits; indicates hypothyroidism
• Weight daily; same clothing, scale,
time of day
• T_3, T_4, which are increased; serum
TSH, which is decreased; free thyroxine
index, which is increased if dosage is too
low; discontinue drug 3-4 wk before
RAIU
⚠ Blood studies: CBC for blood
dyscrasias: leukopenia, thrombocytopenia, agranulocytosis; LFTs
⚠ Overdose: peripheral edema, heat
intolerance, diaphoresis, palpitations,
dysrhythmias, severe tachycardia, in-

creased temp, delirium, CNS irritability
⚠ Hypersensitivity: rash, enlarged cervi-
cal lymph nodes; drug may have to be
discontinued
• Hypoprothrombinemia: bleeding,
petechiae, ecchymosis
• Clinical response: after 3 wk should
include increased weight, pulse; de-
creased T_4
• Bone marrow depression: sore throat,
fever, fatigue
Administer:
• With meals to decrease GI upset
• At same time each day to maintain
drug level
• Lowest dose that relieves symptoms
Perform/provide:
• Storage in light-resistant container
• Fluids to 3-4 L/day, unless contraindi-
cated
Evaluate:
• Therapeutic response: weight gain,
decreased pulse, decreased T_4, de-
creased B/P
Teach patient/family:
• To abstain from breastfeeding after
delivery
• To take pulse daily
• To report redness, swelling, sore
throat, mouth lesions, which indicate
blood dyscrasias
• To keep graph of weight, pulse, mood
• To avoid OTC products that contain
iodine
• That seafood, other iodine products
may be restricted
• Not to discontinue this medication
abruptly; thyroid crisis may occur; stress
response
• That response may take several
months if thyroid is large
• The symptoms/signs of overdose:
periorbital edema, cold intolerance,
mental depression
• The symptoms of inadequate dose:
tachycardia, diarrhea, fever, irritability
• To take medication as prescribed; not
to skip or double dose; missed doses

⚠ Safety alert   *"Tall Man" lettering

should be taken when remembered up to 1 hr before next dose

• To carry emergency ID listing condition, medication

protamine (R)
(proe'ta-meen)
Func. class.: Heparin antagonist
Chem. class.: Low-molecular-weight protein

Action: Binds heparin, making it ineffective
Uses: Heparin overdose, hemorrhage

DOSAGE AND ROUTES

• *Adult and child:* **IV** 1 mg of protamine/100 units heparin given or 100 anti-Xa units of LMWH; administer slowly 1-3 min; not to exceed 50 mg/10 min
Available forms: Inj 10 mg/ml

SIDE EFFECTS

CNS: Lassitude
CV: Hypotension, bradycardia, ***circulatory collapse***
GI: Nausea, vomiting, anorexia
HEMA: Bleeding
INTEG: Rash, dermatitis, urticaria
RESP: Dyspnea, ***pulmonary edema, severe respiratory distress***
SYST: ***Anaphylaxis, angioedema***
Contraindications: Hypersensitivity
Precautions: Pregnancy (C), lactation, children, allergy to salmon, diabetes mellitus

PHARMACOKINETICS

IV: Onset 5 min, duration 2 hr

NURSING CONSIDERATIONS

Assess:
🅰 Hypersensitivity: urticuria, cough, wheezing, have emergency equipment nearby
• Blood studies (Hct, platelets, occult blood in stools) q3mo
• Coagulation tests (APTT, ACT) 15 min after dose, then in several hours

• VS, B/P, pulse after 30 min; plus 3 hr after dose
• Skin rash, urticaria, dermatitis
🅰 Allergy to fish; use with caution; men that have had a vasectomy may be more prone to hypersensitivity
Administer:
• After diluting 50 mg/5 ml sterile bacteriostatic H_2O for inj; shake, give 20 mg or less over 1-3 min; may further dilute with equal volume of NaCl or D_5W and run over 2-3 hr; titrate to APTT, ACT; use infusion pump
Additive compatibilities: Cimetidine, ranitidine, verapamil
Perform/provide:
• Storage at 36°-46° F (2°-8° C)
Evaluate:
• Therapeutic response: reversal of heparin overdose

pseudoephedrine
(otc, R)
(soo-doh-eh-fed'rin)
Afrin, Allermed, Canafed, Cenafed, Children's Congestion Relief, Children's Silfedrine, Congestion Relief, Decofed Syrup, DeFed-60, Dorcol Children's Decongestant, Drixoral Non-Drowsy Formula, Dynafed, Efidac/24, Eltor ✦, Genaphed, Halofed, Mini Thin Pseudo, PediaCare Infant's Decongestant, Pseudo, pseudoephedrine HCl, Pseudogest, Seudotabs, Sinustop Pro, Sudafed, Sudafed 12 Hour, Sudex, Triaminic AM Decongestant Formula
Func. class.: Adrenergic
Chem. class.: Substituted phenylethylamine

Action: Primary activity through α-effects on respiratory mucosal membranes reducing congestion hyperemia, edema; minimal bronchodilation secondary to β-effects

Uses: Nasal decongestant, adjunct in otitis media; with antihistamines

DOSAGE AND ROUTES

• *Adult and child >12 yr:* **PO** 60 mg q6h; **EXT REL** 120 mg q12h or 240 mg q24h
• *Geriatric:* **PO** 30-60 mg q6h prn
• *Child 6-12 yr:* **PO** 30 mg q6h, not to exceed 120 mg/day
• *Child 2-6 yr:* **PO** 15 mg q6h, not to exceed 60 mg/day

Available forms: Caps, ext rel 120, 240 mg; oral sol 15 mg, 30 mg/5 ml; drops 7.5 mg/0.8 ml; tabs 30, 60 mg; caps 60 mg; tabs, ext rel 120, 240 mg

SIDE EFFECTS

CNS: Tremors, anxiety, insomnia, headache, dizziness, hallucinations, *seizures* (elderly)
CV: Palpitations, tachycardia, hypertension, chest pain, *dysrhythmias, CV collapse*
EENT: Dry nose, irritation of nose and throat
GI: Anorexia, nausea, vomiting, dry mouth
GU: Dysuria

Contraindications: Hypersensitivity to sympathomimetics, narrow-angle glaucoma
Precautions: Pregnancy (C), cardiac disorders, hyperthyroidism, diabetes mellitus, prostatic hypertrophy, lactation, hypertension

PHARMACOKINETICS

PO: Onset 15-30 min, duration 4-6 hr, 8-12 hr (ext rel); metabolized in liver, excreted in feces and breast milk

INTERACTIONS

⚠ Do not use with MAOIs or tricyclics; hypertensive crisis may occur
Increase: effect of this drug—urinary alkalizers
Decrease: effect of this drug—

methyldopa, urinary acidifiers, rauwolfia alkaloids

NURSING CONSIDERATIONS

Assess:
• For nasal congestion; auscultate lung sounds; check for tenacious bronchial secretions
• B/P, pulse throughout treatment
• For CNS side effects in the elderly: excitation, seizures, hallucinations
Administer:
• Near bedtime; stimulation can occur
Perform/provide:
• Storage at room temperature
Evaluate:
• Therapeutic response: decreased nasal congestion
Teach patient/family:
• The reason for drug administration
• Not to use continuously, or more than recommended dose; rebound congestion may occur
⚠ To notify prescriber immediately of anxiety; slow, fast heart rate; dyspnea; seizures
• To check with prescriber before using other drugs, as drug interactions may occur
• To avoid taking near bedtime; stimulation can occur
• Not to use if stimulation, restlessness, or tremors occur
• That use in children may cause excessive agitation

⚠ Safety alert   *"Tall Man" lettering

psyllium (otc, ℞)

(sill'ee-um)

Alramucil, Fiberall, Fiberall Natural Flavor and Orange Flavor, Genifiber, Hydrocil Instant, Karacil ✽, Konsyl, Konsyl Orange, Maalox Daily Fiber Therapy, Metamucil, Metamucil Lemon Lime, Metamucil Orange Flavor, Metamucil Sugar Free, Metamucil Sugar Free Orange Flavor, Modane Bulk, Mylanta Natural Fiber Supplement, Natural Fiber Laxative, Natural Fiber Laxative Sugar Free, Natural Vegetable Reguloid, Perdiem, Prodiem Plain ✽, Reguloid Natural, Reguloid Orange, Reguloid Sugar Free Orange, Reguloid Sugar Free Regular, Restore, Restore Sugar Free, Serutan, Syllact, V-Lax

Func. class.: Bulk laxative
Chem. class.: Psyllium colloid

Action: Bulk-forming laxative
Uses: Chronic constipation, ulcerative colitis, irritable bowel syndrome

DOSAGE AND ROUTES

• *Adult:* **PO** 1-2 tsp in 8 oz H_2O bid or tid, then 8 oz H_2O or 1 premeasured packet in 8 oz H_2O bid or tid, then 8 oz H_2O
• *Child >6 yr:* **PO** 1 tsp in 4 oz H_2O at bedtime
Available forms: Chew pieces 1.7, 3.4 g/piece; effervescent powder 3.4, 3.7 g/packet; powder 3.3, 3.4, 3.5, 4.94 g/tsp; granules 2.5, 4.03 g/tsp; wafers 3.4 g/wafer

SIDE EFFECTS

GI: Nausea, vomiting, anorexia, diarrhea, cramps, intestinal esophageal blockage

Contraindications: Hypersensitivity, intestinal obstruction, abdominal pain, nausea/vomiting, fecal impaction
Precautions: Pregnancy (C)

PHARMACOKINETICS

Excreted in feces, not absorbed in GI tract

INTERACTIONS

Decrease: absorption of cardiac glycosides, oral anticoagulants, salicylates
Drug/Herb
Increase: laxative effect—flax, senna

NURSING CONSIDERATIONS

Assess:
• Blood, urine electrolytes if used often
• I&O ratio to identify fluid loss
• Cause of constipation; fluids, bulk, exercise missing
• Cramping, rectal bleeding, nausea, vomiting; drug should be discontinued
Administer:
PO route
• Alone for better absorption, separate from other drugs by 1-2 hr
• In morning or evening (oral dose)
• Immediately after mixing with H_2O
• With 8 oz H_2O or juice followed by another 8 oz of fluid
Evaluate:
• Therapeutic response: decrease in constipation or decreased diarrhea in colitis
Teach patient/family:
• To maintain adequate fluid consumption
• That normal bowel movements do not always occur daily
• Not to use in presence of abdominal pain, nausea, vomiting
• To notify prescriber if constipation unrelieved or if symptoms of electrolyte imbalance occur: muscle cramps, pain, weakness, dizziness, excessive thirst

P

Side effects: *italics* = common; ***bold italics*** = life-threatening

pyrantel (otc)
(pie-ran'tel)
Antiminth, Combantrin ✦,
Pin-Rid, Pin-X, Reese's
Pinworm
Func. class.: Anthelmintic
Chem. class.: Pyrimidine derivative

Action: Causes paralysis in worm by neuroblockade via stimulation of ganglionic receptors; worms expelled by normal peristalsis
Uses: Pinworms, roundworms, hookworms

DOSAGE AND ROUTES
• *Adult and child >2 yr:* **PO** 11 mg/kg as single dose, not to exceed 1 g; repeat in 2 wk for pinworms
Available forms: Oral susp 50 mg/ml; liquid 50 mg/ml; caps, soft gel 180 mg

SIDE EFFECTS
CNS: Dizziness, headache, drowsiness, insomnia, fever, weakness
GI: Nausea, vomiting, anorexia, diarrhea, distention, abdominal cramps
INTEG: Rash
Contraindications: Hypersensitivity
Precautions: Pregnancy (C), seizure disorders, hepatic disease, dehydration, anemia, child <2 yr, malnutrition

PHARMACOKINETICS
PO: Peak 1-3 hr; metabolized in liver; excreted in feces, urine (unchanged/metabolites)

INTERACTIONS
Antagonizes effect of pyrantel: piperazine

NURSING CONSIDERATIONS
Assess:
• Stools during entire treatment; specimens must be sent to lab while still warm
• For diarrhea during expulsion of worms
• For allergic reaction: rash

Administer:
• After meals to avoid GI symptoms
• After shaking suspension
Perform/provide:
• Storage in tight, light-resistant container in cool environment
Evaluate:
• Therapeutic response: expulsion of worms, 3 negative stool cultures after completion of treatment
Teach patient/family:
• Proper hygiene after BM, including hand-washing technique; tell patient not to put fingers in mouth
• That infected person should sleep alone; not to shake bed linen; to change bed linen daily, wash in hot water; that all family members should be treated for pinworms; treat dogs/cats; keep children away from animal's feces
• To clean toilet daily with disinfectant (green soap solution)
• The need for compliance with dosage schedule, duration of treatment
• To drink fruit juice to help expel worms
• To wear shoes, wash all fruits, vegetables well before eating

pyrazinamide (℞)
(peer-a-zin'a-mide)
PMS Pyrazinamide ✦,
pyrazinamide, Tebrazid ✦
Func. class.: Antitubercular agent
Chem. class.: Pyrazinoic acid amine, nicoturimide analog

Action: Bactericidal interference with lipid, nucleic acid biosynthesis
Uses: Tuberculosis, as an adjunct when other drugs are not feasible

DOSAGE AND ROUTES
• *Adult and child:* **PO** 15-30 mg/kg/day not to exceed 2 g/day
Available forms: Tabs 500 mg

SIDE EFFECTS
CNS: Headache

⚠ Safety alert   ✦ "Tall Man" lettering

*GI: **Hepatotoxicity,*** abnormal hepatic studies, peptic ulcer, nausea, vomiting, anorexia, cramps, diarrhea
GU: Urinary difficulty, increased uric acid
*HEMA: **Hemolytic anemia***
INTEG: Photosensitivity, urticaria
Contraindications: Hypersensitivity, severe hepatic damage, acute gout
Precautions: Pregnancy (C), child <13 yr, renal failure, diabetes, porphyria, chronic gout

PHARMACOKINETICS

PO: Peak 2 hr, half-life 9-10 hr; metabolized in liver, excreted in urine (metabolites/unchanged drug)

INTERACTIONS

Drug/Lab Test
Increase: PBI
Decrease: 17-KS

NURSING CONSIDERATIONS

Assess:
• Signs of anemia: Hct, Hgb, fatigue
• Temp; if >101° F (38° C), drug should be reduced
A Hepatic studies qwk: ALT, AST, bilirubin
• Renal status before, qmo: BUN, creatinine, output, sp gr, urinalysis, uric acid
• Hepatic status: decreased appetite, jaundice, dark urine, fatigue
Administer:
• With meals for GI symptoms
• After C&S is completed; qmo to detect resistance
Evaluate:
• Therapeutic response: decreased symptoms of TB, culture negative
Teach patient/family:
• That compliance with dosage schedule, length is necessary
• To avoid alcohol
• To report fever, loss of appetite, malaise, nausea, vomiting, darkened urine, pale stools

---

pyridostigmine (Ŗ)
(peer-id-oh-stig'meen)
Mestinon, Mestinon SR, Mestinon Timespan, Regonol
Func. class.: Cholinergic; anticholinesterase
Chem. class.: Tertiary amine carbamate

Action: Inhibits destruction of acetylcholine, which increases concentration at sites where acetylcholine is released; this facilitates transmission of impulses across myoneural junction
Uses: Nondepolarizing muscle relaxant antagonist, myasthenia gravis

DOSAGE AND ROUTES

Myasthenia gravis
• *Adult:* **PO** 60-180 mg bid-qid, not to exceed 1.5 g/day; **IM/IV** 2 mg or $\frac{1}{30}$ of **PO** dose; **SUS REL** 180-540 mg daily or bid at intervals of at least 6 hr
• *Child:* **PO** 7 mg/kg/day in 5-6 divided doses
Nondepolarizing neuromuscular blocker antagonist
• *Adult:* 0.6-1.2 mg **IV** atropine, then 10-30 mg
• *Child:* **IV** 0.1-0.25 mg/kg/dose
Available forms: Tabs 60 mg; tabs, ext rel 180 mg; syr 60 mg/5 ml; inj 5 mg/ml

SIDE EFFECTS

CNS: Dizziness, headache, sweating, weakness, ***seizures,*** incoordination, ***paralysis,*** drowsiness, LOC
CV: Tachycardia, dysrhythmias, bradycardia, AV block, hypotension, ECG changes, ***cardiac arrest,*** syncope
EENT: Miosis, blurred vision, lacrimation, visual changes
GI: Nausea, diarrhea, vomiting, cramps, increased salivary and gastric secretions, peristalsis
GU: Urinary frequency, incontinence, urgency
INTEG: Rash, urticaria, flushing
*RESP: **Respiratory depression,***

P

♣ Canada only   Side effects: *italics* = common; ***bold italics*** = life-threatening

bronchospasm, constriction, la-ryngospasm, respiratory arrest
Contraindications: Bradycardia; hypotension; obstruction of intestine, renal system; bromide sensitivity
Precautions: Pregnancy (C), seizure disorders, bronchial asthma, coronary occlusion, hyperthyroidism, dysrhythmias, peptic ulcer, megacolon, poor GI motility

PHARMACOKINETICS

PO: Onset 20-30 min, duration 3-6 hr
IM/IV/SUBCUT: Onset 2-15 min, duration 2½-4 hr; metabolized in liver, excreted in urine

INTERACTIONS

Increase: action—decamethonium, succinylcholine
Decrease: action—gallamine, metocurine, pancuronium, tubocurarine, atropine
Decrease: pyridostigmine action—aminoglycosides, anesthetics, procainamide, quinidine, mecamylamine, polymyxin, magnesium, corticosteroids, antidysrhythmics
Drug/Herb
Increase: effect—jaborandi tree, pill-bearing spurge

NURSING CONSIDERATIONS

Assess:
• VS, respiration q8h
• I&O ratio; check for urinary retention or incontinence
• Bradycardia, hypotension, bronchospasm, headache, dizziness, convulsions, respiratory depression; drug should be discontinued if toxicity occurs
Administer:
• Do not break, crush, or chew sus rel tabs
• Only with atropine sulfate available for cholinergic crisis
• Only after all other cholinergics have been discontinued
• Increased doses for tolerance, as ordered

• Larger doses after exercise or fatigue, as ordered
• On empty stomach for better absorption
IV route
• Undiluted, give through Y-tube or 3-way stopcock, give 0.5 mg or less/min
Syringe compatibilities: Glycopyrrolate
Y-site compatibilities: Heparin, hydrocortisone, potassium chloride, vit B/C
Perform/provide:
• Storage at room temperature
Evaluate:
• Therapeutic response: increased muscle strength, hand grasp, improved gait, absence of labored breathing (if severe)
Teach patient/family:
• That drug is not a cure, only relieves symptoms
• To wear emergency ID specifying myasthenia gravis, drugs taken
Treatment of overdose: Discontinue drug, atropine 1-4 mg IV

pyridoxine (vit B$_6$) (℞, otc)

(peer-i-dox'een)
Beesix, Doxine, Nestrex, pyridoxine HCl, Pyri, Rodex, Vitabee 6, vitamin B$_6$
Func. class.: Vit B$_6$, water soluble

Action: Needed for fat, protein, carbohydrate metabolism; enhances glycogen release from liver and muscle tissue; needed as coenzyme for metabolic transformations of a variety of amino acids
Uses: Vit B$_6$ deficiency of inborn errors of metabolism, seizures, isoniazid therapy, oral contraceptives, alcoholic polyneuritis
Investigational uses: Palmar-Plantar erythrodysesthesia syndrome

DOSAGE AND ROUTES
RDA
• *Adult:* **PO** male 1.7-2 mg; female 1.4-1.6 mg

Vit B₆ deficiency

Vit B$_6$ deficiency
- *Adult:* **PO/IM/IV** 5-25 mg daily × 3wk
- *Child:* **PO/IM/IV** 100 mg until desired response

Deficiency caused by isoniazid, cycloSERINE, hydrALAZINE, penicillamine
- *Adult:* **PO** 6-100 mg daily
- *Child:* **PO** 5-25 mg daily

Prevention of deficiency caused by isoniazid, cycloSERINE, hydrALAZINE, penicillamine
- *Adult:* **PO** 6-50 mg daily
- *Child:* **PO** 0.5-1.5 mg daily
- *Infant:* **PO** 0.1-0.5 mg daily

Palmar-Plantar erythrodysesthesia syndrome (off-label)
- *Adult:* **PO** 50-150 mg daily

Available forms: Tabs 10, 25, 50, 100 mg; tabs, ext rel 100 mg; inj 100 mg/ml; ext rel cap 150 mg

SIDE EFFECTS

CNS: Paresthesia, flushing, warmth, lethargy (rare with normal renal function)
INTEG: Pain at inj site
Contraindications: Hypersensitivity
Precautions: Pregnancy (A), lactation, children, Parkinson's disease, patients taking levodopa should avoid supplemental vitamins with >5 mg pyridoxine

PHARMACOKINETICS

PO/Inj: Half-life 2-3 wk, metabolized in liver, excreted in urine

INTERACTIONS

Decrease: effects of levodopa
Decrease: effects of pyridoxine—oral contraceptives, isoniazid, cycloSERINE, hydrALAZINE, penicillamine, chloramphenicol, immunosuppressants

NURSING CONSIDERATIONS

Assess:
- Pyridoxine levels throughout treatment
- Nutritional status: yeast, liver, legumes, bananas, green vegetables, whole grains

Administer:
PO route
Do not break, crush, or chew ext rel tabs, caps
IM route
- Rotate sites; burning or stinging at site may occur
- Z-track to minimize pain
IV route
- Undiluted or added to most IV sol; give 50 mg or less/1 min if undiluted
Syringe compatibilities: Doxapram
Perform/provide:
- Storage in tight, light-resistant container
Evaluate:
- Therapeutic response: absence of nausea, vomiting, anorexia, skin lesions, glossitis, stomatitis, edema, seizures, restlessness, paresthesia
Teach patient/family:
- To avoid vitamin supplements unless directed by prescriber
- To keep out of children's reach
- To increase meat, bananas, potatoes, lima beans, whole grain cereals in diet
- To discuss birth control status with prescriber

pyrimethamine (℞)

(peer-i-meth'a-meen)
Daraprim, Fansidar (with sulfadoxine)
Func. class.: Antimalarial
Chem. class.: Folic acid antagonist

Action: Inhibits folic acid metabolism in parasite, prevents transmission by stopping growth of fertilized gametes
Uses: Malaria prophylaxis, *Plasmodium vivax*
Investigational uses: *Pneumocystis jiroveci* pneumonia as an adjunct

DOSAGE AND ROUTES

Prophylaxis of malaria
- *Adult and child >10 yr:* **PO** 25 mg qwk
- *Child 4-10 yr:* **PO** 12.5 mg qwk
- *Child <4 yr:* **PO** 6.25 mg qwk

Toxoplasmosis
- *Adult:* **PO** 100 mg, then 25 mg daily × 4-5 wk, with 1 g sulfadoxine q6h
- *Child:* **PO** 1 mg/kg/day in 2 divided doses or 2 mg/kg/day × 3 days, then 1 mg/kg/day or divided twice daily × 4 wk, max 25 mg/day

Toxoplasmosis in AIDS patients
- *Adult:* **PO** 100-200 mg/day × 1-2 days, then 50-100 mg/day × 3-6 wk, then 25-50 mg/day for life (given with clinda-mycin or sulfADIAZINE)

Available forms: Tabs 25 mg; combo tabs 500 mg sulfadoxine/25 mg pyri-methamine

SIDE EFFECTS

CNS: Stimulation, irritability, ***seizures***, tremors, ataxia, fatigue
CV: ***Dysrhythmias***
GI: Nausea, vomiting, cramps, anorexia, diarrhea, atrophic glossitis, gas-tritis
*HEMA: **Thrombocytopenia, leukopenia, pancytopenia, megaloblastic anemia,** decreased folic acid, **agranulocytosis***
INTEG: Skin eruptions, photosensitivity
*RESP: **Respiratory failure***
Contraindications: Hypersensitivity, chloroquine-resistant malaria, megalo-blastic anemia caused by folate defi-ciency
Precautions: Pregnancy (C), blood dyscrasias, seizure disorder, lactation, G6PD disease, renal, hepatic disease

PHARMACOKINETICS

PO: Peak 2 hr, half-life 111 hr; metab-olized in liver, highly protein bound, excreted in urine (metabolites)

INTERACTIONS

Synergistic action: folic acid
Increase: bone marrow suppression—bone marrow depressants, radiation therapy

NURSING CONSIDERATIONS
Assess:
- Folic acid level; megaloblastic anemia occurs
🛆 Blood studies, CBC, platelets, since blood dyscrasias occur; twice weekly if dosage is increased
🛆 For toxicity: vomiting, anorexia, sei-zure, blood dyscrasia, glossitis; drug should be discontinued immediately
Administer:
- Leucovorin IM 3-9 mg/day × 3 days if folic acid deficiency occurs
- Before or after meals at same time each day to maintain drug level, to de-crease GI symptoms
Perform/provide:
- Storage in tight, light-resistant con-tainer
Evaluate:
- Therapeutic response: decreased symptoms of malaria
Teach patient/family:
- To report visual problems, fever, fa-tigue, bruising, bleeding; may indicate blood dyscrasias
Treatment of overdose: Gastric lavage, short-acting barbiturate, leucovo-rin, respiratory support if needed

---

quetiapine (℞)
(kwe-tie′a-peen)
Seroquel
Func. class.: Antipsychotic

Action: Functions as an antagonist at multiple neurotransmitter receptors in the brain including $5HT_{1A}$, $5HT_2$, dopa-mine D_1, D_2, H_1, and adrenergic α_1, α_2 receptors
Uses: Psychotic disorders
Research note: Increased dose of quetiapine may be necessary when used with phenytoin

DOSAGE AND ROUTES
- *Adult:* **PO** 25 mg bid, with incremental increases of 25 mg bid-tid on days 2 and

3 to a dose of 300-400 mg daily given bid-tid, max 800 mg/day
Available forms: Tabs 25, 100, 200, 300 mg

SIDE EFFECTS

CNS: EPS, pseudoparkinsonism, akathisia, dystonia, tardive dyskinesia; drowsiness, insomnia, agitation, anxiety, *headache*, **seizures, neuroleptic malignant syndrome**, *dizziness*
CV: Orthostatic hypotension, ***tachycardia***
GI: Nausea, anorexia, constipation, abdominal pain, dry mouth
INTEG: Rash
MISC: Asthenia, back pain, fever, ear pain
RESP: Rhinitis
Contraindications: Hypersensitivity
Precautions: Pregnancy (C), children, hepatic disease, elderly, breast cancer, lactation, long-term use, seizures, dementia

PHARMACOKINETICS

PO: Extensively metabolized by liver half-life ≥6 hr; peak 1½ hr; inhibits P450 CYP3A4 enzyme system

INTERACTIONS

Increase: CNS depression—alcohol, opioid analgesics, sedative/hypnotics, antihistamines
Increase: quetiapine clearance—phenytoin, thioridazine, barbiturates, glucocorticoids, carbamazepine, rifampin
Increase: quetiapine action—fluconazole, itraconazole, ketoconazole
Increase: effects of erythromycin
Decrease: quetiapine clearance—cimetidine
Decrease: effects of DOPamine agonists, levodopa, lorazepam
Drug/Herb
Increase: action—cola tree, hops, nettle, nutmeg
Increase: EPS—betel palm, kava

NURSING CONSIDERATIONS

Assess:
• Mental status before initial administration
• Swallowing of PO medication: check for hoarding or giving of medication to other patients
• I&O ratio; palpate bladder if urinary output is low
• Bilirubin, CBC, hepatic studies qmo
• Urinalysis before, during prolonged therapy
• Affect, orientation, LOC, reflexes, gait, coordination, sleep pattern disturbances
• B/P standing and lying; also pulse, respirations; take these q4h during initial treatment; establish baseline before starting treatment; report drops of 30 mm Hg; watch for ECG changes
• Dizziness, faintness, palpitations, tachycardia on rising
• EPS, including akathisia (inability to sit still, no pattern to movements), tardive dyskinesia (bizarre movements of the jaw, mouth, tongue, extremities), pseudoparkinsonism (rigidity, tremors, pill rolling, shuffling gait)
A For neuroleptic malignant syndrome: hyperthermia, increased CPK, altered mental status, muscle rigidity, seizures, tachycardia, diaphoresis, hyper/hypotension, fatigue; notify prescriber immediately if symptoms occur
• Skin turgor daily
• Constipation, urinary retention daily; if these occur, increase bulk and water in the diet

Administer:
• Reduced dose in elderly
• Antiparkinsonian agent on order from prescriber, to be used for EPS
• Avoid use of CNS depressants

Perform/provide:
• Decreased stimulus by dimming lights, avoiding loud noises
• Supervised ambulation until patient is stabilized on medication; do not involve in strenuous exercise program because

Q

fainting is possible; patient should not stand still for a long time

• Sips of water, sugarless candy, gum for dry mouth

• Storage in tight, light-resistant container

Evaluate:

• Therapeutic response: decrease in emotional excitement, hallucinations, delusions, paranoia; reorganization of patterns of thought, speech

Teach patient/family:

• To rise slowly, to prevent orthostatic hypotension

• To take medication only as prescribed

• If drowsiness occurs, avoid hazardous activities such as driving

• To avoid use of OTC meds unless directed by prescriber

• To notify prescriber if pregnancy is planned, suspected

• To notify prescriber immediately of fever, difficulty breathing, fatigue

---

quinapril (℞)

(kwin′a-pril)
Accupril
Func. class.: Antihypertensive
Chem. class.: Angiotensin-converting enzyme (ACE) inhibitor

Action: Selectively suppresses renin-angiotensin-aldosterone system; inhibits ACE, prevents conversion of angiotensin I to angiotensin II; results in dilation of arterial, venous vessels

Uses: Hypertension, alone or in combination with thiazide diuretics; systolic CHF

DOSAGE AND ROUTES

Hypertension (monotherapy)

• *Adult:* **PO** 10-20 mg daily initially, then 20-80 mg/day divided bid or daily

• *Geriatric:* **PO** 10 mg daily, titrate to desired response

Congestive heart failure

• *Adult:* **PO** 5 mg bid, may increase qwk until 20-40 mg/day in 2 divided doses

Renal dose

• *Adult:* **PO** CCr 30-60 ml/min 5 mg/day initially; CCr <30 ml/min 2.5 mg/day initially

Available forms: Tabs 5, 10, 20, 40 mg

SIDE EFFECTS

CNS: Headache, dizziness, fatigue, somnolence, depression, malaise, nervousness, vertigo

CV: Hypotension, postural hypotension, syncope, palpitations, angina pectoris, *MI, tachycardia,* vasodilation, chest pain

GI: Nausea, diarrhea, constipation, *vomiting,* gastritis, *GI hemorrhage,* dry mouth

GU: Increased BUN, creatinine, decreased libido, impotence

HEMA: Thrombocytopenia, agranulocytosis

INTEG: Angioedema, rash, sweating, photosensitivity, pruritus

META: Hyperkalemia

MISC: Back pain, amblyopia

MS: Myalgia

RESP: Cough, pharyngitis, dyspnea

Contraindications: Pregnancy (D) 2nd/3rd trimester, hypersensitivity to ACE inhibitors, children

Precautions: Pregnancy (C) 1st trimester, impaired renal, hepatic function, dialysis patients, hypovolemia, blood dyscrasias, COPD, bilateral renal stenosis, asthma, elderly, lactation

PHARMACOKINETICS

Bioavailability ≥60%

PO: Onset <1 hr, peak 2-4 hr, duration 24 hr, serum protein binding 97%, half-life 2 hr, metabolized by liver (active metabolites quinaprilat), metabolites excreted in urine (60%)/ feces (37%)

INTERACTIONS

Use caution with vasodilators, hydrALA-ZINE, prazosin, potassium-sparing di-

---

uretics, sympathomimetics, potassium supplements

Increase: hypotension—diuretics, other antihypertensives, ganglionic blockers, adrenergic blockers, phenothiazines, nitrates, acute alcohol ingestion

Increase: toxicity of lithium, digoxin

Decrease: absorption of tetracycline

Decrease: hypotensive effect of quinapril—indomethacin

Drug/Herb

Increase: toxicity, death—aconite

Increase: antihypertensive effect—barberry, betony, black catechu, black cohosh, bloodroot, broom, burdock, cat's claw, dandelion, goldenseal, Irish moss, Jamaican dogwood, kelp, khella, mistletoe, parsley

Increase or decrease: antihypertensive effect—astragalus, cola tree

Decrease: antihypertensive effect—coltsfoot, guarana, khat, licorice

Drug/Lab Test

False positive: Urine acetone, ANA titer

NURSING CONSIDERATIONS

Assess:

⚠ Blood studies: neutrophils, decreased platelets; WBC with differential baseline and periodically q3mo; if neutrophils <1000/mm³, discontinue treatment (recommended in collagen-vascular disease)

• B/P, orthostatic hypotension, syncope

• Renal studies: protein, BUN, creatinine; watch for increased levels; may indicate nephrotic syndrome

• Baselines in renal, hepatic studies before therapy begins and periodically; increased LFTs; uric acid and glucose may be increased

• Potassium levels; hyperkalemia is rare

• Edema in feet, legs daily, weight daily in CHF

⚠ Allergic reactions: rash, fever, pruritus, urticaria; drug should be discontinued if antihistamines fail to help

• Renal symptoms: oliguria, urinary frequency, dysuria

Administer:

• Tabs may be crushed if necessary

Evaluate:

• Therapeutic response: decrease in B/P

Teach patient/family:

• Not to discontinue drug abruptly

• Not to use OTC products (cough, cold, allergy); not to use salt substitutes containing potassium unless directed by prescriber

• To comply with dosage schedule, even if feeling better

• To rise slowly to sitting or standing position to minimize orthostatic hypotension

• To notify prescriber of mouth sores, sore throat, fever, swelling of hands or feet, irregular heartbeat, chest pain, persistent dry cough

• To report excessive perspiration, dehydration, vomiting, diarrhea; may lead to fall in B/P

• That drug may cause dizziness, fainting, light-headedness; may occur during first few days of therapy

• That drug may cause skin rash or impaired taste perception

• How to take B/P, and normal readings for age-group

Treatment of overdose: 0.9% NaCl IV inf

quinidine (℞)
(kwin'i-deen)
quinidine gluconate
Quinaglute Dura-Tabs,
Quinalan, Quinate ✦
quinidine polygalacturonate
Cardioquin
quinidine sulfate
Apo-Quinidine ✦, Cin-Quin,
Novoquinidine ✦, Quinidex
Extentabs, Quinora
Func. class.: Antidysrhythmic (Class IA)
Chem. class.: Quinine dextroisomer

Action: Prolongs duration of action potential and effective refractory period, thus decreasing myocardial excitability; anticholinergic properties
Uses: PVCs, atrial fibrillation, PAT, ventricular tachycardia, atrial flutter, malaria/IV quinidine gluconate

DOSAGE AND ROUTES
Quinidine sulfate
Atrial fibrillation/flutter
• *Adult:* **PO** 200 mg q2-3h × 5-8 doses; may increase daily until sinus rhythm is restored; max 4 g/day given only after digitalization, maintenance 200-300 mg tid-qid or 300-600 mg q8-12h (sus rel)
Paroxysmal supraventricular tachycardia
• *Adult:* **PO** 400-600 mg q2-3h, then 200-300 mg q6-8h or 300-600 mg q8-12h (sus rel)
Premature atrial/ventricular contraction
• *Adult:* **PO** 200-300 mg q6-8h or 300-600 mg (sus rel) q8-12h; max 4 g/day
• *Child:* **PO** 30 mg/kg/day or 900 mg/m^2/day in 5 divided doses
Quinidine gluconate
• *Adult:* **PO** 324-660 mg q6-12h (sus rel); **IM** 600 mg, then 400 mg q2h; **IV** give 16 mg/min
Available forms: *Gluconate* tabs sus rel 324, 330 mg; inj gluconate 80 mg/ml;

sulfate tabs 200, 300 mg; tabs sus rel 300 mg; *polygalacturonate* tabs 275 mg

SIDE EFFECTS
*CNS: **Headache**, **dizziness**,* involuntary movement, confusion, psychosis, restlessness, irritability, syncope, excitement, depression, ataxia
CV: **Hypotension**, *bradycardia*, PVCs, **heart block, cardiovascular collapse, arrest,** torsades de pointes, widening QRS complex, **ventricular tachycardia**
EENT: Cinchonism: tinnitus, blurred vision, hearing loss, mydriasis, disturbed color vision
GI: Nausea, vomiting, anorexia, abdominal pain, *diarrhea,* **hepatotoxicity**
HEMA: **Thrombocytopenia,** hemolytic anemia, agranulocytosis, hypoprothrombinemia
INTEG: Rash, urticaria, **angioedema,** swelling, photosensitivity, flushing with severe pruritus
RESP: Dyspnea, **respiratory depression**
Contraindications: Hypersensitivity, or idiosyncratic response, digitalis toxicity, history of long QT syndrome, drug-induced torsades de pointe, blood dyscrasias, severe heart block, myasthenia gravis
Precautions: Pregnancy (C), lactation, children, renal disease, potassium imbalance, hepatic disease, CHF, respiratory depression, elderly

PHARMACOKINETICS
PO: Peak 0.5-6 hr, duration 6-8 hr; half-life 6-7 hr, metabolized in liver, excreted unchanged (10%-50%) by kidneys, protein bound (80%-90%)

INTERACTIONS
Additive vagolytic effect: anticholinergic blockers
Additive cardiac depression: other antidysrhythmics, phenothiazines, reserpine
Increase: effects of neuromuscular

blockers, digoxin, warfarin, tricyclics, propranolol

Increase: quinidine effects—cimetidine, sodium bicarbonate, carbonic anhydrase inhibitors, antacids, hydroxide suspensions, amiodarone, verapamil

Decrease: quinidine effects—barbiturates, phenytoin, rifampin, nifedipine, sucralfate, cholinergics

Drug/Herb

Hypokalemia, increased antidysrhythmic action: aloe, buckthorn, cascara sagrada, senna

Increase: toxicity, death—aconite

Increase: effect—aloe, broom, chronic buckthorn use, cascara sagrada (chronic use), Chinese rhubarb, figwort, fumitory, goldenseal, kudzu, licorice

Increase: serotonin effect—horehound

Decrease: effect—coltsfoot

Drug/Food

Delayed absorption, decreased metabolism: grapefruit juice

Drug/Lab Test

Increase: CPK

Interference: Triamterene therapy interferes with quinidine test levels

NURSING CONSIDERATIONS

Assess:

⚠ ECG continuously to determine increased PR or QRS segments, QT interval; discontinue or reduce dose

• Blood levels (therapeutic level 2-7 mcg/ml)

• B/P continuously for fluctuations

⚠ For cinchonism: tinnitus, headache, nausea, dizziness, fever, vertigo, tremor; may lead to hearing loss

• Cardiac status: rate, rhythm, character, continuously

• Respiratory status: rate, rhythm, lung fields for crackles; increased respiration, increased pulse; drug should be discontinued

• CNS effects: dizziness, confusion, psychosis, paresthesias, convulsions; drug should be discontinued

Administer:

• AV node blocker (digoxin) before starting quinidine to avoid increased ventricular rate

PO route

• Do not break, crush, or chew ext rel products

• With a full glass of water, on empty stomach; if GI upset occurs, may take with food

• Sus rel forms not interchangeable

IM route

• IM inj in deltoid; aspirate to avoid intravascular administration

IV route

• After diluting 800 mg/50 ml or more D₅; give 16 mg or less over 1 min as inf; use infusion pump

Additive compatibilities: Bretylium, cimetidine, milrinone, ranitidine, verapamil

Y-site compatibilities: Diazepam, milrinone

Evaluate:

• Therapeutic response: decreased dysrhythmias

Teach patient/family:

• That if dizziness, drowsiness occur, avoid driving or hazardous activities

• To use sunglasses; may cause sensitivity to light

• To carry emergency ID stating disease and medication use

• How to take pulse and when to notify prescriber

• To avoid OTC meds unless approved by prescriber

Q

---

quinine (otc, ℞)
(kwye'nine)
Novoquine ✤ quinine sulfate
Func. class.: Antimalarial
Chem. class.: Cinchona tree alkaloid

Action: Inhibits parasite replications, transcription of DNA to RNA by forming complexes with DNA of parasite
Uses: *Plasmodium falciparum*, malaria, nocturnal leg cramps

Side effects: *italics* = common; ***bold italics*** = life-threatening

DOSAGE AND ROUTES

• *Adult:* **PO** 650 mg q8h × 10 days, given with pyrimethamine 25 mg q12h × 3 days, with sulfADIAZINE 500 mg qid × 5 days

• *Child:* **PO** 25 mg/kg/day divided q8h for 3-7 days in conjunction with another agent

Leg cramps

• *Adult:* **PO** 250-300 mg at bedtime

Available forms: Caps 200, 300, 325 mg; tabs 260, 325 mg

SIDE EFFECTS

CNS: Headache, stimulation, fatigue, irritability, **seizures**, bad dreams, dizziness, fever, confusion, anxiety

CV: Angina, dysrhythmias, tachycardia, hypotension, **acute circulatory failure**

EENT: Blurred vision, corneal changes, retinal changes, difficulty focusing, tinnitus, vertigo, deafness, photophobia, diplopia, night blindness

ENDO: Hypoglycemia

GI: Nausea, vomiting, anorexia, diarrhea, epigastric pain

GU: Renal tubular damage, **anuria**

HEMA: **Thrombocytopenia, purpura, hypothrombinemia, hemolysis**

INTEG: Pruritus, pigmentary changes, skin eruptions, lichen planuslike eruptions, flushing, facial edema, sweating

MISC: **Hemolytic uremic syndrome**

RESP: Dyspnea

Contraindications: Pregnancy (X), hypersensitivity, G6PD deficiency, retinal field changes, lactation

Precautions: Blood dyscrasias, severe GI disease, neurologic disease, severe hepatic disease, psoriasis, cardiac dysrhythmias, tinnitus

PHARMACOKINETICS

PO: Peak 1-3 hr, metabolized in liver, excreted in urine, half-life 8-14 hr

INTERACTIONS

Toxicity: $NaHCO_3$, acetaZOLAMIDE

Increase: levels of digoxin, digitoxin, neuromuscular blockers, other anticoagulants

Decrease: absorption—magnesium or aluminum salts

Drug/Lab Test

Increase: 17-KS

Interference: 17-OHCS

NURSING CONSIDERATIONS

Assess:

• B/P, pulse, watch for hypotension, tachycardia

• Hepatic studies qwk: ALT, AST, bilirubin

• Blood studies, CBC, since blood dyscrasias occur

• For cinchonism: nausea, blurred vision, tinnitus, headache, difficulty focusing

Administer:

• Before or after meals at same time each day to maintain level

Perform/provide:

• Storage in tight, light-resistant container

Evaluate:

• Therapeutic response: decreased symptoms of malaria

Teach patient/family:

• Not to breastfeed while taking medication

• To avoid OTC preparations: cold preparations, tonic water

---

rabeprazole (℞)

(rah-bep'rah-zole)

Aciphex

Func. class.: Antiulcer, proton pump inhibitor

Chem. class.: Benzimidazole

Action: Suppresses gastric secretion by inhibiting hydrogen/potassium ATPase enzyme system in gastric parietal cell; characterized as gastric acid pump inhibitor, since it blocks final step of acid production

Uses: Gastroesophageal reflux disease (GERD), severe erosive esophagitis, poorly responsive systemic GERD,

---

pathologic hypersecretory conditions (Zollinger-Ellison syndrome, systemic mastocytosis, multiple endocrine adenomas); treatment of active duodenal ulcers with or without antiinfectives for *Helicobacter pylori;* daytime, nighttime heartburn

DOSAGE AND ROUTES
Healing of duodenal ulcers
• *Adult:* **PO** 20 mg daily × ≤4 wk to be taken after breakfast
Healing of erosive esophagitis or ulcerative GERD
• *Adult:* **PO** 20 mg daily × 4-8 wk
Pathologic hypersecretory conditions
• *Adult:* **PO** 60 mg/day; may increase to 120 mg in 2 divided doses
Available forms: Tabs, del rel 20 mg

SIDE EFFECTS
CNS: Headache, dizziness, asthenia
CV: Chest pain, angina, tachycardia, bradycardia, palpitations, peripheral edema
EENT: Tinnitus, taste perversion
GI: Diarrhea, abdominal pain, vomiting, nausea, constipation, flatulence, acid regurgitation, abdominal swelling, anorexia, irritable colon, esophageal candidiasis, dry mouth
GU: UTI, urinary frequency, increased creatinine, *proteinuria, hematuria,* testicular pain, glycosuria
HEMA: Pancytopenia, thrombocytopenia, neutropenia, leukocytosis, anemia
INTEG: Rash, dry skin, urticaria, pruritus, alopecia
META: Hypoglycemia, increased hepatic enzymes, weight gain
MISC: Back pain, fever, fatigue, malaise
RESP: Upper respiratory infections, cough, epistaxis
Contraindications: Hypersensitivity
Precautions: Pregnancy (C), lactation, children

PHARMACOKINETICS
Eliminated in urine as metabolites and in feces

INTERACTIONS
Increase: serum levels of rabeprazole—benzodiazepines, phenytoin, clarithromycin
Decrease: levels of rabeprazole—sucralfate

NURSING CONSIDERATIONS
Assess:
• GI system: bowel sounds q8h, abdomen for pain, swelling, anorexia
• Hepatic studies: AST, ALT, alk phosphatase during treatment
Administer:
• Do not break, crush, or chew delayed rel tab
• After breakfast daily
Evaluate:
• Therapeutic response: absence of epigastric pain, swelling, fullness
Teach patient/family:
• To report severe diarrhea, drug may have to be discontinued
• That diabetic patient should know hypoglycemia may occur
• To avoid hazardous activities; dizziness may occur
• To avoid alcohol, salicylates, NSAIDs; may cause GI irritation
• To wear sunscreen, protective clothing to prevent burns

radioactive iodine (sodium iodide) ^{131}I (℞)   R
Func. class.: Antithyroid
Chem. class.: Radiopharmaceutical

Action: Converted to protein-bound iodine by thyroid gland for use when needed
Uses:
High dose: Thyroid cancer, hyperthyroidism
Low dose: Visualization to determine thyroid cancer, diagnostic aid in thyroid function studies

DOSAGE AND ROUTES

Thyroid cancer
• *Adult:* **PO** 50-150 mCi, may repeat depending on clinical status
Hyperthyroidism
• *Adult:* **PO** 4-10 mCi, depending on serum thyroxine level
Available forms: Caps 1-50, 0.8-100 mCi; oral sol 7.05 mCi/ml, 3.5-150 mCi/vial

SIDE EFFECTS

EENT: Sore throat, cough
ENDO: Hypothyroidism, ***hyperthyroid adenoma***, transient thyroiditis
GI: Nausea, diarrhea, vomiting
*HEMA: **Eosinophilia, lymphedema, leukemia, bone marrow depression, leukopenia**, anemia*
INTEG: Alopecia
Contraindications: Pregnancy (X), recent MI, lactation, large nodular goiter, age <30 yr, vomiting/diarrhea, acute hyperthyroidism, use of thyroid drugs, lactation

PHARMACOKINETICS

PO: Onset 3-6 days; excreted in urine, sweat, feces, breast milk; crosses placenta; excreted in 56 days

INTERACTIONS

Hypothyroidism: lithium
Decrease: uptake if recent intake of stable iodine, thyroid, antithyroid drugs

NURSING CONSIDERATIONS

Assess:
• Weight daily with same clothing, scale, time of day
• Blood work, including CBC for blood dyscrasias (leukopenia, thrombocytopenia, agranulocytosis)
• Overdose: peripheral edema, heat intolerance, diaphoresis, palpitations, dysrhythmias, severe tachycardia, increased temp, delirium, CNS irritability
• Hypersensitivity: rash, enlarged cervical lymph nodes; drug may have to be discontinued
• Hypoprothrombinemia: bleeding, petechiae, ecchymosis
• Clinical response: after 3 wk should include increased weight, pulse; decreased T_4
• Bone marrow depression: sore throat, fever, fatigue
Administer:
• Only after discontinuing all other antithyroid agents × 5-7 days
• After NPO overnight, food delays action
• During or within 10 days after menstruation
• Do not take antithyroid agents except propranolol, which decreases hyperthyroid symptoms, until total effect of taking ^{131}I has occurred (about 6 wk)
Perform/provide:
• Limited contact with patient ½ hr/day for each person
• Adequate rest after treatment
• Fluids to 3-4 L/day for 48 hr to remove agent from body
Evaluate:
• Therapeutic response: weight gain, decreased pulse, decreased T_4, B/P
Teach patient/family:
• To empty bladder often during treatment; avoid irradiation of gonads
• To report redness, swelling, sore throat, mouth lesions; indicate blood dyscrasias
• To avoid extended contact with children, spouse for 1 wk
• That bathroom may be used by entire family
• To avoid coughing, expectorating for 24 hr (saliva and vomitus are highly radioactive for 6-8 hr)

⚠ Safety alert   *"Tall Man" lettering

raloxifene (℞)

(ral-ox'ih-feen)

Evista

Func. class.: Bone resorption inhibitor, selective estrogen receptor modulator (SERM)

Chem. class.: Benzothiophene

Action: Reduces resorption of bone and decreases bone turnover; mediated through estrogen receptor binding

Uses: Prevention, treatment of osteoporosis in postmenopausal women

DOSAGE AND ROUTES

• *Adult:* **PO** 60 mg daily

Available forms: Tabs 60 mg

SIDE EFFECTS

CNS: Insomnia, migraines, depression, fever

CV: Hot flashes, chest pain

EENT: retinal vein occlusion (rare)

GI: Nausea, vomiting, diarrhea, anorexia, cramps, dyspepsia

GU: Vaginitis, UTI, leukorrhea, cystitis, *hot flashes*

INTEG: Rash, sweating

META: Weight gain, peripheral edema

MS: Arthralgia, myalgia, *leg cramps,* arthritis

RESP: Sinusitis, pharyngitis, increased cough, pneumonia, laryngitis, rhinitis, bronchitis

Contraindications: Pregnancy (X), hypersensitivity, lactation, women with active or history of venous thromboembolic events

Precautions: Venous thromboembolic events, hepatic disease, CV disease, cervical/uterine cancer, elevated triglycerides, pulmonary embolism

PHARMACOKINETICS

Elimination half-life 28-32 hr; excreted in feces; excreted in breast milk; highly bound to plasma proteins

INTERACTIONS

Administer cautiously with other highly protein-bound drugs

Decrease: action of anticoagulants

Decrease: action of raloxifene—ampicillin, cholestyramine

Drug/Lab Test

Increase: Apolipoprotein A_1, corticosteroid-binding globulin, thyroxine-binding globulin (TBG)

Decrease: Calcium, total protein, albumin, platelets, apolipoprotein, fibrinogen, LDL cholesterol, total cholesterol

NURSING CONSIDERATIONS

Assess:

• Weight daily, notify prescriber of weekly weight gain >5 lb

• B/P q4h, watch for increase caused by H_2O and sodium retention

• I&O ratio; decreasing urinary output, increasing edema

• Hepatic studies, including AST, ALT, bilirubin, alk phosphatase

• Bone density test baseline and throughout treatment, bone-specific alk phosphatase, osteocalcin, collagen breakdown

Administer:

• Without regard to meals, vit D

• Add calcium supplement if inadequate

Evaluate:

• Therapeutic response: prevention, treatment of osteoporosis

Teach patient/family:

• To weigh weekly, report gain >5 lb

• To discontinue 72 hr before prolonged bedrest; advise to avoid one position for long periods

• To take calcium supplements, vit D if intake is inadequate

• To increase exercise using weights

• To stop smoking and to decrease alcohol consumption

• That this drug does not help control hot flashes

• To report fever, acute migraine, insomnia, emotional distress; urinary tract infection, or vaginal burning/itching; swelling, warmth, or pain in calves

R

ramelteon
See Appendix A—Selected
New Drugs

ramipril (Ŗ)
(ra-mi'pril)
Altace
Func. class.: Antihypertensive
Chem. class.: Angiotensin-converting
enzyme inhibitor (ACE)

Do not confuse:
Altace/alteplase
Altace/Artane
ramipril/enalapril

Action: Selectively suppresses renin-
angiotensin-aldosterone system; inhibits
ACE, prevents conversion of angiotensin I
to angiotensin II; results in dilation of
arterial, venous vessels

Uses: Hypertension, alone or in combination with thiazide diuretics; CHF (post
MI), reduction in risk of MI, stroke,
death from CV disorders

DOSAGE AND ROUTES

Hypertension
• *Adult:* PO 2.5 mg daily initially, then
2.5-20 mg/day divided bid or daily; *renal impairment:* 1.25 mg daily with
CCr <40 ml/min/1.73 m², increase as
needed to max of 5 mg/day

CHF post-MI
• *Adult:* PO 1.25-2.5 mg bid; may increase to 5 mg bid

**Reduction in risk of MI, stroke,
death**
• *Adult:* PO 2.5 mg daily × 7 days, then
5 mg daily × 21 days; then may increase
to 10 mg/day

Renal dose
• *Adult:* PO CCr <40 ml/min 50% of
dose

Available forms: Caps 1.25, 2.5, 5, 10
mg

SIDE EFFECTS

CNS: Headache, dizziness, anxiety, in-
somnia, paresthesia, *fatigue,* depres-
sion, malaise, vertigo, **seizures**
CV: Hypotension, chest pain, palpita-
tions, angina, syncope, dysrhythmia
EENT: Hearing loss
GI: Nausea, constipation, vomiting, dys-
pepsia, dysphagia, anorexia, diarrhea,
abdominal pain
GU: Proteinuria, increased BUN, creat-
inine, impotence
HEMA: Decreased Hct, Hgb, **eosin-
ophilia, leukopenia**
INTEG: Rash, sweating, photosensitivity,
pruritus
META: Hyperkalemia
MISC: Angioedema
MS: Arthralgia, arthritis, myalgia
RESP: Cough, dyspnea

Contraindications: Pregnancy (D)
2nd/3rd trimester, hypersensitivity to ACE
inhibitors, lactation, children, history of
angioedema

Precautions: Pregnancy (C) 1st trimester, impaired renal, hepatic function;
dialysis patients, hypovolemia, blood
dyscrasias, CHF, COPD, asthma, elderly,
renal artery stenosis

PHARMACOKINETICS

Bioavailability >50%-60%
PO: Onset 1-2 hr, peak 3-6 hr, duration 24%, protein binding 73%, half-
life 1-2 hr, 9-18 hr for active metabolite, metabolized by liver (metabolites
excreted in urine, feces)

INTERACTIONS

Increase: hypotension—diuretics, other
antihypertensives, ganglionic blockers,
adrenergic blockers, nitrates, acute alcohol ingestion
Increase: toxicity—vasodilators, hydrAL-
AZINE, prazosin, potassium-sparing
diuretics, sympathomimetics, potassium
supplements
Increase: serum levels of digoxin, lithium
Decrease: absorption—antacids

Decrease: antihypertensive effect—
indomethacin
Drug/Herb
Increase: toxicity, death—aconite
Increase: antihypertensive effect—
barberry, betony, black catechu, black
cohosh, bloodroot, broom, burdock,
cat's claw, dandelion, goldenseal, Irish
moss, Jamaican dogwood, kelp, khella,
mistletoe, parsley
Increase or decreased: antihypertensive effect—astragalus, cola tree
Decrease: antihypertensive effect—
coltsfoot, guarana, khat, licorice
Drug/Lab Test
False positive: Urine acetone, ANA titer

NURSING CONSIDERATIONS
Assess:
⚠ Blood studies: neutrophils, decreased
platelets; WBC with diff baseline and
periodically q3mo, if neutrophils <1000/
mm^3, discontinue treatment (recommended in collagen-vascular disease)
• B/P, orthostatic hypotension, syncope
• Renal studies: protein, BUN,
creatinine; increased levels may indicate
nephrotic syndrome
• Baselines in renal, hepatic function
tests before therapy begins and
periodically; increased LFTs; uric acid
and glucose may be increased
• Potassium levels, although hyperkalemia rarely occurs
• Dipstick of urine for protein daily in
first morning specimen; if protein is
increased, a 24-hr urinary protein
should be collected
• Edema in feet, legs daily, weight daily
in CHF
⚠ Allergic reactions: rash, fever, pruritus, urticaria; drug should be discontinued if antihistamines fail to help
• Renal symptoms: polyuria, oliguria,
urinary frequency, dysuria
Administer:
• Caps can be opened and added to food
Perform/provide:
• Storage in tight container at 86° F
(30° C) or less
• Supine position for severe hypotension

Evaluate:
• Therapeutic response: decrease in B/P
Teach patient/family:
• Not to discontinue drug abruptly
• Not to use OTC products (cough, cold,
allergy) unless directed by prescriber;
not to use salt substitutes containing
potassium without consulting prescriber
• To comply with dosage schedule, even
if feeling better
• To rise slowly to sitting or standing
position to minimize orthostatic hypotension
• To notify prescriber of mouth sores,
sore throat, fever, swelling of hands or
feet, irregular heartbeat, chest pain
• To report excessive perspiration, dehydration, vomiting, diarrhea; may lead to
fall in B/P
• That drug may cause dizziness, fainting, light-headedness; may occur during
first few days of therapy
• That drug may cause skin rash or
impaired perspiration
• How to take B/P, and normal readings
for age group
Treatment of overdose: 0.9% NaCl
IV inf, hemodialysis

---

ranitidine (R, otc)
(ra-nit'i-deen)
Apo-Ranitidine ✦, Zantac,
Zantac C ✦, Zantac EFFER-
dose, Zantac GELdose
**ranitidine bismuth
citrate**
Tritec
Func. class.: H$_2$-Histamine receptor
antagonist

R

Do not confuse:
Zantac/Xanax
Zantac/Zofran
ranitidine/amantadine
Action: Inhibits histamine at H$_2$-
receptor site in parietal cells, which
inhibits gastric acid secretion
Uses: Duodenal ulcer, Zollinger-Ellison
syndrome, gastric ulcers, hypersecretory

Side effects: *italics* = common; ***bold italics*** = life-threatening

conditions, gastroesophageal reflux disease, stress ulcers, erosive esophagitis (maintenance), active duodenal ulcers with *Helicobacter pylori* in combination with clarithromycin

Investigational uses: Prevention of aspiration pneumonitis, stress ulcers, upper GI bleeding

DOSAGE AND ROUTES

Ranitidine
Renal dose
• *Adult:* CCr <50 ml/min give **PO** q24h give **IM/IV** q8-24h
Duodenal ulcer
• *Adult:* **PO** 150 mg bid, maintenance 150 mg at bedtime
Zollinger-Ellison syndrome
• *Adult:* **PO** 150 mg bid, may increase if needed
Gastric ulcer
• *Adult:* **PO** 150 mg bid × 6 wk, then 150 mg at bedtime
GERD
• *Adult:* **PO** 150 mg bid
Erosive esophagitis
• *Adult:* **PO** 150 mg bid, 300 mg at bedtime; **IM** 50 mg q6-8h; **IV BOL** 50 mg diluted to 20 ml over 5 min q6-8h; **IV INT INF** 50 mg/100 ml D₅ over 15-20 min q6-8h
• *Child:* **PO** 4-5 mg/kg/day divided q8-12h, max 6 mg/kg/day or 300 mg; **IV** 2-4 mg/kg/day divided q6-8h
Ranitidine bismuth citrate
• *Adult:* **PO** 400 mg bid × 4 wk with clarithromycin 500 mg tid × 1st 2 wk
Available forms: Tabs 75, 150, 300 mg; sol for inj 25 mg/ml; tabs, effervescent 75, 150 mg; inj 25 mg/ml; caps 150, 300 mg; syr 15 mg/ml; granules, effervescent 150 mg/packet; ranitidine bismuth citrate: tabs 400 mg

SIDE EFFECTS

CNS: Headache, sleeplessness, dizziness, confusion, agitation, depression, hallucination (elderly)
CV: Tachycardia, bradycardia, PVCs
EENT: Blurred vision, increased ocular pressure

GI: Constipation, abdominal pain, diarrhea, nausea, vomiting, ***hepatotoxicity***
GU: Impotence, gynecomastia
INTEG: Urticaria, rash, fever
Contraindications: Hypersensitivity
Precautions: Pregnancy (B), lactation, child <12 yr, hepatic disease, renal disease

PHARMACOKINETICS

PO: Peak 2-3 hr, duration 8-12 hr; metabolized by liver; excreted in urine, breast milk; half-life 2-3 hr

INTERACTIONS

Increase: absorption, toxicity—anticoagulants, sulfonylureas, procainamide
Decrease: absorption of ranitidine—antacids, diazepam, anticholinergics, metoclopramide

Drug/Lab Test
Increase: AST, ALT, alk phosphatase, creatinine, LDH, bilirubin
False positive: Urine protein

NURSING CONSIDERATIONS

Assess:
• Gastric pH (>5 should be maintained)
• I&O ratio, BUN, creatinine
• Mental status: confusion, dizziness, depression, anxiety, weakness, tremors, psychosis, diarrhea, abdominal discomfort, jaundice; report immediately
• GI complaints: nausea, vomiting, diarrhea, cramps

Administer:
PO route
• With meals for prolonged effect
• Antacids 1 hr before or 1 hr after ranitidine
IV route
• IV after diluting 50 mg/20 ml 0.9% NaCl, D₅W, D₁₀W, LR, NaCO₃ 5% and give 50 mg or less/5 min or more; may dilute 50 mg/50-100 ml of 0.9% NaCl, D₅W, D₁₀W, LR, NaCO₃ 5% and give over 15-20 min

Additive compatibilities: Aceta-ZOLAMIDE, amikacin, aminophylline,

---

chloramphenicol, chlorothiazide, ciprofloxacin, colistimethate, dexamethasone, digoxin, DOBUTamine, DOPamine, doxycycline, epINEPHrine, erythromycin, floxacillin, fluconazole/ondansetron, flumazenil, furosemide, gentamicin, heparin, insulin (regular), isoproterenol, lidocaine, lincomycin, meropenem, methylPREDNISolone, moxalactam, penicillin G potassium, penicillin G sodium, polymyxin B, potassium chloride, protamine, quinidine, sodium nitroprusside, ticarcillin, tobramycin, vancomycin

Syringe compatibilities: Atropine, cyclizine, dexamethasone, dimenhyDRINATE, diphenhydrAMINE, DOBUTamine, DOPamine, fentanyl, glycopyrrolate, hydromorphone, isoproterenol, meperidine, metoclopramide, morphine, nalbuphine, oxymorphone, pentazocine, perphenazine, prochlorperazine, promethazine, scopolamine

Y-site compatibilities: Acyclovir, aldesleukin, allopurinol, amifostine, aminophylline, amsacrine, atracurium, aztreonam, bretylium, cefepime, cefmetazole, ceftazidime, ciprofloxacin, cisatracurium, cisplatin, cladribine, cyclophosphamide, cytarabine, diltiazem, DOBUTamine, DOPamine, DOXOrubicin, DOXOrubicin liposome, enalaprilat, epINEPHrine, esmolol, fentanyl, filgrastim, fluconazole, fludarabine, foscarnet, furosemide, gallium, granisetron, heparin, hydromorphone, idarubicin, labetalol, lorazepam, melphalan, meperidine, methotrexate, midazolam, milrinone, morphine, niCARdipine, nitroglycerin, norepinephrine, ondansetron, paclitaxel, pancuronium, piperacillin, piperacillin/tazobactam, procainamide, propofol, remifentanil, sargramostim, tacrolimus, teniposide, theophylline, thiopental, thiotepa, vecuronium, vinorelbine, warfarin, zidovudine

Perform/provide:
• Storage at room temperature

Evaluate:
• Therapeutic response: decreased abdominal pain

Teach patient/family:
• That gynecomastia, impotence may occur but are reversible
• To avoid driving, other hazardous activities until stabilized on this medication
• To avoid black pepper, caffeine, alcohol, harsh spices, extremes in temperature of food
• That drug must be continued for prescribed time to be effective

---

rasburicase (R)

(rass-burr'i-case)
Elitek
Func. class.: Antineoplastic, antimetabolite
Chem. class.: Recombinant urate-oxidase enzyme

Action: Catalyzes enzymatic oxidation of uric acid into an inactive and a soluble metabolite

Uses: To reduce uric acid levels in children with leukemia, lymphoma, solid tumor malignancies who are receiving chemotherapy

DOSAGE AND ROUTES

• *Adult:* **IV INF** 0.15 or 0.2 mg/kg as a single daily dose given as **IV INF** over ½ hr

Available forms: Powder for inj 1.5 mg/vial

SIDE EFFECTS

CNS: Headache
GI: Nausea, vomiting, anorexia, diarrhea, abdominal pain, constipation, dyspepsia, mucositis
HEMA: **Neutropenia with fever**
SYST: Anaphylaxis, hemolysis, ***methemoglobinemia, sepsis***

Contraindications: Hypersensitivity, G6PD deficiency, hemolytic reactions, or methemoglobinemia reactions to this drug

Precautions: Pregnancy (C), lactation, children <2 yr

R

PHARMACOKINETICS

Elimination half-life 18 hr

NURSING CONSIDERATIONS

Assess:

• Renal studies: BUN, serum uric acid, urine creatinine clearance, electrolytes before and during therapy

• Monitor temp q4h; fever may indicate beginning infection; no rectal temps

• Anaphylaxis, have emergency equipment nearby

• For G6PD deficiency, hemolytic reactions, methemoglobinemia; these patients should not be given this agent

• For toxicity: severe diarrhea, nausea, vomiting

• GI symptoms: frequency of stools, cramping, if severe diarrhea occurs, fluid and electrolytes may need to be given

Administer:

• Antiemetic 30-60 min before giving drug and prn

Evaluate:

• Therapeutic response: decreased uric acid levels

Teach patient/family:

• Reason for therapy, expected results

⚠ High Alert

remifentanil (℞)
(rem-ih-fin'ta-nill)
Ultiva
Func. class.: Opiate agonist analgesic
Chem. class.: μ-Opioid agonist

Controlled Substance Schedule II

Action: Inhibits ascending pain pathways in limbic system, thalamus, midbrain, hypothalamus

Uses: In combination with other drugs in general anesthesia to provide analgesia

DOSAGE AND ROUTES

• *Adult:* Induction **IV** 0.5-1 mcg/kg/min with a hypnotic or volatile agent; maintenance with isoflurane (0.4-1.5 MAC) or propofol (100-200 mcg/kg/min); CONT INF 0.25-0.4 mcg/kg/min

Available forms: Powder for inj lyophilized 1 mg/ml after reconstitution

SIDE EFFECTS

CNS: Drowsiness, *dizziness,* confusion, *headache,* sedation, euphoria, delirium, agitation, anxiety

CV: Palpitations, *bradycardia,* change in B/P, facial flushing, syncope, *asystole*

EENT: Tinnitus, blurred vision, miosis, diplopia

GI: Nausea, vomiting, anorexia, constipation, cramps, dry mouth

GU: Urinary retention, dysuria

INTEG: Rash, urticaria, bruising, flushing, diaphoresis, pruritus

MS: Rigidity

RESP: **Respiratory depression, apnea**

Contraindications: Child <12 yr, hypersensitivity

Precautions: Pregnancy (C), lactation, increased intracranial pressure, acute MI, severe heart disease, renal disease, hepatic disease, asthma, respiratory conditions, convulsive disorders, elderly

PHARMACOKINETICS

Unknown

INTERACTIONS

Respiratory depression, hypotension, profound sedation: alcohol, sedatives, hypnotics, or other CNS depressants; antihistamines, phenothiazines

Drug/Herb
Increase: CNS depression—kava

NURSING CONSIDERATIONS

Assess:

• I&O ratio, check for decreasing output; may indicate urinary retention, especially in elderly

• CNS changes; dizziness, drowsiness, hallucinations, euphoria, LOC, pupil reaction

• Allergic reactions: rash, urticaria

• Respiratory dysfunction: respiratory

---

depression, character, rate, rhythm; notify prescriber if respirations are <12/min; CV status; bradycardia, syncope
• Use pain scoring to determine pain perception

Administer:
• Add 1 ml diluent per mg remifentanil
• Interruption of infusion results in rapid reversal (no residual opioid effect within 5-10 min)

Y-site compatibilities: Acyclovir, alfentanil, amikacin, aminophylline, ampicillin, ampicillin/sulbactam, aztreonam, bretylium, bumetanide, buprenorphine, butorphanol, calcium gluconate, cefazolin, cefepine, cefotaxime, cefotetan, cefoxitin, ceftazidime, ceftizoxime, ceftriaxone, cefuroxime, cimetidine, ciprofloxacin, cisatracurium, cisplatin, clindamycin, dactinomycin, dexamethasone, digoxin, diltiazem, diphenhydrAMINE, DOBUTamine, docetaxel, DOPamine, doxacurium, doxycycline, droperidol, enalaprilat, epINEPHrine, esmolol, etoposide, famotidine, fentanyl, fluconazole, furosemide, ganciclovir, gatiflexacin, gemcitabine, gentamicin, granisetron, haloperidol, heparin, hetastarch, hydrocortisone sodium succinate, hydromorphone, hydrOXYzine, imipenem/cilastatin, inamrinone, isoproterenol, ketorolac, levofloxacin, lidocaine, lorazepam, magnesium sulfate, mannitol, meperidine, methylPREDNISolone sodium succinate, metoclopramide, metronidazole, midazolam, minocycline, morphine, nalbuphine, netilmicin, nitroglycerin, norepinephrine, ofloxacin, ondansetron, paclitaxel, palonsetron, phenylephrine, piperacillin, potassium chloride, procainamide, prochlorperazine, promethazine, ranitidine, sulfentanil, sulfamethoxazole, teniposide, theophylline, thiopental, thiotepa, ticarcillin, ticarcillin/clavulanale, tobramycin, trimethoprim, vancomycin, voriconazole, zidovudine

Solution compatibilities: D$_5$, 0.45% NaCl, LR

Perform/provide:
• Storage in light-resistant area at room temperature

Evaluate:
• Therapeutic response: maintenance of anesthesia

Teach patient/family:
• To call for assistance when ambulating or smoking; drowsiness, dizziness may occur
• To make position changes slowly to prevent orthostatic hypotension

---

repaglinide (R)
(re-pag'lih'nide)
Prandin
Func. class.: Antidiabetic
Chem. class.: Meglitinide

Action: Causes functioning β-cells in pancreas to release insulin, leading to drop in blood glucose levels; closes ATP-dependent potassium channels in the β-cell membrane; this leads to opening of calcium channels; increased calcium influx induces insulin secretion
Uses: Type 2 diabetes mellitus

DOSAGE AND ROUTES
• *Adult:* **PO** 1-2 mg with each meal, max 16 mg/day, adjust at weekly intervals
Available forms: Tabs 0.5, 1, 2 mg

SIDE EFFECTS

CNS: Headache, weakness, paresthesia
ENDO: **Hypoglycemia**
GI: Nausea, vomiting, diarrhea, constipation, dyspepsia
INTEG: Rash, allergic reactions
MISC: Chest pain, UTI, allergy
MS: Back pains, arthralgia
RESP: URI, sinusitis, rhinitis, bronchitis
Contraindications: Hypersensitivity to meglitinides, diabetic ketoacidosis, type 1 diabetes
Precautions: Pregnancy (C), elderly, cardiac disease, severe renal disease, severe hepatic disease, thyroid disease,

R

severe hypoglycemic reactions, lactation, children

PHARMACOKINETICS

PO: Competely absorbed by GI route; onset 30 min, peak 1-1½ hr, duration <4 hr; half-life 1 hr; metabolized in liver; excreted in urine, feces (metabolites); crosses placenta; 98% plasma protein bound

INTERACTIONS

Increase: in both—levonorgestrel/ethinyl estradiol

Increase: repaglinide metabolism—CYP450 inducers: rifampin, barbiturates, carbamazepine

Increase: repaglinide effect—NSAIDs, salicylates, sulfonamides, chloramphenicol, MAOIs, coumarins, β-blockers, probenecid, gemfibrozil, simvastatin

Decrease: repaglinide metabolism—CYP450 inhibitors: antifungals (ketoconazole, miconazole), erythromycin, macrolides

Decrease: repaglinide action—calcium channel blockers, corticosteroids, oral contraceptives, thiazide diuretics, thyroid preparations, estrogens, phenothiazines, phenytoin, rifampin, isoniazid, phenobarbital, sympathomimetics

Drug/Herb

Increase: antidiabetic effect—alfalfa, aloe, basil, bay, bilberry, bitter melon, black catechu, buchu, burdock, coriander, dandelion, eyebright (po), fenugreek, garlic, ginseng, glucomannan, glucosamine, goat's rue, gymnema, horehound, horse chestnut, jambul, myrrh, myrtle

Increase or decrease: hypoglycemic effect—chromium, fenugreek, ginseng

Decrease: hypoglycemic effect—broom, buchu, dandelion, juniper

Decrease: glucose tolerance—karela

Decrease: antidiabetic effect—bee pollen, blue cohosh, broom, chromium, elecampane, eucalyptus, gotu kola

Drug/Food

Decrease: repaglinide level, give before meals

NURSING CONSIDERATIONS

Assess:

⚠ Hypo/hyperglycemic reaction that can occur soon after meals: dizziness, weakness, headache, tremor, anxiety, tachycardia, hunger, sweating, abdominal pain

• $A1_c$, fasting, postprandial glucose during treatment

Administer:

• Up to 15 min before meals; 2, 3, or 4 ×/day preprandially

• Skip dose if meal is skipped; add dose if meal is added

Perform/provide:

• Storage in tight container in cool environment

Evaluate:

• Therapeutic response: decrease in polyuria, polydipsia, polyphagia, clear sensorium, absence of dizziness, stable gait

Teach family/patient:

• Technique of blood glucose monitoring; use blood glucose meter

• The symptoms of hypo/hyperglycemia; what to do about each

• That drug must be continued on daily basis; explain consequences of discontinuing drug abruptly

• To avoid OTC medications unless ordered by prescriber

• That diabetes is a lifelong illness; drug will not cure disease

• That all food included in diet plan must be eaten to prevent hypoglycemia; to have glucagon emergency kit available; take before meals 2, 3, or 4 ×/day

• To carry emergency ID

• To avoid alcohol, explain disulfiram-like reaction

Treatment of overdose: Glucose 25 g IV via dextrose 50% solution, 50 ml or 1 mg glucagon

Rarely Used

reserpine (R)
(re-ser'peen)
Novoreserpine ✦, Reserfia ✦,
reserpine
Func. class.: Antihypertensive, antiadrenergic agent, peripheral action

Uses: Hypertension

DOSAGE AND ROUTES
• *Adult:* **PO** 0.05-0.1 mg daily × 1-2 wk,
then 0.1-0.25 mg daily maintenance
• *Geriatric:* **PO** 0.05 mg daily, increase
by 0.05 weekly to desired dose
Contraindications: Pregnancy (D),
hypersensitivity, depression, suicidal
patients, active peptic ulcer disease,
ulcerative colitis, Parkinson's disease

**Rh$_o$(D) immune
globulin standard dose
IM$_o$** (R)
Gamulin Rh, HydroRho-D,
Rho-GAM

**Rh$_o$(D) globulin
microdose IM** (R)
HypRho-D Mini-Dose,
MiCRhoGAM, Mini-Gamulin

**Rh$_o$(D) globulin
IV** (R)
WinRho SD, WinRho SDF
Func. class.: Immune globulins

Do not confuse:
Gamulin Rh/MICRh$_o$GAM
Action: Suppresses immune response
of nonsensitized Rh$_o$ (D or D^u)-negative
patients who are exposed to Rh$_o$ (D or
D^u)-positive blood
Uses: Prevention of isoimmunization in
Rh-negative women given Rh-positive
blood after abortions, miscarriages,
amniocentesis

DOSAGE AND ROUTES
Prior delivery
• *Adult:* **IM** 1 vial (standard dose) at
26-28 wk, 1 vial (standard dose) 72 hr
after delivery
Pregnancy termination <13 wk
• *Adult:* **IM** 1 vial (microdose) within
72 hr
Pregnancy termination >13 wks
• *Adult:* **IM** 1 vial (standard dose)
within 72 hr
Fetal-maternal hemorrhage
• *Adult:* **IM** packed RBCs volume of
hemorrhage/15 = needed vials (standard
dose)
Following delivery
• *Adult:* **IM** 1 vial (standard dose) if
fetal-packed RBCs <15 ml, or 2 vials if
fetal-packed RBCs >15 ml; give within
72 hr of delivery or miscarriage
Transfusion error
• *Adult:* **IM** (standard dose) give within
72 hr
After 34 wk gestation
• *Adult:* **IM/IV** 120 mcg given within 72
hr (IV dose)
Available forms: Inj single-dose vial
(50 mcg/vial-microdose; 300 mcg/vial-
standard); inj 120, 300 mcg Rh$_o$ (D)
immune globulin IV, human

SIDE EFFECTS
CNS: Lethargy
INTEG: Irritation at inj site, fever
MS: Myalgia
Contraindications: Previous immuni-
zation with this drug, Rh$_o$ (O)-positive/
D^u-positive patient
Precautions: Pregnancy (C)

INTERACTIONS
Decrease: antibody response—live
virus vaccines

NURSING CONSIDERATIONS
Assess:
🄰 Allergies, reactions to immunizations;
previous immunization with this drug
🄰 For intravascular hemolysis: back

R

---

pain, chills, hemoglobinuria, renal insufficiency

• Type, crossmatch mother and newborn's cord blood; if mother is Rh₀ (D) negative, Dᵘ-negative and newborn Rh₀ (D) positive, this medication should be given

Administer:

IM route

• Reconstitute Rh₀(D) immune globulin IV using 1.25 ml of 0.9% NaCl, swirl

• IM inj in deltoid; aspirate within 3 hr if possible

• Only equal lot numbers of drug, crossmatch

• Only MICRhoGAM for abortions or miscarriages <12 wk unless fetus or father is Rh negative; unless patient is Rh₀ (D)-positive, Dᵘ-positive, Rh antibodies are present

• Do not use Rh₀(D) immune globulin or Rh₀(D) immune globulin micro dose by IV

IV, direct route

• Reconstitute Rh₀(D) immune globulin IV using 2.5 ml of 0.9% NaCl, swirl, give over 3-5 min

Perform/provide:

• Storage in refrigerator

Evaluate:

• Rh₀ (D) sensitivity in transfusion error, prevention of erythroblastosis fetalis for normal vision

Teach patient/family:

• How drug works; that drug must be given after subsequent deliveries if subsequent babies are Rh positive

---

riboflavin (vit B₂)
(otc)
(rye′boh-flay-vin)
Func. class.: Vit B₂, water soluble

Action: Needed for respiratory reactions by catalyzing proteins

Uses: Vit B₂ deficiency or polyneuritis; cheilosis adjunct with thiamine

DOSAGE AND ROUTES

Deficiency

• *Adult and child >12 yr:* **PO** 5-25 mg daily

• *Child <12 yr:* **PO** 2-10 mg daily, then 0.6 mg/1000 calories ingested

RDA

• *Adult:* males 1.4-1.8 mg, females 1.2-1.3 mg

Available forms: Tabs 5, 10, 25, 50, 100, 250 mg

SIDE EFFECTS

GU: Yellow discoloration of urine

Precautions: Pregnancy (A)

PHARMACOKINETICS

PO: Half-life 65-85 min, 60% protein bound, unused amounts excreted in urine (unchanged)

INTERACTIONS

Increase: riboflavin need—alcohol, probenecid, tricyclics, phenothiazines

Decrease: action of tetracyclines

Drug/Lab Test

May cause false elevations of urinary catecholamines

NURSING CONSIDERATIONS

Assess:

• Nutritional status: liver, eggs, dairy products, yeast, whole grain, green vegetables

Administer:

• With food for better absorption

Perform/provide:

• Storage in airtight, light-resistant container

Evaluate:

• Therapeutic response: absence of headache, GI problems, cheilosis, skin lesions, depression, burning, itchy eyes, anemia

Teach patient/family:

• That urine may turn bright yellow

• About addition of needed foods that are rich in riboflavin

• To avoid alcohol

---

rifabutin (℞)
(riff'a-byoo-ten)
Mycobutin
Func. class.: Antimycobacterial agent
Chem. class.: Rifamycin S derivative

Do not confuse:
rifabutin/rifampin

Action: Inhibits DNA-dependent RNA polymerase in susceptible strains of *Escherichia coli* and *Bacillus subtilis;* mechanism of action against *Mycobacterium avium* unknown

Uses: Prevention of *M. avium* complex (MAC) in patients with advanced HIV infection

Investigational uses: *Helicobacter pylori* that has not responded to other treatment

DOSAGE AND ROUTES

• *Adult:* 300 mg daily (may take as 150 mg bid)

Available forms: Caps 150 mg

SIDE EFFECTS

CNS: Headache, fatigue, anxiety, confusion, insomnia

GI: Nausea, vomiting, anorexia, diarrhea, heartburn, **hepatitis,** discolored saliva

GU: Hematuria, *discolored urine*

HEMA: **Hemolytic anemia, eosinophilia, thrombocytopenia, leukopenia**

INTEG: Rash

MISC: Flulike symptoms, shortness of breath, chest pressure

MS: Asthenia, arthralgia, myalgia

Contraindications: Hypersensitivity, active TB, WBC <1000/mm³ or platelet count <50,000/mm³

Precautions: Pregnancy (B), lactation, hepatic disease, blood dyscrasias, children

PHARMACOKINETICS

PO: Peak 2-3 hr, duration >24 hr, half-life 3 hr; metabolized in liver (active/inactive metabolites), excreted in urine primarily as metabolites

INTERACTIONS

Increase: levels of rifabutin: ritonavir
Decrease: action of amprenavir, anticoagulants, β-blockers, barbiturates, clofibrate, corticosteroids, cycloSPORINE, dapsone, delavirdine, digoxin, disopyramide, efavirenz, estrogens, fluconazole, indinavir, ketoconazole, nelfinavir, nevirapine, opioid analgesic, oral contraceptives, phenytoin, quinidine, saquinavir, sulfonylureas, theophylline, tocainide, verapamil, zidovudine

Drug/Food
High-fat diet decreases absorption

Drug/Lab Test
Interference: Folate level, vit B_{12}, BSP, gallbladder studies

NURSING CONSIDERATIONS

Assess:

• CBC for neutropenia, thrombocytopenia, eosinophilia

• For acute TB: chest x-ray, sputum culture, blood culture, biopsy of lymph nodes, PPD; drug should not be given for active TB

• Signs of anemia: Hct, Hgb, fatigue

• Hepatic studies qwk: ALT, AST, bilirubin

• Renal status before, qmo: BUN, creatinine, output, specific gravity, urinalysis

• Hepatic status: decreased appetite, jaundice, dark urine, fatigue

Administer:

• With food if GI upset occurs; better to take on empty stomach 1 hr ac or 2 hr pc, high-fat foods slow absorption, may take in 2 divided doses

• Antiemetic if vomiting occurs

• After C&S is completed; qmo to detect resistance

R

Evaluate:

• Therapeutic response: not used for active TB because of risk of development of resistance to rifampin; culture negative

Teach patient/family:

• That patients using oral contraceptives should consider using non-hormonal methods of birth control, since rifabutin may decrease their efficacy

• That compliance with dosage schedule, duration is necessary

• That scheduled appointments must be kept; relapse may occur

• That urine, feces, saliva, sputum, sweat, tears may be colored red-orange; soft contact lenses may be permanently stained

• To report flulike symptoms: excessive fatigue, anorexia, vomiting, sore throat; unusual bleeding, yellowish discoloration of skin, eyes

• To report myositis: muscle or bone pain

---

rifampin (R)

(rif′am-pin)
Rifadin, Rimactane, Rofact ✤
Func. class.: Antitubercular
Chem. class.: Rifamycin B derivative

Do not confuse:
rifampin/rifabutin

Action: Inhibits DNA-dependent polymerase, decreases tubercle bacilli replication

Uses: Pulmonary tuberculosis, meningococcal carriers (prevention)

Research note: Repaglinide given with rifampin resulted in the decrease of repaglinide levels

DOSAGE AND ROUTES

Tuberculosis

• *Adult:* **PO/IV** max 600 mg/day as single dose 1 hr ac or 2 hr pc or 10 mg/kg/day 2-3 ×/wk

• *Child >5 yr:* **PO/IV** 10-20 mg/kg/day as single dose 1 hr ac or 2 hr pc, not to exceed 600 mg/day, with other antituberculars

• 6-mo regimen: 2 mo treatment of isoniazid, rifampin, pyrazinamide and possibly streptomycin or ethambutol; then rifampin and isoniazid × 4 mo

• 9-mo regimen: rifampin and isoniazid supplemented with pyrazinamide, or streptomycin or ethambutol

Meningococcal carriers

• *Adult:* **PO/IV** 600 mg bid × 2 days

• *Child >5 yr:* **PO/IV** 10-20 mg/kg not to exceed 600 mg/dose

• *Infant 3 mo-1 yr:* 5 mg/kg **PO** bid for 2 days

Prevention of H. influenzae *type B infection*

• *Adult:* **PO** 600 mg/day × 4 days

• *Child:* **PO** 20 mg/kg/day × 4 days

Available forms: Caps 150, 300 mg; powder for inj 600 mg/vial

SIDE EFFECTS

CNS: Headache, fatigue, anxiety, drowsiness, confusion

EENT: Visual disturbances

GI: Nausea, vomiting, anorexia, diarrhea, pseudomembranous colitis, heartburn, sore mouth and tongue, *pancreatitis,* increased LFTs

GU: Hematuria, acute renal failure, hemoglobinuria

HEMA: Hemolytic anemia, eosinophilia, thrombocytopenia, leukopenia

INTEG: Rash, pruritus, urticaria

MISC: Flulike symptoms, menstrual disturbances, edema, shortness of breath

MS: Ataxia, weakness

Contraindications: Hypersensitivity

Precautions: Pregnancy (C), lactation, hepatic disease, blood dyscrasias, child <5 yr

PHARMACOKINETICS

PO: Peak 2-3 hr, duration >24 hr, half-life 3 hr; metabolized in liver (active/inactive metabolites), excreted in urine as free drug (30% crosses placenta) and breast milk

---

⚠ Safety alert   *“Tall Man” lettering

INTERACTIONS

Lithium toxicity: lithium
Hepatotoxicity: isoniazid
Incompatible with sodium lactate
Decrease: action of acetaminophen, alcohol, anticoagulants, antidiabetics, β-blockers, barbiturates, benzodiazepines, chloramphenicol, clofibrate, corticosteroids, cycloSPORINE, dapsone, digoxin, diltiazem, doxycycline, fluoroquinolones, haloperidol, hormones, imidazole antifungals, NIFEdipine, oral contraceptives, phenytoin, protease inhibitors, sulfonamides, theophylline, verapamil, zidovudine

Drug/Lab Test

Interference: Folate level, vit B_{12}, gallbladder studies, dexamethasone suppression test

False positive: Direct Coombs' test

NURSING CONSIDERATIONS

Assess:
• For infection: sputum culture, lung sounds
• Signs of anemia: Hct, Hgb, fatigue
• Hepatic studies qmo: ALT, AST, bilirubin
• Renal status before, qmo: BUN, creatinine, output, specific gravity, urinalysis
• Hepatic status: decreased appetite, jaundice, dark urine, fatigue

Administer:
• After C&S is completed; qmo to detect resistance

PO route
• On empty stomach, 1 hr ac or 2 hr pc with a full glass of water
• Antiemetic if vomiting occurs

IV route
• After diluting each 600 mg/10 ml of sterile water for inj (60 mg/ml), agitate, withdraw dose and dilute in 100 ml or 500 ml of D_5W or 0.9% NaCl given as an inf over 3 hr, or if diluted in 100 ml, give over ½ hr; do not admix with other sol or medications

Evaluate:
• Therapeutic response: decreased symptoms of TB, culture negative

Teach patient/family:
• That compliance with dosage schedule, duration is necessary
• That scheduled appointments must be kept; relapse may occur
• To avoid alcohol, hepatotoxicity may occur
• That urine, feces, saliva, sputum, sweat, tears may be colored red-orange; soft contact lenses may be permanently stained
• To report flulike symptoms: excessive fatigue, anorexia, vomiting, sore throat; unusual bleeding, yellowish discoloration of skin, eyes
• To use nonhormonal form of birth control

---

rifapentine (℞)
(riff'ah-pen-teen)
Priftin
Func. class.: Antitubercular
Chem. class.: Rifamycin derivative

Action: Inhibits DNA-dependent polymerase, decreases tubercle bacilli replication

Uses: Pulmonary tuberculosis, must be used with at least one other antitubercular agent

DOSAGE AND ROUTES

Intensive phase
• *Adult:* **PO** 600 mg (four 150-mg tabs 2 ×/wk), with an interval of 72 hr between doses × 2 mo; must be given with at least one other antitubercular agent

Continuation phase
• *Adult:* **PO** 600 mg qwk × 4 mo in combination with isoniazid or other appropriate antitubercular

Available forms: Tabs 150 mg

SIDE EFFECTS

CNS: Headache, fatigue, anxiety, dizziness
EENT: Visual disturbances
GI: Nausea, vomiting, anorexia, diar-

R

rhea, bilirubinemia, hepatitis, increased ALT, AST, *heartburn,* **pancreatitis**
GU: **Hematuria,** pyuria, **proteinuria,** urinary casts, urine discoloration
HEMA: **Thrombocytopenia, leukopenia, neutropenia, lymphopenia,** anemia, **leukocytosis,** purpura, hematoma
INTEG: Rash, pruritus, urticaria, acne
MISC: Edema, aggressive reaction, increased B/P
MS: Gout, arthrosis

Contraindications: Hypersensitivity to rifamycins, porphyria
Precautions: Pregnancy (C), lactation, hepatic disease, blood dyscrasias, children <12 yr, HIV, elderly

PHARMACOKINETICS

PO: Peak 5-6 hr, half-life 13 hr; metabolized in liver (active/inactive metabolites), excreted in urine and feces, excreted in breast milk, protein binding 97%, steady state 10 days, CYP450 3A4, 2C8/9 inducer

INTERACTIONS

Use with extreme caution with protease inhibitors
Decrease: action of amitriptyline, anticoagulants, antidiabetics, barbiturates, β-blockers, chloramphenicol, clarithromycin, clofibrate, corticosteroids, cycloSPORINE, dapsone, delavirdine, diazepam, digoxin, diltiazem, disopyramide, doxycycline, fentanyl, fluconazole, fluoroquinolones, haloperidol, indinavir, itraconazole, ketoconazole, methadone, mexiletine, nelfinavir, NIFEdipine, nortriptyline, oral contraceptives, phenothiazines, phenytoin, progestins, quinidine, quinine, ritonavir, saquinavir, sildenafil, tacrolimus, theophylline, thyroid preparations, tocainide, verapamil, warfarin, zidovudine
Drug/Food
Increase: absorption with food
Drug/Lab Test
Interference: Folate level, vit B_{12}

NURSING CONSIDERATIONS
Assess:
• Baselines in CBC, AST, ALT, bilirubin, platelets
• For infection: sputum culture, lung sounds
• Signs of anemia: Hct, Hgb, fatigue
• Hepatic studies qmo: ALT, AST, bilirubin
• Renal status qmo: BUN, creatinine, output, specific gravity, urinalysis
• Hepatic status: decreased appetite, jaundice, dark urine, fatigue
Administer:
PO route
• May give with food for GI upset
• Antiemetic if vomiting occurs
• After C&S is completed; qmo to detect resistance
Evaluate:
• Therapeutic response: decreased symptoms of TB, culture negative
Teach patient/family:
• That compliance with dosage schedule, duration is necessary
• That scheduled appointments must be kept; relapse may occur
• That urine, feces, saliva, sputum, sweat, tears may be colored red-orange; soft contact lenses, dentures may be permanently stained
• To use alternative method of contraception, oral contraceptive action may be decreased
• To report flulike symptoms: excessive fatigue, anorexia, vomiting, sore throat; unusual bleeding, yellowish discoloration of skin, eyes

---

rifaximin (℞)
(rif-ax′i-min)
Xifaxan
Func. class.: Antiinfective—miscellaneous
Chem. class.: Analog of rifampin

Action: Binds to bacterial DNA–dependent RNA polymerase, thereby inhibiting bacterial R synthesis

---

⚠ Safety alert   *"Tall Man" lettering

Uses: Traveler's diarrhea in those ≥12 yr, caused by *E. coli*

DOSAGE AND ROUTES

• *Adult and child ≥12 yr:* **PO** 200 mg tid × 3 days without regard to meals
Available forms: Tabs 200 mg

SIDE EFFECTS

CNS: Abnormal dreams, dizziness, insomnia
GI: Abdominal pain, constipation, defecation urgency, flatulence, nausea, rectal tenesmus, vomiting
MISC: Headache, pyrexia
Contraindications: Hypersensitivity
Precautions: Pregnancy (C), lactation, children

PHARMACOKINETICS

Half life 6 hr, induces P4503A4 (CYP3A4), excreted in feces

INTERACTIONS

None known

NURSING CONSIDERATIONS
Assess:
• For GI symptoms: amount, character of diarrhea, abdominal pain, nausea, vomiting
A For overgrowth of infection and pseudomembranous colitis
Administer:
• Without regard to food
Evaluate:
• Therapeutic response: absence of infection
Teach patient/family:
• To discontinue rifaximin and notify prescriber if diarrhea persists for more than 24-48 hr, if diarrhea worsens, or if blood is in stools and fever is present

---

riluzole (R)
(rill'you-zole)
Rilutek
Func. class.: ALS agent
Chem. class.: Benzathiazole

Action: May act by modulating the release of glutamate and inactivating voltage-dependent sodium channels
Uses: Amyotropic lateral sclerosis (ALS)

DOSAGE AND ROUTES

• *Adult:* **PO** 50 mg q12h, take 1 hr ac or 2 hr pc
Available forms: Tabs 50 mg

SIDE EFFECTS

CNS: Hypertonia, depression, dizziness, insomnia, somnolence, vertigo
CV: Hypertension, tachycardia, phlebitis, palpitation, postural hypertension
GI: Nausea, vomiting, dyspepsia, anorexia, diarrhea, flatulence, stomatitis, dry mouth, increased LFTs, jaundice
GU: UTI, dysuria
*HEMA: **Neutropenia***
INTEG: Pruritus, eczema, alopecia, ***exfoliative dermatitis***
RESP: Decreased lung function, rhinitis, increased cough
Contraindications: Hypersensitivity
Precautions: Pregnancy (C), neutropenia, renal disease, hepatic disease, elderly, lactation, children, cigarette smoking

PHARMACOKINETICS

Well absorbed, extensively metabolized by the liver, excretion in urine/feces

INTERACTIONS

Increase: elimination of riluzole—cigarette smoking, rifampin, omeprazole, charcoal-broiled food
Increase: hepatic injury—allopurinol, methyldopa, sulfasalazine, leflunomide, methotrexate, tacrine
Increase: LFTs—barbiturates, carbamazepine

R

Side effects: *italics* = common; ***bold italics*** = life-threatening

Decrease: elimination of riluzole—caffeine, theophylline, amitriptyline, quinolones

Drug/Food

High fat meal: decreased absorption

NURSING CONSIDERATIONS

Assess:

• Hepatic studies: AST, ALT, bilirubin, GGT, baseline and qmo × 3 mo, then q3mo; monitor liver chemistries

• For neutropenia <500/mm

Administer:

• 1 hr ac or 2 hr pc; a high-fat meal decreases absorption

Teach patient/family:

• To report febrile illness, which may indicate neutropenia

• The reason for drug and expected results

---

rimantadine (℞)

(ri-man'tah-deen)
Flumadine
Func. class.: Synthetic antiviral
Chem. class.: Tricyclic amine

Do not confuse:

rimantadine/amantadine/ranitidine

Action: Prevents uncoating of nucleic acid in viral cell, preventing penetration of virus to host; causes release of dopamine from neurons

Uses: Prophylaxis or treatment of influenza type A

DOSAGE AND ROUTES

Renal/hepatic dose

• Reduce dose as needed

Influenza type A

Prophylaxis

• *Adult and child >10 yr:* **PO** 100 mg bid; in renal, hepatic disease, lower dose to 100 mg/day

• *Child 1-10 yr:* **PO** 5 mg/kg/day, not to exceed 150 mg

Treatment

• *Adult:* **PO** 100 mg bid; in renal or hepatic disease, lower dose to 100 mg/day; start treatment at onset of symptoms, continue for at least 1 wk

• *Geriatric:* **PO** 100 mg/day × 5-7 days

Available forms: Tabs 100 mg; syr 50 mg/5 ml

SIDE EFFECTS

CNS: Headache, dizziness, fatigue, depression, hallucinations, tremors, *seizures,* insomnia, poor concentration, asthenia, gait abnormalities, *anxiety,* confusion

CV: Pallor, palpitations, edema

EENT: Tinnitus, taste abnormality, eye pain

GI: Nausea, vomiting, constipation, *dry mouth, anorexia, abdominal pain,* diarrhea, dyspepsia

INTEG: Rash

Contraindications: Hypersensitivity to drugs of adamantine class (this drug, amantadine)

Precautions: Pregnancy (C), seizure disorders, hepatic disease, renal disease, lactation, children <1 yr

PHARMACOKINETICS

PO: Peak 6 hr, elimination half-life 25½ hr, plasma protein binding (40%)

INTERACTIONS

Increase: rimantadine concentration—cimetidine

Decrease: peak concentration of rimantadine—acetaminophen, aspirin

NURSING CONSIDERATIONS

Assess:

• Assess for seizures; if seizures occur, drug should be discontinued

• Bowel pattern before, during treatment

• CNS effect in elderly or patients with severe hepatic/renal disease

• Skin eruptions, photosensitivity after administration of drug

• Respiratory status: rate, character, wheezing, tightness in chest

---

- Allergies before initiation of treatment, reaction of each medication; list allergies on chart in bright red letters
- Signs of infection

Administer:
- Within 48 hr of exposure to influenza; continue for 10 days after contact
- At least 4 hr before bedtime to prevent insomnia
- After meals for better absorption, to decrease GI symptoms
- In divided doses to prevent CNS disturbances: headache, dizziness, fatigue, drowsiness

Perform/provide:
- Storage in tight, dry container

Evaluate:
- Therapeutic response: absence of fever, malaise, cough, dyspnea in infection

Teach patient/family:
- About aspects of drug therapy: need to report dyspnea, dizziness, poor concentration, behavioral changes
- To avoid hazardous activities if dizziness occurs

rimexolone ophthalmic
See Appendix C

risedronate (℞)
(rih-sed′roh-nate)
Actonel
Func. class.: Bone resorption inhibitor
Chem. class.: Bisphosphonate

Action: Inhibits bone resorption, absorbs calcium phosphate crystal in bone and may directly block dissolution of hydroxyapatite crystals of bone
Uses: Paget's disease, prevention, treatment of osteoporosis in postmenopausal women, glucocorticoid-induced osteoporosis

DOSAGE AND ROUTES
Paget's disease
- *Adult:* **PO** 30 mg daily × 2 mo; patients with Paget's disease should receive calcium and vit D if dietary intake is lacking; if relapse occurs, retreatment is advised

Postmenopausal osteoporosis
- *Adult:* **PO** 5 mg daily or 35 mg qwk

Glucocorticoid osteoporosis
- *Adult:* **PO** 5 mg daily

Available forms: Tabs 5, 30, 35 mg

SIDE EFFECTS
CNS: Dizziness, headache, depression
CV: Chest pain, hypertension
GI: Abdominal pain, anorexia, diarrhea, nausea, constipation
MISC: Rash, UTI, pharyngitis
MS: Bone pain, arthralgia

Contraindications: Hypersensitivity to bisphosphonates, inability to stand or sit upright for ≥30 min
Precautions: Pregnancy (C), children, lactation, renal disease, active upper GI disorders

PHARMACOKINETICS
Rapidly cleared from circulation, taken up mainly by bones, eliminated primarily through kidneys

INTERACTIONS
Increase: GI irritation—NSAIDs, salicylates
Decrease: absorption of risedronate—calcium supplements, antacids
Drug/Food
Decrease: bioavailability—take ½ hr before food or drinks other than water
Drug/Lab Test
Interference: Bone-imaging agents

NURSING CONSIDERATIONS
Assess:
- Symptoms of Paget's disease: headache, bone pain, increased head circumference
- Electrolytes: renal function studies; Ca, P, Mg, K

R

♣ Canada only   Side effects: *italics* = common; ***bold italics*** = life-threatening

• For hypercalcemia: paresthesia, twitching, laryngospasm, Chvostek's, Trousseau's signs

Administer:

• For 2 months to be effective in Paget's disease

• With a full glass of water, patient should be in upright position for ½ hr

• Supplemental calcium and vit D in Paget's disease

• Give daily ≥30 min ac

Perform/provide:

• Storage in cool environment, out of direct sunlight

Evaluate:

• Therapeutic response: increased bone mass, absence of fractures

Teach patient/family:

• To sit upright for ½ hr after dose to prevent irritation

• To comply with diet

• To notify prescriber if pregnancy is suspected

---

risperidone (Ŗ)

(ris-pehr'ih-dohn)
Risperdal, Risperdal M-TAB
Func. class.: Antipsychotic
Chem. class.: Benzisoxazole derivative

Do not confuse:
Risperdal/reserpine

Action: Unknown; may be mediated through both dopamine type 2 (D_2) and serotonin type 2 (5-HT_2) antagonism

Uses: Psychotic disorders

Research note: Risperidone given with paroxetine resulted in an increase of risperidone levels

DOSAGE AND ROUTES

• *Adult:* **PO** 1 mg bid, with incremental increases of 1 mg bid on days 2 and 3 to a dose of 3 mg bid by day 3; then do not increase dose for at least 1 wk; **PO** (orally disintegrating) Do not open blister pack until ready to use. Tear 1 of the 4 units apart at perforation, bend corner where indicated, peel back foil, do not

push tab through foil, remove from pack and place on the tongue, tab disintegrates in seconds and can be swallowed with or without liquids.

• *Geriatric:* **PO** 0.5 mg daily-bid, increase by 1 mg qwk

Hepatic/renal dose

• *Adult:* **PO** 0.5 mg bid, increase by 0.5 mg bid, increase to 1.5 mg bid

Available forms: Tabs 1, 2, 3, 4 mg; oral sol 1 mg/ml; tabs, orally disintegrating 0.5, 1, 2 mg

SIDE EFFECTS

CNS: EPS, *pseudoparkinsonism, akathisia, dystonia, tardive dyskinesia; drowsiness, insomnia, agitation, anxiety, headache,* **seizures, neuroleptic malignant syndrome,** dizziness

CV: Orthostatic hypotension, **tachycardia**

EENT: Blurred vision

GI: Nausea, vomiting, *anorexia, constipation,* jaundice, weight gain

RESP: Rhinitis

Contraindications: Hypersensitivity, lactation, seizure disorders

Precautions: Pregnancy (C), children, renal disease, hepatic disease, elderly, breast cancer

PHARMACOKINETICS

PO: Extensively metabolized by liver to a major active metabolite, plasma protein binding 90%

INTERACTIONS

Increase: sedation—other CNS depressants, alcohol

Increase: EPS—other antipsychotics

Increase: risperidone excretion—carbamazepine

Decrease: levodopa effect—levodopa

Drug/Herb

Increase: CNS depression—kava

Increase: action—cola tree, hops, nettle, nutmeg

Increase: EPS—betel palm, kava

Drug/Lab Test

Increase: Prolactin levels

⚠ Safety alert   *"Tall Man" lettering

NURSING CONSIDERATIONS

Assess:

• Mental status before initial administration

• Swallowing of PO medication; check for hoarding or giving of medication to other patients

• I&O ratio; palpate bladder if urinary output is low

• Bilirubin, CBC, hepatic studies qmo

• Urinalysis before, during prolonged therapy

• Affect, orientation, LOC, reflexes, gait, coordination, sleep pattern disturbances

• B/P standing and lying; also pulse, respirations; take these q4h during initial treatment; establish baseline before starting treatment; report drops of 30 mm Hg; watch for ECG changes

• Dizziness, faintness, palpitations, tachycardia on rising

• EPS, including akathisia, tardive dyskinesia (bizarre movements of the jaw, mouth, tongue, extremities), pseudoparkinsonism (rigidity, tremors, pill rolling, shuffling gait)

⚠ For neuroleptic malignant syndrome: hyperthermia, increased CPK, altered mental status, muscle rigidity

• Skin turgor daily

• Constipation, urinary retention daily; if these occur, increase bulk and water in diet

Administer:

• Reduced dose in elderly

• Antiparkinsonian agent on order from prescriber, to be used for EPS

• Avoid use with CNS depressants

Perform/provide:

• Decreased stimulus by dimming lights, avoiding loud noises

• Supervised ambulation until patient is stabilized on medication; do not involve in strenuous exercise program because fainting is possible; patient should not stand still for a long time

• Increased fluids to prevent constipation

• Sips of water, candy, gum for dry mouth

• Storage in tight, light-resistant container

Evaluate:

• Therapeutic response: decrease in emotional excitement, hallucinations, delusions, paranoia; reorganization of patterns of thought, speech

Teach patient/family:

• That orthostatic hypotension may occur and to rise from sitting or lying position gradually

• To avoid hot tubs, hot showers, tub baths; hypotension may occur

• To avoid abrupt withdrawal of this drug; EPS may result; drug should be withdrawn slowly

• To avoid OTC preparations (cough, hay fever, cold) unless approved by prescriber; serious drug interactions may occur; avoid use of alcohol; increased drowsiness may occur

• To avoid hazardous activities if drowsy or dizzy

• Compliance with drug regimen

• To report impaired vision, tremors, muscle twitching

• In hot weather, that heat stroke may occur; take extra precautions to stay cool

• To use contraception, inform prescriber if pregnancy is planned or suspected

Treatment of overdose: Lavage if orally ingested; provide airway; *do not induce vomiting*

R

ritodrine (℞)

(rih'toh-dreen)
ritodrine, Yutopar
Func. class.: Tocolytic, uterine relaxant
Chem. class.: β₂-Adrenergic agonist

Action: Reduces frequency, intensity of uterine contractions by stimulation of the β_2-receptors in uterine smooth muscle
Uses: Management of preterm labor

DOSAGE AND ROUTES

• *Adult:* **IV INF** 150 mg/500 ml (0.3 mg/ml) given 0.1 mg/min, increased gradually by 0.05 mg/min q10min until desired response, max 0.35 mg/min

Available forms: Inj 10 mg/ml, 15 mg/ml

SIDE EFFECTS

CNS: Headache, restlessness, anxiety, nervousness, sweating, chills, drowsiness, tremor

CV: Altered maternal, fetal heart rate, B/P, dysrhythmias, palpitations, chest pain, maternal pulmonary edema

GI: Nausea, vomiting, anorexia, malaise, bloating, constipation, diarrhea

META: Hyperglycemia, hypokalemia

MISC: Erythema, rash, dyspnea, hyperventilation, glycosuria, *lactic acidosis*

Contraindications: Hypersensitivity, eclampsia, hypertension, dysrhythmias, thyrotoxicosis, before 20th wk of pregnancy, antepartum hemorrhage, intrauterine fetal death, maternal cardiac disease, pulmonary hypertension, uncontrolled diabetes, pheochromocytoma, bronchial asthma

Precautions: Pregnancy (B), migraine, sulfite sensitivity, pregnancy-induced hypertension, diabetes

PHARMACOKINETICS

IV: Immediate, distribution half-life 6 min, 2nd phase 1½-2½ hr, elimination phase >10 hr; metabolized in liver; 90% excreted in urine; crosses placenta

INTERACTIONS

Pulmonary edema: corticosteroids

Systemic hypertension: atropine

Increase: CV effects of ritodrine—magnesium sulfate, diazoxide, meperidine, potent general anesthetics

Increase: effects of sympathomimetic amines

Decrease: action of ritodrine—β-blockers

Drug/Lab Test

Increase: blood glucose, free fatty acids, insulin, GTT

Decrease: potassium

NURSING CONSIDERATIONS

Assess:

• Maternal, fetal heart tones during infusion; maternal ECG to determine CV disease

• Intensity, length of uterine contractions

• Fluid intake to prevent fluid overload; discontinue if this occurs

• Blood glucose in diabetics

Administer:

• Only clear sol

• After dilution: 150 mg/500 ml D_5W or NS, give at 0.3 mg/ml

• Using infusion pump

• Considered incompatible with any drug in sol or syringe

• In bed during infusion

Perform/provide:

• Positioning of patient in left lateral recumbent position to decrease hypotension, increase renal blood flow

Evaluate:

• Therapeutic response: decreased intensity, length of contraction, absence of preterm labor, decreased B/P

---

ritonavir (℞)

(ri-toe′na-veer)

Norvir

Func. class.: Antiretroviral

Chem. class.: Protease inhibitor

Do not confuse:

ritonavir/retrovir

Action: Inhibits human immunodeficiency virus (HIV-1) protease and prevents maturation of the infectious virus

Uses: HIV-1 in combination with other antiretrovirals

DOSAGE AND ROUTES

• *Adult:* **PO** 600 mg bid. If nausea occurs begin dose at ½ and gradually increase

• *Child 2-16 yr:* **PO** 400 mg/m² bid up to 1200 mg/day

Available forms: Caps 100 mg; oral sol 80 mg/ml

SIDE EFFECTS

CNS: Paresthesia, *headache, seizures,* fever
GI: Diarrhea, buccal mucosa ulceration, abdominal pain, *nausea,* taste perversion, dry mouth, dizziness, insomnia, vomiting, anorexia
INTEG: Rash
MISC: Asthenia, *angioedema, anaphylaxis, Stevens-Johnson syndrome,* increase lipids, lipodystrophy
MS: Pain
Contraindications: Hypersensitivity
Precautions: Pregnancy (B), hepatic disease, lactation, children, pancreatitis, diabetes

PHARMACOKINETICS

Well absorbed; 98% protein binding, hepatic metabolism, peak 2-4 hr, terminal half-life 3-5 hr

INTERACTIONS

⚠ Toxicity: amiodarone, azole antifungals, benzodiazepines, bepridil, buPROPion, clozapine, desipramine, dihydroergotamine, encainide, ergotamine, flecainide, HMG-CoA reductase inhibitors, interleukins, meperidine, midazolam, pimozide, piroxicam, propafenone, propoxyphene, quinidine, saquinavir, terfenadine, triazolam, zolpidem
Increase: ritonavir levels—fluconazole
Increase: level of both drugs—clarithromycin, ddI
Decrease: ritonavir levels—rifamycins, nevirapine, barbiturates, phenytoin
Decrease: levels of anticoagulants, atovaquone, divalproex, ethinyl estradiol, lamotrigine, phenytoin, sulfamethoxazole, theophylline, zidovudine
Drug/Herb
Decrease: ritonavir levels—St. John's wort; avoid concurrent use
Drug/Lab Test
Increase: AST, ALT, CPK, cholesterol, GGT, triglycerides, uric acid
Decrease: Hct, RBC, Hgb, neutrophils, WBC

NURSING CONSIDERATIONS
Assess:
• Signs of infection, anemia
• Hepatic studies: ALT, AST
• Viral load and CD4 baseline and throughout therapy
• C&S before drug therapy; drug may be taken as soon as culture is taken; repeat C&S after treatment; determine the presence of other sexually transmitted diseases
• Bowel pattern before, during treatment; if severe abdominal pain with bleeding occurs, discontinue drug; monitor hydration
• Skin eruptions; rash
• Allergies before treatment, reaction to each medication
Administer:
• With food; mix oral powder with high-calorie drink such as Ensure
• Store caps in refrigerator
Teach patient/family:
• To take as prescribed; if dose is missed, take as soon as remembered up to 1 hr before next dose; do not double dose
• That drug must be taken in equal intervals around the clock to maintain blood levels for duration of therapy
• To take with food; mix liquid formulation with chocolate milk or liquid nutritional supplement
• That drug is not a cure for HIV; opportunistic infections may continue to be acquired
• That redistribution of body fat or accumulation of body fat may occur
• That others may continue to contract HIV from the patient
• Not to use St. John's wort; that it decreases this drug's effect

R

rituximab

(rih-tuks'ih-mab)

Rituxan

Func. class.: Antineoplastic—miscellaneous

Chem. class.: Murine/human monoclonal antibody

Action: Directed against the CD20 antigen that is found on malignant B lymphocytes; CD20 regulates a portion of cell-cycle initiation/differentiation

Uses: Non-Hodgkin's lymphoma (CD20 positive, B-cell), bulky disease (tumors >10 cm)

DOSAGE AND ROUTES

• *Adult:* **IV INF** 375 mg/m^2 qwk × 4 doses; give at 50 mg/hr for 1st inf; if hypersensitivity does not occur, increase rate by 50 mg/hr q½h, max 400 mg/hr; slow/interrupt inf if hypersensitivity occurs; other inf can be given at 100 mg/hr and increased by 100 mg/hr, max 400 mg/hr

Available forms: Inj 10 mg/ml

SIDE EFFECTS

*CV: **Cardiac dysrhythmias***

GI: Nausea, vomiting, anorexia

*GU: **Renal failure***

*HEMA: **Leukopenia, neutropenia, thrombocytopenia***

*INTEG: Irritation at site, rash, **fatal mucocutaneous infections (rare)***

*OTHER: Fever, chills, asthenia, headache, **angioedema**, hypotension, myalgia, **bronchospasm***

*SYST: **Stevens-Johnson syndrome***

Contraindications: Hypersensitivity, murine proteins

Precautions: Pregnancy (C), lactation, children, elderly, cardiac conditions

PHARMACOKINETICS

Half-life 42-79 min

NURSING CONSIDERATIONS

Assess:

⚠ For signs of fatal infusion reaction: hypoxia, pulmonary infiltrates, acute respiratory distress syndrome, MI, ventricular fibrillation, cardiogenic shock; most fatal infusion reactions occur with first infusion; potentially fatal

⚠ For signs of severe mucocutaneous reactions: Stevens-Johnson syndrome, lichenoid dermatitis, toxic epidermal lysis; occur 1-13 wk after drug is given

⚠ Tumor lysis syndrome: acute renal failure requiring hemodialysis, hyperkalemia, hypocalcemia, hyperuricemia, hyperphosphatemia

• CBC, differential, platelet count weekly; withhold drug if WBC is <3500/mm^3, or platelet count <100,000/mm^3; notify prescriber of these results; drug should be discontinued

• Food preferences: list likes, dislikes

• GI symptoms: frequency of stools

• Signs of dehydration: rapid respirations, poor skin turgor, decreased urine output, dry skin, restlessness, weakness

Administer:

IV INF route

• After diluting to a final conc. of 1-4 mg/ml; use 0.9% NaCl, D$_5$W, gently invert bag to mix; do not mix with other drugs

Perform/provide:

• Increase fluid intake to 2-3 L/day for dehydration unless contraindicated

• Changing of IV site q48h

• Nutritious diet with iron, vitamin supplement, low fiber, few dairy products

• Storage of vials at 36°-40° F, protect vials from direct sunlight, inf sol is stable at 36°-46° F × 24 hr and room temperature for another 12 hr

Evaluate:

• Therapeutic response: decrease in tumor size, decrease in spread of cancer

Teach patient/family:

• To report adverse reactions

rivastigmine (℞)
(riv-as-tig′mine)
Exelon
Func. class.: Anti-Alzheimer agent
Chem. class.: Cholinesterase inhibitor

Action: May enhance cholinergic functioning by increasing acetylcholine
Uses: Mild to moderate Alzheimer's dementia

DOSAGE AND ROUTES

• *Adult:* **PO** 1.5 mg bid with food; after 2 wk or more, may increase to 3 mg bid after 2 wk or more; may increase to 4.5 mg bid and thereafter 6 mg bid, max 12 mg/day
Available forms: Caps 1.5, 3, 4.5, 6 mg; solution 2 mg/ml

SIDE EFFECTS

CNS: Tremors, confusion, insomnia, psychosis, hallucination, depression, dizziness, headache, anxiety, somnolence, fatigue, syncope
GI: Nausea, vomiting, anorexia, abdominal distress, flatulence, diarrhea, constipation, dyspepsia
MISC: Urinary tract infection, asthenia, increased sweating, hypertension, flulike symptoms, weight change
Contraindications: Hypersensitivity to this drug, other carbamates; narrow-angle glaucoma, undiagnosed skin lesions
Precautions: Pregnancy (B), renal disease, hepatic disease, respiratory disease, seizure disorder, peptic ulcer, cardiac disease, urinary obstruction, asthma, lactation, children

PHARMACOKINETICS

Rapidly and completely absorbed, metabolized to decarbamylated metabolite, half-life is 1.5 hr, excreted via kidneys (metabolites), clearance is lowered in the elderly, hepatic disease, and increased in nicotine use

INTERACTIONS

Synergistic effect: cholinomimetics, other cholinesterase inhibitors

Drug/Herb
Increase: effect—pill-bearing spurge

NURSING CONSIDERATIONS

Assess:
• Hepatic studies: AST, ALT, alk phosphatase, LDH, bilirubin, CBC
• For severe GI effects: nausea, vomiting, anorexia, weight loss
• B/P, respiration during initial treatment; hypo/hypertension should be reported
• Mental status: affect, mood, behavioral changes, depression; complete suicide assessment
Administer:
• With meals; take with morning and evening meal even though absorption may be decreased
• Discontinue treatment for several doses and restart at same or next lower dosage level, if adverse reactions cause intolerance
• If treatment is interrupted for longer than several days, treatment should be initiated with lowest daily dose and titrated as indicated above
Perform/provide:
• Assistance with ambulation during beginning therapy
Evaluate:
• Therapeutic response: decreased dementia
Teach patient/family:
• The procedure for giving oral solution; use instruction sheet provided
• To notify prescriber of severe GI effects

R

rizatriptan (R)

(rye-zah-trip'tan)
Maxalt, Maxalt-MLT
Func. class.: Migraine agent
Chem. class.: 5-HT$_{1D}$ receptor agonist

Action: Binds selectively to the vascular 5-HT$_{1D}$ receptor subtype, exerts antimigraine effect; causes vasoconstriction in cranial arteries

Uses: Acute treatment of migraine

DOSAGE AND ROUTES:

• *Adult:* **PO** 5-10 mg single dose, redosing separate by 2 hr or more; max 30 mg/24 hr, use 5 mg in patient on propranolol; max 15 mg/24 hr

Available forms: Maxalt: tabs 5, 10 mg; Maxalt-MLT: tabs, orally disintegrating 5, 10 mg

SIDE EFFECTS

CNS: Dizziness, drowsiness, headache, fatigue, warm/cold sensations, flushing
CV: MI, ventricular fibrillation, ventricular tachycardia, coronary artery vasospasm
ENDO: Hot flashes, mild increase in growth hormone
GI: Nausea, dry mouth, diarrhea, abdominal pain
RESP: Chest tightness, pressure, dyspnea

Contraindications: Angina pectoris, history of MI, documented silent ischemia, Prinzmetal's angina, ischemic heart disease, concurrent ergotamine-containing preparations, uncontrolled hypertension, hypersensitivity, basilar or hemiplegic migraine

Precautions: Pregnancy (C), postmenopausal women, men >40 yr, risk factors for CAD, hypercholesterolemia, obesity, diabetes, impaired hepatic or renal function, lactation, children, elderly

PHARMACOKINETICS

Onset of pain relief 10 min-2 hr, peak 1-1½ hr, duration 14-16 hr, 14% plasma protein binding, metabolized in the liver (metabolite), excreted in urine (82%), feces (12%), half-life 2-3 hr

INTERACTIONS

Extended vasospastic effects: ergot, ergot derivatives, other 5-HT receptor agonists
Weakness, hyperreflexia, incoordination: SSRIs
Increase: rizatriptan action—cimetidine, oral contraceptives, MAOIs, nonselective MAOI (type A and B), isocarboxazid, pargyline, phenelzine, propranolol, tranylcypromine
Drug/Herb
Serotonin syndrome: SAM-e, St. John's wort
Increase: effect—butterbur

NURSING CONSIDERATIONS

Assess:
• For stress level, activity, recreation, coping mechanisms
• Neurologic status: LOC, blurring vision, nausea, vomiting, tingling in extremities preceding headache
• Ingestion of tyramine foods (pickled products, beer, wine, aged cheese), food additives, preservatives, colorings, artificial sweeteners, chocolate, caffeine, which may precipitate these types of headaches

Administer:
• Oral disintegrating tab: do not open blister until use; peel blister open with dry hands; place tab on tongue, where it will dissolve, and swallow with saliva (contains phenylalanine)

Perform/provide:
• Quiet, calm environment with decreased stimulation for noise, bright light, excessive talking

Evaluate:
• Therapeutic response: decrease in frequency, severity of headache

Teach patient/family:
• Use of orally disintegrating tab: instruct patient not to open blister until

use, to peel blister open with dry hands, to place tab on tongue, where it will dissolve, and to swallow with saliva (contains phenylalanine)

• To report any side effects to prescriber
• To use alternative contraception while taking drug if oral contraceptives are being used

---

⚠ High Alert

rocuronium (℞)
(ro-kyur-oh′nium)
Zemuron
Func. class.: Neuromuscular blocker (nondepolarizing)
Chem. class.: Biquaternary ammonium ester

Action: Inhibits transmission of nerve impulses by binding with cholinergic receptor sites, antagonizing action of acetylcholine
Uses: Facilitation of endotracheal intubation, skeletal muscle relaxation during mechanical ventilation, surgery, or general anesthesia

DOSAGE AND ROUTES
Intubation
• *Adult and child >3 mo:* **IV** 0.6 mg/kg
Available forms: Inj 10 mg/ml

SIDE EFFECTS
CV: Bradycardia, tachycardia, change in B/P, edema
GI: Nausea, vomiting
INTEG: Rash, flushing, pruritus, urticaria
RESP: **Prolonged apnea, bronchospasm, cyanosis, respiratory depression,** wheezing
Contraindications: Hypersensitivity
Precautions: Pregnancy (C), cardiac disease, lactation, child <2 yr, electrolyte imbalances, dehydration, neuromuscular disease, respiratory disease, renal disease, hepatic disease

PHARMACOKINETICS
Half-life 71-203 min, duration ½ hr, metabolized in liver

INTERACTIONS
Theophylline increases risk of dysrhythmias
Increase: neuromuscular blockade caused by amphotericin B, verapamil, aminoglycosides, clindamycin, enflurane, isoflurane, lincomycin, lithium, opiates, local anesthetics, polymyxin, antiinfectives, quinidine, thiazides

NURSING CONSIDERATIONS
Assess:
• For electrolyte imbalances (K, Mg), before drug is used; electrolyte imbalances may lead to increased action of this drug
• VS (B/P, pulse, respirations, airway) until fully recovered; rate, depth, pattern of respirations, strength of hand grip; patient should be intubated before use
• Recovery: decreased paralysis of face, diaphragm, leg, arm, rest of body; residual weakness and respiratory problems may occur during recovery
• Allergic reactions: rash, fever, respiratory distress, pruritus; drug should be discontinued
Administer:
• Using peripheral nerve stimulator by anesthesiologist to determine neuromuscular blockade; deep tendon reflexes should be monitored during extended use
• Undiluted direct IV over 2 min (only by qualified person, usually anesthesiologist); do not administer IM
• Maintenance q20-45min after 1st dose; titrate to response
Perform/provide:
• Storage in light-resistant area
• Reassurance if communication is difficult during recovery from neuromuscular blockade

R

Evaluate:

• Therapeutic response: paralysis of jaw, eyelid, head, neck, rest of body as evaluated by peripheral nerve stimulator

Teach patient/family:

• About all procedures or treatments; patient will remain conscious if anesthesia is not given also

Treatment of overdose: Edrophonium or neostigmine, atropine, monitor VS; may require mechanical ventilation

---

ropinirole (℞)

(roh-pin'ih-role)

Requip

Func. class.: Antiparkinson agent

Chem. class.: Dopamine-receptor agonist, non-ergot

Action: Selective agonist for D$_2$ receptors (presynaptic/postsynaptic sites); binding at D$_3$ receptor contributes to antiparkinson effects

Uses: Parkinson's disease, restless leg syndrome (RLS)

DOSAGE AND ROUTES

• *Adult:* **PO** 0.25 mg tid, titrate weekly to a max of 24 mg/day

Restless leg syndrome

• *Adult:* **PO** 0.25 mg at bedtime, may increase until symptom's resolved

Available forms: Tabs 0.25, 0.5, 1, 2, 4, 5 mg

SIDE EFFECTS

CNS: Agitation, insomnia, psychosis, hallucination, dystonia, depression, dizziness, somnolence, ***sleep attacks***

CV: Orthostatic hypotension, tachycardia, hypertension, hypotension, syncope, palpitations

EENT: Blurred vision

GI: Nausea, vomiting, anorexia, dry mouth, constipation, dyspepsia, flatulence

GU: Impotence, urinary frequency

*HEMA: **Hemolytic anemia, leukopenia, agranulocytosis***

INTEG: Rash, sweating

RESP: Pharyngitis, rhinitis, sinusitis, bronchitis, dyspnea

Contraindications: Hypersensitivity

Precautions: Pregnancy (C), renal disease, cardiac disease, dysrhythmias, affective disorder, psychosis, hepatic disease

PHARMACOKINETICS

PO: Half-life 6 hr; extensively metabolized by the liver by P450 CYP1A2 enzyme system

INTERACTIONS

Increase: ropinirole effect—cimetidine, ciprofloxacin, diltiazem, enoxacin, erythromycin, fluvoxamine, mexiletine, norfloxacin, tacrine, digoxin, theophylline, L-dopa

Decrease: ropinirole effects—butyrophenones, metoclopramide, phenothiazines, thioxanthenes

Drug/Herb

Decrease: ropinirole action—chaste tree fruit, kava

NURSING CONSIDERATIONS

Assess:

• Involuntary movements in parkinsonism: akinesia, tremors, staggering gait, muscle rigidity, drooling

• B/P, respiration during initial treatment; hypo/hypertension should be reported

⚠ For sleep attacks, drowsiness, falling asleep without warning even during hazardous activities

• Mental status: affect, mood, behavioral changes, depression; complete suicide assessment

Administer:

• Drug until NPO before surgery

• Adjust dosage to patient response

• With meals

Perform/provide:

• Testing for diabetes mellitus, acromegaly if on long-term therapy

Evaluate:

• Therapeutic response: improvement in movement disorder

⚠ Safety alert   *"Tall Man" lettering

Teach patient/family:
• That therapeutic effects may take several weeks to a few months
• To change positions slowly to prevent orthostatic hypotension
• To use drug exactly as prescribed; if drug is discontinued abruptly, parkinsonian crisis may occur

ropivacaine (℞)

(roe-pi'va-kane)

Naropin

Func. class.: Local anesthetic

Chem. class.: Amide

Action: Competes with calcium for sites in nerve membrane that control sodium transport across cell membrane; decreases rise of depolarization phase of action potential
Uses: Peripheral nerve block, caudal anesthesia, central neural block, vaginal, epidural, spinal block

DOSAGE AND ROUTES
Lumbar epidural block for cesarean section
• *Adult:* 20-30 ml of 0.5% sol
• *Adult:* 15-20 ml of 0.75% sol
Thoracic epidural
• *Adult:* 5-15 ml of 0.5% to 0.75% sol
Major nerve block
• *Adult:* 35-50 ml of 0.5% sol
• *Adult:* 10-40 ml of 0.75% sol
Labor pain (epidural)
• *Adult:* 10-20 ml 0.2% sol then 6-14 ml 1 hr
Postop (lumbar or thoracic epidural)
• *Adult:* 6-14 ml/hr of 0.2% sol
Infiltration/minor nerve block
• *Adult:* 1-100 ml of 0.2% sol
• *Adult:* 1-40 ml of 0.5% sol
Available forms: Inj 2, 5, 7.5 mg/ml

SIDE EFFECTS
CNS: Anxiety, restlessness, *convulsions, loss of consciousness,* drowsiness, disorientation, tremors, shivering, paresthesia

*CV: **Myocardial depression, cardiac arrest, dysrhythmias,** bradycardia, hypotension, hypertension, **fetal bradycardia***
EENT: Blurred vision, tinnitus, pupil constriction
ENDO: Hypokelamia
GI: Nausea, vomiting
GU: Urinary retention
INTEG: Rash, urticaria, allergic reactions, edema, burning, skin discoloration at inj site, tissue necrosis
*RESP: **Status asthmaticus, respiratory arrest, anaphylaxis***
Contraindications: Hypersensitivity to amide local anesthetics, child <12 yr, elderly, severe hepatic disease, severe hypotension, complete heart block
Precautions: Pregnancy (B), severe drug allergies, hyperthyroidism, cardiovascular disease; hepatic, neurological disease

PHARMACOKINETICS

Onset varies with inj site, duration varies with inj site; metabolized by liver, excreted in urine (metabolites)

INTERACTIONS

Dysrhythmias: epINEPHrine, halothane, enflurane
Hypertension: MAOIs, tricyclics, phenothiazines
Increase: effect—amiodarone, ciprofloxacin, fluvoxamine, azole antifungal
Decrease: action of ropivacaine—chloroprocaine

NURSING CONSIDERATIONS
Assess:
• B/P, pulse, respiration during treatment
• Fetal heart tones during labor
• Allergic reactions: rash, urticaria, itching
• Cardiac status: ECG for dysrhythmias, pulse, B/P during anesthesia

R

Administer:
• Only with crash cart, resuscitative equipment nearby
• Only drugs without preservatives for epidural or caudal anesthesia

Perform/provide:
• Use of new sol; discard unused portions

Evaluate:
• Therapeutic response: anesthesia necessary for procedure

Treatment of overdose: Airway, O_2, vasopressor, IV fluids, anticonvulsants for seizures

---

rosiglitazone (℞)
(ros-ih-glit'ah-zone)
Avandia
Func. class.: Antidiabetic, oral
Chem. class.: Thiazolidinedione

Action: Improves insulin resistance by hepatic glucose metabolism, insulin receptor kinase activity, insulin receptor phosphorylation

Uses: Type 2 diabetes mellitus, alone or in combination with sulfonylureas, metformin, or insulin

DOSAGE AND ROUTES

Monotherapy
• *Adult:* **PO** 4 mg daily or in 2 divided doses, may increase to 8 mg daily or in 2 divided doses after 12 wk

Combination therapy
• *Adult:* **PO** This drug should be added to metformin, sulfonylurea at the adult dose

Available forms: Tabs 2, 4, 8 mg

SIDE EFFECTS

CNS: Fatigue, headache
ENDO: Hyper/hypoglycemia
MISC: Accidental injury, URI, sinusitis, anemia, back pain, diarrhea, edema

Contraindications: Hypersensitivity to thiazolidinediones, children, lactation, diabetic ketoacidosis

Precautions: Pregnancy (C), elderly, thyroid disease, hepatic, renal disease

PHARMACOKINETICS

Maximal reductions in FBS after 6-12 wk, protein binding 99.8%, excreted in urine, feces, elimination half-life 3-4 hr, may be excreted in breast milk

---

INTERACTIONS

Decrease: effect of oral contraceptives, alternative method advised

Drug/Herb
Hypoglycemia: chromium, coenzyme Q10, fenugreek
Poor glucose control: glucosamine
Increase: antidiabetic effect—alfalfa, aloe, basil, bay, bilberry, bitter melon, black catechu, buchu, burdock, coriander, dandelion, eyebright (po), fenugreek, garlic, ginseng, glucomannan, glucosamine, goat's rue, gymnema, horehound, horse chestnut, jambul, myrrh, myrtle
Decrease: antidiabetic effect—bee pollen, blue cohosh, broom, chromium, elecampane, eucalyptus, gotu kola

NURSING CONSIDERATIONS

Assess:
• For hypoglycemic reactions (sweating, weakness, dizziness, anxiety, tremors, hunger), hyperglycemic reactions soon after meals
• Check LFTs periodically AST, ALT (if ALT >2.5 × ULN, do not use)
• FBS, HbA1c, fasting plasma insulin, plasma lipids/lipoproteins, B/P, body weight during treatment

Administer:
• Once or in 2 divided doses
• Tabs crushed and mixed with food or fluids for patients with difficulty swallowing

Perform/provide:
• Conversion from other oral hypoglycemic agents if needed; change may be made without gradual dosage change; monitor serum or urine glucose and ketones tid during conversion
• Storage in tight container in cool environment

⚠ A Safety alert   *"Tall Man" lettering

Teach patient/family:
• To monitor blood glucose; that periodic LFTs mandatory
• The symptoms of hypo/hyperglycemia, what to do about each
• That the drug must be continued on daily basis; explain consequences of discontinuing drug abruptly
• To avoid OTC medications or herbal preparations unless approved by prescriber
• That diabetes is lifelong illness; that this drug is not a cure; only controls symptoms
• That all food included in diet plan must be eaten to prevent hypoglycemia
• To carry emergency ID and glucagon emergency kit for emergencies
• To report symptoms of hepatic dysfunction (nausea, vomiting, abdominal pain, fatigue, anorexia, dark urine, jaundice)
• That 2 wk is needed to see a reduction in blood glucose and 2-3 months to see full effect
• To notify prescriber if oral contraceptives are used
• Not to use if breast feeding, may be secreted in breast milk
Evaluate:
• Therapeutic response: Decrease in polyuria, polydipsia, polyphagia; clear sensorium; absence of dizziness; stable gait, blood glucose at normal level

---

rosuvastatin (℞)

(roe-soo′va-sta-tin)
Crestor
Func. class.: Antilipemic
Chem. class.: HMG-CoA reductase inhibitor

Action: Inhibits HMG-CoA reductase enzyme, which reduces cholesterol synthesis
Uses: As an adjunct in primary hypercholesterolemia (types IIa, IIb), and mixed dyslipidemia elevated serum triglycerides, homozygous familial hypercholesterolemia (FH)

DOSAGE AND ROUTES
(Patient should first be placed on a cholesterol-lowering diet)
Hypercholesterolemia
• *Adult:* **PO** 5-40 mg daily; initial dose 10 mg daily, reanalyze lipid levels at 2-4 wk and adjust dosage accordingly
Homozygous FH
• *Adult:* **PO** 20 mg daily, max 40 mg
Dose in patients taking cyclosporine
• *Adult:* 5 mg daily
Dose when taken with gemfibrozil
• *Adult:* 10 mg daily
Available forms: Tabs 5, 10, 20, 40 mg

SIDE EFFECTS
CNS: Headache, dizziness, insomnia, paresthesia
GI: Nausea, constipation, abdominal pain, flatus, diarrhea, dyspepsia, heartburn, **kidney failure, liver dysfunction,** vomiting
HEMA: **Thrombocytopenia, hemolytic anemia, leucopenia**
INTEG: Rash, pruritus, photosensitivity
MS: Asthenia, muscle cramps, arthritis, arthralgia, myalgia, **myositis, rhabdomyolysis,** leg, shoulder or localized pain
RESP: Rhinitis, sinusitis, *pharyngitis,* bronchitis, increased cough
Contraindications: Pregnancy (X), hypersensitivity, lactation, active liver disease
Precautions: Past hepatic disease, alcoholism, severe acute infections, trauma, hypotension, uncontrolled seizure disorders, severe metabolic disorders, electrolyte imbalances, children, severe renal impairment, elderly, hypothyroidism

PHARMACOKINETICS
PO: Peak 3-5 hr, minimal live metabolism (about 10%), 88% protein bound; excreted primarily in feces (90%); crosses placenta; half-life 19 hr

R

Side effects: *italics* = common; **bold italics** = life-threatening

INTERACTIONS

Increase: effects of rosuvastatin—bile acid sequestrants

Increase: myalgia, myositis—cycloSPORINE, gemfibrozil, niacin, clofibrate, azole antifungals

Increase: bleeding—warfarin

Drug/Food

Possible toxicity: grapefruit juice

Drug/Lab Test

Increase: CPK, LFTs

NURSING CONSIDERATIONS

Assess:

• Diet, obtain diet history including fat, cholesterol in diet

• Fasting cholesterol, LDL, HDL, triglycerides periodically during treatment

• LFTs q1-2mo during the first 1½ yr of treatment; AST, ALT, LFTs may increase

• Renal function in patients with compromised renal system: BUN, creatinine, I&O ratio

A For muscle pain, tenderness, obtain CPK; if these occur, drug may need to be discontinued

Administer:

• May be taken at any time of day, with or without food

Perform/provide:

• Storage in cool environment in airtight, light-resistant container

Evaluate:

• Therapeutic response: cholesterol at desired level after 8 wk

Teach patient/family:

• To report suspected pregnancy

• That blood work and ophthalmic exam will be necessary during treatment

• To report blurred vision, severe GI symptoms, dizziness, headache, muscle pain, weakness

• To use sunscreen or stay out of the sun to prevent photosensitivity

• That previously prescribed regimen will continue: low-cholesterol diet, exercise program, smoking cessation

---

salmeterol (R)

(sal-met′er-ole)

Serevent

Func. class.: β₂-Adrenergic agonist, bronchodilator

Action: Causes bronchodilation by action on β₂ (pulmonary) receptors by increasing levels of cAMP, which relaxes smooth muscle with very little effect on heart rate, maintains improvement in FEV from 3 to 12 hr; prevents nocturnal asthma symptoms

Uses: Prevention of exercise-induced asthma, bronchospasm, COPD

DOSAGE AND ROUTES

• *Adult:* **INH** 50 mcg (one inhalation as dry powder); exercise-induced bronchospasm: 50 mcg (2 inh) ½-1 hr prior to exercise

• *Child 4-12 yr:* **INH** 50 mcg as dry powder bid; exercise-induced bronchospasm 50 mcg as dry powder ½-1 hr prior to exercise

Available forms: Inhalation powder 50 mcg/blister

SIDE EFFECTS

CNS: Tremors, anxiety, insomnia, headache, dizziness, stimulation, restlessness, hallucinations, flushing, irritability

CV: Palpitations, tachycardia, hypertension, angina, hypotension, dysrhythmias

EENT: Dry nose, irritation of nose and throat

GI: Heartburn, nausea, vomiting

MS: Muscle cramps

*RESP: **Bronchospasm***

Contraindications: Hypersensitivity to sympathomimetics, tachydysrhythmias, severe cardiac disease

Precautions: Pregnancy (C), lactation, cardiac disorders, hyperthyroidism, diabetes mellitus, hypertension, prostatic hypertrophy, narrow-angle glaucoma, seizures, acute asthma, as a substitute to corticosteroids

---

A Safety alert   *"Tall Man" lettering

PHARMACOKINETICS

INH: Onset 5-15 min, peak 4 hr, duration 12 hr, metabolized in liver, excreted in urine, breast milk; crosses placenta; blood-brain barrier

INTERACTIONS

Increase: action of aerosol bronchodilators

Increase: action of salmeterol—tricyclics, MAOIs

Decrease: salmeterol action—other β-blockers

Drug/Herb

Increase: stimulation—betel palm, butterbur, coffee, cola nut, figwort, fumitory, guarana, hawthorn, lily of the valley, motherwort, plantain, tea (black/green), yerba maté

NURSING CONSIDERATIONS

Assess:

• Respiratory function: vital capacity, forced expiratory volume, ABGs, lung sounds, heart rate and rhythm

Administer:

• Gum, sips of water for dry mouth

Perform/provide:

• Storage in foil pouch; do not expose to temperatures over 86° F (30° C); discard 6 wk after removal from foil pouch

Evaluate:

• Therapeutic response: absence of dyspnea, wheezing

Teach patient/family:

• Not to use OTC medications; extra stimulation may occur

• Review package insert with patient

• To avoid getting powder in eyes

• To avoid smoking, smoke-filled rooms, persons with respiratory infections

• Not for treatment of acute exacerbation

Treatment of overdose: β₂-Adrenergic blocker

---

salsalate (℞)

(sal'sah-late)
Amigesic, Anaflex, Disalcid, Marthritic, Mono-Gesic, Salflex, salsalate, Salgesic, Salsitab

Func. class.: Nonopioid analgesic, nonsteroidal antiinflammatory
Chem. class.: Salicylate

Action: Blocks formation of peripheral prostaglandins, which cause pain and inflammation; antipyretic action results from inhibition of hypothalamic heat-regulating center; does not inhibit platelet aggregation

Uses: Mild to moderate pain or fever, including arthritis, juvenile rheumatoid arthritis

DOSAGE AND ROUTES

• *Adult:* **PO** 3 g/day in divided doses
Available forms: Caps 500 mg; tabs 500, 750 mg

SIDE EFFECTS

CNS: Stimulation, drowsiness, dizziness, confusion, ***convulsions,*** headache, flushing, hallucinations, ***coma***
CV: Rapid pulse, ***pulmonary edema***
EENT: Tinnitus, hearing loss
ENDO: Hypoglycemia, hyponatremia, hypokalemia, alteration in acid-base balance
GI: Nausea, vomiting, GI bleeding, diarrhea, heartburn, anorexia, ***hepatotoxicity***
HEMA: ***Thrombocytopenia, agranulocytosis, leukopenia, neutropenia, hemolytic anemia,*** increased protime
INTEG: Rash, urticaria, bruising
RESP: Wheezing, hyperpnea
Contraindications: Hypersensitivity to salicylates, NSAIDs, GI bleeding, bleeding disorders, children <3 yr, vit K deficiency
Precautions: Pregnancy (C) 1st trimester, anemia, hepatic disease, renal

S

---

disease, Hodgkin's disease, lactation, elderly

PHARMACOKINETICS

Metabolized by liver; excreted by kidneys; half-life 1 hr; highly protein bound; crosses blood-brain barrier and placenta slowly

INTERACTIONS

Toxic effects: PABA

Increase: blood loss—alcohol, heparin, NSAIDs, warfarin

Increase: effects of anticoagulants, insulin, methotrexate, probenecid, penicillins, phenytoin

Decrease: effects of spironolactone, sulfinpyrazone, sulfonamides, loop diuretics

Decrease: effects of salsalate—antacids, steroids, urinary alkalizers

Decrease: blood glucose levels—salicylates

Drug/Food

Foods that cause acidic urine, may increase salsalate levels

Drug/Lab Test

Increase: Coagulation studies, hepatic studies, serum uric acid, amylase, CO_2, urinary protein

Decrease: Serum potassium, PBI, cholesterol, blood glucose

Interference: Urine catecholamines, pregnancy test

NURSING CONSIDERATIONS

Assess:

• Pain: frequency, intensity, characteristics; relief of pain after medication

🅐 For asthma, aspirin hypersensitivity, nasal polyps; may develop hypersensitivity to this product

• Hepatic studies: AST, ALT, bilirubin (long-term therapy)

• Renal studies: BUN, urine creatinine (long-term therapy)

• Blood studies: CBC, Hct, Hgb, PT (long-term therapy)

• I&O ratio; decreasing output may indicate renal failure (long-term therapy)

• Hepatotoxicity: dark urine, clay-colored stools; jaundiced skin, sclera; itching, abdominal pain, fever, diarrhea (long-term therapy)

• Allergic reactions: rash, urticaria; drug may have to be discontinued

• Ototoxicity: tinnitus, ringing, roaring in ears; audiometric testing is needed before, after long-term therapy

• Visual changes: blurring, halos, corneal and retinal damage

• Edema in feet, ankles, legs

• Drug history; many interactions

Administer:

• To patient crushed or whole; chewable tablets may be chewed

• With food or milk to decrease gastric symptoms

Evaluate:

• Therapeutic response: decreased pain, fever

Teach patient/family:

• To report any symptoms of hepatotoxicity, renal toxicity, visual changes, ototoxicity, allergic reactions (long-term therapy)

• Not to exceed recommended dosage; acute poisoning may result

• To read label on other OTC drugs; many contain aspirin

• That therapeutic response takes 2 wk (arthritis)

• To avoid alcohol ingestion; GI bleeding may occur

• To watch for signs of bleeding: dark stools

Treatment of overdose: Lavage, activated charcoal, monitor electrolytes, VS

---

saquinavir (℞)

(sa-quen'ah-veer)

Fortovase, Invirase

Func. class.: Antiretroviral

Chem. class.: Protease inhibitor

Action: Inhibits human immunodeficiency virus (HIV-1) protease, which prevents maturation of the infectious virus

Uses: HIV-1 in combination with other antiretrovirals

DOSAGE AND ROUTES

• *Adult:* PO 600 mg (hard cap-Invirase) or 1200 mg (soft cap-Fortovase) tid within 2 hr after a full meal

Available forms: Caps 200 mg (soft); 200, 500 mg (hard)

SIDE EFFECTS

CNS: Paresthesia, headache
GI: Diarrhea, buccal mucosa ulceration, *abdominal pain, nausea,* vomiting
INTEG: Rash
MISC.: Asthenia, hyperglycemia
MS: Pain

Contraindications: Hypersensitivity
Precautions: Pregnancy (B), hepatic disease, lactation, children, diabetes, pancreatitis

PHARMACOKINETICS

Absorption increased with food, protein binding 98%, extensive first-pass metabolism, terminal half-life 12 hr

INTERACTIONS

Avoid use with HMG-CoA reductase inhibitors
Toxicity: ergots, midazolam, triazolam, dapsone, quinidine, calcium channel blockers, clindamycin
⚠ Increase: vasoconstriction—ergots, do not use concurrently
⚠ Increase: CNS depression—midazolam, triazolam, do not use concurrently
Increase: saquinavir levels—ketoconazole, indinavir, delaviridine, nelfinavir, ritonavir, clarithromycin
Decrease: saquinavir levels—rifamycins, carbamazepine, phenobarbital, phenytoin, nevirapine, dexamethasone

Drug/Herb
St. John's wort may decrease saquinavir levels, avoid concurrent use

Drug/Food
Increase: bioavailability after high-fat meal; grapefruit juice increases levels
Drug/Lab Test
CPK, glucose (low)

NURSING CONSIDERATIONS

Assess:
• Signs of infection, anemia
• Hepatic studies: ALT, AST
• C&S before drug therapy; drug may be taken as soon as culture is taken; repeat C&S after treatment; determine the presence of other sexually transmitted diseases
• Bowel pattern before, during treatment; if severe abdominal pain with bleeding occurs, drug should be discontinued; monitor hydration
• Skin eruptions, rash, urticaria, itching
• Allergies before treatment, reaction of each medication

Administer:
• Within 2 hr of meal

Teach patient/family:
• To take as prescribed within 2 hr of a full meal; if dose is missed, take as soon as remembered up to 1 hr before next dose; do not double dose
• That drug must be taken in equal intervals around the clock to maintain blood levels for duration of therapy
• That Invirase and Fortovase are not interchangeable

---

sargramostim (℞)
(sar-gram'oh-stim)
Leukine, rhu GM-CSF
Func. class.: Biologic modifier: cytokine
Chem. class.: Granulocyte macrophage colony-stimulating factor (GM-CSF)

Do not confuse:
Leukine/leucovorin
Leukine/Leukeran
Action: Stimulates proliferation and differentiation of hematopoietic progenitor cells (granulocytes, macrophages)

Uses: Acceleration of myeloid recovery in patients with non-Hodgkin's lymphoma, acute lymphoblastic leukemia, autologous bone marrow transplantation in Hodgkin's disease; bone marrow transplantation failure or engraftment delay, mobilization and transplant of peripheral blood progenitor cells (PBPCs)

Investigational uses: Aplastic anemia, Crohn's disease, ganciclovir- or zidovudine-induced neutropenia

DOSAGE AND ROUTES

Myeloid reconstitution after autologous bone marrow transplantation
• *Adult:* IV 250 mcg/m²/day × 3 wk; give over 2 hr, 2-4 hr after autologous bone marrow infusion, not less than 24 hr after last dose of antineoplastics and 12 hr after last dose of radiotherapy, bone marrow transplantation failure, or engraftment delay

Acceleration of myeloid recovery
• *Adult:* IV 250 mcg/m²/day × 14 days; give over 2 hr; may repeat in 7 days, may repeat 500 mcg/m²/day × 14 days after another 7 days if no improvement

Mobilization of PBPCs
• *Adult:* IV/SUBCUT 250 mcg/m²/day during collection of PBPCs

After PBPC transplantation
• *Adult:* IV/SUBCUT 250 mcg/m²/day until ANC >1500 cells/mm³ × 3 days

Available forms: Powder for inj lyophilized 250, 500 mcg

SIDE EFFECTS

CNS: Fever, malaise, CNS disorder, weakness, chills, dizziness, syncope

CV: **Transient supraventricular tachycardia,** peripheral edema, **pericardial effusion**

GI: Nausea, vomiting, diarrhea, anorexia, **GI hemorrhage,** stomatitis, **liver damage**

GU: Urinary tract disorder, abnormal kidney function

HEMA: **Blood dyscrasias, hemorrhage**

INTEG: Alopecia, rash, peripheral edema

RESP: Dyspnea

Contraindications: Hypersensitivity to GM-CSF, benzyl alcohol, yeast products; excessive leukemic myeloid blast in bone marrow, peripheral blood, neonates

Precautions: Pregnancy (C), lactation, child; renal, hepatic, lung disease; cardiac disease; pleural, pericardial effusions, peripheral edema

PHARMACOKINETICS

Half-life 2 hr, detected within 5 min after administration, peak 2 hr

INTERACTIONS

Do not use this drug concomitantly with antineoplastics

Increase: myeloproliferation—lithium, corticosteroids

NURSING CONSIDERATIONS

Assess:

⚠ Blood studies: CBC, differential count before treatment and twice weekly; leukocytosis may occur (WBC >50,000 cells/mm³, ANC >20,000 cells/mm³), platelets; if ANC >20,000/mm³ or 10,000/mm³ after nadir has occurred, or platelets >500,000/mm³ reduce dose by ½ or discontinue; if blast cells occur, discontinue

• Renal, hepatic studies before treatment: BUN, creatinine, urinalysis; AST, ALT, alk phosphatase; twice weekly monitoring is needed in renal, hepatic disease

• For hypersensitivity, rashes, local inj site reactions; usually transient

• For increased fluid retention in cardiac disease

• For myalgia, arthralgia in legs, feet, use analgesics

Administer:

SUBCUT route
• Use reconstituted sol

IV route
• After reconstituting with 1 ml sterile water for inj without preservative; do not reenter vial; discard unused portion;

⚠ Safety alert   *"Tall Man" lettering

direct reconstitution sol at side of vial; rotate contents; do not shake
• Dilute in 0.9% NaCl inj to prepare IV inf; if final concentration is <10 mcg/ml, add human albumin to make a final concentration of 0.1% to NaCl before adding sargramostim to prevent adsorption; for a final concentration of 0.1% albumin, add 1 mg human albumin/1 ml 0.9% NaCl inj run over 2 hr (bone marrow transplant or failure of graft); over 4 hr (chemotherapy for AML); over 24 hr as cont inf (PBPCs); give within 6 hr after reconstitution

Y-site compatibilities: Amikacin, aminophylline, aztreonam, bleomycin, butorphanol, calcium gluconate, carboplatin, carmustine, cefazolin, cefepime, cefotaxime, cefotetan, ceftizoxime, ceftriaxone, cefuroxime, cimetidine, cisplatin, clindamycin, cyclophosphamide, cycloSPORINE, cytarabine, dacarbazine, dactinomycin, dexamethasone, diphenhydrAMINE, DOPamine, DOXOrubicin, doxycycline, droperidol, etoposide, famotidine, fentanyl, floxuridine, fluconazole, fluorouracil, furosemide, gentamicin, granisetron, heparin, idarubicin, ifosfamide, immune globulin, magnesium sulfate, mannitol, mechlorethamine, meperidine, mesna, methotrexate, metoclopramide, metronidazole, mezlocillin, miconazole, minocycline, mitoxantrone, netilmicin, pentostatin, piperacillin/tazobactam, potassium chloride, prochlorperazine, promethazine, ranitidine, teniposide, ticarcillin, ticarcillin/clavulanate, trimethoprim-sulfamethoxazole, vinBLAStine, vinCRIStine, zidovudine

Perform/provide:
• Storage in refrigerator; do not freeze

Evaluate:
• Therapeutic response: WBC and differential recovery

---

scopolamine (℞)
(skoe-pol′a-meen)
Scopolamine Hydrobromide Injection
Func. class.: Cholinergic blocker
Chem. class.: Belladonna alkaloid

Action: Inhibits acetylcholine at receptor sites in autonomic nervous system, which controls secretions, free acids in stomach; blocks central muscarinic receptors, which decreases involuntary movements
Uses: Reduction of secretions before surgery, motion sickness, parkinsonian symptoms

DOSAGE AND ROUTES
Parkinsonian symptoms
• *Adult:* **IM/SUBCUT/IV** 0.3-0.6 mg tid-qid using dilution provided
Preoperatively
• *Adult:* **SUBCUT** 0.4-0.6 mg
Nausea and vomiting
• *Child:* **SUBCUT** 0.006 mg/kg or 0.2 mg/m^2
Available forms: Inj 0.3, 0.4, 0.86, 1 mg/ml

SIDE EFFECTS
CNS: Confusion, anxiety, restlessness, irritability, delusions, hallucinations, headache, sedation, depression, incoherence, dizziness, excitement, delirium, flushing, weakness
CV: Palpitations, tachycardia, postural hypotension, paradoxic bradycardia
EENT: Blurred vision, photophobia, dilated pupils, difficulty swallowing, mydriasis, cycloplegia
GI: Dryness of mouth, constipation, nausea, vomiting, abdominal distress, *paralytic ileus*
GU: Urinary hesitancy, retention
INTEG: Urticaria
MISC: Suppression of lactation, nasal congestion, decreased sweating
Contraindications: Hypersensitivity, narrow-angle glaucoma, myasthenia

gravis, GI/GU obstruction, hypersensitivity to belladonna, barbiturates

Precautions: Pregnancy (C), elderly, lactation, prostatic hypertrophy, CHF, hypertension, dysrhythmia, children, gastric ulcer

PHARMACOKINETICS

SUBCUT/IM: Peak 30-45 min, duration 7 hr

IV: Peak 10-15 min, duration 4 hr

Excreted in urine, bile, feces (unchanged)

INTERACTIONS

Increase: anticholinergic effect—alcohol, opioids, antihistamines, phenothiazines, tricyclics

Drug/Herb

Increase: anticholinergic effects—henbane, jimsonweed, scopolia

NURSING CONSIDERATIONS

Assess:

• I&O ratio; retention commonly causes decreased urinary output

• Parkinsonism, EPS: shuffling gait, muscle rigidity, involuntary movements

• Urinary hesitancy, retention; palpate bladder if retention occurs

• Constipation; increase fluids, bulk, exercise if this occurs

• For tolerance over long-term therapy; dose may have to be increased or changed

• Mental status: affect, mood, CNS depression, worsening of mental symptoms during early therapy

Administer:

• Parenteral dose with patient recumbent to prevent postural hypotension

• Parenteral dose slowly; keep in bed for at least 1 hr after dose

• With or after meals for GI upset; may give with fluids other than H_2O

• At bedtime to avoid daytime drowsiness in patient with parkinsonism

• With analgesic to avoid behavioral changes when given as a preop

Additive compatibilities: Floxacillin, furosemide, meperidine, succinylcholine

Syringe compatibilities: Atropine, benzquinamide, butorphanol, chlorproMA-ZINE, cimetidine, diamorphine, dimenhyDRINATE, diphenhydrAMINE, droperidol, fentanyl, glycopyrrolate, hydromorphone, hydrOXYzine, meperidine, metoclopramide, midazolam, morphine, nalbuphine, pentazocine, pentobarbital, perphenazine, prochlorperazine, promazine, promethazine, ranitidine, sufentanil, thiopental

Y-site compatibilities: Heparin, hydrocortisone, potassium chloride, propofol, sufentanil, vit B/C

Perform/provide:

• Storage at room temperature in light-resistant container

• Hard candy, frequent drinks, sugarless gum to relieve dry mouth

Evaluate:

• Therapeutic response: decreased secretions

Teach patient/family:

• Not to discontinue this drug abruptly; to taper off over 1 wk

• To avoid driving, other hazardous activities; drowsiness may occur

• To avoid OTC medication: cough, cold preparations with alcohol, antihistamines unless directed by prescriber

scopolamine ophthalmic
See Appendix C

scopolamine (℞) (transdermal)
(skoe-pol′-a-meen)
Transderm-Scop, Transderm-V

Func. class.: Antiemetic, anticholinergic

Chem. class.: Belladonna alkaloid

Action: Competitive antagonism of acetylcholine at receptor site in eye, smooth muscle, cardiac muscle, glandular cells; inhibition of vestibular input to the CNS, resulting in inhibition of vomiting reflex

Uses: Prevention of motion sickness
Investigational uses: Drooling

DOSAGE AND ROUTES

• *Adult:* **PATCH** 1 placed behind ear 4-5 hr before travel, reapply q3d, alternate ears

• Not recommended for children
Drooling (off-label)
• *Adult:* **TD** 1.5 mg patch q3d
Available forms: Patch, 0.5, 1 mg delivered in 72 hr

SIDE EFFECTS

CNS: Dizziness, drowsiness, confusion, disorientation, memory disturbances, hallucinations
EENT: Blurred vision, altered depth perception, *dilated pupils,* photophobia, *dry mouth;* dry, itchy, red eyes; acute narrow-angle glaucoma
GU: Difficult urination
INTEG: Rash, erythema
Contraindications: Hypersensitivity, glaucoma
Precautions: Pregnancy (C), children, elderly; pyloric, urinary, bladder neck, intestinal obstruction; hepatic disease, renal disease

PHARMACOKINETICS

Patch: Onset 4-5 hr, duration 72 hr

INTERACTIONS

Increase: anticholinergic effects—antihistamines, antidepressants

NURSING CONSIDERATIONS

Administer:
• With clean, dry hands. Wash, dry hands before and after applying to surface behind ear

Teach patient/family:
• To avoid hazardous activities, activities requiring alertness; dizziness may occur
• To change patch q72h

• To apply at least 4 hr before traveling
• If blurred vision, severe dizziness, drowsiness occurs, to discontinue use, use another type of antiemetic or rotate the patch to other ear
• To read label of all OTC medications; if any scopolamine is found in product, avoid use
• To keep out of children's reach

Rarely Used ⚠ High Alert

secobarbital (℞)
(see-koe-bar'bi-tal)
Secogen Sodium ✤, Seconal Sodium Pulvules, Seral ✤
Func. class.: Sedative/hypnotic-barbiturate

Controlled Substance Schedule II (USA), Schedule G (CDSA IV) (Canada)
Uses: Insomnia, sedation, preoperative medication, status epilepticus, acute tetanus convulsions

DOSAGE AND ROUTES

Insomnia
• *Adult:* **PO/IM** 100-200 mg at bedtime
• *Child:* **IM** 3-5 mg/kg, not to exceed 100 mg, not to inject >5 ml in one site
Sedation/preoperatively
• *Adult:* **PO** 200-300 mg 1-2 hr preoperatively
• *Child:* **PO** 50-100 mg 1-2 hr preoperatively
Status epilepticus
• *Adult and child:* **IM/IV** 250-350 mg
Acute psychotic agitation
• *Adult and child:* **IM/IV** 5.5 mg/kg q3-4h
Contraindications: Pregnancy (D), hypersensitivity to barbiturates, respiratory depression, addiction to barbiturates, severe liver impairment, porphyria, uncontrolled severe pain

S

selegiline (℞)

(se-le'ji-leen)
Apo-Selegiline, Carbex,
Eldepryl, Gen-Selegiline,
Novo-Selegiline ✦, Nu-
Selegiline, SD-Deprenyl
Func. class.: Antiparkinson agent
Chem. class.: MAOI, type B

Do not confuse:
Eldepryl/enalapril

Action: Increased dopaminergic activity by inhibition of MAO type B activity; not fully understood

Uses: Adjunct management of Parkinson's disease in patients being treated with levodopa/carbidopa who had poor response to therapy

Investigational uses: Alzheimer's disease, depression

DOSAGE AND ROUTES

• *Adult:* **PO** 10 mg/day given with levodopa/carbidopa in divided doses 5 mg at breakfast and lunch; after 2-3 days begin to reduce dose of levodopa/carbidopa 10%-30%

Alzheimer's disease (off-label)
• *Adult:* **PO** 5 mg bid AM, PM

Available forms: Tabs 5 mg, caps 5 mg

SIDE EFFECTS

CNS: Increased tremors, chorea, restlessness, blepharospasm, increased bradykinesia, grimacing, tardive dyskinesia, dystonic symptoms, involuntary movements, increased apraxia, hallucinations, *dizziness,* mood changes, nightmares, delusions, lethargy, apathy, overstimulation, sleep disturbances, headache, migraine, numbness, muscle cramps, confusion, anxiety, tiredness, vertigo, personality change, back/leg pain

CV: Orthostatic hypotension, hypertension, dysrhythmia, palpitations, angina pectoris, hypotension, *tachycardia,* edema, *sinus bradycardia,* syncope, *hypertensive crisis*

EENT: Diplopia, dry mouth, blurred vision, tinnitus

GI: Nausea, vomiting, constipation, weight loss, anorexia, diarrhea, heartburn, rectal bleeding, poor appetite, dysphagia, xerostomia

GU: Slow urination, nocturia, prostatic hypertrophy, urinary hesitation, retention, frequency, sexual dysfunction

INTEG: Increased sweating, alopecia, hematoma, rash, photosensitivity, facial hair

RESP: Asthma, shortness of breath

Contraindications: Hypersensitivity

Precautions: Pregnancy (C), lactation, children

PHARMACOKINETICS

Rapidly absorbed, peak ½-2 hr; rapidly metabolized (active metabolites: *N*-desmethyldeprenyl, amphetamine, methamphetamine), metabolites excreted in urine, half-life 9 min

INTERACTIONS

⚠ **Fatal interaction**—Opioids (especially meperidine); do not administer together

⚠ **Serotonin syndrome** (confusion, seizures, fever, hypertension, agitation)—fluoxetine, paroxetine, sertraline, fluvoxamine (discontinue 5 wk prior to selegiline); do not use together

⚠ **Fatal interaction**—Do not use with tricyclics

Increase: side effects of levodopa/carbidopa

Drug/Herb
Decrease: selegiline action—chaste tree fruit, kava

Drug/Lab Test
Decrease: VMA

False positive: Urine ketones, urine glucose

False negative: Urine glucose (glucose oxidase)

False increase: Uric acid, urine protein

NURSING CONSIDERATIONS

Assess:

• Decreased parkinsonian symptoms: rigidity, unsteady gait, weakness, tremors

• B/P, respiration throughout treatment

• Mental status: affect, mood behavioral changes, depression; perform suicide assessment

Administer:

• Drug until NPO before surgery

• Adjusting dosage to response

• With meals; limit protein taken with drug

• At doses <10 mg/day, because of risks associated with nonselective inhibition of MAO

Perform/provide:

• Assistance with ambulation during beginning therapy

Evaluate:

• Therapeutic response: decrease in akathisia, improved mood

Teach patient/family:

• To change positions slowly to prevent orthostatic hypotension

• To report side effects: twitching, eye spasms; indicate overdose

• To use drug exactly as prescribed; if discontinued abruptly, parkinsonian crisis may occur

• To avoid foods high in tyramine: cheese, pickled products, wine, beer, large amounts of caffeine

• Not to exceed recommended dose of 10 mg; might precipitate hypertensive crisis; report severe headache, other unusual symptoms

Treatment of overdose: IV fluids for hypertension, IV dilute pressure agent for B/P titration

---

selenium topical
See Appendix C

---

senna, sennosides
(**otc**)
(sen'na)
Black Draught, Dr. Caldwell
Dosalax, Ex-Lax Gentle,
Fletcher's Castoria, Gentlax,
Senexon, Senna-Gen,
Senokot, Senokotxtra,
Senolax
Func. class.: Laxative-stimulant
Chem. class.: Anthraquinone

Action: Stimulates peristalsis by action on Auerbach's plexus; softens feces by increasing water, electrolytes in large intestine

Uses: Acute constipation; bowel preparation for surgery or examination

DOSAGE AND ROUTES

• *Adult:* **PO** 1-8 tabs (Senokot)/day or ½ to 4 tsp of granules (1 tsp-4 ml) added to water or juice; **RECT SUPP** 1-2 at bedtime; **SYR** 1-4 tsp at bedtime, 7.5-15 ml (Black Draught) ¾ oz dissolved in 2.5 oz liquid given between 2-4 PM the day before procedure (X-Prep)

• *Child >27 kg:* **PO** ½ adult dose; do not use Black Draught for children

• *Child 1 mo-1 yr:* **SYR** 1.25-2.5 ml (Senokot) at bedtime

Available forms: Supp 625 mg, 30 mg sennosides; powder 662 mg/g, 6, 15 mg sennosides/3 g; tabs 8.6 mg sennosides, 180 mg; oral sol 3 mg sennosides/ml

SIDE EFFECTS

GI: Nausea, vomiting, anorexia, cramps, diarrhea, flatulence
GU: Pink, red or brown, black urine
META: Hypocalcemia, enteropathy, alkalosis, hypokalemia, **tetany**
Contraindications: Hypersensitivity, GI bleeding, obstruction, CHF, lactation, abdominal pain, nausea/vomiting, appendicitis, acute surgical abdomen
Precautions: Pregnancy (C)

S

Side effects: *italics* = common; ***bold italics*** = life-threatening

PHARMACOKINETICS

PO: Onset 6-24 hr; metabolized by liver, excreted in feces

INTERACTIONS

Do not use with disulfiram (Antabuse)

Drug/Herb
Increase: laxative effect—flax, senna

NURSING CONSIDERATIONS

Assess:
• Stool: color, consistency, amount
• Blood, urine electrolytes if drug is used often
• I&O ratio to identify fluid loss
• Cause of constipation; fluids, bulk, exercise missing, constipating drugs
• Cramping, rectal bleeding, nausea, vomiting; drug should be discontinued

Administer:
• In morning or evening (oral dose) with full glass of water
• Dissolve granules in water or juice before administration
• On empty stomach for more rapid results
• Shake oral sol before giving

Evaluate:
• Therapeutic response: decrease in constipation

Teach patient/family:
• That urine, feces may turn yellow-brown to red
• Not to use laxatives for long-term therapy; bowel tone will be lost
• That normal bowel movements do not always occur daily
• Not to use in presence of abdominal pain, nausea, vomiting
• To notify prescriber if constipation unrelieved or of symptoms of electrolyte imbalance: muscle cramps, pain, weakness, dizziness, excessive thirst

sertaconazole topical
See Appendix C

A Safety alert   *"Tall Man" lettering

sertraline (℞)

(ser'tra-leen)
Zoloft
Func. class.: Antidepressant
Chem. class.: SSRI

Do not confuse:
Zoloft/Zocor

Action: Inhibits serotonin reuptake in CNS; increases action of serotonin; does not affect dopamine, norepinephrine
Uses: Major depressive disorder, obsessive-compulsive disorder (OCD), post-traumatic stress disorder (PTSD), panic disorder, social anxiety disorder, premenstrual disphoric disorder (PMDD)

DOSAGE AND ROUTES

• *Adult:* **PO** 50 mg daily; may increase to max of 200 mg/day; do not change dose at intervals of <1 wk; administer daily in AM or PM; or 100 mg 3 ×/wk (off-label)
• *Geriatric:* **PO** 25 mg daily, increase by 25 mg q3 days to desired dose
• *Child 6-12 yr:* **PO** 25 mg daily
• *Child 13-17 yr:* **PO** 50 mg daily
Premenstrual disorders
• *Adult:* **PO** 50-150 mg nightly
Available forms: Tabs 25, 50, 100 mg; oral conc 20 mg/ml

SIDE EFFECTS

CNS: Insomnia, agitation, somnolence, dizziness, headache, tremor, fatigue, paresthesia, twitching, confusion, ataxia, gait abnormality (elderly)
CV: Palpitations, chest pain
EENT: Vision abnormalities
ENDO: SIADH (elderly)
GI: Diarrhea, nausea, constipation, anorexia, dry mouth, dyspepsia, *vomiting, flatulence*
GU: Male sexual dysfunction, micturition disorder
INTEG: Increased sweating, rash, hot flashes

Contraindications: Hypersensitivity to this drug or SSRIs

Precautions: Pregnancy (B), lactation, elderly, hepatic disease, renal disease, epilepsy, recent MI; latex sensitivity (dropper of oral conc)

PHARMACOKINETICS

PO: Peak 4.5-8.4 hr; steady state 1 wk; plasma protein binding 99%, elimination half-life 1-4 days, extensively metabolized, metabolite excreted in urine, bile

INTERACTIONS

Altered lithium levels: lithium

Sertraline is contraindicated with pimozide

Disulfiram reaction: disulfiram and oral conc due to alcohol content

⚠ Fatal reactions: MAOIs

Increase: sertraline levels—cimetidine, warfarin, other highly protein-bound drugs

Increase: effects of antidepressants (tricyclics), diazepam, TOLBUTamide, warfarin, benzodiazepines, sumatriptan

Drug/Herb

Hypertensive crisis: ephedra

Increase: of SSRI, serotonin syndrome—St. John's wort, SAM-e; do not use together

Increase: anticholinergic effect—corkwood, jimsonweed

Increase: CNS effect—hops, lavender

Drug/Lab Test

Increase: AST, ALT

NURSING CONSIDERATIONS

Assess:

• Mental status: mood, sensorium, affect, suicidal tendencies, increase in psychiatric symptoms, depression, panic

• B/P (lying/standing), pulse q4h; if systolic B/P drops 20 mm Hg, hold drug, notify prescriber; VS q4h in patients with cardiovascular disease

• Weight qwk; appetite may decrease with drug

• Urinary retention, constipation, especially in elderly

• Alcohol consumption; hold dose until morning

Administer:

• Increased fluids, bulk in diet for constipation, urinary retention

• With food, milk for GI symptoms

• Crushed if patient is unable to swallow medication whole

• Sugarless gum, hard candy, frequent sips of water for dry mouth

• Oral conc: dilute prior to use with 4 oz (½ cup) of water, orange juice, ginger ale or lemon/lime soda; do not mix with other liquids

• Avoid use with other CNS depressants

Perform/provide:

• Storage at room temperature; do not freeze

• Assistance with ambulation during therapy, since drowsiness, dizziness occur

• Safety measures, including side rails, primarily for elderly

• Checking to see that PO medication is swallowed

Evaluate:

• Therapeutic response: significant improvement in depression, OCS

Teach patient/family:

• That therapeutic effect may take 1 wk or longer

• To use caution in driving, other activities requiring alertness; drowsiness, dizziness, blurred vision may occur

• Not to discontinue medication quickly after long-term use; may cause nausea, headache, malaise

• To avoid alcohol

• To notify prescriber if pregnant or plan to become pregnant or breast-feed

S

Rarely Used

sevelamer (R)
(seh-vel'ah-mer)
Renagel
Func. class.: Polymeric phosphate binder

Uses: End-stage renal disease (ESRD)

DOSAGE AND ROUTES

Reduction of serum phosphorus in adults not taking phosphate binders
- *Adult:* PO initially 800-1600 mg tid with meals based on serum phosphorus level (see below); adjust dose gradually at 2-wk intervals until serum phosphorus 6 mg/dl
- *Adult, serum phosphorus ≥9 mg/dl:* 1600 mg tid with meals
- *Adult, serum phosphorus ≥7.5 and <9 mg/dl:* 1200-1600 mg tid with meals
- *Adult, serum phosphorus >6 and <7.5 mg/dl:* 800 mg tid with meals

Contraindications: Hypophosphatemia, bowel obstruction, hypersensitivity

Rarely Used

sibutramine (R)
(si-byoo'tra-meen)
Meridia
Func. class.: Appetite suppressant

Controlled Substance Schedule IV
Uses: Obesity in conjunction with other treatments

DOSAGE AND ROUTES

- *Adult:* PO 10 mg daily; may be increased to 15 mg daily after 4 wk, or lowered to 5 mg daily depending on response

Contraindications: Hypersensitivity, hypothyroidism, anorexia nervosa, severe hepatic/renal disease, uncontrolled hypertension, history of CAD, CHF, dysrhythmias, lactation, CVA

sildenafil (R)
(sil-den'a-fill)
Viagra
Func. class.: Erectile agent
Chem. class.: Selective inhibitor of cGMP-PDE5

Action: Enhances the effect of nitric oxide (NO) by inhibiting phosphodiesterase type 5 (PDE5), which is necessary for degrading cGMP in the corpus cavernosum
Uses: Treatment of erectile dysfunction

DOSAGE AND ROUTES

- *Adult:* PO 50 mg 1 hr before sexual activity, may be taken ½-4 hr before sexual activity; may be increased to 100 mg or decreased to 25 mg; max once/day
Renal/hepatic dose
- *Adult:* PO 25 mg, take 1 hr before sexual activity; do not use more than 1 ×/day

Available forms: Tabs 25, 50, 100 mg

SIDE EFFECTS

CNS: Headache, flushing, dizziness
CV: **MI, sudden death, CV collapse**
MISC.: Dyspepsia, nasal congestion, UTI, abnormal vision, diarrhea, rash, **NAION (nonarteritic ischemic optic neuropathy)**
Contraindication: Hypersensitivity to nitrates
Precautions: Pregnancy (B), anatomical penile deformities, sickle cell anemia, leukemia, multiple myeloma, retinitis pigmentosa

PHARMACOKINETICS

Rapidly absorbed; bioavailability 40%; metabolized by P45 CYP3A4, 2C9 in the liver (active metabolites); terminal half-life 4 hr, peak ½-1½ hr; reduced absorption with high-fat meal; excreted feces, urine

INTERACTIONS

⚠ Do not use with nitrates; fatal fall in B/P

⚠ Safety alert   *"Tall Man" lettering

Increase: sildenafil levels—cimetidine, erythromycin, ketoconazole, itraconazole, antiretroviral protease inhibitors
Decrease: sildenafil levels—rifampin, barbiturates
Decrease: B/P—α-blockers

NURSING CONSIDERATIONS
Assess:
• For any severe loss of vision while taking this or any similar products; these products should not be used
• Use of organic nitrates that should not be used with this drug
Administer:
• Approximately 1 hr before sexual activity, do not use more than once a day
Teach patient/family:
• That drug does not protect against sexually transmitted diseases, including HIV
• That drug absorption is reduced with a high-fat meal
• That drug should not be used with nitrates in any form
• That tabs may be split
• To notify prescriber immediately and stop taking product if vision loss occurs

---

silver nitrate (R)
Func. class.: Keratolytic

Action: Antiinfective, astringent, caustic
Uses: Cauterization of lesions, warts, burns (low concentrations)

DOSAGE AND ROUTES
• *Adult and child:* **TOP** apply to area to be treated
Available forms: Sticks, sol 10%, 25%, 50%

SIDE EFFECTS
INTEG: Skin discoloration
Contraindications: Hypersensitivity

INTERACTIONS
Not to be used with alkalines, phosphates, thimerosal, benzalkonium chloride, halogenated acids

NURSING CONSIDERATIONS
Administer:
• After moistening stick with water
• To burns using a wet dressing (low concentrations 0.125%)
Perform/provide:
• Storage in cool area
Evaluate:
• Therapeutic response: absence of lesions, healing of burned areas
Teach patient/family:
• To avoid contact with clothing, unaffected areas; discoloration may occur

---

silver nitrate 1%
See Appendix C

---

silver nitrate 1% sulfacetamide sodium ophthalmic
See Appendix C

---

silver protein, mild (R, otc)
Argyrol S.S. 10%, Argyrol S.S. 20%
Func. class.: Disinfectant
Chem. class.: Silver colloidal compound

Action: Destroys gram-positive, gram-negative organisms
Uses: Eye, nose, throat, swelling, infection

DOSAGE AND ROUTES
• *Adult and child:* **TOP** sol use as needed
Available forms: Top sol 5%, 10%, 25%; eyedrops 20%

SIDE EFFECTS
INTEG: Irritation, discolored tissue
Contraindications: Hypersensitivity
Precautions: Pregnancy (C)

R

NURSING CONSIDERATIONS

Administer:
• To area to be treated only; do not apply to healthy skin

Perform/provide:
• Storage in tight container

Evaluate:
• Area of body involved: irritation, rash, breaks, dryness, scales

---

silver sulfADIAZINE topical
See Appendix C

---

simethicone (otc, ℞)
(si-meth'i-kone)
Extra Strength Gas-X, Extra Strength Maalox Anti-Gas, Extra Stength Maalox GRFGas Relief Formula ✿, Flatulex, Gas-Relief, Gas-X, Genasyme, Maalox Anti-Gas, Maalox GRF Gas Relief Formula ✿, Maximum Strength Gas Relief, Maximum Strength Mylanta Gas Relief, Maximum Strength Phazyme, Mylanta Gas, Mylicon, Ovol ✿, Phazyme, Phazyme 95, Phazyme 125
Func. class.: Antiflatulent

Do not confuse:
Mylicon/Mylanta Gas

Action: Disperses, prevents gas pockets in GI system; does not decrease gas production

Uses: Flatulence

Investigational uses: Dyspepsia

DOSAGE AND ROUTES

• *Adult and child >12 yr:* **PO** 40-100 mg pc, at bedtime
• *Child <2 yr:* **PO** 20 mg qid

Available forms: Chew tabs 40, 80, 125 mg; tabs 60, 80, 95 mg; drops 40 mg/0.6 ml, 40 mg/ml, 95 mg/1.425 ml; caps 95, 125 mg; caps, soft gel 125 mg

SIDE EFFECTS

GI: Belching, rectal flatus

Contraindications: Hypersensitivity, GI obstruction/perforation

Precautions: Pregnancy (C), abdominal pain, fistula, hiatal hernia

NURSING CONSIDERATIONS

Assess:
• Reason for excess gas production, decreased bowel sounds, recent surgery, other GI conditions

Administer:
• After meals, at bedtime; shake susp well before giving; chew tabs should be chewed

Evaluate:
• Therapeutic response: absence of flatulence

Teach patient/family:
• That tablets must be chewed
• To shake suspension well before pouring

---

simvastatin (℞)
(sim-va-sta'tin)
Zocor
Func. class.: Antilipidemic
Chem. class.: HMG-CoA reductase inhibitor

Do not confuse:
Zocor/Cozaar
Zocor/Zoloft

Action: Inhibits HMG-CoA reductase enzyme, which reduces cholesterol synthesis

Uses: As an adjunct in primary hypercholesterolemia (types IIa, IIb), isolated hypertriglyceridemia (Frederickson type IV) and type III hyperlipoproteinemia, coronary artery disease

DOSAGE AND ROUTES

• *Adult:* **PO** 20 mg daily in PM initially; usual range 5-40 mg/day in PM, not to exceed 80 mg/day; dosage adjustments

---

⚠ Safety alert   *"Tall Man" lettering

may be made in 4-wk intervals or more; those taking verapamil and amiodarone max 20 mg/day

• *Geriatric/renal disease/those taking cycloSPORINE:* **PO** 5 mg/day, initially
Available forms: Tabs 5, 10, 20, 40, 80 mg

SIDE EFFECTS

CNS: Headache
EENT: Lens opacities
GI: Nausea, constipation, diarrhea, dyspepsia, flatus, abdominal pain, *liver dysfunction,* pancreatitis
INTEG: Rash, pruritus, photosensitivity
MS: Muscle cramps, myalgia, *myositis, rhabdomyolysis*
RESP: Upper respiratory tract infection
Contraindications: Pregnancy (X), hypersensitivity, lactation, active hepatic disease
Precautions: Past hepatic disease, alcoholism, severe acute infections, trauma, severe metabolic disorders, electrolyte imbalances

PHARMACOKINETICS

Metabolized in liver (active metabolites), highly protein bound, excreted primarily in bile, feces (60%)

INTERACTIONS

Increase: effects of warfarin
Increase: myalgia, myositis—cycloSPORINE, gemfibrozil, niacin, erythromycin, clofibrate, clarithromycin, ketoconazole, itraconazole, protease inhibitors
Increase: serum level of digoxin
Drug/Herb

Increase: effect—glucomannan
Decrease: effect—gotu kola
Drug/Lab Test
Increase: CPK, LFTs

NURSING CONSIDERATIONS

Assess:
• 12-hr fasting lipid profile: LDL, HDL, TG, cholesterol at 6-8 wk, and q6mo
• Hepatic studies q1-2mo during the

first 1½ yr of treatment; AST, ALT, LFTs may increase
A For rhabdomyolysis: muscle tenderness, increased CPK levels; therapy should be discontinued
• Renal studies in patients with compromised renal system: BUN, I&O ratio, creatinine
Administer:
• Total daily dose in evening
Perform/provide:
• Storage in cool environment in tight container protected from light
Evaluate:
• Therapeutic response: decrease in cholesterol to desired level after 8 wk
Teach patient/family:
• That blood work and eye exam will be necessary during treatment
• To report blurred vision, severe GI symptoms, dizziness, headache
• That previously prescribed regimen will continue: low-cholesterol diet, exercise program

---

sirolimus (℞)

(seer-oh-lie'mus)
Rapamune
Func. class.: Immunosuppressant
Chem. class.: Macrolide

Action: Produces immunosuppression by inhibiting T-lymphocyte activation and proliferation
Uses: Organ transplants to prevent rejection, recommended use is with cycloSPORINE and corticosteroids
Investigational uses: Psoriasis

DOSAGE AND ROUTES

• *Adult:* **PO** 2 mg daily with a 6 mg loading dose, may use 5 mg daily with a 15 mg loading dose
• *Child >13 yr weighing <40 kg (88 lb):* to 1 mg/m²/day, 3 mg/m² loading dose
Hepatic dose
• *Adult/child ≥13 yr/<40 kg:* **PO** Reduce by 33% in maintenance dose
Available forms: Oral sol 1 mg/ml

Side effects: *italics* = common; ***bold italics*** = life-threatening

S

SIDE EFFECTS

CNS: Tremors, headache, insomnia, paresthesia, chills, fever
CV: Hypertension, *atrial fibrillation, CHF, hypotension, palpitation, tachycardia*
EENT: Blurred vision, photophobia
GI: Nausea, vomiting, diarrhea, constipation
GU: UTIs, *albuminuria, hematuria, proteinuria, renal failure*
HEMA: Anemia, leukopenia, thrombocytopenia, purpura
INTEG: Rash, acne, photosensitivity
META: Hyperglycemia, increased creatinine, edema, hypercholesterolemia, *hyperlipemia,* hypophosphatemia, weight gain, hyperkalemia, hyperuricemia, hypokalemia, hypomagnesemia
RESP: Pleural effusion, atelectasis, dyspnea
SYST: Lymphoma

Contraindications: Hypersensitivity to this drug or to components of the drug, lactation
Precautions: Pregnancy (C), severe renal, hepatic disease; diabetes mellitus, hyperkalemia, hyperuricemia, lymphomas, infection, other malignancies, children <13 yr, hypertension

PHARMACOKINETICS

Rapidly absorbed, peak 1 hr single dose, 2 hr multiple dosing, protein binding 92%; extensively metabolized by CYP3A4 enzyme system

INTERACTIONS

Increase: blood levels—antifungals, calcium channel blockers , cimetidine, danazol, erythromycin, cycloSPORINE, metoclopramide, bromocriptine, HIV-protease inhibitors
Decrease: blood levels—carbamazepine, phenobarbital, phenytoin, rifamycin, rifapentine
Decrease: effect of vaccines

Drug/Food
Alters bioavailability; use consistently with or without food; do not use with grapefruit juice
Drug/Herb
St. John's wort: may decrease the effect of sirolimus
Increase: effect—ginseng, maitake, mistletoe
Decrease: immunosuppression—astragalus, echinacea, melatonin

NURSING CONSIDERATIONS
Assess:
• Blood levels in those that may have altered metabolism, trough level ≥15 ng/ml are associated with increased adverse reactions
• Lipid profile: cholesterol, triglycerides, a lipid-lowering agent may be needed
⚠ For infection and development of lymphoma
⚠ Blood studies: Hgb, WBC, platelets during treatment qmo; if leukocytes <3000/mm³ or platelets <100,000/mm³, drug should be discontinued or reduced; decreased hemoglobulin level may indicate bone marrow suppression
• Hepatic studies: alk phosphatase, AST, ALT, amylase, bilirubin, and for hepatotoxicity: dark urine, jaundice, itching, light-colored stools; drug should be discontinued
Administer:
• Prophylaxis for *Pneumocystis jiroveci* pneumonia for 1 yr after transplantation; prophylaxis for cytomegalovirus (CMV) is recommended for 90 days after transplantation in those at increased risk for CMV
• All medications PO if possible, avoiding IM inj; bleeding may occur
• For 3 days before transplant surgery; patients should be placed in protective isolation
• Use amber oral dose syringe and withdraw amount oral sol needed from the bottle, empty correct dose into plastic/glass container holding 60 ml of water/orange juice, stir vigorously and have

patient drink at once, refill container with additional 120 ml water/orange juice, stir vigorously and drink at once, if using a pouch squeeze entire contents into container and follow above directions

• Store protected from light, refrigerate, stable for 24 mo

Evaluate:

• Therapeutic response: absence of graft rejection; immunosuppression in autoimmune disorders

Teach patient/family:

• To report fever, rash, severe diarrhea, chills, sore throat, fatigue; serious infections may occur; clay-colored stools, cramping (hepatotoxicity)

• To avoid crowds, persons with known infections to reduce risk of infection

• To use contraception before, during and 12 wk after drug has been discontinued, avoid breastfeeding

• Use sunscreen, protective clothing to prevent burns

---

sodium bicarbonate (R̥, otc)

Baking Soda, Bellans, Citrocarbonate, Neut, Soda Mint

Func. class.: Alkalinizer
Chem. class.: NaHCO₃

Action: Orally neutralizes gastric acid, which forms water, NaCl, CO_2; increases plasma bicarbonate, which buffers H^+-ion concentration; reverses acidosis IV
Uses: Acidosis (metabolic), cardiac arrest, alkalinization (systemic/urinary) antacid

DOSAGE AND ROUTES

Acidosis, metabolic
• *Adult and child:* **IV INF** 2-5 mEq/kg over 4-8 hr depending on CO_2, pH
Cardiac arrest
• *Adult and child:* **IV BOL** 1 mEq/kg of 7.5% or 8.4% sol, then 0.5 mEq/kg q10 min, then doses based on ABGs

• *Infant:* **IV INF** not to exceed 8 mEq/kg/day based on ABGs (4.2% sol)
Alkalinization of urine
• *Adult:* **PO** 325 mg-2 g qid or 48 mEq (4g), then 12-24 mEq q4h
• *Child:* **PO** 12-120 mg/kg/day (1-10 mEq/kg)
Antacid
• *Adult:* **PO** 300 mg-2 g chewed, taken with H_2O daily-qid
Available forms: Tabs 300, 325, 600, 650 mg; inj 4.2%, 5%, 7.5%, 8.4%

SIDE EFFECTS

CNS: Irritability, headache, confusion, stimulation, tremors, *twitching, hyper-reflexia, tetany,* weakness, *seizures* of alkalosis
CV: Irregular pulse, ***cardiac arrest,*** water retention, edema, weight gain
GI: Flatulence, *belching, distention, **paralytic ileus,*** acid rebound
GU: Calculi
META: Alkalosis
RESP: Shallow, slow respirations; cyanosis, ***apnea***
Contraindications: Hypertension, peptic ulcer, renal disease, hypocalcemia
Precautions: Pregnancy (C), CHF, cirrhosis, toxemia, renal disease

PHARMACOKINETICS

PO: Onset 2 min, duration 10 min
IV: Onset 15 min, duration 1-2 hr, excreted in urine

INTERACTIONS

Increase: effects—amphetamines, mecamylamine, quinine, quinidine, pseudoephedrine, flecainide, anorexiants
Increase: sodium and decrease potassium—corticosteroids
Decrease: effects—lithium, chlorpropamide, barbiturates, salicylates, benzodiazepines
Drug/Herb
Decrease: action of sodium bicarbonate—oak bark

Side effects: *italics* = common; ***bold italics*** = life-threatening

Drug/Lab Test

Increase: Urinary urobilinogen
False positive: Urinary protein, blood lactate

NURSING CONSIDERATIONS
Assess:

• Respiratory and pulse rate, rhythm, depth, lung sounds; notify prescriber of abnormalities

• Fluid balance (I&O, weight daily, edema); notify prescriber of fluid overload

• Electrolytes, blood pH, PO_2, HCO_3^-, during treatment; ABGs frequently during emergencies

• Urine pH, urinary output, during beginning treatment

• Extravasation with IV administration (tissue sloughing, ulceration, and necrosis)

• Weight daily with initial therapy

• Alkalosis: irritability, confusion, twitching, hyperreflexia stimulation, slow respirations, cyanosis, irregular pulse

• Milk-alkali syndrome: confusion, headache, nausea, vomiting, anorexia, urinary stones, hypercalcemia

• For GI perforation secondary to CO_2 in GI tract; may lead to perforation if ulcer is severe enough
Administer:

• Chew antacid tablets and drink 8 oz water

• Do not take antacid with milk or milk-alkali syndrome may result
IV route

• In prepared sol or diluted in an equal amount of compatible sol given 2-5 mEq/kg over 4-8 hr, not to exceed 50 mEq/hr; slower rate in children

Additive compatibilities: Amikacin, aminophylline, amobarbital, amphotericin B, atropine, bretylium, calcium gluceptate, cefoxitin, ceftazidime, cephalothin, cephapirin, chloramphenicol, chlorothiazide, cimetidine, clindamycin, cytarabine, droperidol/fentanyl, ergonovine, erythromycin, esmolol, floxacillin, furosemide, heparin, hyaluronidase, hydrocortisone, kanamycin, lidocaine, mannitol, metaraminol, methotrexate, methyldopa, multivitamins, nafcillin, nalmefene, netilmicin, nizatidine, ofloxacin, oxacillin, oxytocin, phenobarbital, phenylephrine, phenytoin, phytonadione, potassium chloride, prochlorperazine, thiopental, verapamil

Syringe compatibilities: Milrinone, pentobarbital

Y-site compatibilities: Acyclovir, amifostine, asparaginase, aztreonam, cefepime, cefmetazole, ceftriaxone, cladribine, cyclophosphamide, cytarabine, DAUNOrubicin, dexamethasone, dexchlorpheniramine, DOXOrubicin, etoposide, famotidine, filgrastim, fludarabine, gallium, granisetron, heparin, ifosfamide, indomethacin sodium trihydrate, insulin, melphalan, mesna, methylPREDNISolone, morphine, paclitaxel, piperacillin/tazobactam, potassium chloride, propofol, remifentanil, tacrolimus, teniposide, thiotepa, tolazoline, vancomycin, vit B/C

Evaluate:

• Therapeutic response: ABGs, electrolytes, blood pH, HCO_3^- WNL
Teach patient/family:

• Not to take antacid with milk, or milk-alkali syndrome may result

• Not to use antacid for more than 2 wk

• To notify prescriber if indigestion is accompanied by chest pain, dyspnea, diarrhea, dark, tarry stools

• About sodium-restricted diet; to avoid use of baking soda for indigestion

---

sodium biphosphate/ sodium phosphate
(otc)

Fleet Enema, Phospho-Soda
Func. class.: Laxative, saline

Action: Increases water absorption in the small intestine by osmotic action, laxative effect occurs by increased peristalsis and water retention
Uses: Constipation, bowel or rectal preparation for surgery, exam

---

DOSAGE AND ROUTES

- *Adult:* **PO** 20-30 ml (Phospho-Soda)
- *Child:* **PO** 5-15 ml (Phospho-Soda)
- *Adult and child >12 yr:* **RECT** 1 enema (118 ml)
- *Child 2-12 yr:* **RECT** ½ enema (59 ml)

Available forms: Enema 7 g phosphate/19 g biphosphate/118 ml; oral sol 18 g phosphate/48 g biphosphate/100 ml

SIDE EFFECTS

CV: ***Dysrhythmias, cardiac arrest,*** hypotension, widening QRS complex
GI: Nausea, cramps, diarrhea
META: Electrolyte, fluid imbalances
Contraindications: Hypersensitivity, rectal fissures, abdominal pain, nausea/vomiting, appendicitis, acute surgical abdomen, ulcerated hemorrhoids, sodium-restricted diets, renal failure, hyperphosphatemia, hypocalcemia, hypokalemia, hypernatremia, Addison's disease, CHF, ascites, bowel perforation
Precautions: Pregnancy (C)

PHARMACOKINETICS

Excreted in feces

NURSING CONSIDERATIONS

Assess:
- Stools: color, amount, consistency
- Bowel pattern, bowel sounds, flatulence, distention, fever, dietary patterns, exercise
- Blood, urine electrolytes if drug is used often by patient
- Cramping, rectal bleeding, nausea, vomiting; if these symptoms occur, drug should be discontinued

Administer:
- Alone for better absorption; do not take within 1-2 hr of other drugs

Evaluate:
- Therapeutic response: decrease in constipation

Teach patient/family:
- Not to use laxatives for long-term therapy; bowel tone will be lost

- That normal bowel movements do not always occur daily
- Not to use in presence of abdominal pain, nausea, vomiting
- To notify prescriber if constipation unrelieved or if symptoms of electrolyte imbalance occur: muscle cramps, pain, weakness, dizziness, excessive thirst
- To maintain fluid consumption

---

sodium polystyrene sulfonate (℞)
(po-lee-stye′reen)
Kayexalate, K-Exit ✦, Kionex, PMS Sodium Polystyrene Sulfonate ✦, SPS
Func. class.: Potassium-removing resin
Chem. class.: Cation exchange resin

Action: Removes potassium by exchanging sodium for potassium in body primarily in large intestine
Uses: Hyperkalemia in conjunction with other measures

DOSAGE AND ROUTES

- *Adult:* **PO** 15 g daily-qid; **RECT** enema 30-50 g/100 ml of sorbitol warmed to body temp q6h
- *Child:* **PO/RECT** 1 mEq of potassium exchanged/g of resin, approximate dose 1 g/kg q6h

Available forms: Susp 15 g polystyrene sulfonate, 21.5 ml sorbitol, 15 g (65 mEq) Na/60 ml; powder 15 g/4 level tsp

SIDE EFFECTS

GI: Constipation, anorexia, nausea, vomiting, diarrhea (sorbitol), fecal impaction, gastric irritation
META: Hypocalcemia, hypokalemia, hypomagnesemia, sodium retention
Contraindications: Hypersensitivity to saccharin or parabens that may be in some products, ileus
Precautions: Pregnancy (C), renal failure, CHF, severe edema, severe hyper-

S

tension, elderly, sodium restriction, constipation

INTERACTIONS

Increase: hypokalemia—loop diuretics
Decrease: effect of sodium polystyrene—antacids, laxatives

NURSING CONSIDERATIONS
Assess:

• Hyperkalemia: confusion, dyspnea, weakness, dysrhythmias
• ECG for spiked T waves, depressed ST segments, prolonged QT and widening QRS complex
• Bowel function daily, note consistency of stools, times/day
• Hypotension: confusion, irritability, muscular pain, weakness
• Serum K, Ca, Mg, Na, acid-base balance
• I&O ratio, weight daily

Administer:

• Oral dose as susp mixed with H_2O or syr (20-100 ml)
• Mild laxative as ordered to prevent constipation, fecal impaction
• Sorbitol as ordered to prevent constipation
• Retention enema after mixing with warm water; introduce by gravity, continue stirring, flush with 100 ml of fluid, clamp, and leave in place

Perform/provide:

• Retention of enema for at least ½-1 hr
• Irrigation of colon after enema with 1-2 qt nonsodium sol, drain
• Storage of freshly prepared sol 24 hr at room temperature

Evaluate:

• Therapeutic response: potassium level 3.5-5 mg/dl

Teach patient/family:

• Reason for medication and expected results

---

solifenacin (℞)
(sol-i-fen'a-sin)
VESIcare
Func. class.: Overactive bladder product, anticholinergic
Chem. class.: Muscarinic receptor antagonist

Action: Relaxes smooth muscles in urinary tract by inhibiting acetylcholine at postganglionic sites
Uses: Overactive bladder (urinary frequency, urgency, incontinence)

DOSAGE AND ROUTES

• *Adult:* **PO** 5 mg daily, max 10 mg daily
Renal/hepatic dose
• *Adult:* **PO** CCr <30 ml/min 5 mg daily
Available forms: Tabs 5, 10 mg

SIDE EFFECTS

CNS: Anxiety, paresthesia, fatigue, *dizziness,* headache
CV: Chest pain, hypertension
EENT: Vision abnormalities, xerophthalmia
GI: Nausea, vomiting, anorexia, abdominal pain, *constipation,* dry mouth, dyspepsia
GU: Dysuria, urinary retention, frequency, UTI
INTEG: Rash, pruritus
RESP: Bronchitis, cough, pharyngitis, upper respiratory tract infection
Contraindications: Hypersensitivity, uncontrolled narrow-angle glaucoma, urinary retention, gastric retention
Precautions: Pregnancy (C), lactation, children, renal/hepatic disease, controlled narrow-angle glaucoma

PHARMACOKINETICS

Rapidly absorbed, 98% highly protein bound, extensively metabolized by CYP3A4, excreted in urine/feces, terminal half-life 45-68 hr

---

A Safety alert   *"Tall Man" lettering

INTERACTIONS

Increase: action of solifenacin (dose >5 mg is not recommended)—CYP3A4 inducers (ketoconazole)

NURSING CONSIDERATIONS

Assess:

• Urinary patterns: distention, nocturia, frequency, urgency, incontinence
• Allergic reactions: rash; if this occurs, drug should be discontinued

Evaluate:

• Urinary status: dysuria, frequency, nocturia, incontinence

Teach patient/family:

• To avoid hazardous activities; dizziness may occur
• Constipation, blurred vision may occur
• Call prescriber if severe abdominal pain or constipation lasts for 3 or more days
• Heat prostration may occur if used in a hot environment

---

somatropin (℞)

(soe-ma-troe′pin)
Genotropin, Humatrope, Norditropin, Nutropin, Nutropin Depot, Nutropin AQ, Saizen, Serostim
Func. class.: Pituitary hormone
Chem. class.: Growth hormone

Action: Stimulates growth; somatropin similar to natural growth hormone; both preparations developed by recombinant DNA

Uses: Pituitary growth hormone deficiency (hypopituitary dwarfism), children with human growth hormone deficiency, AIDS wasting syndrome, cachexia, adults with somatropin deficiency syndrome (SDS)

DOSAGE AND ROUTES

Genotropin
• *Child:* **SUBCUT** 0.16-0.24 mg/kg/wk divided into 6 or 7 inj, give in abdomen, thigh, buttocks

• *Adult:* **SUBCUT** 0.4-0.8 mg/kg/wk divided in 6-7 daily doses
Humatrope
• *Child:* **SUBCUT/IM** 0.18 mg/kg divided into equal doses either on 3 alternate days or 6 ×/wk, max wk dose is 0.3 mg/kg
• *Adult:* **IM** 0.018 U/kg/day, max 0.0375 U/kg/day
Nutropin/Nutropin AQ (growth hormone deficiency)
SUBCUT 0.3 mg/kg/wk
Serostim
• *Adult:* **SUBCUT** at bedtime >55 kg, 6 mg; 45-55 kg, 5 mg; 35-45 kg, 4 mg
Norditropin
SUBCUT 0.024-0.034 mg/kg 6-7 ×/wk
Available forms: Powder for inj (lyophilized) 1.5 mg (4 international units/ml), 4 mg (12 international units/vial), 5 mg (13 international units/vial), 5 mg (15 international units/vial), 5 mg (15 international units/vial) rDNA origin, 5.8 mg (15 international units/ml), 6 mg (18 international units/ml), 8 mg (24 international units/vial), 10 mg (26 international units/vial); inj 10 mg (30 international units/vial), 5 mg/1.5 ml, 10 mg/1.5 ml, 15 mg/1.5 ml

SIDE EFFECTS

CNS: Headache, growth of intracranial tumor
ENDO: **Hyperglycemia, ketosis, hypothyroidism**
GU: Hypercalciuria
INTEG: Rash, urticaria, pain; inflammation at inj site
MS: Tissue swelling, joint and muscle pain
SYST: **Antibodies to growth hormone**

Contraindications: Hypersensitivity to benzyl alcohol, closed epiphyses, intracranial lesions

Precautions: Pregnancy (C), lactation, diabetes mellitus, hypothyroidism

PHARMACOKINETICS

Half-life 15-60 min, duration 7 days; metabolized in liver

INTERACTIONS

Epiphyseal closure: androgens, thyroid hormones

Decrease: growth—glucocorticosteroids

NURSING CONSIDERATIONS

Assess:

• Growth hormone antibodies if patient fails to respond to therapy

• Thyroid function tests: T_3, T_4, T_7, TSH to identify hypothyroidism

• Allergic reaction: rash, itching, fever, nausea, wheezing

• Hypercalciuria: urinary stones; groin, flank pain; nausea, vomiting, urinary frequency, hematuria, chills

• Growth rate of child at intervals during treatment

Administer:

IM route

• Rotate inj site

• Norditropin: after reconstituting 4 or 8 mg/2 ml diluent

• Humatrope: 5 mg/1.5-5 ml diluent, do not shake

• Nutropin/Nutropin AQ: reconstitute 5 mg/1-5 ml or 10 mg/1-10 ml bacteriostatic water for inj (benzyl alcohol preserved)

Perform/provide:

• Storage in refrigerator for <1 mo, if reconstituted <1 wk; do not use discolored or cloudy sol

Evaluate:

• Therapeutic response: growth in children

Teach patient/family:

• That treatment may continue for years; regular assessments are required

• Maintain a growth record, report knee, hip pain or limping

• That treatment is very expensive

sorafenib

See Appendix A—Selected New Drugs

sotalol (R̥)

(sot'ah-lahl)
Betapace, Betapace AF,
Sotacar ✦
Func. class.: Antidysrhythmic group III
Chem. class.: Nonselective β-blocker

Action: Blockade of β_1- and β_2-receptors leads to antidysrhythmic effect, prolongs action potential in myocardial fibers without affecting conduction, prolongs QT interval, no effect on QRS duration

Uses: Life-threatening ventricular dysrhythmias; Betapace AF: to maintain sinus rhythm in symptomatic atrial fibrillation/flutter

DOSAGE AND ROUTES

• *Adult:* **PO** initial 80 mg bid, may increase to 240-320 mg/day

Renal dose

• *Adult:* **PO** *CCr 30-60 ml/min:* Give q24h; *CCr 10-29 ml/min:* give q36-48h; *CCr <10 ml/min:* individualize dose

Betapace AF

• *Adult:* **PO** initial 80 mg bid, titrate upward to 120 mg bid during initial hospitalization

Renal dose (Betapace AF)

• *Adult:* **PO** *CCr >60 ml/min:* Give q12h; *CCr 40-60 ml/min:* give q24h; *CCr <40 ml/min:* do not use

Available forms: Tabs 80, 120, 160, 240 mg; Betapace AF 80, 120, 160 mg

SIDE EFFECTS

CNS: Dizziness, mental changes, drowsiness, fatigue, headache, catatonia, depression, anxiety, nightmares, paresthesia, lethargy, insomnia, decreased concentration

CV: ***Prodysrhythmia,*** orthostatic hypotension, bradycardia, ***CHF,*** chest pain, ventricular dysrhythmias, AV block, peripheral vascular insufficiency, palpitations, torsades de pointes; ***life-***

threatening ventricular dysrhythmias (Betapace AF)

EENT: Tinnitus, visual changes, sore throat, double vision; dry, burning eyes

GI: Nausea, vomiting, diarrhea, dry mouth, flatulence, constipation, anorexia

GU: Impotence, dysuria, ejaculatory failure, urinary retention

HEMA: **Agranulocytosis, thrombocytopenic purpura** (rare), **thrombocytopenia, leukopenia**

INTEG: Rash, alopecia, urticaria, pruritus, fever

MISC: Facial swelling, decreased exercise tolerance, weight change, Raynaud's disease

MS: Joint pain, arthralgia, muscle cramps, pain

RESP: **Bronchospasm**, dyspnea, wheezing, nasal stuffiness, pharyngitis

Contraindications: Hypersensitivity to β-blockers, cardiogenic shock, heart block (2nd or 3rd degree), sinus bradycardia, CHF, bronchial asthma, congenital or acquired long QT syndrome, CCr <40 ml/min

Precautions: Pregnancy (B), major surgery, lactation, diabetes mellitus, renal disease, thyroid disease, COPD, well-compensated heart failure, CAD, nonallergic bronchospasm, electrolyte disturbances, bradycardia, cardiac dysrhythmias, peripheral vascular disease

PHARMACOKINETICS

PO: Onset 1-2 hr, peak 2-4 hr, duration 8-12 hr, half-life 12 hr; excreted unchanged in urine, crosses placenta, excreted in breast milk, protein binding 0%

INTERACTIONS

Increase: hypoglycemia effect—insulin

Increase: effects of lidocaine

Increase: hypotension—diuretics, other antihypertensives, nitroglycerin

Decrease: β-blocker effects—sympathomimetics

Decrease: bronchodilating effects of theophylline, β₂-agonists

Decrease: hypoglycemic effects of sulfonylureas

Drug/Herb

Hypokalemia, increased antidysrhythmic effect: aloe, buckthorn, cascara sagrada, senna

Increase: toxicity, death—aconite

Increase: effect—aloe, broom, chronic buckthorn use, cascara sagrada (chronic use), Chinese rhubarb, figwort, fumitory, goldenseal, kudzu, licorice

Increase: serotonin effect—horehound

Decrease: effect—coltsfoot

Drug/Lab Test

False increase: Urinary catecholamines

Interference: Glucose, insulin tolerance tests

NURSING CONSIDERATIONS

Assess:

• I&O, weight daily; edema in feet, legs daily

• B/P, pulse q4h; note rate, rhythm, quality

⚠ Apical/radial pulse before administration: notify prescriber of any significant changes; monitor ECG continuously (Betapace AF); use QT interval to determine patient eligibility; baseline QT must be ≤450 msec

• Baselines in renal studies before therapy begins

• Skin turgor, dryness of mucous membranes for hydration status

Administer:

• PO ac, at bedtime; tablet may be crushed or swallowed whole, give 1 hr ac or 2 hr pc

• Reduced dosage in renal dysfunction

• Betapace and Betapace AF are not interchangeable

Perform/provide:

• Storage in dry area at room temperature; do not freeze

Evaluate:

• Therapeutic response: absence of life-threatening dysrhythmias

Teach patient/family:

• Not to discontinue drug abruptly; taper over 2 wk or may precipitate angina, take exactly as prescribed

S

• Not to use OTC products containing α-adrenergic stimulants (nasal decongestants, OTC cold preparations) unless directed by prescriber

• To report bradycardia, dizziness, confusion, depression, fever

• To take pulse at home; advise when to notify prescriber

• To avoid alcohol, smoking, sodium intake

• To carry emergency ID to identify drug being taken, allergies

• To avoid hazardous activities if dizziness is present

• To report symptoms of CHF including: difficulty in breathing, especially on exertion or when lying down; night cough, swelling of extremities

• To wear support hose to minimize effects of orthostatic hypotension

Treatment of overdose: Lavage, IV atropine for bradycardia, IV theophylline for bronchospasm, digitalis, O_2, diuretic for cardiac failure; hemodialysis is useful for removal; administer vasopressor (norepinephrine) for hypotension, isoproterenol for heart block

---

sparfloxacin
(spar-floks'a-sin)
Zagam
Func. class.: Antiinfective
Chem. class.: Fluoroquinolone

Action: Interferes with conversion of intermediate DNA fragments into high-molecular-weight DNA in bacteria; DNA-gyrase inhibitor

Uses: Community-acquired pneumonia; chronic bronchitis caused by *Klebsiella pneumoniae, Haemophilus influenzae, Haemophilus parainfluenzae, Moraxella catarrhalis*

DOSAGE AND ROUTES

• *Adult:* **PO** 400 mg loading dose, then 200 mg q24h × 10 days
Renal dose
• *Adult:* CCr <50 ml/min day 400 mg on

1st day then 200 mg q48h for a total of 1200 ml over 10 days
Available forms: Tabs 200 mg

SIDE EFFECTS

CNS: Headache, dizziness, insomnia
CV: QT interval prolongation, vasodilation
GI: Nausea, flatulence, *vomiting,* diarrhea, *abdominal pain,* **pseudomembranous colitis**
HEMA: **Leukopenia,** eosinophilia, anemia
INTEG: Rash, pruritus, photosensitivity
SYST: **Anaphylaxis, Stevens-Johnson syndrome**
Contraindications: Hypersensitivity to quinolones, photosensitivity
Precautions: Pregnancy (C), lactation, children, renal disease, seizure disorders

PHARMACOKINETICS

Slow, erratic absorption, widely distributed; metabolized by liver, excreted in urine, feces; half-life 20 hr

INTERACTIONS

Nephrotoxicity may occur with cyclo-SPORINE
Torsades de pointes: amiodarone, bepridil, disopyramide, erythromycin, pentamidine, phenothiazines, tricyclics, class Ia antidysrhythmics, class III antidysrhythmics
Increase: warfarin level
Decrease: absorption of sparfloxacin—antacids with aluminum, magnesium, iron products, zinc, sucralfate, give 4 hr apart
Drug/Herb
Increase: effect—cola tree
Drug/Lab Test
Increase: AST, ALT

NURSING CONSIDERATIONS
Assess:

• For previous sensitivity reaction
• For signs and symptoms of infection: characteristics of sputum, WBC >10,000/ mm^3, fever; obtain baseline information before and during treatment

---

• C&S before beginning drug therapy to identify if correct treatment has been initiated

⚠ For allergic reactions, anaphylaxis: rash, urticaria, pruritus, chills, fever, joint pain; may occur a few days after therapy begins; epINEPHrine and resuscitation equipment should be available for anaphylactic reaction

• Blood studies: LFTs if patient is on long-term therapy

• Bowel pattern daily; if severe diarrhea occurs, drug should be discontinued

• For overgrowth of infection: perineal itching, fever, malaise, redness, pain, swelling, drainage, rash, diarrhea, change in cough, sputum

Administer:

• As directed only

• 4 hr before or 4 hr after antacids, zinc, calcium

Perform/provide:

• An increase of fluid intake to 2 L/day to prevent crystalluria

Evaluate:

• Therapeutic response: absence of signs/symptoms of infection (WBC <10,000/mm^3, temp WNL, C&S negative for organism)

Teach patient/family:

• To avoid hazardous activities until response is known

• To contact prescriber if vaginal itching, loose, foul-smelling stools, furry tongue occur (may indicate superinfection); report itching, rash, pruritus, urticaria

• To take all medication prescribed for the length of time ordered; drug must be taken as directed to maintain blood levels; do not give medication to others

• To notify prescriber of diarrhea with blood or pus

• To increase fluid intake to 2 L/day to prevent crystalluria

• To take 4 hr before or 4 hr after antacids, dairy products, zinc products

• To avoid direct sunlight or use sunscreen to prevent phototoxicity

• To use frequent rinsing of mouth, sugarless candy, or gum for dry mouth

---

spironolactone (℞)

(speer'on-oh-lak'tone)

Aldactone, Novo-Spiroton ✦

Func. class.: Potassium-sparing diuretic

Chem. class.: Aldosterone antagonist

Action: Competes with aldosterone at receptor sites in distal tubule, resulting in excretion of sodium chloride, water, retention of potassium, phosphate

Uses: Edema of CHF, hypertension, diuretic-induced hypokalemia, primary hyperaldosteronism (diagnosis, short-term treatment, long-term treatment), edema of nephrotic syndrome, cirrhosis of the liver with ascites

Investigational uses: CHF

DOSAGE AND ROUTES

Edema/hypertension

• *Adult:* PO 25-400 mg/daily in single or divided doses

CHF

• *Adult:* PO 12.5-25 mg/day

Edema

• *Child:* PO 3.3 mg/kg/day in single or divided doses

Hypertension

• *Child:* PO 1-2 mg/kg bid

Hypokalemia

• *Adult:* PO 25-100 mg/day; if **PO**, potassium supplements must not be used

Primary hyperaldosteronism diagnosis

• *Adult:* PO 400 mg/day × 4 days or 4 wk depending on test, then 100-400 mg/day maintenance

Available forms: Tabs 25, 50, 100 mg

SIDE EFFECTS

CNS: Headache, confusion, drowsiness, lethargy, ataxia

ELECT: Hyperchloremic metabolic acidosis, ***hyperkalemia***, hyponatremia

ENDO: Impotence, gynecomastia, irregular menses, amenorrhea, postmenopausal bleeding, hirsutism, deepening voice

GI: Diarrhea, cramps, ***bleeding***, gastritis, *vomiting*, anorexia, nausea

S

HEMA: **Agranulocytosis**
INTEG: *Rash, pruritus,* urticaria
Contraindications: Pregnancy (D), hypersensitivity, anuria, severe renal disease, hyperkalemia
Precautions: Dehydration, hepatic disease, lactation, renal impairment, electrolyte imbalances

PHARMACOKINETICS

PO: Onset 24-48 hr, peak 48-72 hr; metabolized in liver, excreted in urine, crosses placenta

INTERACTIONS

Increase: action of antihypertensives, digitalis, lithium
Increase: hyperkalemia—potassium-sparing diuretics, potassium products, ACE inhibitors, salt substitutes
Decrease: effect of anticoagulants
Decrease: effect of spironolactone—ASA
Drug/Herb

Hypokalemia: bearberry, gossypol
Severe photosensitivity: St. John's wort
⚠ **Fatal hypokalemia:** arginine
Increase: effect—cucumber, dandelion, horsetail, licorice, nettle, pumpkin, Queen Anne's lace
Increase: hypotension—khella
Drug/Lab Test

Interference: 17-OHCS, 17-KS, radioimmunoassay, digoxin assay

NURSING CONSIDERATIONS

Assess:

• Electrolytes: Na, Cl, K, BUN, serum creatinine, ABGs, CBC
• Weight, I&O daily to determine fluid loss; effect of drug may be decreased if used daily; ECG periodically (long-term therapy)
• Signs of metabolic acidosis: drowsiness, restlessness
• Rashes, temp daily
• Confusion, especially in elderly; take safety precautions if needed
• Hydration: skin turgor, thirst, dry mucous membranes

Administer:

• In AM to avoid interference with sleep
• With food; if nausea occurs, absorption may be decreased slightly
Evaluate:

• Therapeutic response: improvement in edema of feet, legs, sacral area daily if medication is being used in CHF
Teach patient/family:

• To avoid foods with high potassium content: oranges, bananas, salt substitutes, dried apricots, dates; avoid potassium salt substitutes

• That drowsiness, ataxia, mental confusion may occur; observe caution in driving

• To notify prescriber of cramps, diarrhea, lethargy, thirst, headache, skin rash, menstrual abnormalities, deepening voice, breast enlargement

Treatment of overdose: Lavage if taken orally; monitor electrolytes, administer IV fluids, monitor hydration, renal, CV status

---

stavudine (℞)

(sta'vyoo-deen)
d4t, Zerit
Func. class.: Antiretroviral
Chem. class.: Nucleoside reverse transcriptase inihibitor

Action: Prevents replication of HIV by the inhibition of the enzyme reverse transcriptase, causes DNA chain termination
Uses: Treatment of HIV-1 in combination with other antiretrovirals

DOSAGE AND ROUTES

• *Adult >60 kg:* **PO** 40 mg q12h
• *Adult <60 kg:* **PO** 30 mg q12h
• *Child <30 kg:* **PO** 1 mg/kg q12h
• *Child ≥30 kg ≤60 kg:* **PO** 30 mg q12h
• *Child >60 kg:* **PO** 40 mg q12h
Renal dose
• *Adult: >60 kg:* **PO** CCr 26-50 ml/min 20 mg q12h; CCr 10-25 ml/min 20 mg q24h
• *Adult: <60 kg:* **PO** CCr 26-50 ml/min

---

15 mg q12h; CCr 10-25 ml/min 15 mg
q24h

Available forms: Caps 15, 20, 30, 40
mg; powder for oral sol 1 mg/ml

SIDE EFFECTS

CNS: Peripheral neuropathy, insomnia,
anxiety, neuropathy, depression, dizziness, confusion, headache, chills/fever,
malaise

CV: Chest pain, vasodilation, hypertension

EENT: Conjunctivitis, abnormal vision

*GI: **Hepatotoxicity,*** diarrhea, nausea,
vomiting, anorexia, dyspepsia, constipation, stomatitis, ***pancreatitis***

*HEMA: **Bone marrow suppression***

INTEG: Rash, sweating, pruritus, benign
neoplasms

*MISC: **Lactic acidosis,*** asthenia, lipodystrophy

MS: Myalgia, arthralgia

RESP: Dyspnea, pneumonia, asthma

Contraindications: Hypersensitivity
to this drug or zidovudine, didanosine,
zalcitabine; severe peripheral neuropathy

Precautions: Pregnancy (C), advanced
HIV infection, lactation, bone marrow
suppression, renal disease, hepatic disease, peripheral neuropathy, osteoporosis

PHARMACOKINETICS

Excreted in urine, breast milk; peak 1
hr; half-life: elimination: 1-1.6 hr,
intracellular: 3-3.5 hr

INTERACTIONS

Increase: myelosuppression—other
myelosuppressants

Increase: peripheral neuropathy—
lithium, dapsone, chloramphenicol didanosine, ethambutol, hydrALAZINE, phenytoin, vinCRIStine, zalcitabine

Decrease: stavudine effect—methadone

NURSING CONSIDERATIONS

Assess:

⚠ For lactic acidosis and severe hepatomegaly with steatosis, death may result

- Blood studies: WBC, differential, RBC,
Hct, Hgb, platelets
- Renal tests: urinalysis, protein, blood
- C&S before drug therapy; drug may be
given as soon as culture is taken
- Bowel pattern before, during treatment
- Weakness, tremors, confusion,
dizziness; drug may have to be decreased
or discontinued
- Viral load and CD4 counts baseline
and throughout treatment
- For peripheral neuropathy: tingling,
pain, in extremities; discontinue drug
⚠ For pancreatitis: severe upper abdominal pain, nausea, vomiting throughout treatment, discontinue drug

Administer:

- With or without meals; absorption
does not appear to be lowered when
taken with food
- Every 12 hr around the clock

Teach patient/family:

- The signs of peripheral neuropathy:
burning, weakness, pain, prickling feeling in the extremities
- That drug should not be given with
antineoplastics
- That drug is not a cure for AIDS, but
will control symptoms
- To call prescriber if sore throat, swollen lymph nodes, malaise, fever occur;
other drugs may be needed to prevent
other infections
- That even with this drug, patient may
pass AIDS virus to others
- That follow-up visits are necessary;
serious toxicity may occur; blood counts
must be done q2wk
- That serious drug interactions may
occur if other medications are ingested;
see prescriber before taking chloramphenicol, dapsone, cisplatin, didanosine,
ethambutol, lithium, antifungals, antineoplastics
- That drug may cause fainting or dizziness

Evaluate:

- Therapeutic response: decreased
symptoms of HIV

S

⚠ High Alert

streptokinase (℞)

(strep-toe-kye′nase)
Kabikinase, Streptase
Func. class.: Thrombolytic enzyme
Chem. class.: β-Hemolytic strepto-
coccus filtrate (purified)

Action: Activates conversion of plasminogen to plasmin (fibrinolysin): plasmin breaks down clots (fibrin), fibrinogen, factors V, VII; occlusion of venous
access lines

Uses: Deep-vein thrombosis, pulmonary
embolism, arterial thrombosis, arterial
embolism, arteriovenous cannula occlusion, lysis of coronary artery thrombi
after MI, acute evolving transmural MI

DOSAGE AND ROUTES

Lysis of coronary artery thrombi
• *Adult:* **IC** 20,000 international units,
then 2000 international units/min over 1
hr as **IV INF**

Arteriovenous cannula occlusion
• *Adult:* **IV INF** 250,000 international
units/2 ml sol into occluded limb of cannula run over ½ hr; clamp for 2 hr; aspirate contents; flush with NaCl sol and
reconnect

Thrombosis/embolism/DVT/
pulmonary embolism
• *Adult:* **IV INF** 250,000 international
units over ½ hr, then 100,000 international units/hr for 72 hr for deep-vein
thrombosis; 100,000 international
units/hr over 24-72 hr for pulmonary
embolism; 100,000 international units/hr
× 24-72 hr for arterial thrombosis or
embolism

Acute evolving transmural MI
• *Adult:* **IV INF** 1,500,000 international
units diluted to a volume of 45 ml; give
within 1 hr; intracoronary **INF** 20,000
international units by **BOL,** then 2000
international units/min × 1 hr, total dose
140,000 international units

Available forms: Powder for inj, ly-

ophilized, 250,000, 600,000, 750,000,
1,500,000 international units/vial

SIDE EFFECTS

CNS: Headache, fever
CV: Dysrhythmias, hypotension, noncar-
diogenic pulmonary edema, ***pulmonary embolism***
EENT: Periorbital edema
GI: Nausea
HEMA: Decreased Hct, ***bleeding***
INTEG: Rash, urticaria, phlebitis at IV inf
site, itching, flushing
MS: Low back pain
RESP: Altered respirations, SOB, ***bronchospasm***
SYST: ***GI, GU, intracranial, retroperitoneal bleeding, surface bleeding, anaphylaxis***
Contraindications: Hypersensitivity,
active internal bleeding, recent CVA,
intracranial, intrapleural surgery, intraspinal surgery, CNS neoplasms, uncontrolled severe hypertension, lactation,
children
Precautions: Pregnancy (C), arterial
emboli from left side of heart, ulcerative
colitis, enteritis, severe renal disease,
hepatic disease, hypocoagulation, COPD,
subacute bacterial endocarditis, rheumatic valvular disease, cerebral embo-
lism/thrombosis/hemorrhage, intraarterial diagnostic procedure or surgery (10
days), recent major surgery

PHARMACOKINETICS

IV: Onset immediate, duration <12 hr;
half-life <20 min; excreted in bile,
urine

INTERACTIONS

Bleeding potential: aspirin, indomethacin, phenylbutazone, anticoagulants,
other NSAIDs, abciximab, eptifibatide,
tirofiban, clopidogrel, ticlopidine, some
cephalosporins, plicamycin, valproic
acid, dipyridamole, GP IIb, IIIa inhibitors

Drug/Lab Test
Increase: PT, aPTT, TT
Decrease: Plasminogen, fibrinogen

NURSING CONSIDERATIONS
Assess:
• Allergy: fever, rash, itching, chills; mild reaction may be treated with antihistamines

⚠ For bleeding during 1st hr of treatment; hematuria, hematemesis, bleeding from mucous membranes, epistaxis, ecchymosis; may require tranfusion (rare), continue to assess for bleeding for 24 hr

• Blood studies (Hct, platelets, PTT, PT, TT, aPTT) before starting therapy; PT or aPTT must be less than 2× control before starting therapy; PTT or PT q3-4h during treatment

⚠ For hypersensitive reactions: fever, rash, dyspnea, facial swelling; drug should be discontinued; for streptokinase reactions previously; notify prescriber immediately, stop drug, keep resuscitative equipment nearby

• VS, B/P, pulse, respirations, neurologic signs, temp at least q4h; temp >104° F (40° C) indicates internal bleeding; systolic pressure increase >25 mm Hg should be reported to prescriber; assess neurologic status, neurologic change may indicate intracranial bleeding

⚠ For neurologic changes that may indicate intracranial bleeding

⚠ Retroperitoneal bleeding: back pain, leg weakness, diminished pulses

• For Guillain-Barré syndrome that may occur after treatment with this drug

• ECG continuously, cardiac enzymes, radionuclide myocardial scanning/coronary angiography

• For respiratory depression

Administer:
IV route
• As soon as thrombi identified; not useful for thrombi over 1 wk old

• Cryoprecipitate or fresh frozen plasma if bleeding occurs

• Loading dose at beginning of therapy; may require increased loading doses

• Heparin after fibrinogen level >100 mg/dl; heparin infusion to increase PTT to 1.5-2 × baseline for 3-7 days; IV heparin with loading dose is recommended after discontinuing streptokinase to prevent redevelopment of thrombi

• After reconstituting with 5 ml NS or D₅W; do not shake; further dilute to total volume of 45 ml; may be diluted to 500 ml in 45 ml increments; may dilute vial in 15 ml NS, further dilute 750,000 international units/50 ml NS or D₅W; further dilute 1,500,000 international units dose/100 ml or more

• About 10% patients have high streptococcal antibody titers requiring increased loading doses

• IV therapy using 0.8-μm filter

Y-site compatibilities: DOBUTamine, DOPamine, heparin, lidocaine, nitroglycerin

Perform/provide:
• Storage of reconstituted sol in refrigerator; discard after 24 hr

• Bed rest during entire course of treatment

• Avoid venous or arterial puncture, inj, rectal temp; any invasive treatment

• Treatment of fever with acetaminophen or aspirin

• Pressure for 30 sec to minor bleeding sites; inform prescriber if this does not attain hemostasis; apply pressure dressing

Evaluate:
• Therapeutic response: resolution of thrombosis, embolism

Teach patient/family:
• Reason for medication and expected results

---

streptomycin (℞)
(strep-toe-mye′sin)
Func. class.: Antiinfective/antitubercular
Chem. class.: Aminoglycoside

Action: Interferes with protein synthesis in bacterial cell by binding to ribosomal subunit, causing inaccurate peptide sequence to form in protein chain, causing bacterial death

---

Side effects: *italics* = common; ***bold italics*** = life-threatening

Uses: Sensitive strains of *Mycobacterium tuberculosis,* nontuberculous infections caused by sensitive strains of *Yersinia pestis, Brucella, Haemophilus influenzae, Klebsiella pneumoniae, Escherichia coli, Enterobacter aerogenes, Streptococcus viridans, Francisella tularensis, Proteus*

DOSAGE AND ROUTES
Tuberculosis
• *Adult:* IM 15 mg/kg (max 1 g) daily × 2-3 mo, then 1 g 2-3 ×/week with other antitubercular drugs
• *Child:* IM 20-40 mg/kg/day in divided doses with other antitubercular drugs; max 15 mg/kg/day
Streptococcal endocarditis
• *Adult:* IM 1 g q12h × 1 wk with penicillin, then 500 mg bid × 1 wk
Enterococcal endocarditis
• *Adult:* IM 1 g q12h × 2 wk, then 500 mg q12h × 4 wk with penicillin, max 15 mg/kg/day
Available forms: Inj 500 mg ✿, 1 g/ml

SIDE EFFECTS
CNS: Confusion, depression, numbness, tremors, *convulsions,* muscle twitching, *neurotoxicity,* dizziness
CV: Hypotension, myocarditis, palpitations
EENT: **Ototoxicity,** deafness, visual disturbances, tinnitus
GI: Nausea, vomiting, anorexia, increased ALT, AST, bilirubin; hepatomegaly, *hepatic necrosis,* splenomegaly
GU: Oliguria, hematuria, renal damage, azotemia, renal failure, nephrotoxicity
HEMA: Agranulocytosis, thrombocytopenia, leukopenia, eosinophilia, anemia
INTEG: Rash, burning, urticaria, dermatitis, alopecia
Contraindications: Pregnancy (D), severe renal disease, hypersensitivity
Precautions: Neonates, mild renal disease, myasthenia gravis, lactation,

hearing deficit, elderly, Parkinson's disease

PHARMACOKINETICS
IM: Onset rapid, peak 1-2 hr; plasma half-life 2-2½ hr; not metabolized, excreted unchanged in urine, crosses placental barrier, poor penetration into CSF, small amounts enter breast milk

INTERACTIONS
Increase: ototoxicity, neurotoxicity, nephrotoxicity—other aminoglycosides, amphotericin B, polymyxin, vancomycin, ethacrynic acid, furosemide, mannitol, methoxyflurane, cisplatin, cephalosporins, bacitracin
Increase: streptomycin effects—nondepolarizing muscle relaxants, succinylcholine, warfarin
Drug/Herb
Increase: toxicity—lysine (large amounts)

NURSING CONSIDERATIONS
Assess:
• Weight before treatment; calculation of dosage is usually based on ideal body weight, but may be calculated on actual body weight
• I&O ratio, urinalysis daily for proteinuria, cells, casts; report sudden change in urine output
• Serum peak 20-30 min after IM inj, trough level drawn 8 hr; acceptable levels—peak 5-25 mcg/ml, trough should not be >5 mcg/ml
• Renal impairment by collecting urine for CCr testing, BUN, serum creatinine; lower dosage should be given in renal impairment (CCr <80 ml/min), monitor electrolytes: K, Na, Cl, Mg
• Deafness by audiometric testing, ringing, roaring in ears, vertigo; assess hearing before, during, after treatment
• Dehydration: high specific gravity, decrease in skin turgor, dry mucous membranes, dark urine
• Overgrowth of infection: fever, malaise, redness, pain, swelling, perineal

⚠ Safety alert   *"Tall Man" lettering

itching, diarrhea, stomatitis, change in
cough, sputum
• C&S before starting treatment to identify infecting organism
• Vestibular dysfunction: nausea, vomiting, dizziness, headache; drug should be
discontinued if severe
• Inj sites for redness, swelling,
abscesses; use warm compresses at site

Administer:
• IM inj in large muscle mass; rotate inj
sites
• Drug in evenly spaced doses to main-
tain blood level
Additive compatibilities: Bleomycin
Syringe compatibilities: Penicillin G
sodium
Y-site compatibilities: Esmolol
Perform/provide:
• Adequate fluids of 2-3 L/day unless
contraindicated to prevent irritation of
tubules
• Supervised ambulation, other safety
measures with vestibular dysfunction
Evaluate:
• Therapeutic effect: absence of fever,
draining wounds, negative C&S after
treatment
Teach patient/family:
• To report headache, dizziness, symp-
toms of overgrowth of infection, renal
impairment
• To report loss of hearing, ringing,
roaring in ears, fullness in head
Treatment of overdose:
Hemodialysis; monitor serum levels of
drug

---

succimer (℞)
(sux′i-mer)
Chemet
Func. class.: Heavy metal antagonist
Chem. class.: Chelating agent

Action: Binds with ions of lead to form
a water-soluble complex excreted by
kidneys
Uses: Lead poisoning in children with
lead levels above 45 mcg/dl; may be
beneficial in mercury, arsenic poisoning

DOSAGE AND ROUTES
• *Child:* **PO** 10 mg/kg or 350 mg/m²
q8h × 5 days, then 10 mg/kg or 350
mg/m² q12h × 2 wk; another course may
be required depending on lead levels;
allow 2 wk between courses
Available forms: Caps 100 mg

SIDE EFFECTS
CNS: Drowsiness, dizziness, paresthesia,
sensorimotor neuropathy
EENT: Otitis media, watery eyes, film in
eyes, plugged ears
*GI: Nausea, vomiting, diarrhea, metal-
lic taste, anorexia*
GU: **Proteinuria,** decreased urination,
voiding difficulties
HEMA: **Increased platelets, inter-
mittent eosinophilia**
INTEG: Rash, urticaria, pruritus
META: Increased AST, ALT, alk phospha-
tase, cholesterol
RESP: Sore throat, rhinorrhea, nasal con-
gestion, cough
SYST: Back, stomach, head, rib, flank
pain; abdominal cramps, chills, fever,
flulike symptoms, head cold, headache
Contraindications: Hypersensitivity
Precautions: Pregnancy (C), lactation,
children <1 yr

PHARMACOKINETICS
PO: Peak 1-2 hr, 49% excreted (39%
in feces, 9% urine, 1% as CO₂ from
lungs)

INTERACTIONS
Not recommended concurrently with
other chelating agents

NURSING CONSIDERATIONS
Assess:
• Renal, hepatic studies: ALT, AST, alk
phosphatase, BUN, creatinine, serum
lead level
• I&O
• For lead sources in home, school
• Allergic reactions: rash, pruritus,
urticaria; drug should be discontinued if
antihistamines fail to help

Administer:
• To children who cannot swallow capsule by separating the capsule and sprinkling content on food or in a spoon followed by a drink, administer immediately after preparation

Perform/provide:
• Adequate fluids; check hydration status daily

Evaluate:
• Therapeutic response: decrease in serum lead level

Teach patient/family:
• That therapeutic effect may take 1-3 mo
• To report urticaria, rash
• To increase fluid intake

⚠ High Alert

succinylcholine (℞)
(suk-sin-ill-koe'leen)
Anectine, Anectine Flo-Pack, Quelicin, succinylcholine chloride, Sucostrin, Suxamethonium
Func. class.: Neuromuscular blocker (depolarizing–ultra short)

Action: Inhibits transmission of nerve impulses by binding with cholinergic receptor sites, antagonizing action of acetylcholine; causes release of histamine
Uses: Facilitation of endotracheal intubation, skeletal muscle relaxation during orthopedic manipulations

DOSAGE AND ROUTES

• *Adult:* **IV** 0.3-1.1 mg/kg, then 0.5-10 kg/min; **IM** 3-4 mg/kg
• *Child:* **IV/IM** 1-4 mg/kg
Available forms: Inj 20, 50, 100 mg/ml; powder for inj 100, 500 mg/vial, 1 g/vial

SIDE EFFECTS

CV: Bradycardia, tachycardia; increased, decreased B/P; *sinus arrest, dysrhythmias*
EENT: Increased secretions, increased intraocular pressure

HEMA: Myoglobulinemia
INTEG: Rash, flushing, pruritus, urticaria
MS: Weakness, muscle pain, fasciculations, prolonged relaxation
RESP: Prolonged apnea, bronchospasm, cyanosis, respiratory depression, wheezing

Contraindications: Hypersensitivity, malignant hyperthermia, decreased plasma pseudocholinesterase, penetrating eye injuries, acute narrow-angle glaucoma
Precautions: Pregnancy (C), cardiac disease, severe burns, fractures—fasciculations may increase damage—lactation, children <2 yr, electrolyte imbalances, dehydration, neuromuscular disease, respiratory disease, collagen diseases, glaucoma, eye surgery, elderly or debilitated patients, renal/hepatic disease

PHARMACOKINETICS

IV: Onset 1 min, peak 2-3 min, duration 6-10 min
IM: Onset 2-3 min
Hydrolyzed in blood, excreted in urine (active/inactive metabolites)

INTERACTIONS

Dysrhythmias: theophylline
Increase: neuromuscular blockade—aminoglycosides, β-blockers, cardiac glycosides, clindamycin, lincomycin, procainamide, quinidine, local anesthetics, polymyxin antibiotics, lithium, opioids, thiazides, enflurane, isoflurane, magnesium salts, oxytocin
Drug/Herb
Blocks succinylcholine: melatonin

NURSING CONSIDERATIONS

Assess:
• For electrolyte imbalances (K, Mg); may lead to increased action of this drug
• VS (B/P, pulse, respirations, airway) until fully recovered; rate, depth, pattern of respirations, strength of hand grip
• I&O ratio; check for urinary retention, frequency, hesitancy

---

⚠ Safety alert   *"Tall Man" lettering

• Recovery: decreased paralysis of face, diaphragm, leg, arm, rest of body
• Allergic reactions: rash, fever, respiratory distress, pruritus; drug should be discontinued

Administer:
• Deep IM inj, preferably high in deltoid muscle

IV route
• Using nerve stimulator by anesthesiologist to determine neuromuscular blockade
• Anticholinesterase to reverse neuromuscular blockade
• IV inf; dilute 1-2 mg/ml in D_5, isotonic saline sol, give 0.5-10 mg/min, titrate to response; may be given directly over 1 min

Additive compatibilities: Amikacin, cephapirin, isoproterenol, meperidine, methyldopa, morphine, norepinephrine, scopolamine

Syringe compatibilities: Heparin

Y-site compatibilities: Etomidate, heparin, potassium chloride, propofol, vit B/C

Perform/provide:
• Storage in refrigerator, powder at room temperature; close tightly
• Reassurance if communication is difficult during recovery from neuromuscular blockade; postoperative stiffness is normal, soon subsides

Evaluate:
• Therapeutic response: paralysis of jaw, eyelid, head, neck, rest of body

Treatment of overdose: Edrophonium or neostigmine, atropine, monitor VS; may require mechanical ventilation

---

sucralfate (℞)
(soo-kral'fate)
Carafate, Sulcrate ✤
Func. class.: Protectant, antiulcer
Chem. class.: Aluminum hydroxide, sulfated sucrose

Do not confuse:
Carafate/Cafergot

Action: Forms a complex that adheres to ulcer site, adsorbs pepsin

Uses: Duodenal ulcer, oral mucositis, stomatitis after radiation of head and neck

Investigational uses: Gastric ulcers, gastroesophageal reflux

DOSAGE AND ROUTES
Duodenal ulcers
• *Adult:* **PO** 1 g qid 1 hr ac, at bedtime
• *Child:* **PO** 40-80 mg/kg/day
GERD
• *Adult:* **PO** 1 g qid 1 hr ac and at bedtime
• *Child:* **PO** 500 mg-1 g qid, 1 hr ac and at bedtime

Available forms: Tabs 1 g; oral susp 1 g/10 ml

SIDE EFFECTS
CNS: Drowsiness, dizziness
GI: Dry mouth, constipation, nausea, gastric pain, vomiting
INTEG: Urticaria, rash, pruritus

Contraindications: Hypersensitivity
Precautions: Pregnancy (B), lactation, children, renal failure

PHARMACOKINETICS
PO: Duration up to 6 hr

INTERACTIONS
Decrease: action of tetracyclines, phenytoin, fat-soluble vitamins, cimetidine, digoxin, ketoconazole, ranitidine, theophylline
Decrease: absorption of fluoroquinolones
Decrease: absorption of sucralfate—antacids

NURSING CONSIDERATIONS
Assess:
• Gastric pH (>5 should be maintained); blood in stools

Administer:
PO route
• Do not crush or chew tabs; tabs may be broken or dissolved in water

---

Side effects: *italics* = common; ***bold italics*** = life-threatening

S

• Do not take antacids 30 min before or after sucralfate
• On an empty stomach, 1 hr before meals and at bedtime

Perform/provide:
• Storage at room temperature

Evaluate:
• Therapeutic response: absence of pain, GI complaints

Teach patient/family:
• To take on empty stomach
• To take full course of therapy, not to use over 8 wk, to avoid smoking
• To avoid antacids within ½ hr of drug

---

*sulfADIAZINE (℞)
(sul-fa-dye′a-zeen)
Coptin, sulfADIAZINE
Func. class.: Antiinfective
Chem. class.: Sulfonamide, intermediate acting

Do not confuse:
sulfADIAZINE/sulfiSOXAZOLE
Action: Interferes with bacterial biosynthesis of proteins by competitive antagonism of PABA
Uses: UTIs, rheumatic fever prophylaxis, with pyrimethamine for *Toxoplasma gondii* encephalitis, chancroid, inclusion conjunctivitis, malaria, meningitis, *Haemophilus influenzae,* meningococeal meningitis, nocardiosis, acute otitis media, trachoma, chloroquine-resistant malaria

DOSAGE AND ROUTES
Meningococcal carriers (asymptomatic)
• *Adult:* **PO** 1 g q12h × 2 days
• *Child 1-12 yr:* **PO** 500 mg q12h × 2 days
• *Child 2-12 mo:* **PO** 500 mg daily × 2 days
Rheumatic fever prophylaxis
• *Child >30 kg:* **PO** 1 g daily
• *Child <30 kg:* **PO** 500 mg daily
Available forms: Tabs 500 mg

SIDE EFFECTS
CNS: Headache, insomnia, hallucinations, depression, vertigo, fatigue, anxiety, *convulsions,* drug fever, chills, drowsiness
CV: Allergic myocarditis
GI: Nausea, vomiting, abdominal pain, stomatitis, *hepatitis,* glossitis, pancreatitis, diarrhea, *enterocolitis,* anorexia
GU: Renal failure, toxic nephrosis, increased BUN, creatinine, crystalluria, hematuria, proteinuria
HEMA: Leukopenia, thrombocytopenia, agranulocytosis, hemolytic anemia, aplastic anemia
INTEG: Rash, dermatitis, urticaria, *Stevens-Johnson syndrome,* erythema, photosensitivity, alopecia
SYST: Anaphylaxis
Contraindications: Hypersensitivity to sulfonamides, sulfonylureas, thiazide and loop diuretics, salicylates, sunscreens with PABA, lactation, infants <2 mo (except congenital toxoplasmosis), pregnancy at term, porphyria
Precautions: Pregnancy (C), impaired hepatic function, severe allergy, bronchial asthma, renal dysfunction

PHARMACOKINETICS
PO: Rapidly absorbed, onset ½ hr; peak 3-6 hr, 30%-50% bound to plasma proteins, half-life 8-10 hr; excreted in urine, breast milk; crosses placenta, metabolized in liver

INTERACTIONS
Increase: hypoglycemic response—sulfonylurea agents
Increase: anticoagulant effects—warfarin
Increase: effects of barbiturates, TOLBUTamide, uricosurics
Increase: free-drug concentrations—indomethacin, probenecid, salicylates
Increase: thrombocytopenia—thiazide diuretics
Increase: nephrotoxicity—cycloSPORINE
Decrease: renal excretion of methotrexate

Decrease: hepatic clearance of phenytoin

Drug/Lab Test
False positive: Urinary glucose test (Benedict's method, Chemstrip uG)

NURSING CONSIDERATIONS

Assess:

• I&O ratio; note color, character, pH of urine if drug administered for UTIs; output should be 800 ml less than intake; if urine is highly acidic, alkalization may be needed

• Renal studies: BUN, creatinine, urinalysis (long-term therapy)

• Blood dyscrasias: skin rash, fever, sore throat, bruising, bleeding, fatigue, joint pain, monitor CBC before and periodically

• Allergic reaction: rash, dermatitis, urticaria, pruritus, dyspnea, bronchospasm

Administer:

• On an empty stomach

• With full glass of H_2O to maintain adequate hydration; increase fluids to 2 L/day to decrease crystallization in kidneys

• Medication after C&S; repeat C&S after full course of medication

Perform/provide:

• Storage in tight, light-resistant container at room temperature

Evaluate:

• Therapeutic response: absence of pain, fever, C&S negative

Teach patient/family:

• To take each oral dose with full glass of water to prevent crystalluria

• To complete full course of treatment to prevent superinfection

• To avoid sunlight or use sunscreen to prevent burns

• To avoid OTC medication (aspirin, vit C) unless directed by prescriber

• To notify prescriber of skin rash, sore throat, fever, mouth sores, unusual bruising, bleeding

---

sulfamethoxazole (R)

(sul-fa-meth-ox′a-zole)
Apo-Sulfamethoxazole ✦,
Gantanol, Urobak
Func. class.: Antiinfective
Chem. class.: Sulfonamide, intermediate acting

Action: Interferes with bacterial biosynthesis of proteins by competitive antagonism of PABA

Uses: UTIs, chancroid, inclusion conjunctivitis, malaria, meningococcal meningitis, nocardiosis, acute otitis media, toxoplasmosis, trachoma

DOSAGE AND ROUTES

• *Adult:* **PO** 2 g, then 1 g bid or tid for 7-10 days

• *Child >2 mo:* **PO** 50-60 mg/kg × 1 dose then 25-30 mg/kg bid, not to exceed 75 mg/kg/day

Renal dose

• *Adult:* **PO** CCr <50 ml/min give 50% of dose

Available forms: Tabs 500 mg, oral susp 500 mg/5 ml

SIDE EFFECTS

CNS: Headache, insomnia, hallucinations, depression, vertigo, fatigue, anxiety, ***convulsions, drug fever,*** chills, drowsiness

CV: ***Allergic myocarditis***

GI: *Nausea, vomiting, abdominal pain,* stomatitis, ***hepatitis***, glossitis, pancreatitis, diarrhea, ***enterocolitis***, anorexia

GU: ***Renal failure, toxic nephrosis,*** increased BUN, creatinine, crystalluria, hematuria, proteinuria

HEMA: ***Leukopenia, thrombocytopenia, agranulocytosis, hemolytic anemia, aplastic anemia***

INTEG: Rash, dermatitis, urticaria, ***Stevens-Johnson syndrome,*** erythema, photosensitivity, alopecia

SYST: ***Anaphylaxis***

Contraindications: Hypersensitivity to sulfonamides, sulfonylureas, thiazide

S

---

and loop diuretics, salicylates, sunscreens with PABA, infants <2 mo (except congenital toxoplasmosis), pregnancy at term, porphyria, lactation, G6PD deficiency

Precautions: Pregnancy (C), impaired hepatic/renal function, severe allergy, bronchial asthma

PHARMACOKINETICS

PO: Poorly absorbed, peak 3-4 hr, 50%-70% bound to plasma proteins, half-life 7-12 hr; excreted in urine (unchanged 90%), breast milk; crosses placenta

INTERACTIONS

Increase: effects of barbiturates, uricosurics
Increase: drug-free concentrations—indomethacin, probenecid, salicylates
Increase: thrombocytopenia—thiazide diuretics
Increase: nephrotoxicity—cyclo-SPORINE
Increase: hypoglycemic response—sulfonylurea agents
Increase: anticoagulant effects—warfarin
Decrease: renal excretion of methotrexate
Decrease: hepatic clearance of phenytoin
Drug/Lab Test
False positive: Urinary glucose test (Benedict's method)

NURSING CONSIDERATIONS

Assess:
• I&O ratio; note color, character, pH of urine if drug administered for UTIs; output should be 800 ml less than intake; if urine is highly acidic, alkalization may be needed
• Renal studies: BUN, creatinine, urinalysis (long-term therapy)
• Blood dyscrasias: skin rash, fever, sore throat, bruising, bleeding, fatigue, joint pain, monitor CBC before and periodically

⚠ Allergic reaction: rash, dermatitis, urticaria, pruritus, dyspnea, bronchospasm

Administer:
PO route
• On empty stomach
• With full glass of H_2O to maintain adequate hydration; increase fluids to 2 L/day to decrease crystallization in kidneys
• Medication after C&S; repeat C&S after full course of medication

Perform/provide:
• Storage in tight, light-resistant container at room temperature

Evaluate:
• Therapeutic response: absence of pain, fever, C&S negative

Teach patient/family:
• To take each oral dose with full glass of H_2O to prevent crystalluria
• To complete full course of treatment to prevent superinfection
• To avoid sunlight or use sunscreen to prevent burns
• To avoid OTC medication (aspirin, vit C) unless directed by prescriber
⚠ To notify prescriber of skin rash, sore throat, fever, mouth sores, unusual bruising, bleeding

---

sulfasalazine (℞)

(sul-fa-sal'a-zeen)
Azulfidine, Azulfidine EN-tabs, PMS-Sulfasalazine ✦, S.A.S. ✦, Salazopyrin ✦, sulfasalazine
Func. class.: GI antiinflammatory, antirheumatic (DMARD)
Chem. class.: Sulfonamide

Do not confuse:
sulfasalazine/sulfiSOXAZOLE
Action: Prodrug to deliver sulfapyridine and 5-aminosalicylic acid to colon; antiinflammatory in connective tissue also
Uses: Ulcerative colitis; rheumatoid arthritis; juvenile, rheumatoid arthritis (Azulfidine EN-tabs)

⚠ Safety alert   *"Tall Man" lettering

Investigational uses: Ankylosing spondylitis, Crohn's disease, granulomatous colitis, regional enteritis

DOSAGE AND ROUTES
Bowel disease
• *Adult:* **PO** 3-4 g/day in divided doses; maintenance 2 g/day in divided doses q6h
• *Child ≥6 yr:* **PO** 40-60 mg/kg/day in 4-6 divided doses, then 30 mg/kg/day in 4 doses, max 2 g/day
Rheumatoid arthritis
• *Adult:* **PO** 2 g/day in evenly divided doses, initiate treatment with a lower dose of enteric-coated tab
Juvenile rheumatoid arthritis
• *Child ≥6 yr:* **PO** 30-50 mg/kg/24 hr, divided into 2 doses
Renal dose
• *Adult:* **PO** CCr 10-30 ml/min give bid; CCr <10 ml/min give daily
Available forms: Tabs 500 mg; oral susp 250 mg/5 ml; tabs, del rel 500 mg

SIDE EFFECTS
CNS: Headache, confusion, insomnia, hallucinations, depression, vertigo, fatigue, anxiety, ***convulsions,*** drug fever, chills
CV: ***Allergic myocarditis***
GI: *Nausea, vomiting, abdominal pain,* stomatitis, ***hepatitis,*** glossitis, pancreatitis, diarrhea
GU: ***Renal failure, toxic nephrosis,*** increased BUN, creatinine, crystalluria
HEMA: ***Leukopenia, neutropenia, thrombocytopenia, agranulocytosis, hemolytic anemia***
INTEG: Rash, dermatitis, urticaria, ***Stevens-Johnson syndrome,*** erythema, photosensitivity
SYST: ***Anaphylaxis***
Contraindications: Hypersensitivity to sulfonamides or salicylates, pregnancy at term, child <2 yr, intestinal, urinary obstruction, porphyria
Precautions: Pregnancy (C), lactation, impaired hepatic function, severe allergy, bronchial asthma, impaired renal function, megaloblastic anemia

PHARMACOKINETICS
PO: Partially absorbed, peak 1½-6 hr, duration 6-12 hr, half-life 6 hr, excreted in urine as sulfasalazine (15%), sulfapyridine (60%), 5-aminosalicylic acid and metabolites (20%-33%), in breast milk; crosses placenta

INTERACTIONS
Increase: leukopenia risk—thiopurines (azathioprine, mercaptopurine)
Increase: hypoglycemic response—oral hypoglycemics
Increase: anticoagulant effects—oral anticoagulants
Decrease: effect of cycloSPORINE, digoxin, folic acid
Decrease: renal excretion of methotrexate
Drug/Food
Decrease: iron/folic acid absorption
Drug/Lab Test
False positive: Urinary glucose test

NURSING CONSIDERATIONS
Assess:
• Renal studies: BUN, creatinine, urinalysis (long-term therapy)
🅐 Blood dyscrasias: skin rash, fever, sore throat, bruising, bleeding, fatigue, joint pain; monitor CBC before and q3mo
🅐 Allergic reaction: rash, dermatitis, urticaria, pruritus, dyspnea, bronchospasm
Administer:
• Do not break, crush, or chew delayed rel tabs
• With full glass of H_2O to maintain adequate hydration; increase fluids to 2 L/day to decrease crystallization in kidneys
• Total daily dose in evenly spaced doses and after meals to help minimize GI intolerance
Perform/provide:
• Storage in tight, light-resistant container at room temperature
Evaluate:
• Therapeutic response: absence of fever, mucus in stools, pain in joints

S

Side effects: *italics* = common; ***bold italics*** = life-threatening

Teach patient/family:
- To take each oral dose with full glass of H_2O to prevent crystalluria
- That contact lens, urine/skin may be yellow-orange
- To avoid sunlight or use sunscreen to prevent burns
- To notify prescriber of skin rash, sore throat, fever, mouth sores, unusual bruising, bleeding

---

sulfinpyrazone (Rx)
(sul-fin-peer'a-zone)
Anturan ✤, Anturane, sulfinpyrazone
Func. class.: Uricosuric
Chem. class.: Pyrazolone

Action: Inhibits tubular reabsorption of urates, with increased excretion of uric acid; inhibits prostaglandin synthesis, which decreases platelet aggregation
Uses: Gout, gouty arthritis

DOSAGE AND ROUTES
Gout/gouty arthritis
- *Adult:* **PO** 100-200 mg bid × 1 wk, then 200-400 mg bid, not to exceed 800 mg/day
- *Child:* **PO** 10 mg/kg/day in 3-4 divided doses
Renal dose
- CCr <50 ml/min; avoid use
Available forms: Tabs 100 mg; caps 200 mg

SIDE EFFECTS
CNS: Dizziness, **convulsions, coma**
EENT: Tinnitus
GI: Gastric irritation, nausea, vomiting, anorexia, **hepatic necrosis, GI bleeding**
GU: Renal calculi, hypoglycemia
HEMA: **Agranulocytosis** (rare)
INTEG: Rash, dermatitis, pruritus, fever, photosensitivity
RESP: **Apnea**, irregular respirations
Contraindications: Hypersensitivity to pyrazolone derivatives, salicylates, blood dyscrasias, CCr <50 ml/min, active peptic ulcer, GI inflammation, nephrolithiasis
Precautions: Pregnancy (C), renal disease, NSAIDs hypersensitivity

PHARMACOKINETICS
PO: Peak 1-2 hr, duration 4-6 hr, half-life 4 hr; metabolized by liver, excreted in urine

INTERACTIONS
Increase: toxicity—acetaminophen
Increase: effects of warfarin, TOLBUTamide
Increase: bleeding risk—NSAIDs
Decrease: effects of verapamil, theophylline
Decrease: effects of sulfinpyrazone—salicylates, niacin
Drug/Lab Test
Increase: PSP, aminohippuric acid
False positive: Clinitest

NURSING CONSIDERATIONS
Assess:
- Uric acid levels (3-7 mg/dl); joint mobility, pain, swelling
- Respiratory rate, rhythm, depth; notify prescriber of abnormalities
- Renal function
- Bleeding tendencies, RBC, Hct
- I&O
- Electrolytes, CO_2 before, during treatment
- Urine pH, output, glucose during beginning treatment
Administer:
- With glass of milk
- With food for GI symptoms
- Increased fluids to prevent calculi; alkalinization of urine may be required
Evaluate:
- Therapeutic response: absence of pain, stiffness in joints
Teach patient/family:
- To avoid aspirin, NSAIDs, alcohol, high-purine diet

---

*sulfiSOXAZOLE (℞)

(sul-fi-sox'a-zole)
Gantrisin, Novo-Soxazole ♣,
sulfiSOXAZOLE, Gantrisin
Pediatric
Func. class.: Antiinfective
Chem. class.: Sulfonamide, short
acting

Do not confuse:
sulfiSOXAZOLE/sulfasalazine
sulfiSOXAZOLE/ sulfADIAZINE
Action: Interferes with bacterial biosynthesis of proteins by competitive antagonism of PABA
Uses: Urinary tract, systemic infections; chancroid; trachoma; toxoplasmosis; acute otitis media, malaria, *Haemophilus influenzae* meningitis, meningococcal meningitis, nocardiosis, eye infections

DOSAGE AND ROUTES
UTIs, other systemic infections
• *Adult:* PO 2-4 g loading dose, then 1-2 g qid × 7-10 days
• *Child >2 mo:* PO 75 mg/kg or 2 g/m^2 loading dose, then 120-150 mg/kg/day or 4 g/m^2/day in divided doses q6h, not to exceed 6 g/day
Chlamydia trachomatis
• *Adult:* PO 500 mg-1 g qid × 3 wk
Renal dose
• *Adult:* PO CCr 10-50 ml/min give q8-12h; CCr <10 ml/min give q12-24h
Available forms: Tabs 500 mg; sulfiSOXAZOLE acetyl: liquid 500 mg/5 ml

SIDE EFFECTS
CNS: Headache, insomnia, hallucinations, depression, vertigo, fatigue, anxiety, **seizures,** drug fever, chills, drowsiness
*CV: **Allergic myocarditis***
GI: Nausea, vomiting, abdominal pain, stomatitis, ***hepatitis,*** glossitis, pancreatitis, diarrhea, ***enterocolitis,*** anorexia
*GU: **Renal failure, toxic nephrosis,*** increased BUN, creatinine, crystalluria, hematuria, proteinuria
*HEMA: **Leukopenia, thrombocytope-***nia, agranulocytosis, hemolytic anemia, aplastic anemia*
INTEG: Rash, dermatitis, urticaria, ***Stevens-Johnson syndrome,*** erythema, photosensitivity, alopecia
*SYST: **Anaphylaxis***
Contraindications: Hypersensitivity to sulfonamides and sulfonylureas, thiazide and loop diuretics, salicylates; sunscreen with PABA, lactation, infants <2 mo (except congenital toxoplasmosis), pregnancy at term, porphyria
Precautions: Pregnancy (C), lactation, impaired hepatic/renal function, severe allergy, bronchial asthma

PHARMACOKINETICS
PO: Rapidly absorbed, peak 2-4 hr, 85% protein bound; half-life 4-7 hr, excreted in urine, crosses placenta

INTERACTIONS
Increase: effects of barbiturates, TOLBUTamide, uricosurics
Increase: free-drug concentrations—indomethacin, probenecid, salicylates
Increase: thrombocytopenia—thiazides
Increase: nephrotoxicity—cyclo-SPORINE
Increase: hypoglycemic response—sulfonylurea agents
Increase: anticoagulant effect—warfarin
Decrease: renal excretion of methotrexate
Decrease: hepatic clearance of phenytoin
Drug/Lab Test
False positive: Urinary glucose test

NURSING CONSIDERATIONS
Assess:
• I&O ratio; note color, character, pH of urine if drug administered for UTIs; output should be 800 ml less than intake; if urine is highly acidic, alkalization may be needed
• Renal studies: BUN, creatinine, urinalysis (long-term therapy)
⚠ Blood dyscrasias: skin rash, fever,

S

sore throat, bruising, bleeding, fatigue, joint pain, monitor CBC before and periodically

A Allergic reaction: rash, dermatitis, urticaria, pruritus, dyspnea, bronchospasm

Administer:

• On an empty stomach

• With full glass of H_2O to maintain adequate hydration; increase fluids to 2 L/day to decrease crystallization in kidneys

• Medication after C&S; repeat C&S after full course of medication

Perform/provide:

• Storage in tight, light-resistant container at room temperature

Evaluate:

• Therapeutic response: absence of pain, fever, C&S negative

Teach patient/family:

• To take each oral dose with full glass of H_2O to prevent crystalluria

• To complete full course of treatment to prevent superinfection

• To avoid sunlight or use sunscreen to prevent burns; avoid hazardous activities if dizziness occurs

• To avoid OTC medication (aspirin, vit C) unless directed by prescriber

• To notify prescriber of skin rash, sore throat, fever, mouth sores, unusual bruising, bleeding

---

sulfiSOXAZOLE dicolamine ophthalmic
See Appendix C

---

sulindac (R)
(sul-in'dak)
Apo-Sulin ✦, Clinoril,
NovoSundac ✦, sulindac
Func. class.: Nonsteroidal antiinflammatory, antirheumatic
Chem. class.: Indeneacetic acid derivative

Do not contuse:
Clinoril/Clozaril
Clinoril/Oruvail

Action: Inhibits prostaglandin synthesis by decreasing an enzyme needed for biosynthesis; analgesic, antiinflammatory, antipyretic

Uses: Mild to moderate pain, osteoarthritis; rheumatoid, gouty arthritis; ankylosing spondylitis, bursitis, juvenile arthritis

DOSAGE AND ROUTES

Arthritis

• *Adult:* **PO** 150 mg bid, may increase to 200 mg bid

• *Child:* **PO** 2-4 mg/kg/day in divided doses, max 6 mg/kg/day or 200 mg bid whichever is less (safe and effective dose not established)

Bursitis/acute arthritis

• *Adult:* **PO** 200 mg bid × 1-2 wk, then reduce dose

Available forms: Tabs 150, 200 mg

SIDE EFFECTS

CNS: Dizziness, drowsiness, fatigue, tremors, confusion, insomnia, anxiety, depression, headache

CV: Tachycardia, peripheral edema, palpitations, dysrhythmias

EENT: Tinnitus, hearing loss, blurred vision

GI: Nausea, anorexia, vomiting, diarrhea, jaundice, ***cholestatic hepatitis,*** constipation, flatulence, cramps, dry mouth, peptic ulcer, ***bleeding, ulceration, perforation***

*GU: **Nephrotoxicity: dysuria, hematuria, oliguria, azotemia***

*HEMA: **Blood dyscrasias*** with prolonged use

INTEG: Purpura, *rash, pruritus,* sweating, photosensitivity

Contraindications: Hypersensitivity, asthma, severe renal disease, severe hepatic disease, active ulcers

Precautions: Pregnancy (C) 1st trimester, lactation, children, bleeding disorders, GI disorders, cardiac disorders, hypersensitivity to other antiinflammatory agents, renal disease

---

PHARMACOKINETICS

PO: Peak 2 hr, half-life 3-3½ hr; metabolized in liver; excreted in urine (metabolites), breast milk; 93% protein binding

INTERACTIONS

GI side effects: aspirin, corticosteroids, other NSAIDs

Increase: bleeding risk—anticoagulants, thrombolytics, plicamycin, tirofiban, eptifibatide, clopidogrel, ticlopidine, valproic acid, some cephalosporins

Increase: nephrotoxicity—cycloSPORINE

Increase: toxicity—methotrexate, sulfonamides, sulfonylureas, probenecid

Decrease: sulindac effect—diflunisal, do not use together

Drug/Herb

Increase: gastric irritation—arginine, gossypol

Increase: NSAIDs effect—bearberry, bilberry

Increase: bleeding risk—bogbean, chondroitin

NURSING CONSIDERATIONS

Assess:

• Pain: frequency, intensity, characteristics, relief after med

⚠ Asthma, aspirin hypersensitivity, nasal polyps; increased hypersensitivity

• Renal, hepatic studies: BUN, creatinine, AST, ALT, Hgb, before treatment, periodically thereafter

• Have B/P checked qmo; drug causes sodium retention

• Audiometric, ophthalmic exam before, during, after treatment

• For eye, ear problems: blurred vision, tinnitus may indicate toxicity

Administer:

• With food to decrease GI symptoms; take on empty stomach to facilitate absorption; tablet may be crushed

• With a full glass of water

Perform/provide:

• Storage at room temperature

Evaluate:

• Therapeutic response: decreased pain, stiffness, swelling in joints, ability to move more easily

Teach patient/family:

• To report blurred vision or ringing, roaring in ears (may indicate toxicity)

• To avoid driving, other hazardous activities if dizzy or drowsy

• To report change in urine pattern, weight increase, edema, pain increase in joints, fever, blood in urine (indicates nephrotoxicity)

• That therapeutic effects may take up to 1 mo

• To avoid alcohol and aspirin

• To take with full glass of water

• To use sunscreen

---

sumatriptan (℞)

(soo-ma-trip'tan)

Imitrex

Func. class.: Antimigraine agent

Chem. class.: 5-HT$_{1P}$ receptor agonist

Action: Binds selectively to the vascular 5-HT$_{1p}$ receptor subtype, exerts antimigraine effect; causes vasoconstriction in cranial arteries

Uses: Acute treatment of migraine with or without aura and cluster headache

DOSAGE AND ROUTES

• *Adult:* **SUBCUT** 6 mg or less; may repeat in 1 hr; not to exceed 12 mg/24 hr; **PO** 25 mg with fluids, if no relief in 2 hr, give another dose, max 200 mg/day; **NASAL** one dose of 5, 10, or 20 mg in one nostril, may repeat in 2 hr, max 40 mg/24 hr

Hepatic dose

• *Adult:* **PO** 25 mg, if no response after 2 hr, give up to 50 mg

Available forms: Inj 12 mg/ml; tabs 25, 50, 100 mg, nasal spray 5 mg/100 mcl-U dose spray device, 20 mg/100 mcl-U

SIDE EFFECTS

CNS: Tingling, hot sensation, burning, feeling of pressure, tightness, numbness, dizziness, sedation, headache, anxiety, fatigue, cold sensation

R

CV: Flushing, **MI**
EENT: Throat, mouth, nasal discomfort; vision changes
GI: Abdominal discomfort
INTEG: Inj site reaction, sweating
MS: Weakness, neck stiffness, myalgia
RESP: Chest tightness, pressure
Contraindications: Angina pectoris, history of MI, documented silent ischemia, Prinzmetal's angina, ischemic heart disease, IV use, concurrent ergotamine-containing preparations, uncontrolled hypertension, hypersensitivity, basilar or hemiplegic migraine
Precautions: Pregnancy (C), postmenopausal women, men >40 yr, risk factors for CAD, hypercholesterolemia, obesity, diabetes, impaired hepatic or renal function, lactation, children <18 yr, elderly

PHARMACOKINETICS

Onset of pain relief 10 min-2 hr, peak 10-20 min, 10%-20% plasma protein binding, metabolized in the liver (metabolite), excreted in urine, feces

INTERACTIONS

Extended vasospastic effects: ergot, ergot derivatives
Increase: sumatriptan effect—MAOIs, SSRIs
Drug/Herb
Serotonin syndrome: SAM-e, St. John's wort
Increase: effect—butterbur

NURSING CONSIDERATIONS

Assess:
• B/P; signs/symptoms of coronary vasospasms
• Tingling, hot sensation, burning, feeling of pressure, numbness, flushing, inj site reaction
• For stress level, activity, recreation, coping mechanisms
• Neurologic status: LOC, blurring vision, nausea, vomiting, tingling in extremities preceding headache
• Ingestion of tyramine foods (pickled products, beer, wine, aged cheese), food additives, preservatives, colorings, artificial sweeteners, chocolate, caffeine, which may precipitate these types of headaches
Administer:
• Swallow tabs whole; do not break, crush, or chew
• SUBCUT only just below the skin; avoid IM or IV administration, use only for actual migraine attack
• Take tabs with fluids as soon as symptoms appear; may take a second dose >4 hr; max 200 mg/24 hr
Perform/provide:
• Quiet, calm environment with decreased stimulation for noise, bright light, excessive talking
Evaluate:
• Therapeutic response: decrease in frequency, severity of migraine
Teach patient/family:
• To report chest pain, tightness; sudden, severe abdominal pain to prescriber immediately
• To use contraception while taking drug
• To use nasal spray: one spray in one nostril, may repeat if headache returns, do not repeat if pain continues after 1st dose
• To have dark, quiet environment

---

suprofen ophthalmic
See Appendix C

---

tacrine (℞)
(tack'rin)
Cognex
Func. class.: Anti-Alzheimer agent
Chem. class.: Reversible cholinesterase inhibitor

Do not confuse:
Cognex/Corgard
Action: Elevates acetylcholine concentrations (cerebral cortex) by slowing degradation of acetylcholine released in cholinergic neurons; does not alter underlying dementia

---

⚠ Safety alert   *"Tall Man" lettering

Uses: Treatment of mild to moderate dementia in Alzheimer's disease

DOSAGE AND ROUTES

• *Adult:* **PO** 10 mg qid × 4 wk, then 20 mg qid × 4 wk, increase at 4-wk intervals if patient tolerating drug well and if transaminase is WNL, then titrate to higher doses (30-40 mg qid) at 4-wk intervals
Available forms: Caps 10, 20, 30, 40 mg

SIDE EFFECTS

CNS: Dizziness, confusion, insomnia, tremor, *ataxia, somnolence, anxiety, agitation, depression, hallucinations, hostility, abnormal thinking,* chills, fever, headache, *seizures*
CV: Hypotension or hypertension, ***bradycardia, heart block***
GI: Nausea, vomiting, anorexia, abdominal pain, constipation, dyspepsia, flatulence, ***hepatotoxicity, GI bleeding,*** diarrhea
GU: Urinary frequency, UTI, *incontinence*
INTEG: Rash, flushing
OTHER: Myalgia
RESP: Rhinitis, URI, cough, pharyngitis
Contraindications: Hypersensitivity to this drug or acridine derivatives, patients treated with this drug who developed jaundice with a total bilirubin of >3 mg/dl
Precautions: Pregnancy (C), sick sinus syndrome, history of ulcers, GI bleeding, hepatic disease, bladder obstruction, asthma, lactation, children, seizure disorders, history of bradyarrhythmias

PHARMACOKINETICS

Rapidly absorbed PO, 55% bound to plasma proteins, extensively metabolized to metabolites by CYP450 enzyme system, elimination half-life 2-4 hr

INTERACTIONS

Synergistic effect: succinylcholine, cholinesterase inhibitors, cholinergic agonists

Smoking may decrease drug level
Increase: bleeding risk—NSAIDs
Increase: tacrine levels—cimetidine, ciprofloxacin, fluvoxamine, ritonavir
Increase: elimination half-life of theophylline
Decrease: activity of anticholinergics
Drug/Food:
May delay absorption, give 1 hr ac

NURSING CONSIDERATIONS

Assess:
• B/P: hypotension, hypertension
• Mental status: affect, mood, behavioral changes, depression; complete suicide assessment; hallucinations, confusion
• GI status: nausea, vomiting, anorexia, constipation, abdominal pain; add bulk, increase fluids for constipation
• GU status: urinary frequency, incontinence
• Jaundice confirmed by significant increase bilirubin (>3 mg/dl) and/or those with hypersensitivity (rash/fever) with increase ALT, should be immediately, permanently discontinued
• Serum ALT every other week, × 4-16 wk, then q3mo
Administer:
• Between meals; may be given with meals for GI symptoms
• Dosage adjusted to response no more than q4wk
Perform/provide:
• Assistance with ambulation during beginning therapy; dizziness, ataxia may occur
Evaluate:
• Therapeutic response: decrease in confusion, improved mood
Teach patient/family:
• To report side effects; severe nausea, vomiting, sweating, salivation, bradycardia, hypotension, collapse, seizures; indicate overdose
• To use drug exactly as prescribed: at regular intervals, preferably between meals; may be taken with meals for GI upset; drug is not a cure
• To notify prescriber of nausea, vomiting, diarrhea (dose increase or begin-

T

ning treatment), or rash; very dark or very light stools, jaundice (delayed onset)

• Not to increase or abruptly decrease dose; serious consequences may result

Treatment of overdose: Withdraw drug, administer tertiary anticholinergics, provide supportive care

---

tacrolimus (Rx)
(tak-roe-li′mus)
Prograf
tacrolimus topical
Protopic
Func. class.: Immunosuppressant
Chem. class.: Macrolide

Action: Produces immunosuppression by inhibiting T-lymphocytes

Uses: Organ transplants to prevent rejection; topical: atopic dermatitis

Investigational uses: Autoimmune diseases, severe recalcitrant psoriasis

DOSAGE AND ROUTES

• *Adult and child:* **IV** 0.03-0.05 mg/kg/day × 3 days then **PO** 0.15 mg/kg bid; adjust dose in renal impairment

• *Adult:* **TOP** apply ointment bid × 7 days

• *Child ≥2-15 yr:* apply ointment bid × 7 days

Available forms: Inj 5 mg/ml; caps 0.5, 1, 5 mg; ointment 0.03%, 0.1%

SIDE EFFECTS

CNS: Tremors, *headache,* insomnia, paresthesia, chills, fever, *seizures*
CV: Hypertension
EENT: Blurred vision, photophobia
GI: Nausea, vomiting, diarrhea, constipation, *GI bleeding*
GU: UTIs, *albuminuria, hematuria, proteinuria, renal failure*
HEMA: **Anemia, leukocytosis, thrombocytopenia, purpura**
INTEG: Rash, flushing, itching, alopecia
META: Hirsutism, hyperglycemia, hyperkalemia, hyperuricemia, hypokalemia, hypomagnesemia

RESP: **Pleural effusion, atelectasis,** dyspnea
SYST: **Anaphylaxis**

Contraindications: Hypersensitivity to this drug or to some kinds of castor oil

Precautions: Pregnancy (C), severe renal, hepatic disease; diabetes mellitus, hyperkalemia, hyperuricemia, lymphomas, lactation, children <12, hypertension

PHARMACOKINETICS

Extensively metabolized, half-life 10 hr, 75% protein binding

INTERACTIONS

Increase: toxicity—aminoglycosides, cisplatin, cycloSPORINE
Increase: blood levels—antifungals, calcium channel blockers, cimetidine, danazol, erythromycin, mycophenolate, mofetil
Decrease: blood levels—carbamazepine, phenobarbital, phenytoin, rifamycin
Decrease: effect of vaccines
Drug/Herb
Decrease: immunosuppression—astragalus, echinacea, melatonin
Decrease: effect—ginseng, maitake, mistletoe

NURSING CONSIDERATIONS

Assess:

• Blood studies: Hgb, WBC, platelets during treatment qmo; if leukocytes <3000/mm^3 or platelets <100,000/mm^3, drug should be discontinued or reduced; decreased hemoglobulin level may indicate bone marrow suppression

• Hepatic studies: alk phosphatase, AST, ALT, amylase, bilirubin, and for hepatotoxicity: dark urine, jaundice, itching, light-colored stools; drug should be discontinued

Administer:

• All medications PO if possible, avoiding IM inj; bleeding may occur

• With meals to reduce GI upset; nausea is common

🅐 Safety alert   *"Tall Man" lettering

• For several days before transplant surgery, patients should be placed in protective isolation

⚠ Anaphylaxis: rash, pruritus, wheezing, laryngeal edema; stop infusion, initiate emergency procedures

IV route

• After diluting in 0.9% NaCl or D$_5$W to 0.004 to 0.02 mg/ml as a continuous infusion

Additive compatibilities: Cimetidine

Y-site compatibilities: Acyclovir, aminophylline, amphotericin B, ampicillin, ampicillin/sulbactam, benztropine, calcium gluconate, cefazolin, cefotetan, ceftazidime, ceftriaxone, cefuroxime, chloramphenicol, cimetidine, ciprofloxacin, clindamycin, dexamethasone, digoxin, diphenhydrAMINE, DOBUTamine, DOPamine, doxycycline, erythromycin, esmolol, fluconazole, furosemide, ganciclovir, gentamicin, haloperidol, heparin, hydrocortisone, imipenem/cilastatin, insulin (regular), isoproterenol, leucovorin, lorazepam, methylPREDNISolone, metoclopramide, metronidazole, mezlocillin, multivitamins, nitroglycerin, oxacillin, penicillin G potassium, perphenazine, phenytoin, piperacillin, potassium chloride, propranolol, ranitidine, sodium bicarbonate, sodium nitroprusside, trimethoprim-sulfamethoxazole, vancomycin

Evaluate:

• Therapeutic response: absence of graft rejection; immunosuppression in autoimmune disorders

Teach patient/family:

• To report fever, rash, severe diarrhea, chills, sore throat, fatigue; serious infections may occur; clay-colored stools, cramping (hepatotoxicity)

• To avoid crowds, persons with known infections to reduce risk of infection

• To avoid exposure to natural or artificial sunlight

• Not to breastfeed while taking this medication

---

tadalafil (℞)
(tah-dal'a-fil)
Cialis
Func. class.: Impotence agent
Chem. class.: Phosphodiesterase type 5 inhibitor

Action: Inhibits phosphodiesterase type 5 (PDE5); enhances erectile function by increasing the amount of cGMP which causes smooth muscle relaxation and increased blood flow into the corpus cavernosum; improves erectile function for up to 36 hr

Uses: Treatment of erectile dysfunction

DOSAGE AND ROUTES

• *Adult:* **PO** 10 mg, taken prior to sexual activity, dose may be reduced to 5 mg or increased to a max of 20 mg; usual max dosing frequency is once per day

Renal dose

• *Adult (CCr 31-50 ml/min):* **PO** 5 mg/daily, max 10 mg q 48 hr; CCr <30 ml/min, max 5 mg

Hepatic dose

• *Adult (Child-Pugh class A, B):* **PO** max 10 mg daily; (Child-Pugh class C), not recommended

Concomitant medications

• Ketoconazole, ritonavir, max 10 mg q72h

Available forms: Tabs 5, 10, 20 mg

SIDE EFFECTS

CNS: Headache, flushing, dizziness
CV: **MI, sudden death, CV collapse**
MISC: Back pain/myalgia, *dyspepsia, nasal congestion, UTI,* blurred vision, changes in color vision, *diarrhea,* pruritus, priapism, **NAION (nonarteritic ischemic optic neuropathy)**

Contraindications: Hypersensitivity, patients taking organic nitrates either regularly and/or intermittently, patients taking any α-adrenergic antagonist other than 0.4 mg once daily tamsulosin

Precautions: Anatomical penile deformities, sickle cell anemia, leukemia,

T

---

multiple myeloma. Tadalafil is not indicated for use in newborns, children, or women.

PHARMACOKINETICS

Rapidly absorbed; metabolized by liver; terminal half-life 17.5 hr, peak ½-6 hr; excreted primarily as metabolites feces, urine; plasma concentration 61% in feces, 36% in urine; 94% protein bound; rate and extent of absorption of tadalafil are not influenced by food.

INTERACTIONS

⚠ Do not use with nitrates because of unsafe drop in B/P which could result in MI or stroke

Increase: tadalafil levels—ketoconazole, ritonavir (although not studied, may also include other HIV protease inhibitors)

Decrease: B/P—antihypertensives

NURSING CONSIDERATIONS

Assess:

• Use of organic nitrates that should not be used with this drug

• For any severe loss of vision, while taking this or any similar products

Administer:

• Give prior to sexual activity; do not use more than once a day

• That drug should not be used with nitrates in any form

Teach patient/family:

• That drug does not protect against sexually transmitted diseases, including HIV

• To tell physician if patient has a bleeding problem

• That drug has no effect in the absence of sexual stimulation

• To seek medical help if an erection lasts more than 4 hours

• To tell physician of all medicines, vitamins, and herbs patient is taking, especially ritonavir, indinavir, ketoconazole, itraconazole, erythromycin, nitrates, α-blockers

• That tadalafil is contraindicated for use with α-blockers except 0.4 mg/daily tamsulosin

• To notify prescriber immediately, and stop taking product if vision loss occurs

---

tamoxifen (℞)
(ta-mox'i-fen)
Alpha-Tamoxifen ✦, Med Tamoxifen ✦, Nolvadex, Nolvadex-D ✦, Novo-Tamoxifen ✦, Tamofen ✦, Tamone ✦, Tamoplex ✦
Func. class.: Antineoplastic
Chem. class.: Antiestrogen hormone

Action: Inhibits cell division by binding to cytoplasmic estrogen receptors; resembles normal cell complex but inhibits DNA synthesis and estrogen response of target tissue

Uses: Advanced breast carcinoma not responsive to other therapy in estrogen-receptor-positive patients (usually postmenopausal), prevention of breast cancer, following breast surgery/radiation in ductal carcinoma in situ

Investigational uses: Mastalgia, to reduce pain/size of gynecomastia, ovulation stimulation, malignant carcinoid tumor, carcinoid syndrome

DOSAGE AND ROUTES

Breast cancer

• *Adult:* **PO** 20-40 mg daily; doses >20 mg/day, divide AM/PM

High risk for breast cancer

• *Adult:* **PO** 20 mg daily × 5 yr

DCIS

• *Adult:* **PO** 20 mg daily × 5 yr

Available forms: Tabs 10, 20 mg

SIDE EFFECTS

CNS: Hot flashes, headache, lightheadedness, depression

CV: Chest pain

EENT: Ocular lesions, retinopathy, corneal opacity, blurred vision (high doses)

GI: Nausea, vomiting, altered taste (anorexia)

⚠ Safety alert   *"Tall Man" lettering

GU: Vaginal bleeding, pruritus vulvae
*HEMA: **Thrombocytopenia, leukopenia,** DVT, PE*
INTEG: Rash, alopecia
META: Hypercalcemia
Contraindications: Pregnancy (D), hypersensitivity, lactation
Precautions: Leukopenia, thrombocytopenia, cataracts

PHARMACOKINETICS

PO: Peak 4-7 hr, half-life 7 days (1 wk terminal), excreted primarily in feces

INTERACTIONS

Increase: chance of bleeding—anticoagulants
Increase: tamoxifen levels—bromocriptine
Increase: thromboembolic events—cytotoxics
Decrease: tamoxifen levels—aminoglutethimide, medroxyprogesterone, rifamycin
Decrease: letrozole levels—letrozole
Drug/Lab Test
Increase: serum calcium

NURSING CONSIDERATIONS

Assess:
• CBC, differential, platelet count qwk; withhold drug if WBC is <3500 or platelet count is <100,000; notify prescriber
• Bleeding q8h: hematuria, guaiac, bruising, petechiae, mucosa or orifices
• Effects of alopecia on body image; discuss feelings about body changes
⚠ For uterine malignancies, symptoms of stroke, pulmonary embolism that may occur in women with ductal carcinoma in situ (DCIS) and women at high risk for breast cancer
⚠ Symptoms indicating severe allergic reactions: rash, pruritus, urticaria, purpuric skin lesions, itching, flushing
Administer:
• Do not break, crush, or chew tabs
• Antacid before oral agent; give drug after evening meal, before bedtime

• Antiemetic 30-60 min before giving drug to prevent vomiting
Perform/provide:
• Liquid diet, if needed, including cola, Jell-O; dry toast or crackers may be added if patient is not nauseated or vomiting
• Increase fluid intake to 2-3 L/day to prevent dehydration
• Nutritious diet with iron, vitamin supplements as ordered
• Storage in light-resistant container at room temperature
Evaluate:
• Therapeutic response: decreased tumor size, spread of malignancy
Teach patient/family:
• To report any complaints, side effects to prescriber
• To increase fluids to 2 L/day unless contraindicated
• To wear sunscreen, protective clothing, sunglasses
• That vaginal bleeding, pruritus, hot flashes are reversible after discontinuing treatment
• To report immediately decreased visual acuity, which may be irreversible; stress need for routine eye exams; care providers should be told about tamoxifen therapy
• To report vaginal bleeding immediately
• That tumor flare—increase in size of tumor, increased bone pain—may occur and will subside rapidly; may take analgesics for pain
• That premenopausal women must use mechanical birth control because ovulation may be induced
• That hair may be lost during treatment; a wig or hairpiece may make patient feel better; new hair may be different in color, texture

T

tamsulosin (℞)

(tam-sue-lo'sen)

Flomax

Func. class.: Selective α_1-adrenergic blocker

Chem. class.: Sulfamoylphenethylamine derivative

Do not confuse:

Flomax/Fosamax/Volmax

Action: Binds preferentially to α_{1A}-adrenoceptor subtype located mainly in the prostate

Uses: Symptoms of benign prostatic hyperplasia

DOSAGE AND ROUTES

• *Adult:* **PO** 0.4 mg daily, increasing up to 0.8 mg daily if required

Available forms: Caps 0.4 mg

SIDE EFFECTS

CNS: Dizziness, headache, asthenia, insomnia

CV: Chest pain

EENT: Amblyopia

GI: Nausea, diarrhea

GU: Decreased libido, abnormal ejaculation

MS: Back pain

RESP: Rhinitis, pharyngitis, cough

Contraindications: Hypersensitivity

Precautions: Pregnancy (B), children, lactation, hepatic disease, coronary artery disease, severe renal disease

PHARMACOKINETICS

PO: Unknown, peak 4-5 hr, duration 9-15 hr; half-life 14 hr; metabolized in liver; excreted via urine; extensively protein bound (98%)

INTERACTIONS

Not to be taken with: prazosin, terazosin, doxazosin, β-blockers, vardenafil

Increase: toxicity—cimetidine

Drug/Food

Decrease: absorption with food

NURSING CONSIDERATIONS

Assess:

• Prostatic hyperplasia: change in urinary patterns, baseline and throughout treatment

• CBC with diff and LFTs; B/P and heart rate

• BUN, uric acid, urodynamic studies (urinary flow rates, residual volume)

• I&O ratios, weight daily, edema, report weight gain or edema

Administer:

• Swallow caps whole; do not break, crush, or chew

• Give ½ hr after same meal each day

Perform/provide:

• Storage in tight container in cool environment

Evaluate:

• Therapeutic response: decreased symptoms of benign prostatic hyperplasia

Teach patient/family:

• Not to drive or operate machinery for 4 hr after first dose or after dosage increase

tegaserod (℞)

(teg-as'er-odd)

Zelnorm

Func. class.: 5-HT$_4$ receptor partial agonist, misc. GI agent, prokinetic

Action: A 5-HT$_4$ receptor partial agonist that binds 5-HT$_4$ receptors, stimulating peristalsis and intestinal secretion

Uses: Irritable bowel syndrome (IBS) where primary bowel symptom is constipation, chronic constipation not associated with IBS

DOSAGE AND ROUTES

• *Adult:* **PO** 6 mg bid before meals × 4-6 wk, another 4-6-wk course may be used

Available forms: Tabs 2, 6 mg

SIDE EFFECTS

CNS: Headache, dizziness, depression, vertigo, fatigue, suicide attempt, poor concentration
CV: Hypotension, angina, ***dysrrhythmias, bundle branch block, supraventricular tachycardia***
GI: Nausea, abdominal pain, increased appetite, eructation, increased AST, increased ALT, diarrhea, irritable colon, tenesmus, flatulence
GU: Polyuria, renal pain, ovarian cyst, miscarriage, albuminuria
MISC: Pain, facial edema, increased CPK, asthma, breast carcinoma
MS: Back pain, arthralgia
*SYST: **Anaphylaxis***

Contraindications: Hypersensitivity, severe renal disease, moderate to severe hepatic disease, history of bowel obstruction, gallbladder disease, abdominal adhesions, sphincter of Oddi dysfunction, hypotension
Precautions: Pregnancy (B), lactation, children, diarrhea

PHARMACOKINETICS

Peak 1 hr, 98% protein binding, terminal half-life 11 hr, ⅔ excreted unchanged in feces, remainder in urine as metabolite

INTERACTIONS

Decrease: effect of digoxin, oral contraceptives
Decrease: tegaserod effect—antimuscarinics
Drug/Food
Food decreases absorption, but is minimized when taken ½ hr before meal

NURSING CONSIDERATIONS
Assess:
• GI symptoms: nausea, abdominal pain
• CV status: B/P, pulse, chest pain
Administer:
• Before meals, bid
Perform/provide:
• Store at room temperature

Evaluate:
• Therapeutic response: Decreased constipation in IBS
Teach patient/family:
• To notify prescriber of GI symptoms, hypersensitivity reactions

---

telithromycin (℞)
(teh-lih-throw-my´sin)
Ketek
Func. class.: Antiinfective
Chem. class.: Ketolides

Action: Binds to 50S ribosomal subunits of susceptible bacteria and suppresses protein synthesis
Uses: Acute bacterial exacerbation of chronic bronchitis caused by *Streptococcus pneumoniae, Haemophilus influenzae, Moraxella catarrhalis*; acute bacterial sinusitis caused by *S. pneumoniae, H. influenzae, M. catarrhalis, Staphylococcus aureus*, community-acquired pneumonic

DOSAGE AND ROUTES
Acute bacterial exacerbation of bronchitis
• *Adult:* **PO** 800 mg daily × 5 days
Acute bacterial sinusitis
• *Adult:* **PO** 800 mg daily × 5 days
Community-acquired pneumonia
• *Adult:* **PO** 800 mg daily × 7-10 days
Available forms: Tabs 400 mg

SIDE EFFECTS
CNS: Dizziness, headache, insomnia, increased sweating
EENT: Blurred vision, diplopia, difficulty focusing
GI: Nausea, vomiting, diarrhea, hepatitis, abdominal pain/distention, stomatitis, anorexia
GU: Vaginitis, moniliasis
INTEG: Rash, urticaria
MISC: Atrial dysrhythmias
MS: Muscle cramps
*SYST: **Anaphylaxis***
Contraindications: Hypersensitivity

Precautions: Pregnancy (C), lactation, children, elderly, myasthenia gravis, ongoing prodysrhythmias, hepatic disease

PHARMACOKINETICS

Peak 1 hr; metabolized in liver; excreted in bile, feces; protein binding 60%-70%

INTERACTIONS

⚠ Serious dysrhythmias: pimozide; do not use together

Increase: action, toxicity of atorvastatin, digoxin, ergots, lovastatin, metoprolol, midazolam, simvastatin, theophylline

Increase: telithromycin—itraconazole, ketoconazole

Decrease: action of telihrymycin—rifampin, phenytoin, carbamazepine, phenobarbital

Decrease: action of sotalol

Drug/Herb

Do not use acidophilus with antiinfectives

Drug/Lab Test

Increase: AST/ALT

NURSING CONSIDERATIONS

Assess:

• For infection: temp, sputum, WBCs, baseline and periodically

• Oliguria in renal disease

• Hepatic studies: AST, ALT, if patient is on long-term therapy

• C&S before drug therapy; drug may be given as soon as culture is taken; C&S may be repeated after treatment

• Bowel pattern before, during treatment

• Skin eruptions, itching

Administer:

• May take without regard to food

• Do not use this drug if using class 1A or III antidysrhythmics

Perform/provide:

• Storage at room temperature

• Adequate intake of fluids (2 L) during diarrhea episodes

Evaluate:

• Therapeutic response: decreased symptoms of infection

Teach patient/family:

• To report sore throat, fever, fatigue (could indicate superinfection)

• To notify nurse of diarrhea stools, dark urine, pale stools, jaundice of eyes or skin, and severe abdominal pain

• To report blurred vision, if interfering with daily activities

• To avoid driving, hazardous activities if blurred vision occurs

• To take as prescribed, do not double or skip doses

• To avoid simvastatin, lovastatin, or atorvastatin

• May take without regard to meals

Treatment of hypersensitivity:

• Withdraw drug; maintain airway; administer epINEPHrine, aminophylline, O₂, IV corticosteroids

---

telmisartan (R)
(tel-mih-sar'tan)
Micardis
Func. class.: Antihypertensive
Chem. class.: Angiotensin II receptor (Type AT₁)

Action: Blocks the vasoconstrictor and aldosterone-secreting effects of angiotensin II; selectively blocks the binding of angiotensin II to the AT₁ receptor found in tissues

Uses: Hypertension, alone or in combination

Investigational uses: Heart failure

Research note: Telmisartan administered with digoxin resulted in an increased digoxin level

DOSAGE AND ROUTES

• *Adult:* **PO** 40 mg daily; range 20-80 mg

Available forms: Tabs 20, 40, 80 mg

SIDE EFFECTS

CNS: Dizziness, insomnia, *anxiety,* headache, fatigue

⚠ Safety alert   *"Tall Man" lettering

GI: Diarrhea, dyspepsia, *anorexia, vomiting*
MS: Myalgia, pain
RESP: Cough, *upper respiratory infection,* sinusitis, pharyngitis
Contraindications: Pregnancy (D) 2nd/3rd trimesters, hypersensitivity
Precautions: Pregnancy (C) 1st trimester, hypersensitivity to ACE inhibitors: lactation, children, elderly

PHARMACOKINETICS

Extensively metabolized, terminal half-life 24 hr, highly bound to plasma proteins, excreted feces >97%

INTERACTIONS

Increase: digoxin peak/trough concentrations—digoxin
Increase: antihypertensive action—diuretics, other antihypertensives
Increase: hyperkalemia—potassium-sparing diuretics, potassium salt substitutes

Drug/Herb
Increase: toxicity, death—aconite
Increase: antihypertensive effect—barberry, betony, black catechu, black cohosh, bloodroot, broom, burdock, cat's claw, dandelion, goldenseal, Irish moss, Jamaican dogwood, kelp, khella, mistletoe, parsley
Increase or decrease: antihypertensive effect—astragalus, cola tree
Decrease: antihypertensive effect—coltsfoot, guarana, khat, licorice

NURSING CONSIDERATIONS

Assess:
• B/P, pulse q4h; note rate, rhythm, quality
• Electrolytes: K, Na, Cl
• Baselines in renal, hepatic studies before therapy begins
• Edema in feet, legs daily
• Skin turgor, dryness of mucous membranes for hydration status

Administer:
• Without regard to meals
• Increased dose to African-American

patients, B/P response may be reduced
Evaluate:
• Therapeutic response: decreased B/P
Teach patient/family:
• To comply with dosage schedule, even if feeling better
• To notify prescriber of mouth sores, fever, swelling of hands or feet, irregular heartbeat, chest pain
• That excessive perspiration, dehydration, vomiting, diarrhea may lead to fall in blood pressure; consult prescriber if these occur
• That drug may cause dizziness, fainting; light-headedness may occur
• To use contraception while taking this drug
• To notify prescriber of all prescriptions, OTC, and supplements taken

---

temazepam (℞)
(te-maz′e-pam)
Razepam, Restoril, temazepam
Func. class.: Sedative-hypnotic
Chem. class.: Benzodiazepine

Controlled Substance Schedule IV (USA), Schedule F (Canada)
Action: Produces CNS depression at limbic, thalamic, hypothalamic levels of the CNS; may be mediated by neurotransmitter γ-aminobutyric acid (GABA); results are sedation, hypnosis, skeletal muscle relaxation, anticonvulsant activity, anxiolytic action
Uses: Insomnia

DOSAGE AND ROUTES

• *Adult:* **PO** 15-30 mg at bedtime
• *Geriatric:* **PO** 7.5 mg at bedtime
Available forms: Caps 7.5, 15, 30 mg

SIDE EFFECTS

CNS: Lethargy, drowsiness, daytime sedation, dizziness, confusion, light-headedness, headache, anxiety, irritability
CV: Chest pain, pulse changes
GI: Nausea, vomiting, diarrhea, heart-

T

burn, abdominal pain, constipation, anorexia

*HEMA: **Leukopenia, granulocytope-nia*** (rare)

Contraindications: Pregnancy (X), hypersensitivity to benzodiazepines, lactation, intermittent porphyria

Precautions: Anemia, hepatic disease, renal disease, suicidal individuals, drug abuse, elderly, psychosis, children <15 yr, acute narrow-angle glaucoma, seizure disorders

PHARMACOKINETICS

PO: Onset 30-45 min, duration 6-8 hr, half-life 10-20 hr; metabolized by liver, excreted by kidneys, crosses placenta, excreted in breast milk

INTERACTIONS

Increase: effects of cimetidine, disulfiram, oral contraceptives

Increase: action of both drugs—alcohol, CNS depressants

Decrease: effect of antacids, theophylline, rifampin

Drug/Herb

Increase: CNS depression—catnip, chamomile, clary, cowslip, hops, kava, lavender, mistletoe, nettle, pokeweed, poppy, Queen Anne's lace, senega, skullcap, valerian

Increase: hypotension—black cohosh

Drug/Lab Test

Increase: ALT, AST, serum bilirubin

Decrease: RAI uptake

False increase: Urinary 17-OHCS

NURSING CONSIDERATIONS

Assess:

• Blood studies: Hct, Hgb, RBCs (long-term therapy)

• Hepatic studies: AST, ALT, bilirubin (long-term therapy)

• Mental status: mood, sensorium, affect, memory (long, short)

⚠ Blood dyscrasias: fever, sore throat, bruising, rash, jaundice, epistaxis (rare)

• Type of sleep problem: falling asleep, staying asleep

Administer:

• After removal of cigarettes to prevent fires

• After trying conservative measures for insomnia

• ½-1 hr before bedtime for sleeplessness

• On empty stomach for fast onset, but may be taken with food if GI symptoms occur

• Avoid use with CNS depressants; serious CNS depression may result

Perform/provide:

• Assistance with ambulation after receiving dose

• Safety measures: night-light, call bell within easy reach

• Checking to see if PO medication has been swallowed

• Storage in tight container in cool environment

Evaluate:

• Therapeutic response: ability to sleep at night, decreased early morning awakening if taking drug for insomnia

Teach patient/family:

• To avoid driving, other activities requiring alertness until stabilized

• To avoid alcohol ingestion

• That effects may take 2 nights for benefits to be noticed

• Alternative measures to improve sleep: reading, exercise several hours before bedtime, warm bath, warm milk, TV, self-hypnosis, deep breathing

• That hangover, memory impairment are common in elderly but less common than with barbiturates

• To use contraception while taking this product

Treatment of overdose: Lavage, activated charcoal; monitor electrolytes, VS

temozolomide (℞)

(tem-oh-zole'oh-mide)

Temodar

Func. class.: Antineoplastic-alkylating agent

Chem. class.: Imidazotetrazine derivative

Action: A prodrug that undergoes conversion to MTIC. MTIC action prevents DNA transcription

Uses: Anaplastic astrocytoma with relapse, glioblastoma multiforme

Investigational uses: Metastatic melanoma

DOSAGE AND ROUTES

Anaplastic astrocytoma

• *Adult:* **PO** Adjust dose based on nadir neutrophil and platelet counts 150 mg/m^2/day × 5 days during a 28-day cycle

Glioblastoma multiforme

• *Adult:* **PO** 75 mg/m^2/day × ×42 days with focal radiotherapy; then maintenance of 6 cycles

Available forms: Caps 5, 20, 100, 250 mg

SIDE EFFECTS

*CNS: **Seizures**, hemiparesis, dizziness, poor coordination, amnesia, insomnia, paresthesia, somnolence, paresis, ataxia, anxiety, dysphagia, depression, confusion*

GI: Nausea, anorexia, vomiting

GU: Urinary incontinence, UTI, frequency

*HEMA: **Thrombocytopenia, leukopenia**, anemia*

INTEG: Rash, pruritus

MISC: Headache, fatigue, asthenia, fever, edema, back pain, weight increase, diplopia

RESP: URI, pharyngitis, sinusitis, coughing

Contraindications: Pregnancy (D), hypersensitivity to this drug or carbazine, lactation

Precautions: Radiation therapy, renal, hepatic disease

PHARMACOKINETICS

Absorption complete, rapid; crosses blood-brain barrier, excreted urine/feces, half-life 1.8 hr, peak 1 hr

INTERACTIONS

Increase: myelosuppression—radiation, other antineoplastics

Decrease: antibody reaction—live virus vaccines

NURSING CONSIDERATIONS

Assess:

• CBC on day 22 (21 days after 1st dose), CBC weekly until recovery if ANC is <1.5 × 10^9/L and platelets <100 × 10^9/L, do not administer to patients that do not tolerate 100 mg/m^2, myelosuppression usually occurs late in the treatment cycle

• For seizures throughout treatment

• Monitor temp q4h (may indicate beginning infection)

• Hepatic studies before, during therapy (bilirubin, AST, ALT, LDH), as needed or monthly

• Bleeding: hematuria, guaiac, bruising or petechiae, mucosa or orifices q8h

Administer:

• Do not break, crush, chew, or open caps

• Antiemetic 30-60 min before giving drug to prevent vomiting

• Caps one at a time with 8 oz of water at same time of day

• Fluids IV or PO before chemotherapy to hydrate patient

• If accidentally damaged, do not allow contact with skin, or inhale

• Give on empty stomach to prevent nausea/vomiting

Perform/provide:

• Storage in light-resistant container, dry area

Evaluate:

• Therapeutic response: decreased tumor size, spread of malignancy

Teach patient/family:

• To report signs of infection: fever, sore throat, flulike symptoms

T

- To report signs of anemia: fatigue, headache, faintness, shortness of breath, irritability
- To report bleeding; avoid use of razors, commercial mouthwash
- To avoid use of aspirin products or ibuprofen

⚠ High Alert

tenecteplase (℞)

(ten-ek′ta-place)
TNKase
Func. class.: Thrombolytic enzyme
Chem. class.: Tissue plasminogen activator

Action: Activates conversion of plasminogen to plasmin (fibrinolysin): plasmin breaks down clots (fibrin), fibrinogen, factors V, VII; occlusion of venous access lines

Uses: Acute myocardial infarction

DOSAGE AND ROUTES

- *Adult <60 kg:* **IV BOL** 30 mg, give over 5 sec
- *Adult ≥60-<70 kg:* **IV BOL** 35 mg, give over 5 sec
- *Adult ≥70-<80 kg:* **IV BOL** 40 mg, give over 5 sec
- *Adult ≥80-<90 kg:* **IV BOL** 45 mg, give over 5 sec
- *Adult ≥90 kg:* **IV BOL** 50 mg, give over 5 sec

Available forms: Powder for inj, lyophilized 50 mg

SIDE EFFECTS

CV: Dysrhythmias, hypotension, pulmonary edema, *pulmonary embolism, cardiogenic shock, cardiac arrest, heart failure, myocardial reinfarction, myocardial rupture, tamponade, pericarditis, pericardial effusion, thrombosis*
HEMA: Decreased Hct, *bleeding*
INTEG: Rash, urticaria, phlebitis at IV inf site, itching, flushing

SYST: **GI, GU, intracranial, retroperitoneal bleeding, surface bleeding, anaphylaxis**

Contraindications: Hypersensitivity, arteriovenous malformation, aneurysm, active bleeding, intracranial, intraspinal surgery, CNS neoplasms, severe hypertension, severe renal disease, hepatic disease, history of CVA

Precautions: Pregnancy (C), arterial emboli from left side of heart, lactation, children, hypocoagulation, COPD, subacute bacterial endocarditis, rheumatic valvular disease, cerebral embolism/thrombosis/hemorrhage, intraarterial diagnostic procedure or surgery (10 days), recent major surgery, ulcerative colitis, enteritis, elderly

PHARMACOKINETICS

IV: Onset immediate, half-life 20-24 min; metabolized by the liver

INTERACTIONS

Bleeding potential: aspirin, indomethacin, phenylbutazone, anticoagulants, antithrombolytics, glycoprotein IIb, IIIa inhibitors, dipyridamole
Drug/Herb
Increase: risk of bleeding—agrimony, alfalfa, angelica, anise, basil, bay, bilberry, black haw, bogbean, bromelain, buchu, chondroitin, cinchona bark, dong quai, fenugreek, feverfew, garlic, ginger, ginkgo, ginseng, horse chestnut, Irish moss, kelp, kelpware, khella, lovage, lungwort, meadowsweet, motherwort, mugwort, nettle, papaya, parsley (large amts), pau d'arco, pineapple, poplar, prickly ash, safflower, saw palmetto, tonka bean, turmeric, wintergreen, yarrow
Decrease: anticoagulant effect—chamomile, coenzyme Q10, flax, glucomannan, goldenseal, guar gum
Drug/Lab Test
Increase: PT, aPTT, TT
Decrease: Plasminogen, fibrinogen

⚠ Safety alert   *"Tall Man" lettering

NURSING CONSIDERATIONS

Assess:

• Allergy: fever, rash, itching, chills; mild reaction may be treated with antihistamines

A For bleeding during 1st hr of treatment; hematuria, hematemesis, bleeding from mucous membranes, epistaxis, ecchymosis; may require tranfusion (rare), continue to assess for bleeding for 24 hr

• Blood studies (Hct, platelets, PTT, PT, TT, aPTT) before starting therapy; PT or aPTT must be less than 2× control before starting therapy; PTT or PT q3-4h during treatment

• For hypersensitive reactions: fever, rash, dyspnea; drug should be discontinued

• VS, B/P, pulse, respirations, neurologic signs, temp at least q4h; temp >104° F (40° C) indicates internal bleeding; systolic pressure increase >25 mm Hg should be reported to prescriber

A For neurologic changes that may indicate intracranial bleeding

A Retroperitoneal bleeding: back pain, leg weakness, diminished pulses

Administer:

IV route

• As soon as thrombi identified; not useful for thrombi over 1 wk old

• Cryoprecipitate or fresh frozen plasma if bleeding occurs

• Heparin after fibrinogen level >100 mg/dl; heparin infusion to increase PTT to 1.5-2 × baseline for 3-7 days; IV heparin with loading dose is recommended

• Aseptically withdraw 10 ml of sterile H_2O for inj from diluent vial, use red cannula syringe-filling device, inject all contents of syringe into drug vial, direct into powder, swirl, withdraw correct dose, discard any unused solution; stand the shield with dose vertically on flat surface and passively recap the red cannula, remove entire shield assembly by twisting counter-clockwise, give by **IV BOL**

• IV therapy: use upper extremity vessel that is accessible to manual compression

Perform/provide:

• Bed rest during entire course of treatment

• Avoidance of venous or arterial puncture, inj, rectal temp; any invasive treatment

• Treatment of fever with acetaminophen or aspirin

• Pressure for 30 sec to minor bleeding sites; inform prescriber if this does not attain hemostasis; apply pressure dressing

Evaluate:

• Therapeutic response: resolution of myocardial infarction

Teach patient/family:

• Proper tooth brushing to avoid bleeding

• Notify prescriber immediately of sudden severe headache

• Notify prescriber of bleeding, hypersensitivity

Rarely Used

teniposide (℞)

(ten-i-poe′side)
Vumon, VM 26
Func. class.: Antineoplastic

Uses: Childhood acute lymphoblastic leukemia (ALL), refractory childhood acute lymphocytic leukemia

DOSAGE AND ROUTES

• *Child:* **IV INF** combo teniposide 165 mg/m² and cytarabine 300 mg/m² 2 ×/wk × 8-9 doses or combo teniposide 250 mg/m² and vinCRIStine 1.5 mg/m² qwk × 4-8 wk and predniSONE 40 mg/m² **PO** × 28 days

Contraindications: Pregnancy (D), hypersensitivity, bone marrow depression, severe hepatic disease, severe renal disease, bacterial infection

T

tenofovir (R)

(ten-oh-foh'veer)

Viread

Func. class.: Antiretroviral

Chem. class.: Nucleoside analog reverse transcriptase inhibitor

Action: Inhibits replication of HIV virus by competing with the natural substrate and then incorporating into cellular DNA by viral reverse transcriptase, thereby terminating cellular DNA chain

Uses: HIV-1 infection with other antiretrovirals

DOSAGE AND ROUTES

• *Adult:* **PO** 300 mg with meal; if used with didanosine, give tenofovir 2 hr before or 1 hr after didanosine

Renal dose

• CCr 30-49 ml/min 300 mg q48h

• CCr 10-29 ml/min 300 mg 2 ×/wk

• CCr <10 ml/min not recommended

Available forms: Tabs 300 mg (300 mg of fumarate salt equivalent to 245 mg tenofovir disoproxil)

SIDE EFFECTS

CNS: Headache

GI: Nausea, vomiting, diarrhea, anorexia, *flatulence, abdominal pain*

SYST: Change in body fat distribution

Contraindications: Hypersensitivity

Precautions: Pregnancy (B), lactation, children, elderly, renal disease, hepatic insufficiency, CCr <60 ml/min, osteoporosis

PHARMACOKINETICS

Rapidly absorbed, distributed to extravascular space, excreted unchanged in urine, 70%-80%; terminal half-life 17 hr

INTERACTIONS

Increase: tenofovir level—cidofovir, acyclovir, valacyclovir, ganciclovir, valganciclovir

Increase: level of didanosine when given with tenofovir

Increase: tenofovir level—any drug that decreases renal function

NURSING CONSIDERATIONS

Assess:

• Hepatic studies: AST, ALT, bilirubin; amylase, lipase, triglycerides periodically during treatment

• For bone, renal toxicity: if bone abnormalities are suspected, obtain tests; serum phosphorus, creatinine

⚠ For lactic acidosis, severe hepatomegaly with steatosis

Administer:

• PO daily with meal

• This drug 2 hr before or 1 hr after taking didanosine (if used)

Perform/provide:

• Storage at 25° C (77° F)

Evaluate:

• Therapeutic response: Decrease in signs/symptoms of HIV

Teach patient/family:

• To take with meal

• That GI complaints resolve after 3-4 wk of treatment

• Not to breastfeed while taking this drug

• That drug must be taken daily even if patient feels better

• That follow-up visits must be continued because serious toxicity may occur; blood counts must be done q2wk

• That drug will control symptoms but is not a cure for HIV; patient is still infectious, may pass HIV virus on to others

• That other drugs may be necessary to prevent other infections

• That changes in body fat distribution may occur

terazosin (R)

(ter-ay'zoe-sin)
Hytrin
Func. class.: Antihypertensive
Chem. class.: α-Adrenergic blocker

Action: Decreases total vascular resistance, which is responsible for a decrease in B/P; this occurs by blockade of α_1-adrenoreceptors

Uses: Hypertension, as a single agent or in combination with diuretics or β-blockers, BPH

DOSAGE AND ROUTES

Hypertension

• *Adult:* **PO** 1 mg at bedtime, may increase dose slowly to desired response; not to exceed 20 mg/day

Benign prostatic hyperplasia

• *Adult:* **PO** 1 mg at bedtime, gradually increase up to 5-10 mg

Available forms: Tabs 1, 2, 5, 10 mg

SIDE EFFECTS

CNS: Dizziness, headache, drowsiness, anxiety, depression, vertigo, weakness, fatigue

CV: Palpitations, orthostatic hypotension, tachycardia, edema, rebound hypertension

EENT: Blurred vision, epistaxis, tinnitus, dry mouth, red sclera, nasal congestion, sinusitis

GI: Nausea, vomiting, diarrhea, constipation, abdominal pain

GU: Urinary frequency, incontinence, impotence, priapism

RESP: Dyspnea, cough, pharyngitis

Contraindications: Hypersensitivity

Precautions: Pregnancy (C), children, lactation

PHARMACOKINETICS

Peak 1 hr, half-life 9-12 hr, highly bound to plasma proteins; metabolized in liver, excreted in urine, feces

INTERACTIONS

Increase: hypotensive effects—β-blockers, nitroglycerin, verapamil, other antihypertensives, alcohol

Decrease: hypotensive effects—estrogens, NSAIDs, sympathomimetics

NURSING CONSIDERATIONS

Assess:

• Urinary symptoms associated with BPH
• Orthostatic B/P, pulse, jugular venous distention q4h
• BUN, uric acid if on long-term therapy
• Weight daily, I&O
• Skin turgor, dryness of mucous membranes for hydration status
• Crackles, dyspnea, orthopnea q30min

Administer

• Dose at bedtime or do not operate machinery; fainting may occur

Perform/provide:

• Cool storage in tight container

Evaluate:

• Therapeutic response: decreased B/P, edema in feet, legs, decreased symptoms of BPH

Teach patient/family:

• That fainting occasionally occurs after first dose; not to drive or operate machinery for 4 hr after first dose or after an increase in dose; or take first dose at bedtime
• To rise slowly from sitting/lying position

terbinafine (R)

(ter-bin'a-feen)
Lamisil
Func. class.: Antifungal
Chem. class.: Synthetic allylamine derivative

Action: Interferes with cell membrane permeability in fungi such as *Trichophyton rubrum, Trichophyton mentagrophytes, Trichophyton tonsurans, Epidermophyton floccosum, Microsporum canis, Microsporum audouinii, Microsporum gypseum, Candida,* broad-spectrum antifungal

Side effects: *italics* = common; ***bold italics*** = life-threatening

Uses: (TOP) Tinea cruris, tinea corporis, tinea pedis; (oral) onychomycosis of the toenail or fingernail due to dermatophytes

Investigational uses: Cutaneous candidiasis, tinea versicolor

DOSAGE AND ROUTES

Topical

• Massage into affected area, surrounding area daily or bid, continue for 7-14 days, not to exceed 4 wk

Oral

• *Fingernail:* 250 mg/day × 6 wk
• *Toenail:* 250 mg/day × 12 wk

Available forms: Cream 1%, tabs 250 mg

SIDE EFFECTS

Topical

INTEG: Burning, stinging, dryness, itching, local irritation

Oral

GI: Diarrhea, dyspepsia, abdominal pain, nausea, hepatitis

HEMA: **Neutropenia**

INTEG: Rash, pruritus, urticaria, ***Stevens-Johnson syndrome***

MISC: Headache, hepatic enzyme changes, taste, visual disturbance

Contraindications: Hypersensitivity, chronic/active hepatic disease, renal disease GFR ≤50 ml/min

Precautions: Pregnancy (B), lactation, children, renal disease

INTERACTIONS

Increase: levels of dextromethorphan
Increase: terbinafine clearance—rifampin
Increase: clearance of cycloSPORINE
Decrease: terbinafine clearance—cimetidine

Drug/Herb

Side effects: cola nut, guarana, yerba maté, tea (black, green) coffee

NURSING CONSIDERATIONS

Assess:

• Hepatic studies (ALT, AST) prior to beginning treatment; do not use in presence of liver disease
• CBC in treatment >6 wk
• For continuing infection: increased size, number of lesions

Administer:

• To affected area, surrounding area; do not cover with occlusive dressings

Perform/provide:

• Storage below 25° C (77° F)

Evaluate:

• Therapeutic response: decrease in size, number of lesions

Teach patient/family:

Topical

• To wear cotton clothing
• To use clean towel, dry well
• To avoid contact with mucous membranes
• Not to cover areas unless directed by prescriber
• To report excessive itching, burning
• How to apply; massage cream into affected area and surrounding skin in AM, PM; effects observed within 1 wk, continue 1-2 wk after symptoms decrease

Oral

• To notify prescriber of nausea, vomiting, fatigue, jaundice, dark urine, clay-colored stool, RUQ pain, that may indicate hepatic dysfunction

---

terbinafine topical
See Appendix C

---

terbutaline (R)
(ter-byoo'te-leen)
Brethine, Bricanyl
Func. class.: Selective β₂-agonist; bronchodilator
Chem. class.: Catecholamine

Action: Relaxes bronchial smooth muscle by direct action on β₂-adrenergic receptors through accumulation of cAMP at β-adrenergic receptor sites; bronchodilation, diuresis, CNS, cardiac stimulation occur; relaxes uterine smooth muscle

Uses: Bronchospasm, hyperkalemia
Investigational uses: Premature labor

DOSAGE AND ROUTES

Bronchodilation
• *Adult and child >15 yr:* 2.5-5 mg q6h during the day, max 15 mg/24 hr
• *Child 12-15 yr:* **PO** 2.5 mg tid q6h
Bronchospasm
• *Adult and child >12 yr:* **INH** 2 puffs q1min, then q4-6h; **PO** 2.5-5 mg q8h; **SUBCUT** 0.25 mg q15-30min, max 0.5 mg in 4 hr
Tocolytic (preterm labor) (off-label)
• *Adult:* **PO** 2.5 mg q4-6h until delivery
Renal dose
• *Adult:* **PO** GFR 10-50 ml/min 50% of dose
Severe renal failure
• Avoid GFR if <10 ml/min
Available forms: Tabs 2.5, 5 mg; aerosol 0.2 mg/actuation; inj 1 mg/ml

SIDE EFFECTS

CNS: Tremors, anxiety, insomnia, headache, dizziness, stimulation
CV: Palpitations, tachycardia, hypertension, dysrhythmias, ***cardiac arrest***
GI: Nausea, vomiting
Contraindications: Hypersensitivity to sympathomimetics, narrow-angle glaucoma, tachydysrhythmias
Precautions: Pregnancy (B), cardiac disorders, hyperthyroidism, diabetes mellitus, prostatic hypertension, lactation, elderly, hypertension, seizure disorder

PHARMACOKINETICS

PO: Onset ½ hr, peak 1-2 hr, duration 4-8 hr
SUBCUT: Onset 6-15 min, peak ½-1 hr, duration 1½-4 hr
INH: Onset 5-30 min, peak 1-2 hr, duration 3-6 hr

INTERACTIONS

Incompatible with bleomycin
Hypertensive crisis: MAOIs
Increase: effects of both drugs—other sympathomimetics
Decrease: action—β-blockers
Drug/Herb
Increase: effect—green tea (large amounts), guarana

NURSING CONSIDERATIONS

Assess:
• Respiratory function: vital capacity, forced expiratory volume, ABGs, B/P, pulse, respiratory pattern, lung sounds, sputum before and after treatment
• Tolerance over long-term therapy; dose may have to be changed; monitor for rebound bronchospasm
⚠ Paradoxical bronchospasm: dyspnea, wheezing, keep emergency equipment nearby
• Labor: maternal heart rate, B/P, contraction, fetal heart rate
Administer:
• With food; may be crushed
• 2 hr before bedtime to avoid sleeplessness
IV route
• IV after diluting each 5 mg/1 L D₅W for inf
• IV, run 5 mcg/min; may increase 5 mcg q10min, titrate to response; after ½-1 hr taper dose by 5 mcg; switch to PO as soon as possible
Additive compatibilities: Aminophylline
Syringe compatibilities: Doxapram
Y-site compatibilities: Insulin (regular)
Perform/provide:
• Storage at room temperature; do not use discolored sol
• An increase in fluids of >2 L/day
Evaluate:
• Therapeutic response: absence of dyspnea, wheezing
Teach patient/family:
• Not to use OTC medications; extra stimulation may occur

T

• The use of inhaler; review package insert with patient

• To avoid getting aerosol in eyes; burning, stinging will occur

• To wash inhaler in warm water and dry daily, rinse mouth after use

• All aspects of drug; avoid smoking, smoke-filled rooms, persons with respiratory infections

• To increase fluids >2 L/day; allow 15 min between inhalation of this drug and inhaler containing steroid

• To take on time; if missed, do not make up after 1 hr; wait until next dose

Treatment of overdose: Administer an α-blocker, then norepinephrine for severe hypotension

---

terconazole vaginal antifungal
See Appendix C

---

teriparatide (℞)
(tah-ree-par′ah-tide)
Forteo
Func. class.: Parathyroid hormone (rDNA)

Action: Contains human recombinant parathyroid hormone, to stimulate new bone growth

Uses: Postmenopausal women with osteoporosis, men with primary or hypogonadal osteoporosis who are at high risk for fracture

DOSAGE AND ROUTES

• *Adult:* **SUBCUT** 20 mcg daily
Available forms: Prefilled pen delivery device (delivers 20 mcg/day)

SIDE EFFECTS

CNS: Dizziness, headache, insomnia, depression, vertigo
CV: Hypertension, angina, syncope
GI: Nausea, diarrhea, dyspepsia, vomiting, constipation

INTEG: Rash, sweating
MISC: Pain, asthenia
MS: Arthralgia, leg cramps
RESP: Rhinitis, cough, pharyngitis, pneumonia, dyspnea

Contraindications: Hypersensitivity, increased baseline risk of osteosarcoma (Paget's disease, open epiphyses; previous bone radiation), bone metastases, history of skeletal malignancies, other metabolic bone diseases, preexisting hypercalcemia

Precautions: Pregnancy (C), lactation, urolithiasis, hypotension, use >2 yr

PHARMACOKINETICS

SUBCUT: Extensively and rapidly absorbed, metabolized by liver, excreted by kidneys

INTERACTIONS

Increase: digoxin toxicity: digoxin
Drug/Lab Test
Increase: Calcium

NURSING CONSIDERATIONS
Assess:

• Uric acid, chloride, magnesium, electrolytes, urine pH, vit D, phosphate for normal serum levels. Serum calcium may be transiently increased after dosing (max at 4-6 hr post-dose)

• For bone pain, headache, fatigue, changes in LOC, leg cramps

• For signs of persistent hypercalcemia: nausea, vomiting, constipation, lethargy, muscle weakness

• Nutritional status: diet for sources of vit D (milk, some seafood); calcium (dairy products, dark green vegetables), phosphates (dairy products)
Administer:
SUBCUT route

• Give by SUBCUT only, rotate inj sites
Perform/provide:

• Store refrigerated, do not freeze
Evaluate:

• Therapeutic response: increased bone mineral density

⚠ Safety alert   *"Tall Man" lettering

Teach patient/family:

- The symptoms of hypercalcemia
- About foods rich in calcium
- How to use delivery device, dispose of needles, not to share pen with others
- To sit or lie down if dizziness or fast heartbeat occurs after the first few doses
- To rotate administration sites

---

testolactone (℞)

(tess-toe-lak'tone)

Teslac

Func. class.: Antineoplastic
Chem. class.: Androgen hormone

Controlled Substance Schedule III

Action: Acts on adrenal cortex to suppress activity; reduces estrone synthesis

Uses: Advanced breast carcinoma in postmenopausal women; prostatic cancer

DOSAGE AND ROUTES

- *Adult:* **PO** 250 mg qid

Available forms: Tabs 50 mg

SIDE EFFECTS

CNS: Paresthesias, dizziness

CV: Orthostatic hypertension, edema

EENT: Deepening voice

GI: Nausea, vomiting, anorexia, glossitis

GU: Urinary retention, ***renal failure***

INTEG: Rash, nail changes, facial hair growth

META: Hypercalcemia

Contraindications: Hypersensitivity, premenopausal women, carcinoma of male breast, lactation

Precautions: Pregnancy (C), renal disease, hypercalcemia, cardiac disease

PHARMACOKINETICS

None known

INTERACTIONS

Enhanced effects of oral anticoagulants

Drug/Lab Test
Increase: Urinary 17-OHCS
Decrease: Estradiol

NURSING CONSIDERATIONS

Assess:

- Calcium levels
- B/P q4h; tell patient to rise slowly from sitting or lying down
- Food preferences; list likes, dislikes
- Edema in feet; joint, stomach pain; shaking

A Symptoms indicating severe allergic reaction: rash, pruritus, urticaria, purpuric skin lesions, itching, flushing

- Anorexia, nausea, vomiting, constipation, weakness, loss of muscle tone (indicating hypercalcemia)

Administer:

- For 3 mo or longer for desired response

Evaluate:

- Therapeutic response: decreased tumor size, spread of malignancy

Teach patient/family:

- To recognize and report signs of hepatotoxicity, hypercalcemia, virilization (in females), bleeding if on anticoagulants

T

testosterone cypionate (℞)

Andro-Cyp, Andronate, depAndro, Depotest, Depo-Testosterone, Dura-test, T-Cypionate, Testa-C, Testred, Testoject-LA, Virilon IM

testosterone enanthate (℞)

Andro LA, Andropository, Andryl, Delatest, Delatestryl, Everone, Malog-x ✦, Testone LA, Testrin-PA

testosterone gel (℞)

AndroGel 1%, Testim

testosterone, long-acting (℞)

testosterone pellets (℞)

Testopel

testosterone transdermal (℞)

Androderm, Testoderm, Testoderm TTS, Testoderm with Adhesive

testosterone buccal (℞)

Striant

Func. class.: Androgenic anabolic steroid

Chem. class.: Halogenated testosterone derivative

Controlled Substance Schedule III

Action: Increases weight by building body tissue, increases potassium, phosphorus, chloride, nitrogen levels, bone development

Uses: Female breast cancer, eunuchoidism, male climacteric, oligospermia, impotence, osteoporosis, weight loss in AIDS patients, vulvar dystrophies, low testosterone levels, delayed male puberty (inj)

DOSAGE AND ROUTES

Replacement
• *Adult:* **IM** 25-50 mg 2-3 ×/wk (base or propionate) or 50-400 mg q2-4wk (enanthate or cypionate)
• *Adult:* **Trans Testoderm** 4-6 mg applied q24h; **Androderm, AndroGel** 5 mg applied q24h; once daily (gel); **Buccal** 1 buccal system (30 mg) to the gum region q12h ac/PM

Breast cancer
• *Adult:* **IM** 50-100 mg 3 ×/wk (propionate) or 200-400 mg q2-4wk (cypionate or enanthate)

Delayed male puberty
• *Child >12 yr:* **IM** up to 100 mg/mo for up to 6 mo

Available forms: Enanthate: inj 200 mg/ml; *cypionate:* inj 100, 200 mg/ml; pellets 75 mg; transdermal 2.5, 4, 5, 6 mg/24 hr; gel 1%; buccal system 30 mg

SIDE EFFECTS

CNS: Dizziness, headache, fatigue, tremors, paresthesias, flushing, sweating, anxiety, lability, insomnia, carpal tunnel syndrome
CV: Increased B/P
EENT: Conjunctival edema, nasal congestion
ENDO: Abnormal GTT
GI: Nausea, vomiting, constipation, weight gain, *cholestatic jaundice*
GU: Hematuria, amenorrhea, vaginitis, decreased libido, decreased breast size, clitoral hypertrophy, testicular atrophy
INTEG: Rash, acneiform lesions, oily hair and skin, flushing, sweating, acne vulgaris, alopecia, hirsutism
MS: Cramps, spasms

Contraindications: Pregnancy (X), severe renal, severe cardiac, severe hepatic disease, hypersensitivity, lactation, genital bleeding (rare)

Precautions: Diabetes mellitus, CV disease, MI

PHARMACOKINETICS

PO: Metabolized in liver, excreted in urine, breast milk; crosses placenta

INTERACTIONS

Edema: ACTH, adrenal steroids
Increase: effects of oxyphenbutazone
Increase: PT—anticoagulants
Decrease: glucose levels may alter need for oral antidiabetics, insulin
Drug/Lab Test
Increase: Serum cholesterol, blood glucose, urine glucose
Decrease: Serum calcium, serum potassium, T_4, T_3, thyroid ^{131}I uptake test, urine 17-OHCS, 17-KS, PBI

NURSING CONSIDERATIONS

Assess:
• Weight daily; notify prescriber if weekly weight gain is >5 lb
• B/P q4h
• I&O ratio; be alert for decreasing urinary output, increasing edema
• Growth rate in children; growth rate may be uneven (linear/bone growth) with extended use
• Electrolytes: K, Na, Cl, Ca; cholesterol
• Hepatic studies: ALT, AST, bilirubin
• Edema, hypertension, cardiac symptoms, jaundice
• Mental status: affect, mood, behavioral changes, aggression
• Signs of masculinization in female: increased libido, deepening of voice, decreased breast tissue, enlarged clitoris, menstrual irregularities; male: gynecomastia, impotence, testicular atrophy
• Hypercalcemia: lethargy, polyuria, polydipsia, nausea, vomiting, constipation; drug may have to be decreased
• Hypoglycemia in diabetics; oral antidiabetic action is increased
Administer:
• Titrated dose; use lowest effective dose
• IM inj deep into upper outer quadrant of gluteal muscle
• Transdermal patches: Testoderm to skin of scrotum; Androderm to skin of

back, upper arms, thighs, abdomen; area must be dry-shaved; may be reapplied after bathing, swimming
• Gel: apply daily to clean, dry area on shoulders, upper arms or abdomen
Buccal system route
• Do not chew or swallow buccal system
• Rotate sites, place above incisor tooth on either side of mouth
• Open packet, place rounded side of surface against the gum and hold firmly in place with finger over lip for 30 sec; if it falls off, replace with new system, discard in trash can away from children or pets
Perform/provide:
• Diet with increased calories, protein; decrease sodium if edema occurs
Evaluate:
• Therapeutic response: 4-6 wk in osteoporosis
Teach patient/family:
• That drug must be combined with complete health plan: diet, rest, exercise
• To notify prescriber if therapeutic response decreases; if edema occurs
• About changes in sex characteristics
• That women should report menstrual irregularities, voice changes, acne, facial hair growth, if pregnancy is planned or suspected
• That 1-3-mo course is necessary for response in breast cancer
• The proper application of patches

---

tetracaine (℞)
(tet′ra-kane)
Pontocaine
Func. class.: Local anesthetic
Chem. class.: Ester

Action: Competes with calcium for binding sites in nerve membrane that control sodium transport across cell membrane; decreases rise of depolarization phase of action potential
Uses: Spinal anesthesia, epidural and peripheral nerve block, perineum, lower extremities

---

Side effects: *italics* = common; ***bold italics*** = life-threatening

DOSAGE AND ROUTES

Varies with route of anesthesia

Available forms: Inj 0.2%, 0.3%, 1%; powder

SIDE EFFECTS

CNS: Anxiety, restlessness, ***convulsions, LOC,*** drowsiness, disorientation, tremors, shivering

CV: ***Myocardial depression, cardiac arrest, dysrhythmias,*** bradycardia, hypo/hypertension, fetal bradycardia

EENT: Blurred vision, tinnitus, pupil constriction

GI: Nausea, vomiting

INTEG: Rash, urticaria, allergic reactions, edema, burning, skin discoloration at inj site, tissue necrosis

RESP: ***Status asthmaticus, respiratory arrest, anaphylaxis***

Contraindications: Hypersensitivity, sulfite allergy, severe liver disease, heart block

Precautions: Pregnancy (C), elderly, severe drug allergies, lactation, children <12 yr

PHARMACOKINETICS

Onset MS 3 min; spinal 3-8 min; duration 1.5-3 hr; metabolized by liver, excreted in urine (metabolites)

INTERACTIONS

Dysrhythmias: epINEPHrine, halothane, enflurane

Hypertension: MAOIs, tricyclics, phenothiazines

Decrease: action of tetracaine—chloroprocaine

Decrease: action of sulfonamides

NURSING CONSIDERATIONS

Assess:
• B/P, pulse, respiration during treatment
• Fetal heart tones during labor
• Allergic reactions: rash, urticaria, itching
• Cardiac status: ECG for dysrhythmias, pulse, B/P, during anesthesia

Administer:
• Only if not cloudy, does not contain precipitate
• Only with crash cart, resuscitative equipment nearby
• Only without preservatives for epidural or caudal anesthesia

Perform/provide:
• Use of new sol, discard unused portions, store in refrigerator, avoid freezing

Evaluate:
• Therapeutic response: anesthesia necessary for procedure

Treatment of overdose: Maintain adequate airway, O_2, vasopressor, IV fluids, anticonvulsants for seizures

---

tetracaine ophthalmic
See Appendix C

---

tetracaine topical
See Appendix C

---

tetracycline (℞)

(tet-ra-sye′kleen)
Achromycin V, Actisite (dental product), Apo-Tetra ✦, Novotetra ✦, Nu-Tetra ✦, Panmycin, Robitet, Sumycin, Teline, Tetracap, tetracycline HCl, Tetracyn, Tetralan, Tetram

Func. class.: Broad-spectrum antiinfective

Chem. class.: Tetracycline

Action: Inhibits protein synthesis and phosphorylation in microorganisms; bacteriostatic

Uses: Syphilis, *Chlamydia trachomatis,* gonorrhea, lymphogranuloma venereum; uncommon gram-positive, gram-negative organisms; rickettsial infections

---

A Safety alert   *"Tall Man" lettering

DOSAGE AND ROUTES

Susceptible gram-positive/gram-negative infections
- *Adult:* **PO** 250-500 mg q6h
- *Child >8 yr:* **PO** 25-50 mg/kg/day in divided doses q6h

Gonorrhea
- *Adult:* **PO** 1.5 g, then 500 mg q6h for a total of 9 g over 7 days

Chlamydia trachomatis
- *Adult:* **PO** 500 mg qid × 7 days

Syphilis
- *Adult and adolescent:* **PO** 500 mg qid × 2 wk; if syphilis duration >1 yr, must treat 30 days

Brucellosis
- *Adult:* **PO** 500 mg q6h × 3 wk with 1 g streptomycin **IM** q12h × 1 wk, and 1 ×/day the 2nd wk

Urethral, endocervical, rectal infections (C. trachomatis)
- *Adult:* **PO** 500 mg qid × 7 days

Acne
- *Adult and adolescent:* **PO** 250 mg q6h, then 125-500 mg daily or every other day

Available forms: Oral susp 125 mg/5 ml; caps 250, 500 mg

SIDE EFFECTS

CNS: Fever, headache, paresthesia
CV: Pericarditis
EENT: Dysphagia, glossitis, decreased calcification, discoloration of deciduous teeth, oral candidiasis, oral ulcers
GI: Nausea, abdominal pain, *vomiting, diarrhea,* anorexia, enterocolitis, **hepatotoxicity,** flatulence, abdominal cramps, epigastric burning, stomatitis
GU: Increased BUN
HEMA: **Eosinophilia, neutropenia, thrombocytopenia, leukocytosis, hemolytic anemia**
INTEG: Rash, urticaria, *photosensitivity, increased pigmentation,* **exfoliative dermatitis,** pruritus, **angioedema**

Contraindications: Pregnancy (D), hypersensitivity to tetracyclines, children <8 yr, lactation

Precautions: Renal disease, hepatic disease

PHARMACOKINETICS

PO: Peak 2-3 hr, duration 6 hr, half-life 6-10 hr; excreted in urine, breast milk; crosses placenta; 20%-60% protein bound

INTERACTIONS

Nephrotoxicity: methoxyflurane
Increase: effect of warfarin, digoxin
Decrease: effect of tetracycline—antacids, NaHCO₃, dairy products, alkali products, iron, cimetidine
Decrease: effect of penicillins, oral contraceptives
Drug/Herb
Photosensitivity: dong quai
Drug/Lab Test
False increase: Urinary catecholamines

NURSING CONSIDERATIONS

Assess:
- Signs of anemia: Hct, Hgb, fatigue
- I&O ratio
- Blood studies: PT, CBC, AST, ALT, BUN, creatinine
- Allergic reactions: rash, itching, pruritus, angioedema
- Nausea, vomiting, diarrhea; administer antiemetic, antacids as ordered
- Overgrowth of infection: fever, malaise, redness, pain, swelling, drainage, perineal itching, diarrhea, changes in cough or sputum

Administer:
- After C&S obtained
- 2 hr before or after iron products; 3 hr after antacid products
- Should be given on an empty stomach

Perform/provide:
- Storage in tight, light-resistant container at room temperature

Evaluate:
- Therapeutic response: decreased temp, absence of lesions, negative C&S

Teach patient/family:
- To avoid sun exposure; sunscreen does not seem to decrease photosensitivity

---

♣ Canada only

Side effects: *italics* = common; **bold italics** = life-threatening

• That all prescribed medication must be taken to prevent superinfection

• To avoid milk products, antacids, or separate by 2 hr; take with a full glass of water

tetrahydrozoline nasal agent
See Appendix C

tetrahydrozoline ophthalmic
See Appendix C

theophylline (℞)
(thee-off'i-lin)
Accurbron, Aquaphyllin, Asmalix, Bronkodyl, Elixomin, Elixophyllin, Lanophyllin, Quibron-T Dividose, Quibron-T/SR Dividose, Respbid, Slo-bid Gyrocaps, Slo-Phyllin, Sustaire, Theo-24, Theobid Duracaps, Theochron, Theoclear-80, Theoclear L.A., Theo-Dur, Theolair-SR, Theo-Sav, Theospan-SR, Theostat 80, Theovent, Theo-X, T-Phyl, Uni-Dur, Uniphyl
Func. class.: Spasmolytic
Chem. class.: Xanthine, ethylenediamide

Action: Relaxes smooth muscle of respiratory system by blocking phosphodiesterase, which increases cAMP
Uses: Bronchial asthma, bronchospasm of COPD, chronic bronchitis

DOSAGE AND ROUTES
Hepatic dose
• *Adult:* **PO** 6 mg/kg loading dose, then 2 mg/kg q8h × 2 doses, then 1-2 mg/kg q12h; **IV** 4.7 mg/kg, then 0.39 mg/kg/hr

for 12 hr, then 0.08-0.16 mg/kg/hr maintenance
Bronchospasm, bronchial asthma
• *Adult:* **PO** 100-200 mg q6h; dosage must be individualized; **RECT** 250-500 mg q8-12h
• *Child:* **PO** 50-100 mg q6h, not to exceed 12 mg/kg/24 hr
COPD, chronic bronchitis
• *Adult:* **PO** 330-660 mg q6-8h pc
• *Child 1-9 yr:* **PO** 5 mg/kg loading dose, then 4 mg/kg q6h
• *Child 9-16 yr:* **PO** 5 mg/kg loading dose, then 3 mg/kg q6h
Apnea of prematurity
• *Neonate:* 2-10 mg/kg/day divided q8-12h (usual loading dose is 4 mg/kg **PO**)
Available forms: Caps 50, 100, 200, 250 mg; tabs 100, 125, 200, 225, 250, 300 mg; tabs, time rel 100, 200, 250, 300, 400, 500 mg; caps, time rel 50, 65, 100, 125, 130, 200, 250, 260, 300, 400, 500 mg; elix 80, 11.25 mg/15 ml; sol 80 mg/15 ml; liquid 80, 150, 160 mg/15 ml; susp 300 mg/15 ml

SIDE EFFECTS
*CNS: Anxiety, restlessness, insomnia, dizziness, **seizures,** headache, light-headedness, muscle twitching, tremors*
*CV: Palpitations, sinus tachycardia, hypotension, **dysrhythmias,** fluid retention with tachycardia*
ENDO: Hyperglycemia
GI: Nausea, vomiting, anorexia, diarrhea, bitter taste, dyspepsia, gastric distress
INTEG: Flushing, urticaria
RESP: Increased rate
Contraindications: Hypersensitivity to xanthines, tachydysrhythmias
Precautions: Pregnancy (C), elderly, CHF, cor pulmonale, hepatic disease, active peptic ulcer disease, diabetes mellitus, hyperthyroidism, hypertension, children

---

A Safety alert   *"Tall Man" lettering

PHARMACOKINETICS

PO: Peak 2 hr
SOL: Peak 1 hr
Metabolized in liver, excreted in urine and breast milk, crosses placenta

INTERACTIONS

Cardiotoxicity: β-blockers
Increase: theophylline action—cimetidine, propranolol, erythromycin, ciprofloxacin, oral contraceptives, influenza vaccine, fluoroquinones, mexiletine, corticosteroids, disulfiram, fluvoxamine, interferons
Increase: effects of anticoagulants
Decrease: theophylline level—phenytoin, phenobarbital, carbamazepine, rifampin, smoking
Decrease: effect of lithium

Drug/Herb

Toxicity: ephedra (ma huang), cola nut, guarana, yerba maté, tea (black, green), coffee
Decrease: theophylline levels—St. John's wort

NURSING CONSIDERATIONS

Assess:

A Theophylline blood levels (therapeutic level is 5-15 mcg/ml); toxicity may occur with small increase above 20 mcg/ml
• Monitor I&O; diuresis occurs; elderly or child may be dehydrated
• Signs of toxicity: irritability, insomnia, restlessness, tremors, nausea, vomiting
• Respiratory rate, rhythm, depth; auscultate lung fields bilaterally; notify prescriber of abnormalities
• Allergic reactions: rash, urticaria; drug should be discontinued

Administer:

• Do not break, crush, chew or dissolve time-release products
• PO with 8 oz of water for GI symptoms; avoid food; absorption may be affected; take dose consistently; do not take Theo-24 with meals
• Contents of bead-filled capsule sprinkled over food for children's use

IV route

• Loading dose over 20-30 min, max 20-25 mg/min; do not give by rapid IV, use only cont inf
Additive compatibilities: Cefepime, chlorproMAZINE, fluconazole, furosemide, hydrocortisone, lidocaine, methylprednisolone, verapamil
Y-site compatibilities: Acyclovir, ampicillin, ampicillin/sulbactam, aztreonam, cefazolin, cefotetan, ceftazidime, ceftriaxone, cimetidine, cisatracurium, clindamycin, dexamethasone, diltiazem, DOBUTamine, DOPamine, doxycycline, erythromycin, famotidine, fluconazole, gentamicin, haloperidol, heparin, hydrocortisone, lidocaine, methyldopate, methylPREDNISolone, metronidazole, midazolam, nafcillin, nitroglycerin, penicillin G potassium, piperacillin, potassium chloride, ranitidine, remifentanil, sodium nitroprusside, ticarcillin, ticarcillin/clavulanate, tobramycin, vancomycin

Evaluate:

• Therapeutic response: ability to breathe more easily

Teach patient/family:

• To check OTC medications, current prescription medications for epHEDrine, which will increase stimulation; to avoid alcohol, caffeine
• To avoid hazardous activities; dizziness may occur
• That if GI upset occurs, to take drug with 8 oz H_2O; avoid food; absorption may be decreased
• To notify prescriber of toxicity: nausea, vomiting, anxiety, insomnia, convulsions
• To notify prescriber of change in smoking habit; dosage may have to be changed

T

thiamine (vit B₁)
(PO-OTC, IV, IM-℞)
Betalin S, Betaxin ✦, Biamine,
Revitonus, Thiamilate,
thiamine HCl
Func. class.: Vit B₁
Chem. class.: Water soluble

Do not confuse:
thiamine/Tenormin
Action: Needed for pyruvate metabolism, carbohydrate metabolism
Uses: Vit B₁ deficiency or polyneuritis, cheilosis adjunct with thiamine beriberi, Wernicke-Korsakoff syndrome, pellagra, metabolic disorders

DOSAGE AND ROUTES
RDA
- *Adult:* Males 1.2-1.5 mg; females 1.1 mg; pregnancy 1.5 mg; lactation 1.6 mg
- *Child 7-10 yr:* 1.3 mg
- *Child 4-6 yr:* 0.9 mg
- *Child 1-3 yr:* 0.7 mg
- *Infants 6 mo-1 yr:* 0.4 mg
- *Neonates and infants to 6 mo:* 0.3 mg
Beriberi
- *Adult:* **IM** 10-20 mg tid × 2 wk, then 5-10 mg daily × 1 mo
Beriberi with cardiac failure
- *Adult and child:* **IV** 10-30 mg tid
Available forms: Tabs 50, 100, 250, 500 mg; inj 100 mg/ml; enteric coated tabs 20 mg

SIDE EFFECTS
CNS: Weakness, restlessness
CV: **Collapse, pulmonary edema,** hypotension
EENT: Tightness of throat
GI: Hemorrhage, *nausea, diarrhea*
INTEG: **Angioneurotic edema,** cyanosis, sweating, warmth
SYST: **Anaphylaxis**
Contraindications: Hypersensitivity
Precautions: Pregnancy (A)

PHARMACOKINETICS
PO/INJ: Unused amounts excreted in urine (unchanged)

NURSING CONSIDERATIONS
Assess:
- Nutritional status: yeast, beef, liver, whole or enriched grains, legumes
Administer:
IM route
- By IM inj; rotate sites if pain and inflammation occur; do not mix with alkaline sols; Z-track to minimize pain
IV route
- Undiluted over 5 min or diluted with IV sol and given as an inf at 100 mg or less/5 min or more
Syringe compatibilities: Doxapram
Y-site compatibilities: Famotidine
Perform/provide:
- Storage in tight, light-resistant container
- Application of cold to help decrease pain
Evaluate:
- Therapeutic response: absence of nausea, vomiting, anorexia, insomnia, tachycardia, paresthesias, depression, muscle weakness
Teach patient/family:
- The necessary foods to be included in diet: yeast, beef, liver, legumes, whole grain

thiethylperazine (℞)
(thye-eth-il-per′a-zeen)
Norzine, Torecan
Func. class.: Antiemetic
Chem. class.: Phenothiazine, piperazine derivative

Do not confuse:
Torecan/Toradol
Action: Acts centrally by blocking chemoreceptor trigger zone, which in turn acts on vomiting center; dopamine blocker
Uses: Nausea, vomiting

⚠ Safety alert   ✦ "Tall Man" lettering

DOSAGE AND ROUTES

• *Adult:* **PO/IM** 10 mg/daily-tid
Available forms: Tabs 10 mg; inj 5 mg/ml

SIDE EFFECTS

CNS: Euphoria, depression, restlessness, tremor, EPS, **seizures,** drowsiness, confusion, **neuroleptic malignant syndrome**
CV: **Circulatory failure, tachycardia,** postural hypotension, ECG changes
GI: Nausea, vomiting, anorexia, dry mouth, diarrhea, constipation, weight loss, metallic taste, cramps
GU: Urinary retention, dark urine
HEMA: **Agranulocytosis, leukopenia**
RESP: **Respiratory depression**
Contraindications: Pregnancy (X), hypersensitivity to phenothiazines, coma, seizure, encephalopathy, bone marrow depression
Precautions: Children <2 yr, elderly, lactation, Parkinson's disease

PHARMACOKINETICS

PO: Onset 45-60 min
RECT: Onset 45-60 min, metabolized by liver, crosses placenta, excreted in urine, breast milk

INTERACTIONS

Avoid use with phenothiazines, seizures may occur
Increase: anticholinergic action— anticholinergics, antiparkinson drugs, tricyclic antidepressants
Increase: sedation—barbiturates, general anesthetics, ethanol, anxiolytics, sedatives, hypnotics, benzodiazepines, opiate agonists
Decrease: effect of thiethylperazine— barbiturates, antacids

NURSING CONSIDERATIONS

Assess:
• VS, B/P; check patients with cardiac disease more often
⚠ For neuroleptic malignant syndrome: dyspnea, fever, seizures, diaphoresis, fatigue, loss of urinary control, tachycardia; have emergency equipment nearby
• Respiratory status before, during, after administration of emetic; check rate, rhythm, character; respiratory depression can occur rapidly with elderly or debilitated patients
Administer:
• IM inj in large muscle mass; aspirate to avoid IV administration; patient should remain recumbent 1 hr after inj
Syringe compatibilities: Butorphanol, hydromorphone, midazolam, ranitidine
Y-site compatibilities: Aldesleukin
Evaluate:
• Therapeutic response: absence of nausea, vomiting
Teach patient/family:
• To avoid hazardous activities, activities requiring alertness; dizziness may occur

Rarely Used

thioguanine (6-TG) (℞)

(thye-oh-gwah'neen)
thioguanine, Lanvis ✦
Func. class.: Antineoplastic-antimetabolite

Uses: Acute leukemias, chronic granulocytic leukemia, lymphomas, multiple myeloma, solid tumors

DOSAGE AND ROUTES

• *Adult and child:* **PO** 2 mg/kg/day, then increase slowly to 3 mg/kg/day after 4 wk
Contraindications: Pregnancy (D), prior drug resistance, leukopenia (<2500/mm^3), thrombocytopenia (<100,000/mm^3), anemia

T

⚠ High Alert

thiopental (℞)
(thye-oh-pen′tal)
Pentothal, thiopental sodium
Func. class.: General anesthetic
Chem. class.: Barbiturate

Controlled Substance Schedule III

Action: Acts in reticular-activating system to produce anesthesia, raises seizure threshold

Uses: Short, general anesthesia; narcoanalysis, induction anesthesia before other anesthetics

Investigational uses: Increased intracranial pressure

DOSAGE AND ROUTES
Induction and anesthesia
• *Adult:* IV 25-75 mg test dose, observe for 60 min; initial dose 50-70 mg given at 20-40 sec interval; additional 25-50 mg as needed
Rapid induction
• *Adult:* 210-280 mg or 3-5 mg/kg in 2-4 divided doses
• *Child:* 3-5 mg/kg over 20-30 sec, then 1 mg/kg as needed
Narcoanalysis
• *Adult:* IV 100 mg/min, not to exceed 50 ml/min
Sedation or narcosis
• *Adult:* RECT 12-20 mg/lb
Available forms: Powder for inj 2%, 2.5% (20 mg/ml, 25 mg/ml)

SIDE EFFECTS
CNS: Retrograde amnesia, prolonged somnolence
CV: Tachycardia, hypotension, ***myocardial depression, dysrhythmias***
EENT: Sneezing, coughing
INTEG: Chills, *shivering,* necrosis, pain at inj site
MS: Muscle irritability
RESP: ***Respiratory depression, bronchospasm***
Contraindications: Hypersensitivity, status asthmaticus, porphyrias

Precautions: Pregnancy (C), severe cardiovascular disease, renal disease, hypotension, hepatic disease, myxedema, myasthenia gravis, asthma, increased intracranial pressure

PHARMACOKINETICS
IV: Onset 30-60 sec; duration 4-15 min; half-life 11½ hr; crosses placenta

INTERACTIONS
Increase: action—CNS depressants
Drug/Herb
Increase: CNS depression—kava

NURSING CONSIDERATIONS
Assess:
• VS q3-5min during IV administration, after dose, q4h postoperatively
• Extravasation; if it occurs, apply moist heat and 1% procaine to affected area
• Dysrhythmias or myocardial depression

Administer:
• Only with crash cart, resuscitative equipment nearby
Intermittent IV route
• Dilute to 20-50 mg/ml, give by slow injection over 20-30 sec, max 25 mg/min
CONT INF route
• Dilute to 2-4 mg/ml
Additive compatibilities: Chloramphenicol, hydrocortisone sodium succinate, oxytocin, pentobarbital, phenobarbital, potassium chloride, sodium bicarbonate
Solution compatibilities: D_5/0.45% NaCl, D_5W, multiple electrolyte sol, 0.45% NaCl, 0.9% NaCl, 1/6 M sodium lactate
Syringe compatibilities: Aminophylline, hyaluronidase, hydrocortisone sodium succinate, neostigmine, pentobarbital, propofol, scopolamine, tubocurarine
Y-site compatibilities: Doxacurium, fentanyl, heparin, milrinone, mivacurium, nitroglycerin, ranitidine, remifentanil

⚠ Safety alert   *"Tall Man" lettering

Evaluate:
• Therapeutic response: maintenance of anesthesia

---

thioridazine (R)

(thye-or-rid'a-zeen)
Apo-Thioridazine ✦, Mellaril,
Mellaril Concentrate,
Mellaril-5, Novo-Ridazine ✦,
PMS-Thioridazine ✦,
thioridazine HCl
Func. class.: Antipsychotic, neuroleptic
Chem. class.: Phenothiazine piperidine

Do not confuse:
Mellaril/Elavil
Action: Depresses cerebral cortex, hypothalamus, limbic system, which control activity, aggression; blocks neurotransmission produced by dopamine at synapse; exhibits strong α-adrenergic, anticholinergic blocking action; mechanism for antipsychotic effects is unclear
Uses: Psychotic disorders, schizophrenia, behavioral problems in children, anxiety, major depressive disorders, organic brain syndrome, dementia in elderly

DOSAGE AND ROUTES
Psychosis
• *Adult:* PO 25-100 mg tid, max dose 800 mg/day; dose is gradually increased to desired response, then reduced to minimum maintenance
Depression/behavioral problems/ organic brain syndrome
• *Adult:* PO 25 mg tid, range from 10 mg bid-qid to 50 mg tid-qid
• *Geriatric:* PO 10-25 mg daily-bid, increase 4-7 days by 10-25 mg to desired dose
• *Child 2-12 yr:* PO 0.5-3 mg/kg/day in divided doses
Available forms: Tabs 10, 15, 25, 50, 100, 150, 200 mg; conc 30, 100 mg/ml; susp 25, 100 mg/5 ml; syr 10 mg/15 ml

SIDE EFFECTS
CNS: EPS (rare): *pseudoparkinsonism, akathisia, dystonia, tardive dyskinesia,* **seizures,** *headache,* confusion, **neuroleptic malignant syndrome,** dizziness
CV: Orthostatic hypotension, **cardiac arrest,** ECG changes, **tachycardia**
EENT: Blurred vision, glaucoma, dry eyes
GI: *Dry mouth, nausea, vomiting, anorexia, constipation,* diarrhea, jaundice, weight gain
GU: Urinary retention, urinary frequency, enuresis, impotence, amenorrhea, gynecomastia
HEMA: Anemia, **leukopenia, leukocytosis, agranulocytosis**
INTEG: *Rash,* photosensitivity, dermatitis
RESP: **Laryngospasm,** dyspnea, **respiratory depression**
Contraindications: Hypersensitivity, blood dyscrasias, coma, children <2 yr, brain damage, bone marrow depression
Precautions: Pregnancy (C), lactation, seizure disorders, hypertension, hepatic disease, cardiac disease

PHARMACOKINETICS
PO: Onset erratic, peak 2-4 hr; metabolized by liver, excreted in urine, breast milk; crosses placenta, half-life 26-36 hr

INTERACTIONS
Oversedation: other CNS depressants, alcohol, barbiturate anesthetics
Increase: anticholinergic effects—anticholinergics
Decrease: thioridazine effect—lithium, barbiturates
Decrease: antihypertensive effect—centrally acting antihypertensives
Decrease: absorption—aluminum hydroxide, magnesium hydroxide antacids
Drug/Herb
Increase: CNS depression—kava
Increase: EPS—betel palm, kava
Increase: effect—cola tree, hops, nettle, nutmeg

T

Drug/Lab Test

Increase: LFTs, cardiac enzymes, cholesterol, blood glucose, prolactin, bilirubin, PBI, cholinesterase, ^{131}I

Decrease: Hormones (blood, urine)

False positive: Pregnancy test, PKU

False negative: Urinary steroid, pregnancy test

NURSING CONSIDERATIONS

Assess:

• Mental status before first dose

• Swallowing of PO medication; check for hoarding or giving of medication to other patients

• I&O ratio; palpate bladder if low urinary output occurs, urinary retention may be the cause

• Bilirubin, CBC, LFTs qmo

• Urinalysis is recommended before and during prolonged therapy

• Affect, orientation, LOC, reflexes, gait, coordination, sleep pattern disturbances

• B/P standing and lying; also include pulse and respirations q4h during initial treatment; establish baseline before starting treatment; report drops of 30 mm Hg

• Dizziness, faintness, palpitations, tachycardia on rising

• EPS including akathisia (inability to sit still, no pattern to movements), tardive dyskinesia (bizarre movements of jaw, mouth, tongue, extremities), pseudoparkinsonism (rigidity, tremors, pill rolling, shuffling gait)

A For neuroleptic malignant syndrome: altered mental status, muscle rigidity, increased CPK, hyperthermia, dyspnea, fatigue

• Skin turgor daily

• Constipation, urinary retention daily; increase bulk, water in diet

Administer:

• Antiparkinsonian agent on order from prescriber for EPS

• Concentrate mixed in citrus juices or distilled or acidified tap water

• Decreased dose in elderly

• Remain lying down after IM inj for at least 30 min

• Avoid use with CNS depressants

Perform/provide:

• Decreased sensory input by dimming lights, avoiding loud noises

• Supervised ambulation until stabilized on medication if needed; do not involve in strenuous exercise program because fainting is possible; patient should not stand still for long periods

• Increased fluids to prevent constipation

• Sips of water, candy, gum for dry mouth

• Storage in tight, light-resistant container; avoid contact with skin

Evaluate:

• Therapeutic response: decrease in emotional excitement, hallucinations, delusions, paranoia, reorganization of patterns of thought, speech

Teach patient/family:

• That orthostatic hypotension occurs frequently, to rise from sitting or lying position gradually; to avoid hazardous activities until stabilized on medication

• To avoid hot tubs, hot showers, tub baths; hypotension may occur

• To avoid abrupt withdrawal of thioridazine, or EPS may result; drug should be withdrawn slowly

• To avoid OTC preparations (cough, hay fever, cold) unless approved by prescriber; serious drug interactions may occur; avoid use with alcohol; increased drowsiness may occur

• To use sunscreen to prevent burns

• About compliance with drug regimen

• About the necessity for meticulous oral hygiene, since oral candidiasis may occur

• To report sore throat, malaise, fever, bleeding, mouth sores; if these occur, CBC should be drawn and drug discontinued; may cause vision impairment, report to prescriber

• That in hot weather, heat stroke may occur; take extra precautions to stay cool

• May cause discoloration of urine

Treatment of overdose: Lavage if orally ingested, provide an airway; do not induce vomiting, CV monitoring, continuous EKG

Rarely Used

thiotepa (℞)
(thye-oh-tep′a)
Thioplex
Func. class.: Antineoplastic

Uses: Hodgkin's disease, lymphomas; breast, ovarian, lung, bladder cancer; neoplastic effusions

DOSAGE AND ROUTES

• *Adult:* **IV** 0.3-0.4 mg/kg at 1-4 wk intervals
Neoplastic effusions
• *Adult:* **INTRACAVITY** 0.6-0.8 mg/kg
Bladder cancer
• *Adult:* **INSTILL** 60 mg/30-60 ml water for inj instilled in bladder for 2 hr once weekly × 4 wk
Contraindications: Pregnancy (D), hypersensitivity

Rarely Used

thiothixene (℞)
(thye-oh-thix′een)
Navane, thiothixene
Func. class.: Antipsychotic, neuroleptic

Do not confuse:
Navane/Norvasc
Uses: Psychotic disorders, schizophrenia, acute agitation

DOSAGE AND ROUTES

• *Adult:* **PO** 2-5 mg bid-qid depending on severity of condition; dose gradually increased to 15-30 mg if needed; **IM** 4 mg bid-qid; max dose 30 mg daily; administer **PO** dose as soon as possible
• *Geriatric:* **PO** 1-2 mg daily-bid, increase by 1-2 mg q4-7d to desired dose
Contraindications: Hypersensitivity, blood dyscrasias, child <12 yr, bone marrow depression, circulatory collapse, CNS depression, coma, alcoholism, CV disease, hepatic disease, Reye's syndrome, narrow-angle glaucoma

**thyroid USP
(desiccated)** (℞)
(thye′roid)
Armour Thyroid, Thyrar, Thyroid Strong, Westhroid
Func. class.: Thyroid hormone
Chem. class.: Active thyroid hormone in natural state and ratio

Do not confuse:
Thyrar/Thyrolar
Action: Increases metabolic rates, increases cardiac output, O_2 consumption, body temp, blood volume, growth, development at cellular level
Uses: Hypothyroidism, cretinism (juvenile hypothyroidism), myxedema

DOSAGE AND ROUTES

Hypothyroidism
• *Adult:* **PO** 65 mg daily, increased by 65 mg q30d until desired response; maintenance dose 65-195 mg daily
• *Geriatric:* **PO** 7.5-15 mg daily, double dose q6-8wk until desired response
Cretinism/juvenile hypothyroidism
• *Child over 1 yr:* **PO** up to 180 mg daily titrated to response
• *Child 4-12 mo:* **PO** 30-60 mg daily
• *Child 1-4 mo:* **PO** 15-30 mg daily; may increase q2wk; titrated to response; maintenance dose 30-45 mg daily
Myxedema
• *Adult:* **PO** 16 mg daily, double dose q2wk, maintenance 65-195 mg/day
Available forms: Tabs 16, 32, 65, 98, 130, 195, 260, 325 mg; tabs enteric coated 32, 65, 130 mg; sugarcoated tabs 32, 65, 130, 195 mg; caps 65, 130, 195, 325 mg

SIDE EFFECTS

CNS: Insomnia, tremors, headache, ***thyroid storm***
CV: Tachycardia, palpitations, angina, dysrhythmias, hypertension, ***cardiac arrest***
GI: Nausea, diarrhea, increased or decreased appetite, cramps

T

Side effects: *italics* = common; ***bold italics*** = life-threatening

MISC: Menstrual irregularities, weight loss, sweating, heat intolerance, fever

Contraindications: Adrenal insufficiency, MI, thyrotoxicosis

Precautions: Pregnancy (A), elderly, angina pectoris, hypertension, ischemia, cardiac disease, lactation

PHARMACOKINETICS

PO: Peak 12-48 hr, half-life 6-7 days

INTERACTIONS

Increase: effects of anticoagulants, sympathomimetics, tricyclics, catecholamines

Decrease: thyroid absorption—bile acid sequestrants

Decrease: effects of digoxin, insulin, hypoglycemics

Decrease: thyroid effects—estrogens

Drug/Herb

Decrease: thyroid effect—agar, bugleweed, carnitine, kelpware, soy, spirulina

Drug/Lab Test

Increase: CPK, LDH, AST, PBI, blood glucose

Decrease: Thyroid function tests

NURSING CONSIDERATIONS

Assess:
• B/P, pulse before each dose
• I&O ratio
• Weight daily in same clothing, using same scale, at same time of day
• Height, growth rate of child
• T_3, T_4, which are decreased; radioimmunoassay of TSH, which is increased; radio uptake, which is decreased if dosage is too low
• PT may require decreased anticoagulant; check for bleeding, bruising
• Increased nervousness, excitability, irritability; may indicate too high dose of medication, usually after 1-3 wk of treatment
• Cardiac status: angina, palpitation, chest pain, change in VS

Administer:
• In AM if possible as a single dose to decrease sleeplessness
• At same time each day to maintain drug level
• Only for hormone imbalances; not to be used for obesity, male infertility, menstrual disorders, lethargy
• Lowest dose that relieves symptoms

Perform/provide:
• Removal of medication 4 wk before RAIU test

Evaluate:
• Therapeutic response: absence of depression; increased weight loss, diuresis, pulse, appetite; absence of constipation, peripheral edema, cold intolerance; pale, cool, dry skin; brittle nails, alopecia, coarse hair, menorrhagia, night blindness, paresthesias, syncope, stupor, coma, rosy cheeks

Teach patient/family:
• That hair loss will occur in child, is temporary
• To report excitability, irritability, anxiety; indicates overdose
• Not to switch brands unless directed by prescriber
• That hypothyroid child will show almost immediate behavior/personality change
• That treatment drug is not to be taken to reduce weight
• To avoid OTC preparations with iodine; read labels
• To avoid iodine food, iodized salt, soybeans, tofu, turnips, some seafood, some bread

---

tiagabine (℞)
(tie-ah-ga′been)
Gabitril
Func. class.: Anticonvulsant

Action: Mechanism unknown; may increase seizure threshold; structurally similar to GABA; tiagabine binding sites in neocortex, hippocampus

Uses: Adjunct treatment of partial seizures

⚠ Safety alert   *"Tall Man" lettering

DOSAGE AND ROUTES

• *Adult:* **PO** 4 mg daily, may increase by 4-8 mg qwk until desired response, max 56 mg/day

• *Child 12-18 yr:* **PO** 4 mg daily, may increase by 4 mg at beginning of wk 2; may increase by 4-8 mg qwk until desired response; max 32 mg/day

Available forms: Tabs 2, 4, 12, 16 mg

SIDE EFFECTS

CNS: Dizziness, anxiety, somnolence, ataxia, confusion, *asthenia,* unsteady gait, depression

CV: Vasodilation

GI: Nausea, vomiting, diarrhea

INTEG: Pruritus, rash

RESP: Pharyngitis, coughing

Contraindications: Hypersensitivity to this drug

Precautions: Pregnancy (C), hepatic disease, renal disease, lactation, children <12 yr, elderly

PHARMACOKINETICS

Absorption >95%, half-life 7-9 hr

INTERACTIONS

Lower doses may be needed when used with valproate

Increase: CNS depression—CNS depressants

Decrease: effect—carbamazepine, phenobarbital, phenytoin, primidone

Drug/Food

High fat meal decreases rate of absorption

NURSING CONSIDERATIONS

Assess:

• Renal studies: urinalysis, BUN, urine creatinine q3mo

• Hepatic studies: ALT, AST, bilirubin

• Description of seizures: location, duration, presence of aura

• Mental status: mood, sensorium, affect, behavioral changes; if mental status changes, notify prescriber

Administer:

• With food

Perform/provide:

• Storage at room temperature away from heat and light

• Assistance with ambulation during early part of treatment; dizziness occurs

• Seizure precautions: padded side rails; move objects that may harm patient

Evaluate:

• Therapeutic response: decreased seizure activity; document on patient's chart

Teach patient/family:

• To carry emergency ID stating patient's name, drugs taken, condition, prescriber's name and phone number

• To avoid driving, other activities that require alertness

• Not to discontinue medication quickly after long-term use

• To take with food

Treatment of overdose: Lavage, VS

ticarcillin (℞)
(tye-kar-sill'in)
Ticar
Func. class.: Broad-spectrum antiinfective
Chem. class.: Extended-spectrum penicillin

Action: Interferes with cell wall replication of susceptible organisms; osmotically unstable cell wall swells, bursts from osmotic pressure

Uses: Respiratory, soft tissue, urinary tract infections, bacterial septicemia; effective for gram-positive cocci *(Staphylococcus aureus, Streptococcus faecalis, Streptococcus pneumoniae),* gram-negative cocci *(Neisseria gonorrhoeae),* gram-positive bacilli *(Clostridium perfringens, Clostridium tetani),* gram-negative bacilli *(Bacteroides, Fusobacterium nucleatum, Escherichia coli, Proteus mirabilis, Salmonella, Morganella morganii, Proteus rettgeri, Enterobacter, Pseudomonas aeruginosa, Serratia);* and *Peptococcus, Peptostreptococcus, Eubacterium*

DOSAGE AND ROUTES

Bacterial septicemia, respiratory, skin, soft tissue, intraabdominal, reproductive infections

• *Adult:* **IV INF** 200-300 mg/kg/day in divided doses q4-6h

• *Child <40 kg:* **IV INF** 200-300 mg/kg/day in divided doses q4-6h

Urinary tract complicated infections

• *Adult/child:* **IV INF** 150-200 mg/kg/day in divided doses q4-6h

Uncomplicated urinary infections

• *Adult:* **IV Direct/IM** 1 g q6h

• *Child <40 kg:* **IV Direct/IM** 50-100 mg/kg/day q6-8h

Severe infections (Pseudomonas, Proteus, E. coli)

• *Neonates:* **IM/IV** <2 kg: 75 mg/kg q8-12h; **IM/IV** >2 kg: 75-100 mg/kg q8h

Renal dose/hepatic dose

• CCr >60 ml/min 3 g q4h; CCr 30-60 ml/min 2 g q4h; CCr 10-30 ml/min 2 g q8h; CCr <10 ml/min 2 g q12h or 1 g q6h; CCr <10 ml/min and hepatic dysfunction 2 g q24h or 1 g q12h

Available forms: Inj 1, 3, 6, 20, 30 g

SIDE EFFECTS

CNS: Lethargy, hallucinations, anxiety, depression, twitching, *coma, seizures*

GI: Nausea, vomiting, diarrhea; increased AST, ALT; abdominal pain, glossitis, colitis

GU: Oliguria, proteinuria, hematuria, *vaginitis, moniliasis, glomerulonephritis*

HEMA: Anemia, increased bleeding time, *bone marrow depression, granulocytopenia*

INTEG: Rash

META: Hypokalemia

SYST: **Anaphylaxis**

Contraindications: Hypersensitivity to penicillins

Precautions: Pregnancy (B), hypersensitivity to cephalosporins, lactation, renal disease

PHARMACOKINETICS

IM: Peak 1 hr, duration 4-6 hr

IV: Peak 30-45 min, duration 4 hr, half-life 70 min; small amount metabolized in liver; excreted in urine, breast milk

INTERACTIONS

Increase: effect of neuromuscular blockers, heparin

Increase: ticarcillin concentrations—aspirin, probenecid

Decrease: effect—oral contraceptives, erythromycins

Decrease: antimicrobial effect of ticarcillin—tetracyclines, aminoglycosides IV

Drug/Lab Test

False positive: Urine glucose, urine protein

NURSING CONSIDERATIONS

Assess:

• I&O ratio; report hematuria, oliguria, since penicillin in high doses is nephrotoxic

⚠ Any patient with compromised renal system, since drug is excreted slowly in poor renal system function; toxicity may occur rapidly

⚠ For anaphylaxis: wheezing, rash, pruritus, laryngeal edema, keep emergency equipment nearby

• Hepatic studies: AST, ALT

• Blood studies: WBC, RBC, Hgb, Hct, bleeding time

• Renal tests: urinalysis, protein, blood, BUN, creatinine

• C&S before drug therapy; drug may be given as soon as culture is taken

• Bowel pattern before, during treatment

• Skin eruptions after administration of penicillin to 1 wk after discontinuing drug

• Allergies before initiation of treatment, reaction of each medication

Administer:

• Drug after C&S has been completed

⚠ Safety alert   *"Tall Man" lettering

IM route

• Inject into well-developed muscle

• Reconstitute ticarcillin 1 g/2 ml sterile water for inj, NaCl inj, 1% lidocaine HCl without epINEPHrine (385 mg/ml)

IV route

• After diluting 1 g or less/4 ml sterile H_2O for inj; dilute further with 10-20 ml or more D_5W, NS, or sterile H_2O for inj sol; give 1 g or less/5 min or more or by intermittent inf over ½-2 hr or by continuous inf at prescribed rate

Y-site compatibilities: Acyclovir, allopurinol, amifostine, aztreonam, cisatracurium, cyclophosphamide, diltiazem, DOXOrubicin, famotidine, filgrastim, fludarabine, granisetron, heparin, hydromorphone, IL-2, insulin (regular), magnesium sulfate, melphalan, meperidine, morphine, ondansetron, perphenazine, propofol, remifentanil, sargramostim, teniposide, theophylline, thiotepa, verapamil, vinorelbine

Perform/provide:

• EpINEPHrine, suction, tracheostomy set, endotracheal intubation equipment

• Adequate fluid intake (2 L) during diarrhea episodes

• Scratch test to assess allergy on order from prescriber; done when penicillin is only drug of choice

• Storage at room temperature, reconstituted sol 72 hr at room temperature

Evaluate:

• Therapeutic response: absence of fever, purulent drainage, redness, inflammation

Teach patient/family:

• That culture may be taken after completed course of medication

• To report sore throat, fever, fatigue (may indicate superinfection)

• To wear or carry emergency ID if allergic to penicillins

• To notify nurse of diarrhea

Treatment of overdose: Withdraw drug, maintain airway, administer epINEPHrine, aminophylline, O_2, IV corticosteroids for anaphylaxis

---

ticarcillin/ clavulanate (℞)

Timentin

Func. class.: Broad-spectrum antiinfective

Chem. class.: Extended-spectrum penicillin

Action: Interferes with cell wall replication of susceptible organisms; osmotically unstable cell wall swells, bursts from osmotic pressure

Uses: Respiratory, soft tissue, and urinary tract infections, bacterial septicemia; effective for gram-positive cocci *(Staphylococcus aureus, Streptococcus faecalis, Streptococcus pneumoniae)*, gram-negative cocci *(Neisseria gonorrhoeae)*, gram-positive bacilli *(Clostridium perfringens, Clostridium tetani)*, gram-negative bacilli *(Bacteroides, Fusobacterium nucleatum, Escherichia coli, Proteus mirabilis, Salmonella, Morganella morganii, Proteus rettgeri, Enterobacter, Pseudomonas aeruginosa, Serratia);* and *Peptococcus, Peptostreptococcus, Eubacterium*

DOSAGE AND ROUTES

Systemic/urinary tract infections, serious infections

• *Adult ≥60 kg:* **IV INF** 3.1 g q4-6h

• *Adult <60 kg:* **IV INF** 200-300 mg/kg/day q4-6h

• *Child >60 kg:* **IV INF** 3.1 g q4h

• *Child <60 kg:* **IV INF** 300 mg/kg/day q4h

Mild/moderate infections

• *Child ≥60 kg:* **IV INF** 3.1 g q6h

• *Child <60 kg:* **IV INF** 200 mg/kg/day q6h

Renal dose

• CCr 60 ml/min 3.1 g q4h; CCr 30-60 ml/min 2 g q4h; CCr 10-30 ml/min 2 g q8h; CCr <10 ml/min 2 g q12h; CCr <10 ml/min with hepatic dysfunction 2 g q24h

Available forms: Inj 3 g ticarcillin, 0.1 g clavulanate; IV inf 3 g ticarcillin, 0.1 g

T

---

clavulanate; powder for inj 3 g ticarcillin, 0.1 g clavulanate

SIDE EFFECTS

CNS: Lethargy, hallucinations, anxiety, depression, twitching, ***coma, seizures***
GI: *Nausea, vomiting, diarrhea;* increased AST, ALT; abdominal pain, glossitis, colitis
GU: Oliguria, proteinuria, hematuria, *vaginitis, moniliasis,* ***glomerulonephritis***
HEMA: Anemia, increased bleeding time, ***bone marrow depression, granulocytopenia***
META: Hyperkalemia, hypokalemia, alkalosis, hypernatremia
SYST: ***Anaphylaxis***

Contraindications: Hypersensitivity to penicillins; neonates
Precautions: Pregnancy (B), hypersensitivity to cephalosporins, renal disease

PHARMACOKINETICS

IV: Peak 30-45 min, duration 4 hr, half-life 64-68 min; excreted in urine

INTERACTIONS

Increase: effect of neuromuscular blockers, heparin
Increase: ticarcillin concentrations—aspirin, probenecid
Decrease: antimicrobial effect of ticarcillin—tetracyclines, aminoglycosides IV
Decrease: effect—oral contraceptives, erythromycin
Drug/Lab Test
False positive: Urine glucose, urine protein, Coombs' test

NURSING CONSIDERATIONS

Assess:
• I&O ratio; report hematuria, oliguria, since penicillin in high doses is nephrotoxic
⚠ Any patient with compromised renal system, since drug is excreted slowly in poor renal system function; toxicity may occur rapidly

⚠ For anaphylaxis: wheezing, rash, laryngeal edema; have emergency equipment nearby
• Hepatic studies: AST, ALT
• Blood studies: WBC, RBC, Hct, Hgb, bleeding time
• Renal studies: urinalysis, protein, blood, BUN, creatinine
• C&S before drug therapy; drug may be given as soon as culture is taken
• Bowel pattern before, during treatment
• Skin eruptions after administration of penicillin to 1 wk after discontinuing drug
• Allergies before initiation of treatment, reaction of each medication
Administer:
• Drug after C&S
IV route
• After diluting 3.1 g or less/13 ml of sterile H_2O or NaCl (200 mg/ml), shake; may further dilute in 50-100 ml or more NS, D_5W, or LR sol and run over ½ hr
Y-site compatibilities: Allopurinol, amifostine, aztreonam, cefepime, cyclophosphamide, diltiazem, DOXOrubicin liposome, famotidine, filgrastim, fluconazole, fludarabine, foscarnet, gallium, granisetron, heparin, insulin (regular), melphalan, meperidine, morphine, ondansetron, perphenazine, propofol, remifentanil, sargramostim, teniposide, theophylline, thiotepa, vinorelbine
Perform/provide:
• EpINEPHrine, suction, tracheostomy set, endotracheal intubation equipment
• Adequate fluid intake (2 L) during diarrhea episodes
• Scratch test to assess allergy on order from prescriber; usually done when penicillin is only drug of choice
• Storage of reconstituted sol 12-24 hr at room temperature, or 3-7 days refrigerated
Evaluate:
• Therapeutic response: absence of fever, purulent drainage, redness, inflammation
Teach patient/family:
• To report persistent diarrhea

⚠ Safety alert   *"Tall Man" lettering

• That culture may be taken after completed course of medication
• To report sore throat, fever, fatigue (may indicate superinfection)
• To wear or carry emergency ID if allergic to penicillins

Treatment of overdose: Withdraw drug, maintain airway, administer epINEPHrine, O_2, IV corticosteroids for anaphylaxis

---

ticlopidine (℞)
(tye-cloe'pi-deen)
Ticlid
Func. class.: Platelet aggregation inhibitor
Chem. class.: Thienopyridine compound

Action: Irreversible inhibition of platelet aggregation through antagonism of ADP

Uses: Reducing the risk of stroke in high-risk patients

Investigational uses: Intermittent claudication, chronic arterial occlusion, subarachnoid hemorrhage, uremic patients with AV shunts/fistulas, open heart surgery, coronary artery bypass grafts, primary glomerulonephritis, sickle cell disease, diabetic retinopathy

DOSAGE AND ROUTES

• *Adult:* PO 250 mg bid with food
Available forms: Tabs 250 mg

SIDE EFFECTS

CNS: Dizziness
GI: Nausea, vomiting, *diarrhea,* GI discomfort, ***cholestatic jaundice, hepatitis,*** increased cholesterol, LDL, VLDL, TG
HEMA: ***Bleeding (epistaxis, hematuria, conjunctival hemorrhage, GI bleeding), agranulocytosis, neutropenia, thrombocytopenia, thrombotic thombocytopenic purpura***
INTEG: *Rash,* pruritus

Contraindications: Hypersensitivity, severe hepatic disease, blood dyscrasias, active bleeding, coagulopathy

Precautions: Pregnancy (B), past hepatic disease, renal disease, elderly, lactation, children, increased bleeding risk, anemia, peptic ulcer disease, surgery

PHARMACOKINETICS

Peak 1-3 hr, metabolized by liver, excreted in urine, feces; half-life increases with repeated dosing, initially 12-36 hr, antiplatelet effect 2-5 days, 98% protein binding

INTERACTIONS

Increase: levels of phenytoin
Increase: bleeding tendencies— anticoagulants, salicylates, thrombolytics, NSAIDs, abciximab, eptifibatide, tirofiban, ticlopidine
Increase: effects of ticlopidine— cimetidine
Increase: effects of theophylline
Decrease: plasma levels of ticlopidine—antacids
Decrease: plasma levels of digoxin

NURSING CONSIDERATIONS

Assess:
• Hepatic studies: AST, ALT, bilirubin, creatinine (long-term therapy)
⚠ Blood studies: CBC; CBC q2wk × 3 mo, Hct, Hgb, PT (long-term therapy)
⚠ Bleed time baseline and throughout, levels may be 2-5 × normal limit
Administer:
• With food to decrease gastric symptoms
Evaluate:
• Therapeutic response: absence of stroke
Teach patient/family:
• That blood work will be necessary during treatment
• To report any unusual bleeding to prescriber
• To report side effects such as diarrhea, skin rashes, subcutaneous bleeding,

T

signs of cholestasis (jaundiced skin and sclera, dark urine, light-colored stools)

tigecycline
See Appendix A—Selected New Drugs

tiludronate (℞)
(till-oo'droe-nate)
Skelid
Func. class.: Bone resorption inhibitor
Chem. class.: Bisphosphonate

Action: Decreases bone resorption and new bone development

Uses: Paget's disease in those with alk phosphatase at 2× upper limit, patients at risk for future complications of Paget's disease

DOSAGE AND ROUTES
• *Adult:* **PO** 400 mg daily, with 8 oz water × 3 mo
Available forms: Tabs 240 mg (equivalent to 200 mg tiludronic acid)

SIDE EFFECTS
CNS: Headache, somnolence, dizziness, anxiety, vertigo, nervousness, involuntary movements
CV: Chest pain, edema, hypertension, peripheral edema
ENDO: Hyperparathyroidism
GI: Nausea, diarrhea, dry mouth, gastritis, vomiting, flatulence, gastric ulcers, gastritis, dyspepsia
GU: **Nephrotoxicity,** UTI
INTEG: Rash, epidermal necrosis, pruritus, sweating
MS: Bone pain, decreased mineralization of nonaffected bones, pathologic fractures
RESP: Rhinitis, bronchitis, crackles, sinusitis, URI

Contraindications: Hypersensitivity to bisphosphonates, severe renal disease with creatinine >5 mg/dl

Precautions: Pregnancy (C), renal disease, lactation, restricted vit D/calcium, GI disease

PHARMACOKINETICS
Onset up to several wk, protein binding 90%, excreted by kidneys; half-life 150 hr

INTERACTIONS
Increase: tiludronate effect—indomethacin
Decrease: tiludronate absorption—antacids, mineral supplements with magnesium, calcium, aluminum, aspirin, separate by ≥2 hr

NURSING CONSIDERATIONS
Assess:
• GI symptoms, polyuria, flushing, head swelling, tingling, headache—may indicate hypercalcemia; nervousness, irritability, twitching, seizures, spasm, paresthesia indicates hypocalcemia at start of treatment
• Nutritional status; evaluate diet for sources of vit D (milk, some seafood), calcium (dairy products, dark green vegetables), phosphates
• BUN, creatinine, uric acid, chloride, electrolytes, urine pH, urinary calcium, magnesium, phosphate, urinalysis (calcium should be kept at 9-10 mg/dl), albumin, alk phosphatase baseline and q3-6mo; check urine sediment for casts throughout treatment
• For increased drug level—toxic reactions occur rapidly; have calcium chloride or gluconate on hand if calcium level drops too low; check for tetany
Administer:
• On empty stomach to improve absorption (2 hr ac), with 6-8 oz water
• Take calcium or mineral supplements 2 hr before or 2 hr after tiludronate
• Take aluminum or magnesium antacids ≥2 hr after tiludronate
• Do not take indomethacin within 2 hr
• Tabs from foil strip immediately before use

Evaluate:
• Therapeutic response: calcium levels 9-10 mg/dl; decreasing symptoms of Paget's disease

Teach patient/family:
• To notify prescriber of hypercalcemic relapse: renal calculi, nausea, vomiting, thirst, lethargy, deep bone or flank pain
• To follow a low-calcium diet as prescribed (Paget's disease, hypercalcemia)
• To notify prescriber of diarrhea, nausea; dose may be divided to lessen these symptoms

---

timolol (Ꭱ)

(tye'moe-lole)
Apo-Timol ✚, Blocadren, Novo-Timol ✚, timolol maleate
Func. class.: Antihypertensive
Chem. class.: Nonselective β-blocker

Do not confuse:
Timoptic/Viroptic

Action: Competitively blocks stimulation of β-adrenergic receptor within vascular smooth muscle (decreases rate of SA node discharge, increases recovery time), slows conduction of AV node, decreases heart rate, which decreases O_2 consumption in myocardium; also decreases renin-aldosterone-angiotensin system, at high doses inhibits $β_2$-receptors in bronchial system

Uses: Mild to moderate hypertension

Investigational uses: Mitral valve prolapse, hypertrophic cardiomyopathy, thyrotoxicosis, tremors, anxiety, pheochromocytoma, tachydysrhythmias, angina pectoris

DOSAGE AND ROUTES

Hypertension
• *Adult:* **PO** 10 mg bid, or 20 mg daily, may increase by 10 mg q7d, not to exceed 60 mg/day

Myocardial infarction
• *Adult:* **PO** 10 mg bid beginning 1-4 wk after MI

Migraine headache prevention
• *Adult:* **PO** 10 mg bid or 20 mg daily; may increase to 30 mg/day, 20 mg in AM, 10 mg in PM, discontinue if not effective after 8 wk

Available forms: Tabs 5, 10, 20 mg

SIDE EFFECTS

CNS: Insomnia, dizziness, hallucinations, anxiety, fatigue, depression
CV: Hypotension, bradycardia, **CHF,** edema, chest pain, claudication, angina, AV block, ventricular dysrhythmias
EENT: Visual changes, sore throat, *double vision,* dry burning eyes
GI: Nausea, vomiting, **ischemic colitis,** diarrhea, *abdominal pain,* **mesenteric arterial thrombosis,** flatulence, constipation
GU: Impotence, urinary frequency
HEMA: **Agranulocytosis, thrombocytopenia, purpura**
INTEG: Rash, alopecia, pruritus, fever
META: Hypoglycemia
MUSC: Joint pain, muscle pain
RESP: **Bronchospasm,** dyspnea, cough, crackles, nasal stuffiness

Contraindications: Hypersensitivity to β-blockers, cardiogenic shock, heart block (2nd or 3rd degree), sinus bradycardia, CHF, cardiac failure, severe COPD

Precautions: Pregnancy (C), major surgery, lactation, diabetes mellitus, renal disease, thyroid disease, COPD, well-compensated heart failure, CAD, nonallergic bronchospasm, peripheral vascular disease, hepatic disease

PHARMACOKINETICS

PO: Peak 1-2 hr; half-life 4 hr; metabolized by liver; excreted in urine, breast milk, protein binding <10%

INTERACTIONS

Increase: hypotension, bradycardia—reserpine, hydrALAZINE, methyldopa, prazosin, anticholinergics, alcohol, reserpine, nitrates
Increase: effects of β-blockers, calcium channel blockers

Decrease: antihypertensive effects—NSAIDs, sympathomimetics, thyroid
Decrease: hypoglycemic effects—insulin, sulfonylureas
Decrease: bronchodilation—theophyllines

Drug/Herb

Increase: toxicity, death—aconite
Increase: antihypertensive effect—barberry, betony, black catechu, black cohosh, bloodroot, broom, burdock, cat's claw, dandelion, goldenseal, Irish moss, Jamaican dogwood, kelp, khella, mistletoe, parsley
Increase or decrease: antihypertensive effect—astragalus, cola tree
Decrease: antihypertensive effect—coltsfoot, guarana, khat, licorice

Drug/Lab Test

Increase: Renal, hepatic studies, potassium, uric acid
Decrease: Hct, Hgb, HDL
Interference: Glucose, insulin tolerance test

NURSING CONSIDERATIONS

Assess:

• Headaches: location, severity, duration, frequency baseline and throughout treatment
• I&O, weight daily
• B/P during initial treatment, periodically thereafter, pulse q4h; note rate, rhythm, quality
• Apical/radial pulse before administration; notify prescriber of any significant changes
• Baselines in renal, hepatic studies before therapy begins
• Edema in feet, legs daily
• Skin turgor, dryness of mucous membranes for hydration status

Administer:

• PO ac, at bedtime; tablet may be crushed or swallowed whole
• Reduced dosage in renal dysfunction

Perform/provide:

• Dry storage at room temperature; do not freeze

Evaluate:

• Therapeutic response: decreased B/P after 1-2 wk

Teach patient/family:

• To take with or immediately after meals
• Not to discontinue drug abruptly; taper over 2 wk; may cause precipitate angina
• Not to use OTC products containing α-adrenergic stimulants (nasal decongestants, cold preparations) unless directed by prescriber
• To report bradycardia, dizziness, confusion, depression, fever, sore throat, shortness of breath to prescriber
• To take pulse at home; advise when to notify prescriber
• To avoid alcohol, smoking, sodium intake
• To comply with weight control, dietary adjustments, modified exercise program
• To carry emergency ID to identify drug, allergies
• To avoid hazardous activities if dizziness is present
• To report symptoms of CHF: difficulty breathing, especially on exertion or when lying down; night cough; swelling of extremities
• To take medication at bedtime and wear support hose to minimize effect of orthostatic hypotension

Treatment of overdose: Lavage, IV atropine for bradycardia, IV theophylline for bronchospasm, digitalis, O$_2$, diuretic for cardiac failure, hemodialysis; administer vasopressor (norepinephrine)

---

timolol ophthalmic
See Appendix C

---

tinidazole (R)
(tye-ni'da-zole)
Tindamax
Func. class.: Antiprotozoal
Chem. class.: Nitroimidazole derivative

Action: Interferes with DNA/RNA synthesis in protozoa
Uses: Amebiasis, giardiasis, trichomoniasis

DOSAGE AND ROUTES
Amebiasis
• *Adult:* **PO** 2 g/day × 3-5 days
• *Child >3 yr:* **PO** 50 mg/kg/day × 3-5 days, max 2 g
Giardiasis
• *Adult:* **PO** 2 g as a single dose
• *Child >3 yr:* **PO** 50 mg/kg as a single dose, max 2 g
Trichomoniasis
• *Adult:* **PO** 2 g as a single dose
Available forms: Tabs 250, 500 mg

SIDE EFFECTS
CNS: Dizziness, headache, **seizures,** *peripheral neuropathy*
GI: Nausea, vomiting, anorexia, increased AST and ALT, constipation, abdominal pain
HEMA: **Leukopenia,** neutropenia
INTEG: Pruritus, urticaria, *rash,* oral monilia
SYST: **Angioedema**
Contraindications: Hypersensitivity to this product or nitroimidazole derivative, pregnancy 1st trimester
Precautions: Pregnancy (C), hepatic disease, lactation, children, elderly, CNS depression

PHARMACOKINETICS
Metabolized extensively in the liver; excreted unchanged (20%-25%) in urine, (12%) feces; half-life 12-14 hr; crosses blood-brain barrier

INTERACTIONS
Do not use within 2 wk of taking disulfiram
CYP3A4 inducers (phenobarbital, rifampin, phenytoin); cholestyramine, oxytetracycline: decrease action of tinidazole
CYP3A4 inhibitors (cimetidine, ketoconazole): increase action of tinidazole
Increase: action of anticoagulants, cycloSPORINE, tacrolimus, fluorouracil, hydantoins, lithium

NURSING CONSIDERATIONS
Assess:
• Signs of infection, anemia
• Bowel pattern before, during treatment
Administer:
• Administer to those over 3 yr old
• With food to increase plasma concentrations, minimize epigastric distress and other GI effects
Evaluate:
• Therapeutic response: decreased in infection as evidenced by negative culture
Teach patient/family:
• To take with food to increase plasma concentrations, minimize epigastric distress and other GI effects; not to use alcoholic beverages during or for 3 days afterward
• Trichomoniasis: both partners should be treated

⚠ High Alert

tinzaparin (R)
(tin-zay-par'in)
Innohep
Func. class.: Anticoagulant
Chem. class.: Unfractionated porcine heparin

Action: Prevents conversion of fibrinogen to fibrin and prothrombin to thrombin by enhancing inhibitory effects of antithrombin III; produces higher ratio of antifactor Xa to antifactor IIa

Side effects: *italics* = common; **bold italics** = life-threatening

Uses: Treatment of deep-vein thrombosis, pulmonary emboli when given with warfarin

DOSAGE AND ROUTES

• *Adult:* SUBCUT 175 anti-Xa international units/kg daily ≥6 days and until adequate anticoagulation with warfarin (INR ≥2 for 2 consecutive days)

Available forms: Inj 40,000 international units/2 ml

SIDE EFFECTS

CNS: Fever, confusion, dizziness, insomnia

CV: Angina, dysrhythmias, peripheral edema

GI: Nausea, constipation, flatulence, dyspepsia, *hepatitis*

GU: UTI, hematuria, urinary retention, dysuria

HEMA: Hemorrhage, *hypochromic anemia, thrombocytopenia,* bleeding

INTEG: Ecchymosis

MISC: Headache, chest pain

Contraindications: Hypersensitivity to this drug, heparin, pork or benzyl alcohol, sulfites; hemophilia, leukemia with bleeding, peptic ulcer disease, thrombocytopenic purpura, heparin-induced thrombocytopenia

Precautions: Pregnancy (C), alcoholism, elderly, hepatic disease (severe), renal disease (severe), blood dyscrasias, severe, uncontrolled hypertension, subacute bacterial endocarditis, acute nephritis, lactation, children

PHARMACOKINETICS

Maximum antithrombin activity (3-5 hr), elimination half-life 4.5 hr

INTERACTIONS

Do not mix with other drugs or infusion fluids

Increase: action of tinzaparin—oral anticoagulants, salicylates, thrombolytics, NSAIDs, platelet inhibitors, ticlopidine

Drug/Herb

Increase: risk of bleeding—agrimony, alfalfa, angelica, anise, basil, bay, bilberry, black haw, bogbean, bromelain, buchu, chondroitin, cinchona bark, dong quai, fenugreek, feverfew, garlic, ginger, ginkgo, ginseng, horse chestnut, Irish moss, kelp, kelpware, khella, lovage, lungwort, meadowsweet, motherwort, mugwort, nettle, papaya, parsley (large amts), pau d'arco, pineapple, poplar, prickly ash, safflower, saw palmetto, tonka bean, turmeric, wintergreen, yarrow

Decrease: anticoagulant effect—chamomile, coenzyme Q10, flax, glucomannan, goldenseal, guar gum

NURSING CONSIDERATIONS

Assess:

• Blood studies (Hct, platelets, occult blood in stools), anti-Xa; thrombocytopenia may occur

• Bleeding gums, petechiae, ecchymosis, black tarry stools, hematuria

Administer:

• Only after screening patient for bleeding disorders

• SUBCUT only; do not give IM

• To recumbent patient; give SUBCUT; rotate inj sites (left/right anterolateral, left-right posterolateral abdominal wall)

• Insert whole length of needle into skin fold held with thumb and forefinger

🅰 Only this drug when ordered; not interchangeable with heparin or LMWHs

• At same time each day to maintain steady blood levels

• Do not massage area or aspirate when giving SUBCUT inj

• Avoiding all IM inj that may cause bleeding

Perform/provide:

• Storage at 77° F (25° C); do not freeze

Evaluate:

• Therapeutic response: resolution of deep vein thrombosis

Teach patient/family:

• To use soft-bristle toothbrush to avoid bleeding gums, to use electric razor

---

🅰 Safety alert   *"Tall Man" lettering

• To report any signs of bleeding: gums, under skin, urine, stools
Treatment of overdose: Protamine 1 mg/100 anti-Xa international units of tinzaparin

---

tioconazole vaginal antifungal
See Appendix C

---

tiotropium (℞)
(ty-oh'tro-pee-um)
Spiriva
Func. class.: Anticholinergic, bronchodilator
Chem. class.: Synthetic quaternary ammonium compound

Action: Inhibits interaction of acetylcholine at receptor sites on the bronchial smooth muscle, resulting in decreased cGMP and bronchodilation
Uses: COPD, for long-term treatment, once-daily maintenance of bronchospasm, associated with COPD, including chronic bronchitis and emphysema

DOSAGE AND ROUTES
• *Adult:* INH content of 1 cap daily using HandiHaler inhalation device
Available forms: Powder for inhalation 18 mcg in blister packs containing 6 caps with inhaler

SIDE EFFECTS
CNS: Depression
CV: Chest pain, increased heart rate
EENT: Dry mouth, blurred vision, glaucoma
GI: Vomiting, abdominal pain, constipation, dyspepsia
INTEG: Rash
MISC: Urinary difficulty, urinary retention
RESP: Cough, worsening of symptoms, sinusitis, upper respiratory tract infection, epistaxis, pharyngitis
Contraindications: Hypersensitivity to this drug, atropine or its derivatives

Precautions: Pregnancy (C), lactation, children, narrow-angle glaucoma, prostatic hypertrophy, bladder neck obstruction, elderly

PHARMACOKINETICS
Half-life 5-6 days in animals; does not cross blood-brain barrier, very little metabolized in the liver, excreted in urine

INTERACTIONS
Anticholinergics: avoid use with other anticholinergics
Drug/Herb
Increase: constipation—black catechu
Increase: anticholinergic effect—butterbur, jimsonweed
Increase: bronchodilator effect—green tea (large amounts), guarana
Decrease: anticholinergic effect—jaborandi tree, pill-bearing spurge

NURSING CONSIDERATIONS
Assess:
• For tolerance over long-term therapy; dose may have to be increased or changed
Administer:
• Caps are for INH only; do not swallow
• Immediately before administration, peel back foil until cap is visible; until "stop" line, open dust cap of HandiHaler by pulling upward, then open mouthpiece
• Place cap in center chamber; firmly close mouthpiece until it clicks, leaving dust cap open
• Remove used capsule and dispose; close the mouthpiece and dust cap; store
Evaluate:
• Therapeutic response: ability to breathe easier
Teach patient/family:
• Signs of narrow-angle glaucoma
• That drug is used for long-term maintenance, not for immediate relief of breathing problems

T

• To avoid getting the powder in the eyes; may cause blurred vision and pupil dilation

• Hold HandiHaler with mouthpiece upward; press button in once, completely, and release; this allows for medication to be released

• Breathe out completely; do not breathe into mouthpiece at any time

• Raise device to mouth and close lips tightly around mouthpiece

• With head upright, breathe in slowly/deeply, but allow the cap to vibrate; breathe until lungs fill; hold breath and remove mouthpiece; resume normal breathing

• Repeat

---

tipranavir
See Appendix A—Selected New Drugs

⚠ High Alert

tirofiban (℞)
(tie-roh-fee′ban)
Aggrastat
Func. class.: Antiplatelet
Chem. class.: Glycoprotein IIb/IIIa inhibitor

Action: Antagonist of platelet glycoprotein (GP) IIb/IIIa receptor that leads to binding of fibrinogen and von Willebrand's factor, which inhibits platelet aggregation

Uses: Acute coronary syndrome in combination with heparin

DOSAGE AND ROUTES

• *Adult:* IV 0.4 mcg/kg/min × 30 min, then 0.1 mcg/kg/min for 12-24 hr after angioplasty or atherectomy
Renal dose
• *Adult:* IV CCr <30 ml/min 0.2 mcg/kg/min × 30 min, then 0.05 mcg/kg/min, during angiography and for up to 24 hr after angioplasty

Available forms: Inj for sol 250 mcg/ml, inj 50 mcg/ml

SIDE EFFECTS

CNS: Dizziness, headache
CV: Bradycardia, hypotension
GI: Nausea, vomiting
HEMA: **Bleeding, thrombocytopenia**
INTEG: *Rash*
OTHER: Dissection, coronary artery edema, pain in legs/pelvis, sweating

Contraindications: Hypersensitivity, active internal bleeding, stroke, major surgery, severe trauma, intracranial neoplasm, aneurysm, hemorrhage, acute pericarditis, platelets <100,000/mm³, history of thrombocytopenia, coagulopathy

Precautions: Pregnancy (B), lactation, elderly, renal disease, bleeding tendencies, children, hypertension

Pharmocokinetics: Half-life 2 hr, excretion via urine/feces; plasma clearance 20%-25% lower in elderly with coronary artery disease; renal insufficiency decreases plasma clearance

INTERACTIONS

Increase: bleeding—aspirin, heparin, NSAIDs, abciximab, eptifibatide, clopidogrel, ticlopidine, dipyridamole, cefamandole, cefotetan, cefoperazone, valproic acid

Drug/Herb

Increase: risk of bleeding—agrimony, alfalfa, angelica, anise, basil, bay, bilberry, black haw, bogbean, bromelain, buchu, chondroitin, cinchona bark, dong quai, fenugreek, feverfew, garlic, ginger, ginkgo, ginseng, green tea, horse chestnut, Irish moss, kelp, kelpware, khella, lovage, lungwort, meadowsweet, motherwort, mugwort, nettle, papaya, parsley (large amts), pau d'arco, pineapple, poplar, prickly ash, safflower, saw palmetto, tonka bean, turmeric, wintergreen, yarrow

Decrease: anticoagulant effect—chamomile, coenzyme Q10, flax, glucomannan, goldenseal, guar gum

---

NURSING CONSIDERATIONS

Assess:

⚠️ Platelet counts, Hct, Hgb, prior to treatment, within 6 hr of loading dose and at least daily thereafter; watch for bleeding from puncture sites, catheters or in stools, urine

Administer:

IV route

• Dilute inj: withdraw and discard 100 ml from a 500 ml bag of sterile 0.9% NaCl or D₅W and replace this vol with 100 ml of tirofiban inj from two vials

• Tirofiban inj for sol is premixed in containers of 500-ml 0.9% NaCl (50 mg/ml)

• Minimize other arterial/venous punctures; IM inj, catheter use, intubation, to reduce bleeding risks

Y-site compatibility: Heparin

Evaluate:

• Therapeutic response: treatment of acute coronary syndrome

Teach patient/family:

• That it is necessary to quit smoking to prevent excessive vasoconstriction

---

tizanidine

(ti-za'nih-deen)
Zanaflex
Func. class.: Skeletal muscle relaxant, α₂-adrenergic agonist
Chem. class.: Imidazoline

Action: Increases presynaptic inhibition of motor neurons and reduces spasticity by α₂-adrenergic agonism

Uses: Acute/intermittent management of increased muscle tone associated with spasticity

DOSAGE AND ROUTES

• *Adult:* **PO** 4 mg q6-8h, increase gradually by 2-4 mg increments q6-8h, may repeat dose q6-8h, max 36 mg/24 hr

Available forms: Tabs 2, 4 mg; caps 2, 4, 6 mg

SIDE EFFECTS

CNS: Somnolence, dizziness, speech disorder, dyskinesia, nervousness, hallucination, psychosis

CV: Hypotension, bradycardia

GI: Dry mouth, vomiting, increased ALT, abnormal LFTs, constipation

OTHER: Blurred vision, urinary frequency, pharyngitis, rhinitis, tremor, rash, muscle weakness

Contraindications: Hypersensitivity

Precautions: Pregnancy (C), hypotension, liver disease, lactation, elderly, children, renal disease

PHARMACOKINETICS

Completely absorbed, widely distributed, peak 1-2 hr; duration 3-6 hr; half-life 2.5 hr; protein binding 30%; metabolized by liver, excreted in urine, feces

INTERACTIONS

Increase: CNS depression—alcohol, other CNS depressants

Decrease: clearance of tizanidine—oral contraceptives

Drug/Lab Test

Increase: Alk phosphatase, AST, ALT, serum glucose

NURSING CONSIDERATIONS

Assess:

• For muscle spasticity baseline and throughout treatment

• For hypotension, gradual dosage increase should lessen hypotensive effects; have patient rise slowly from supine to upright; watch those patients receiving antihypertensives for increased effects

• For increased sedation, dizziness, hallucinations, psychosis; drug may need to be discontinued

• Vision by ophthalmic exam, corneal opacities may occur

• Hepatic studies: 1, 3, 6 mo during treatment and periodically thereafter

Administer

• Consistantly either with or without food; food may affect absorption

---

Side effects: *italics* = common; **bold italics** = life-threatening

- Titrate doses carefully
- Avoid use with other CNS depressants

Teach patient/family:

- To rise slowly from lying or sitting to upright position
- To ask for assistance if dizziness, sedation occur; to avoid drinking alcohol, to avoid operating machinery or driving until effects are known
- To avoid use of alcohol
- Discontinue gradually

---

tobramycin (℞)

(toe-bra-mye′sin)

Nebcin, TOBI, tobramycin sulfate

Func. class.: Antiinfective

Chem. class.: Aminoglycoside

Action: Interferes with protein synthesis in bacterial cell by binding to ribosomal subunit, causing inaccurate peptide sequence to form in protein chain, causing bacterial death

Uses: Severe systemic infections of CNS, respiratory, GI, urinary tract, bone, skin, soft tissues caused by *Pseudomonas aeruginosa, Escherichia coli, Enterobacter, Providencia, Citrobacter, Staphylococcus, Proteus, Klebsiella, Serratia;* cystic fibrosis (nebulizer) for *Pseudomonas aeruginosa*

DOSAGE AND ROUTES

- *Adult:* **IM/IV** 3 mg/kg/day in divided doses q8h; may give up to 5 mg/kg/day in divided doses q6-8h; once daily dosing is an option
- *Child:* **IM/IV** 6-7.5 mg/kg/day in 3-4 equal divided doses
- *Child ≥6 yr:* **NEB** 300 mg bid in repeating cycles of 28 days on/28 days off of drug; give **INH** over 10-15 min using a handheld PARI LC PLUS reusable nebulizer with a DeVilbiss Pulmo-Aid compressor
- *Neonate <1 wk:* **IM** up to 4 mg/kg/day in divided doses q12h; **IV** up to 4 mg/kg/day in divided doses q12h diluted in 50-100 mg NS or D_5W; give over 30-60 min

Renal dose

- *Adult:* **IM/IV** 1 mg/kg, then dose determined by blood levels

Available forms: Inj 10, 40 mg/ml; powder for inj 1.2 g; neb sol 300 mg/5 ml

SIDE EFFECTS

CNS: Confusion, depression, numbness, tremors, ***convulsions,*** muscle twitching, ***neurotoxicity,*** dizziness, vertigo

CV: Hypo/hypertension, palpitation

EENT: ***Ototoxicity,*** deafness, visual disturbances, tinnitus

GI: Nausea, vomiting, anorexia; increased ALT, AST, bilirubin, hepatomegaly, ***hepatic necrosis,*** splenomegaly

GU: ***Oliguria, hematuria, renal damage, azotemia, renal failure, nephrotoxicity***

HEMA: ***Agranulocytosis, thrombocytopenia, leukopenia, eosinophilia,*** anemia

INTEG: ***Rash,*** burning, urticaria, dermatitis, alopecia

Contraindications: Pregnancy (D), severe renal disease, hypersensitivity to aminoglycosides

Precautions: Neonates, mild renal disease, myasthenia gravis, lactation, hearing deficits, Parkinson's disease, elderly

PHARMACOKINETICS

IM: Onset rapid, peak 1 hr

IV: Onset immediate, peak 1 hr

Plasma half-life 2-3 hr prolonged in neonates; not metabolized, excreted unchanged in urine, crosses placental barrier, poor penetration into CSF

INTERACTIONS

Increase: ototoxicity, neurotoxicity, nephrotoxicity—other aminoglycosides, amphotericin B, polymyxin, vancomycin, ethacrynic acid, furosemide, mannitol, methoxyflurane, cisplatin, cephalosporins, bacitracin, acyclovir, penicillins

---

Drug/Herb

Toxicity: lysine (large amounts)

NURSING CONSIDERATIONS
Assess:

• Weight before treatment; dosage is usually based on ideal body weight, but may be calculated on actual body weight

• I&O ratio, urinalysis daily for proteinuria, cells, casts; report sudden change in urine output

• VS during infusion; watch for hypotension, change in pulse

• IV site for thrombophlebitis, including pain, redness, swelling q30min; change site if needed; apply warm compresses to discontinued site

• Serum peak, drawn at 30-60 min after IV infusion or 60 min after IM inj, trough drawn just before next dose, peak 4-12 mcg/ml, trough 1-2 mcg/ml

• Renal impairment by securing urine for CCr testing, BUN, serum creatinine; lower dosage should be given in renal impairment (CCr <80 ml/min); monitor electrolytes: potassium, sodium, chloride, magnesium monthly, if patient is on long-term therapy

• Deafness by audiometric testing; ringing, roaring in ears; vertigo; assess hearing before, during, after treatment

• Dehydration: high specific gravity, decrease in skin turgor, dry mucous membranes, dark urine

• Overgrowth of infection: fever, malaise, redness, pain, swelling, perineal itching, diarrhea, stomatitis, change in cough, sputum

• C&S before starting treatment to identify infecting organism

• Vestibular dysfunction: nausea, vomiting, dizziness, headache; drug should be discontinued if severe

• Inj sites for redness, swelling, abscesses; use warm compresses at site
Administer:

• Drug in evenly spaced doses to maintain blood level; separate aminoglycosides and penicillins by ≥1 hr

IM route

• IM inj in large muscle mass; rotate inj sites
Nebulizer

• Give as close to q12hr apart as possible; do not use <6 hr apart

• Do not mix with dornase alfa in the nebulizer

• Have patient inhale sitting or standing, breathe normally through mouthpiece; may use noseclips
IV route

• Diluted in 50-100 ml 0.9% NaCl or D_5W (adult), infuse over 20-60 min

• Do not admix

Syringe compatibilities: Doxapram

Y-site compatibilities: Acyclovir, amifostine, amiodarone, amsacrine, aztreonam, ciprofloxacin, cisatracurium, cyclophosphamide, diltiazem, doxorubicin liposome, enalaprilat, esmolol, filgrastim, fluconazole, fludarabine, foscarnet, furosemide, granisetron, hydromorphone, IL-2, insulin (regular), labetalol, magnesium sulfate, melphalan, meperidine, midazolam, morphine, perphenazine, remifentanil, tacrolimus, teniposide, theophylline, thiotepa, tolazoline, vinorelbine, zidovudine
Perform/provide:

• Adequate fluids of 2-3 L/day unless contraindicated to prevent irritation of tubules

• Flush of IV line with NS or D_5W after infusion

• Supervised ambulation, other safety measures with vestibular dysfunction
Evaluate:

• Therapeutic response: absence of fever, draining wounds, negative C&S after treatment
Teach patient/family:

• To report headache, dizziness, symptoms of overgrowth of infection, renal impairment

• To report loss of hearing; ringing, roaring in ears; feeling of fullness in head
Nebulizer

• To use multiple therapies first, then tobramycin

Side effects: *italics* = common; ***bold italics*** = life-threatening

Treatment of overdose:
Hemodialysis; monitor serum levels of
drug

---

tobramycin ophthalmic
See Appendix C

---

tocainide (℞)
(toe-kay'nide)
Tonocard
Func. class.: Antidysrhythmic (Class
Ib)
Chem. class.: Lidocaine analog

Action: Produces dose-dependent decreases in sodium and potassium conduction, thereby decreasing the excitability of myocardial cells; does not affect
heart rate or B/P
Uses: Life-threatening ventricular dysrhythmias (multifocal/unifocal PVCs),
ventricular tachycardia

DOSAGE AND ROUTES
• *Adult:* **PO** 400 mg q8h, may increase
to 1.2-1.8 g/day in divided doses q8-12h
Available forms: Tabs 400, 600 mg

SIDE EFFECTS

CNS: Headache, dizziness, involuntary
movement, confusion, psychosis, restlessness, irritability, paresthesias, tremors, *seizures*
CV: Hypotension, bradycardia, angina,
PVCs, *heart block, cardiovascular
collapse, sinus arrest, CHF,* chest
pain, tachycardia, prodysrhythmia
EENT: Tinnitus, blurred vision, hearing
loss
GI: Nausea, vomiting, anorexia, diarrhea,
hepatitis
*HEMA: Blood dyscrasias: leukope-
nia, agranulocytosis, hypoplastic
anemia, thrombocytopenia, bone
marrow depression*
INTEG: Rash, urticaria, lupus, alopecia,
sweating
RESP: Dyspnea, *respiratory depres-*
sion, pulmonary fibrosis, pulmonary edema, interstitial pneumonitis
pneumonia
Contraindications: Hypersensitivity
to amides, severe heart block
Precautions: Pregnancy (C), lactation,
children, renal disease, hepatic disease,
CHF, pulmonary depression, myasthenia
gravis, blood dyscrasias, hypokalemia,
atrial flutter/fibrillation, elderly

PHARMACOKINETICS
PO: Peak 0.5-3 hr; half-life 10-17 hr;
metabolized by liver, excreted in urine,
40% unchanged

INTERACTIONS
Increase: tocainide effects—metoprolol
Decrease: tocainide effects—cimeti-
dine, rifampin
Drug/Herb
Increase: toxicity, death—aconite
Increase: effect—aloe, broom, chronic
buckthorn use, cascara sagrada (chronic
use), Chinese rhubarb, figwort, fumitory,
goldenseal, kudzu, licorice
Increase: serotonin effect—horehound
Decrease: effect—coltsfoot
Drug/Lab Test
Increase: CPK
False positive: ANA titer

NURSING CONSIDERATIONS
Assess:
⚠ Chest x-ray film, pulmonary function
tests, hepatic enzymes during treatment,
monitor for lung sounds, sputum, SOB
after 3-18 wk
• CBC, with differential and platelet
count during beginning treatment and
q3mo
• I&O ratio; check for decreasing output
• Blood levels (therapeutic level 4-10
mcg/ml)
• B/P continuously for fluctuations
• Lung fields; bilateral crackles may
occur in CHF patient
• Increased respiration, increased
pulse; drug should be discontinued
• Toxicity: fine tremors, dizziness

⚠ Safety alert   *"Tall Man" lettering

• Blood dyscrasias: fatigue, sore throat, fever, bruising
• Cardiac status, respiration: rate, rhythm, character

Administer:
• With meals to decrease GI symptoms

Evaluate:
• Therapeutic response: decreased dysrhythmia

Teach patient/family:
• Of reason for medication and expected results
• Method for taking pulse at home and what to report to prescriber
• To avoid hazardous activities until drug response is known; dizziness, confusion, sedation may occur
• To use a bracelet or other emergency ID indicating medications taken, condition, and prescriber's name and phone number
• To report bleeding, bruising, respiratory symptoms, chills, fever, sore throat to prescriber

Treatment of overdose: O_2, artificial ventilation, ECG; administer DOPamine for circulatory depression, diazepam or thiopental for convulsions

---

tolcapone (℞)
(toll′cah′pone)
Tasmar
Func. class.: Antiparkinson agent
Chem. class.: Catecholamine inhibitor (comt)

Action: Selective, reversible inhibitor of catecholamine; used as adjunct to levodopa/carbidopa therapy
Uses: Parkinson's disease

DOSAGE AND ROUTES
• *Adult:* PO 100-200 mg tid, with levodopa/carbidopa therapy; max 600 mg/day, discontinue if no benefit in 3 wk
Renal dose
• *Adult:* PO Use 100 mg tid or less
Available forms: Tabs 100, 200 mg

SIDE EFFECTS
CNS: Dystonia, dyskinesia, dreaming, *fatigue, headache, confusion,* psychosis, hallucination, dizziness
CV: Orthostatic hypotension, chest pain, hypotension
EENT: Cataract, eye inflammation
GI: Nausea, vomiting, anorexia, abdominal distress, diarrhea, constipation, *fatal liver failure,* increased LFTs
GU: UTI, urine discoloration, uterine tumor, micturition disorder, hematuria
HEMA: **Hemolytic anemia, leukopenia, agranulocytosis**
INTEG: Sweating, alopecia
Contraindications: Hypersensitivity
Precautions: Pregnancy (C), renal disease, cardiac disease, hepatic disease, hypertension, asthma, lactation

PHARMACOKINETICS
Rapidly absorbed, peak 2 hr, protein binding 99%, extensively metabolized, half-life 2-3 hr, excreted in urine (60%), feces (40%)

INTERACTIONS
May influence pharmacokinetics of α-methyldopa, DOBUTamine, apomorphine, isoproterenol
Inhibition of normal catecholamine metabolism: MAOIs, MAO-B inhibitor may be used

Drug/Herb
Decrease: effect—kava

NURSING CONSIDERATIONS
Assess:
• Hepatic studies: AST, ALT, alk phosphatase, LDH, bilirubin, CBC, monitor ALT, AST q2wk × 1 yr, then q4wk × 6 mo, and q8wk thereafter; if LFTs are elevated, this drug should not be used
• Involuntary movements in parkinsonism: akinesia, tremors, staggering gait, muscle rigidity, drooling
• B/P, respiration during initial treatment; hypo/hypertension should be reported

---

• Mental status: affect, mood, behavioral changes

Administer:

• Within 1 hr before or 2 hr after food PO tid with levodopa/carbidopa therapy, only to be used if levodopa/carbidopa does not provide satisfactory result

Evaluate:

• Therapeutic response: decrease in akathisia, increased mood

Teach patient/family:

• To change positions slowly to prevent orthostatic hypotension

• That urine, sweat may change color

• That food taken within 1 hr ac or 2 hr pc decreases action of drug by 20%

• To report signs of hepatic injury: clay-colored stools, jaundice, fatigue, appetite loss, lethargy

• To report nausea, vomiting, anorexia

---

tolnaftate topical
See Appendix C

---

tolterodine (℞)
(toll-tehr′oh-deen)
Detrol, Detrol LA
Func. class.: Overactive bladder product
Chem. class.: Muscarinic receptor antagonist

Action: Relaxes smooth muscles in urinary tract by inhibiting acetylcholine at postganglionic sites

Uses: Overactive bladder (urinary frequency, urgency), urinary incontinence

DOSAGE AND ROUTES

• *Adult and elderly:* **PO** 2 mg bid, hepatic disease 1 mg bid; 4 mg daily, may decrease to 2 mg if needed, max 4 mg/day

Renal dose

• *Adult:* **PO** CCr ≤30 ml/min reduce by 50%

Available forms: Tabs 1, 2 mg; cap, ext rel 2, 4 mg

SIDE EFFECTS

CNS: Anxiety, paresthesia, fatigue, *dizziness,* headache
CV: Chest pain, hypertension
EENT: Vision abnormalities, xerophthalmia
GI: *Nausea, vomiting, anorexia,* abdominal pain, constipation, dry mouth, dyspepsia
GU: Dysuria, urinary retention, frequency, UTI
INTEG: Rash, pruritus
RESP: Bronchitis, cough, pharyngitis, URI

Contraindications: Hypersensitivity, uncontrolled narrow-angle glaucoma, urinary retention, gastric retention

Precautions: Pregnancy (C), lactation, children, renal disease, hepatic disease, controlled narrow-angle glaucoma

PHARMACOKINETICS

Rapidly absorbed, highly protein bound, extensively metabolized, excreted in urine/feces

INTERACTIONS

Increase: action of tolterodine—antiretroviral protease inhibitors, macrolide antiinfectives, azole antifungals
Increase: anticholinergic effect—antimuscarinics
Increase: urinary frequency—diuretics

Drug/Food
Food increases the bioavailability of tolterodine

NURSING CONSIDERATIONS

Assess:

• Urinary patterns: distention, nocturia, frequency, urgency, incontinence

• Allergic reactions: rash; if this occurs, drug should be discontinued

Evaluate:

• Urinary status: dysuria, frequency, nocturia, incontinence

Teach patient/family:

• To avoid hazardous activities; dizziness may occur

---

topiramate (℞)

(toh-pire'ah-mate)

Topamax

Func. class.: Anticonvulsant, miscellaneous

Chem. class.: Monosaccharide derivative

Action: Mechanism of action unknown; may prevent seizure spread as opposed to an elevation of seizure threshold

Uses: Partial seizures in adults and children 2-16 yr old; tonic-clonic seizures; seizures in Lennox-Gastaut syndrome

Investigational uses: Cluster headache, infantile spasms

DOSAGE AND ROUTES

Adjunctive therapy

• *Adult:* **PO** 25-50 mg/day initially, titrate by 25-50 mg/wk, up to 400 mg/day in 2 divided doses

Renal dose

• CCr <70 ml/min give ½ dose

Available forms: Tabs 25, 100, 200 mg; sprinkle cap 15, 25 mg

SIDE EFFECTS

CNS: Dizziness, fatigue, cognitive disorder, insomnia, anxiety, depression, paresthesia

EENT: Diplopia, vision abnormality

GI: Diarrhea, anorexia, nausea, dyspepsia, abdominal pain, constipation, dry mouth

GU: Breast pain, dysmenorrhea, menstrual disorder

INTEG: Rash

MISC: Weight loss, leukopenia

RESP: URI, pharyngitis

Contraindications: Hypersensitivity

Precautions: Pregnancy (C), hepatic, renal disease, acute myopia, secondary angle closure glaucoma, lactation, children

PHARMACOKINETICS

Well absorbed, terminal half-life 19-25 hr; excreted in urine (55%-97% unchanged), crosses placenta, excreted in breast milk, protein binding (9%-17%); steady state 4 days

INTERACTIONS

Kidney stones: carbonic anhydrase inhibitors

Increase: CNS depression—alcohol, CNS depressants

Increase: topiramate levels—metformin

Decrease: levels of oral contraceptives, digoxin, valproic acid

Decrease: topiramate levels—phenytoin, carbamazepine, valproic acid

Drug/Herb

Increase: effect—gingko

Decrease: effect—ginseng, santonica

NURSING CONSIDERATIONS

Assess:

• Renal studies: urinalysis, BUN, urine creatinine q3mo; symptoms of renal colic

• Hepatic studies: ALT, AST, bilirubin if on long-term treatment

• CBC during long-term therapy

• Description of seizures: location, type, duration, aura

• Mental status: mood, sensorium, affect, behavioral changes; if mental status changes, notify prescriber

• Body weight, evidence of cognitive disorder

Administer:

• Swallow tabs whole; do not break, crush, or chew tabs; very bitter

• May take without regard to meals

• Sprinkle cap can be given whole or opened and sprinkled on soft food; do not chew

Perform/provide:

• Storage at room temperature away from heat and light

• Assistance with ambulation during early part of treatment; dizziness occurs

• Seizure precautions: padded side rails, move objects that may harm patient

T

Evaluate:
• Therapeutic response: decreased seizure activity

Teach patient/family:
• To carry emergency ID stating patient's name, drugs taken, condition, prescriber's name, phone number
• To avoid driving, other activities that require alertness
• Not to discontinue medication quickly after long-term use
• To notify prescriber immediately of blurred vision, periorbital pain
• To maintain adequate fluid intake
• To use nonhormonal contraceptive; effect of oral contraceptives is decreased

---

⚠ High Alert

topotecan
(toh-poh-tee'kan)
Hycamtin
Func. class.: Antineoplastic hormone
Chem. class.: Semisynthetic derivative of camptothecin (topoisomerase inhibitor)

Action: Antitumor drug with topoisomerase I–inhibitory activity topoisomerase I relieves torsional strain in DNA by causing single-strand breaks; causes double-strand DNA damage
Uses: Metastatic carcinoma of the ovary after failure of traditional chemotherapy, relapsed small cell lung cancer

DOSAGE AND ROUTES
• *Adult:* **IV INF** 1.5 mg/m² over 30 min daily × 5 days starting on day 1 of a 21-day course × 4 courses; may be reduced to 0.25 mg/m² for subsequent courses if severe neutropenia occurs
Renal dose
• *Adult:* **IV** CCr 20-39 ml/min 0.75 mg/m²/day × 5 days starting on day 1 of a 21 day course
Available forms: Lyophilized powder for inj 4 mg

SIDE EFFECTS
CNS: Arthralgia, asthenia, headache, myalgia, pain
GI: Abdominal pain, constipation, diarrhea, obstruction, nausea, stomatitis, vomiting; increased ALT, AST; anorexia
*HEMA: **Neutropenia, leukopenia, thrombocytopenia, anemia, sepsis***
INTEG: Total alopecia
RESP: Dyspnea
Contraindications: Pregnancy (D), hypersensitivity, lactation, severe bone marrow depression
Precautions: Children

PHARMACOKINETICS
Rapidly and completely absorbed; excreted in urine and feces as metabolites; half-life 6 hr, geriatric half-life 8 hr; 94% bound to plasma proteins

INTERACTIONS
Increase: duration of neutropenia when used with G-CSF
Increase: myelosuppression when used with cisplatin

NURSING CONSIDERATIONS
Assess:
• Hepatic studies: AST, ALT, alk phosphatase, which may be elevated
• For CNS symptoms: drowsiness, confusion, depression, anxiety
• CBC, differential, platelet count weekly; withhold drug if WBC is <3500/mm³ or platelet count is <100,000/mm³; notify prescriber of these results; drug should be discontinued
• Buccal cavity q8h for dryness, sores or ulceration, white patches, oral pain, bleeding, dysphagia
• GI symptoms: frequency of stools, cramping
• Signs of dehydration: rapid respiration, poor skin turgor, decreased urine output, dry skin, restlessness, weakness
Administer:
• Changing of IV site q48h

Perform/provide:

• Increased fluid intake to 2-3 L/day to prevent dehydration, unless contraindicated

• Rinsing of mouth tid-qid with water, club soda; brushing of teeth bid-tid with soft brush or cotton-tipped applicator for stomatitis; use unwaxed dental floss

• Nutritious diet with iron, vit K supplements, low fiber, few dairy products

Evaluate:

• Therapeutic response: decreased tumor size, spread of malignancy

Teach patient/family:

• That total alopecia may occur; hair grows back, but is different in color and texture

• To avoid foods with citric acid or hot or rough texture if stomatitis is present; to drink adequate fluids

• To report stomatitis; any bleeding, white spots, ulcerations in mouth; tell patient to examine mouth daily; report symptoms

• To report signs of anemia: fatigue, headache, faintness, shortness of breath, irritability

• To use effective contraception during treatment, avoid breastfeeding

---

toremifene (℞)

(tor-em′ih-feen)

Fareston

Func. class.: Antineoplastic

Chem. class.: Antiestrogen hormone

Action: Inhibits cell division by binding to cytoplasmic estrogen receptors; resembles normal cell complex but inhibits DNA synthesis and estrogen response of target tissue

Uses: Advanced breast carcinoma not responsive to other therapy in estrogen-receptor-positive patients (usually postmenopausal)

DOSAGE AND ROUTES

• *Adult:* **PO** 60 mg daily

Available forms: Tabs 60 mg

SIDE EFFECTS

CNS: Hot flashes, headache, lightheadedness, depression

*CV: **CHF, MI, pulmonary embolism,*** chest pain

EENT: Ocular lesions, retinopathy, corneal opacity, blurred vision (high doses)

GI: Nausea, vomiting, altered taste (anorexia)

GU: Vaginal bleeding, pruritus vulvae

*HEMA: **Thrombocytopenia, leukopenia***

INTEG: Rash, alopecia

META: Hypercalcemia

Contraindications: Pregnancy (D), hypersensitivity, history of thromboembolism

Precautions: Leukopenia, thrombocytopenia, lactation, cataracts

PHARMACOKINETICS

PO: Peak 3 hr, excreted primarily in feces

INTERACTIONS

May increase the effect of warfarin

Drug/Lab Test

Increase: serum calcium

NURSING CONSIDERATIONS

Assess:

• CBC, differential, platelet count qwk; withhold drug if WBC is <3500/mm^3 or platelet count is <100,000/mm^3; notify prescriber

• Bleeding: hematuria, guaiac, bruising, petechiae, mucosa or orifices q8h

• Effects of alopecia on body image; discuss feelings about body changes

⚠ Symptoms indicating severe allergic reactions: rash, pruritus, urticaria, purpuric skin lesions, itching, flushing

Administer:

• Antacid before oral agent; give drug after evening meal, before bedtime

• Antiemetic 30-60 min before giving drug to prevent vomiting

Perform/provide:

• Liquid diet, if needed, including cola, Jell-O; dry toast or crackers may be

---

Side effects: *italics* = common; ***bold italics*** = life-threatening

added if patient is not nauseated or vomiting

• Increase fluid intake to 2-3 L/day to prevent dehydration

• Nutritious diet with iron, vitamin supplements as ordered

• Storage in light-resistant container at room temperature

Evaluate:

• Therapeutic response: decreased tumor size, spread of malignancy

Teach patient/family:

• To report any complaints, side effects to prescriber

• That vaginal bleeding, pruritus, hot flashes are reversible after discontinuing treatment

• To report immediately decreased visual acuity, which may be irreversible; stress need for routine eye exams; care providers should be told about tamoxifen therapy

• To report vaginal bleeding immediately

• That tumor flare—increase in size of tumor, increased bone pain—may occur and will subside rapidly; may take analgesics for pain

• That premenopausal women must use mechanical birth control because ovulation may be induced

• That hair may be lost during treatment; a wig or hairpiece may make patient feel better; new hair may be different in color, texture

---

torsemide (℞)

(tor′suh-mide)

Demadex

Func. class.: Loop diuretic

Chem. class.: Sulfonamide derivative

Action: Acts on loop of Henle, proximal, distal tubule by inhibiting absorption of chloride, sodium, water

Uses: Treatment of hypertension and edema in CHF, hepatic disease, renal disease

DOSAGE AND ROUTES

CHF

• *Adult:* **PO/IV** 10-20 mg/day, may increase as needed up to 200 mg/day

Chronic renal failure

• *Adult:* **PO/IV** 20 mg/day, may increase up to 200 mg/day

Hepatic cirrhosis

• *Adult:* **PO/IV** 5-10 mg/day may increase as needed up to 40 mg/day

Hypertension

• *Adult:* **PO** 5 mg/day may increase to 10 mg/day

Available forms: Tabs 5, 10, 20, 100 mg; inj 10 mg/ml

SIDE EFFECTS

CNS: Headache, dizziness, asthenia, insomnia, nervousness

CV: Orthostatic hypotension, chest pain, ECG changes, ***circulatory collapse,*** ventricular tachycardia

EENT: Loss of hearing, ear pain, tinnitus, blurred vision

ELECT: Hypokalemia, hypochloremic alkalosis, hypomagnesemia, hypocalcemia, hyponatremia, metabolic alkalosis

ENDO: Hyperglycemia, hyperuricemia

GI: Nausea, diarrhea, dyspepsia, GI hemorrhage, rectal bleeding, cramps

GU: Polyuria, **renal failure,** glycosuria

INTEG: Rash, photosensitivity

MS: Cramps, stiffness

RESP: Rhinitis, cough increase

Contraindications: Hypersensitivity to sulfonamides, anuria, hypovolemia, infants, lactation, electrolyte depletion

Precautions: Pregnancy (B), diabetes mellitus, dehydration, severe renal disease

PHARMACOKINETICS

PO: Rapidly absorbed; duration 6 hr; excreted in urine, feces, breast milk; crosses placenta; half-life 2-4 hr, plasma protein binding 97%-99%

⚠ Safety alert *"Tall Man" lettering

INTERACTIONS

Incompatible with acidic sol, vit C, corticosteroids, diphenhydrAMINE, DOBUTamine, esmolol, epINEPHrine, gentamicin, meperidine, milrinone, netilmicin, norepinephrine, reserpine, spironolactone, tetracyclines in sol

Incompatible with any drug in syringe

Increase: toxicity—lithium, nondepolarizing skeletal muscle relaxants, digitalis

Increase: action of antihypertensives, oral anticoagulants, nitrates

Increase: ototoxicity—aminoglycosides, cisplatin, vancomycin

Decrease: antihypertensive effect of torsemide—indomethacin, metolazone

Drug/Herb

Severe photosensitivity: St. John's wort

Increase: effect—aloe, cucumber, dandelion, horsetail, pumpkin, Queen Anne's lace

Increase: hypotension khella

Drug/Lab Test

Interference: GTT

NURSING CONSIDERATIONS

Assess:

• Hearing when giving high doses

• Weight, I&O daily to determine fluid loss; effect of drug may be decreased if used daily

• Rate, depth, rhythm of respiration, effect of exertion

• B/P lying, standing; postural hypotension may occur

• Electrolytes: K, Na, Cl; include BUN, blood glucose, CBC, serum creatinine, blood pH, ABGs, uric acid, Ca, Mg

• Glucose in urine of diabetic

• Signs and symptoms of metabolic alkalosis: drowsiness, restlessness

• Signs and symptoms of hypokalemia: postural hypotension, malaise, fatigue, tachycardia, leg cramps, weakness

• Rashes, temp elevation daily

• Confusion, especially in elderly; take safety precautions if needed

Administer:

• In AM to avoid interference with sleep if using drug as a diuretic

• Potassium replacement if potassium <3 mg/dl

• With food or milk if nausea occurs; absorption may be decreased slightly

Evaluate:

• Therapeutic response: improvement in edema of feet, legs, sacral area daily if medication is being used in CHF

Teach patient/family:

• To rise slowly from lying, sitting position

• To recognize adverse reactions: muscle cramps, weakness, nausea, dizziness, tinnitus

• To take with food or milk for GI symptoms; to limit alcohol use

• To take early in day to prevent nocturia

Treatment of overdose: Lavage if taken orally; monitor electrolytes, administer dextrose in saline; monitor hydration, CV, renal status

---

trace elements (℞)

Concentrated Multiple Trace Elements, ConTE-PAK-4, M.T.E.-4, M.T.E.-4 Concentrated, M.T.E.-5, M.T.E.-5 Concentrated, M.T.E.-6, M.T.E.-6 Concentrated, M.T.E.-7, MulTE-PAK-4, MulTE-PAK-5, Multiple Trace Element, Multiple Trace Element Neonatal, Multiple Trace Element Pediatric, Neotrace 4, PedTE-PAK-4, Pedtrace-4, P.T.E.-4, P.T.E.-5

Func. class.: Mineral supplements

T

Action: Needed for adequate absorption and synthesis of amino acids

Uses: Prevention of trace element deficiency

Side effects: *italics* = common; ***bold italics*** = life-threatening

DOSAGE AND ROUTES

Usual dosage may be given in TPN sol

Chromium
- *Adult:* IV 10-15 mcg daily
- *Child:* IV 0.14-0.20 mcg/kg/day

Copper
- *Adult:* IV 0.5-1.5 mg/day
- *Child:* IV 0.05-0.2 mg/kg/day

Iodine
- *Adult:* IV 1 mcg/kg/day

Manganese
- *Adult:* IV 1-3 mg/day

Selenium
- *Adult:* 40-120 mcg/day
- *Child:* 3 mcg/kg/day

Zinc
- *Adult:* IV 2-4 mg/day
- *Child:* IV 0.05 mg/kg/day

Available forms: Many forms available—see particular elements

SIDE EFFECTS

CHROMIUM: **Seizures, coma,** nausea, vomiting, ulcers, renal/hepatic toxicity

COPPER: Personality changes, diarrhea, weakness, photophobia, muscle weakness

IODINE: Headache, edema of eyelids, acne, metallic taste, sore mouth, running nose

MANGANESE: Incoordination, headache, irritability, lability, slurred speech, impotence

SELENIUM: Alopecia, depression, vomiting, GI cramping, nervousness, garlic smell

ZINC: Vomiting, oliguria, hypothermia, vision changes, tachycardia, jaundice, **coma**

Precautions: Pregnancy (C), hepatic, biliary disease, lactation, vomiting, diarrhea

NURSING CONSIDERATIONS

Assess:
• Trace element levels; notify prescriber if low; copper 0.07-0.15 mg/ml, zinc 0.05-0.15 mg/100 ml, manganese 4-20 mcg/100 ml, selenium 0.1-0.19 mcg/ml

• Trace element deficiency of patient receiving TPN for extended period

Administer:
• By IV infusion, often mixed with TPN solution

Evaluate:
• Therapeutic response: absence of element deficiency

---

tramadol (℞)
(tram'a-dole)
Ultram
Func. class.: Central analgesic

Do not confuse:
tramadol/Toradol

Action: Not completely understood, binds to opioid receptors, inhibits re-uptake of norepinephrine, serotonin; does not cause histamine release or affect heart rate

Uses: Management of moderate to severe pain

DOSAGE AND ROUTES

• *Adult:* PO 50-100 mg prn q4-6h; not to exceed 400 mg/day

• *Geriatric >75 years:* PO <300 mg/day in divided doses

Renal dose
• CCr <30 ml/min give q12h, max 200 mg/day

Hepatic impairment
• PO 50 mg q12h

Available forms: Tabs 50 mg

SIDE EFFECTS

CNS: Dizziness, CNS stimulation, somnolence, headache, anxiety, confusion, euphoria, **seizures,** hallucinations

CV: Vasodilation, orthostatic hypotension, tachycardia, hypertension, abnormal ECG

GI: Nausea, constipation, vomiting, dry mouth, diarrhea, abdominal pain, anorexia, flatulence, *GI bleeding*

GU: Urinary retention/frequency, menopausal symptoms, dysuria, menstrual disorder

INTEG: Pruritus, rash, urticaria, vesicles

Contraindications: Hypersensitivity, acute intoxication with any CNS depressant

Precautions: Pregnancy (C), seizure disorder, lactation, children, elderly, renal disease, hepatic disease, respiratory depression, head trauma, increased intracranial pressure, acute abdominal condition, drug abuse

PHARMACOKINETICS

Rapidly and almost completely absorbed, steady state 2 days, may cross blood-brain barrier, extensively metabolized, 30% excreted in the urine as unchanged drug

INTERACTIONS

Inhibition of norepinephrine and serotonin reuptake: MAO inhibitors, use together with caution
Increase: CNS depression—alcohol, sedatives, hypnotics, opiates
Increase: serotonin syndrome—SSRIs
Decrease: levels of tramadol—carbamazepine

Drug/Herb
Increase: CNS depression—chamomile, hops, kava, skullcap, valerian

Drug/Lab Test
Increase: Creatinine, hepatic enzymes
Decrease: Hgb

NURSING CONSIDERATIONS

Assess:
• Pain: location, type, character, give before pain becomes extreme
• I&O ratio: check for decreasing output; may indicate urinary retention
• Need for drug
• Bowel pattern; for constipation increase fluids, bulk in diet
• CNS changes: dizziness, drowsiness, hallucinations, euphoria, LOC, pupil reaction
• Allergic reactions: rash, urticaria
• For increased side effects in hepatic, renal disease

Administer:
• With antiemetic for nausea, vomiting

• When pain is beginning to return; determine dosage interval by patient response

Perform/provide:
• Storage in cool environment, protected from sunlight
• Assistance with ambulation
• Safety measures: side rails, night-light, call bell within easy reach

Evaluate:
• Therapeutic response: decrease in pain

Teach patient/family:
• To report any symptoms of CNS changes, allergic reactions
• That drowsiness, dizziness, and confusion may occur, to call for assistance
• To make position changes slowly, orthostatic hypotension may occur
• To avoid OTC medications and alcohol unless approved by prescriber

---

trandolapril (℞)
(tran-doe'la-prill)
Mavik
Func. class.: Antihypertensive
Chem. class.: Angiotension-converting enzyme inhibitor

Action: Selectively suppresses renin-angiotensin-aldosterone system; inhibits ACE; prevents conversion of angiotensin I to angiotensin II, dilates arterial and venous vessels, lowers B/P

Uses: Hypertension, heart failure, post-MI/left ventricular dysfunction post MI

DOSAGE AND ROUTES

Hypertension
• *Adult:* **PO** 1 mg/day, 2 mg/day in African-Americans, make dosage adjustment ≥wk; up to 8 mg/day

Heart failure post-MI/left ventricular dysfunction post MI
• *Adult:* **PO** 1 mg/day, titrate upward to 4 mg/day if tolerated

Renal/hepatic dose
• CCr <30 ml/min give 0.5 mg/day, may increase gradually up to 4 mg/day

Available forms: Tabs 1, 2, 4 mg

T

SIDE EFFECTS

CNS: Dizziness, syncope, paresthesias, headache, fatigue, drowsiness, depression, sleep disturbances, anxiety

CV: Hypotension, MI, palpitations, angina, TIAs, *stroke, bradycardia,* dysrhythmias

GI: Nausea, vomiting, cramps, diarrhea, constipation, pancreatitis, *dyspepsia*

GU: Proteinuria, renal failure

HEMA: Agranulocytosis, neutropenia, leukopenia, anemia

INTEG: Rash, purpura, pruritus

MISC: Hyperkalemia, hyponatremia, impotence, *myalgia, angioedema,* muscle cramps, *asthenia,* hypocalcemia, gout

RESP: Dyspnea, *cough*

Contraindications: Pregnancy (D) 2nd/3rd trimester, hypersensitivity, history of angioedema

Precautions: Pregnancy (C) 1st trimester, hyperkalemia, hepatic disease, bilateral renal stenosis, post–kidney transplant, aorta/mitral valve stenosis, cirrhosis, severe renal disease, untreated CHF, autoimmune disease, severe hypertension

PHARMACOKINETICS

PO: Peak 4-8 hr, duration 24 hr; half-life 6 h; metabolized by liver (active metabolite trandolaprilat), excreted in urine, protein binding 80%

INTERACTIONS

Effects increase: phenothiazines, diuretics

Severe hypotension: diuretics, other antihypertensives

Increase: potassium levels—salt substitutes, potassium-sparing diuretics, potassium supplements

Increase: effects of ergots, neuromuscular blocking agents, antihypertensives, hypoglycemics, barbiturates, reserpine, levodopa

Decrease: effects of trandolapril—antacids

Drug/Herb

Increase: toxicity, death—aconite

Increase: antihypertensive effect—barberry, betony, black catechu, black cohosh, bloodroot, broom, burdock, cat's claw, dandelion, goldenseal, Irish moss, Jamaican dogwood, kelp, khella, mistletoe, parsley

Increase or decrease: antihypertensive effect—astragalus, cola tree

Decrease: antihypertensive effect—coltsfoot, guarana, khat, licorice

NURSING CONSIDERATIONS

Assess:

• B/P, pulse q4h; note rate, rhythm, quality

• Electrolytes: K, Na, Cl

• Baselines in renal, hepatic studies before therapy begins

• Edema in feet, legs daily

• Skin turgor, dryness of mucous membranes for hydration status

• Symptoms of CHF: edema, dyspnea, wet crackles

Evaluate:

• Therapeutic response: decreased B/P

Teach patient/family:

• Not to use OTC (cough, cold, or allergy) products unless directed by prescriber

• To avoid sunlight or wear sunscreen for photosensitivity

• To comply with dosage schedule, even if feeling better

• To notify prescriber of mouth sores, sore throat, fever, swelling of hands or feet, irregular heartbeat, chest pain, signs of angioedema

• That excessive perspiration, dehydration, vomiting, diarrhea may lead to fall in blood pressure; consult prescriber if these occur

• That drug may cause dizziness, fainting; light-headedness may occur during 1st few days of therapy

• That drug may cause skin rash or impaired perspiration

⚠ Safety alert   *"Tall Man" lettering

• Not to discontinue drug abruptly
• To rise slowly to sitting or standing position to minimize orthostatic hypotension

---

tranylcypromine (℞)

(tran-ill-sip′roe-meen)
Parnate
Func. class.: Antidepressant-MAOI
Chem. class.: Nonhydrazine

Action: Increases concentrations of endogenous epinephrine, norepinephrine, serotonin, dopamine in storage sites in CNS by inhibition of MAO; increased concentration reduces depression
Uses: Depression, when uncontrolled by other means
Investigational uses: Bulimia, cocaine addiction, migraines, seasonal affective disorder, panic disorder

DOSAGE AND ROUTES

• *Adult:* **PO** 10 mg bid; may increase to 30 mg/day after 2 wk; up to 60 mg/day
Available forms: Tabs 10 mg

SIDE EFFECTS

CNS: Dizziness, drowsiness, confusion, headache, anxiety, tremors, stimulation, weakness, hyperreflexia, mania, insomnia, fatigue
CV: Orthostatic hypotension, hypertension, dysrhythmias, **hypertensive crisis**
EENT: Blurred vision
ENDO: **SIADH-like syndrome**
GI: Constipation, dry mouth, nausea, vomiting, *anorexia,* diarrhea, weight gain
GU: Change in libido, urinary frequency
HEMA: Anemia
INTEG: Rash, flushing, increased perspiration
Contraindications: Hypersensitivity to MAOIs, elderly, uncontrolled hypertension, CHF, severe hepatic disease, pheochromocytoma, severe renal disease, severe cardiac disease

Precautions: Pregnancy (C), suicidal patients, convulsive disorders, severe depression, schizophrenia, hyperactivity, diabetes mellitus, lactation, child <16 yr

PHARMACOKINETICS

Metabolized by liver, excreted by kidneys, crosses placenta, excreted in breast milk

INTERACTIONS

⚠ *Serotonin-syndrome:* fluoxetine, fluvoxamine, sertraline, paroxetine
⚠ *Hypertensive crisis:* tricyclics, meperidine, dibenzazepine agents, methylphenidate, dextromethorphan, nasal decongestants, sinus medications, appetite suppressants, asthma inhalants
Increase: pressor effects—guanethidine, clonidine, indirect-acting sympathomimetics (epHEDrine), busPIRone
Increase: effects of direct-acting sympathomimetics (epINEPHrine), alcohol, barbiturates, benzodiazepines, CNS depressants, levodopa, β-blockers, antidiabetics, sulfonamide, rauwolfia alkaloids, methyldopa, thiazide diuretics, sumatriptan

Drug/Herb

Hypertensive crisis: betel palm, butcher's broom, capsicum peppers, galanthamine, green tea (large amounts), guarana (large amounts), night-blooming cereus
Mania: ginseng
Serotonin syndrome: parsley

Drug/Food

Tyramine foods; avoid all

NURSING CONSIDERATIONS

Assess:

• B/P (lying, standing), pulse; if systolic B/P drops 20 mm Hg, stop drug, notify prescriber
• Blood studies: CBC, leukocytes, cardiac enzymes (long-term therapy)
• Hepatic studies: ALT, AST, bilirubin; hepatotoxicity may occur

---

Side effects: *italics* = common; ***bold italics*** = life-threatening

T

A Toxicity: increased headache, palpitation; discontinue drug immediately; prodromal signs of hypertensive crisis

• Mental status changes: mood, sensorium, affect, memory (long, short), increase in psychiatric symptoms

• Urinary retention, constipation, edema: take weight weekly

• Withdrawal symptoms: headache, nausea, vomiting, muscle pain, weakness

Administer:

• Increased fluids, bulk in diet if constipation occurs

• With food or milk for GI symptoms

• Crushed if patient is unable to swallow medication whole

• Dosage at bedtime if oversedation occurs during day

• Gum, hard candy, frequent sips of water for dry mouth

• Phentolamine for severe hypertension

• Avoid use of CNS depressants

Perform/provide:

• Cool storage in tight container

• Assistance with ambulation during beginning therapy for drowsiness/dizziness

• Safety measures including side rails

• Checking to see if PO medication swallowed

Evaluate:

• Therapeutic response: decreased depression

Teach patient/family:

• That therapeutic effects may take 48 hr-3 wk

• To avoid driving, other activities requiring alertness

• To avoid alcohol ingestion, OTC medications: cold, weight loss, hay fever, cough syrup; increased effects may occur

• Not to discontinue medication quickly after long-term use

A To avoid high-tyramine foods: cheese (aged), sour cream, yogurt, beer, wine, pickled products, liver, raisins, bananas, figs, avocados, meat tenderizers, chocolate, increased caffeine, ginseng; give complete list of tyramine foods

• To report headache, palpitation, neck stiffness

• To rise slowly to prevent postural hypotension

Treatment of overdose: Lavage, activated charcoal; monitor electrolytes, vital signs; diazepam IV, $NaHCO_3$

⚠ High Alert

trastuzumab (℞)

(tras-tuz′uh-mab)
Herceptin
Func. class.: Antineoplastic—miscellaneous
Chem. class.: Humanized monoclonal antibody

Action: DNA-derived monoclonal antibody selectively binds to extracellular portion of human epidermal growth factor receptor 2; it inhibits proliferation of cancer cells

Uses: Breast cancer; metastatic with overexpression of HER2

DOSAGE AND ROUTES

• *Adult:* **IV** 4 mg/kg given over 90 min, then maintenance 2 mg/kg given over 30 min; do not give as IV push or BOL

Available forms: Lyophilized powder 440 mg

SIDE EFFECTS

CNS: Dizziness, numbness, paresthesias, depression, insomnia, neuropathy, peripheral neuritis

*CV: **Tachycardia, CHF***

GI: Nausea, vomiting, anorexia, diarrhea

HEMA: Anemia, ***leukopenia***

INTEG: Rash, acne, herpes simplex

META: Edema, peripheral edema

MISC: Flulike symptoms; fever, headache, chills

MS: Arthralgia, bone pain

RESP: Cough, dyspnea, pharyngitis, rhinitis, sinusitis

*SYST: **Anaphylaxis, angioedema***

Contraindications: Hypersensitivity to this drug, Chinese hamster ovary cell protein
Precautions: Pregnancy (B), lactation, children, elderly, cardiac disease, anemia, leukopenia

PHARMACOKINETICS
Half-life 1.7-12 days

INTERACTIONS
Increase: chance of cardiomyopathy—anthracyclines, cyclophosphamide, avoid use

NURSING CONSIDERATIONS
Assess:
🅐 CHF and other cardiac symptoms: dyspnea, coughing; gallop; obtain a full cardiac workup including ECG, echo, MUGA
• For symptoms of infection; may be masked by drug
• CNS reaction: LOC, mental status, dizziness, confusion
🅐 For hypersensitive reactions, anaphylaxis
🅐 For infusion reactions that may be fatal: fever, chills, nausea, vomiting, pain, headache, dizziness, hypotension, discontinue drug
Administer:
• Acetaminophen as ordered to alleviate fever and headache
IV route
• After reconstituting vial with 20 ml bacteriostatic water for inj, 1.1% benzyl alcohol preserved (supplied) to yield 21 mg/ml, mark date on vial 28 days from reconstitution date, if patient is allergic to benzyl alcohol, reconstitute with sterile water for inj—use immediately
• Do not mix or dilute with other drugs or dextrose sol
Perform/provide:
• Increased fluid intake to 2-3 L/day
Evaluate:
• Therapeutic response: decrease in size of tumors

Teach patient/family:
• To take acetaminophen for fever
• To avoid hazardous tasks, since confusion, dizziness may occur
• To report signs of infection: sore throat, fever, diarrhea, vomiting
• Emotional lability is common; notify prescriber if severe or incapacitating

---

travoprost ophthalmic
See Appendix C

---

trazodone (℞)
(tray´zoe-done)
Desyrel, Desyrel Dividose, trazodone HCl, Trazon, Trialodine
Func. class.: Antidepressant—miscellaneous
Chem. class.: Triazolopyridine

Action: Selectively inhibits serotonin, norepinephrine uptake by brain, potentiates behavorial changes
Uses: Depression
Investigational uses: Chronic pain

DOSAGE AND ROUTES
• *Adult:* **PO** 150 mg/day in divided doses; may increase by 50 mg/day q3-4d, not to exceed 600 mg/day
• *Child 6-18 yr:* **PO** 1.5-2 mg/kg/day in divided dose, may increase q3-4d, up to 6 mg/kg/day
• *Geriatric:* **PO** 25-50 mg at bedtime, increase by 25-50 mg q3-7d to desired dose, usual 75-150 mg/day
Available forms: Tabs 50, 100, 150, 300 mg

SIDE EFFECTS
CNS: Dizziness, drowsiness, confusion, headache, anxiety, tremors, stimulation, weakness, insomnia, nightmares, EPS (elderly), increase in psychiatric symptoms

---

Side effects: *italics* = common; ***bold italics*** = life-threatening

*CV: Orthostatic hypotension, ECG changes, tachycardia, **hypertension**, palpitations*

EENT: Blurred vision, tinnitus, mydriasis

*GI: Diarrhea, dry mouth, nausea, vomiting, **paralytic ileus**, increased appetite, cramps, epigastric distress, jaundice, **hepatitis**, stomatitis, constipation*

*GU: Urinary retention, **acute renal failure**, priapism*

*HEMA: **Agranulocytosis, thrombocytopenia, eosinophilia, leukopenia***

INTEG: Rash, urticaria, sweating, pruritus, photosensitivity

Contraindications: Hypersensitivity to tricyclics, recovery phase of MI, convulsive disorders, prostatic hypertrophy

Precautions: Pregnancy (C), suicidal patients, severe depression, increased intraocular pressure, narrow-angle glaucoma, urinary retention, cardiac disease, hepatic disease, hyperthyroidism, electroshock therapy, elective surgery

PHARMACOKINETICS

Metabolized by liver, excreted by kidneys, feces; half-life 4.4-7.5 hr

INTERACTIONS

⚠ Hyperpyretic crisis, convulsions, hypertensive episode: MAOI (pargyline [Eutonyl])

Increase: toxicity—fluoxetine

Increase: effects of direct-acting sympathomimetics (epINEPHrine), alcohol, barbiturates, benzodiazepines, CNS depressants, digoxin, phenytoin

Decrease: effects of guanethidine, clonidine, indirect-acting sympathomimetics (epHEDrine)

Drug/Herb

Serotonin syndrome: SAM-e, St. John's wort

Increase: CNS depression—chamomile, hops, kava, lavender, skullcap, valerian

Increase: anticholinergic effect—corkwood, jimsonweed

Drug/Lab Test

Increase: Serum bilirubin, blood glucose, alk phosphatase

Decrease: VMA, 5-HIAA

False increase: Urinary catecholamines

NURSING CONSIDERATIONS

Assess:

• Pain: location, duration, intensity before and 1-2 hr after medication

• B/P (lying, standing), pulse q4h; if systolic B/P drops 20 mm Hg, hold drug, notify prescriber; take vital signs q4h in patients with cardiovascular disease

• Blood studies: CBC, leukocytes, differential, cardiac enzymes if patient is receiving long-term therapy

• Hepatic studies: AST, ALT, bilirubin

• Weight qwk; appetite may increase with drug

• ECG for flattening of T wave, bundle branch block, AV block, dysrhythmias in cardiac patients

• EPS, primarily in elderly: rigidity, dystonia, akathisia

• Mental status changes: mood, sensorium, affect, suicidal tendencies, increase in psychiatric symptoms, depression, panic

• Urinary retention, constipation; constipation most likely in children

• Withdrawal symptoms: headache, nausea, vomiting, muscle pain, weakness; not usual unless drug discontinued abruptly

• Alcohol consumption; hold dose until morning

Administer:

• Increased fluids, bulk in diet if constipation occurs, especially in elderly

• With food, milk for GI symptoms

• Dosage at bedtime for oversedation during day; may take entire dose at bedtime; elderly may not tolerate daily dosing

• Gum, hard candy, frequent sips of water for dry mouth

• Avoid use of CNS depressants

Perform/provide:

• Storage in tight, light-resistant container at room temperature

• Assistance with ambulation during beginning therapy for drowsiness/dizziness

---

⚠ Safety alert   *"Tall Man" lettering

- Safety measures, including side rails, primarily for elderly
- Checking to see if PO medication swallowed

Evaluate:
- Therapeutic response: decreased depression

Teach patient/family:
- That therapeutic effects may take 2-3 wk
- To use caution in driving, other activities requiring alertness because of drowsiness, dizziness, blurred vision
- To avoid alcohol ingestion
- Not to discontinue medication quickly after long-term use; may cause nausea, headache, malaise
- To report urinary retention immediately
- To wear sunscreen or large hat, since photosensitivity occurs
- Signs of suicidal ideation

Treatment of overdose: ECG monitoring; induce emesis; lavage, activated charcoal; administer anticonvulsant

---

treprostinil (℞)
(treh-prah′stin-ill)
Remodulin
Func. class.: Antiplatelet agent
Chem. class.: Tricyclic benzidine prostacyclin analog

Action: Direct vasodilation of pulmonary, systemic arterial vascular beds, inhibition of platelet aggregation
Uses: Pulmonary arterial hypertension (PAH) NYHA class II through IV

DOSAGE AND ROUTES

- *Adult:* SUBCUT INF 1.25 ng/kg/min by **CONT INF**, may reduce to 0.625 mg if not tolerated; may increase by 1.25 ng/kg/min qwk for first 4 wk, then 2.5 ng/kg/min/wk for remainder of infusion
Hepatic dose
- *Adult:* SUBCUT INF 0.625 ng/kg ideal body weight/min and increase cautiously

Available forms: Inj 1, 2.5, 5, 10 mg/ml

SIDE EFFECTS

CNS: Dizziness, headache
CV: Vasodilation, hypotension, edema
GI: Nausea, *diarrhea*
INTEG: Rash, pruritus
OTHER: Jaw pain
SYST: Infusion site reactions, infusion site pain
Contraindications: Hypersensitivity
Precautions: Pregnancy (B), past hepatic disease, renal disease, elderly, lactation, children, thromboembolic disease

PHARMACOKINETICS

Metabolized by liver, excreted in urine, feces; terminal half-life 2-4 hr, 90% protein binding

INTERACTIONS

Excessive hypotension: diuretics, antihypertensives, vasodilators
Increased bleeding tendencies—anticoagulants, aspirin

NURSING CONSIDERATIONS
Assess:
- Hepatic studies: AST, ALT, bilirubin, creatinine (long-term therapy)
⚠ Blood studies: CBC; CBC q2wk × 3 mo, Hct, Hgb, PT (long-term therapy)
⚠ Bleed time baseline and throughout; levels may be 2-5 × normal limit
Administer:
- By continuous infusion, SUBCUT or surgically placed indwelling central venous catheter using infusion pump
Evaluate:
- Therapeutic response: decreased pulmonary arterial hypertension (PAH)
Teach patient/family:
- That blood work will be necessary during treatment
- To report side effects such as diarrhea, skin rashes
- That therapy will be needed for prolonged periods of time, sometimes years

T

• To prevent infection, aseptic technique must be used in preparing and administration of treprostinil

tretinoin (vit A acid, retinoic acid) (℞)

(tret′i-noyn)
Retin-A, Stievaa ✦, Tretinoin LF, IV, Vesanoid
Func. class.: Vit A acid, acne product; antineoplastic (miscellaneous)
Chem. class.: Tretinoin derivative

Action: Decreases cohesiveness of follicular epithelium, decreases microcomedone formation (TOP); induces maturation of acute promyelocytic leukemia, exact action is unknown (PO)
Uses: Acne vulgaris (grades 1-3) (TOP); (PO) acute promyelocytic leukemia, facial wrinkles, photoaging
Investigational uses: Acne rosacea, actinic keratosis, ichthyosis, Kaposi's sarcoma, keloids, keratosis follicularis, melasma

DOSAGE AND ROUTES

• *Adult and child:* **TOP** cleanse area, apply at bedtime; cover lightly
Promyelocytic leukemia
• *Adult:* **PO** 45 mg/m²/day given as 2 evenly divided doses until remission, discontinue treatment 30 days after remission or 90 days of treatment, whichever is first
Available forms: Cream 0.01%, 0.05%; gel 0.01%, 0.025%; liquid 0.05%; caps 10 mg

SIDE EFFECTS

Oral
CNS: *Headache, fever, sweating*
GI: *Nausea, vomiting, **hemorrhage**, abdominal pain, diarrhea, constipation, dyspepsia, distention, hepatitis*
INTEG: (TOP) Rash, stinging, warmth, redness, erythema, blistering, crusting, peeling, contact dermatitis, hypopigmentation, hyperpigmentation
Contraindications: Pregnancy (D) (PO), hypersensitivity to retinoids or sensitivity to parabens
Precautions: Pregnancy (C) (TOP), lactation, eczema, sunburn

PHARMACOKINETICS
TOP: Poor systemic absorption

INTERACTIONS
Use with caution: medicated, abrasive soaps, cleansers that have drying effect, products with high concentrations of alcohol astringents (TOP)
Increase: peeling—medication containing agents such as sulfur, benzoyl peroxide, resorcinol, salicylic acid (TOP)
Increase: plasma concentrations of tretinoin—ketoconazole (oral)
Increase: ICP, risk of pseudotumor cerebri—tetracyclines, do not use together
Increase: photosensitivity—retinoids, quinolones, phenothiazines, sulfonamides, sulfonylureas, thiazide diuretics

NURSING CONSIDERATIONS
Assess:
Topical
• Area of body involved, what helps or aggravates condition; cysts, dryness, itching; lesions may worsen at beginning of treatment
Oral
• Hepatic function, coagulation, hematologic parameters, also cholesterol, triglyceride
Administer:
Topical
• Once daily before bedtime; cover area lightly using gauze; use gloves to apply
Perform/provide:
Topical
• Storage at room temperature
• Hand washing after application
Evaluate:
• Therapeutic response: decrease in size and number of lesions

---

A Safety alert   *"Tall Man" lettering

Teach patient/family:
Topical

• To avoid application on normal skin, getting cream in eyes, nose, other mucous membranes

• To avoid sunlight, sunlamps, or use protective clothing, sunscreen

• That treatment may cause warmth, stinging, dryness, peeling will occur

• That cosmetics may be used over drug; not to use shaving lotions

• That rash may occur during first 1-3 wk of therapy

• That drug does not cure condition; only relieves symptoms

• That therapeutic results may be seen in 2-3 wk but may not be optimal until after 6 wk

---

triamcinolone (℞)

(trye-am-sin'oh-lone)
Amcort, Aristocort, Aristocort Forte, Aristocort Intralesional, Aristospan Intra-Articular, Aristospan Intralesional, Articulose L.A., Atolone, Azmacort, Cenocort A-40, Cenocort Forte, Kenacort, Kenaject-40, Kenalog, Kenalog-10, Kenalog-40, Tac-3, Tac-40, Triam-A, triamcinolone, triamcinolone acetonide, Triam Forte, Triamolone 40, Triamonide 40, Tri-Kort, Trilog, Trilone, Trisoject

Func. class.: Corticosteroid, synthetic

Chem. class.: Glucocorticoid, intermediate-acting

Action: Decreases inflammation by suppression of migration of polymorphonuclear leukocytes, fibroblasts, reversal of increased capillary permeability and lysosomal stabilization

Uses: Severe inflammation, immunosuppression, neoplasms, asthma (steroid dependent), collagen, respiratory, dermatologic disorders

DOSAGE AND ROUTES

• *Adult:* **PO** 4-12 mg/day in divided doses daily-qid; **IM** 40 mg qwk (acetonide, or diacetate), 5-48 mg into neoplasms (diacetate, acetonide), 2-40 mg into joint or soft tissue (diacetate, acetonide), 0.5 mg/in^2 of affected intralesional skin (hexacetonide), 2-20 mg into joint or soft tissue (hexacetonide)

• *Child:* **PO** 117 mcg/kg/day in divided doses

Asthma

• *Adult:* **INH** 2 tid-qid, not to exceed 16 **INH**/day

• *Child 6-12 yr:* **INH** 1-2 tid-qid, not to exceed 12 **INH**/day

Available forms: Tabs 1, 2, 4, 8 mg; syr 2 mg/5 ml, 4.85 mg/5 ml; inj 25, 40 mg/ml diacetate; inj 3, 10, 40 mg/ml acetonide; inj 20, 5 mg/ml hexacetonide; aerosol actuation/100 mcg (acetonide)

SIDE EFFECTS

CNS: Depression, flushing, sweating, headache, mood changes
*CV: Hypertension, **circulatory collapse, thrombophlebitis, embolism,** tachycardia, edema
EENT: Fungal infections, increased intraocular pressure, blurred vision
*GI: Diarrhea, nausea, abdominal distention, **GI hemorrhage,** increased appetite, **pancreatitis**
*HEMA: **Thrombocytopenia***
INTEG: Acne, poor wound healing, ecchymosis, petechiae
MS: Fractures, osteoporosis, weakness

Contraindications: Psychosis, hypersensitivity, idiopathic thrombocytopenia, acute glomerulonephritis, amebiasis, fungal infections, nonasthmatic bronchial disease, child <2 yr, AIDS, TB, adrenal insufficiency

Precautions: Pregnancy (C), diabetes mellitus, glaucoma, osteoporosis, seizure disorders, ulcerative colitis, CHF, myasthenia gravis, renal disease, esophagitis,

T

Side effects: *italics* = common; ***bold italics*** = life-threatening

peptic ulcer, lactation, acne, cataracts, coagulopathy

PHARMACOKINETICS

PO/IM: Peak 1-2 hr, half-life 2-5 hr

INTERACTIONS

Increase: side effects—alcohol, salicylates, indomethacin, amphotericin B, digitalis, cycloSPORINE, diuretics

Increase: action of triamcinolone—salicylates, estrogens, indomethacin, oral contraceptives, ketoconazole, macrolide antiinfectives

Decrease: action of triamcinolone—cholestyramine, colestipol, barbiturates, rifampin, epHEDrine, phenytoin, theophylline

Decrease: effects of anticoagulants, anticonvulsants, antidiabetics, ambenonium, neostigmine, isoniazid, toxoids, vaccines, anticholinesterases, salicylates, somatrem

Drug/Herb

Hypokalemia: aloe, buckthorn, cascara, Chinese rhubarb, senna

Drug/Lab Test

Increase: Cholesterol, sodium, blood glucose, uric acid, calcium, urine glucose

Decrease: Ca, K, T_4, T_3, thyroid ^{131}I uptake test, urine 17-OHCS, 17-KS, PBI

False negative: Skin allergy tests

NURSING CONSIDERATIONS

Assess:

• Potassium, blood glucose, urine glucose while on long-term therapy; hypokalemia and hyperglycemia

• Weight daily; notify prescriber if weekly gain >5 lb

• B/P q4h, pulse; notify prescriber if chest pain occurs

• I&O ratio; be alert for decreasing urinary output, increasing edema

• Plasma cortisol levels during long-term therapy (normal level: 138-635 nmol/L SI units when drawn at 8 AM)

• Infection: increased temp, WBC, even after withdrawal of medication; drug masks infection

• Potassium depletion: paresthesias, fatigue, nausea, vomiting, depression, polyuria, dysrhythmias, weakness

• Edema, hypertension, cardiac symptoms

• Mental status: affect, mood, behavioral changes, aggression

Administer:

• After shaking susp (parenteral)

• Titrated dose; use lowest effective dose

• IM inj deep in large muscle mass; rotate sites; avoid deltoid; use 21G needle

• In one dose in AM to prevent adrenal suppression; avoid SUBCUT administration; may damage tissue

• With food or milk to decrease GI symptoms, tablet may be crushed

Perform/provide:

• Assistance with ambulation for patient with bone tissue disease to prevent fractures

• Use of spacer device for elderly patients with inhaler

Evaluate:

• Therapeutic response: ease of respirations, decreased inflammation

Teach patient/family:

• That emergency ID as steroid user should be carried

• To notify prescriber if therapeutic response decreases; dosage adjustment may be needed

• Not to discontinue abruptly; adrenal crisis can result

• To avoid OTC products: salicylates, alcohol in cough products, cold preparations unless directed by prescriber

• About cushingoid symptoms

• The symptoms of adrenal insufficiency: nausea, anorexia, fatigue, dizziness, dyspnea, weakness, joint pain

---

triamcinolone nasal agent
See Appendix C

---

triamcinolone topical
See Appendix C

triamcinolone
(topical-oral) (otc)
(trye-am-sin'oh-lone)
Kenalog in Orabase, Oralone
Dental
Func. class.: Topical anesthetic
Chem. class.: Synthetic fluorinated
adrenal corticosteroid

Action: Binds with steroid receptors,
decreases inflammation
Uses: Oral pain

DOSAGE AND ROUTES
• *Adult and child:* **TOP** press ¼ inch
into affected area until film appears,
repeat bid-tid
Available forms: Paste 0.1%

SIDE EFFECTS
INTEG: Rash, irritation, sensitization
Contraindications: Hypersensitivity,
infants <1 yr, application to large areas,
presence of fungal, viral, or bacterial
infections of mouth or throat
Precautions: Pregnancy (C), child <6
yr, sepsis, denuded skin

NURSING CONSIDERATIONS
Assess:
• Allergy: rash, irritation, reddening,
swelling
• Infection: if affected area is infected,
do not apply
Administer:
• After cleansing oral cavity after meals
Evaluate:
• Therapeutic response: absence of pain
in affected area
Teach patient/family:
• To report rash, irritation, redness,
swelling
• How to apply paste

triamterene (℞)
(trye-am'ter-een)
Dyrenium
Func. class.: Potassium-sparing
diuretic
Chem. class.: Pteridine derivative

Action: Acts on distal tubule to inhibit
reabsorption of sodium, chloride; increase potassium retention
Uses: Edema, may be used with other
diuretics; hypertension

DOSAGE AND ROUTES
• *Adult:* **PO** 100 mg bid pc, not to ex-
ceed 300 mg/day
• *Geriatric:* **PO** 50 mg daily, max 100
mg/day
Available forms: Caps 50, 100 mg

SIDE EFFECTS
CNS: Weakness, headache, dizziness,
fatigue
ELECT: Hyperkalemia, hyponatremia,
hypochloremia
GI: Nausea, diarrhea, vomiting, dry
mouth, jaundice, ***hepatic disease***
*GU: **Azotemia, interstitial nephritis,*** increased BUN, creatinine, renal
stones, bluish discoloration of urine
*HEMA: **Thrombocytopenia, megaloblastic anemia,*** low folic acid levels
INTEG: Photosensitivity, rash
Contraindications: Hypersensitivity,
anuria, severe renal disease, severe hepatic disease, hyperkalemia, lactation
Precautions: Pregnancy (B), dehydration, hepatic disease, CHF, renal disease,
cirrhosis

PHARMACOKINETICS
PO: Onset 2 hr, peak 6-8 hr, duration
12-16 hr; half-life 3 hr; metabolized in
liver, excreted in bile and urine

INTERACTIONS
Nephrotoxicity: indomethacin
Increase: effects of antihypertensives,
amantadine

T

Increase: hyperkalemia—other potassium-sparing diuretics, potassium products, ACE inhibitors, salt substitutes
Decrease: renal clearance of triamterene—cimetidine

Drug/Herb
Fatal hypokalemia: arginine
Hypokalemia: bearberry, gossypol
Severe photosensitivity: St. John's wort
Increase: diuretic—cucumber, dandelion, horsetail, licorice, nettle, pumpkin, Queen Anne's lace

Drug/Lab Test
Interference: Quinidine serum levels, LDH

NURSING CONSIDERATIONS

Assess:
• Weight, I&O daily to determine fluid loss; effect of drug may be decreased if used daily
• Electrolytes: K, Na, Cl; include BUN, blood glucose, CBC, serum creatinine, blood pH, ABGs, LFTs
• Improvement in CVP q8h
• Signs of metabolic acidosis: drowsiness, restlessness
• Rashes, temp daily
• Confusion, especially in elderly; take safety precautions if needed
• Hydration: skin turgor, thirst, dry mucous membranes

Administer:
• In AM to avoid interference with sleep
• With food if nausea occurs; absorption may be decreased slightly

Evaluate:
• Therapeutic response: improvement in edema of feet, legs, sacral area daily if medication is being used in CHF

Teach patient/family:
• To take medication after meals for GI upset
• To avoid prolonged exposure to sunlight; photosensitivity may occur; may turn urine blue
• To avoid foods high in potassium: oranges, bananas, salt substitutes, dried apricots, dates
• To notify prescriber of weakness, headache, nausea, vomiting, dry mouth, fever, sore throat, mouth sores, unusual bleeding or bruising

Treatment of overdose: Lavage if taken orally; monitor electrolytes; administer IV fluids, dialysis; monitor hydration, CV, renal status

---

triazolam (R)
(trye-ay'zoe-lam)
Apo-Triazo ✦, Gen-Triazolam ✦,
Halcion, Novo-Triolam ✦,
Nu-Triazol ✦
Func. class.: Sedative-hypnotic,
antianxiety
Chem. class.: Benzodiazepine

Controlled Substance Schedule IV (USA), Targeted (CDSA IV) (Canada)
Action: Produces CNS depression at limbic, thalamic, hypothalamic levels of CNS; may be mediated by neurotransmitter γ-aminobutyric acid (GABA); results are sedation, hypnosis, skeletal muscle relaxation, anticonvulsant activity, anxiolytic action
Uses: Insomnia, sedative, hypnotic

DOSAGE AND ROUTES

• *Adult:* **PO** 0.125-0.5 mg at bedtime
• *Geriatric:* **PO** 0.625-0.125 mg at bedtime
Available forms: Tabs 0.125, 0.25 mg

SIDE EFFECTS

CNS: Headache, lethargy, drowsiness, daytime sedation, dizziness, confusion, light-headedness, anxiety, irritability, amnesia, poor coordination
CV: Chest pain, pulse changes
GI: Nausea, vomiting, diarrhea, heartburn, abdominal pain, constipation
HEMA: Leukopenia, granulocytopenia (rare)
Contraindications: Pregnancy (X), hypersensitivity to benzodiazepines, lactation, intermittent porphyria
Precautions: Anemia, hepatic disease, renal disease, suicidal individuals, drug abuse, elderly, psychosis, child <15 yr,

---

⚠ Safety alert   *"Tall Man" lettering

acute narrow-angle glaucoma, seizure disorders

PHARMACOKINETICS

PO: Onset 30-45 min, duration 6-8 hr; metabolized by liver, excreted by kidneys (inactive metabolites), crosses placenta, excreted in breast milk; half-life 2-3 hr

INTERACTIONS

Smoking may decrease hypnotic effect
⚠ Increase: effects of cimetidine, disulfiram, erythromycin, macrolides, probenecid, isoniazid, oral contraceptives; do not use concurrently
Increase: action of both drugs—alcohol, CNS depressants
Decrease: effect of antacids, theophylline, rifampin, smoking
Drug/Herb
Increase: CNS depression—catnip, chamomile, clary, cowslip, hops, kava, lavender, mistletoe, nettle, pokeweed, poppy, Queen Anne's lace, senega, skullcap, valerian
Increase: hypotension—black cohosh
Drug/Lab Test
Increase: ALT, AST, serum bilirubin
Decrease: RAI uptake
False increase: Urinary 17-OHCS

NURSING CONSIDERATIONS
Assess:
• Blood studies: Hct, Hgb, RBC if blood dyscrasias suspected (rare)
• Hepatic studies: AST, ALT, bilirubin if hepatic damage has occurred
• Mental status: mood, sensorium, affect, memory (long, short)
• Blood dyscrasias: fever, sore throat, bruising, rash, jaundice, epistaxis (rare)
• Type of sleep problem: falling asleep, staying asleep
Administer:
• After removal of cigarettes to prevent fires
• After trying conservative measures for insomnia
• ½ hr before bedtime for sleeplessness

• On empty stomach for fast onset, but may be taken with food if GI symptoms occur
• Avoid use with CNS depressants; serious CNS depression may result
Perform/provide:
• Assistance with ambulation after receiving dose
• Safety measures: side rails, night-light, call bell within easy reach
• Checking to see if PO medication has been swallowed
• Cool storage in tight container
Evaluate:
• Therapeutic response: ability to sleep at night, decreased amount of early morning awakening if taking drug for insomnia
Teach patient/family:
• That dependence is possible after long-term use
• To avoid driving, other activities requiring alertness until drug is stabilized
• To avoid alcohol ingestion
• That effects may take 2 nights for benefits to be noticed; for short-term use only
• Alternative measures to improve sleep: reading, exercise several hours before bedtime, warm bath, warm milk, TV, self-hypnosis, deep breathing
• That hangover is common in elderly but less common than with barbiturates; rebound insomnia may occur for 1-2 nights after discontinuing drug
Treatment of overdose: Lavage, activated charcoal; monitor electrolytes, VS

T

trifluoperazine (℞)

(trye-floo-oh-per′a-zeen)
Apo-Trifluoperazine ♣,
Novofluorazine ♣, Solazine ♣,
Suprazine, Terfluzine,
trifluoperazine HCl, Triflurin
Func. class.: Antipsychotic, neuroleptic
Chem. class.: Phenothiazine, piperazine

Do not confuse:

trifluoperazine/trihexyphenidyl

Action: Depresses cerebral cortex, hypothalamus, limbic system, which control activity, aggression; blocks neurotransmission produced by dopamine at synapse; exhibits strong α-adrenergic, anticholinergic blocking action; mechanism for antipsychotic effects is unclear

Uses: Psychotic disorders, nonpsychotic anxiety, schizophrenia

DOSAGE AND ROUTES

Psychotic disorders

• *Adult:* **PO** 2-5 mg bid, usual range 15-20 mg/day, may require 40 mg/day or more; **IM** 1-2 mg q4-6h

• *Geriatric:* **PO** 0.5-1 mg daily-bid, increase q4-7d by 0.5-1 mg/day to desired dose

• *Child >6 yr:* **PO** 1 mg daily or bid; **IM** not recommended for children, but 1 mg may be given daily or bid

Nonpsychotic anxiety

• *Adult:* **PO** 1-2 mg bid, not to exceed 6 mg/day; do not give longer than 12 wk

Available forms: Tabs 1, 2, 5, 10 mg; conc 10 mg/ml; inj 2 mg/ml

SIDE EFFECTS

*CNS: EPS: pseudoparkinsonism, akathisia, dystonia, tardive dyskinesia, **seizures**, headache, **neuroleptic malignant syndrome**, dizziness*

*CV: Orthostatic hypotension, hypertension, **cardiac arrest**, ECG changes, **tachycardia***

EENT: Blurred vision, glaucoma, dry eyes

GI: Dry mouth, nausea, vomiting, anorexia, constipation, diarrhea, jaundice, weight gain

GU: Urinary retention, urinary frequency, enuresis, impotence, amenorrhea, gynecomastia

HEMA: Anemia, **leukopenia, leukocytosis, agranulocytosis**

INTEG: Rash, photosensitivity, dermatitis

*RESP: **Laryngospasm**, dyspnea, **respiratory depression***

Contraindications: Hypersensitivity, cardiovascular disease, coma, blood dyscrasias, severe hepatic disease, child <6 yr, narrow-angle glaucoma

Precautions: Pregnancy (C), breast cancer, seizure disorders, lactation, diabetes mellitus, respiratory conditions, prostatic hypertrophy, elderly

PHARMACOKINETICS

PO: Onset rapid, peak 2-3 hr, duration 12 hr
IM: Onset immediate, peak 1 hr, duration 12 hr
Metabolized by liver, excreted in urine, breast milk; crosses placenta

INTERACTIONS

Oversedation: other CNS depressants, alcohol, barbiturate anesthetics
Increase: effects of both drugs—β-adrenergic blockers, alcohol
Increase: anticholinergic effects—anticholinergics
Decrease: absorption—aluminum hydroxide, magnesium hydroxide antacids
Decrease: effects of lithium, levodopa, anticonvulsants

Drug/Herb
Increase: EPS—betel palm, kava
Increase: action—cola tree, hops, nettle, nutmeg
Increase: CNS depression—chamomile, hops, kava, skullcap, valerian

Drug/Lab Test
Increase: LFTs, cardiac enzymes, cholesterol, blood glucose, prolactin, bilirubin, PBI, cholinesterase, ^{131}I

⚠ Safety alert   *"Tall Man" lettering

Decrease: Hormones (blood, urine)
False positive: Pregnancy tests, PKU
False negative: Urinary steroids, 17-OHCS, pregnancy tests

NURSING CONSIDERATIONS

Assess:

A For neuroleptic malignant syndrome: seizures, hyper/hypotension, dyspnea, diaphoresis, fatigue, muscle stiffness; notify prescriber immediately

• Mental status before initial administration

• Swallowing of PO medication; check for hoarding or giving of medication to other patients

• I&O ratio; palpate bladder if low urinary output occurs, urinary retention may be the cause

• Bilirubin, CBC, LFTs qmo

• Urinalysis is recommended before and during prolonged therapy

• Affect, orientation, LOC, reflexes, gait, coordination, sleep pattern disturbances

• For hypo/hyperglycemia; appetite patterns

• B/P standing and lying; also include pulse, respirations q4h during initial treatment; establish baseline before starting treatment; report drops of 30 mm Hg

• Dizziness, faintness, palpitations, tachycardia on rising

• EPS including akathisia (inability to sit still, no pattern to movements), tardive dyskinesia (bizarre movements of jaw, mouth, tongue, extremities), pseudoparkinsonism (rigidity, tremors, pill rolling, shuffling gait)

• Skin turgor daily

• Constipation, urinary retention daily; if these occur increase bulk, water in diet

Administer:

• Reduced dose in elderly

• Antiparkinsonian agent on order from prescriber for EPS

• Lying down after IM injection for at least 30 min

• Avoid use with CNS depressants

PO route

• Conc in 60 ml of tomato or fruit juice, milk, carbonated beverage, coffee, tea, water, or semisolid foods (soup, pudding)

Perform/provide:

• Decreased stimulus by dimming lights, avoiding loud noises

• Supervised ambulation until stabilized on medication if needed; do not involve in strenuous exercise program because fainting is possible; patient should not stand still for long periods

• Increased fluids and bulk in diet to prevent constipation

• Sips of water, candy, gum for dry mouth

• Storage in tight, light-resistant container, oral sol in amber bottles; slight yellowing of inj or conc is common, does not affect potency

Evaluate:

• Therapeutic response: decrease in emotional excitement, hallucinations, delusions, paranoia, reorganization of patterns of thought, speech

Teach patient/family:

• That orthostatic hypotension occurs frequently, and to rise from sitting or lying position gradually; avoid hazardous activities until stabilized on medication

• To avoid hot tubs, hot showers, tub baths; hypotension may occur

• To avoid abrupt withdrawal of this drug or EPS may result; drug should be withdrawn slowly

• To avoid OTC preparations (cough, hay fever, cold) unless approved by prescriber, since serious drug interactions may occur; avoid use with alcohol; increased drowsiness may occur

• To use sunscreen

• About compliance with drug regimen

• About the necessity for meticulous oral hygiene; oral candidiasis may occur

• To report sore throat, malaise, fever, bleeding, mouth sores; CBC should be drawn and drug discontinued

A That in hot weather, heat stroke may occur; take extra precautions to stay cool

Treatment of overdose: Lavage if orally ingested; provide an airway; do not induce vomiting

---

trifluridine ophthalmic
See Appendix C

---

trihexyphenidyl (℞)
(trye-hex-ee-fen'i-dill)
Apo-Trihex ✦, Artane, Artane
Sequels, Novohexidyl ✦,
PMS-Trihexyphenidyl ✦,
Trihexane, Trihexy-2,
Trihexy-5, trihexyphenidyl HCl
Func. class.: Cholinergic blocker
Chem. class.: Synthetic tertiary
amine

Do not confuse:
tryhexyphenidyl/trifluoperazine
Artane/Altace

Action: Blocks central muscarinic receptors, which decreases involuntary
movements, sweating, salivation
Uses: Parkinson's symptoms, drug-
induced EPS
Investigational uses: Hypersalivation

DOSAGE AND ROUTES
Parkinson symptoms
• *Adult:* **PO** 1 mg, increased by 2 mg
q3-5d to a total of 6-10 mg/day, given in
3-4 divided doses; give **EXT REL** q12h
Drug-induced EPS
• *Adult:* **PO** 1 mg/day; usual dose 5-15
mg/day, in 3-4 divided doses; give **EXT
REL** q12h
Available forms: Tabs 2, 5 mg; caps
ext rel 5 mg; elix 2 mg/5 ml

SIDE EFFECTS

CNS: Confusion, anxiety, restlessness,
irritability, delusions, hallucinations,
headache, sedation, depression, incoherence, dizziness, flushing, weakness
CV: Palpitations, tachycardia, postural
hypotension
EENT: Blurred vision, photophobia, dilated pupils, difficulty swallowing, dry
eyes, increased intraocular tension,
angle-closure glaucoma

GI: Dryness of mouth, constipation,
nausea, vomiting, abdominal distress,
paralytic ileus
GU: Urinary hesitancy, retention, dysuria
INTEG: Urticaria, rash
MISC: Suppression of lactation, nasal
congestion, decreased sweating, increased temp, hyperthermia, heat stroke,
numbness of fingers
MS: Weakness, cramping
Contraindications: Hypersensitivity,
narrow-angle glaucoma, myasthenia
gravis, GI/GU obstruction, myocardial
ischemia, unstable CV disease, prostatic
hypertrophy
Precautions: Pregnancy (C), elderly,
lactation, tachycardia, abdominal obstruction, infection, children, gastric
ulcer

PHARMACOKINETICS

PO: Onset 1 hr, peak 2-3 hr, duration
6-12 hr, excreted in urine, half-life
5-10 hr

INTERACTIONS

Increase: anticholinergic effects—
antihistamines, phenothiazines, amantadine
Increase: CNS depression—analgesics,
alcohol, sedatives/hypnotics, antihistamines, opioids
Increase: levels of digoxin
Decrease: action of haloperidol

NURSING CONSIDERATIONS
Assess:
• For Parkinson's and EPS baseline and
throughout treatment
• I&O ratio; retention commonly causes
decreased urinary output
• B/P, pulse frequently while dose is
being determined
• Urinary hesitancy, retention; palpate
bladder if retention occurs
• Constipation; increase fluids, bulk,
exercise
• For tolerance over long-term therapy;
dosage may have to be increased or medication changed

⚠ Safety alert   *"Tall Man" lettering

• Mental status: affect, mood, CNS depression, worsening of mental symptoms during early therapy

Administer:

• With or after meals for GI upset; may give with fluids other than water
• At bedtime to avoid daytime drowsiness in patient with parkinsonism

Perform/provide:

• Storage at room temperature in light-resistant container
• Hard candy, frequent drinks, sugarless gum to relieve dry mouth

Evaluate:

• Therapeutic response: parkinsonism: shuffling gait, muscle rigidity, involuntary movements

Teach patient/family:

• Not to discontinue this drug abruptly; to taper off over 1 wk
• To avoid driving, other hazardous activities; drowsiness may occur
• To avoid OTC medications: cough, cold preparations with alcohol, antihistamines unless directed by prescriber
• To avoid sudden position changes
• To avoid hot climates; overheating may occur

---

trimethobenzamide (℞)

(trye-meth-oh-ben'za-mide)
Arrestin, Benzacot, Brogan,
Stemetic, T-Gen, Tebamide,
Ticon, Tigan, Tiject-20, Triban,
Trimazide, Trimethobenzamide, trimethobenzamide HCl
Func. class.: Antiemetic, anticholinergic
Chem. class.: Ethanolamine derivative

Action: Acts centrally by blocking chemoreceptor trigger zone, which in turn acts on vomiting center
Uses: Nausea, vomiting, prevention of postoperative vomiting

DOSAGE AND ROUTES

Postoperative vomiting

• *Adult:* **IM/RECT** 200 mg before or during surgery; may repeat 3 hr after

Discontinuing anesthesia

• *Child 13-40 kg:* **PO/RECT** 100-200 mg tid-qid
• *Child <13 kg:* **PO/RECT** 100 mg tid-qid

Nausea/vomiting

• *Adult:* **PO** 250-300 mg tid-qid; **IM/RECT** 200 mg tid-qid

Available forms: Caps 100, 250, 300 mg; supp 100 (pediatric), 200 (adult) mg; inj 100 mg/ml

SIDE EFFECTS

CNS: Drowsiness, restlessness, headache, dizziness, insomnia, confusion, nervousness, tingling, *vertigo,* EPS
CV: Hypertension, hypotension, palpitation
EENT: Dry mouth, blurred vision, diplopia, nasal congestion, photosensitivity
GI: Nausea, anorexia, diarrhea, vomiting, constipation
INTEG: Rash, urticaria, fever, chills, flushing

Contraindications: Hypersensitivity to opioids, shock, children (parenterally)

Precautions: Pregnancy (C), children, cardiac dysrhythmias, elderly, asthma, prostatic hypertrophy, bladder-neck obstruction, narrow-angle glaucoma, stenosing peptic ulcer, pyloroduodenal obstruction

PHARMACOKINETICS

PO: Onset 20-40 min, duration 3-4 hr
IM: Onset 15 min, duration 2-3 hr
Metabolized by liver, excreted by kidneys

INTERACTIONS

May mask ototoxic symptoms associated with antibiotics
Increase: effect—CNS depressants

NURSING CONSIDERATIONS

Assess:

• For nausea, vomiting before, after treatment

• VS, B/P; check patients with cardiac disease more often

• Signs of toxicity of other drugs or masking of symptoms of disease: brain tumor, intestinal obstruction

• Observe for drowsiness, dizziness

Administer:

PO route

• Tablets may be swallowed whole, chewed, allowed to dissolve

Rectal route

• Do not use suppositories in newborns or premature infants

• Suppositories 100 mg is for pediatric use, 200 mg for adult use

IM route

• Inj in large muscle mass; aspirate to avoid IV administration; inj is not to be used in children or infants

Syringe compatibilities: Glycopyrrolate, hydromorphone, midazolam, nalbuphine

Y-site compatibilities: Heparin, hydrocortisone, potassium chloride, vit B/C

Evaluate:

• Therapeutic response: decreased nausea, vomiting

Teach patient/family:

• To avoid hazardous activities, activities requiring alertness; dizziness may occur; to request assistance with ambulation

• To avoid alcohol, other depressants

• To keep out of children's reach

---

trimethoprim (R)

(trye-meth'oh-prim)
Primsol, Proloprim,
trimethoprim, Trimpex
Func. class.: Urinary antiinfective
Chem. class.: Folate antagonist

Action: Prevents bacterial synthesis by blocking enzyme reduction of dihydrofolic acid

Uses: *Escherichia coli, Proteus mirabilis, Klebsiella, Enterobacter* UTIs

DOSAGE AND ROUTES

Urinary tract infection

• *Adult:* **PO** 100 mg q12h × 10 days

Otitis media

• *Child >6 mo:* **PO** 5 mg/kg q12h

Pneumocystis jiroveci pneumonia

• *Adult:* **PO** 20 mg/kg/day with 100 mg dapsone × 21 days

Renal dose

• *Adult:* **PO** CCr 15-30 ml/min 50 mg q12h; CCr <15 ml/min avoid use

Available forms: Tabs 100, 200 mg

SIDE EFFECTS

CNS: Fever

GI: Nausea, vomiting, abdominal pain, abnormal taste, increased AST, ALT, bilirubin, creatinine

HEMA: **Thrombocytopenia, leukopenia, neutropenia, megaloblastic anemia** (rare)

INTEG: **Exfoliative dermatitis,** pruritus, rash

Contraindications: Hypersensitivity, CCr <15 ml/min, megaloblastic anemia

Precautions: Pregnancy (C), folate deficiency, lactation, fragile X chromosome, child <12 yr old, renal disease, hepatic disease

PHARMACOKINETICS

PO: Peak 1-4 hr, half-life 8-11 hr; metabolized in liver, excreted in urine (unchanged 60%), breast milk; crosses placenta

INTERACTIONS

Increase: action of phenytoin

NURSING CONSIDERATIONS

Assess:

• For symptoms of UTI: fever, frequency, burning or pain when urinating; baseline and throughout

• Nocturia; may indicate drug resistance

• Signs of infection, anemia

⚠ Safety alert   *"Tall Man" lettering

- AST, ALT, BUN, bilirubin, creatinine, urine cultures
- C&S; drug may be given as soon as culture is obtained
- Skin eruptions

Administer:
- With full glass of water
- Drug in equal intervals around clock to maintain blood levels

Perform/provide:
- Storage in tight, light-resistant container
- Adequate intake of fluids (2 L) to decrease bacteria in bladder

Evaluate:
- Therapeutic response: absence of pain in bladder area, negative C&S

Teach patient/family:
- All aspects of drug therapy: need to complete entire course of medication to ensure organism death (10-14 days); culture may be taken after completed course of medication
- That drug must be taken in equal intervals around clock to maintain blood levels
- To notify nurse of nausea, vomiting, rash, severe fatigue, sore throat

---

trimethoprim-sulfamethoxazole (R)
(trye-meth'oh-prim–sul-fa-meth-ox'a-zole)
Apo-Sulfatrim ✤, Apo-Sulfatrim DS ✤, Bactrim, Bactrim IV, Bethaprim, Cotrim, Novo-Trimel ✤, Novo-Trimel DS ✤, Nu-Cotrimox ✤, Nu-Cotrimox DS ✤, Roubac ✤, Septra, Septra DS, SMZ/TMP, Sulfatrim
Func. class.: Antiinfective
Chem. class.: sulfonamide—miscellaneous

Action: Sulfamethoxazole (SMZ) interferes with bacterial biosynthesis of proteins by competitive antagonism of PABA when adequate levels are maintained;

trimethoprim (TMP) blocks synthesis of tetrahydrofolic acid; combination blocks 2 consecutive steps in bacterial synthesis of essential nucleic acids, protein
Uses: UTI, otitis media, acute and chronic prostatitis, shigellosis, *Pneumocystis jiroveci* pneumonitis, chronic bronchitis, chancroid, traveler's diarrhea

DOSAGE AND ROUTES
Based on TMP content
UTI
- *Adult:* **PO** 160 mg TMP q12h × 10-14 days
- *Child:* **PO** 8 mg/kg TMP daily in 2 divided doses q12h
Otitis media
- *Child:* **PO** 8 mg/kg TMP daily in 2 divided doses q12h × 10 days
Chronic bronchitis
- *Adult:* **PO** 160 mg TMP q12h × 14 days
Pneumocystis jiroveci pneumonitis
- *Adult and child:* **PO** 20 mg/kg TMP daily in 4 divided doses q6h × 14 days; **IV** 15-20 mg/kg/day (based on TMP) in 3-4 divided doses for up to 14 days
- Dosage reduction necessary in moderate to severe renal impairment (CCr <30 ml/min)
Available forms: Tabs 80 mg trimethoprim/400 mg sulfamethoxazole, 160 mg trimethoprim/800 mg sulfamethoxazole; susp 40 mg/200 mg/5 ml; IV 16 mg/80 mg/ml

SIDE EFFECTS
CNS: Headache, insomnia, hallucinations, depression, vertigo, fatigue, anxiety, ***convulsions, drug fever,*** chills, ***aseptic meningitis***
CV: ***Allergic myocarditis***
GI: Nausea, vomiting, *abdominal pain,* stomatitis, ***hepatitis,*** glossitis, pancreatitis, diarrhea, ***enterocolitis,*** anorexia
GU: ***Renal failure, toxic nephrosis;*** increased BUN, creatinine; crystalluria
HEMA: ***Leukopenia, neutropenia, thrombocytopenia, agranulocytosis, hemolytic anemia, hypopro-***

T

thrombinemia, Henoch-Schönlein purpura, methemoglobinemia, eosinophilia I

INTEG: Rash, dermatitis, urticaria, *Stevens-Johnson syndrome*, erythema, photosensitivity, pain, inflammation at inj site, *toxic epidermal necrolysis, erythema multiforme*

RESP: Cough, shortness of breath

SYST: **Anaphylaxis, SLE**

Contraindications: Hypersensitivity to trimethoprim or sulfonamides, pregnancy at term, megaloblastic anemia, infants <2 mo, CCr <15 ml/min, lactation, porphyria

Precautions: Pregnancy (C), renal disease, elderly, G6PD deficiency, impaired hepatic/renal function, possible folate deficiency, severe allergy, bronchial asthma

PHARMACOKINETICS

PO: Rapidly absorbed, peak 1-4 hr; half-life 8-13 hr, excreted in urine (metabolites and unchanged), breast milk; crosses placenta; 68% bound to plasma proteins; TMP achieves high levels in prostatic tissue and fluid

INTERACTIONS

Thrombocytopenia: thiazide diuretics

Increase: hypoglycemic response—sulfonylurea agents

Increase: anticoagulant effects—oral anticoagulants

Increase: bone marrow depressant effects—methotrexate

Decrease: hepatic clearance of phenytoin

Decrease: response—cycloSPORINE

Drug/Lab Test

Increase: Alk phosphatase, creatinine, bilirubin

NURSING CONSIDERATIONS

Assess:

• Allergic reactions: rash, fever (AIDS patients more susceptible)

• I&O ratio; note color, character, pH of urine if drug administered for UTI; output should be 800 ml less than intake; if urine is highly acidic, alkalization may be needed

• Renal studies: BUN, creatinine, urinalysis (long-term therapy)

• Type of infection; obtain C&S before starting therapy

• Blood dyscrasias, skin rash, fever, sore throat, bruising, bleeding, fatigue, joint pain

• Allergic reaction: rash, dermatitis, urticaria, pruritus, dyspnea, bronchospasm

Administer:

PO route

• Medication after C&S; repeat C&S after full course of medication

• With resuscitative equipment, epI-NEPHrine available; severe allergic reactions may occur

• On an empty stomach 1 hr ac, 2 hr pc

• With full glass of water to maintain adequate hydration; increase fluids to 2 L/day to decrease crystallization in kidneys

IV route

• After diluting 5 ml of drug/125 ml D_5W, run over 1-1½ hr

Syringe compatibilities: Heparin

Y-site compatibilities: Acyclovir, aldesleukin, allopurinol, amifostine, amphotericin B cholesteryl, atracurium, aztreonam, cefepime, cyclophosphamide, diltiazem, DOXOrubicin liposome, enalaprilat, esmolol, filgrastim, fludarabine, gallium, granisetron, hydromorphone, labetalol, lorazepam, magnesium sulfate, melphalan, meperidine, morphine, pancuronium, perphenazine, piperacillin/tazobactam, remifentanil, sargramostim, tacrolimus, teniposide, thiotepa, vecuronium, zidovudine

Perform/provide:

• Storage in tight, light-resistant container at room temperature

Evaluate:

• Therapeutic response: absence of pain, fever, C&S negative

Teach patient/family:

• To take each oral dose with full glass of water to prevent crystalluria; drink

---

8-10 glasses of water/day; to take on an empty stomach 1 hr ac, 2 hr pc
• To complete full course of treatment to prevent superinfection
• To avoid sunlight or use sunscreen to prevent burns
• To avoid OTC medications (aspirin, vit C) unless directed by prescriber
• To use alternative contraceptive measures; decreased effectiveness of oral contraceptives may result
• To notify prescriber if skin rash, sore throat, fever, mouth sores, unusual bruising, bleeding occur

---

trimipramine (℞)

(tri-mip′ra-meen)
Apo-Trimip ✦,
Novo-Tripramine ✦,
Rhotrimine, Surmontil
Func. class.: Antidepressant—tricyclic
Chem. class.: Tertiary amine

Action: Selectively inhibits serotonin uptake by brain; potentiates behavioral changes
Uses: Depression, enuresis in children

DOSAGE AND ROUTES

• *Adult:* **PO** 50-150 mg/day in divided doses, may be increased to 200 mg/day
• *Geriatric:* **PO** 25 mg at bedtime, increase by 25 mg q3-7d, max 100 mg/day
• *Child >6 yr:* 25 mg at bedtime, may increase to 50 mg in child <12 yr or 75 mg in child >12 yr
Available forms: Caps 25, 50, 100 mg

SIDE EFFECTS

CNS: Dizziness, drowsiness, confusion, headache, anxiety, tremors, stimulation, weakness, insomnia, nightmares, EPS (elderly), increase in psychiatric symptoms
CV: Orthostatic hypotension, ECG changes, tachycardia, **hypertension,** palpitations
EENT: Blurred vision, tinnitus, mydriasis
GI: Diarrhea, *dry mouth,* nausea, vomit-

ing, ***paralytic ileus,*** increased appetite, cramps, epigastric distress, jaundice, ***hepatitis,*** stomatitis, *constipation,* taste change
GU: Urinary retention, ***acute renal failure***
HEMA: ***Agranulocytosis, thrombocytopenia, eosinophilia, leukopenia***
INTEG: Rash, urticaria, sweating, pruritus, photosensitivity

Contraindications: Hypersensitivity to tricyclics, recovery phase of MI, convulsive disorders, prostatic hypertrophy
Precautions: Pregnancy (C), suicidal patients, severe depression, increased intraocular pressure, narrow-angle glaucoma, urinary retention, cardiac disease, hepatic disease, renal disorders, hyperthyroidism, electroshock therapy, elective surgery, elderly

PHARMACOKINETICS

Metabolized by liver, excreted by kidneys, steady state 2-6 days; half-life 20-26 hr

INTERACTIONS

⚠ Hyperpyretic crisis, convulsions, hypertensive episode: MAOIs
Increase: effects of direct-acting sympathomimetics (epINEPHrine), alcohol, barbiturates, benzodiazepines, CNS depressants, cimetidine, methylphenidate
Decrease: effects of guanethidine, clonidine, indirect-acting sympathomimetics (epHEDrine)
Drug/Herb
Serotonin syndrome: SAM-e, St. John's wort
Increase: anticholinergic effect—belladonna, corkwood, henbane, jimsonweed
Increase: hypertension—yohimbe
Increase: antidepressant action—scopolia
Drug/Lab Test
Increase: Serum bilirubin, blood glucose, alk phosphatase
Decrease: VMA, 5-HIAA
False increase: Urinary catecholamines

T

NURSING CONSIDERATIONS
Assess:
• B/P (lying, standing), pulse q4h; if systolic B/P drops 20 mm Hg, hold drug, notify prescriber; take VS q4h in patients with cardiovascular disease

• Blood studies: CBC, leukocytes, differential, cardiac enzymes if patient is receiving long-term therapy

• Hepatic studies: AST, ALT, bilirubin, creatinine

• Weight qwk; appetite may increase with drug

• ECG for flattening of T wave, bundle branch block, AV block, dysrhythmias in cardiac patients

• EPS primarily in elderly: rigidity, dystonia, akathisia

• Mental status changes: mood, sensorium, affect, suicidal tendencies, increase in psychiatric symptoms, depression, panic

• Urinary retention, constipation; constipation is more likely to occur in children, elderly

• Withdrawal symptoms: headache, nausea, vomiting, muscle pain, weakness; not usual unless drug is discontinued abruptly

• Alcohol consumption; hold dose until morning

Administer:
• Increased fluids, bulk in diet for constipation, urinary retention

• With food, milk for GI symptoms

• Dosage at bedtime for oversedation during day; may take entire dose at bedtime; elderly may not tolerate once/day dosing

• Gum, hard candy, or frequent sips of water for dry mouth

• Avoid use with CNS depressants

Perform/provide:
• Storage in tight, light-resistant container at room temperature

• Assistance with ambulation during beginning therapy for drowsiness/dizziness

• Safety measures, including side rails, primarily for elderly

• Checking to see if PO medication swallowed

Evaluate:
• Therapeutic response: decreased depression or enuresis

Teach patient/family:
• That therapeutic effects may take 2-3 wk

• To use caution in driving, other activities requiring alertness because of drowsiness, dizziness, blurred vision

• That appetite and weight may increase

• That urine may turn blue-green; to report urinary retention

• To avoid alcohol ingestion

• Not to discontinue medication quickly after long-term use; may cause nausea, headache, malaise

• To wear sunscreen or large hat, since photosensitivity occurs

Treatment of overdose:
ECG monitoring; induce emesis; lavage, activated charcoal; administer anticonvulsant

---

triptorelin (R̄)
(trip-toe'rel-in)
Trelstar Depot
Func. class.: Gonadotropin-releasing hormone
Chem. class.: Synthetic decapeptide analog of LHRH

Action: Inhibitor of pituitary gonadotropin secretion; initially increases LH and FSH, with increases in testosterone, reduction in sex steroid levels

Uses: Advanced prostate cancer

DOSAGE AND ROUTES
• *Adult:* **IM** 3.75 mg qmo

Available forms: Microgranules, depot inj 3.75 mg

SIDE EFFECTS
CNS: Headache, insomnia, dizziness, lability, fatigue
CV: Hypertension
ENDO: Gynecomastia, breast tenderness, hot flashes

GI: Nausea, vomiting, diarrhea

GU: Impotence, urinary retention, UTI

INTEG: Rash, pain on inj, pruritus, hypersensitivity

*MISC: **Anaphylaxis, angioedema***

MS: Osteoneuralgia

Contraindications: Pregnancy (X), hypersensitivity to this product or other LHRH agonists or LHRH, lactation

PHARMACOKINETICS

Metabolism may be by CYP450, eliminated by liver, kidneys; terminal half-life is 3 hr in healthy males

Drug/Lab Test

Increase: Alk phosphatase, estradiol, FSH, LH, testosterone levels

Decrease: Testosterone levels, progesterone

NURSING CONSIDERATIONS

Assess:

• Severe hypersensitivity: discontinue drug and give antihistamines, have emergency equipment nearby

• I&O ratios; palpate bladder for distention in urinary obstruction

• For relief of bone pain (back pain)

• Assess levels of testosterone and PSA

Administer:

• IM using implant, inserted by qualified person

• Using syringe with 20G needle, withdraw 2 ml sterile water for inj, inject into vial, shake well, withdraw vial contents, inject immediately

Evaluate:

• Therapeutic response: more normal levels of prostate-specific antigen, acid phosphatase, alk phosphatase; testosterone level of <25 ng/dl

Teach patient/family:

• That postmenopausal symptoms may occur but will decrease after treatment is discontinued

• That disease flare may occur at beginning of therapy

• To report allergic reaction immediately

---

tromethamine (℞)

(troe-meth′a-meen)

Tham

Func. class.: Alkalinizer

Chem. class.: Amine

Action: Proton acceptor that corrects acidosis by combining with hydrogen ions to form bicarbonate and buffer; acts as diuretic (osmotic)

Uses: Acidosis (metabolic) associated with cardiac disease, COPD, cardiac bypass surgery, neonatal respiratory distress syndrome (RDS)

DOSAGE AND ROUTES

• *Adult:* **IV** 0.3 M required = kg of weight × HCO_3^- deficit (mEq/L)

• *Child:* **IV** same as above given over 3-6 hr, not to exceed 40 ml/kg

Available forms: Inj 18 g/500 ml

SIDE EFFECTS

CV: Irregular pulse, ***cardiac arrest***

*GI: **Hepatic necrosis***

INTEG: Infection at inj site, extravasation, phlebitis

META: Alkalosis, hypoglycemia, ***hyperkalemia with oliguria***

RESP: Shallow, slow respirations, cyanosis, ***apnea***

Contraindications: Hypersensitivity, anuria, uremia

Precautions: Pregnancy (C), severe respiratory disease/respiratory depression, cardiac edema, renal disease, infants

PHARMACOKINETICS

IV: Excreted in urine

INTERACTIONS

Drug/Herb

Decrease: alkaline effect—oak bark

NURSING CONSIDERATIONS

Assess:

• Respiratory rate, rhythm, depth; notify prescriber of abnormalities that may indicate acidosis

---

Side effects: *italics* = common; ***bold italics*** = life-threatening

- Electrolytes, blood glucose, chloride; CO_2, before, during treatment
- Urine pH, urinary output, urine glucose during beginning treatment
- I&O ratio, report large increase or decrease
- IV site for extravasation, phlebitis, thrombosis
- For signs of potassium depletion

Administer:
- IV slowly to avoid pain at infusion site and toxicity
- IV undiluted as inf or added to priming fluid or ACD blood; give 5 ml or less/min

Evaluate:
- Therapeutic response: decreased metabolic acidosis

Teach patient/family:
- To increase potassium in diet: bananas, oranges, cantaloupe, honeydew, spinach, potatoes, dried fruit

---

tropicamide ophthalmic
See Appendix C

---

trospium (℞)
(trose'pee-um)
Sanctura
Func. class.: Anticholinergic, overactive bladder product
Chem. class.: Muscarinic receptor antagonist

Action: Relaxes smooth muscles in bladder by inhibiting acetylcholine effect on muscarinic receptors
Uses: Overactive bladder (urinary frequency, urgency)

DOSAGE AND ROUTES
- *Adult:* **PO** 20 mg bid, give 5 ml ≥1 hr before meals

Renal dose
- *Adult:* **PO** CCr <30 ml/min 20 mg daily at bedtime
- *Geriatric ≥75 yr:* **PO** titrate down to 20 mg daily based on response and tolerance

Available forms: Tabs 20 mg

SIDE EFFECTS

CNS: Fatigue, dizziness, headache
EENT: Dry eyes, vision abnormalities
GI: Flatulence, abdominal pain, *constipation, dry mouth,* dyspepsia
Contraindications: Hypersensitivity, uncontrolled narrow-angle glaucoma, urinary retention, gastric retention
Precautions: Pregnancy (C), lactation, children, renal/hepatic disease, controlled narrow-angle glaucoma, ulcerative colitis, intestinal atony, myasthenia gravis

PHARMACOKINETICS

Rapidly absorbed (10%), protein bound (50%-85%), metabolism in humans not fully understood, extensively metabolized, excreted in urine (6%), feces (85%), excreted in urine by active tubular secretion

INTERACTIONS
Increase: drowsiness—alcohol
Drug/Food
Decrease: absorption—high-fat meal

NURSING CONSIDERATIONS
Assess:
- Urinary patterns: distention, nocturia, frequency, urgency, incontinence

Administer:
- 1 hr before meals or on empty stomach

Evaluate:
- Therapeutic response: correction of urinary status: absence of dysuria, frequency, nocturia, incontinence

Teach patient/family:
- To avoid hazardous activities; dizziness may occur
- Alcohol may increase drowsiness
- Define anticholinergic effects that may occur

⚠ Safety alert   *"Tall Man" lettering

⚠ High Alert

tubocurarine (℞)
(too-boe-kyoor-ar'een)
Tubarine ✤, Tubocuraine
Func. class.: Neuromuscular
blocker, nondepolarizing
Chem. class.: Curare alkaloid

Action: Inhibits transmission of nerve impulses by binding with cholinergic receptor sites, antagonizing action of acetylcholine
Uses: Facilitation of endotracheal intubation, skeletal muscle relaxation during mechanical ventilation, surgery, or general anesthesia

DOSAGE AND ROUTES

• *Adult:* IV BOL 0.2-0.6 mg/kg, then 0.04-0.1 mg/kg 20-45 min after 1st dose if needed for long procedures
Available forms: Inj 3 mg/ml, 20 units/ml

SIDE EFFECTS

CV: Bradycardia, tachycardia, increased, decreased B/P
EENT: Increased secretions
INTEG: Rash, flushing, pruritus, urticaria
RESP: **Prolonged apnea, bronchospasm, cyanosis, respiratory depression,** wheezing
Contraindications: Hypersensitivity
Precautions: Pregnancy (C), cardiac disease, lactation, children <2 yr, electrolyte imbalances, dehydration, neuromuscular disease, respiratory disease, renal/hepatic disease

PHARMACOKINETICS

IV: Onset 3-5 min, dose dependent, peak 2-3 min, duration ½-1½ hr; half-life 1-3 hr; degraded in liver, kidney (minimally); excreted in urine (unchanged) crosses placenta

INTERACTIONS

Dysrhythmias: theophylline
Increase: neuromuscular blockade—aminoglycosides, amphotericin B, clindamycin, loop diuretics, lincomycin, quinidine, local anesthetics, polymyxin antiinfectives, lithium, opioid analgesics, thiazides, enflurane, isoflurane, trimethaphan, magnesium salts, verapamil

NURSING CONSIDERATIONS

Assess:
• For electrolyte imbalances (K, Mg); may lead to increased action of this drug
• VS (B/P, pulse, respirations, airway) q15min until fully recovered; rate, depth, pattern of respirations, strength of hand grip
• I&O ratio; check for urinary retention, frequency, hesitancy
• Recovery: decreased paralysis of face, diaphragm, leg, arm, rest of body; allow to recover fully before completing neurologic assessment
• Allergic reactions: rash, fever, respiratory distress, pruritus; drug should be discontinued

Administer:
• With diazepam or morphine when used for therapeutic paralysis; provides no sedation alone
• Using nerve stimulator by anesthesiologist to determine neuromuscular blockade
• Anticholinesterase to reverse neuromuscular blockade
• IV undiluted 3 mg/ml; give single dose over 1-1½ sec by qualified person; diluted to 4 ml in NS given 0.5 ml/2 min for myasthenia testing
Solution compatibilities: D₅, D₁₀W, 0.9% NaCl, 0.45% NaCl, Ringer's, LR, dextrose/Ringer's or dextrose/LR combinations
Syringe compatibilities: Pentobarbital, thiopental
Perform/provide:
• Storage in light-resistant area; use only fresh sol
• Reassurance if communication is difficult during recovery from neuromuscular blockade

Evaluate:

• Therapeutic response: paralysis of jaw, eyelid, head, neck, rest of body

Treatment of overdose: Edrophonium or neostigmine, atropine, monitor VS; may require mechanical ventilation

undecylenic acid topical
See Appendix C

unoprostone ophthalmic
See Appendix C

urea (℞)
(yoor-ee′a)
Ureaphil
Func. class.: Diuretic, osmotic
Chem. class.: Carbonic acid diamide salt

Action: Elevates plasma osmolality, increasing flow of water into plasma from ocular and cranial fluids
Uses: To decrease intracranial pressure, intraocular pressure

DOSAGE AND ROUTES

• *Adult:* IV 1-1.5 g/kg of 30% sol over 1-3 hr, not to exceed 4 ml/min; do not exceed 120 g/day
• *Child >2 yr:* IV 0.5-1.5 g/kg, not to exceed 4 ml/min
• *Child <2 yr:* IV 0.1 g/kg, not to exceed 4 ml/min
Available forms: Inj 40 g/150 ml

SIDE EFFECTS

CNS: Dizziness, disorientation, fever, syncope, *headache*
GI: Nausea, vomiting
INTEG: Venous thrombosis, phlebitis, extravasation
Contraindications: Severe renal disease, active intracranial bleeding, marked dehydration, liver failure, sickle cell disease with CNS involvement
Precautions: Pregnancy (C), hepatic disease, renal disease, electrolyte imbalances, lactation

PHARMACOKINETICS

IV: Onset ½-1 hr, peak 1 hr, duration 3-10 hr (diuresis), 5-6 hr (intraocular pressure); half-life 1 hr; excreted in urine, breast milk; crosses placenta

INTERACTIONS

Incompatible with whole blood, alkalies in sol or syringe
Increase: renal excretion of lithium

NURSING CONSIDERATIONS

Assess:

• Weight, I&O daily to determine fluid loss; effect of drug may be decreased if used daily; for hourly urinary output
• Rate, depth, rhythm of respiration, effect of exertion
• B/P lying, standing, postural hypotension may occur
• Electrolytes: K, Na, Cl; include BUN, blood glucose, CBC, serum creatinine, blood pH, ABGs, LFTs
• Fever, signs of extravasation
• Confusion, especially in elderly; take safety precautions if needed
• Hydration: skin turgor, thirst, dry mucous membranes

Administer:

• IV after diluting 30 g/100 ml diluent with D_5, D_{10}; run 30% sol over 1-2 hr; check for extravasation; do not exceed 4 ml/min; may cause bleeding; use IV filter
• Within minutes of reconstitution; sol becomes ammonia on standing

Evaluate:

• Therapeutic response: improvement in edema of feet, legs, sacral area daily in CHF

Teach patient/family:

• That drug will cause diuresis in ½ hr

Treatment of overdose: Lavage if taken orally; monitor electrolytes, administer IV fluids, monitor BUN, hydration, CV status

---

🛆 Safety alert   *"Tall Man" lettering

⚠ High Alert

urokinase (℞)

(yoor-oh-kin'ase)
Abbokinase, Abbokinase
Open-Cath

Func. class.: Thrombolytic enzyme
Chem. class.: β-Hemolytic streptococcus filtrate (purified)

Action: Promotes thrombolysis by directly converting plasminogen to plasmin
Uses: Venous thrombosis, pulmonary
embolism, arterial thrombosis, arterial
embolism, arteriovenous cannula occlusion, lysis of coronary artery thrombi
after MI

DOSAGE AND ROUTES

Lysis of pulmonary emboli
• *Adult and child:* **IV** 4400 international
units/kg/hr × 12-24 hr, not to exceed
200 ml; then **IV** heparin, then anticoagulants
Coronary artery thrombosis
• *Adult:* **INSTILL** 6000 international
units/min into occluded artery for 1-2 hr
after giving **IV BOL** of heparin 2500-
10,000 units
• May also give as **IV INF** 2 million-3
million units over 45-90 min
Venous catheter occlusion
• *Adult and child:* **INSTILL** 5000 international units into line, wait 5 min, then
aspirate, repeat aspiration attempts
q5min × ½ hr; if occlusion has not been
removed, cap line and wait ½-1 hr, then
aspirate; may need 2nd dose if still occluded
Available forms: Powder for inj,
lyophilized: 250,000 international units/
vial; powder for catheter clearance

SIDE EFFECTS

CNS: Headache, fever
CV: Hypotension, dysrhythmias
GI: Nausea, vomiting
HEMA: Decreased Hct, ***bleeding***
INTEG: Rash, urticaria, phlebitis at IV inf
site, itching, flushing

MS: Low back pain
RESP: Altered respirations, SOB, ***bronchospasm,*** cyanosis
SYST: ***GI, GU, intracranial, retroperitoneal bleeding,*** surface bleeding,
anaphylaxis (rare)
Contraindications: Hypersensitivity,
internal active bleeding, intraspinal surgery, neoplasms of CNS, ulcerative colitis/
enteritis, severe uncontrolled hypertension, renal disease, hepatic disease,
hypocoagulation, COPD, subacute bacterial endocarditis, rheumatic valvular
disease, cerebral embolism/thrombosis/
hemorrhage, intraarterial diagnostic
procedure or surgery (10 days), recent
major surgery/trauma, aneurysm AV
malformation
Precautions: Pregnancy (B), arterial
emboli from left side of heart, hepatic
disease

PHARMACOKINETICS

IV: Half-life 10-20 min; small amounts
excreted in urine

INTERACTIONS

Bleeding potential: aspirin, indomethacin, phenylbutazone, anticoagulants,
other NSAIDs, abciximab, eptifibatide,
tirofiban, clopidogrel, ticlopidine, some
cephalosporins, plicamycin, valproic
acid, dipyridamole, glycoprotein IIb, IIIa
inhibitors
Drug/Lab Test
Increase: PT, APTT, TT

NURSING CONSIDERATIONS

Assess:
• VS, B/P, pulse, resp, neurologic signs,
temp at least q4h; temp >104° F (40° C)
is an indicator of internal bleeding; cardiac rhythm following intracoronary
administration
• For neurologic changes that may indicate intracranial bleeding
• Retroperitoneal bleeding: back pain,
leg weakness, diminished pulses
• Peripheral pulses, lung sounds, respiratory function

U

Side effects: *italics* = common; ***bold italics*** = life-threatening

• Hypersensitivity: fever, rash, itching, chills, facial swelling, dyspnea; mild reaction may be treated with antihistamines; notify prescriber of severe reactions, stop drug, keep resuscitative equipment nearby

• Bleeding during 1st hr of treatment (hematuria, hematemesis, bleeding from mucous membranes, epistaxis, ecchymosis)

• Blood studies (Hct, platelets, PTT, PT, TT, APTT) before starting therapy; PT or APTT must be less than 2 × control before starting therapy TT; or PT q3-4h during treatment

• ECG continuously, cardiac enzymes, radionuclide myocardial scanning/coronary angiography

Administer:
IV route
• Using infusion pump, terminal filter (0.45 μm or smaller)

• Reconstituting only with 5.2 ml sterile water for inj (not bacteriostatic water), and roll (not shake) to enhance reconstitution; further dilute with 190 ml; give as intermittent inf or give to clear cannula by using 1 ml of diluted drug; inject into cannula slowly, clamp 5 min, aspirate clot; avoid excessive pressure when urokinase is injected into catheter; force could rupture catheter or expel clot into circulation

• As soon as thrombi identified; not useful for thrombi over 1 wk old

• Cryoprecipitate or fresh frozen plasma if bleeding occurs

• Loading dose at beginning of therapy; may require increased loading doses

• Heparin therapy after thrombolytic therapy is discontinued, TT or APTT less than 2 × control (about 3-4 hr)

Y-site compatibilities: TPN 55, 56
Perform/provide:
• Storage in refrigerator; use immediately after reconstitution

• Bed rest during entire course of treatment; use caution in handling patients

• Avoidance of venous, arterial puncture procedures, inj, rectal temp

• Treatment of fever with acetaminophen or aspirin

• Placement of sign above patient's bed stating urokinase therapy

• Pressure for 30 sec to minor bleeding sites; 30 min to sites of arterial puncture followed by pressure dressing; inform prescriber if hemostasis not attained, apply pressure dressing

Evaluate:
• Therapeutic response: decreased clotting, thrombosis, embolism

Teach patient/family:
• To report immediately any sign of bleeding

• That bed rest is needed during treatment

• Reasons for treatment and expected results

---

ursodiol (℞)
(ur-soh-die'-ohl)
Actigall, Urso
Func. class.: Gallstone solubilizing agent
Chem. class.: Ursodeoxycholic acid

Action: Suppresses hepatic synthesis, secretion of cholesterol; inhibits intestinal absorption of cholesterol
Uses: Dissolution of radiolucent, noncalcified gallbladder stones (less than 20 mm in diameter) in which surgery is not indicated, biliary cirrhosis, gallstone prophylaxis
Investigational uses: Severe pruritus, cystic fibrosis, intrahepatic cholestasis of pregnancy (ICP), nonalcoholic steatosis-hepatitis (NASH)

DOSAGE AND ROUTES
• *Adult:* **PO** 8-10 mg/kg/day in 2-3 divided doses using gallbladder ultrasound q6mo; determine if stones have dissolved; if so, continue therapy, repeat ultrasound within 1-3 mo
Gallstone prophylaxis in rapid weight loss
• *Adult:* **PO** 300 mg bid
Available forms: Caps 300 mg

SIDE EFFECTS

CNS: Headache, anxiety, depression, insomnia, fatigue

GI: Diarrhea, nausea, vomiting, abdominal pain, constipation, stomatitis, flatulence, dyspepsia, biliary pain

INTEG: Pruritus, rash, urticaria, dry skin, sweating, alopecia

MS: Arthralgia, myalgia, back pain

OTHER: Cough, rhinitis

Contraindications: Calcified cholesterol stones, radiopaque stones, radiolucent bile pigment stones, chronic hepatic disease, hypersensitivity, biliary obstruction, pancreatitis

Precautions: Pregnancy (B), lactation, children

PHARMACOKINETICS

80% excreted in feces, 20% metabolized, excreted into bile, lost in feces

INTERACTIONS

Increase: risk of stone formation—clofibrate, gemfibrozil, estrogens, oral contraceptives

Decrease: action of ursodiol—cholestyramine, colestipol, aluminum-based antacids

NURSING CONSIDERATIONS

Assess:
• GI status: diarrhea, abdominal pain, nausea, vomiting; drug may have to be discontinued if side effects are severe
• Skin for pruritus, rash, urticaria, dry skin; provide soothing lotion to lesions
• Musculoskeletal status: aches or stiffness in joints

Administer:
• For up to 9-12 mo; if no improvement is seen, discontinue drug

Evaluate:
• Therapeutic response: decreasing size of stones on ultrasound

Teach patient/family:
• That anxiety, depression, insomnia are side effects and are reversible after discontinuing drug

---

valacyclovir (Ⓡ)
(val-a-sye′kloh-vir)
Valtrex
Func. class.: Antiviral
Chem. class.: Acyclic purine nucleoside analog

Do not confuse:
valtrex/valcyte
valacyclovir/valganciclovir

Action: Interferes with DNA synthesis by conversion to acyclovir, causing decreased viral replication, time of lesional healing

Uses: Treatment or suppression of herpes zoster, genital herpes, herpes labialis

Investigational uses: Prevention of CMV in advanced HIV, posttransplant patients

DOSAGE AND ROUTES

Genital herpes (suppressive, initial)
• *Adult:* **PO** 1 g bid × 10 days initially

Genital herpes (recurrent episodes)
• *Adult:* **PO** 500 mg bid × 3 days

Genital herpes (suppressive therapy)
• *Adult:* **PO** 1 g daily with normal immune function; 500 mg daily for those with ≤9 recurrences/yr; 500 mg bid in HIV-infected patients with CD4 ≥100

Herpes zoster
• *Adult:* **PO** 1 g tid × 1 wk

Herpes labialis
• *Adult:* **PO** 2 g bid × 1 day

Renal dose
• *Adult:* **PO** CCr 30-49 ml/min 1 g q12h (herpes zoster); 1 g q12h × 1 day (herpes labialis); CCr 10-29 ml/min 1 g q24h (genital herpes/herpes zoster); 500 mg q24h (recurrent genital herpes); CCr <10 ml/min 500 mg q24h (genital herpes/herpes zoster), 500 mg q24h (recurrent genital herpes)

Available forms: Tabs 500 mg, 1 g

SIDE EFFECTS

CNS: Tremors, lethargy, *dizziness, head-ache,* weakness, *depression*
ENDO: Dysmenorrhea
GI: Nausea, vomiting, diarrhea, ab-dominal pain, constipation, increased AST
*HEMA: **Thrombocytopenic purpura, hemolytic uremic syndrome***
INTEG: Rash

Contraindications: Hypersensitivity to this drug or acyclovir
Precautions: Pregnancy (B), lactation, hepatic disease, renal disease, electrolyte imbalance, dehydration, elderly

PHARMACOKINETICS

PO: Onset unknown, terminal half-life 2½-3½ hr; converted to acyclovir that crosses placenta and enters breast milk, excreted in urine primarily as acyclovir

INTERACTIONS

Increase: blood levels of valacyclovir—cimetidine, probenecid

NURSING CONSIDERATIONS
Assess:
• Signs of infection; characteristics of lesions; therapy should be started at first sign or symptom of herpes and is most effective within 72 hr of outbreak
A For thrombocytopenic purpura, hemolytic uremic syndrome; may be fatal
• C&S before drug therapy; drug may be taken as soon as culture is taken; repeat C&S after treatment; determine the presence of other sexually transmitted diseases
• Bowel pattern before, during treatment
• Skin eruptions: rash
• Allergies before treatment, reaction of each medication
Administer:
• Within 72 hr of outbreak
• Orally before infection occurs

Evaluate:
• Therapeutic response: absence of itching, painful lesions; crusting and healed lesions
Teach patient/family:
• To take as prescribed; if dose is missed, take as soon as remembered up to 2 hr before next dose; do not double dose
• That drug may be taken orally before infection occurs; drug should be taken when itching or pain occurs, usually before eruptions
• That partners need to be told that patient has herpes; they can become infected; condoms must be worn to prevent reinfections
• That drug does not cure infection, just controls symptoms and does not prevent infection of others
Treatment of overdose: Discontinue drug, hemodialysis, resuscitate if needed

valganciclovir (R)
(val-gan-sy′kloh-veer)
Valcyte
Func. class.: Antiviral
Chem. class.: Synthetic nucleoside analog

Do not confuse:
Valcyte/Valtrex
valganciclovir/valacyclovir
Action: Valganciclovir is metabolized to ganciclovir; inhibits replication of human cytomegalovirus in vivo and in vitro by selective inhibition of viral DNA synthesis
Uses: Cytomegalovirus (CMV) retinitis in immunocompromised persons, including those with AIDS, after indirect ophthalmoscopy confirms diagnosis, prevention of CMV in transplantation

DOSAGE AND ROUTES
Treatment of CMV
• *Adult:* **PO** induction 900 mg bid × 21 days with food; maintenance 900 mg daily with food

Transplant
• *Adult:* **PO** 900 mg daily with food starting within 10 days of transplantation until day 100 of post transplantation
Renal dose
• *Adult:* **PO** CCr ≥60 ml/min same as above; CCr 40-59 ml/min 450 mg bid, then 450 mg daily; CCr 25-39 ml/min 450 mg daily, then 450 mg q2 days; CCr 10-24 ml/min 450 mg q2 days, then 450 mg 2×/week
Available form: Tab 450 mg

SIDE EFFECTS

CNS: Fever, chills, **coma, confusion,** abnormal thoughts, dizziness, bizarre dreams, *headache,* psychosis, tremors, somnolence, *paresthesia, weakness,* **seizures**
EENT: Retinal detachment in CMV retinitis
GI: Abnormal LFTs, *nausea, vomiting, anorexia, diarrhea, abdominal pain,* **hemorrhage**
GU: **Hematuria,** *increased creatinine, BUN*
HEMA: **Granulocytopenia, thrombocytopenia, irreversible neutropenia, anemia, eosinophilia**
INTEG: **Rash,** alopecia, *pruritus,* urticaria, pain at site, phlebitis, **Stevens-Johnson syndrome**
MISC: Local and systemic infections and sepsis
Contraindications: Hypersensitivity to acyclovir or ganciclovir, absolute neutrophil count <500, platelet count <25,000, hemodialysis
Precautions: Pregnancy (C), preexisting cytopenias, renal function impairment, lactation, children <6 mo, elderly

PHARMACOKINETICS

Metabolized to ganciclovir, which has a half-life of 3-4½ hr, excreted by kidneys (unchanged); crosses blood-brain barrier, CSF

INTERACTIONS

Severe granulocytopenia: zidovudine, antineoplastics, radiation; do not give together
Increase: toxicity—dapsone, pentamidine, flucytosine, vinCRIStine, vinBLAStine, adriamycin, DOXOrubicin, amphotericin B, trimethoprim-sulfamethoxazole combinations or other nucleoside analogs, cycloSPORINE
Increase: seizures—imipenem/cilastatin
Decrease: effect of didanosine
Decrease: renal clearance of valganciclovir—probenecid

NURSING CONSIDERATIONS
Assess:
• For leukopenia/neutropenia/thrombocytopenia: WBCs, platelets q2d during 2 ×/day dosing and then q1wk
• For leukopenia with daily WBC count in patients with prior leukopenia with other nucleoside analogs or for whom leukopenia counts are <1000 cells/mm³ at start of treatment
• Serum creatinine or CCr ≥q2wk
Administer:
• With food
Evaluate:
• Therapeutic response: decreased symptoms of CMV
Teach patient/family:
• That drug does not cure condition; regular ophthalmologic and blood tests are necessary
• That major toxicities may necessitate discontinuing drug
• To use contraception during treatment and that infertility may occur; men should use barrier contraception for 90 days after treatment
• To take with food
⚠ To report infection: fever, chills, sore throat; blood dyscrasias: bruising, bleeding, petechiae
• To avoid crowds, persons with respiratory infections
• To use sunscreen to prevent burns

V

---

valproate
(val′proh-ate)
Depacon
valproic acid
(val′proh-ik)
Depakene, Myproic acid
divalproex sodium
(dye-val′proh-ex)
Depakote, Depakote ER,
Epival ✦
Func. class.: Anticonvulsant
Chem. class.: Carboxylic acid derivative

Action: Increases levels of γ-aminobutyric acid (GABA) in brain, which decreases seizure activity

Uses: Simple (petit mal), complex (petit mal) absence, mixed, manic episodes associated with bipolar disorder, prophylaxis of migraine, adjunct in schizophrenia, tardive dyskinesia, aggression in children with ADHD, organic brain syndrome mania, migraines

Investigational uses: Tonic-clonic (grand mal), myoclonic seizures; rectal (valproic acid)

DOSAGE AND ROUTES
Epilepsy
• *Adult and child:* **PO** 10-15 mg/kg/day divided in 2-3 doses, may increase by 5-10 mg/kg/day qwk, not to exceed 60 mg/kg/day in 2-3 divided doses; **IV** ≤20 mg/min over 1 hr
Mania (divalproex sodium)
• *Adult:* **PO** 750 mg daily in divided doses, max 60 mg/kg/day
Migraine (divalproex sodium)
• *Adult:* **PO** 250 mg bid, may increase to 1000 mg/day if needed or 500 mg (Depakote ER) daily × 7 days, then 1000 mg daily

Available forms: Valproic acid: caps 250 mg; divalproex: tabs delayed rel 125, 250, 500 mg; ext rel tabs 250, 500 mg; sprinkle cap 125 mg; valproate: inj 100 mg/ml; syr 250 mg/5 ml

SIDE EFFECTS
CNS: Sedation, drowsiness, dizziness, headache, incoordination, depression, hallucinations, behavioral changes, tremors, aggression, weakness
EENT: Visual disturbances, taste perversion
GI: Nausea, vomiting, constipation, diarrhea, dyspepsia, anorexia, cramps, ***hepatic failure, pancreatitis, toxic hepatitis,*** stomatitis
GU: Enuresis, irregular menses
*HEMA: **Thrombocytopenia, leukopenia, lymphocytosis,*** increased PT, bruising, epistaxis
INTEG: Rash, alopecia, photosensitivity, dry skin
Contraindications: Pregnancy (D), hypersensitivity, hepatic disease
Precautions: Lactation, child <2 yr, elderly

PHARMACOKINETICS
PO: Onset 15-30 min, peak 1-4 hr, duration 4-6 hr
Metabolized by liver; excreted by kidneys, breast milk; crosses placenta; half-life 9-16 hr

INTERACTIONS
Increase: valproic acid level—erythromycin, felbamate
Increase: CNS depression—alcohol, opioids, barbiturates, antihistamines, MAOIs, sedative/hypnotics
Increase: toxicity of valproic acid—salicylates
Increase: action of phenytoin, tricyclic antidepressants, carbamazepine, ethosuximide, barbiturates, zidovudine
Increase: bleeding—antiplatelets, NSAIDs, tirofiban, eptifibatide, abciximab, cefamandole, cefoperazone, cefotetan, heparin, thrombolytics
Increase: toxicity of carbamazepine ethosuximide, lamotrigine, zidovudine
Decrease: metabolism of valproic acid—cimetidine
Decrease: valproic acid level—rifampin carbamazepine, lamotrigine

Drug/Lab Test
False positive: Ketones, urine
Interference: Thyroid function tests

NURSING CONSIDERATIONS

Assess:

• Seizure disorder: location, aura, activity, duration; seizure precautions should be in place

• Bipolar disorder: mood, activity, sleeping/eating, behavior

• Migraines: frequency, intensity, alleviating factor

• Blood studies: Hct, Hgb, RBC, serum folate, PT, platelets, vit D if on long-term therapy

• Hepatic studies: AST, ALT, bilirubin, hepatic failure

• Blood levels: therapeutic level 50-100 mcg/ml, in seizures

• Respiratory dysfunction: respiratory depression, character, rate, rhythm; hold drug if respirations are <12/min or if pupils are dilated

Administer:

PO route

• Swallow tabs or caps whole; do not break, crush, or chew ER tabs

• Elixir alone; do not dilute with carbonated beverage; do not give syrup to patients on sodium restriction

• Give with food or milk to decrease GI symptoms

Evaluate:

• Therapeutic response: decreased seizures

Teach patient/family:

• That physical dependency may result from extended use

• To avoid driving, other activities that require alertness

• Not to discontinue medication quickly after long-term use; convulsions may result

• To report visual disturbances, rash, diarrhea, abdominal pain, light-colored stools, jaundice, protracted vomiting to prescriber

---

valsartan (Rx)
(val'sahr-tan)
Diovan
Func. class.: Antihypertensive
Chem. class.: Angiotensin II receptor antagonist (Type AT_1)

Action: Blocks the vasoconstrictor and aldosterone-secreting effects of angiotensin II; selectively blocks the binding of angiotensin II to the AT_1 receptor found in tissues

Uses: Hypertension, alone or in combination, CHF

DOSAGE AND ROUTES

Hypertension

• *Adult:* **PO** 80-160 mg daily alone or in combination with other antihypertensives, may increase to 320 mg

CHF

• *Adult:* **PO** 40 mg bid, up to 60 mg bid

Available forms: Tabs 80, 160, 320 mg

SIDE EFFECTS

CNS: Dizziness, insomnia, drowsiness, vertigo, headache, fatigue
CV: Angina pectoris, 2nd-degree AV block, ***cerebrovascular accident,*** hypotension, ***myocardial infarction, dysrhythmias***
EENT: Conjunctivitis
GI: Diarrhea, abdominal pain, nausea, ***hepatotoxicity***
GU: Impotence, ***nephrotoxicity***
HEMA: Anemia, neutropenia
META: Hyperkalemia
MS: Cramps, myalgia, pain, stiffness
RESP: Cough

Contraindications: Pregnancy (D) 2nd/3rd trimester, hypersensitivity, severe hepatic disease, bilateral renal artery stenosis

Precautions: Hypersensitivity to ACE inhibitors: congestive heart failure, hypertrophic cardiomyopathy aortic/mitral valve stenosis, CAD; lactation, children, elderly

V

PHARMACOKINETICS

Peak 2 hr, duration >24 hr, extensively metabolized, half-life 6 hr; excreted in feces, urine, breast milk

INTERACTIONS

Drug/Herb

Increase: toxicity, death—aconite
Increase: antihypertensive effect—barberry, betony, black catechu, black cohosh, bloodroot, broom, burdock, cat's claw, dandelion, goldenseal, Irish moss, Jamaican dogwood, kelp, khella, mistletoe, parsley
Increase or decrease: antihypertensive effect—astragalus, cola tree
Decrease: antihypertensive effect—coltsfoot, guarana, khat, licorice

NURSING CONSIDERATIONS

Assess:

• B/P, pulse q4h; note rate, rhythm, quality
• Blood studies; BUN, creatinine, LFTs before treatment
• Electrolytes: K, Na, Cl, total CO_2
• Baselines in renal, hepatic studies before therapy begins
• Edema in feet, legs daily
• Skin turgor, dryness of mucous membranes for hydration status

Administer:

• Without regard to meals

Evaluate:

• Therapeutic response: decreased B/P

Teach patient/family:

• To comply with dosage schedule, even if feeling better
• To notify prescriber of fever, swelling of hands or feet, irregular heartbeat, chest pain
• That excessive perspiration, dehydration, diarrhea may lead to fall in blood pressure; consult prescriber if these occur
• That drug may cause dizziness, fainting; light-headedness may occur
• To rise slowly to sitting or standing position to minimize orthostatic hypotension

• Not to take this medication if pregnant or breastfeeding, or have had an allergic reaction to this drug
• That if a dose is missed, to take it as soon as possible, unless it is within an hour before next dose

---

vancomycin (℞)

(van-koe-mye′sin)
Lyphocin, Vancocin, Vancoled, vancomycin HCl
Func. class.: Antiinfective, misc.
Chem. class.: Tricyclic glycopeptide

Action: Inhibits bacterial cell wall synthesis

Uses: Resistant staphylococcal infections, pseudomembranous colitis, staphylococcal enterocolitis, endocarditis prophylaxis for dental procedures, diphtheroid endocarditis

DOSAGE AND ROUTES

Serious staphylococcal infections

• *Adult:* IV 500 mg q6-8h or 1 g q12h
• *Child:* IV 40 mg/kg/day divided q6-8h
• *Neonate:* IV 15 mg/kg initially followed by 10 mg/kg q8-24h

Pseudomembranous/staphylococcal enterocolitis

• *Adult:* PO 500 mg/day in divided doses for 7-10 days
• *Child:* PO 40 mg/kg/day divided q6h, not to exceed 2 g/day

Endocarditis prophylaxis

• *Adult:* IV 1 g over 1 hr, 1 hr before procedure
• *Child:* IV 20 mg/kg over 1 hr, 1 hr prior to procedure

Available forms: Pulvules 125, 250 mg; powder for oral sol 1, 10 g; powder for inj 500 mg, 1, 5, 10 g

SIDE EFFECTS

CV: **Cardiac arrest, vascular collapse** (rare)
EENT: Ototoxicity, permanent deafness, tinnitus
GI: **Nausea, pseudomembranous colitis**

A Safety alert   *"Tall Man" lettering

GU: **Nephrotoxicity,** *increased BUN, creatinine, albumin,* **fatal uremia**
HEMA: **Leukopenia, eosinophilia, neutropenia**
INTEG: Chills, fever, rash, thrombophlebitis at inj site, urticaria, pruritus, necrosis (Red man syndrome)
RESP: Wheezing, dyspnea
SYST: **Anaphylaxis**
Contraindications: Hypersensitivity, previous hearing loss
Precautions: Pregnancy (C), renal disease, lactation, elderly, neonates

PHARMACOKINETICS

IV: Peak 5 min; half-life 4-8 hr; excreted in urine (active form)
PO: Absorption: poor

INTERACTIONS

Ototoxicity or nephrotoxicity: aminoglycosides, cephalosporins, colistin, polymyxin, bacitracin, cisplatin, amphotericin B, nondepolarizing muscle relaxants

NURSING CONSIDERATIONS

Assess:
• I&O ratio; report hematuria, oliguria; nephrotoxicity may occur
⚠ Any patient with compromised renal system; drug is excreted slowly in poor renal system function; toxicity may occur rapidly; BUN, creatinine
• Blood studies: WBC
• Serum levels: peak 1 hr after 1 hr inf 25-40 mg/ml, trough prior to next dose 5-10 mg/ml
• C&S; drug may be given as soon as culture is taken
• Auditory function during, after treatment
• B/P during administration; sudden drop may indicate Red man syndrome
• Signs of infection
• Hearing loss, ringing, roaring in ears; drug should be discontinued
• Skin eruptions
• Respiratory status: rate, character, wheezing, tightness in chest

• Allergies before treatment, reaction of each medication
Administer:
• Antihistamine if Red man syndrome occurs: decreased B/P, flushing of neck, face
• Dose based on serum concentration
IV route
• After reconstitution with 10 ml sterile water for injection (500 mg/10 ml); further dilution is needed for IV, 500 mg/100 ml 0.9%NaCl, D₅W given as int inf over 1 hr; decrease rate of infusion if Red man's syndrome occurs
Y-site compatibilities: Acyclovir, allopurinol, amifostine, amiodarone, amsacrine, atracurium, cisatracurium, cyclophosphamide, diltiazem, DOXOrubicin liposome, enalaprilat, esmolol, filgrastim, fluconazole, fludarabine, gallium, granisetron, hydromorphone, insulin (regular), labetalol, lorazepam, magnesium sulfate, melphalan, meperidine, meropenem, midazolam, morphine, ondansetron, paclitaxel, pancuronium, perphenazine, propofol, remifentanil, sodium bicarbonate, tacrolimus, teniposide, theophylline, thiotepa, tolazoline, vecuronium, vinorelbine, warfarin, zidovudine
Perform/provide:
• Storage at room temperature for up to 2 wk after reconstitution
• EpINEPHrine, suction, tracheostomy set, endotracheal intubation equipment on unit; anaphylaxis may occur
• Adequate intake of fluids (2 L/day) to prevent nephrotoxicity
Evaluate:
• Therapeutic response: absence of fever, sore throat; negative culture
Teach patient/family:
• All aspects of drug therapy: need to complete entire course of medication to ensure organism death (7-10 days); culture may be taken after completed course of medication
• To report sore throat, fever, fatigue; could indicate superinfection

V

• That drug must be taken in equal intervals around clock to maintain blood levels

---

vardenafil (R)
(var-den'a-fil)
Levitra
Func. class.: Impotence agent
Chem. class.: Phosphodiesterase type 5 inhibitor

Action: Inhibits phosphodiesterase type 5 (PDE5), enhances erectile function by increasing the amount of cGMP which in turn causes smooth muscle relaxation and increased blood flow into the corpus cavernosum

Uses: Treatment of erectile dysfunction

DOSAGE AND ROUTES

• *Adult:* PO 10 mg, taken 1 hr before sexual activity, dose may be reduced to 5 mg or increased to a max of 20 mg; max dosing frequency is once daily
• *Geriatric >65 yr:* PO 5 mg initially
Hepatic dose (Child-Pugh B)
• *Adult:* PO 5 mg, max 10 mg
Concomitant medications
• Ritonavir, max 2.5 mg q72hr; for indinavir, ketoconazole 400 mg/day and itraconazole 400 mg/day, max 2.5 mg/day; for ketoconazole 200 mg/day, itraconazole 200 mg/day and erythromycin max 5 mg/day
Available forms: Tabs 2.5, 5, 10, 20 mg

SIDE EFFECTS

CNS: Headache, flushing, dizziness, insomnia
CV: Hypertension, ***MI, CV collapse***
EENT: Conjunctivitis, tinnitus, photophobia, diminished vision, glaucoma
GU: Abnormal ejaculation, priapism
MISC: Rash, GERD, GGTP increased, ***NAION (nonarteritic ischemic optic neuropathy)***
MS: Myalgia, arthralgia, neck pain
RESP: Rhinitis, sinusitis, dyspnea, pharyngitis, epistaxis

Contraindications: Hypersensitivity, coadministration of α-blockers or nitrates, renal failure

Precautions: Pregnancy (B), hepatic impairment, retinis pigmentosa, cardiovascular disease including congenital or acquired QT prolongation, anatomical penile deformities, sickle cell anemia, leukemia, multiple myeloma, not indicated for women, children, or newborns

PHARMACOKINETICS

Rapidly absorbed; bioavailability 15%; protein binding 95%; metabolized by liver; terminal half-life 4-5 hr, onset 20 min, peak ½-1½ hr, duration <5 hr, reduced absorption with high-fat meal; primarily excreted in feces (91-95%)

INTERACTIONS

Hypotension: α-blockers, protease inhibitors, do not use concurrently
Do not use with class III antidysrhythmics (amiodarone, dofetilide, ibutilide, sotalol) or class IA antidysrhythmics (disopyramide, quinidine, procainamide)
A Do not use with nitrates because of unsafe decrease in B/P which could result in MI or stroke
Increase: vardenafil levels—erythromycin, azole antifungals (ketoconazole, intraconazole), cimetidine, antiretroviral protease inhibitors
Decrease: B/P—NIFEdipine, α-blockers

NURSING CONSIDERATIONS

Assess:
• If any severe loss of vision occurs while taking this or any similar products, these products should not be used
• Use of organic nitrates that should not be used with this drug

Administer:
• Approximately 1 hr before sexual activity, do not use more than once a day
• Do not use with nitrates in any form

A Safety alert   *"Tall Man" lettering

Teach patient/family:

• That drug does not protect against sexually transmitted diseases, including HIV

• That drug absorption is reduced with a high-fat meal

• That drug should not be used with nitrates in any form

• That drug has no effect in the absence of sexual stimulation

• That patient should seek immediate medical attention if erections last for more than 4 hr

• To inform physician of all medications being taken

• To notify prescriber immediately and stop taking product if vision loss occurs

---

vasopressin (℞)

(vay-soe-press'in)
Pitressin Synthetic
Func. class.: Pituitary hormone
Chem. class.: Lysine vasopressin

Action: Promotes reabsorption of water by action on renal tubular epithelium; causes vasoconstriction

Uses: Diabetes insipidus (nonnephrogenic/nonpsychogenic), abdominal distention postoperatively, bleeding esophageal varices

DOSAGE AND ROUTES

Diabetes insipidus

• *Adult:* **IM/SUBCUT** 5-10 units bid-qid as needed; **IM/SUBCUT** 2.5-5 units q2-3d (Pitressin Tannate) for chronic therapy

• *Child:* **IM/SUBCUT** 2.5-10 units bid-qid as needed; **IM/SUBCUT** 1.25-2.5 units q2-3d (Pitressin Tannate) for chronic therapy

Abdominal distention

• *Adult:* **IM** 5 units, then q3-4h, increasing to 10 units if needed (aqueous)

Available forms: Inj 20, 5 units/ml (tannate), spray, cotton pledgets

SIDE EFFECTS

CNS: Drowsiness, headache, lethargy, flushing
CV: Increased B/P
EENT: Nasal irritation, congestion, rhinitis
GI: Nausea, heartburn, cramps
GU: Vulval pain, uterine cramping
MISC: Tremor, sweating, vertigo, urticaria, bronchial constriction

Contraindications: Hypersensitivity, chronic nephritis

Precautions: Pregnancy (C), lactation, CAD

PHARMACOKINETICS

Nasal: Onset 1 hr, duration 3-8 hr, half-life 15 min; metabolized in liver, kidneys; excreted in urine

NURSING CONSIDERATIONS

Assess:

• Nasal mucosa if given by intranasal spray; for irritation

• Pulse, B/P, when giving drug IV or IM

• I&O ratio, weight daily; check for edema in extremities; if water retention is severe, diuretic may be prescribed

• H_2O intoxication: lethargy, behavioral changes, disorientation, neuromuscular excitability

Evaluate:

• Therapeutic response: absence of severe thirst, decreased urine output, osmolality

Teach patient/family:

• To measure and record I&O

• To avoid alcohol, all OTC medications unless approved by prescriber

V

⚠ High Alert

vecuronium (Ⓡ)
(vek-yoo-roe'nee-um)
Norcuron
Func. class.: Neuromuscular
blocker, nondepolarizing
Chem. class.: Monoquaternary analog of pancuronium

Do not confuse:

Nocuron/Narcan

Action: Inhibits transmission of nerve
impulses by binding with cholinergic
receptor sites, antagonizing action of
acetylcholine

Uses: Facilitation of endotracheal intubation, skeletal muscle relaxation during
mechanical ventilation, surgery, general
anesthesia

DOSAGE AND ROUTES

• *Adult and child >9 yr:* **IV BOL** 0.08-
0.10 mg/kg, then 0.01-0.015 mg/kg for
prolonged procedures
Available forms: 10 mg/5 ml vial

SIDE EFFECTS

CNS: Skeletal muscle weakness or paralysis (rare)
INTEG: Urticaria
RESP: **Prolonged apnea, possible
respiratory paralysis,** bronchospasm, tachycardia, flushing, wheezing
SYST: **Anaphylaxis**
Contraindications: Hypersensitivity
Precautions: Pregnancy (C), cardiac
disease, lactation, children <2 yr, electrolyte imbalances, dehydration, neuromuscular disease, respiratory disease,
hepatic disease

PHARMACOKINETICS

IV: Onset 2-3 min, peak 3-5 min,
duration 15-25 (recovery index) min;
half-life 65-75 min; not metabolized;
excreted in urine/feces; crosses placenta

INTERACTIONS

Dysrhythmias: theophylline
Increased neuromuscular blockade—
aminoglycosides, amphotericin B, clindamycin, lincomycin, quinidine, local
anesthetics, polymyxin antibiotics, lithium, opioid analgesics, phenytoin, piperacillin, thiazides, enflurane, isoflurane,
succinylcholine, verapamil

NURSING CONSIDERATIONS

Assess:

• VS (B/P, pulse, respirations, airway)
q15min until fully recovered; rate, depth,
pattern of respirations, strength of hand
grip
• I&O ratio; check for urinary retention,
frequency, hesitancy
• Recovery: decreased paralysis of face,
diaphragm, leg, arm, rest of body; allow
to recover fully before completing neurologic assessment
• Allergic reactions: rash, fever, respiratory distress, pruritus; drug should be
discontinued

Administer:

• With diazepam or morphine when
used for therapeutic paralysis; provides
no sedation alone
• Using nerve stimulator by anesthesiologist to determine neuromuscular blockade
• Anticholinesterase to reverse neuromuscular blockade
• IV after diluting with diluent provided;
give by direct IV over 1 min; may give as
continuous inf 10-20 mg/100 ml; titrate
to patient response (only by qualified
person)

Y-site compatibilities: Aminophylline, cefazolin, cefuroxime, cimetidine, diltiazem, DOBUTamine, DOPamine, epINEPHrine, esmolol, fentanyl,
fluconazole, gentamicin, heparin, hydrocortisone, hydromorphone, isoproterenol, labetalol, lorazepam, midazolam,
milrinone, morphine, niCARdipine, nitroglycerin, norepinephrine, propofol,
ranitidine, sodium nitroprusside,

trimethoprim-sulfamethoxazole, vancomycin

Perform/provide:
• Storage in refrigerator; discard in 24 hr
• Reassurance if communication is difficult during recovery from neuromuscular blockade

Evaluate:
• Therapeutic response: paralysis of jaw, eyelid, head, neck, rest of body

Treatment of overdose: Edrophonium or neostigmine, atropine, monitor VS; may require mechanical ventilation

---

venlafaxine (℞)
(ven-la-fax′een)
Effexor, Effexor-XR
Func. class.: Antidepressant (misc)

Action: Potent inhibitor of neuronal serotonin and norepinephrine uptake, weak inhibitor of dopamine; no muscarinic, histaminergic, or α-adrenergic receptors in vitro

Uses: Prevention/treatment of major depression, to treat depression at end of life, long-term treatment of general anxiety disorder; social anxiety disorder

Investigational uses: Hot flashes, obsessive-compulsive disorder (OCD), premenstrual dysphoria disorder (PMDD), posttraumatic stress disorder (PTSD)

DOSAGE AND ROUTES
Renal dose
• Mild-moderate impairment, 75% of dose
Hepatic dose
• Moderate impairment, 50% of dose
Depression
• *Adult:* **PO** 75 mg/day in 2 or 3 divided doses; taken with food, may be increased to 150 mg/day; if needed, may be further increased to 225 mg/day; increments of 75 mg/day at intervals of no less than 4 days; some hospitalized patients may require up to 375 mg/day in 3 divided

doses; **EXT REL** 37.5-75 mg PO daily, max 225 mg/day; give XR daily
Hot flashes (Investigational)
• *Adult:* **PO** 12.5 mg bid × 4 wk or **EXT REL** 37.5 mg × 4 wk

Available forms: Tabs scored 25, 37.5, 50, 75, 100 mg (Effexor); cap ext rel 37.5, 75, 150 mg (Effexor XR)

SIDE EFFECTS

CNS: Emotional lability, vertigo, apathy, ataxia, CNS stimulation, euphoria, hallucinations, hostility, increased libido, hypertonia, hypotonia, psychosis, insomnia, anxiety, *suicidal ideation in children/adolescents, seizures*
CV: Migraine, angina pectoris, hypertension, extrasystoles, postural hypotension, syncope, thrombophlebitis
EENT: Abnormal vision, taste, *ear pain,* cataract, conjunctivitis, corneal lesions, dry eyes, otitis media, photophobia
GI: Dysphagia, eructation, nausea, anorexia, dry mouth, colitis, gastritis, gingivitis, *rectal hemorrhage,* stomatitis, stomach and mouth ulceration
GU: Anorgasmia, abnormal ejaculation, *dysuria, hematuria, metrorrhagia, vaginitis, impaired urination,* albuminuria, amenorrhea, kidney calculus, cystitis, nocturia, breast and bladder pain, polyuria, *uterine hemorrhage, vaginal hemorrhage,* moniliasis
HEMA: Agranulocytosis, aplastic anemia, neutropenia, pancytopenia
INTEG: Ecchymosis, acne, alopecia, brittle nails, dry skin, photosensitivity
META: Peripheral edema, weight loss or gain, diabetes mellitus, edema, glycosuria, hyperlipemia, hypokalemia
MS: Arthritis, bone pain, bursitis, myasthenia tenosynovitis, arthralgia
RESP: Bronchitis, dyspnea, asthma, chest congestion, epistaxis, hyperventilation, laryngitis
SYST: Malaise, neck pain, enlarged abdomen, cyst, facial edema, hangover, hernia

Contraindications: Hypersensitivity, bipolar disorder

Precautions: Pregnancy (C), mania, lactation, children, elderly, hypertension, seizure disorder, recent MI, cardiac disease

PHARMACOKINETICS

Well absorbed, extensively metabolized in the liver to an active metabolite; 87% of drug recovered in urine; 27% protein binding; half-life 5-7, 11-13 hr (active metabolite) respectively

INTERACTIONS

⚠ Hyperthermia, rigidity, rapid fluctuations of vital signs, mental status changes, neuroleptic malignant syndrome: MAOIs

Increase: venlafaxine effect—cimetidine

Increase: CNS depression—alcohol, opioids, antihistamines, sedative/hypnotics

Increase: levels of clozapine, desipramine, haloperidol, warfarin

Increase: serotonin syndrome—sibutramine, sumatriptan, trazadone

Decrease: effect of indinavir

Decrease: venlafaxine effect—cyproheptadine

Drug/Herb

Serotonin syndrome: SAM-e, St. John's wort

Increase: CNS depression—chamomile, hops, kava, lavender, skullcap, valerian

Increase: anticholinergic effect—corkwood, jimsonweed

Increase: hypertension—yohimbe

Drug/Lab Test

Increase: ALK phosphatase, bilirubin, AST, ALT, BUN, creatinine, serum cholesterol, CPK, LDH

NURSING CONSIDERATIONS

Assess:

• B/P lying, standing; pulse q4h; if systolic B/P drops 20 mm Hg, hold drug, notify prescriber; take VS q4h in patients with cardiovascular disease

• Electrolytes: Hypo/hyperkalemia, hypo/hyperphosphatemia, hyponatremia, hyperuricemia, hypo/hyperglycemia can occur

• Blood studies: CBC, leukocytes, differential cardiac enzymes if patient is receiving long-term therapy

• Hepatic studies: AST, ALT, bilirubin

• Weight qwk; weight loss or gain; appetite may increase; peripheral edema may occur

• With food, milk for GI symptoms

• Sugarless gum, hard candy, frequent sips of water for dry mouth

• Mental status: mood, sensorium, affect, increase in psychiatric symptoms; depression, panic; assess for suicidal ideation in children/adolescents

• Withdrawal symptoms: headache, nausea, vomiting, muscle pain, weakness; not usual unless drug is discontinued abruptly

Administer:

• Avoid use with CNS depressants

• In small amounts because of suicide potential, especially in the beginning of therapy

Perform/provide:

• Storage in tight container at room temperature; do not freeze

• Assistance with ambulation during beginning therapy, since drowsiness, dizziness occur

• Checking to see if PO medication swallowed

Evaluate:

• Therapeutic response; decreased depression

Teach patient/family:

• To notify prescriber of rash, hives or allergic reactions

• To use with caution when driving or other activities requiring alertness because of drowsiness, dizziness, blurred vision

• To avoid alcohol ingestion

• Not to discontinue medication quickly after long-term use; may cause nausea, headache, malaise

• To wear sunscreen or large hat, since photosensitivity occurs

• To avoid pregnancy or lactation while taking this product

Treatment of overdose: ECG monitoring; induce emesis; lavage, activated charcoal; administer anticonvulsant

verapamil (℞)

(ver-ap′a-mill)
Apo-Verap ✦, Calan, Calan SR, Covera-HS, Isoptin, Isoptin SR, verapamil HCl, verapamil HCl SR, Verelan PM
Func. class.: Calcium channel blocker; antihypertensive; antianginal
Chem. class.: Diphenylalkylamine

Action: Inhibits calcium ion influx across cell membrane during cardiac depolarization; produces relaxation of coronary vascular smooth muscle; dilates coronary arteries; decreases SA/AV node conduction; dilates peripheral arteries

Uses: Chronic stable, vasospastic, unstable angina; dysrhythmias, hypertension, supraventricular tachycardia, atrial flutter or fibrillation

Investigational uses: Prevention of migraine headaches, ventricular outflow obstruction in hypertrophic cardiomyopathy, recumbent nocturnal leg cramps

DOSAGE AND ROUTES

Angina
• *Adult:* PO 80-120 mg tid, increase qwk

Dysrhythmias
• *Adult:* PO 240-320 mg/day in 3-4 divided doses in digitalized patients
• *Adult:* IV BOL 5-10 mg (0.075-0.15 mg/kg) over 2 min, may repeat 10 mg (0.15 mg/kg) ½ hr after 1st dose
• *Child 1-15 yr:* IV BOL 0.1-0.3 mg/kg over 2 min or more, repeat in 30 min, not to exceed 5 mg in a single dose
• *Child 0-1 yr:* IV BOL 0.1-0.2 mg/kg over ≥2 min, may repeat after 30 min

Hypertension
• *Adult:* PO 80 mg tid, may titrate

upward; **EXT REL** 120-240 mg/day as a single dose, may increase to 240-480 mg/day

Available forms: Tabs 40, 80, 120 mg; ext rel tabs 120, 180, 240 mg; inj 2.5 mg/ml; caps, ext rel 100, 200, 240, 300 mg

SIDE EFFECTS

CNS: Headache, drowsiness, dizziness, anxiety, depression, weakness, insomnia, confusion, light-headedness, asthenia, fatigue
CV: Edema, CHF, bradycardia, hypotension, palpitations, AV block
GI: Nausea, diarrhea, gastric upset, *constipation,* increased LFTs
GU: Impotence, gynecomastia, nocturia, polyuria
INTEG: Rash, bruising
MISC: Gingival hyperplasia
SYST: Stevens-Johnson syndrome
Contraindications: Sick sinus syndrome, 2nd- or 3rd-degree heart block, hypotension <90 mm Hg systolic, cardiogenic shock, severe CHF
Precautions: Pregnancy (C), CHF, hypotension, hepatic injury, lactation, children, renal disease, concomitant β-blocker therapy, elderly

PHARMACOKINETICS

IV: Onset 3 min, peak 3-5 min, duration 10-20 min
PO: Onset variable, peak 3-4 hr, duration 17-24 hr, half-life (biphasic) 4 min, 3-7 hr (terminal)
Metabolized by liver, excreted in urine (70% as metabolites)

INTERACTIONS

Increase: hypotension—prazosin, quinidine, fentanyl, other antihypertensives, nitrates
Increase: effects of verapamil—β-blockers, cimetidine
Increase: levels of digoxin, theophylline, cycloSPORINE, carbamazepine, nondepolarizing muscle relaxants
Decrease: effects of lithium

V

Decrease: antihypertensive effects—NSAIDs

Drug/Herb

Increase: effect—barberry, betel palm, burdock, goldenseal, khat, lily of the valley, plantain

Decrease: effect—yohimbe

Drug/Food

Increase: hypotensive effects—grapefruit juice

Drug/Lab Test

Increase: AST, ALT, alk phosphatase, BUN, creatinine, serum cholesterol

NURSING CONSIDERATIONS

Assess:

• Cardiac status: B/P, pulse, respiration, ECG intervals (PR, QRS, QT)

🛆 I&O ratios, weight daily; CHF: crackles, weight gain, dyspnea, jugular vein distention

• Renal, hepatic studies during long-term treatment, serum potassium: periodically

Administer:

PO route

• Do not crush or chew ext rel, sus rel products; cap may be opened and contents sprinkled on food; do not dissolve chew cap contents

• Before meals, at bedtime; sus rel give with food

IV route

• Undiluted through Y-tube or 3-way stopcock of compatible sol; give over 2 min, or 3 min elderly, discard unused solution

Additive compatibilities: Amikacin, amiodarone, ascorbic acid, atropine, bretylium, calcium chloride, calcium gluconate, cefamandole, cefazolin, cefotaxime, cefoxitin, cephapirin, chloramphenicol, cimetidine, clindamycin, dexamethasone, diazepam, digoxin, DOPamine, epINEPHrine, erythromycin, gentamicin, heparin, hydrocortisone sodium phosphate, hydrocortisone, hydromorphone, insulin (regular), isoproterenol, lidocaine, magnesium sulfate, mannitol, meperidine, metaraminol, methicillin, methyldopa, methylPRED-NISolone, metoclopramide, mezlocillin, morphine, moxalactam, multivitamins, naloxone, nitroglycerin, norepinephrine, oxytocin, pancuronium, penicillin G potassium, penicillin G sodium, pentobarbital, phenobarbital, phentolamine, phenytoin, piperacillin, potassium chloride, potassium phosphates, procainamide, propranolol, protamine, quinidine, sodium bicarbonate, sodium nitroprusside, theophylline, ticarcillin, tobramycin, tolazoline, vancomycin, vasopressin, vit B/C

Syringe compatibilities: Amrinone, heparin, milrinone

Y-site compatibilities: Amrinone, ciprofloxacin, DOBUTamine, DOPamine, famotidine, hydrALAZINE, meperidine, methicillin, milrinone, penicillin G potassium, piperacillin, propofol, ticarcillin

Evaluate:

• Therapeutic response: decreased anginal pain, decreased B/P, dysrhythmias

Teach patient/family:

• To increase fluids/fiber to counteract constipation

• How to take pulse before taking drug; to keep record or graph

• To avoid hazardous activities until stabilized on drug, dizziness no longer a problem

• To limit caffeine consumption; no alcohol products

• To avoid OTC drugs unless directed by prescriber

• To comply with all areas of medical regimen: diet, exercise, stress reduction, drug therapy

• To change positions slowly to prevent syncope

Treatment of overdose: Defibrillation, atropine for AV block, vasopressor for hypotension, IV calcium

---

vidarabine ophthalmic
See Appendix C

⚠ High Alert

vinBLAStine (VLB) (℞)
(vin-blast'een)
Velban, Velbe ✤, vinblastine
sulfate
Func. class.: Antineoplastic
Chem. class.: Vinca rosea alkaloid

Do not confuse:
vinBLAStine/vinCRIStine

Action: Inhibits mitotic activity, arrests
cell cycle at metaphase; inhibits RNA
synthesis, blocks cellular use of glutamic
acid needed for purine synthesis; a vesicant

Uses: Breast, testicular cancer, lymphomas, neuroblastoma; Hodgkin's, non-
Hodgkin's lymphomas; mycosis fungoides, histiocytosis, Kaposi's sarcoma

DOSAGE AND ROUTES

• *Adult:* IV 0.1 mg/kg or 3.7 mg/m² qwk
or q2wk, not to exceed 0.5 mg/kg or
18.5 mg/m² qwk
• *Child:* 2.5 mg/m² then 3.75, 5, 6.25,
7.5 at 7-day intervals
Available forms: Inj, powder 10 mg
for 10 ml IV

SIDE EFFECTS

CNS: Paresthesias, peripheral neuropathy,
depression, headache, ***convulsions***
CV: Tachycardia, orthostatic hypotension
GI: Nausea, vomiting, ileus, *anorexia,
stomatitis,* constipation, abdominal
pain, ***GI, rectal bleeding, hepatotoxicity,*** pharyngitis
GU: Urinary retention, ***renal failure***
*HEMA: **Thrombocytopenia, leukopenia, myelosuppression***
HEMA: Agranulocytosis, granulocytosis,
aplastic anemia, neutropenia, pancytopenia
INTEG: Rash, alopecia, photosensitivity
META: SIADH

*RESP: **Fibrosis, pulmonary infiltrate, bronchospasm***
Contraindications: Pregnancy (D),
hypersensitivity, infants, leukopenia,
granulocytopenia, lactation
Precautions: Renal disease, hepatic
disease

PHARMACOKINETICS

Half-life (triphasic) 35 min, 53 min, 19
hr; metabolized in liver, excreted in
urine, feces; crosses blood-brain barrier

INTERACTIONS

Synergism: bleomycin
Bronchospasm: mitomycin
Do not use with radiation
Increase: toxicity, bone marrow
suppression—antineoplastics
Increase: action of methotrexate
Increase: adverse reactions—live virus
vaccines
Decrease: phenytoin level—phenytoin

NURSING CONSIDERATIONS

Assess:
⚠ CBC, differential, platelet count qwk;
withhold drug if WBC is <2000/mm³ or
platelet count is <75,000/mm³; notify
prescriber
• Pulmonary function tests, chest x-ray
studies before, during therapy; chest
x-ray film should be obtained q2wk during treatment
• Neurologic status: sensory-vibratory
evaluation if side effects occur
• Renal studies: BUN, serum uric acid,
urine CCr, electrolytes before, during
therapy
• I&O ratio; report fall in urine output of
30 ml/hr
• Monitor temp q4h; may indicate beginning infection
• Hepatic studies before, during therapy
(bilirubin, AST, ALT, LDH) as needed or
qmo
• RBC, Hct, Hgb, since these may be
decreased

- Bleeding: hematuria, guaiac, bruising or petechiae, mucosa of orifices q8h
- Dyspnea, crackles, unproductive cough, chest pain, tachypnea, fatigue, increased pulse, pallor, lethargy
- Effects of alopecia on body image; discuss feelings about body changes
- Sensitivity of feet/hands, which precedes neuropathy
- Jaundiced skin, sclera; dark urine, clay-colored stools, itchy skin, abdominal pain, fever, diarrhea
- Buccal cavity q8h for dryness, sores or ulceration, white patches, oral pain, bleeding, dysphagia
- Local irritation, pain, burning, discoloration at inj site
- Symptoms indicating severe allergic reaction: rash, pruritus, urticaria, purpuric skin lesions, itching, flushing
- Frequency of stools and characteristics: cramping; acidosis; signs of dehydration: rapid respirations, poor skin turgor, decreased urine output, dry skin, restlessness, weakness

Administer:
- Antiemetic 30-60 min before giving drug and prn to prevent vomiting
- Transfusion for anemia

IV route
- After diluting 10 mg/10 ml NaCl; give through Y-tube or 3-way stopcock or directly over 1 min
- Hyaluronidase 150 units/ml in 1 ml NaCl, warm compress for extravasation for vesicant activity treatment

Additive compatibilities: Bleomycin
Syringe compatibilities: Bleomycin, cisplatin, cyclophosphamide, droperidol, fluorouracil, leucovorin, methotrexate, metoclopramide, mitomycin, vinCRIStine
Y-site compatibilities: Allopurinol, amifostine, amphotericin B cholesteryl, aztreonam, bleomycin, cisplatin, cyclophosphamide, DOXOrubicin, DOXOrubicin liposome, droperidol, filgrastim, fludarabine, fluorouracil, granisetron, heparin, leucovorin, melphalan, methotrexate, metoclopramide, mitomycin, ondansetron, paclitaxel, piperacillin/

tazobactam, sargramostim, teniposide, thiotepa, vinCRIStine, vinorelbine
Perform/provide:
- Deep-breathing exercises with patient 3-4 ×/day; place in semi-Fowler's position
- Liquid diet: cola, Jell-O; dry toast or crackers may be added if patient is not nauseated or vomiting
- Increase fluid intake to 2-3 L/day to prevent urate deposits, calculi formation
- Rinsing of mouth tid-qid with water
- Brushing of teeth bid-tid with soft brush or cotton-tipped applicators for stomatitis; use unwaxed dental floss
- Nutritious diet with iron, vitamin supplements
- HOB raised to facilitate breathing

Evaluate:
- Therapeutic response: decreased tumor size, spread of malignancy

Teach patient/family:
- To report any complaints or side effects to nurse or prescriber
- To report any changes in breathing or coughing; to avoid exposure to persons with infection
- That hair may be lost during treatment, a wig or hairpiece may make patient feel better; tell patient that new hair may be different in color, texture
- To report change in gait or numbness in extremities; may indicate neuropathy
- To avoid foods with citric acid, hot or rough texture
- To report any bleeding, white spots or ulcerations in mouth to prescriber; to examine mouth daily
- To wear sunscreen, protective clothing, sunglasses
- To avoid receiving vaccinations
- To use effective contraception, avoid breastfeeding

⚠ Safety alert   *"Tall Man" lettering

⚠ High Alert

vinCRIStine (VCR) (℞)
(vin-kris'teen)
Oncovin, Vincasar PFS, vincristine sulfate
Func. class.: Antineoplastic—
miscellaneous
Chem. class.: Vinca alkaloid

Do not confuse:
vinCRIStine/vinBLAStine

Action: Inhibits mitotic activity, arrests
cell cycle at metaphase; inhibits RNA
synthesis, blocks cellular use of glutamic
acid needed for purine synthesis; a vesicant

Uses: Breast, lung cancer, lymphomas,
neuroblastoma, Hodgkin's disease, acute
lymphoblastic and other leukemias,
rhabdomyosarcoma, Wilms' tumor, osteogenic and other sarcomas

DOSAGE AND ROUTES
• *Adult:* **IV** 1-2 mg/m^2/wk, not to exceed 2 mg
• *Child:* **IV** 1.5-2 mg/m^2/wk, not to
exceed 2 mg
Available forms: Inj 1 mg/ml; powder
for inj 5 mg/vial

SIDE EFFECTS
*CNS: Decreased reflexes, numbness,
weakness, motor difficulties,* CNS depression, cranial nerve paralysis, **seizures**
CV: Orthostatic hypotension
*GI: Nausea, vomiting, anorexia, stoma-
titis, constipation, paralytic ileus,
abdominal pain, hepatotoxicity*
*HEMA: Thrombocytopenia, leukope-
nia, myelosuppression, anemia*
INTEG: Alopecia

Contraindications: Pregnancy (D),
hypersensitivity, infants, radiation therapy, lactation
Precautions: Renal disease, hepatic
disease, hypertension, neuromuscular
disease

PHARMACOKINETICS
Half-life (triphasic) 0.85 min, 7.4 min,
164 min; metabolized in liver; excreted
in bile, feces; crosses placental barrier,
blood-brain barrier

INTERACTIONS
Neurotoxicity: peripheral nervous system
drugs
Do not use with radiation
Acute pulmonary reactions: mitomycin-c
Increase: action of methotrexate, anti-
coagulants
Decrease: digoxin level—digoxin
Decrease: action of vinCRIStine—L-aspa-
raginase

NURSING CONSIDERATIONS
Assess:
• CBC, differential, platelet count qwk;
withhold drug if WBC is <4000/mm^3 or
platelet count is <75,000/mm^3; notify
prescriber
• Renal studies: BUN, serum uric acid,
urine CCr, electrolytes before, during
therapy
• I&O ratio, report fall in urine output of
30 ml/hr
• Monitor temp q4h; may indicate beginning infection
• Hepatic studies before, during therapy
(bilirubin, AST, ALT, LDH) as needed or
monthly
• RBC, Hct, Hgb; may be decreased
• Deep tendon reflexes; drug is neuro-
toxic
• Sensitivity of feet/hands, which precedes neuropathy
• Bleeding: hematuria, guaiac, bruising
or petechiae, mucosa of orifices q8h
• Effects of alopecia on body image,
discuss feelings about body changes
• Jaundiced skin, sclera; dark urine,
clay-colored stools, itchy skin, abdominal pain, fever, diarrhea
• Buccal cavity q8h for dryness, sores or
ulceration, white patches, oral pain,
bleeding, dysphagia
• Symptoms indicating severe allergic

V

Side effects: *italics* = common; ***bold italics*** = life-threatening

reaction: rash, pruritus, urticaria, purpuric skin lesions, itching, flushing

• Frequency of stools, characteristics: cramping, acidosis; signs of dehydration: rapid respirations, poor skin turgor, decreased urine output, dry skin, restlessness, weakness

Administer:

• Agents to prevent constipation
• Antiemetic 30-60 min before giving drug and prn
• Transfusion for anemia
• Antispasmodic for GI symptoms

IV route

• After diluting with diluent provided or 1 mg/10 ml of sterile H_2O or NaCl; give through Y-tube or 3-way stopcock or directly over 1 min
• Hyaluronidase 150 units/ml in 1 ml NaCl; apply warm compress for extravasation

Additive compatibilities: Bleomycin, cytarabine, fluorouracil, methotrexate

Syringe compatibilities: Bleomycin, cisplatin, cyclophosphamide, doxapram, DOXOrubicin, droperidol, fluorouracil, heparin, leucovorin, methotrexate, metoclopramide, mitomycin, vinBLAStine

Y-site compatibilities: Allopurinol, amifostine, amphotericin B cholesteryl, aztreonam, bleomycin, cisplatin, cladribine, cyclophosphamide, DOXOrubicin, DOXOrubicin liposome, droperidol, filgrastim, fludarabine, fluorouracil, granisetron, heparin, leucovorin, melphalan, methotrexate, metoclopramide, mitomycin, ondansetron, paclitaxel, piperacillin/tazobactam, sargramostim, teniposide, thiotepa, vinBLAStine, vinorelbine

Perform/provide:

• Liquid diet: cola, Jell-O; dry toast or crackers may be added if patient is not nauseated or vomiting
• Rinsing of mouth tid-qid with water
• Brushing of teeth bid-tid with soft brush or cotton-tipped applicators for stomatitis; use unwaxed dental floss
• Nutritious diet with iron, vitamin supplements

Evaluate:

• Therapeutic response: decreased tumor size, spread of malignancy

Teach patient/family:

• To report change in gait or numbness in extremities; may indicate neuropathy
• To report any complaints or side effects to nurse or prescriber
• To report any bleeding, white spots or ulcerations in mouth to prescriber; to examine mouth daily
• To increase bulk, fluids, exercise to prevent constipation
• To avoid persons with infections
• To avoid vaccinations
• That hair may be lost; hair will grow back but different texture, color
• To use effective contraception, avoid breastfeeding

> ### ⚠ High Alert
>
> ## vinorelbine (℞)
> (vi-nor'el-bine)
> Navelbine
> *Func. class.:* Antineoplastic—miscellaneous
> *Chem. class.:* Semisynthetic vinca alkaloid

Action: Inhibits mitotic activity, arrests cell cycle at metaphase; inhibits RNA synthesis, blocks cellular use of glutamic acid needed for purine synthesis; a vesicant

Uses: Unresectable advanced non–small cell lung cancer (NSCLC) stage IV; may be used alone or in combination with cisplatin for stage III or IV NSCLC breast cancer

DOSAGE AND ROUTES

• *Adult:* IV 30 mg/m² qwk

Hepatic dose

• *Adult:* IV total bilirubin 2.1-3 mg/dl 15 mg/m² qwk; total bilirubin ≥3 mg/dl 7.5 mg/m² daily

Available forms: Inj 10 mg/ml

SIDE EFFECTS

CNS: Paresthesias, peripheral neuropathy, depression, headache, ***convulsions,*** weakness, jaw pain

CV: Chest pain

GI: Nausea, vomiting, ileus, *anorexia, stomatitis,* constipation, abdominal pain, diarrhea, ***hepatotoxicity***

HEMA: **Neutropenia, anemia, thrombocytopenia, granulocytopenia**

INTEG: Rash, alopecia, photosensitivity

META: SIADH

MS: Myalgia

RESP: Shortness of breath

Contraindications: Pregnancy (D), hypersensitivity, infants, granulocyte count <1000 cells/mm³ pretreatment, lactation

Precautions: Renal, hepatic disease, elderly, children

PHARMACOKINETICS

Half-life 27-43 hr, peak 1-2 hr

INTERACTIONS

Possible increased toxicity: fluorouracil

NURSING CONSIDERATIONS

Assess:

• B/P (baseline and q15min) during administration

• CBC, differential, platelet count weekly; withhold drug if WBC is <4000/mm³ or platelet count is <75,000/mm³; notify prescriber of results, recovery will take 3 wk

• For dyspnea, crackles, unproductive cough, chest pain, tachypnea

• Renal studies: BUN, serum uric acid, urine CCr before, during therapy; I&O ratio; report fall in urine output to <30 ml/hr; for decreased hyperuricemia

• For cold, fever, sore throat (may indicate beginning infection); notify prescriber if these occur; effects of alopecia on body image

• For bleeding: hematuria, guaiac, bruising or petechiae, mucosa or orifices

q8h, no rectal temps; avoid IM inj; use pressure to venipuncture sites

• Nutritional status: an antiemetic may be needed

A For symptoms of severe allergic reactions: rash, pruritus, urticaria, itching, flushing, bronchospasm, hypotension, epINEPHrine and crash cart should be nearby

Administer:

• Antiemetic 30-60 min before giving drug and prn to prevent vomiting

IV route

• Hyaluronidase 150 units/ml in 1 ml NaCl, warm compress for extravasation for vesicant activity treatment

• By cont inf: 40 mg/m² q3wk after an IV bol of 8 mg/m²; may be given in combination with DOXOrubicin, fluorouracil, cisplatin

Y-site compatibilities: Amikacin, aztreonam, bleomycin, bumetanide, buprenorphine, butorphanol, calcium gluconate, carboplatin, carmustine, cefotaxime, ceftazidime, ceftizoxime, chlorproMAZINE, cimetidine, cisplatin, clindamycin, cyclophosphamide, cytarabine, dacarbazine, dactinomycin, DAUNOrubicin, dexamethasone, diphenhydrAMINE, DOXOrubicin, DOXOrubicin liposome, doxycycline, droperidol, enalaprilat, etoposide, famotidine, filgrastim, floxuridine, fluconazole, fludarabine, gallium, gentamicin, granisetron, haloperidol, heparin, hydrocortisone, hydromorphone, hydrOXYzine, idarubicin, ifosfamide, imipenem-cilastatin, lorazepam, mannitol, mechlorethamine, melphalan, meperidine, mesna, methotrexate, metoclopramide, metronidazole, minocycline, mitoxantrone, morphine, nalbuphine, netilmicin, ondansetron, plicamycin, streptozocin, teniposide, ticarcillin, ticarcillin/clavulanate, tobramycin, vancomycin, vinBLAStine, vinCRIStine, zidovudine

Perform/provide:

• Liquid diet: cola, Jell-O; dry toast or crackers if patient not nauseated or vomiting

• Brushing of teeth bid-tid with soft

Side effects: *italics* = common; **bold italics** = life-threatening

brush or cotton-tipped applicators for stomatitis; unwaxed dental floss
• Nutritious diet with iron, vitamin supplements

Evaluate:
• Therapeutic response: decreased tumor size, spread of malignancy

Teach patient/family:
• To report change in gait or numbness in extremities; may indicate neuropathy
• To report any complaints or side effects to nurse or prescriber
• To examine mouth daily for bleeding, white spots, ulcerations; notify prescriber
• To avoid crowds, people with infections, vaccinations
• To use effective contraception, avoid breastfeeding
• That hair may be lost; hair will grow back, but different texture, color

---

vitamin A (R, otc)

Aquasol A, Del-Vi-A, Vitamin A
Func. class.: Vitamin, fat soluble
Chem. class.: Retinol

Action: Needed for normal bone, tooth development, visual dark adaptation, skin disease, mucosa tissue repair, assists in production of adrenal steroids, cholesterol, RNA

Uses: Vit A deficiency

DOSAGE AND ROUTES

• *Adult and child >8 yr:* **PO** 100,000-500,000 international units daily × 3 days, then 50,000 daily × 2 wk; dose based on severity of deficiency; maintenance 10,000-20,000 international units for 2 mo
• *Child 1-8 yr:* **IM** 5000-15,000 international units daily × 10 days
• *Infant <1 yr:* **IM** 5000-15,000 international units × 10 days

Maintenance
• *Child 4-8 yr:* **IM** 15,000 international units daily × 2 mo

• *Child <4 yr:* **IM** 10,000 international units daily × 2 mo

Available forms: Caps 10,000, 25,000, 50,000 international units; drops 5000 international units; inj 50,000 international units/ml; tabs 10,000, 25,000, 50,000 international units

SIDE EFFECTS

CNS: Headache, *increased intracranial pressure, intracranial hypertension,* lethargy, malaise
EENT: Gingivitis, papilledema, exophthalmos, inflammation of tongue and lips
GI: Nausea, vomiting, anorexia, abdominal pain, *jaundice*
INTEG: Drying of skin, pruritus, increased pigmentation, night sweats, alopecia
META: Hypomenorrhea, hypercalcemia
MS: Arthralgia, retarded growth, hard areas on bone

Contraindications: Hypersensitivity to vit A, malabsorption syndrome (PO)
Precautions: Pregnancy (C), lactation, impaired renal function

PHARMACOKINETICS

Stored in liver, kidneys, fat; excreted (metabolites) in urine, feces

INTERACTIONS

Increase: levels of vit A—corticosteroids, oral contraceptives
Decrease: absorption of vit A—mineral oil, cholestyramine, colestipol
Drug/Lab Test
False increase: Bilirubin, serum cholesterol

NURSING CONSIDERATIONS

Assess:
• Nutritional status: yellow and dark green vegetables, yellow/orange fruits, vit A–fortified foods, liver, egg yolks
• Vit A deficiency: decreased growth, night blindness, dry, brittle nails; hair loss; urinary stones; increased infection, hyperkeratosis of skin; drying of cornea

---

Administer:
PO route
- With food (PO) for better absorption
- Do not administer IV because of risk of anaphylactic shock, IM only
- Oral preparations are not indicated for vitamin A deficiency in those with malabsorption syndrome

Perform/provide:
- Storage in tight, light-resistant container

Evaluate:
- Therapeutic response: increased growth rate, weight; absence of dry skin and mucous membranes, night blindness

Teach patient/family:
- That if dose is missed, it should be omitted
- That ophthalmic exams may be required periodically throughout therapy
- Not to use mineral oil while taking this drug
- To notify prescriber of nausea, vomiting, lip cracking, loss of hair, headache
- Not to take more than the prescribed amount

Treatment of overdose: Discontinue drug

---

vitamin D (cholecalciferol, vitamin D₃ or ergocalciferol, vitamin D₂) (℞, otc)

Calciferol, Delta-D, Drisdol, Radiostol ✹, Radiostol Forte ✹, Vitamin D, Vitamin D₃
Func. class.: Vit D
Chem. class.: Fat soluble

Do not confuse:
Calciferol/calcitriol
Action: Needed for regulation of calcium, phosphate levels, normal bone development, parathyroid activity, neuromuscular functioning
Uses: Vit D deficiency, rickets, renal osteodystrophy, hypoparathyroidism, hypophosphatemia, psoriasis, rheumatoid arthritis

DOSAGE AND ROUTES
Deficiency
- *Adult:* **PO/IM** 12,000 international units daily, then increased to 500,000 international units/day
- *Child:* **PO/IM** 1500-5000 international units daily × 2-4 wk, may repeat after 2 wk or 600,000 international units as single dose

Hypoparathyroidism
- *Adult and child:* **PO/IM** 200,000 international units given with 4 g calcium tab

Available forms: Tabs 400, 1000, 50,000 international units; caps 25,000, 50,000 international units; liq 8000 international units/ml; inj 500,000 international units/ml, 500,000 international units/5 ml

SIDE EFFECTS
CNS: Fatigue, weakness, drowsiness, ***convulsions,*** headache, psychosis
CV: Hypertension, dysrhythmias
GI: Nausea, vomiting, anorexia, cramps, diarrhea, constipation, metallic taste, dry mouth
GU: Polyuria, nocturia, ***hematuria, albuminuria, renal failure,*** decreased libido
INTEG: Pruritus, photophobia
MS: Decreased bone growth, early joint pain, early muscle pain
Contraindications: Hypersensitivity, hypercalcemia, renal dysfunction, hyperphosphatemia
Precautions: Pregnancy (C), cardiovascular disease, renal calculi

PHARMACOKINETICS
Half-life 12-22 hr; stored in liver, duration 2 mo; excreted in bile (metabolites) and urine

INTERACTIONS
Increase: toxicity—diuretics (thiazides), antacids, verapamil
Decrease: effects of vit D—cholestyramine, colestipol, phenobarbital, phenytoin

V

NURSING CONSIDERATIONS

Assess:
- Vit D levels q2wk during treatment
- Calcium, PO_4, magnesium, BUN, alk phosphatase, urine Ca, creatinine
- In children, monitor height and weight
- Nutritional status: egg yolk, fortified dairy products, cod, halibut, salmon, sardines

Administer:
- IM inj deep in large muscle mass; administer slowly; aspirate carefully; rotate inj sites; avoid IV administration
- A decrease of antacids and laxatives containing magnesium

Evaluate:
- Therapeutic response: absence of rickets/osteomalacia, adequate calcium/phosphate levels, decrease in bone pain

Teach patient/family:
- That if dose is missed, to omit
- The necessary foods in diet
- To avoid vitamin supplements unless directed by prescriber
- To keep appointments with health care providers; line between therapeutic and toxic doses is narrow
- To report weakness, lethargy, headache, anorexia, loss of weight
- To report nausea, vomiting, abdominal cramps, diarrhea, constipation, excessive thirst, polyuria, muscle and bone pain
- To decrease intake of antacids and laxatives containing magnesium

---

vitamin E (OTC)

Amino-Opti-E, Aquasol E, Daltose ✦, E-Complex-600, E-Ferol, E-Vitamin Succinate, E-200 I.U. Softgels, Gordo-Vite E, Tocopherol, Vitamin E, Vita-Plus E Softgells, Vitec

Func. class.: Vit E
Chem. class.: Fat soluble

Action: Needed for digestion and metabolism of polyunsaturated fats, decreases platelet aggregation, decreases blood clot formation, promotes normal growth and development of muscle tissue, prostaglandin synthesis

Uses: Vit E deficiency, impaired fat absorption, hemolytic anemia in premature neonates, prevention of retrolental fibroplasia, sickle cell anemia, supplement in malabsorption syndrome

DOSAGE AND ROUTES

Deficiency
- *Adult:* **PO** 60-75 international units daily
- *Child:* **PO** 1 mg/0.6 g of dietary fat

Prevention of deficiency
- *Adult:* **PO** 30 international units/day; **TOP** apply to affected areas
- *Infants:* **PO** 5 international units/day

Available forms: Caps 100, 200, 400, 500, 600, 1000 international units; tabs 100, 200, 400 international units; drops 50 mg/ml; chew tabs 400 units; ointment, cream, lotion, oil

SIDE EFFECTS

CNS: Headache, fatigue
CV: Increased risk of thrombophlebitis
EENT: Blurred vision
GI: Nausea, cramps, diarrhea
GU: Gonadal dysfunction
INTEG: Sterile abscess, contact dermatitis
META: Altered metabolism of hormones: thyroid, pituitary, adrenal; altered immunity
MS: Weakness

Contraindications: IV use in infants
Precautions: Pregnancy (A)

PHARMACOKINETICS

PO: Metabolized in liver, excreted in bile

INTERACTIONS

Increase: action of oral anticoagulants
Decrease: absorption—cholestyramine, colestipol, mineral oil, sucralfate

NURSING CONSIDERATIONS

Assess:
- Nutritional status: wheat germ, dark green leafy vegetables, nuts, eggs, liver, vegetable oils, dairy products, cereals

---

⚠ Safety alert   ✦"Tall Man" lettering

Administer:

PO route

- Administer with or after meals
- Chew chewable tabs well
- Sol may be dropped in mouth or mixed with food

TOP route

- To moisturize dry skin

Perform/provide:

- Storage in tight, light-resistant container

Evaluate:

- Therapeutic response: absence of hemolytic anemia, adequate vit E levels, improvement in skin lesions, decreased edema

Teach patient/family:

- The necessary foods in diet
- To omit if dose is missed
- To avoid vitamin supplements unless directed by prescriber

---

voriconazole (R)

(vohr-i-kahn'a-zol)
Vfend
Func. class.: Antifungal, systemic
Chem. class.: Triazole derivative

Action: Inhibits fungal CYP 450-mediation demethylation, needed for biosynthesis

Uses: Invasive aspergillosis, serious fungal infections (*Scedosporium apiospermum, Fusarium* sp.)

DOSAGE AND ROUTES

- *Adult:* **PO** Give 1 hr ac or pc; ≥40 kg: 200 mg q12h; <40 kg: 100 mg q12h
- *Adult:* **IV** Loading dose 6 mg/kg q12h × 2 dose, then 4 mg/kg q12h; may switch to oral dosing

Available forms: Tabs 50, 200 mg; powder for inj, lyophilized 200 mg voriconazole, 3200 mg sulfobutyl ester β-cyclodextrin sodium (SBECD), powder for oral susp 45 g (40 mg/ml after reconstitution)

SIDE EFFECTS

CNS: Headache, paresthesias, peripheral neuropathy, hallucinations, psychosis, EPS, depression, Guillain-Barré syndrome, insomnia, suicidal ideation, dizziness

CV: Tachycardia, hyper/hypotension, vasodilation, *atrial arrhythmias, atrial fibrillation, AV block, bradycardia, CHF, MI*

EENT: Blurred vision, eye hemorrhage

GI: Nausea, vomiting, anorexia, diarrhea, cramps, *hemorrhagic gastroenteritis, acute hepatic failure, hepatitis, intestinal perforation, pancreatitis*

GU: Hypokalemia, azotemia, *renal tubular necrosis, permanent renal impairment, anuria, oliguria*

HEMA: Anemia, *eosinophilia,* hypomagnesemia, *thrombocytopenia, leukopenia, pancytopenia*

INTEG: Burning, irritation, pain, necrosis at inj site with extravasation, dermatitis, rash, photosensitivity

MISC: Respiratory disorder

SYST: Stevens-Johnson syndrome, toxic epidermal necrolysis, sepsis

Contraindications: Pregnancy (D), hypersensitivity, severe bone marrow depression, lactation, children, severe hepatic disease

Precautions: Renal disease (IV)

PHARMACOKINETICS

By P45 enzymes, protein binding 58%; max serum conc 1-2 hr after dosing; eliminated via hepatic metabolism

INTERACTIONS

Increase: effects of benzodiazepines, calcium channel blockers, cycloSPORINE, ergots, HMG-CoA reductase inhibitors, pimozide, quinidine, predniso-LONE, sirolimus, sulfonylureas, tacrolimus, vinca alkaloids, warfarin, rifabutin, proton pump inhibitors, NNRTIs, protease inhibitors, phenytoin

Increase: nephrotoxicity—other nephrotoxic antibiotics (aminoglycosides,

V

cisplatin, vancomycin, cycloSPORINE, polymyxin B)
Increase: hypokalemia—corticosteroids, digitalis, skeletal muscle relaxants, thiazides
Drug/Herb
Increase: possibility of nephrotoxicity—gossypol
Drug/Food
Avoid use with high-fat meals

NURSING CONSIDERATIONS

Assess:
• VS q15-30min during first infusion; note changes in pulse, B/P
• I&O ratio; watch for decreasing urinary output, change in specific gravity; discontinue drug to prevent permanent damage to renal tubules
• Blood studies: CBC, K, Na, Ca, Mg q2wk, BUN, creatinine weekly
• Weight weekly; if weight increases over 2 lb/wk, edema is present; renal damage should be considered
⚠ For renal toxicity: increasing BUN, serum creatinine; if BUN is >40 mg/dl or if serum creatinine >3 mg/dl, drug may be discontinued or dosage reduced
⚠ For hepatotoxicity: increasing AST, ALT, alk phosphatase, bilirubin
• For allergic reaction: dermatitis, rash; drug should be discontinued, antihistamines (mild reaction) or epINEPHrine (severe reaction) administered
• For hypokalemia: anorexia, drowsiness, weakness, decreased reflexes, dizziness, increased urinary output, increased thirst, paresthesias
• For ototoxicity: tinnitus (ringing, roaring in ears), vertigo, loss of hearing (rare); visual disturbance
Administer:
PO route
• Oral susp: tap bottle, add 46 ml of water to bottle, shake well, remove cap, push bottle adaptor into neck of bottle, replace cap, write expiration date (14 days); shake well before each use, administer using only oral dispenser supplied
• 1 hr before or after meals

IV route
• Drug only after C&S confirms organism, drug needed to treat condition; make sure drug is used in life-threatening infections
• Reconstitute powder with 19 ml water for inj to 10 mg/ml, shake until dissolved; infuse over 1-2 hr at a conc of 5 mg/ml or less; do not admix with other drugs, 4.2% sodium bicarbonate inf
• Store at room temp (powder, tabs)
Evaluate:
• Therapeutic response: decreased fever, malaise, rash, negative C&S for infecting organism
Teach patient/family:
• That long-term therapy may be needed to clear infection (2 wk–3 mo depending on type of infection)
• To notify prescriber of bleeding, bruising, or soft tissue swelling
• Take 1 hr before or after meal
• Do not drive at night because of vision changes
• Avoid strong, direct sunlight
• Women of childbearing age should use effective contraceptive

---

⚠ High Alert

warfarin (℞)
(war'far-in)
Coumadin, warfarin sodium, Warfilone ✦
Func. class.: Anticoagulant

Do not confuse:
Coumadin/Cardura
Coumadin/Compazine
Action: Interferes with blood clotting by indirect means; depresses hepatic synthesis of vit K–dependent coagulation factors (II, VII, IX, X)
Uses: Pulmonary emboli, deep-vein thrombosis; prevention or treatment of venous thrombosis, pulmonary embolism, thromboembolic complications associated with atrial fibrillation, or cardiac valve replacement; after MI to reduce risk of death

---

⚠ Safety alert   *"Tall Man" lettering

DOSAGE AND ROUTES

• *Adult:* **PO/IV** 2.5-10 mg/day × 3 days, then titrated to prothrombin time or INR daily
• *Geriatric:* **PO/IV** 2-10 mg/day
• *Child:* 0.1 mg/kg/day titrated to INR
Available forms: Tabs 1, 2, 2.5, 3, 4, 5, 6, 7.5, 10 mg; inj 5.4 mg powder for inj

SIDE EFFECTS

CNS: Fever
GI: Diarrhea, nausea, vomiting, anorexia, stomatitis, cramps, ***hepatitis***
*GU: **Hematuria***
*HEMA: **Hemorrhage, agranulocytosis, leukopenia, eosinophilia***
INTEG: Rash, dermatitis, urticaria, alopecia, pruritus
Contraindications: Pregnancy (X), hypersensitivity, hemophilia, leukemia with bleeding, peptic ulcer disease, thrombocytopenic purpura, hepatic disease (severe), malignant hypertension, subacute bacterial endocarditis, acute nephritis, blood dyscrasias, eclampsia, preeclampsia, lactation
Precautions: Alcoholism, elderly, CHF

PHARMACOKINETICS

PO: Onset 12-24 hr, peak 1½-4 days, duration 3-5 days, effective half-life 1½-2½ days; metabolized in liver, excreted in urine/feces (active/inactive metabolites), crosses placenta, 99% bound to plasma proteins

INTERACTIONS

Increase: warfarin action—allopurinol, chloramphenicol, furosemide, HMG-CO reductase inhibitors, SSRIs, amiodarone, diflunisal, heparin, steroids, cimetidine, disulfiram, thyroid, glucagon, metronidazole, quinidine, sulindac, sulfinpyrazone, sulfonamides, clofibrate, salicylates, ethacrynic acids, indomethacin, mefenamic acid, oxyphenbutazones, phenylbutazone, penicillins, cefamandole, chloral hydrate, cotrimoxazole, erythromycin, quinolone antiinfectives, isoniazid, thrombolytic agents, tricyclics, NSAIDs, COX-2 selective inhibitors
Increase: toxicity—oral sulfonylureas, phenytoin
Decrease: warfarin action—barbiturates, griseofulvin, ethchlorvynol, carbamazepine, rifampin, oral contraceptives, dicloxacillin, nafcillin, phenytoin, estrogens, vit K, sucralfate, vit K foods
Drug/Herb
Increase: risk of bleeding—agrimony, alfalfa, angelica, anise, basil, bay, bilberry, black haw, bogbean, bromelain, buchu, chondroitin, cinchona bark, dong quai, fenugreek, feverfew, garlic, ginger, ginkgo, ginseng, horse chestnut, Irish moss, kelp, kelpware, khella, lovage, lungwort, meadowsweet, motherwort, mugwort, nettle, papaya, parsley (large amts), pau d'arco, pineapple, poplar, prickly ash, safflower, saw palmetto, tonka bean, turmeric, wintergreen, yarrow
Decrease: anticoagulant effect—chamomile, coenzyme Q10, flax, glucomannan, goldenseal, guar gum, St. John's wort
Drug/Lab Test
Increase: T_3 uptake
Decrease: Uric acid

NURSING CONSIDERATIONS

Assess:
• Blood studies (Hct, platelets, occult blood in stools) q3mo
• PT, which should be 1½-2 × control; PT often done daily initially or INR
• Bleeding gums, petechiae, ecchymosis, black tarry stools, hematuria
🅰 Fever, skin rash, urticaria
• Needed dosage change q1-2wk; when stable, PT q3wk
Administer:
• At same time each day to maintain steady blood levels
• Tabs whole or crushed
• Avoiding all IM inj that may cause bleeding
IV route
• Reconstitute with 2.7 ml of sterile

W

Side effects: *italics* = common; ***bold italics*** = life-threatening

water for inj; do not use solution that is discolored or has particulates

• Give over 1-2 min into peripheral vein

Y-site compatibilities: Cefazolin, ceftriaxone, DOPamine, heparin, lidocaine, morphine, nitroglycerin, potassium chloride, ranitidine

Perform/provide:

• Storage in tight container

Evaluate:

• Therapeutic response: decrease of deep-vein thrombosis

Teach patient/family:

• To avoid OTC preparations that may cause serious drug interactions unless directed by prescriber

• To use soft-bristle toothbrush to avoid bleeding gums, and to use electric razor

• To carry emergency ID identifying drug taken

• The importance of compliance

• To report any signs of bleeding: gums, under skin, urine, stools

• To avoid hazardous activities (football, hockey, skiing), dangerous work

• The importance of avoiding unusual changes in vitamin intake, diet, or lifestyle

• To inform dentists and other physicians of anticoagulant intake

• To limit foods high in vit K (green leafy vegetables) may impair anticoagulation

Treatment of overdose: Administer vit K

---

xylometazoline nasal agent

See Appendix C

---

zafirlukast (℞)

(za-feer′loo-cast)

Accolate

Func. class.: Bronchodilator

Chem. class.: Leukotriene receptor antagonist

Action: Antagonizes the contractile action of leukotrienes (LTC$_4$, LTD$_4$, LTE$_4$)

in airway smooth muscle; inhibits bronchoconstriction caused by antigens

Uses: Prophylaxis and chronic treatment of asthma in adults/children >5 yr

Investigational uses: Chronic urticaria

DOSAGE AND ROUTES

• *Adult/child ≥12 yr:* **PO** 20 mg bid, take 1 hr ac or 2 hr pc

• *Child 5-11 yr:* **PO** 10 mg bid

Available forms: Tabs 10, 20 mg

SIDE EFFECTS

CNS: Headache, dizziness

GI: Nausea, diarrhea, abdominal pain, vomiting, dyspepsia

OTHER: Infections, pain, asthenia, myalgia, fever, increased ALT, urticaria, rash, **angioedema**

Contraindications: Hypersensitivity

Precautions: Pregnancy (B), elderly, lactation, children, hepatic disease

PHARMACOKINETICS

Rapidly absorbed, peak 3 hr, 99% protein binding (albumin), extensively metabolized; inhibits P450 2C9 and 3A4 enzyme systems; excreted in feces, clearance is reduced in the elderly, hepatic impairment, half-life 10 hr

INTERACTIONS

Increase: plasma levels of zafirlukast—aspirin

Increase: PT—warfarin

Decrease: plasma levels of zafirlukast—erythromycin, theophylline

Drug/Herb

Increase: effect—green tea (large amounts), guarana

Drug/Food

Decrease: bioavailability

NURSING CONSIDERATIONS

Assess:

⚠ Adult patients carefully for symptoms of Churg-Strauss syndrome (rare), including eosinophilia, vasculitic rash,

---

worsening pulmonary symptoms, cardiac complications, and/or neuropathy
• Respiratory rate, rhythm, depth; auscultate lung fields bilaterally; notify prescriber of abnormalities

Administer:
• 1 hr ac or 2 hr pc; absorption may be decreased if given with food
• With water if GI upset occurs

Evaluate:
• Therapeutic response: ability to breathe more easily

Teach patient/family:
• To check OTC medications, current prescription medications, which will increase stimulation
• To avoid hazardous activities; dizziness may occur
• That if GI upset occurs, to take drug with 8 oz water; avoid food if possible, absorption may be decreased
• To notify prescriber of nausea, vomiting, diarrhea, abdominal pain, fatigue, jaundice, anorexia, flulike symptoms (hepatic dysfunction)
• Not to use for acute asthma episodes
• Not to take if breastfeeding
• To take even if symptom free

---

zalcitabine (℞)

(zal-sit′a-bin)
ddC, dideoxycytidine, HIVID
Func. class.: Antiretroviral
Chem. class.: (NRTI) Nucleoside
reverse transcriptase inhibitor

Action: Inhibits HIV-1 replication by the conversion of this drug by cellular enzymes to an active antiviral metabolite, a chain terminator

Uses: HIV-1 infections in combination in adults, children >13 yr

DOSAGE AND ROUTES
• *Adult:* PO 0.75 mg q8h in combination with other antiretrovirals, in presence of peripheral neuropathy initiate dose at 0.375 mg q8h of zalcitabine

Renal dose
• *Adult:* PO CCr 10-40 ml/min 0.75 mg q12h; CCr <10 ml/min 0.75 mg q24h
Available forms: Tabs 0.375, 0.75 mg

SIDE EFFECTS
CNS: Headache, peripheral neuropathy, **seizures**, confusion, anxiety, hypertonia, abnormal thinking, asthenia, insomnia, CNS depression, pain, *dizziness*, chills, *fever*
CV: Hypertension, vasodilation, dysrhythmia, syncope, palpitation, tachycardia, **cardiomyopathy, CHF**
EENT: Ear pain, otitis, photophobia, visual impairment
ENDO: Hypoglycemia, hyponatremia, hyperbilirubinemia, hyperglycemia
GI: **Pancreatitis**, *diarrhea, nausea, vomiting*, abdominal pain, constipation, stomatitis, dysplasia, hepatic abnormalities, *oral ulcers*, flatulence, taste perversion, dry mouth, oral thrush, melena, *increased ALT, AST, alk phosphatase, amylase*
GU: Uric acid, **toxic nephropathy**, polyuria
HEMA: **Leukopenia, granulocytopenia, thrombocytopenia**, anemia
INTEG: Rash, pruritus, alopecia, sweating, acne
MS: Myalgia, arthritis, myopathy, muscular atrophy
RESP: Cough, pneumonia, dyspnea, asthma, hypoventilation
SYST: **Lactic acidosis**
Contraindications: Hypersensitivity
Precautions: Pregnancy (C), renal, hepatic disease, lactation, child <13 yr, peripheral neuropathy, heart failure

PHARMACOKINETICS
PO: Peak 0.5-2 hr, elimination half-life 1-3 hr; elimination via kidneys

INTERACTIONS
Increase: risk of pancreatitis with agents that can cause pancreatitis (ddI, d4T)
Increase: risk of peripheral neuropathy with other agents that can cause periph-

Z

eral neuropathy—aminoglycosides, amphotericin B, chloramphenicol, cimetidine, cisplatin, dapsone, disulfiram, ethionamide, foscarnet, glutethimide, gold, hydrALAZINE, iodoquinol, isoniazid, metronidazole, nitrofurantoin, phenytoin, probenecid, ribavirin, vinCRIStine, other nucleoside analogs

Decrease: absorption—ketoconazole, dapsone, food, antacids, metoclopramide

NURSING CONSIDERATIONS
Assess:
• Neuropathy: tingling or pain in hands and feet, distal numbness

🅐 Pancreatitis: abdominal pain, nausea, vomiting, elevated hepatic enzymes; drug should be discontinued, since condition can be fatal

🅐 For lactic acidosis, severe hepatomegaly with steatosis that can be fatal, drug should be discontinued

• Children by dilated retinal exam q6mo to rule out retinal depigmentation

• Viral load CD4 baseline and throughout treatment

• CBC, differential, platelet count qwk; withhold drug if WBC is <4000/mm³ or platelet count is <75,000/mm³; notify prescriber

• Renal studies: BUN, serum uric acid, urine CCr before, during therapy

• Temp q4h; may indicate beginning infection

• Hepatic studies before, during therapy (bilirubin, AST, ALT), triglycerides, amylase prn or qmo

Administer:
• 1 hr ac or 2 hr pc

Perform/provide:
• Strict medical asepsis, protective isolation if WBC levels are low

Evaluate:
• Therapeutic response: absence of infection; symptoms of HIV

Teach patient/family:
• To report signs of infection: fever, sore throat, flulike symptoms

• To report signs of anemia: fatigue,

headache, faintness, shortness of breath, irritability

• To report bleeding; avoid use of razors, commercial mouthwash

• That hair may be lost during therapy; a wig or hairpiece may make patient feel better

---

zaleplon (℞)
(zal'eh-plon)
Sonata
Func. class.: Sedative/hypnotic, antianxiety
Chem. class.: Pyrazolopyrimidine

Controlled Substance Schedule IV
Action: Binds selectively to omega-1 receptor of the GABA$_A$ receptor complex; results are sedation, hypnosis, skeletal muscle relaxation, anticonvulsant activity, anxiolytic action
Uses: Insomnia

DOSAGE AND ROUTES
• *Adult:* PO 10 mg at bedtime; may increase dose to 20 mg at bedtime if needed; 5 mg may be used in low-weight persons
• *Geriatric:* PO 15 mg at bedtime; may increase if needed
Available forms: Caps 5, 10 mg

SIDE EFFECTS
CNS: Lethargy, drowsiness, daytime sedation, dizziness, confusion, anxiety, amnesia, depersonalization, hallucinations, hypesthesia, paresthesia, somnolence, tremor, vertigo
EENT: Vision change, ear/eye pain, hyperacusis, parosmia
GI: Nausea, abdominal pain, constipation, anorexia, colitis, dyspepsia, dry mouth
MISC: Asthenia, fever, headache, myalgia, dysmenorrhea
Contraindications: Hypersensitivity
Precautions: Pregnancy (C), hepatic disease, renal disease, elderly, psychosis, child <15 yr, lactation

---

PHARMACOKINETICS

PO: Rapid onset, metabolized by liver extensively; excreted by kidneys (inactive metabolites); half-life 1 hr

INTERACTIONS

Increase: effects of zaleplon—cimetidine

Decrease: effect of zaleplon—rifampin

Drug/Herb

Increase: CNS depression—catnip, chamomile, clary, cowslip, hops, kava, lavender, mistletoe, nettle, pokeweed, poppy, Queen Anne's lace, senega, skullcap, valerian

Increase: hypotension—black cohosh

Drug/Food

Prolonged absorption, sleep onset reduced: high-fat/heavy meal

NURSING CONSIDERATIONS

Assess:

• Mental status: mood, sensorium, affect, memory (long, short)

• Type of sleep problem: falling asleep, staying asleep

Administer:

• After removal of cigarettes to prevent fires

• After trying conservative measures for insomnia

• Immediately before bedtime for sleeplessness

• On empty stomach for fast onset

• Avoid use with CNS depressants

Perform/provide:

• Assistance with ambulation after receiving dose

• Safety measure: nightlight, call bell within easy reach

• Checking to see if PO medication has been swallowed

• Storage in tight container in cool environment

Evaluate:

• Therapeutic response: ability to sleep at night, decreased amount of early morning awakening

Teach patient/family:

• To avoid driving or other activities requiring alertness until drug is stabilized

• To avoid alcohol ingestion

• Alternative measures to improve sleep: reading, exercise several hr before bedtime, warm bath, warm milk, TV, self-hypnosis, deep breathing

• That drug may cause memory problems, dependence (if used for longer periods of time), changes in behavior/thinking

• That drug is for short-term use only

• To take immediately before going to bed

• Not to ingest a high-fat/heavy meal before taking

---

zanamivir (℞)
(zan'ah-mih-veer)
Relenza
Func. class.: Antiviral
Chem. class.: Neuramidase inhibitor

Action: Inhibits neuramidase enzyme needed for influenza virus replication

Uses: Treatment of influenza types A and B for those that have been symptomatic for no more than 2 days

Investigational uses: Prophylaxis against influenza and biinfections; avian flu (H3N1)

DOSAGE AND ROUTES

• *Adult and child >7 yr:* **INH** 2 inhalations (two 5 mg blisters) q12h × 5 days, on the 1st day 2 doses should be taken with at least 2 hr between doses

Available forms: Blisters of powder for inhalation: 5 mg

SIDE EFFECTS

CNS: Headache, *dizziness,* fatigue
EENT: Ear, nose, throat infections
GI: *Nausea, vomiting,* diarrhea
RESP: Nasal symptoms, cough, sinusitis, bronchitis

Contraindications: Hypersensitivity

Z

Precautions: Pregnancy (C), lactation, children <7 yr, respiratory disease, elderly

PHARMACOKINETICS

Half-life 2½-5 hr, not metabolized, excreted in urine unchanged

INTERACTIONS

None known

NURSING CONSIDERATIONS

Assess:

• Bowel pattern before, during treatment

• Skin eruptions, photosensitivity after administration of drug

• Respiratory status: rate, character, wheezing, tightness in chest

• Allergies before initiation of treatment, reaction of each medication

• Signs of infection

Administer:

• Within 2 days of symptoms of influenza; continue for 5 days

• Give patient "Patient's Instruction for Use" and review all points before using delivery system

Perform/provide:

• Storage in tight, dry container

Evaluate:

• Therapeutic response: absence of fever, malaise, cough, dyspnea in infection

Teach patient/family:

• That this drug does not reduce transmission risk of influenza to others

• Patients with asthma or COPD to carry a fast-acting inhaled bronchodilator since bronchospasm may occur; to use scheduled inhaled bronchodilators before using this drug

• To avoid hazardous activities if dizziness occurs

• To take drug exactly as prescribed

---

zidovudine (R̲)
(zye-doe'-vue-deen)
Apo-Zidovudine ✤,
Azidothymidine, AZT,
Novo-AZT ✤, Retrovir
Func. class.: Antiretroviral
Chem. class.: Nucleoside reverse transcriptase inhibitor (NRTI)

Action: Inhibits replication of HIV-1 virus by incorporating into cellular DNA by viral reverse transcriptase, thereby terminating the cellular DNA chain
Uses: Used in combination with other antiretrovirals for HIV-1 infection

DOSAGE AND ROUTES

• *Adult:* **PO** 600 mg daily in divided doses, either 200 mg tid or 300 mg bid in combination with other antiretrovirals; **IV** 1-2 mg/kg q4h, initiate **PO** as soon as possible up to 1000 mg

• *Child 6 wk-12 yr:* **PO** 160 mg/m^2 q8h (480 mg/m^2/day, max 200 mg q8h) in combination with other antiretrovirals; **IV** same as adult

• *Neonates:* **PO** 2-3 mg/kg/dose q6h; **IV** 1.5 mg/kg infused over 30 min q6h

Prevention of maternal-fetal HIV transmission

• *Neonatal:* **PO** 2 mg/kg/dose q6h × 6 wk beginning 8-12 hr after birth; **IV** 1.5 mg/kg/dose over 30 min q6h until able to take **PO**

• *Maternal (>14 wk gestation):* **PO** 100 mg 5 ×/day until start of labor, then during labor/delivery **IV** 2 mg/kg over 1 hr followed by **IV INF** 1 mg/kg/hr until umbilical cord clamped

Symptomatic HIV infection

• *Adult:* **PO** 100 mg q4h; **IV** 1-2 mg/kg over 1 hr q4h

• *Child 3 mo to 12 yr:* **PO** 90-180 mg/m^2 q6h (max 200 mg q6h); **IV** 1-2 mg/kg over 1 hr q4h

Prevention of HIV following needle-stick

• *Adult:* **PO** 200 mg tid plus lamivudine 150 mg bid, plus a protease inhibitor for

---

high-risk exposure; begin within 2 hr of exposure

Available forms: Caps 100; tabs 300 mg; inj 200 mg/20 ml; oral syr 50 mg/5 ml

SIDE EFFECTS

CNS: Fever, headache, malaise, diaphoresis, *dizziness, insomnia,* paresthesia, somnolence, chills, tremor, twitching, anxiety, confusion, depression, lability, vertigo, loss of mental acuity, ***seizures***

EENT: Taste change, hearing loss, photophobia

GI: Nausea, vomiting, diarrhea, anorexia, cramps, *dyspepsia,* constipation, dysphagia, *flatulence,* rectal bleeding, mouth ulcer, abdominal pain

GU: Dysuria, polyuria, urinary frequency, hesitancy

*HEMA: **Granulocytopenia, anemia***

INTEG: Rash, acne, pruritus, urticaria

MS: Myalgia, arthralgia, muscle spasm

RESP: Dyspnea

Contraindications: Hypersensitivity

Precautions: Pregnancy (C), granulocyte count <1000/mm^3 or Hgb <9.5 g/dl, lactation, child, severe renal disease, impaired hepatic function, anemia

PHARMACOKINETICS

PO: Rapidly absorbed from GI tract, peak ½-1½ hr, metabolized in liver (inactive metabolites), excreted by kidneys, protein binding 38%, terminal half-life ½-3 hr

INTERACTIONS

Toxicity: probenecid, fluconazole

Increase: bone marrow depression—antineoplastics, radiation, ganciclovir, valganciclovir, SMX/TMP

Increase: zidovudine level—methadone

NURSING CONSIDERATIONS

Assess:

• Blood counts q2wk; watch for decreasing granulocytes, Hgb; if low, therapy may have to be discontinued and restarted after hematologic recovery; blood transfusions may be required; viral load, CD4 counts baseline and throughout

Administer:

• By mouth; capsules should be swallowed whole

• Bid or tid

• Trimethoprim-sulfamethoxazole, pyrimethamine, or acyclovir as ordered to prevent opportunistic infections; if these drugs are given, watch for neurotoxicity

IV route

• After diluting each 1 mg/0.25 ml or more D$_5$W to 4 mg/ml or less; give over 1 hr

Y-site compatibilities: Acyclovir, allopurinol, amifostine, amikacin, amphotericin B, amphotericin B cholesteryl, aztreonam, cefepime, ceftazidime, ceftriaxone, cimetidine, cisatracurium, clindamycin, dexamethasone, DOBUTamine, DOPamine, DOXOrubicin liposome, erythromycin, filgrastim, fluconazole, fludarabine, gentamicin, granisetron, heparin, imipenem/cilastatin, lorazepam, melphalan, metoclopramide, morphine, nafcillin, ondansetron, oxacillin, paclitaxel, pentamidine, phenylephrine, piperacillin, piperacillin/tazobactam, potassium chloride, ranitidine, remifentanil, sargramostim, teniposide, thiotepa, tobramycin, trimethoprim-sulfamethoxazole, trimetrexate, vancomycin, vinorelbine

Perform/provide:

• Storage in cool environment; protect from light

Evaluate:

• Blood dyscrasias (anemia, granulocytopenia): bruising, fatigue, bleeding, poor healing

Teach patient/family:

• That GI complaints and insomnia resolve after 3-4 wk of treatment

• That drug is not cure for AIDS but will control symptoms

• To notify prescriber of sore throat, swollen lymph nodes, malaise, fever; other infections may occur

• That patient is still infective, may pass AIDS virus on to others

Z

• That follow-up visits must be continued since serious toxicity may occur; blood counts must be done q2wk
• That drug must be taken bid or tid
• That serious drug interactions may occur if OTC products are ingested; check with prescriber before taking aspirin, acetaminophen, indomethacin
• That other drugs may be necessary to prevent other infections
• That drug may cause fainting or dizziness

zinc (R, OTC)

Orazinc, PMS Egozine ✥, Verazinc, Zinca-Pak, Zincate, Zinc 15, Zinc-220, zinc sulfate
Func. class.: Trace element; nutritional supplement

Action: Needed for adequate healing, bone and joint development (23% zinc)
Uses: Prevention of zinc deficiency, adjunct to vit A therapy
Investigational uses: Wound healing

DOSAGE AND ROUTES

Dietary supplement
• *Adult:* **PO** 25-50 mg/day
Nutritional supplement (IV)
• *Adult:* **IV** 2.5-4 mg/day; may increase by 2 mg/day if needed
• *Child 1-5 yr:* **IV** 100 mcg/kg/day
• *Infant <1.5-3 kg:* **IV** 300 mcg/kg/day
Wound healing
• *Adult:* **PO** 50 mg daily × 1-2 mo
Available forms: Tabs 66, 110 mg; caps 220 mg; inj 1 mg, 5 mg/ml

SIDE EFFECTS

GI: Nausea, vomiting, cramps, heartburn, ulcer formation
OVERDOSE: Diarrhea, rash, dehydration, restlessness
Precautions: Pregnancy (A)

INTERACTIONS

Decrease: absorption of fluoroquinolones tetracyclines

NURSING CONSIDERATIONS
Assess:
• Zinc levels during treatment
Administer:
• With meals to decrease gastric upset; avoid dairy products
Evaluate:
• Therapeutic response: absence of zinc deficiency
Teach patient/family:
• That element must be taken for 2-3 mo to be effective
• To report immediately nausea, diarrhea, rash, severe vomiting, restlessness, abdominal pain, tarry stools

ziprasidone (R)

(zi-praz'ih-dohn)
Geodon
Func. class.: Antipsychotic/neuroleptic
Chem. class.: Benzisoxazole derivative

Action: Unknown; may be mediated through both dopamine type 2 (D_2) and serotonin type 2 (5-HT_2) antagonism
Uses: Schizophrenia, acute agitation

DOSAGE AND ROUTES

• *Adult:* **PO** 20 mg bid with food, adjust dosage every 2 days upward to max of 80 mg bid; **IM** 10-20 mg; may give 10 mg q2h; doses of 20 mg may be given q4h; max 40 mg/day
Available forms: Tabs 20, 40, 60, 80 mg; inj 20 mg/ml

SIDE EFFECTS

*CNS: EPS, pseudoparkinsonism, akathisia, dystonia, tardive dyskinesia; drowsiness, insomnia, agitation, anxiety, headache, **seizures, neuroleptic malignant syndrome**, dizziness, tremor*
*CV: Orthostatic hypotension, **tachycardia, prolonged QT/QTc, sudden death**, hypertension*
EENT: Blurred vision

GI: Nausea, vomiting, *anorexia, constipation,* jaundice, weight gain, diarrhea, dry mouth, abdominal pain

RESP: Rhinitis, dyspnea

Contraindications: Hypersensitivity, lactation, seizure disorders

Precautions: Pregnancy (C), children, renal disease, hepatic disease, elderly, breast cancer

PHARMACOKINETICS

PO: Extensively metabolized by liver to a major active metabolite, plasma protein binding 90%

INTERACTIONS

Increase: sedation—other CNS depressants, alcohol

Increase: EPS—other antipsychotics, lithium

Increase: ziprasidone excretion—carbamazepine

Increase: ziprasidone level—ketoconazole

Increase: hypotension—antihypertensives

Drug/Herb

Increase: CNS depression—chamomile, hops, kava, skullcap, valerian

Increase: EPS—betel palm, kava

Increase: action—cola tree, hops, nettle, nutmeg

Drug/Lab Test

None

NURSING CONSIDERATIONS

Assess:

• Mental status before initial administration

• Swallowing of PO medication; check for hoarding or giving of medication to other patients

• I&O ratio; palpate bladder if urinary output is low

• Bilirubin, CBC, LFTs qmo

• Urinalysis before, during prolonged therapy

• Affect, orientation, LOC, reflexes, gait, coordination, sleep pattern disturbances

• B/P standing and lying; also pulse, respirations; take these q4h during initial treatment; establish baseline before starting treatment; report drops of 30 mm Hg; watch for ECG changes

• Dizziness, faintness, palpitations, tachycardia on rising

• EPS, including akathisia (inability to sit still, no pattern to movements), tardive dyskinesia (bizarre movements of the jaw, mouth, tongue, extremities), pseudoparkinsonism (rigidity, tremors, pill rolling, shuffling gait)

⚠ For neuroleptic malignant syndrome: hyperthermia, increased CPK, altered mental status, muscle rigidity

• Skin turgor daily

• Constipation, urinary retention daily; if these occur, increase bulk and water in diet

Administer:

PO route

• Reduced dose in elderly

• Antiparkinsonian agent on order from prescriber, to be used for EPS

• Avoid use with CNS depressants

IM route

• Add 1.2 ml sterile water for inj to vial, shake vigorously until drug is dissolved, do not admix

Perform/provide:

• Decreased stimulus by dimming lights, avoiding loud noises

• Supervised ambulation until patient is stabilized on medication; do not involve in strenuous exercise program because fainting is possible; patient should not stand still for a long time

• Increased fluids to prevent constipation

• Sips of water, candy, gum for dry mouth

• Storage in tight, light-resistant container

Evaluate:

• Therapeutic response: decrease in emotional excitement, hallucinations, delusions, paranoia; reorganization of patterns of thought, speech

Teach patient/family:

• That orthostatic hypotension may

occur and to rise from sitting or lying position gradually

• To avoid hot tubs, hot showers, tub baths; hypotension may occur

• To avoid abrupt withdrawal of this drug; EPS may result; drug should be withdrawn slowly

• To avoid OTC preparations (cough, hay fever, cold) unless approved by prescriber, since serious drug interactions may occur; avoid use with alcohol; increased drowsiness may occur

• To avoid hazardous activities if drowsy or dizzy

• Compliance with drug regimen

• To report impaired vision, tremors, muscle twitching

• In hot weather, that heat stroke may occur; take extra precautions to stay cool

Treatment of overdose: Lavage if orally ingested; provide airway; *do not induce vomiting*

---

zoledronic acid (℞)
(zoh'leh-drah'nick ass'id)
Zometa
Func. class.: Bone-resorption inhibitor
Chem. class.: Bisphosphonate

Action: Inhibits normal and abnormal bone resorption, potent inhibitor of osteoclastic bone resorption; inhibits osteoclastic activity, inhibits skeletal calcium release caused by stimulating factors released by tumors; reduction of abnormal bone resorption is responsible for therapeutic effect in hypercalcemia; may directly block dissolution of hydroxyapatite bone crystals

Uses: Moderate to severe hypercalcemia associated with malignancy; multiple myeloma; bone metastases from solid tumors (used with antineoplastics)

DOSAGE AND ROUTES
Hypercalcemia of malignancy
• *Adult:* **IV INF** 4 mg, given as a single infusion over ≥15 min; may re-treat with

4 mg if serum calcium does not return to normal within 1 wk

Multiple myeloma/metastatic bone lesions
• *Adult:* **IV INF** 4 mg, give over 15 min q3-4wk; may continue treatment for 9-15 months, depending on condition

Available form: Powder for inj 4 mg

SIDE EFFECTS
CNS: Dizziness, headache, anxiety, confusion, insomnia, agitation
CV: Hypotension, leg edema
GI: Abdominal pain, anorexia, constipation, nausea, diarrhea, vomiting, mucositis
GU: UTI, possible reduced renal function
META: Anemia, hypokalemia, hypomagnesemia, hypophosphatemia, hypocalcemia, increased serum creatinine
MISC: Fever, chills, flulike symptoms
MS: Bone pain, *arthralgias, myalgias*

Contraindications: Pregnancy (D), hypersensitivity to this drug or bisphosphonates

Precautions: Children, nursing mothers, renal dysfunction, aspirin sensitive asthmatic patients

PHARMACOKINETICS
Rapidly cleared from circulation and taken up mainly by bones, not metabolized, eliminated primarily by kidneys; approximately 50% is eliminated in urine within 24 hr of administration; max effect 7 days

INTERACTIONS
Hypomagnesemia, hypokalemia: digoxin
Do not mix with calcium-containing infusion sol such as lactated Ringer's sol
Decrease: effect of zoledronic acid—calcium, vit D
Decrease: serum calcium, aminoglycosides, loop diuretics

NURSING CONSIDERATIONS
Assess:
• Renal tests and Ca, P, Mg, K; creatinine, if creatinine is elevated hold treatment

---

• For hypercalcemia: paresthesia, twitching, laryngospasm; Chvostek's, Trousseau's signs

Administer:

• Saline hydration must be performed before administration; urine output should be 2 L/day during treatment, do not overhydrate

IV route

• Administer after reconstituting by adding 5 ml of sterile water for inj to each vial, then add to ≥100 ml of sterile 0.9% NaCl, D$_5$W; run over ≥15 min

• Administer in separate IV line from all other drugs

Perform/provide:

• Sol reconstituted with sterile water may be stored under refrigeration for up to 24 hr

Evaluate:

• Therapeutic response: decreased calcium levels

Teach patient/family:

• To report hypercalcemic relapse: nausea, vomiting, bone pain, thirst

• To continue with dietary recommendations including calcium and vit D; take a multiple vitamin daily, 500 mg of calcium, 400 international units vit D in multiple myeloma

• If nausea/vomiting occur, eat small frequent meals, use lozenges or chewing gum

• If bone pain occurs, notify prescriber to obtain analgesics

• Avoid use in pregnancy

---

zolmitriptan (R)

(zole-mih-trip'tan)
Zomig, Zomig-ZMT
Func. class.: Migraine agent
Chem. class.: 5-HT$_{1B}$/5HT$_{1D}$ receptor agonist

Action: Binds selectively to the vascular 5-HT$_{1B}$/5HT$_{1D}$ receptor subtype, exerts antimigraine effect; causes vasoconstriction in cranial arteries

Uses: Acute treatment of migraine with or without aura

DOSAGE AND ROUTES

• *Adult:* **PO** Start on 2.5 mg or lower (tab may be broken), may repeat after 2 hr, max 10 mg/24 hr; **NASAL** 1 spray in each nostril at onset of migraine, repeat in 2 hr, if no relief

Available forms: Tabs 2.5, 5 mg; orally disintegrating tab 2.5, 5 mg; nasal spray 5 mg

SIDE EFFECTS

CNS: Tingling, hot sensation, burning, feeling of pressure, tightness, numbness, dizziness, sedation
CV: Palpitations, chest pain
GI: Abdominal discomfort, nausea, dry mouth, dyspepsia, dysphagia
MISC: Odd taste (spray)
MS: Weakness, neck stiffness, myalgia
RESP: Chest tightness, pressure

Contraindictions: Angina pectoris, history of MI, documented silent ischemia, ischemic heart disease, concurrent ergotamine-containing preparations, uncontrolled hypertension, hypersensitivity, basilar or hemiplegic migraine, risk of CV events

Precautions: Pregnancy (C), postmenopausal women, men >40 yr, risk factors for CAD, hypercholesterolemia, obesity, diabetes, impaired hepatic or renal function, lactation, children, elderly

PHARMACOKINETICS

Duration 2-3½ hr, 25% plasma protein binding, half-life 3-3½ hr, metabolized in the liver (metabolite), excreted in urine, feces

INTERACTIONS

⚠ Extended vasospastic effects: ergot, ergot derivatives
⚠ Do not use within 2 wk of MAOIs
⚠ Weakness, hyperreflexia, incoordination: SSRIs (fluoxetine, fluvoxamine, paroxetine, sertraline)
Increase: half-life of zolmitriptan— cimetidine, oral contraceptives

Z

Drug/Herb
Serotonin syndrome: SAM-e, St. John's wort
Increase: effect—butterbur

NURSING CONSIDERATIONS
Assess:
• Tingling, hot sensation, burning, feeling of pressure, numbness, flushing
• For stress level, activity, recreation, coping mechanisms
• Neurologic status: LOC, blurring vision, nausea, vomiting, tingling in extremities preceding headache
• Ingestion of tyramine foods (pickled products, beer, wine, aged cheese), food additives, preservatives, colorings, artifical sweeteners, chocolate, caffeine, which may precipitate these types of headaches
• For serotonin syndrome, if also taking an SSRI
Administer:
• Take with fluids as soon as symptoms of migraine occur
Perform/provide:
• Quiet, calm environment with decreased stimulation for noise, bright light, excessive talking
Evaluate:
• Therapeutic response: decrease in frequency, severity of headache
Teach patient/family:
• To report any side effects to prescriber
• To use contraception while taking drug

---

zolpidem (℞)
(zole'pih-dem)
Ambien
Func. class.: Sedative-hypnotic
Chem. class.: Nonbenzodiazepine of imidazopyridine class

Controlled Substance Schedule IV
Action: Produces CNS depression at limbic, thalamic, hypothalamic levels of CNS; may be mediated by neurotransmitter γ-aminobutyric acid (GABA); results are sedation, hypnosis, skeletal muscle relaxation, anticonvulsant activity, anxiolytic action
Uses: Insomnia, short-term treatment

DOSAGE AND ROUTES
• *Adult:* **PO** 10 mg at bedtime × 7-10 days only; total dose should not exceed 10 mg
• *Geriatric:* **PO** 5 mg at bedtime
Available forms: Tabs 5, 10 mg

SIDE EFFECTS
CNS: Headache, lethargy, drowsiness, daytime sedation, dizziness, confusion, light-headedness, anxiety, irritability, amnesia, poor coordination
CV: Chest pain, palpitation
GI: Nausea, vomiting, diarrhea, heartburn, abdominal pain, constipation
HEMA: ***Leukopenia, granulocytopenia*** (rare)
Contraindications: Hypersensitivity to benzodiazepines
Precautions: Pregnancy (B), anemia, hepatic disease, renal disease, suicidal individuals, drug abuse, elderly, psychosis, child <18 yr, seizure disorders, lactation

PHARMACOKINETICS
PO: Onset 1.5 hr, metabolized by liver, excreted by kidneys (inactive metabolites), crosses placenta, excreted in breast milk; half-life 2-3 hr

INTERACTIONS
Increase: action of both drugs—alcohol, CNS depressants
Drug/Herb
Increase: CNS depression—chamomile, hops, kava, skullcap, valerian
Drug/Lab Test
Increase: ALT, AST, serum bilirubin
Decrease: RAI uptake
False increase: Urinary 17-OHCS

NURSING CONSIDERATIONS
Assess:
• Blood studies: Hct, Hgb, RBC, if blood dyscrasias are suspected (rare)

🅰 Safety alert   *"Tall Man" lettering

- Hepatic studies: AST, ALT, bilirubin if hepatic damage has occurred
- Mental status: mood, sensorium, affect, memory (long, short)
- Blood dyscrasias: fever, sore throat, bruising, rash, jaundice, epistaxis (rare)
- Type of sleep problem: falling asleep, staying asleep

Administer:
- After removal of cigarettes to prevent fires
- After trying conservative measures for insomnia
- ½-1 hr before bedtime for sleeplessness
- On empty stomach for fast onset but may be taken with food if GI symptoms occur
- Avoid use with CNS depressants; serious CNS depression may result

Perform/provide:
- Assistance with ambulation after receiving dose
- Safety measures: side rails, night-light, call bell within easy reach
- Checking to see if PO medication has been swallowed
- Storage in tight container in cool environment

Evaluate:
- Therapeutic response: ability to sleep at night, decreased amount of early morning awakening if taking drug for insomnia

Teach patient/family:
- That dependence is possible after long-term use
- To avoid driving or other activities requiring alertness until drug is stabilized
- To avoid alcohol ingestion
- That effects may take 2 nights for benefits to be noticed
- Alternative measures to improve sleep: reading, exercise several hours before bedtime, warm bath, warm milk, TV, self-hypnosis, deep breathing
- That hangover is common in elderly but less common than with barbiturates; rebound insomnia may occur for 1-2 nights after discontinuing drug

Treatment of overdose: Lavage, activated charcoal; monitor electrolytes, VS

---

zonisamide (R̶)
(zone-is′a-mide)
Zonegran
Func. class.: Anticonvulsant
Chem. class.: Sulfonamides

Action: May act through action at sodium and calcium channels, but exact action is unknown

Uses: Epilepsy, adjunctive therapy of partial seizures

DOSAGE AND ROUTES

- *Adults and child >16 yr:* 100 mg daily, may increase after 2 wk to 200 mg/day, may increase q2wk, maximum dose 600 mg/day

Available forms: Caps 25, 50, 100 mg

SIDE EFFECTS

CNS: Dizziness, insomnia, paresthesias, depression, fatigue, headache, confusion, somnolence, agitation, irritability

EENT: Diplopia, verbal difficulty, speech abnormalities, taste perversion

GI: Nausea, constipation, anorexia, weight loss, diarrhea, dyspepsia

HEMA: ***Aplastic anemia, granulocytopenia*** (rare)

INTEG: Rash

SYST: ***Stevens-Johnson syndrome***

Contraindications: Hypersensitivity to this drug or sulfonamides, psychiatric condition, hepatic failure

Precautions: Pregnancy (C), allergies, hepatic disease, renal disease, elderly, lactation, child <16 yr

PHARMACOKINETICS

Peak 2-6 hr, half-life 63 hr
Metabolized by liver, excreted by kidneys

Z

INTERACTIONS

Decrease: half-life of zonisamide—drugs inducing CYP 450 enzymes (carbamazepine, phenytoin, phenobarbital)

NURSING CONSIDERATIONS

Assess:
• For seizures: duration, type, intensity precipitating factors
• Renal function: albumin conc
• Mental status: mood, sensorium, affect, memory (long, short)

Evaluate:
• Therapeutic response; decrease in severity of seizures

Teach patient/family:
• Not to discontinue drug abruptly; seizures may occur
• To avoid hazardous activities until stabilized on drug
• To carry emergency ID stating drug use
• To notify prescriber of rash immediately; also, back pain, abdominal pain, blood in urine, increase fluid intake to reduce risk of kidney stones
• To notify prescriber if pregnancy is planned or suspected

Bibliography

Drug information: Bethesda, American Hospital Formulary Service.

Facts and comparisons: St Louis, updated monthly.

Gahart BL: *Intravenous medications,* ed 22, St Louis, 2006, Mosby.

Hardman JG, et al: *Goodman and Gilman's the pharmacological basis of therapeutics,* ed 10, New York, 2002, McGraw-Hill.

McKenry LM, Salerno E: *Mosby's pharmacology in nursing,* ed 21, St Louis, 2003, Mosby.

Mediphor Editorial Group: *Drug interaction facts,* Philadelphia, updated quarterly, JB Lippincott.

Review of natural products: Philadelphia, updated monthly, *Facts and Comparisons.*

Appendixes

Appendix a

Selected new drugs

abatacept (℞)
(ab-a-ta'sept)
Orencia
Func. class.: Antirheumatic agent
(disease modifying); biologic response modifier

Action: A selective costimulation modulator, inhibits T-lymphocytes, inhibits tumor necrosis factor (TNF-α), interferon-γ, interleukin-2, which are involved in immune and inflammatory reactions

Uses: Acute, chronic rheumatoid arthritis that has not responded to other disease-modifying agents, may use in combination with DMARDs; do not use with TNF antagonists (adalimumab, etanercept, infliximab); anakinra

DOSAGE AND ROUTES
• *Adult >100 kg:* **IV INF** 1 g
• *Adult 60-100 kg:* **IV INF** 750 mg
• *Adult <60 kg:* **IV INF** 500 mg over 30 min; give 2-4 wk after 1st **INF**, then q4wk
Available forms: Lyophilized powder, single use vials 250 mg

SIDE EFFECTS
CNS: Headache, asthenia, dizziness
CV: Hypertension, hypotension
GI: Abdominal pain, dyspepsia, nausea
INTEG: Rash, *inj site reaction,* flushing, urticaria, pruritus
RESP: Pharyngitis, cough, URI, non-URI, *rhinitis,* wheezing
SYST: Anaphylaxis, malignancies, angioedema
Contraindications: Hypersensitivity, TB
Precautions: Pregnancy (C), lactation, children, elderly, recurrent infections, COPD

PHARMACOKINETICS
Terminal half-life 13-16 days, steady state 60 days

INTERACTIONS
Do not give concurrently with vaccines; immunizations should be brought up to date before treatment
Do not use with TNF antagonists: (adalimumab, etanercept, infliximab); anakinra
Do not use with corticosteroids, immunosuppressives

NURSING CONSIDERATIONS
Assess:
• For latent/active TB before beginning treatment
• Pain, stiffness, ROM, swelling of joints during treatment
• For inj site pain, swelling
• Patient's overall health on each visit; product should not be given with active infections
Administer:
• To reconstitute, remove plastic flip top from vial and wipe the top with alcohol wipe; insert syringe needle into vial and direct stream of sterile water for inj on the wall of vial; rotate vial until mixed; vent with needle to rid foam after reconstitution 25 mg/ml; further dilute in 100 ml from a 100-ml infusion bag/bottle; withdraw the needed volume (2 vials remove 20 mg; 3 vials remove 30 ml, 4 vials remove 40 ml); slowly add the reconstituted Orencia sol from each vial into the infusion bag/bottle using the same disposable syringe supplied; mix gently, discard unused portions of vials;

A Safety alert   *"Tall Man" lettering

do not use if particulate is present or discolored; give over 30 min; use non–protein binding filter (0.2-1.2 mcg)
• Do not admix with other sol or medications

Perform/provide:
• Storage in refrigerator; do not use expired vials

Evaluate:
• Therapeutic response: decreased inflammation, pain in joints; decreased erythrocyte sedimentation rate (ESR)

Teach patient/family:
• That drug must be continued for prescribed time to be effective
• To use caution when driving; dizziness may occur
• Not to have vaccinations while taking this product
• Regarding patient information included in packaging

---

entecavir (℞)
(en-te′ka-veer)
Baraclude
Func. class.: Antiviral
Chem. class.: Guanosine nucleoside analog

Action: Inhibits hepatitis B virus DNA polymerase by competing with natural substrates and by causing DNA termination after its incorporation into viral DNA; causes viral DNA death
Uses: Chronic hepatitis B (HBV)

DOSAGE AND ROUTES
Chronic hepatitis B (nucleoside treatment–naive)
• *Adult and adolescents ≥16 yr:* **PO** 0.5 mg daily
Chronic hepatitis B while receiving lamivudine or known lamivudine-resistant mutations
• *Adult and adolescents ≥16 yr:* **PO** 1 mg daily
Renal dose
• *Adult:* **PO** CCr ≥50 ml/min 0.5 mg daily; CCr 30-49 ml/min 0.25 mg daily, 0.5 mg daily for lamivudine-refractory

patient; CCr 10-29 ml/min 0.15 daily, 0.3 for lamivudine-refractory patient; CCr <10 ml/min 0.05 mg PO daily, 0.1 mg for lamivudine-refractory patient
Available forms: Tabs, film coated 0.5, 1 mg; oral sol 0.05 mg/ml

SIDE EFFECTS
CNS: Headache, fatigue, dizziness, insomnia
GI: Dyspepsia, nausea, vomiting, diarrhea
*SYST: **Lactic acidosis, severe hepatomegaly with stenosis***
Contraindications: Hypersensitivity
Precautions: Pregnancy (C), lactation, child, severe renal disease, elderly

PHARMACOKINETICS
Peak 0.5-1.5 hr, steady state 6-10 days, 100% bioavailability, extensively distributed to tissues, protein binding 13%, terminal half-life 128-149 hr, excreted unchanged (62%-73%) via kidneys

INTERACTIONS
None known
Drug/Lab Test
Increase: ALT, AST, total bilirubin, amylase, lipase, creatinine, blood glucose, urine glucose
Decrease: Platelets, albumin

NURSING CONSIDERATIONS
Assess:
• For nephrotoxicity: increasing CCr, BUN
• For HIV before beginning treatment, because HIV resistance may occur in chronic hepatitis B patients
⚠ For lactic acidosis, severe hepatomegaly with stenosis
• Elderly patients more carefully; may develop renal, cardiac symptoms more rapidly
• For exacerbations of hepatitis after discontinuing treatment, monitor LFTs

---

Administer:
• By mouth on empty stomach 2 hr before or after food
Perform/provide:
• Storage in cool environment; protect from light
Evaluate:
• Therapeutic response: decreased symptoms of chronic hepatitis B, improving LFTs
Teach patient/family:
• Not to take with food
• To take exactly as prescribed
• Do not stop medication without approval of prescriber
• That optimal duration of treatment is unknown
• To avoid use with other medications unless approved by prescriber
• To notify prescriber of decreased urinary output, blood in urine
• Symptoms of lactic acidosis: muscle pain, severe tiredness, weakness, trouble breathing, stomach pain with nausea/vomiting, coldness in arms/legs, fast/irregular heartbeat, dizziness
• Symptoms of hepatotoxicity: eyes/skin turns yellow, dark urine, light bowel movements, no appetite for days, nausea, stomach pain
• That product does not cure, but lowers the amount of HBV in body
• That product does not stop you from spreading HBV to others by sex, sharing needles or being exposed to blood

exenatide (R)
(ex-en′a-tide)
Byetta
Func. class.: Antidiabetic
Chem. class.: Incretin mimetic

Action: Binds and activates known human GLP-1 receptor, mimics natural physiology for self-regulating glycemic control
Uses: Type 2 diabetes mellitus given in combination with metformin or a sulfonylurea

DOSAGE AND ROUTES
• *Adult:* **SUBCUT** 5 mcg bid 1 hr before morning and evening meal; may increase to 10 mcg bid after 1 mo of therapy
Available forms: Inj 250 mcg/ml pen injector

SIDE EFFECTS
CNS: Headache, dizziness, feeling jittery, restlessness, weakness
ENDO: **Hypoglycemia**
GI: Nausea, vomiting, diarrhea, dyspepsia, anorexia, gastroesophageal reflux, weight loss
Contraindications: Hypersensitivity
Precautions: Pregnancy (C), elderly, severe renal disease, severe hepatic disease, severe GI disease

PHARMACOKINETICS
Peak 2.1 hr, elimination by glomerular filtration

INTERACTIONS
May increase the effect of acetaminophen
Do not use with erythromycin, metoclopramide
Increase: exenatide action
Increase: hypoglycemia—ACE inhibitors, corticosteroids, disopyramide, anabolic steroids, androgens, fibric acid derivatives, alcohol
Increase: hyperglycemia—phenothiazines
Decrease: action of digoxin, lovastatin, acetaminophen (elixir)
Decrease: hypoglycemia—niacin, dextrothyroxine, thiazide diuretics, triamterene, estrogens, progestins, oral contraceptives, MAOIs

NURSING CONSIDERATIONS
Assess:
• Fasting blood, glucose, A1c levels, postprandial glucose during treatment to determine diabetes control
• Hypo/hyperglycemic reaction that can occur soon after meals; for severe hypo-

glycemia give IV D$_{50}$W, then IV dextrose solution

Administer:

• Drug 1 hr before meals; if patient is NPO, may need to hold dose to prevent hypoglycemia

Perform/provide:

• Storage in refrigerator

Evaluate:

• Therapeutic response: decrease in polyuria, polydipsia, polyphagia, clear sensorium, improving A1c, weight; absence of dizziness, stable gait

Teach patient/family:

• The symptoms of hypo/hyperglycemia, what to do about each; to have glucagon emergency kit available; to carry a glucose source (candy, sugar cube) to treat hypoglycemia

• That drug must be continued on daily basis; explain consequences of discontinuing drug abruptly

• That diabetes is a lifelong illness; drug will not cure disease

• That all food in diet plan must be eaten to prevent hypoglycemia

• To carry emergency ID with prescriber and medications

• To continue weight control, dietary restrictions, exercise, hygiene

• That regular blood glucose monitoring and A1c testing is needed

• To notify prescriber if pregnant or intend to become pregnant

• To read "Information for the Patient" and "Pen User Manual"

Rarely Used

galsulfase (℞)
(gal-sul′face)
Naglazyme
Func. class.: Miscellaneous drug

Uses: Mucopolysaccharidosis VI (MPS VI); Maroteaux-Lamy syndrome

DOSAGE AND ROUTES

• *Adult and child ≥5 yr:* IV 1 mg/kg infused over ≥4 hr once per week
Contraindications: Hypersensitivity

⚠ High Alert

insulin, inhaled (℞)
Exubera
Func. class.: Antidiabetic, pancreatic hormone, inhaled
Chem. class.: Exogenous unmodified insulin

Action: Decreases blood glucose; by transport of glucose into cells and the conversion of glucose to glycogen, indirectly increases blood pyruvate and lactate, decreases phosphate and potassium; processed by recombinant DNA technologies
Uses: Adult patients with type 1 or type 2 diabetes mellitus

DOSAGE AND ROUTES

• *Adult:* INH insert dose in handheld inhalation device and inhale 10 min before meal
Available forms: Inhaled, dry powder 1, 3 mg unit dose blisters (3 of the 1 mg blister packs is not equal to 1, 3 mg blister pack)

SIDE EFFECTS

EENT: Blurred vision, dry mouth, cough
GI: Nausea, vomiting, weight gain
META: Hypoglycemia, insulin resistance
*RESP: **Bronchospasm,*** laryngitis, dyspnea, epistaxis, rhinitis, sinusitis
*SYST: **Anaphylaxis,*** antibody formation
Contraindications: Hypersensitivity; poorly controlled, unstable lung disease; smokers; those who have quit smoking within the last 6 mo, diabetic ketoacidosis, hyperosmolar hyperglycemic state (HHs), hypoglycemia, mannitol hypersensitivity
Precautions: Pregnancy (C); chronic lung disorders (asthma, bronchitis, emphysema); hepatic, renal disease; cystic fibrosis

PHARMACOKINETICS

INH: Onset 10-20 min, peak 49 min, range 30-90 min, duration 6 hr, mean bioavailability is 10% of regular insulin (SUBCUT)

INTERACTIONS

Increase: hypoglycemia—salicylate, alcohol, β-blockers, anabolic steroids, sulfinpyrazone, guanethidine, oral hypoglycemics, MAOIs, ACE inhibitors, fibric acid derivatives

Decrease: hypoglycemia—thiazides, thyroid hormones, oral contraceptives, corticosteroids, estrogens, atypical psychotics, progestins

NURSING CONSIDERATIONS

Assess:

• Fasting blood glucose, 2 hr PP (80-150 mg/dl, normal fasting level; 70-130 mg/dl, normal 2 hr level); also A1C may be drawn to identify treatment effectiveness

• For hypoglycemic reaction that can occur during peak time (sweating, weakness, dizziness, chills, confusion, headache, nausea, rapid weak pulse, fatigue, tachycardia, memory lapses, slurred speech, staggering gait, anxiety, tremors, hunger)

• For hyperglycemia: acetone breath, polyuria, fatigue, polydipsia, flushed, dry skin, lethargy

Administer:

• 10 min before meal

• 1 mg and 3 mg blisters are used in combination, consecutive inhalation of 3 (1 mg blisters) is associated with 30%-40% greater insulin exposure than 1 (3 mg blister); they are not interchangeable

• SUBCUT regular insulin 3 units = 1 mg Exubera (1 blister pack)

Evaluate:

• Therapeutic response: decrease in polyuria, polydipsia, polyphagia, clear sensorium, absence of dizziness, stable gait; improving A1c

Teach patient/family:

• That if blurred vision occurs, not to change corrective lens until vision is stabilized 1-2 mo

• To keep insulin, equipment available at all times

• That drug does not cure diabetes but controls symptoms

• To carry emergency ID as diabetic

• To recognize hypoglycemia reaction: headache, tremors, fatigue, weakness

• The dosage, route, mixing instructions, if any diet restrictions, disease process

• To carry candy or lump sugar to treat hypoglycemia

• The symptoms of ketoacidosis: nausea, thirst, polyuria, dry mouth, decreased B/P, dry, flushed skin, acetone breath, drowsiness, Kussmaul respirations

• That a plan is necessary for diet, exercise; all food on diet should be eaten; exercise routine should not vary

• About blood glucose testing; make sure patient is able to determine glucose level in order to self monitor

• To avoid OTC drugs unless directed by prescriber

Treatment of overdose: Glucose 25 g IV, via dextrose 50% sol, 50 ml or glucagon 1 mg

mecasermin (℞)

(mec-a′sir-men)
Increlex
Func. class.: Biologic response modifier; insulin-like growth factor

Action: Stimulates growth; IGF-1 is the principal hormonal mediator of statural growth. GH binds to its receptor in the liver and other tissues

Uses: Growth failure in children with severe primary insulin-like growth factor-1 (IGF-1) deficiency (primary IGFD) or with growth hormone (GH) gene deletion who have developed neutralizing antibodies to GH

Investigational uses: ALS

A Safety alert   *"Tall Man" lettering

DOSAGE AND ROUTES

- *Child:* **SUBCUT** 0.04-0.08 mg/kg (40-80 mcg/kg) bid; if well tolerated for 1 wk, may increase by 0.04 mg/kg/dose, max 0.12 mg/kg bid

Available forms: Inj 10 mg/ml

SIDE EFFECTS

CNS: Headache, *seizures,* dizziness, cardiac valvulopathy
CV: Cardiac murmur
EENT: Ear pain, otitis media, abnormal tympanometry, papilledema, visual impairment
ENDO: **Hypoglycemia, ketosis, hypothyroidism**
GU: Vomiting
HEMA: Thymus hypertrophy
META: Hypoglycemic
MISC: Bruising, lipohypertrophy, hypersensitivity reactions
MS: Arthralgia, joint pain
RESP: Snoring, tonsillar hypertrophy, *apnea*
SYST: **Antibodies to growth hormone**

Contraindications: Hypersensitivity, benzyl alcohol, closed epiphyses, active/suspected neoplasia, IV use
Precautions: Pregnancy (C), diabetes mellitus, hypothyroidism, lactation, child <2 yr, increased intracranial pressure, malnutrition, scoliosis, sleep apnea

PHARMACOKINETICS

Bioavailability almost 100%, metabolism liver/kidney, half-life 5.8 hr

INTERACTIONS

Increase: hypoglycemia—antidiabetics, corticosteroids

NURSING CONSIDERATIONS

Assess:

- Monitor preprandial glucose at beginning of treatment and until well tolerated
- By funduscopic exam at beginning and periodically during treatment
- For allergic reactions; if present, interrupt treatment and notify prescriber
- Growth rate of child at intervals during treatment

Administer:
SUBCUT route

- Rotate inj site; use sterile, disposable syringe/needles; use small-volume syringe for accurate measurement
- Shortly before or after a meal or snack to lessen hypoglycemia

Perform/provide:

- Storage in refrigerator before opening, avoid freezing; after opening, stable for 30 days after initial vial entry, store in refrigerator, do not use if particulate matter is present, avoid direct light, do not use after expiration date

Evaluate:

- Therapeutic response: growth in children

Teach patient/family:

- That treatment may continue for years; regular assessments are required
- To avoid hazardous activities, driving within 2-3 hr of dosing
- Correct administration and needle disposal

---

nelarabine (℞)
(nella-ra'ben)
Arranon
Func. class.: Antineoplastic
Chem. class.: Purine analog

Action: Leukemic blasts allow for incorporation into DNA, thus interfering with cell replication lending to cell death
Uses: T-cell lymphoblastic leukemia, T-cell lymphoblastic lymphoma post relapse or treatment failure with at least two chemotherapeutic agents

DOSAGE AND ROUTES

- *Adult:* **IV** 1500 mg/m^2 over 2 hr on days 1, 3, 5, repeated q 21 days
- *Child:* **IV** 650 mg/m^2 over 1 hr daily × 5 days, repeated q 21 days

Available forms: Sol for inj 5 mg/ml

SIDE EFFECTS

CNS: Dizziness, *fatigue,* insomnia, rigors,

seizures, peripheral neuropathy, *paralysis,* confusion, headache
CV: Edema
GI: Nausea, vomiting, anorexia, diarrhea, stomatitis, constipation
*HEMA: **Neutropenia,** leukopenia, **thrombocytopenia,** anemia*
META: Decreased potassium, calcium, magnesium, glucose, albumin, bilirubin, AST, ALT, hyperuricemia; increased glucose
MS: Myalgia, arthralgia, back pain, weakness
*RESP: **Pleural effusion,** cough, dyspnea, wheezing, epistaxis*
Contraindications: Pregnancy (D), hypersensitivity, severe neurotoxicity
Precautions: Renal disease, hepatic disease, lactation, children, elderly

PHARMACOKINETICS

Metabolized in the liver, excreted kidneys, half-life 30 min-3 hr

INTERACTIONS

• Do not use with live virus vaccinations

NURSING CONSIDERATIONS

Assess:
• CBC (RBC, Hct, Hgb), differential platelet count weekly; withhold drugs if WBC is <4000/mm^3, platelet count is <75,000/mm^3, or RBC, Hct, Hgb low; notify prescriber of these results
• Renal studies: BUN, serum uric acid, urine CCr, electrolytes before and during therapy
• Monitor temp q4h; fever may indicate beginning infection; no rectal temps
• Hepatic studies before and during therapy: bilirubin, ALT, AST, alk phosphatase as needed or monthly
• Bleeding: hematuria, heme-positive stools, bruising or petechiae, mucosa or orifices q8h
• Neurotoxicity: somnolence, confusion, seizures, ataxia, paresthesias, hypoesthesia, coma, status epilepticus, craniospinal demyelination; contact prescriber immediately

• Dyspnea, crackles, unproductive cough, chest pain, tachypnea, fatigue, increased pulse, pallor, lethargy, personality changes
• Buccal cavity q8h for dryness, sores or ulceration, white patches, oral pain, bleeding, dysphagia
• GI symptoms: frequency of stools, cramping, if severe diarrhea occurs, fluid and electrolytes may need to be given
Administer:
• IV hydration, and allopurinol in risk of hyperuricemia
• Use procedures for proper handling/ disposal of anticancer drugs
Perform/provide:
• Rinsing of mouth tid-qid with water, club soda; brushing of teeth bid-tid with soft brush or cotton-tipped applicators for stomatitis; use unwaxed dental floss
• Storage at room temp
Evaluate:
• Therapeutic response: decreased spread of malignancy
Teach patient/family:
• To avoid foods with citric acid, hot or rough texture if stomatitis is present
• Use contraception while taking this product
• To avoid using while lactating
• To report signs of infection: increased temp, sore throat, flulike symptoms
• To report signs of anemia: fatigue, headache, faintness, shortness of breath, irritability
• To report bleeding; to avoid use of razors, commercial mouthwash
• That seizures may occur, do not operate machinery or drive until effects are known
• Not to receive vaccinations while taking this product

⚠ Safety alert   *"Tall Man" lettering

pramlintide (℞)
(pram'lin-tide)
Symlin
Func. class.: Antidiabetic
Chem. class.: Synthetic human amylin analog

Action: Modulates and slows stomach emptying, prevents postprandial rise in plasma glucagon, decreases appetite, leads to decreased caloric intake and weight loss

Uses: Type 1 diabetes mellitus, type 2 diabetes mellitus as an adjunct to insulin therapy with uncontrolled type 1 or type 2 diabetes

DOSAGE AND ROUTES
• *Adult:* **SUBCUT** 15 mcg, may increase by 15 mcg to 30-60 mcg, max 120 mcg/dose

Available forms: Inj 5-ml vials (0.6 mg/ml)

SIDE EFFECTS
CNS: Headache, fatigue, dizziness
GI: Nausea, vomiting, anorexia, abdominal pain
INTEG: Inj site reactions
META: Hypoglycemia (while used with insulin)
MS: Arthralgia
RESP: Cough, pharyngitis
SYST: Systemic allergy

Contraindications: Hypersensitivity to this product or metacresol, gastroparesis

Precautions: Pregnancy (C), lactation

PHARMACOKINETICS
Absorption 30%-40%, extensively bound to blood cells or albumin, half-life 48 min, metabolized by kidneys

INTERACTIONS
May increase effect of acetaminophen
Do not use with erythromycin, metoclopramide
Increase: pramlintide action—

antimuscarinics, α-glucosidase inhibitors, diphenoxylate, loperamide, octreotide, opiate agonist, tricyclic antidepressants
Increase: hypoglycemia—ACE inhibitors, disopyramide, anabolic steroids, androgens, fibric acid derivatives, alcohol, corticosteroids
Increase: hyperglycemia—phenothiazines
Decrease: hypoglycemia—niacin, dextrothyroxine, thiazide diuretics, triamterene, estrogens, progestins, oral contraceptives, MAOIs

NURSING CONSIDERATIONS
Assess:
• Fasting blood glucose, 2 hr PP (80-150 mg/dl, normal fasting level; 70-130 mg/dl, normal 2 hr level); A1c may also be drawn to identify treatment effectiveness; also monitor weight, appetite
• For hypoglycemic reaction (sweating, weakness, dizziness, chills, confusion, headache, nausea, rapid weak pulse, fatigue, tachycardia, memory lapses, slurred speech, staggering gait, anxiety, tremors, hunger)
• For hyperglycemia: acetone breath, polyuria, fatigue, polydipsia, flushed, dry skin, lethargy
Administer:
SUBCUT route
• Take prior to mealtime, or if 30 g of carbohydrates will be consumed
• Do not use if a meal is skipped
• Do not use if discolored
Syringe compatibilities: Do not mix with insulin, give separately
Perform/provide:
• Storage at room temperature, keep away from heat and sunlight; refrigerate all other supply
Evaluate:
• Therapeutic response: decrease in polyuria, polydipsia, polyphagia, clear sensorium, absence of dizziness, stable gait ; improving A1c
Teach patient/family:
• That drug does not cure diabetes but controls symptoms

- To carry emergency ID as diabetic
- To recognize hypoglycemia reaction: headache, fatigue, weakness
- The dosage, route, mixing instructions, if any diet restrictions, disease process
- To carry a glucose source (candy or lump sugar) to treat hypoglycemia
- The symptoms of ketoacidosis: nausea, thirst, polyuria, dry mouth, decreased B/P, dry, flushed skin, acetone breath, drowsiness, Kussmaul respirations
- That a plan is necessary for diet, exercise; all food on diet should be eaten; exercise routine should not vary
- About blood glucose testing; make sure patient is able to determine glucose level
- To avoid OTC drugs unless directed by prescriber, alcohol
- Not to operate machinery or drive until effect is known

Treatment of overdose: Glucose 25 g IV, via dextrose 50% sol, 50 ml or glucagon 1 mg SUBCUT

---

pregabalin (℞)
(pre-gab'a-lin)
Lyrica
Func. class.: Anticonvulsant

Controlled Substance Schedule V
Action: Binds to high-voltage–gated calcium channels in CNS tissues; this may lead to anticonvulsant action, similar to the inhibitory neurotransmitter GABA, anxiolytic, analgesics, and antiepileptic properties
Uses: Neuropathic pain associated with diabetic peripheral neuropathy, partial-onset seizures, postherpetic neuralgia
Investigational uses: Generalized anxiety disorder (GAD), moderate pain, social anxiety disorder

DOSAGE AND ROUTES
Diabetic peripheral neuropathic pain
- *Adult:* PO 50 mg tid, may increase to 300 mg/day (max) within 1 wk, adjust in renal disease

Partial onset seizures
- *Adult:* PO 75 mg bid or 50 mg tid; may increase to 600 mg/day (max)

Postherpetic neuralgia
- *Adult:* PO 75-150 mg bid or 50-100 mg tid in patient with CCr ≥60 ml/min, initially give 75 mg bid or 50 mg tid and may increase to 600 mg/day (max) within 1 wk

Available forms: Caps 25, 50, 75, 100, 150, 200, 225, 300 mg

SIDE EFFECTS

CNS: Dizziness, fatigue, confusion, euphoria, incoordination, nervousness, neuropathy, tremor, vertigo, somnolence, ataxia, amnesia, abnormal thinking
EENT: Dry mouth, blurred vision, nystagmus, amblyopia
GI: Constipation, flatulence, abdominal pain, weight gain
HEMA: Ecchymosis
MS: Back pain
OTHER: Pruritus, impotence
RESP: Dyspnea

Contraindications: Hypersensitivity, abrupt discontinuation
Precautions: Pregnancy (C), renal disease, lactation, children <12 yr, elderly, PR interval prolongation, creatine kinase elevations, CHF (class III, IV), decreased platelets, drug abuse, dependence, glaucoma, myopathy

PHARMACOKINETICS

Well absorbed, absorption decreased with food, 90% recovered in urine unchanged, negligible metabolism, not bound to plasma proteins, half-life 6 hr

INTERACTIONS

Increase: weight gain/fluid retention—thiazolidinedione, avoid use if possible
Increase: CNS depression—anxiolytics, sedatives, hypnotics, barbiturates, general anesthetics, opiate agonists, phenothiazines, sedating H_1 blockers, thiazolidinediones, tricyclic antidepressants

---

A Safety alert *"Tall Man" lettering

NURSING CONSIDERATIONS
Assess:
• Seizures: aura, location, duration, activity at onset
• Pain: location, duration, characteristics if using for diabetic neuropathy
• Renal studies: urinalysis, BUN, urine creatinine q3mo, creatine kinase; if markedly increased, discontinue
• Mental status: mood, sensorium, affect, behavioral changes; if mental status changes, notify prescriber
Administer:
• Do not crush, or chew caps; caps may be opened and contents put in applesauce or dissolved in juice
• Give without regard to meals
• Gradually withdraw over 7 days; abrupt withdrawal may precipitate seizures
Perform/Provide
• Storage at room temperature away from heat and light
• Hard candy, frequent rinsing of mouth, gum for dry mouth
• Assistance with ambulation during early part of treatment; dizziness occurs
• Seizure precautions: padded side rails; move objects that may harm patient
• Increased fluids, bulk in diet for constipation
Evaluate:
• Therapeutic response: decreased seizure activity; decrease in neuropathic pain
Teach patient/family:
• To carry emergency ID stating patient's name, drugs taken, condition, prescriber's name, and phone number
• To avoid driving, other activities that require alertness: dizziness, drowsiness may occur
• Not to discontinue medication quickly after long-term use, taper over ≥1 wk; withdrawal-precipitated seizures may occur, not to double doses if dose is missed, take if 2 hr or more before next dose
• To notify prescriber if pregnancy

planned or suspected; avoid breastfeeding
• To report muscle pain, tenderness, weakness, when accompanied by fever, malaise
• To avoid alcohol
Treatment of overdose: Lavage, VS, hemodialysis

---

ramelteon (R)
(rah-mel'tee-on)
Rozerem
Func. class.: Sedative/hypnotic, antianxiety
Chem. class.: Melatonin receptor agonist

Action: Binds selectively to melatonin receptors (MT_1, MT_2). Thought to be involved in circadian rhythm and the normal sleep/wake cycle
Uses: Insomnia

DOSAGE AND ROUTES
• *Adult:* **PO** 8 mg at bedtime
Hepatic Dose
• Do not use in severe hepatic disease; use with caution in mild to moderate hepatic disease
Available forms: Tabs 8 mg

SIDE EFFECTS
CNS: Dizziness, somnolence, fatigue, headache, insomnia, depression
GI: Nausea, diarrhea, dysgeusia, vomiting
MISC: Myalgia, arthralgia, decreased blood cortisol, influenza, upper RI
Contraindications: Hypersensitivity, children, infants, lactation, alcohol intoxication, hepatic encephalopathy
Precautions: Pregnancy (C), hepatic disease, alcoholism, COPD, seizure disorder, sleep apnea, suicidal ideation

PHARMACOKINETICS
Absorbed rapidly, peak 0.75 hr, protein binding 82%, rapid first pass metabolism via liver, 84% excreted in urine, 4% feces, half-life 2-5 hr

---

Side effects: *italics* = common; ***bold italics*** = life-threatening

INTERACTIONS

Possible toxicity: antiretroviral protease inhibitors

Increase: ramelteon effect—alcohol, azole antifungals (ketoconazole, fluconazole), fluvoxamine, anxiolytics, sedatives, hypnotics, barbiturates

Decrease: effect of ramelteon—rifampin

Drug/Herb

Do not use with melatonin

Increase: CNS depression—catnip, chamomile, clary, cowslip, hops, kava, lavender, mistletoe, nettle, pokeweed, poppy, Queen Anne's lace, senega, skullcap, valerian

Drug/Food

• Food: prolonged absorption, sleep onset reduced—high-fat/heavy meal

NURSING CONSIDERATIONS

Assess:

• Mental status: mood, sensorium, affect, memory (long, short)
• Type of sleep problem: falling asleep, staying asleep

Administer:

• After removal of cigarettes to prevent fires
• After trying conservative measures for insomnia
• Within 30 min of bedtime for sleeplessness
• On empty stomach for fast onset

Perform/provide:

• Assistance with ambulation after receiving dose
• Safety measure: nightlight, call bell within easy reach
• Checking to see if PO medication has been swallowed
• Storage in tight container in cool environment

Evaluate:

• Therapeutic response: ability to sleep at night, decreased amount of early morning awakening

Teach patient/family:

• To avoid driving or other activities requiring alertness until drug is stabilized
• To avoid alcohol ingestion or CNS depressants
• Alternative measures to improve sleep: reading, exercise several hr before bedtime, warm bath, warm milk, TV, self-hypnosis, deep breathing
• To take immediately before going to bed
• Not to ingest a high-fat/heavy meal before taking
• To report cessation of menses, galactorrhea (women), decreased libido, infertility; worsening of insomnia, or behavioral changes

---

rotavirus vaccine (℞)

(rota-vi′rus vak′seen)
RotaTeq
Func. class: Vaccine, rotavirus

Action: A live, oral vaccine; protects against serotypes G1, G2, G3, G4, P1

Uses: Prevents rotavirus gastroenteritis in infants

DOSAGES AND ROUTES

• *Infants:* **PO** Three doses given between 6 and 32 wk of age; the first dose should be given between 6-12 wk, subsequent doses every 4-10 wk

Available forms: Single dose (PO)

SIDE EFFECTS

EENT: Runny nose, sore throat, ear infection

GI: Diarrhea, vomiting, ***gastroenteritis***

GU: ***Urinary tract infection***

RESP: Wheezing, coughing, ***pneumonia, pyrexia***

Contraindications: Hypersensitivity, immunocompromised; bone marrow, lymphatic disorders; blood products given within 6 wk

PHARMACOKINETICS

Unknown

INTERACTIONS

• Do not give with antineoplastics, radiation therapy, corticosteroids

NURSING CONSIDERATIONS

Assess:

• For age of infant; should only be given between 6 and 32 wk of age

• For urinary tract infection, pneumonia, that can be serious

• For intussusception, that was associated with a previously licensed product

Administer:

• Only during 6-32 wk of age

• May be given during well baby checks at 2, 4, 6 mo

Evaulate:

• Therapeutic response: Absence of rotavirus infection

Teach patient/family:

• To report coughing, wheezing, painful or scant urination

---

sorafenib (R)

(sore-ah-fen'ib)
Nexavar
Func. class.: Antineoplastic—miscellaneous
Chem. class.: Multikinase inhibitor, signal transduction inhibitor

Action: Multikinase inhibitor that decreases tumor cell proliferation
Uses: Advanced/metastatic murine renal cell carcinoma

DOSAGE AND ROUTES

• *Adult:* **PO** 400 mg bid without food, continue until no longer benefiting or until unacceptable toxicity occurs
Available forms: Tabs 200 mg

SIDE EFFECTS

CNS: Fatigue, weight loss, headache
CV: **Hypertension, cardiac ischemia, infarction**
GI: Nausea, diarrhea, vomiting, anorexia, **pancreatitis,** mouth ulceration, abdominal pain, constipation

HEMA: **Hemorrhage, leukopenia, lymphopenia, anemia, neutropenia, thrombocytopenia**
INTEG: Rash, pruritus, *dry skin,* erythema, hand-foot rash, **exfoliative dermatitis,** acne, flushing, alopecia
META: Hypophosphatemia
MS: Arthralgia, myalgia
RESP: Hoarseness
Contraindications: Pregnancy (D), hypersensitivity
Precautions: Lactation, children, elderly, hepatic disease

PHARMACOKINETICS

Bioavailability 38%-49%, elimination half-life 25-48 hr, peak 3 hr, high-fat meal decreases bioavailability, plasma protein binding 99.5%, metabolized in the liver, oxidative metabolism by CYP3A4, glucuronidation by UGT1A9, 77% excreted in feces

INTERACTIONS

May decrease sorafenib levels: phenytoin, rifampin, cimetidine, ranitidine, sodium bicarbonate, carbamazepine, dexamethasone, phenobarbital
Increase: effect of UGT1A1 (irinotecan, DOXOrubicin, gemcitabine, oxaliplatin)
Drug/Lab Test
Increase: lipase, amylase

NURSING CONSIDERATIONS

Assess:

• For skin toxicities: grade 1, continue therapy, topical treatment for relief; grade 2 (1st episode), continue therapy, if no improvement after 7 days, delay treatment until resolved to grade ≤1, resume dose by one dose level; grade 2 (2nd or 3rd episode), delay treatment until resolved to grade ≤1, resume dose by one dose level; grade 2 (4th episode), discontinue therapy; grade 3 (1st or 2nd episode), delay treatment until resolved to grade ≤1, resume dose by one dose level; grade 3 (3rd episode), discontinue therapy

---

Side effects: *italics* = common; ***bold italics*** = life-threatening

Administer:
- Swallow tab whole; do not break, crush, or chew
- On empty stomach 1 hr before or 2 hr after meal

Perform/provide:
- Storage in room temp, in dry place

Evaluate:
- Therapeutic response: decrease in renal cell carcinoma progression

Teach patient/family:
- ⚠ To report adverse reactions immediately
- Reason for treatment, expected results
- Use contraception during treatment, birth defects may occur, avoid breastfeeding
- To not double dose if missed

---

tigecycline (℞)
(tye-ge-sye′kleen)
Tygacil
Func. class.: Broad-spectrum antiinfective
Chem. class.: Glycylcyclines

Action: Inhibits protein synthesis and phosphorylation in microorganisms; bacteriostatic structurally similar to the tetracyclines

Uses: Complicated skin/skin structure infections (*Escherichia coli, Enterococcus faecalis* (vancomycin-susceptible only) *Staphylococcus aureus, Streptococcus agalactiae, S. anginosus* group, *S. pyogenes, Bacteroides fragilis;* complicated intraabdominal infections (*Citrobacter freundii*) *Enterobacter cloacae, E. coli, Klebsiella oxytoca, K. pneumoniae, E. faecalis* (vancomycin-susceptible only), *S. aureus* (methicillin-susceptible only), *S. anginosus* group, *B. fragilis, Bacteroides thetaiotaomicron, B. uniformis, B. vulgatus, Clostridium perfringens, Peptostreptococcus micros*

DOSAGE AND ROUTES
- *Adult:* **IV** 100 mg, then 50 mg q12h, **IV INF** is given over 30 min-60 min

q12h; given for 5-14 days depending on infection

Hepatic dose (Child-Pugh C)
- *Adult:* **IV** 100 mg, then 25 mg q12h

Available forms: Powder for inj, lyophilized 50 mg

SIDE EFFECTS

CNS: Headache, dizziness, insomnia
CV: Hyper/hypotension, phlebitis
GI: Nausea, vomiting, diarrhea, anorexia, constipation, dyspepsia
*HEMA: **Anemia, leukocytosis, thrombocytopenia***
INTEG: Rash, pruritus, sweating, photosensitivity
META: Increased ALT, AST, BUN, lactic acid, alk phosphatase, amylase, hyperglycemia, hypokalemia, hypoproteinemia, bilirubinemia
MISC: Back pain, fever, abnormal healing, abdominal pain, abscess, asthenia, infection, pain, peripheral edema, local reactions
RESP: Cough, dyspnea

Contraindications: Pregnancy (D), hypersensitivity to tigecycline, children <18 yr, lactation

Precautions: Renal disease, hepatic disease, hypersensitivity to tetracyclines

PHARMACOKINETICS

Not extensively metabolized, 22% of unchanged drug is excretion in urine, terminal half-life 42 hr, primarily biliary excreted

INTERACTIONS

Increase: effect of warfarin
Decrease: effect of oral contraceptives

NURSING CONSIDERATIONS
Assess:
- ⚠ For pseudomembranous colitis
- Signs of anemia: Hct, Hgb, fatigue
- Blood studies: PT, CBC, AST, ALT, BUN creatinine

⚠ Safety alert   *"Tall Man" lettering

• Allergic reactions: rash, itching, pruritus, angioedema
• Nausea, vomiting, diarrhea; administer antiemetic, antacids as ordered
• Overgrowth of infection: fever, malaise, redness, pain, swelling, drainage, perineal itching, diarrhea, changes in cough or sputum

Administer:
• After C&S obtained

IV route
• Reconstitute each vial with 5.3 ml of 0.9% NaCl, or D_5 (10 mg/ml); swirl to dissolve; immediately withdraw 5 ml of the reconstituted sol and add to a 100 ml IV bag for inf (1 mg/ml); may be yellow or orange, if not, sol should be discarded; do not give if particulate matter is present

Perform/provide:
• Storage in tight, light-resistant container at room temperature

Evaluate:
• Therapeutic response: decreased temp, absence of lesions, negative C&S

Teach patient/family:
• To avoid sun exposure; sunscreen does not seem to decrease photosensitivity
• To avoid pregnancy while taking this product; fetal harm may occur

---

tipranavir (℞)
(ti-pran'a-veer)
Aptivus
Func. class.: Antiretroviral
Chem. class.: Protease inhibitor

Action: Inhibits human immunodeficiency virus (HIV) protease; this prevents the maturation of virus

Uses: HIV in combination with other antiretrovirals

DOSAGE AND ROUTES
• Reduce dose in mild/moderate hepatic impairment and ketoconazole coadministration

• *Adult:* **PO** 500 mg coadministered with ritonavir 200 mg bid with food
Available forms: Caps 250 mg

SIDE EFFECTS
CNS: Headache, insomnia, dizziness, somnolence, fatigue
GI: Diarrhea, abdominal pain, nausea, vomiting, anorexia, dry mouth, ***hepatitis B or C, fatalities when given with ritonavir***
GU: Nephrolithiasis
INTEG: Rash
MS: Pain
OTHER: Asthenia, ***insulin-resistant hyperglycemia,*** hyperlipidemia, ***ketoacidosis***

Contraindications: Hypersensitivity, hepatic disease (Child-Pugh B to C)
Precautions: Pregnancy (C), lactation, children, renal disease, history of renal stones, sulfa allergy, hemophilia, diabetes mellitus

PHARMACOKINETICS
Terminal half-life 6 hr, plasma protein binding 99.9%, steady state 7-10 days, metabolism CYP3A4, 80% fecal excretion

INTERACTIONS
⚠ Life threatening dysrhythmias: ergots, midazolam, rifampin, triazolam
Increase: myopathy—lovastatin, simvastatin
Increase: tipranavir levels—ketoconazole, delavirdine, itraconazole
Increase: levels of both drugs—clarithromycin, zidovudine
Increase: levels of isoniazid—oral contraception
Decrease: tipranavir levels—rifamycins, fluconazole, nevirapine, efavirenz

Drug/Herb
Decrease: tipranavir levels—St. John's wort; avoid concurrent use

Drug/Food
Decrease: tipranavir absorption—

---

grapefruit juice, high-fat, high-protein foods

NURSING CONSIDERATIONS

Assess:

• For complaints of lower back, flank pain, indicates kidney stones
• Signs of infection, anemia, the presence of other sexually transmitted diseases
• Hepatic studies: ALT, AST; total bilirubin, amylase, all may be elevated
• Viral load, CD4 during treatment
• Bowel pattern before, during treatment; if severe abdominal pain with bleeding occurs, drug should be discontinued; monitor hydration
• Skin eruptions; rash, urticaria, itching
• Allergies before treatment, reaction of each medication; place allergies on chart

Administer:

• Swallow cap whole; do not break, crush, or chew
• After meals
• In equal intervals around the clock to maintain blood levels

Teach patient/family:

• To take as prescribed; if dose is missed, take as soon as remembered up to 1 hr before next dose; do not double dose
• That drug must be taken in equal intervals around the clock to maintain blood levels for duration of therapy
⚠ That hyperglycemia may occur; watch for increased thirst, weight loss, hunger, dry, itchy skin; notify prescriber
• To increase fluids to prevent kidney stones, if stone formation occurs, treatment may need to be interrupted
• That drug does not cure AIDS, only controls symptoms; not to donate blood

⚠ Safety alert   *"Tall Man" lettering

Appendix b

Recent FDA drug approvals

Generic name	Trade name	Use
lenalidomide	Revlimid	Transfusion-dependent anemia
nitisinone	Orfadin	Hereditary tyrosinemia type 1
conivaptan	Vaprisol	Euvolemic hyponutremia
lubiprostone	Amitiza	Chronic idiopathic constipation
ranolazine	Ranexa	Chronic angina
sunitinib	Sutent	GI treatment of stomal tumor, advanced renal carcinoma

Appendix c

Ophthalmic, otic, nasal, and topical products

OPHTHALMIC PRODUCTS

α-ADRENERGIC BLOCKER
dapiprazole (℞)
(da-pip'ra-zole)
Rev-Eyes

ANESTHETICS
proparacaine (℞)
(proe-par'a-kane)
Alcaine, Diocane ✿,
Ophthaine, Ophthestic
tetracaine (℞)
(tet'ra-kane)
Pontocaine, Tetracaine

ANTIHISTAMINES
azelastine (℞)
(ay-zell'ah-steen)
Optivar
emedastine (℞)
(ee-med'ah-steen)
Emadine
epinastine (℞)
(ep-een'as-teen)
Elestat
ketotifen (℞)
(kee-toh-tif'en)
Zaditor
olopatadine (℞)
(oh-loh-pat'ah-deen)
Patanol

ANTIINFECTIVES
chloramphenicol (℞)
(klor-am-fen'i-kole)
AK-Chlor, Chloramphenicol,
Chloromycetin Ophthalmic,
Chloroptic, Chloroptic S.O.P.,
Fenicol ✿, Isopto Fenical ✿,
Pentamycin ✿
ciprofloxacin (℞)
(sip-ro-floks'a-sin)
Ciloxan
erythromycin (℞)
(er-ith-roe-mye'sin)
Erythromycin, Ilotycin
fomivirsen (℞)
(foh-muh-vir'sun)
Vitravene
ganciclovir (℞)
(gan-sye'kloe-vir)
Vitrasert
gatifloxacin (℞)
(gat-i-flox'a-sin)
Zymar
gentamicin (℞)
(jen-ta-mye'sin)
Garamycin Ophthalmic,
Genoptic Ophthalmic,
Genoptic S.O.P., Gentacidin,
Gentamicin Ophthalmic,
Gentak
idoxuridine-IDU (℞)
(eye-dox-yoor'i-deen)
Herplex
levofloxacin (℞)
(lee-voh-floks'a-sin)
Quixin

moxifloxacin (℞)
(mox-i-flox′a-sin)
Vigamox

natamycin (℞)
(nat-a-mye′sin)
Natacyn

norfloxacin (℞)
(nor-floks′a-sin)
Chibroxin

ofloxacin (℞)
(oh-flox′a-sin)
Ocuflox

polymyxin B (℞)
(pol-ee-mix′in)
Polymyxin B Sulfate Sterile

silver nitrate 1% (℞)
silver nitrate
sulfacetamide
sodium (℞)
(sul-fa-seet′a-mide)
AK-Sulf, Bleph-10, Bleph-10
S.O.P., Cetamide, Isopto
Cetamide, Ocusulf-10,
Sodium Sulamyd, Sodium
Sulfacetamide, Storzsulf, Sulf-
10, Sulster

* **sulfiSOXAZOLE**
diolamine (℞)
(sul-fih-sox′ah-zohl)
Gantrisin

tobramycin (℞)
(toe-bra-mye′sin)
AKTob, Defy, Tobrex

trifluridine (℞)
(trye-floor′i-deen)
Viroptic

vidarabine (℞)
(vye-dare′a-been)
Vira-A

β-ADRENERGIC BLOCKERS
betaxolol (℞)
(beh-tax′oh-lole)
Betoptic, Betoptic 5
carteolol (℞)
(kar-tee′oh-lole)
Carteolol HCl, Ocupress
levobetaxolol (℞)
(lee-voh-beh-tax′oh-lole)
Betaxon
levobunolol (℞)
(lee-voe-byoo′no-lole)
AKBeta, Betagen
metipranolol (℞)
(met-ee-pran′oh-lole)
OptiPranolol
timolol (℞)
(tye′moe-lole)
Apo-Timop 🍁, Betimol,
Timoptic, Timoptic-XE[3]

CARBONIC ANHYDRASE
INHIBITORS
brinzolamide (℞)
(brin-zoh′la-mide)
Azopt
dorzolamide (℞)
(dor-zol′a-mide)
Trusopt

CHOLINERGICS
(Direct-acting)
acetylcholine (℞)
(ah-see-til-koe′leen)
Miochol-E
carbachol (℞)
(kar′ba-kole)
Carbastat, Carboptic, Iosopto
Carbachol, Miostat
pilocarpine (℞)
(pye-loe-kar′peen)
Adsorbocarpine, Akarpine,
Isopto Carpine, Ocu-Carpine,

Ocusert Pilo-20, Ocusert
Pilo-40, Pilagan, Pilocar,
pilocarpine, Pilopine HS,
Piloptic-½, Piloptic-1,
Piloptic-2, Piloptic-3,
Piloptic-4, Piloptic-6, Pilostat,
Pilopto-Carpine

CHOLINESTERASE INHIBITORS
demecarium (R)
(dem-e-kare'ee-um)
Humorsol

ecothiophate (R)
(ek-oh-thye'eh-fate)
Phospholine Iodide

CORTICOSTEROIDS
dexamethasone (R)
(dex-a-meth'a-sone)
AK-Dex, Decadron
Phosphate, Dexamethasone
Ophthalmic Suspension,
Maxidex

fluorometholone (R)
(flure-oh-meth'oh-lone)
Flarex, Fluor-Op, FML, FML
Forte, FML S.O.P.

loteprednol (R)
(loe-tee-pred'nole)
Alrex, Lotemax

medrysone (R)
(me'dri-sone)
HMS

*### prednisoLONE (R)
(pred-niss'oh-lone)
Econopred, Econopred Plus,
AK-Pred, Inflamase Forte,
Inflamase Mild, Pred-Forte

rimexolone (R)
(ri-mex'a-lone)
Vexol

MYDRIATICS
atropine (R)
(a'troe-peen)
Atropine-1, Atropine Care,
Atropine Sulfate Ophthalmic,
Atropisol, Isopto Atropine

cyclopentolate (R)
(sye-kloe-pen'toe-late)
AK-Pentolate, Cyclogly,
Cyclopentolate HC

homatropine (R)
(home-a'troe-peen)
Homatrine HBr, Isopto
Homatropine, Minims
Homatropine ✿

hydroxyamphetamine HBr (R)
(hy-drox-ee-am-fet'a-meen)
Paredrine

phenylephrine (OTC)
(fen-ill-ef'rin)
AK-Dilate, AK-Nefrin, Isopto
Frin, Neo-Synephrine 2.5%,
Neo-Synephrine 10%,
phenylephrine HCl, 2.5%
Mydfrin, Phenoptic Relief,
Prefrin

scopolamine (R)
(skoe-pol'a-meen)
Isopto Hyoscine

tropicamide (R)
(troe-pik'a-mide)
Mydriacyl, Opticyl, Tropicacyl,
Tropicamide

NONSTEROIDAL ANTIINFLAMMATORIES
diclofenac (R)
(dye-kloe'fen-ak)
Voltaren

flurbiprofen (R)
(flure-bih-proh'fen)
Ocufen

⚠ Safety alert   *"Tall Man" lettering

ketorolac (℞)
(kee-toe'role-ak)
Acular
suprofen (℞)
(soo-proe'fen)
Profenal

SYMPATHOMIMETICS
apraclonidine (℞)
(a-pra-klon'i-deen)
Lopidine
brimonidine (℞)
(brih-moh'nih-deen)
Alphagan, Alphagan P
dipivefrin (℞)
(dye-pi'vef-rin)
Propine, AKPro
*** epINEPHrine/
epinephryl borate** (℞)
(ep-i-nef'rin)
Epifrin, Glaucon/Epinal,
Eppy ✤

**OPHTHALMIC
DECONGESTANTS/
VASOCONSTRICTORS**
levocabastine (℞)
(lee-voh-cab'ah-steen)
Livostin
lodoxamide
(loe-dox'a-mide)
Alomide
naphazoline (ᴏᴛᴄ, ℞)
(naf-az'oh-leen)
20/20 Eye Drops, Allergy
Drops, AK-Con, Albalon,
Allerest Eye Drops, Clear
Eyes, Clear Eyes ACR,
Comfort Eye Drops, Degest
2, Maximum Strength Allergy
Drops, Nafazair, naphazoline

HCl, Naphcon, Naphcon
Forte, Opcon, Vasoclear,
Vasocon Regular
oxymetazoline (℞)
(ox-i-meth'oh-lone)
OcuClear, Visine L.R.
tetrahydrozoline (ᴏᴛᴄ)
(tet-ra-hye-dro'zoe-leen)
Collyrium Fresh, Eyesine,
Geneye, Geneye Extra,
Mallazine Eye Drops, Murine
Plus, Optigene 3,
tetrahydrozoline HCl,
Tetrasine, Tetrasine Extra,
Visine Moisturizing

**MISCELLANEOUS
OPHTHALMICS**
bimatoprost (℞)
(by-mat'oh-prahst)
Lumigan
brinzolamide (℞)
(brin-zole'a-mide)
Azopt
dorzolamide (℞)
(dor-zol'a-mide)
Trusopt
latanoprost (℞)
(la-tan'oh-proest)
Xalatan
travoprost (℞)
(trav'oh-prahst)
Travatan
unoprostone (℞)
(un-oh-proe'stone)
Rescula

Pregnancy categories: Demecarium, isoflurophate (X); apraclonidine, cyclopentolate, ecothiophate, glucocorticoids, levobunalol, metipranolol, pilocarpine, proparacaine, suprofen, tetracaine (C); dapiprazole, dipivefrin (B)
β-*Adrenergic blockers*
Action: Reduces production of aqueous humor by unknown mechanism

---

Side effects: *italics* = common; ***bold italics*** = life-threatening

Uses: Ocular hypertension, chronic open-angle glaucoma

Anesthetics
Action: Decreases ion permeability by stabilizing neuronal membrane
Uses: Cataract extraction, tonometry, gonioscopy, removal of foreign objects, corneal suture removal, glaucoma surgery (ophthalmic); pruritus, sunburn, toothache, sore throat, cold sores, oral pain, rectal pain and irritation, control of gagging (topical)

Antiinfectives
Action: Inhibits folic acid synthesis by preventing PABA use, which is necessary for bacterial growth
Uses: Conjunctivitis, superficial eye infections, corneal ulcers, prophylaxis against infection after removal of foreign matter from the eye

Antiinflammatories
Action: Decreases inflammation, resulting in decreased pain, photophobia, hyperemia, cellular infiltration
Uses: Inflammation of eye, eyelids, conjunctiva, cornea; uveitis, iridocyclitis, allergic conditions, burns, foreign bodies, postoperatively in cataract

Carbonic anhydrase inhibitor
Action: Converted to epINEPHrine, which decreases aqueous production and increases outflow
Uses: Open-angle glaucoma, ocular hypertension

Direct-acting miotic
Action: Acts directly on cholinergic receptor sites; induces miosis, spasm of accommodation, fall in intraocular pressure, caused by stimulation of ciliary, pupillary sphincter muscles, which leads to pulling away of iris from filtration angle, resulting in increased outflow of aqueous humor

Uses: Primary glaucoma, early stages of wide-angle glaucoma (less useful in advanced stages), chronic open-angle glaucoma, acute narrow-angle glaucoma before emergency surgery; also neutralizes mydriatics used during eye exam; may be used alternately with mydriatics to break adhesions between iris and lens

SIDE EFFECTS

CNS: Headache
CV: Hypertension, tachycardia, dysrhythmias
EENT: Burning, stinging
GI: Bitter taste
Contraindications: Hypersensitivity
Precautions: Pregnancy, lactation, children, aphakia, hypersensitivity to carbonic anhydrase inhibitors, sulfonamides, thiazide diuretics, ocular inhibitors, hepatic and renal insufficiency

NURSING CONSIDERATIONS

Assess:
• Ophth exams and intraocular pressure readings
• Blood counts; hepatic, renal function tests and serum electrolytes during long-term treatment

Perform/provide:
• Storage at room temperature away from light

Evaluate:
• Positive therapeutic response
• Absence of increased intraocular pressure

Teach patient/family:
• How to instill drops
• That drug may cause burning, itching, blurring, dryness of eye area

---

⚠ Safety alert *"Tall Man" lettering

NASAL AGENTS

NASAL DECONGESTANTS
azelastine (℞)

(ay-zell'ah-steen)

Astelin

desoxyephedrine (OTC)

(des-oxy-e-fed'rin)

Vicks Inhaler

***epHEDrine** (OTC)

(e-fed'rin)

Pretz-D

***epINEPHrine** (OTC)

(ep-i-neff'rin)

Adrenalin

naphazoline (OTC)

(naff-a-zoe'leen)

Privine

oxymetazoline (OTC)

(ox-i-met-az'oh-leen)

12-Hour Nasal, Afrin 12-Hour Original, Afrin 12-Hour Original Pump Mist, Afrin Severe Congestion with Menthol, Afrin Sinus with Vapornase, Afrin No-Drip 12-Hour, Afrin No-Drip 12-Hour Extra Moisturizing, Dristan, Duramist Plus, Duration, Genasal, Nafrine ♣, Nasal Relief, Neo-Synephrine 12 Hour, Nostrilla, oxymetazoline HCl, Nasal Decongestant, Maximum Strength, Vicks Sinex 12-Hour Long-Acting, Vicks Sinex 12-Hour Ultra Fine Mist for Sinus Relief

phenylephrine (OTC)

(fen-ill-eff'rin)

Alconefrin 12, Children's Nostril, Neo-Synephrine, Sinex

propylhexadrine (OTC)

(proe-pil-hex'a-dreen)

Benzedrex Inhaler

tetrahydrozoline (OTC)

(tet-ra-hye-dro'zoe-leen)

Tyzine, Tyzine Pediatric

xylometazoline (OTC)

(zye-loh-meh-tazz'oh-leen)

Natru-vent, Otrivin, Otrivin Pediatric Nasal

NASAL STEROIDS
beclomethasone (℞)

(be-kloe-meth'a-sone)

Beconase AQ Nasal, Beconase Inhalation, Vancenase AQ Nasal, Vancenase Pocket Inhaler

budesonide (℞)

(byoo-des'oh-nide)

Rhinocort, Rhinocort Aqua

flunisolide (℞)

(floo-niss'oh-lide)

Nasalide, Nasarel

fluticasone (℞)

(floo-tic'a-son)

Flonase

mometasone (℞)

(mo-met'a-sone)

Nasonex

triamcinolone (℞)

(trye-am-sin'oh-lone)

Nasacort AQ

Pregnancy category: C

Action: Produces vasoconstriction (rapid, long acting) of arterioles, thereby decreasing fluid exudation, mucosal engorgement by stimulation of α-adrenergic receptors in vascular smooth muscle

Uses: Nasal congestion

DOSAGE AND ROUTES
Desoxyephedrine

• *Adult and child >6 yr:* 1-2 **INH** in each nostril q2h or less

APPENDIX

EpHEDrine
• *Adult:* Fill dropper to the level marked, then use in each nostril q4h or less
EpINEPHrine
• *Adult and child >6 yr:* Apply with swab, drops, spray prn
Naphazoline
• *Adult and child >6 yr:* 1-2 drops/spray q6h or less
Oxymetazoline
• *Adult and child >6 yr:* **INSTILL** 2-3 gtt or sprays to each nostril bid
• *Child 2-6 yr:* **INSTILL** 2-3 gtt or sprays 0.025 sol bid, not to exceed 3 days
Phenylephrine
• *Adult and child >12 yr:* 2-3 drops/spray (0.25-0.5) in each nostril q3-4h or less; or 2-3 drops/spray (1%) in each nostril q4h or less
• *Child 6-12 yr:* 2-3 drops/spray (0.25%) in each nostril q3-4h
• *Infant >6 mo:* 1-2 drops (0.16%) in each nostril q3h
Propylhexadrine
• *Adult and child >6 yr:* 1-2 **INH** in each nostril q2h or less
Tetrahydrozoline
• *Adult and child >6 yr:* 2-4 drops (0.1%) q3-4h prn or 3-4 sprays in each nostril q4h prn
• *Child 2-6 yr:* 2-3 drops (0.05%) in each nostril q4-6h prn
Xylometazoline
• *Adult and child >12 yr:* 2-3 drops/spray (0.1%) in each nostril q8-10h
• *Child 2-12 yr:* 2-3 drops (0.05%) in each nostril q8-10h
Available forms: Nasal sol 0.025%, 0.05%

SIDE EFFECTS

CNS: Anxiety, restlessness, tremors, weakness, insomnia, dizziness, fever, headache
EENT: Irritation, burning, sneezing, stinging, dryness, rebound congestion
GI: Nausea, vomiting, anorexia
INTEG: Contact dermatitis
Contraindications: Hypersensitivity to sympathomimetic amines

Precautions: Pregnancy (C), children <6 yr, elderly, diabetes, cardiovascular disease, hypertension, hyperthyroidism, increased intracranial pressure, prostatic hypertrophy, glaucoma

NURSING CONSIDERATIONS

Assess:
• For redness, swelling, pain in nasal passages before and during treatment
• For systemic absorption; hypertension, tachycardia; notify prescriber; systemic absorption occurs at high doses or after prolonged use
Administer:
• Having patient tilt head back, squeeze bulb to create a vacuum, and draw correct amount of sol into dropper; insert 2 gtt of sol into nostril; repeat in other nostril
• Store in light-resistant container; do not expose to high temp or let sol come into contact with aluminum
• For <4 consecutive days
• Environmental humidification to decrease nasal congestion, dryness
Evaluate:
• Therapeutic response: decreased nasal congestion
Teach patient/family:
• That stinging may occur for several applications; drying of mucosa may be decreased by environmental humidification
• To notify prescriber if irregular pulse, insomnia, dizziness, or tremors occur
• Proper administration to avoid systemic absorption
• To rinse dropper with very hot water to prevent contamination

TOPICAL GLUCOCORTICOIDS

alclometasone (R)
(al-kloe-met′a-sone)
Adovate
amcinonide (R)
(am-sin′oh-nide)
Cyclocort

betamethasone (℞)
(bay-ta-meth'a-sone)
Alphatrex, Beben ✤,
Betacort ✤, Betatrex, Beta-Val,
Bethovate ✤, Celestoderm ✤,
Diprosone, Ectosonel ✤,
Luxiq, Maxivate, Metaderm ✤,
Psorion, Valisone

**betamethasone
(augmented)** (℞)
(bay-ta-meth'a-sone)
Diprolene, Diprolene AF

clobetasol (℞)
(kloe-bay'ta-sol)
Cormax, Dermovate ✤,
Embeline E 0.05%, Temovate

clocortolone (℞)
(kloe-kore'toe-lone)
Cloderm

desonide (℞)
(dess'oh-nide)
Desonide, DesOwen,
Tridesilon

desoximetasone (℞)
(dess-ox-i-met'a-sone)
Topicort, Topicort LP

dexamethasone (℞)
(dex-a-meth'a-sone)
Aeroseb-Dex, Decaspray

diflorasone (℞)
(dye-flor'a-sone)
Florone, Maxiflor, Psorcon

fluocinolone (℞)
(floo-oh-sin'oh-lone)
Fluocin, Licon, Lidemol ✤,
Lidex, Lyderm ✤, Topsyn ✤,
Vasoderm

flurandrenolide (℞)
(flure-an-dren'oh-lide)
Cordran, Cordran SP,
Drenison 1/4 ✤, Drenison
Tape ✤

fluticasone (℞)
(floo-tik'a-sone)
Cutivate

halcinonide (℞)
(hal-sin'oh-nide)
Halog, Halog-E

halobetasol (℞)
(hal-oh-bay'ta-sol)
Ultravate

hydrocortisone (℞)
(hye-droe-kor'ti-sone)
Actiocort, Aeroseb-HC, Ala-
Cort, Allercort, Alphaderm,
Anusol HC, Bactine,
Barriere-HC ✤, Calde-CORT
Anti-Itch, Carmol HC,
Cetacort, Cortacet ✤,
Cortaid, Cortate ✤, Cort-
Dome, Cortef ✤, Corticaine,
Corticreme ✤, Cortifair, Corti-
zone, Cortoderm ✤, Cortril,
Delcort, Dermacort,
DemiCort, Dermtex HC,
Emo-Cort, Epifoam,
FoilleCort, Gly-Cort,
Gynecort, Hi-Cor, Hycort,
Hyderm ✤, Hydro-Tex,
Hytone, Lacti-Care-HC,
Lanacort, Lemoderm, Locoid,
My Cort, Novoehydrocort ✤,
Nutracort Pharm,
Pharmacort, Pentacort,
Rederm, Rhulicort S-T Cort,
Synacort, Sarna HC ✤, Texa-
Cort, Unicort ✤, Westcort

methylPREDNISolone
(℞)
(meth-il-pred-niss'oh-lone)

mometasone (℞)
(moe-met'a-sone)
Elocon

prednicarbate (℞)
(pred-ni-kar'bate)
Dermatop

Side effects: *italics* = common; ***bold italics*** = life-threatening

triamcinolone (℞)

(trye-am-sin'oh-lone)
Aristocort, Delta-Tritex, Flutex, Kenac, Kenalog, Kenonel, Triaderm, Trianide ❧, Triderm, Trymex

Pregnancy category: C
Action: Antipruritic, antiinflammatory
Uses: Psoriasis, eczema, contact dermatitis, pruritus; usually reserved for severe dermatoses that have not responded to less potent formulation

DOSAGE AND ROUTES

• *Adult and child:* Apply to affected area

SIDE EFFECTS

INTEG: Acne, atrophy, epidermal thinning, purpura, striae
Contraindications: Hypersensitivity, viral infections, fungal infections
Precautions: Pregnancy (C)

NURSING CONSIDERATIONS

Assess:
• Temp; if fever develops, drug should be discontinued
• For systemic absorption, increased temp, inflammation, irritation
Administer:
• Only to affected areas; do not get in eyes
• Leaving site uncovered or lightly covered; occlusive dressing is not recommended—systemic absorption may occur
• Use only on dermatoses; do not use on weeping, denuded, or infected area
• Cleansing before application of drug
• Continuing treatment for a few days after area has cleared
• Store at room temperature
Evaluate:
• Therapeutic response: absence of severe itching, patches on skin, flaking
Teach patient/family:
• To avoid sunlight on affected area, burns may occur
• To limit treatment to 14 days

TOPICAL ANTIFUNGALS

amphotericin B (OTC)

(am-foe-ter'i-sin)
Fungizone

butenafine (℞)

(byoo-tin'a-feen)
Lotrimin Ultra, Mentex

ciclopirox (OTC)

(sye-kloe-peer'ox)
Loprox, Penlac Nail Lacquer

clioquinol (OTC)

(klye-oh-kwin'ole)
Vioform

clotrimazole (OTC)

(kloe-trye'ma-zole)
Canestew ❧, Clotrimaderm ❧, Clotrimazole, Cruex, Desenex, Lotrimin AF, Myclo ❧, Neozol ❧

econazole (OTC)

(ee-kon'a-zole)
Spectazole

haloprogin (OTC)

(hal-oh-proe'jin)
Halotex

ketoconazole (OTC)

(kee-toe-kon'a-zole)
Nizoral

miconazole (OTC)

(mye-kon'a-zole)
Absorbine Antifungal Foot Powder, Breeze Mist Antifungal, Fungoid Tincture, Lotrimin AF, Maximum Strength Desenex Antifungal, Micatin, Monistat-Derm, Onyclear, Tetterine, Zeasorb-AF

naftifine (OTC)

(naff'ti-feen)
Naftin

nystatin (OTC)

(nye-stat'in)
Mycostatin, Nodostine ❧, Nilstat, Nyoderm ❧, Nystex

🅰 Safety alert   *"Tall Man" lettering

oxiconazole (OTC)

(ox-i-kon'a-zole)

Oxistat

selenium (OTC)

(see-leen'ee-um)

Exsel, Head and Shoulders Intensive Treatment, Selenium Sulfide, Selsun, Selsun Blue

sertaconazole (Rx)

(ser-tah-koe'-na-zole)

Ertaczo

terbinafine (OTC)

(ter-bin'a-feen)

Lamisil

tolnaftate (OTC)

(tole-naf'tate)

Absorbine Athlete's Foot Cream, Aftate for Athlete's Foot, Aftate for Jock Itch, Genaspor, Quinsana Plus, Tinactin, Ting, tolnaftate

undecylenic acid (OTC)

(un-deh-sih-len'ik)

Blis-To-Sol, Breeze Mist, Caldesene, Cruex, Decylenes, Desenex, Desenex Maximum Strength, Pedi-Pro, Phicon F, Protectol

Pregnancy category: B

Action: Interferes with fungal cell membrane permeability

Uses: Tinea cruris, tinea pedis, diaper rash, minor skin irritations; amphotericin B is used for *Candida* infections

DOSAGE AND ROUTES

• Massage into affected area, surrounding area daily or bid, continue for 7-14 days, not to exceed 4 wk

SIDE EFFECTS

INTEG: Burning, stinging, dryness, itching, local irritation

Contraindications: Hypersensitivity

Precautions: Pregnancy (B), lactation, children

Interactions: None

NURSING CONSIDERATIONS

Assess:

• Skin for fungal infections; peeling, dryness, itching before and throughout treatment

• For continuing infection; increased size, number of lesions

Administer:

Topical route

• To affected area, surrounding area; do not cover with occlusive dressings

• Store below 30° C (86° F)

Evaluate:

• Therapeutic response: decrease in size, number of lesions

Teach patient/family:

• To apply with glove to prevent further infection; not to cover with occlusive dressings

• That long-term therapy may be needed to clear infection (2 wk-6 mo depending on organism); compliance is needed even after feeling better

• Proper hygiene; hand-washing technique, nail care, use of concomitant top agents if prescribed

• To avoid use of OTC creams, ointments, lotions unless directed by prescriber

• To use medical asepsis (hand washing) before, after each application; to change socks and shoes once a day during treatment of tinea pedis

• To report to health care prescriber if infection persists or recurs; if blisters, burning, oozing, swelling occur

• To avoid alcohol because nausea, vomiting, hypertension may occur

• To use sunscreen or avoid direct sunlight to prevent photosensitivity

• To notify healthcare prescriber of sore throat, fever, skin rash, which may indicate overgrowth of organisms

---

TOPICAL ANTIINFECTIVES

azelaic acid (R)
(a-zuh-lay'ic)
Azelex, Finacen

bacitracin (OTC)
(bass-i-tray'sin)
Bacitin ✿, Bacitracin

clindamycin (R)
(klin-da-my'sin)
Cleocin T, Clindagel,
ClindaMax, Clindets

erythromycin (OTC)
(er-ith-roe-mye'sin)
A/T/S, Akne-Mycin, Eryderm,
Erygel, Erythromycin,
Staticin, T-Statd

gentamicin (R)
(jen-ta-mye'sin)
Gentamicin

mafenide (R)
(ma'fe-nide)
Sulfamylon

metronidazole (R)
(met-roh-nye'da-zole)
MetroGel, MetroCream,
MetroLotion, Noritate

mupirocin (R)
(myoo-peer'oh-sin)
Bactroban

neomycin (OTC)
(nee-oh-mye'sin)
Neomycin Sulfate

nitrofurazone (R)
(nye-troe-fyoor'a-zone)
Furacin, Nitrofurazone

* **silver sulfADIAZINE** (R)
(sul-fa-dye'a-zeen)
Flamazine ✿, Silvadene, SSD,
SSD AF, Thermazine

Pregnancy category: C
Action: Interferes with bacterial protein
synthesis

Uses: Skin infections, minor burns,
wounds, skin grafts, primary pyodermas,
otitis externa

SIDE EFFECTS

INTEG: Rash, urticaria, scaling, redness
Contraindications: Hypersensitivity,
large areas, burns, ulcerations
Precautions: Pregnancy (C), lactation,
impaired renal function, external ear or
perforated eardrum

NURSING CONSIDERATIONS

Assess:
• Allergic reaction: burning, stinging,
swelling, redness
• For signs of nephrotoxicity or ototoxic-
ity
Administer:
• Enough medication to cover lesions
completely
• After cleansing with soap, water before
each application; dry well
• To less than 20% of body surface area
when patient has impaired renal function
Perform/provide:
• Storage at room temperature in dry
place
Evaluate:
• Therapeutic response: decrease in
size, number of lesions

TOPICAL ANTIVIRALS

acyclovir (R)
(ay-sye'kloe-ver)
Zovirax

penciclovir (R)
(pen-sye'kloe-ver)
Denavir

Pregnancy category: C
Action: Interferes with viral DNA replication
Uses: Simple mucocutaneous herpes
simplex, in immunocompromised clients
with initial herpes genitalis

SIDE EFFECTS

INTEG: Rash, urticaria, stinging, burning,
pruritus, vulvitis

⚠ Safety alert   *"Tall Man" lettering

Contraindications: Hypersensitivity
Precautions: Pregnancy (C), lactation

NURSING CONSIDERATIONS
Assess:
• Allergic reaction: burning, stinging, swelling, redness, rash, vulvitis, pruritus
Administer:
• Using finger cot or rubber glove to prevent further infection
• Enough medication to cover lesions completely
• After cleansing with soap, water before each application; dry well
Perform/provide:
• Storage at room temperature in dry place
Evaluate:
• Therapeutic response: decrease in size, number of lesions
Teach patient/family:
• Not to use in eyes or when there is no evidence of infection
• To apply with glove to prevent further infection
• To avoid use of OTC creams, ointments, lotions unless directed by prescriber
• To use medical asepsis (hand washing) before, after each application and avoid contact with eyes
• To adhere strictly to prescribed regimen to maximize successful treatment outcome
• To begin taking drug when symptoms arise

TOPICAL ANESTHETICS

benzocaine (otc)
(ben'zoe-kane)
Americaine Anesthetic, Anbesol Maximum Strength, Baby Anbesol, Biozene, Boil-Ease, Children's Chloraseptic, Dermoplast, Foille, Foille Plus, Hurraccaine, Lanacaine, Medamint, Orabase, Oracin, Ora-Jel

dibucaine (otc)
(dye'byoo-kane)
Dibucaine, Nupercainal
lidocaine (otc, ℞)
(lye'doe-kane)
Anestacon, Burn-O-Jel, Derma Flex, Dentipatch, ELA-Max, Lidocaine HCl Topical, Lidocaine Viscous, Numby Stuff, Solarcaine Aloe Extra Burn Relief, Xylocaine, Xylocaine 10% oral, Xylocaine Viscous, Zilactin-L
pramoxine (otc)
(pra-mox'een)
Itch-X, PrameGel, Prax, Tronothane
tetracaine (otc, ℞)
(tet'ra-cane)
Pontocaine, Viractin

Pregnancy category: C
Action: Inhibits conduction of nerve impulses from sensory nerves
Uses: Oral irritation, sore throat, toothache, cold sore, canker sore, sunburn, minor cuts, insect bites, pain, itching

DOSAGE AND ROUTES
• *Adult and child:* **TOP** apply qid as needed; **RECT** insert tid and after each BM

SIDE EFFECTS
INTEG: Rash, irritation, sensitization
Contraindications: Hypersensitivity, infants <1 yr, application to large areas
Precautions: Pregnancy (C), child <6 yr, sepsis, denuded skin

NURSING CONSIDERATIONS
Assess:
• Pain: location, duration, characteristics before and after administration
• For infection: redness, drainage, inflammation; this drug should not be used until infection is treated
Perform/provide:
• Storage in tight, light-resistant

container; do not freeze, puncture, or
incinerate aerosol container
Evaluate:
• Therapeutic response: decreased
redness, swelling, pain
Teach patient/family:
• To avoid contact with eyes
• Not to use for prolonged periods: use
for <1 wk; if condition remains, pre-
scriber should be contacted

TOPICAL MISCELLANEOUS

docosanol (otc)
(doe-koe′san-ole)
Abreva
pimecrolimus (R)
(pim-eh-croh′lim-us)
Elidel

VAGINAL ANTIFUNGALS

butoconazole (otc)
(byoo-toh-kone′ah-zole)
Femstat-3, Gynazol-1,
Mycelex-3
clotrimazole (otc)
(kloe-trye′ma-zole)
Canesten ♣, Clotrimazole,
Gyne-Lotrimin 3, Gyne-
Lotrimin 7, Mycelex 7,
Myclo ♣
miconazole (otc)
(mye-kon′a-zole)
Femizole-M, Monistat,
Monistat 3, Monistat 7,
Monistat Dual Pak, M-Zole 7
Dual Pack
nystatin (otc)
(nye-stat′in)
Nystatin
terconazole (otc)
(ter-kone′ah-zole)
Terazol 7, Terazol 3

tioconazole (otc)
(tye-oh-kone′ah-zole)
Gyne-Trosyd ♣, Monistat 1,
Vagistat-1

Pregnancy category: Nystatin (A);
clotrimazole (B); butoconazole, terconazole, tioconazole (C)
Action: Interferes with fungal DNA
replication; binds sterols in fungal cell
membranes, which increases permeability, leaking of nutrients
Uses: Vaginal, vulval, vulvovaginal candidiasis (moniliasis)

DOSAGE AND ROUTES
Butoconazole
• *Adult:* **VAG** 5 g (1 applicator) at bed-
time × 3-6 days
Clotrimazole
• *Adult:* 100 mg (1 vag tab, 100 mg) at
bedtime × 1 wk, or 200 mg (2 vag tab,
100 mg) at bedtime × 3 nights, or 500
mg (1 vag tab, 500 mg); or 5 g (1 appli-
cator) at bedtime × 1-2 wk
Miconazole
• *Adult:* 200 mg supp at bedtime × 3
days or 100 mg supp × 1 wk
Nystatin
• *Adult:* 100,000 units daily × 2 wk
Terconazole
• *Adult:* **VAG** 5 g (1 applicator) at bed-
time × 7 days
Tioconazole
• *Adult:* 1 applicator at bedtime × 1 wk

SIDE EFFECTS
GU: Vulvovaginal burning, itching, pelvic
cramps
INTEG: Rash, urticaria, stinging, burning
MISC: Headache, body pain
Contraindications: Hypersensitivity
Precautions: Children <2 yr, preg-
nancy, lactation
Interactions: None

NURSING CONSIDERATIONS
Assess:
• For allergic reaction: burning, sting-
ing, itching, discharge, soreness

⚠ Safety alert   *"Tall Man" lettering

Administer:

Topical route

• One full applicator every night high into the vagina

• Store at room temperature in dry place

Evaluate:

• Therapeutic outcome: decrease in itching or white discharge (vaginal)

Teach patient/family:

• About asepsis (hand-washing) before, after each application

• To apply with applicator only; to avoid use of any other vaginal product unless directed by prescriber; sanitary napkin may prevent soiling of undergarments

• To abstain from sexual intercourse until treatment is completed; reinfection and irritation may occur

• To notify prescriber if symptoms persist

OTIC ANTIINFECTIVES

---

boric acid
Auro-Dri, Dri/Ear, Ear Dry
chloramphenicol (℞)
(klor-am-fen'i-kole)
Chloromycetin Otic

Action: Inhibits protein synthesis in susceptible microorganisms

Uses: Ear infection (external), short-term use

SIDE EFFECTS

EENT: Itching, irritation in ear

INTEG: Rash, urticaria

Contraindications: Hypersensitivity, perforated eardrum

Precautions: Pregnancy (C)

NURSING CONSIDERATIONS

Assess:

• For redness, swelling, fever, pain in ear, which indicates superinfection

Administer:

• After removing impacted cerumen by irrigation

• After cleaning stopper with alcohol

• After restraining child if necessary

• After warming sol to body temp

Evaluate:

• Therapeutic response: decreased ear pain

Teach patient/family:

• The correct method of instillation using aseptic technique, including not touching dropper to ear

• That dizziness may occur after instillation

Appendix d

Commonly used antiinfectives in adults and children

amoxicillin

Adult: **PO** 750 mg-1.5 g daily in divided doses q8h

Child: **PO** 20-50 mg/kg/day in divided doses q8h

ampicillin

Adult and child ≥40 kg: **PO** 1-2 g daily in divided doses q6h

IM/IV 2-8 g daily in divided doses q4-6h

Child <40 kg: **PO** 25-100 mg/kg/day in divided doses q6h

IM/IV 25-50 mg/kg/day in divided doses q8h

cefaclor

Adult: **PO** 250-500 mg q8h, not to exceed 4 g/day or 375-500 mg (ext rel) q12h × 7-10 days

Child >1 mo: **PO** 20-40 mg/kg/day in divided doses q8h, or total daily dose may be divided and given q12h, not to exceed 1 g/day

cephalexin

Adult: **PO** 250-500 mg q6h

Child: **PO** 25-50 mg/kg/day in 4 equal doses

chloramphenicol

Adult and child: **PO/IV** 50-75 mg/kg/day in divided doses q6h, 100 mg/kg/day (for meningitis only) max 4 g/day

Premature infants and neonates: **PO/IV** 25 mg/kg/day in divided doses q12-24h

clindamycin

Adult: **PO** 150-450 mg q6h, max 1.8 g/day

IM/IV 1.2-1.8 g/day in 2-4 divided doses, not to exceed 4800 mg/day

Child >1 mo: **PO** 8-25 mg/kg/day in divided doses q6-8h

IM/IV 20-40 mg/kg/day in divided doses q6-8h, (3-4 equal doses)

Child <1 mo: **IM/IV** 15-20 mg/kg/day divided q6-8h

erythromycin

Adult: **PO** 250-500 mg q6h (base, estolate, stearate); **PO** 400-800 mg q6h (ethylsuccinate); **IV INF** 15-20 mg/kg/day (lactobionate) divided q6h

Child: **PO** 30-50 mg/kg/day in divided doses q6h (salts); **IV** 20-40 mg/kg/day in divided doses q6h (lactobionate), max adult dose

gentamicin

Adult: **IV INF** 3-5 mg/kg/day in 3 divided doses q8h; dilute in 50-200 ml 0.9% NaCl or D_5W given over 30 min-1 hr; **IM** 3 mg/kg/day in divided doses q8h

Child: **IV/IM** 2-2.5 mg/kg q8h

Neonate and infant: **IV/IM** 2.5 mg/kg q8-12h

Neonate <1 wk: **IM/IV** 2.5 mg/kg q12-24h

A Safety alert   *"Tall Man" lettering

kanamycin

Adult and child: **IV INF** 15 mg/kg/day in divided doses q8-12h; diluted 500 mg/200 ml of NS or D_5W given over 30-60 min, not to exceed 1.5 g/day; **IM** 15 mg/kg/day in divided doses q8-12h, not to exceed 1.5 g/day, irrigation not to exceed 1.5 g/day; **INH** 250 mg qid

nafcillin

Adult: **IV** 500-1000 mg q4h

Child and infant >1 mo: **IV** 50-200 mg/kg/day in divided doses q4-6h

Neonates >7 days (weight >2 kg): **IV** 25 mg/kg q8h

Neonates ≤7 days (weight <2 kg): **IV** 25 mg/kg q12h

nitrofurantoin

Adult and child >12 yr: **PO** 50-100 mg qid pc or 50-100 mg at bedtime for long-term treatment

Child 1 mo-3 yr: **PO** 5-7 mg/kg/day in 4 divided doses; 1-3 mg/kg/day for long-term treatment

oxacillin

Adult: **PO** 2-6 g/day in divided doses q4-6h

IM/IV 2-12 g/day in divided doses q4-6h

Child: **PO** 50-100 mg/kg/day in divided doses q6h

IM/IV 50-100 mg/kg/day in divided doses q4-6h

penicillin G benzathine

Adult: **IM** 1.2 million units in single dose

Child >27 kg: **IM** 900,000 units in single dose

Child <27 kg: **IM** 300,000-600,000 units in single dose

penicillin G

Adult: **IM/IV** 5-24 million units in divided doses q4-6h

Child <12 yr: **IV** 150,000 units/kg/day in 4-6 divided doses

penicillin G procaine

Adult and child: **IM** 600,000-1.2 million units in 1-2 doses/day for 10 days to 2 wk

Newborn: Avoid use in newborns

sulfiSOXAZOLE

Adult: **PO** 2-4 g loading dose, then 1-2 g qid × 7-10 days

Child >2 mo: **PO** 75 mg/kg or 2 g/m² loading dose, then 120-150 mg/kg/day or 4 g/m²/day in divided doses q6h, not to exceed 6 g/day

ticarcillin

Adult: **INF** 200-300 mg/kg/day in divided doses q4-6h

Child <40 kg: **IV** 200-300 mg/kg/day in divided doses q4-6h

---

Appendix e Vaccines and toxoids

GENERIC NAME	TRADE NAME	USES	DOSAGE AND ROUTES	CONTRAINDICATIONS
BCG vaccine	TICE BCG	TB exposure	Adult/child >1 mo: 0.2-0.3 ml Child <1 mo: Reduce dose by 50% using 2 ml of sterile water after reconstituting	Hypersensitivity, hypogammaglobulinemia, positive TB test, burns
cholera vaccine	No trade name	Immunization for cholera in other countries	Adult/child >10 yr: IM/SUBCUT 2× of 0.5 ml, 7-30 days before traveling to cholera areas Booster is used q6mo 0.5 ml prn	Hypersensitivity, acute febrile illness
diphtheria and tetanus toxoids, adsorbed	No trade name	Induces antitoxins to provide immunity to diphtheria and tetanus	Adult/child ≥7 yr: IM (adult strength) 0.5 ml q4-8wk × 2 doses, then 3rd dose 6-12 mo after 2nd dose, booster IM 0.5 ml q10yr Child 1-6 yr: IM (pediatric strength) 0.5 ml q4wk × 2 doses, booster 6-12 mo after 2nd dose Infant 6 wk-1 yr: IM (pediatric strength) 0.5 ml q4wk × 3 doses, booster 6-12 mo after 3rd dose	Hypersensitivity to mercury, thimerosal; immunocompromised patients; radiation; corticosteroids; acute illness
diphtheria and tetanus toxoids and whole-cell pertussis vaccine (DPT, DTP) diphtheria and tetanus toxoids and acellular pertussis vaccine	DTwP, Tr-Immunol Acel-Imune, DTaP, Tripedia	Prevention of diphtheria, tetanus, pertussis	Adult: Booster dose q10yr Child >6 wk-6 yr: IM 0.5 ml at 2, 4, 6 mo, 1½ yr; booster needed 0.5 ml at age 6	Hypersensitivity, active infection, poliomyelitis outbreak, immunosuppression, febrile illness
haemophilus b conjugate vaccine, diphtheria CRM$_{197}$ protein conjugate (HbOC)	HibTITER	Polysaccharide immunization of children 2-6 yr against *H. influenzae* b, conjugate	**HibTITER (IM only)** Child: IM 0.5 ml Child 2-6 mo: 0.5 ml q2mo × 3 inj	Hypersensitivity, febrile illness, active infection

haemophilus b conjugate vaccine, meningococcal protein conjugate (PRP-OMP)	PedvaxHIB	Immunization of child 2, 4, 6 mo	Child 7-11 mo: Previously unvaccinated 0.5 ml q2mo inj; Child 12-14 mo: Previously unvaccinated 0.5 ml × 1 inj; **PedvaxHIB (IM only)** Child 2-14 mo: 0.5 ml × 2 inj at 2, 4 mo of age (6 mo dose not needed), then booster at 12-18 mo against invasive disease; Child ≥15 mo: Previously unvaccinated 0.5 ml inj	Hypersensitivity
hepatitis A vaccine, inactivated	Havrix, Vaqta	Active immunization against hepatitis A virus	Adults: IM 1440 EL units (Havrix) or 50 units (Vaqta) as a single dose; booster dose is the same given at 6, 12 mo; Child 2-18 yr: IM 720 EL units (Havrix) or 25 units (Vaqta) as a single dose, booster dose is the same given at 6, 12 mo	Hypersensitivity to this vaccine or yeast
hepatitis B vaccine, recombinant	Engerix-B, Recombivax HB	Immunization against all subtypes of hepatitis B virus	Varies widely	
influenza virus vaccine, trivalent A and B (whole virus/split virus)	Fluogen, FluShield, Fluviral*, Fluvirin, Fluzone, influenza virus vaccine, trivalent	Prevention of Russian, Chilean, Philippine influenza	Adult/child >12 yr: IM 0.5 ml in 1 dose; Child 3-12 yr: IM 0.5 ml, repeat in 1 mo (split) unless 1978-1985 vaccine was given; Child 6 mo to 3 yr: IM 0.25 ml, repeat in 1 mo (split) unless 1978-1985 vaccine was given	Hypersensitivity, active infection, chicken egg allergy, Guillain-Barré syndrome, active neurologic disorders
Japanese encephalitis virus vaccine, inactivated	JE-VAX	Active immunity against Japanese encephalitis (JE)	Adult/child ≥3 yr: SUBCUT 1 ml, days 0, 7, 30; booster SUBCUT 1 ml 2 yr after last dose; Child 1-3 yr: SUBCUT 0.5 ml, days 0, 7, 30; booster SUBCUT 0.5 ml 2 yr after last dose	Hypersensitivity to murine, thimerosal; allergic reactions to previous dose
Lyme disease vaccine (recombinant OspA)	LYMErix	Immunization against Lyme disease	Adult and adolescent 15-70: IM 30 mcg in deltoid, repeat at 1, 12 mo after first dose	Hypersensitivity, antibiotic refractory Lyme arthritis

*Canada only.

Continued

Appendix e Vaccines and toxoids—cont'd

GENERIC NAME	TRADE NAME	USES	DOSAGE AND ROUTES	CONTRAINDICATIONS
measles and rubella virus vaccine, live attenuated	M-R-Vax II	Immunity to measles and rubella by antibody production	Adult/child ≥15 mo: SUBCUT 0.5 ml (1000 units)	Hypersensitivity, immunocompromised patients, active untreated TB, cancer, blood dyscrasias, radiation, corticosteroids, pregnancy; allergic reactions to neomycin, eggs
measles, mumps, and rubella vaccine, live	M-M-R-II	Prevention of measles, mumps, rubella	Adult: SUBCUT 1 vial; 2 vials separated by 1 mo, in person born after 1957 Child >15 mo and adult: SUBCUT 0.5 ml	Hypersensitivity, blood dyscrasias, anemia, active infection, immunosuppression; egg, chicken allergy; pregnancy, febrile illness, neomycin allergy, neoplasms
measles virus vaccine, live attenuated	Attenuvax	Immunity to measles by antibody production	Adult/child ≥15 mo: SUBCUT 0.5 ml (1000 units), 1 dose 15 mo, 2nd dose age 4-6 or 11, or 12	Hypersensitivity to eggs, neomycin; cancer, radiation, corticosteroids, pregnancy, immunocompromised patients, blood dyscrasias, active untreated TB
meningococcal polysaccharide vaccine	Menomune-A/C/Y/W-135	Prophylaxis to meningococcal meningitis	Adult/child >2 yr: SUBCUT 0.5 ml	Hypersensitivity to thimerosal, pregnancy, acute illness
mumps virus vaccine, live	Mumpsvax	Active immunity to mumps	Adult/child ≥1 yr: SUBCUT 0.5 ml (20,000 units)	Hypersensitivity to eggs, neomycin; cancer, radiation, corticosteroids, pregnancy, immunocompromised patients, blood dyscrasias, active untreated TB
plague vaccine	No trade name	Active immunity to *Yersinia pestis* plague	Adult: IM 1 ml, then 0.2 ml in 4-12 wk, then 0.2 ml 5-6 mo after 2nd dose; booster 0.1-0.2 ml q6mo when in plague area	Hypersensitivity to phenol, sulfites, formaldehyde, beef, soy, casein; pregnancy, coagulation disorders

Vaccine	Trade name	Use	Dosage	Contraindications
pneumococcal 7-valent conjugate vaccine	Prevnar	Immunity against *Streptococcus pneumoniae*	Child: IM 0.5 ml × 3 doses (7-11 mo); × 2 doses (12-23 mo); × 1 dose >2-9 yr	Hypersensitivity to diphtheria toxoid or this product
pneumococcal vaccine, polyvalent	Pneumovax 23, Pnu-Imune 23	Pneumococcal immunization	Adult/child >2 yr: IM/SUBCUT 0.5 ml	Hypersensitivity, Hodgkin's disease, ARDS
poliovirus vaccine, live, oral, trivalent (TOPV) poliovirus vaccine (IPV)	Orimune, IPOL	Prevention of polio	Adult/child >2 yr: PO 0.5 ml, given q8wk × 2 doses, then 0.5 ml ½-1 yr after dose 2 Infant: PO 0.5 ml at 2, 4, 18 mo; booster at 4-6 yr; may also be given: IPV at 2, 4 mo, then TOPV at 12-18 mo, booster at 4-6 yr	Hypersensitivity, active infection, allergy to neomycin/streptomycin, immunosuppression, vomiting, diarrhea
rabies vaccine, adsorbed	No trade name	Active immunity to rabies	**Preexposure** Adult/child: IM 1 ml day 0, 7, 21, or 28 days (total 3 doses); booster IM 1 ml prn q2-5 yr **Postexposure** Adult/child not vaccinated: IM 20 international units/kg of human rabies immune globulin (HRIG), give 5 total doses of 1-ml inj of rabies vaccine on days 0, 3, 7, 14, 28	Severe hypersensitivity to previous inj of vaccine, thimerosol
rabies vaccine, human diploid cell (HDCV)	Imovax Rabies, Imovax Rabies I.D.	Active immunity to rabies	**Preexposure** Adult/child: IM 1 ml day 0, 7, 21 or 28 (total 4 doses) **Postexposure** Adult/child: IM 1 ml on day 0, 3, 7, 14, 28 (total 5 doses)	No contraindications
rubella and mumps virus vaccine, live	Biavax II	Immunity to rubella and mumps by antibody production	Adult/child ≥1 yr: SUBCUT 0.5 ml	Hypersensitivity to eggs, neomycin; cancer, radiation, corticosteroids, pregnancy, immunocompromised patients, blood dyscrasias, active untreated TB

*Canada only.

Continued

Appendix e   Vaccines and toxoids—cont'd

GENERIC NAME	TRADE NAME	USES	DOSAGE AND ROUTES	CONTRAINDICATIONS
rubella virus vaccine, live attenuated (RA 27/3)	Meruvax II	Immunity to rubella by antibody production	Adult/child ≥1 yr: SUBCUT 0.5 ml (1000 units)	Hypersensitivity to eggs, neomycin; cancer, radiation, corticosteroids
tetanus toxoid, adsorbed/tetanus toxoid	No trade name	Tetanus toxoid: Used for prophylactic treatment of wounds	Adult/child: IM 0.5 ml q4-6wk × 2 doses, then 0.5 ml 1 yr after dose 2 (adsorbed); SUBCUT/IM 0.5 ml q4-8wk × 3 doses, then 0.5 ml ½-1 yr after dose 3, booster dose 0.5 ml q10yr	Hypersensitivity, active infection, poliomyelitis outbreak, immunosuppression
typhoid vaccine, parenteral typhoid vaccine, oral	No trade name Vivotif Berna Vaccine	Active immunity to typhoid fever	Adult: PO 1 cap 1 hr before meals × 4 doses, booster q5yr Adult/child >10 yr: SUBCUT 0.5 ml, repeat in 4 wk, booster q3yr Child 6 mo-10 yr: SUBCUT 0.25 ml, repeat in 4 wk, booster q3yr	Parenteral: Systemic or allergic reaction, acute respiratory or other acute infection, intensive physical exercise in high temperatures Oral: Hypersensitivity, acute febrile illness, suppressive or antibiotic drugs
typhoid Vi polysaccharide vaccine	Typhim Vi	Active immunity to typhoid fever	Adult/child ≥2 yr: IM 0.5 ml as a single dose, reimmunize q2yr 0.5 ml IM, if needed	Hypersensitivity, chronic typhoid carriers
varicella virus vaccine	Varivax	Prevention of varicella-zoster (chickenpox)	Adult/child ≥13 yr: SUBCUT 0.5 ml, 2nd dose SUBCUT 0.5 ml 4-8 wk later	Hypersensitivity to neomycin; blood dyscrasias, immunosuppression, active untreated TB, acute illness, pregnancy, diseases of lymphatic system
yellow fever vaccine	YF-Vax	Active immunity to yellow fever	Adult/child ≥9 mo: SUBCUT 0.5 ml deeply, booster q10yr Child 6-9 mo: same as above if exposed	Hypersensitivity to egg or chicken embryo protein, pregnancy, child <6 mo, immunodeficiency

*Canada only.

Appendix f Antitoxins and antivenins

GENERIC NAME	TRADE NAME	USE	DOSAGE AND ROUTES	CONTRAINDICATIONS
Black widow spider antivenin (*Lactrodectus mactans*)	No trade name	Black widow spider bite	Adult/child: IM 2.5 ml, 2nd dose may be given if severe; give in anterolateral thigh, obtain test for sensitivity before inj	Hypersensitivity to this product or horse serum
Crotalidae antivenom, polyvalent	No trade name	Rattlesnake bite	Adult/child: IV 20-150 ml depending on seriousness of bite, may give additional doses based on response	Hypersensitivity
Diphtheria antitoxin, equine	No trade name	Diphtheria	Adult/child: IM/slow IV 20,000-120,000 units, may give additional doses after 24 hr	Hypersensitivity
Micrurus fulvius antivenin	No trade name	East/Texas coral snake bite	Adult/child: IV 30-50 ml, give through running IV line of normal saline, give 1st 1-2 ml over 4-5 min, watch for allergic reaction	Hypersensitivity

Appendix g Less frequently used antihistamines

GENERIC NAME	TRADE NAME(S)	USES	DOSAGES AND ROUTES	AVAILABLE FORMS	INTERACTIONS	CONTRAINDICATIONS
acrivastine/pseudoephedrine (℞)	Semprex-D	• Rhinitis • Allergy symptoms • Chronic idiopathic urticaria	• Adult, child >12 yr: PO 8 mg q4-6h	• Caps 8 mg/60 mg	• Increased CNS depression: alcohol, opiates, sedatives, hypnotics • Hypertensive crisis: MAOIs • May increase CNS depression: kava • May increase anticholinergic effect: henbane leaf	• Hypersensitivity to this drug or triprolidine • Severe hypertension • Cardiac disease
azatadine (℞)	Optimine	• Allergy symptoms • Rhinitis • Chronic urticaria	• Adult: PO 1-2 mg bid, not to exceed 4 mg/day • Geriatric: PO 1 mg daily-bid	• Tabs 1 mg	• Increased CNS depression: barbiturates, opiates, hypnotics, tricyclics, alcohol • Decreased effect of: oral anticoagulants • Increased effect of azatadine: MAOIs • Increased CNS depression: kava • Increased anticholinergic effect: henbane leaf	• Hypersensitivity to H_1-receptor antagonists • Acute asthma attack • Lower respiratory tract disease • Child <12 yr
buclizine (℞)	Bucladin-S, Softabs	• Motion sickness • Dizziness • Nausea • Vomiting • Antihistamine	• Adult: PO 25-50 mg prn ½ hr before travel; may be repeated q4-6h prn	• Tabs 50 mg	• Increased anticholinergic effect: henbane leaf • Increased CNS depression: kava	• Hypersensitivity to cyclizines • Shock

clemastine (B)	Contac Allergy 12 Hour, Tavist, Antihist-1	• Allergy symptoms • Rhinitis • Angioedema • Urticaria • Common cold	• Adult/child >12 yr: PO 1.34-2.68 mg bid-tid, not to exceed 8.04 mg/day	• Tabs 1.34, 2.68 mg • Syr 0.67 mg/ml	• Increased CNS depression: barbiturates, opiates, hypnotics, tricyclics, alcohol • Increased effect of clemastine: MAOIs • Increased CNS depression: kava • Increased anticholinergic effect: henbane leaf	• Hypersensitivity to H_1-receptor antagonists • Acute asthma attack • Lower respiratory tract disease
cyclizine (otc, B)	Marezine	• Motion sickness • Prevention of postoperative vomiting • Antihistamine	*Vomiting* • Adult: IM 25-50 mg ½ hr before termination of surgery, then q4-6h prn (lactate) • Child: IM 3 mg/kg divided in 3 equal doses *Motion sickness* • Adult: PO 50 mg then q4-6h prn, not to exceed 200 mg/day (HCl) • Child: PO 25 mg q4-6h prn	• Tabs 50 mg • Inj 50 mg/ml	• May increase CNS effect: alcohol, tranquilizers, opiates • Increased CNS depression: kava	• Hypersensitivity to cyclizines • Shock
dexchlorpheniramine (B)	Dexchlor, dexchlorpheniramine maleate, Poladex, Polaramine	• Allergy symptoms • Rhinitis • Pruritus • Contact dermatitis	• Adult: PO 1-2 mg tid-qid; repeat action 4-6 mg bid-tid • Child 6-11 yr: PO 1 mg q4-6h, or timerel 4 mg at bedtime	• Tabs 2 mg • Repeat action tabs 4, 6 mg • Syr 2 mg/5 ml	• Increased CNS depression: barbiturates, opiates, hypnotics, tricyclics, alcohol • Decreased effect: oral	• Hypersensitivity to H_1-receptor antagonists • Acute asthma attack • Lower respiratory tract disease

Continued

*Canada only.

Appendix g Less frequently used antihistamines—cont'd

GENERIC NAME	TRADE NAME(S)	USES	DOSAGES AND ROUTES	AVAILABLE FORMS	INTERACTIONS	CONTRAINDICATIONS
					anticoagulants, heparin • Increased effect of dexchlorpheniramine: MAOIs • Increased anticholinergic effect: henbane leaf	
trimeprazine (B)	Panectyl*, Temaril	• Pruritus	• Adult: PO 2.5 mg qid; time-rel 5 mg bid • Geriatric: PO 2.5 mg bid • Child 3-12 yr: PO 2.5 mg tid or at bedtime • Child 6 mo-1 yr: PO 1.25 mg tid or at bedtime	• Tabs 2.5 mg • Time-rel spanules 5 mg • Syr 2.5 mg/5 ml	• Increased CNS depression: barbiturates, opiates, hypnotics, tricyclics, alcohol • Decreased effect of oral anticoagulants, heparin • Increased effect of trimeprazine: MAOIs • Increased anticholinergic effect: henbane leaf	• Hypersensitivity to H_1-receptor antagonists • Acute asthma attack • Lower respiratory tract disease
tripelennamine (B)	PBZ, PBZ-SR, Pelamine, tripelennamine HCl	• Rhinitis • Allergy symptoms	• Adults: PO 25-50 mg q4-6h, not to exceed 600 mg/day; time-rel 100 mg bid-tid, not to exceed 600 mg/day • Child >5 yr: PO time-rel 50 mg q8-12h, not to exceed 300 mg/day • Child <5 yr: PO 5 mg/kg/day in 4-6 divided doses, not to exceed 300 mg/day	• Tabs 25, 50 mg • Time-rel tabs 100 mg • Elix 37.5 mg/5 ml	• Increased CNS depression: barbiturates, opiates, hypnotics, tricyclics, alcohol • Decreased effect of oral anticoagulants, heparin • Increased effect of tripelennamine: MAOIs • Increased anticholinergic effect: henbane leaf	• Hypersensitivity to H_1-receptor antagonists • Acute asthma attack • Lower respiratory tract disease

*Canada only.

Appendix h

Herbal products

acidophilus

Uses: Diarrhea, vaginal and other candida infections, urinary tract infections, atopic dermatitis (eczema), atopic disease, IBS, respiratory tract infections

alfalfa

Uses:
• *External:* Boils and insect bites
• *Internal:* Constipation, arthritis, increase blood clotting, diuretic, relieve inflammation of the prostate, treat acute or chronic cystitis, nutrient source

aloe

Uses of aloe vera gel: Minor burns, skin irritations, minor wounds, frostbite, radiation-caused injuries

angelica

Uses: Poor blood flow to the extremities, headaches, backaches, osteoporosis, asthma, allergies, skin disorders, diuretic, antispasmodic, cholagogue, stomach cancer, mild antiseptic, expectorant, bronchitis, ease rheumatic pains, stomach cramps, muscle spasms

anise

Uses:
• *External:* Treat catarrhs of respiratory system (asthma, bronchitis), cancer, cholera, colic, dysmenorrheal, epilepsy, indigestion, insomnia, lice, migraine, nausea, neuralgia, rash, scabies; given to children to reduce gas, colic, and respiratory symptoms
• *Internal:* Expectorant, bronchitis, emphysema, whooping cough, antibacterial, antispasmodic, abortifacient (large quantities), diaphoretic, diuretic, stimulant, tonic, flavoring in food

astragalus

Uses: Bronchitis, COPD, colds, flu, gastrointestinal conditions, weakness, fatigue, chronic hepatitis, ulcers, hypertension and viral myocarditis, immune stimulant, aphrodisiac, and improve sperm motility

bilberry

Uses: Improve night vision, prevent cataracts, macular degeneration, glaucoma, varicose veins, hemorrhoids, diabetic retinopathy, myopia, mild diarrhea, dyspepsia in adults or children, controlling insulin levels, diuretic, urinary antiseptic

Adapted from Skidmore-Roth L: *Mosby's Handbook of Herbs & Natural Supplements, ed 3*, St. Louis, 2006, Elsevier.

black cohosh

Uses: Smooth-muscle relaxant, antispasmodic, antitussive, astringent, diuretic, antidiarrheal, antiarthritic, hormone balancer in perimenopausal women, decrease uterine spasms in first trimester of pregnancy, antiabortion agent, dysmenorrheal

buckthorn

Uses: Powerful laxative

capsicum peppers

Uses:
- *External:* Diabetic neuropathy, psoriasis, postmastectomy pain, Raynaud's disease, herpes zoster, arthritic, muscular pain, poor peripheral circulation
- *Internal:* Cardiovascular health, CAD, reduce cholesterol and blood clotting, peptic ulcer disease, cold, flu

cascara

Uses: Laxative

chamomile

Uses:
- *External:* As an antiseptic and soothing agent for inflamed skin and minor wounds
- *Internal:* As an antispasmodic, antianxiety, gas-relieving, and antiinflammatory agent for the treatment of digestive problems; light sleep aid and sedative

chondroitin

Uses: Alone or in combination with glucosamine for joint conditions, as an antithrombotic, extravasation therapy agent, for ischemic heart disease, hyperlipidemia

chromium

Uses: Essential trace mineral required for proper metabolic functioning, decreases glucose tolerance, arteriosclerosis, elevated cholesterol, glaucoma, hypoglycemia, diabetes, obesity

coenzyme Q10

Uses: Ischemic heart disease, congestive heart failure (CHF), angina pectoris, hypertension, arrhythmias, diabetes mellitus, deafness, Bell's palsy, decreased immunity, mitral valve prolapse, periodontal disease, infertility

dong quai

Uses: Menopausal symptoms, menstrual irregularities, headache neuralgia, herpes infections, malaria, vitiligo, anemia

echinacea

Uses:
- *External:* Wound healing, bruises, burns, scratches, leg ulcers
- *Internal:* Immune stimulant, prophylaxis for colds, influenzae, other infections

⚠ Safety alert   *"Tall Man" lettering

eyebright

Uses: Internally and externally to relieve eye fatigue, redness, sty and eye infections, nasal catarrh in sinusitis and hay fever

feverfew

Uses: Menstrual irregularities, threatened spontaneous abortion, arthritis, fever

flax

Uses:
• *External*: Inflammatory
• *Internal*: Laxative anticholesteremic

garlic

Uses: Antilipidemic, antimicrobial, antiasthmatic, antiinflammatory, possible antihypertensive, treatment for some heavy metal poisonings

ginger

Uses: Antioxidant, nausea, motion sickness, vomiting, sore throat, migraine headaches

ginkgo

Uses: Poor circulation, age-related decline in cognition, memory; vascular disease, antioxidant, depressive mood disorders, sexual dysfunction, asthma, glaucoma, menopausal symptoms, multiple sclerosis, headaches, tinnitus, dizziness, arthritis, altitude sickness, intermittent claudication

ginseng

Uses: Physical and mental exhaustion, stress, sluggishness, fatigue, weak immunity, as a tonic

goldenseal

Uses: Gastritis, gastrointestinal ulceration, peptic ulcer disease, mouth ulcer, bladder infection, sore throat, postpartum hemorrhage, skin disorders, cancer, tuberculosis, wound healing, antiinflammatory, in combination with echinacea for cold and flu

green tea

Uses: Antioxidant, anticancer agent, diuretic, stimulant, antibacterial, antilipidemic, antiatherosclerotic

hops

Uses: Analgesic, hyperactivity, anthelmintic, mild sedative, insomnia, menopausal symptoms

kava

Uses: Anxiolytic, antiepileptic, antidepressant, antipsychotic, nervous anxiety, hyperactivity, restlessness, sleep disturbances, headache, muscle relaxant, wound healing

khat

Uses: Fatigue, obesity, gastric ulcers, depression

lemon balm

Uses:
• *External:* Cold sores
• *Internal:* Insomnia, anxiety, gastric conditions, psychiatric conditions, Graves' disease, attention deficit disorder (ADD)

licorice

Uses: Allergies, arthritis, asthma, constipation, esophagitis, gastritis, hepatitis, inflammatory conditions, peptic ulcers, poor adrenal function, poor appetite

lysine

Uses: Cold sores, herpes infections, Bell's palsy, rheumatoid arthritis, detoxify opiates

maitake

Uses: Diabetes, hypertension, high cholesterol, obesity, cancer

melatonin

Uses: Insomnia, inhibit cataract formation, increase longevity, epilepsy, hypertension, various cancers, jet lag, cancer protection, oral contraceptive

panax ginseng

Uses: Physical and mental exhaustion, stress, sluggishness, fatigue, weak immunity, as a tonic

papaya

Uses:
• *External:* Debridement of worms
• *Internal:* Intestinal worms, gastrointestinal disorders, injection in a herniated lumbar intervertebral disk

raspberry

Uses:
• *External:* Leaves promote diuresis, treat inflammation, cough, wounds
• *Internal:* UTIs, renal calculi, antimicrobial action, morning sickness and speed, ease labor in pregnancy

red clover

Uses: Antispasmodic, expectorant, sedative, psoriasis, eczema, amenorrhea

St. John's wort

Uses:
• *External:* Antiinflammatory, relieve hemorrhoids, treat vitiligo, burns
• *Internal:* Depression, anxiety

SAM-e

Uses: Depression, Alzheimer's disease, migraine headache, hypersensitivity, chronic liver disease, fibromyalgia pain, inflammation in osteoarthritis

saw palmetto

Uses: Benign prostatic hypertrophy, mild diuretic, chronic and subacute cystitis, increase breast size, sperm count, sexual potency

senna

Uses: Laxative

siberian ginseng

Uses: Increase immunity, energy and performance, decrease inflammation and insomnia

turmeric

Uses: Menstrual disorders, colic, inflammation, bruising, dyspepsia, hematuria, flatulence

valerian

Uses: Sedative

wintergreen

Uses:
• *External:* Sore, inflamed muscles and joints
• *Internal:* Bladder inflammation, urinary tract diseases, diseases of prostate and kidney

yohimbe

Uses: Aphrodisiac, hallucinogenic

Appendix i

Combination products

A-200 Shampoo:
0.33% pyrethrins
4% piperonyl butoxide
Uses: Scabicide, pediculicide

Accuretic 10/12.5:
quinapril 10 mg
hydrochlorthiazide 12.5 mg
Uses: Antihypertensive

Accuretic 20/12.5:
quinapril 20 mg
hydrochlorthiazide 12.5 mg
Uses: Antihypertensive

Accuretic 20/25:
quinapril 20 mg
hydrochlorthiazide 25 mg
Uses: Antihypertensive

Aceta w/Codeine:
acetaminophen 300 mg
codeine 30 mg
Uses: Opioid analgesic

Acid-X:
acetaminophen 500 mg
calcium carbonate 250 mg
Uses: Analgesic, antacid

Actagen C Cough Syrup:
Per 5 ml:
triprolidine 1.25 mg
pseudoephedrine 30 mg
codeine 10 mg
Uses: Antihistamine, adrenergic, antitussive

Actifed:
pseudoephedrine 60 mg
triprolidine 2.5 mg
Uses: Decongestant

Actifed Allergy, Daytime:
pseudoephedrine 30 mg
Uses: Adrenergic

Actifed Allergy, Nighttime:
pseudoephedrine 30 mg
diphenhydrAMINE 25 mg
Uses: Decongestant, antihistamine

Actifed with Codeine:
pseudoephedrine 30 mg
triprolidine 1.25 mg
codeine 10 mg
Uses: Adrenergic, antihistamine, antitussive

Actifed with Codeine Cough Syrup:
Per 3 ml:
pseudoephedrine 30 mg
triprolidine 1.25 mg
codeine 10 mg
Uses: Adrenergic, antihistamine, antitussive

Actifed Cold and Allergy:
pseudoephedrine 60 mg
triprolidine 2.5 mg
Uses: Adrenergic, antihistamine

Actifed Cold and Sinus:
chlorpheniramine 2 mg
pseudoephedrine 30 mg
acetaminophen 500 mg
Uses: antihistamine, adrenergic, analgesic

Actifed Plus:
pseudoephedrine 30 mg
triprolidine 1.25 mg
acetaminophen 500 mg
Uses: Decongestant, antihistamine

Actifed Plus ES Caplets:
pseudoephedrine 60 mg
triprolidine 2.5 mg
acetaminophen 500 mg
Uses: Adrenergic, antihistamine, analgesic

Actifed Sinus Daytime:
pseudoephedrine 30 mg
acetaminophen 500 mg
Uses: Decongestant

Actifed Sinus Nighttime:
pseudoephedrine 30 mg
diphenhydrAMINE 25 mg
acetaminophen 500 mg
Uses: Decongestant, antihistamine

Actifed Syrup:
Per 5 ml:
triprolidine 1.25 mg
pseudoephedrine 30 mg
Uses: Antihistamine, adrenergic

Activella Tablets:
estriol 1 mg
norethindrone 0.5 mg
Uses: Menopause

Adderall 5 mg:
dextroamphetamine sulfate 1.25 mg
dextroamphetamine saccharate 1.25 mg
amphetamine sulfate 1.25 mg
amphetamine aspartate 1.25 mg
Uses: CNS stimulant

Adderall 10 mg:
dextroamphetamine sulfate 5 mg
dextroamphetamine saccharate 2.5 mg
amphetamine sulfate 2.5 mg
amphetamine aspartate 2.5 mg
Uses: CNS stimulant

Adderall 20 mg:
dextroamphetamine sulfate 5 mg
dextroamphetamine saccharate 5 mg
amphetamine sulfate 5 mg
amphetamine aspartate 5 mg
Uses: CNS stimulant

Adderall 30 mg:
dextroamphetamine sulfate 7.5 mg
dextroamphetamine saccharate 7.5 mg
amphetamine sulfate 7.5 mg
amphetamine aspartate 7.5 mg
Uses: CNS stimulant

Adderall XR 10 mg:
dextroamphetamine sulfate 2.5 mg
dextroamphetamine saccharate 2.5 mg
amphetamine sulfate 2.5 mg
amphetamine aspartate 2.5 mg
Uses: CNS stimulant

Adderall XR 20 mg:
dextroamphetamine sulfate 5 mg
dextroamphetamine saccharate 5 mg
amphetamine sulfate 5 mg
amphetamine aspartate 5 mg
Uses: CNS stimulant

Adderall XR 30 mg:
dextroamphetamine sulfate 7.5 mg
dextroamphetamine saccharate 7.5 mg
amphetamine sulfate 7.5 mg
amphetamine aspartate 7.5 mg
Uses: CNS stimulant

Advair Diskus 100:
fluticasone 100 mcg
salmeterol 50 mcg
Uses: Corticosteroid, bronchodilator

Advair Diskus 250:
fluticasone 250 mcg
salmeterol 50 mcg
Uses: Corticosteroid, bronchodilator

Advair Diskus 500:
fluticasone 500 mcg
salmeterol 50 mcg
Uses: Corticosteroid, bronchodilator

Advicor 500:
niacin 500 mg
lovastatin 20 mg
Uses: Antilipidemic

Advicor 750:
niacin 750 mg
lovastatin 20 mg
Uses: Antilipidemic

Advicor 1000:
niacin 1000 mg
lovastatin 20 mg
Uses: Antilipidemic

Advil Cold & Sinus Caplets:
pseudoephedrine 30 mg
ibuprofen 200 mg
Uses: Decongestant

Aggrenox:
200 mg ext rel dipyridamole
25 mg aspirin
Uses: Antiplatelet

**AK-Cide Ophthalmic Suspension/
  Ointment:**
10% sulfacetamide sodium
0.5% prednisoLONE acetate

✤ Canada only   Side effects: *italics* = common; ***bold italics*** = life-threatening

Uses: Ophthalmic antiinfective,
antiinflammatory

Aldactazide 25/25:
spironolactone 25 mg
hydrochlorothiazide 25 mg
Uses: Diuretic

Aldactazide 50/50:
spironolactone 50 mg
hydrochlorothiazide 50 mg
Uses: Diuretic

Aldoclor-150:
methyldopa 250 mg
chlorothiazide 150 mg
Uses: Antihypertensive

Aldoclor-250:
methyldopa 250 mg
chlorothiazide 250 mg
Uses: Antihypertensive

Aldori 15:
methyldopa 250 mg
hydrochlorothiazide 15 mg
Uses: Antihypertensive

Aldoril 25:
methyldopa 250 mg
hydrochlorothiazide 25 mg
Uses: Antihypertensive

Aldoril D30
hydrochlorothiazide 30 mg
methyldopa 500 mg
Uses: Antihypertensive

Aldoril D50:
hydrochlorothiazide 50 mg
methyldopa 500 mg
Uses: Antihypertensive

Aleve Cold & Sinus:
naproxen 200 mg
ER pseudoephedrine 120 mg
Uses: Analgesic, adrenergic

Alka-Seltzer Cold:
sodium bicarbonate 958 mg
citric acid 832 mg
potassium bicarbonate 312 mg
Uses: Antacid, adsorbent

Alka-Seltzer Effervescent, Original:
sodium bicarbonate 1916 mg

citric acid 1000 mg
aspirin 325 mg
Uses: Antacid, adsorbent, antiflatulent

Alka-Seltzer Plus Cold & Cough Effervescent Tablets:
dextromethorphan 10 mg
chlorpheniramine 2 mg
phenylephrine 5 mg
Uses: Antitussive, antihistamine, decongestant

Alka-Seltzer Plus Cold & Flu Liqui-Gels:
dextromethorphan 10 mg
pseudoephedrine 30 mg
acetaminophen 325 mg
Uses: Antitussive, decongestant, analgesic

Alka-Seltzer Plus Cold Liqui-Gels:
pseudoephedrine 30 mg
chlorpheniramine 2 mg
acetaminophen 250 mg
Uses: Decongestant, antihistamine

Alka-Seltzer Plus Flu Liqui-Gels
dextromethorphan 10 mg
pseudoephedrine 30 mg
acetaminophen 325 mg
Uses: Antitussive, decongestant, analgesic

Alka-Seltzer Plus Night-Time Cold Effervescent Tablets:
dextromethorphan 10 mg
doxylamine 6.25 mg
phenylephrine 5 mg
Uses: Antitussive, antihistamine, decongestant

Alka-Seltzer Plus Night-Time Cold Liqui-Gels:
doxylamine 6.25 mg
dextromethorphan 10 mg
pseudoephedrine 30 mg
acetaminophen 325 mg
Uses: Antitussive, decongestant, antihistamine, analgesic

Allegra-D:
fexofenadine 60 mg
pseudoephedrine 120 mg
Uses: Antihistamine, adrenergic

Allercon Tablets:
triprolidine 2.5 mg
pseudoephedrine 60 mg
Uses: Antihistamine, adrenergic

Allerest Headache Strength Advanced Formula:
pseudoephedrine 30 mg
chlorpheniramine 2 mg
acetaminophen 325 mg
Uses: Decongestant, antihistamine

Allerest Maximum Strength Tablets:
pseudoephedrine 30 mg
chlorpheniramine 2 mg
Uses: Decongestant, antihistamine

Allerest No-Drowsiness:
pseudoephedrine 30 mg
acetaminophen 325 mg
Uses: Decongestant, analgesic

Allerest Sinus Pain Formula:
pseudoephedrine 30 mg
chlorpheniramine 2 mg
acetaminophen 500 mg
Uses: Decongestant, antihistamine, analgesic

Allerfrim Syrup:
Per 5 ml:
triprolidine 1.25 mg
pseudoephedrine 30 mg
Uses: Antihistamine, adrenergic

Allerfrim Tablets:
triprolidine 2.5 mg
pseudoephedrine 60 mg
Uses: Antihistamine, adrenergic

All-Nite Cold Formula Liquid:
Per 5 ml:
pseudoephedrine 10 mg
doxylamine 1.25 mg
dextromethorphan 5 mg
acetaminophen 167 mg
Uses: Decongestant, antihistamine, analgesic

Alor 5/500:
hydrocodone 5 mg
aspirin 500 mg
Uses: Analgesic

Amaphen:
acetaminophen 325 mg
butalbital 50 mg
caffeine 40 mg
Uses: Analgesic, barbiturates

Ambenyl Cough Syrup:
Per 5 ml:
bromodiphenhydramine 12.5 mg
codeine 10 mg
5% alcohol
Uses: Antihistamine, opioid analgesic

Anacin:
aspirin 400 mg
caffeine 32 mg
Uses: Analgesic

Anacin Maximum Strength:
aspirin 500 mg
caffeine 32 mg
Uses: Analgesic

Anacin PM (Aspirin Free):
diphenhydrAMINE 25 mg
acetaminophen 500 mg
Uses: Analgesic

Anacin w/Codeine:
aspirin 325 mg
codeine 8 mg
caffeine 32 mg
Uses: Opioid analgesic

Anaplex HD Syrup:
Per 5 ml:
hydrocodone 1.7 mg
phenylephrine 5 mg
chlorpheniramine 2 mg
Uses: Analgesic, adrenergic, antihistamine

Anaplex Liquid:
Per 5 ml:
chlorpheniramine 2 mg
pseudoephedrine 30 mg
Uses: Antihistamine, decongestant

Anatuss LA:
pseudoephedrine 120 mg
guaifenesin 400 mg
Uses: Adrenergic, expectorant

Anexsia 5/500:
hydrocodone 5 mg
acetaminophen 500 mg

Uses: Analgesic

Anexsia 7.5/650:

hydrocodone 7.5 mg

acetaminophen 650 mg

Uses: Analgesic

Apresazide 25/25:

hydrALAZINE 25 mg

hydrochlorothiazide 25 mg

Uses: Antihypertensive

Apresazide 50/50:

hydrALAZINE 50 mg

hydrochlorothiazide 50 mg

Uses: Antihypertensive

Apri:

desorgestrel 0.15 mg

ethinyl estradiol 30 mcg

Uses: Estrogen, progestin

Arthritis Pain Formula:

aspirin 500 mg

aluminum hydroxide 27 mg

magnesium hydroxide 100 mg

Uses: Analgesic, antacid

Arthrotec:

diclofenac 50 or 75 mg

misoprostol 200 mcg

Uses: NSAID, gastric protectant

Ascriptin:

aspirin 325 mg

magnesium hydroxide 50 mg

aluminum hydroxide 50 mg

calcium carbonate 50 mg

Uses: Nonopioid analgesic, antipyretic

Ascriptin A/D:

aspirin 325 mg

aluminum hydroxide 75 mg

magnesium hydroxide 75 mg

calcium carbonate 75 mg

Uses: Analgesic

Aspirin-Free Bayer Select Allergy Sinus:

pseudoephedrine 30 mg

chlorpheniramine 2 mg

acetaminophen 500 mg

Uses: Adrenergic, antihistamine, analgesic

Aspirin Free Excedrin:

acetaminophen 500 mg

caffeine 65 mg

Uses: Analgesic

Aspirin Free Excedrin Dual:

acetaminophen 500 mg

calcium carbonate 111 mg

magnesium carbonate 64 mg

magnesium oxide 30 mg

Uses: Analgesic, antacid

Atacand HCT 16:

candesartan 16 mg

hydrochlorthiazide 12.5 mg

Uses: Antihypertensive

Atacand HCT 32:

candesartan 32 mg

hydrochlorthiazide 12.5 mg

Uses: Antihypertensive

Augmentin 250:

amoxicillin 250 mg

clavulanic acid 125 mg

Uses: Antiinfective

Augmentin 500:

amoxicillin 500 mg

clavulanic acid 125 mg

Uses: Antiinfective

Augmentin 875:

amoxicillin 875 mg

clavulanic acid 125 mg

Uses: Antiinfective

Augmentin 125 Chewable:

amoxicillin 125 mg

clavulanic acid 31.25 mg

Uses: Antiinfective

Augmentin 200 Chewable:

amoxicillin 200 mg

clavulanic acid 28.5 mg

Uses: Antiinfective

Augmentin 250 Chewable:

amoxicillin 250 mg

clavulanic acid 62.5 mg

Uses: Antiinfective

Augmentin 400 Chewable:

amoxicillin 400 mg

clavulanic acid 57 mg

Uses: Antiinfective

Augmentin 125 mg/5 ml Suspension:
Per 5 ml:
amoxicillin 125 mg
clavulanic acid 31.25 mg
Uses: Antiinfective
Augmentin 200 mg/5 ml Suspension:
Per 5 ml:
amoxicillin 200 mg
clavulanic acid 28.5 mg
Uses: Antiinfective
Augmentin 250 mg/5 ml Suspension:
Per 5 ml:
amoxicillin 250 mg
clavulanic acid 62.5 mg
Uses: Antiinfective
Augmentin 400 mg/5 ml Suspension:
Per 5 ml:
amoxicillin 400 mg
clavulanic acid 57 mg
Uses: Antiinfective
Auralgan Otic Solution:
5.4% antipyrine
1.4% benzocaine
Uses: Otic analgesic
Avalide:
hydrochlorthiazide 12.5 mg
irbesartan 150 mg
Uses: Antihypertensive
Avalide 300:
hydrochlorthiazide 12.5 mg
irbesartan 300 mg
Uses: Antihypertensive
Avandamet:
rosiglitazone/metformin
1 mg/500 mg
2 mg/500 mg
2 mg/1000 mg
4 mg/500 mg
4 mg/1000 mg
Uses: Diabetes mellitus
Azo-Gantanol:
sulfamethoxazole 500 mg
phenazopyridine 100 mg
Uses: Sulfonamide
Azo-Gantrisin:
sulfiSOXAZOLE 500 mg

phenazopyridine 50 mg
Uses: Sulfonamide
Azo-Sulfamethoxazole:
sulfamethoxazole 500 mg
phenazopyridine 100 mg
Uses: Sulfonamide
Azo-SulfiSOXAZOLE:
sulfiSOXAZOLE 500 mg
phenazopyridine 50 mg
Uses: Sulfonamide
B&O Supprettes No. 15A Supps:
belladonna extract 15 mg
opium 30 mg
Uses: Anticholinergic, opioid analgesic
B&O Supprettes No. 16A Supps:
belladonna extract 16.2 mg
opium 60 mg
Uses: Anticholinergic, opioid analgesic
Bactrim:
trimethoprim 80 mg
sulfamethoxazole 400 mg
Uses: Antiinfective
Bactrim DS:
trimethoprim 160 mg
sulfamethoxazole 800 mg
Uses: Antiinfective
Bactrim I.V.:
Per 5 ml:
trimethoprim 80 mg
sulfamethoxazole 400 mg
Uses: Antiinfective
Bancap HC:
acetaminophen 500 mg
hydrocodone 5 mg
Uses: Analgesic
Bayer Plus, Extra Strength:
aspirin 500 mg
calcium carbonate 250 mg
Uses: Analgesic, antacid
Bayer Select Chest Cold:
dextromethorphan 15 mg
acetaminophen 500 mg
Uses: Antitussive, analgesic
Bayer Select Flu Relief:
acetaminophen 500 mg
pseudoephedrine 30 mg

dextromethorphan 15 mg

chlorpheniramine 2 mg

Uses: Analgesic, adrenergic, antitussive, antihistamine

Bayer Select Head Cold:

pseudoephedrine 30 mg

acetaminophen 500 mg

Uses: Adrenergic, analgesic

Bayer Select Maximum Strength Headache:

acetaminophen 500 mg

caffeine 65 mg

Uses: Nonopioid analgesic

Bayer Select Maximum Strength Menstrual:

acetaminophen 500 mg

pamabrom 25 mg

Uses: Nonopioid analgesic

Bayer Select Maximum Strength Night-Time Pain Relief:

acetaminophen 500 mg

diphenhydrAMINE 25 mg

Uses: Analgesic, antihistamine

Bayer Select Maximum Strength Sinus Pain Relief:

acetaminophen 500 mg

pseudoephedrine 30 mg

Uses: Analgesic, adrenergic

Bayer Select Night Time Cold:

acetaminophen 500 mg

pseudoephedrine 30 mg

dextromethorphan 15 mg

triprolidine 1.25 mg

Uses: Analgesic, adrenergic, antitussive, antihistamine

Bellatal:

phenobarbital 16.2 mg

hyoscyamine sulfate 0.1037 mg

atropine sulfate 0.0194 mg

scopolamine hydrobromide 0.0065 mg

Uses: Barbiturate, anticholinergic

Bellergal-S:

ergotamine 0.6 mg

belladonna alkaloids 0.2 mg

phenobarbital 40 mg

Uses: α-Adrenergic blocker, anticholinergic, barbiturate

Bel-Phen-Ergot-SR:

phenobarbital 40 mg

ergotamine tartrate 0.6 mg

belladonna alkaloids 0.2 mg

Uses: α-Adrenergic blocker, anticholinergic, barbiturate

Benadryl Allergy Decongestant Liquid:

Per 5 ml:

diphenhydrAMINE 12.5 mg

pseudoephedrine 30 mg

Uses: Antihistamine, adrenergic

Benadryl Allergy/Sinus Headache Caplets:

diphenhydrAMINE 12.5 mg

pseudoephedrine 30 mg

acetaminophen 500 mg

Uses: Antihistamine, adrenergic, analgesic

Benadryl Decongestant Allergy:

pseudoephedrine 60 mg

diphenhydrAMINE 25 mg

Uses: Adrenergic, antihistamine

Benylin Expectorant Liquid:

Per 5 ml:

dextromethorphan 5 mg

guaifenesin 100 mg

5% alcohol

Uses: Expectorant, antitussive

Benylin Multi-Symptom Liquid:

Per 5 ml:

dextromethorphan 5 mg

pseudoephedrine 15 mg

guaifenesin 100 mg

Uses: Antitussive, adrenergic, expectorant

Benzamycin:

benzoyl peroxide 5%

erythromycin 3%

Uses: Antiinfective

BenzaClin:

clindamycin 10%

benzoyl peroxide 5%

Uses: Antiinfective

A Safety alert   *"Tall Man" lettering

BiDil:
isosorbide 20 mg
hydrALAZINE 37.5 mg
Uses: Vasodilator

Blephamide Ophthalmic Suspension/ Ointment:
0.2% prednisoLONE
10% sodium sulfacetamide
Uses: Ophthalmic antiinfective, antiinflammatory

Bromfed Capsules:
pseudoephedrine 120 mg
brompheniramine 12 mg
Uses: Antihistamine, adrenergic

Bromfed-PD Capsules:
pseudoephedrine 60 mg
brompheniramine 6 mg
Uses: Adrenergic, antihistamine

Bromfed Tablets:
pseudoephedrine 60 mg
brompheniramine 4 mg
Uses: Antihistamine, adrenergic

Bromfenex:
brompheniramine 12 mg
pseudoephedrine 120 mg
Uses: Antihistamine, adrenergic

Bromfenex PD:
brompheniramine 6 mg
pseudoephedrine 60 mg
Uses: Antihistamine, adrenergic

Bromo-Seltzer:
sodium bicarbonate 2781 mg
acetaminophen 325 mg
citric acid 2224 mg
Uses: Antacid, analgesic

Bufferin:
aspirin 325 mg
calcium carbonate 158 mg
magnesium oxide 63 mg
magnesium carbonate 34 mg
Uses: Analgesic, antacid

Bufferin AF Nite-Time:
acetaminophen 500 mg
diphenhydrAMINE 38 mg
Uses: Analgesic, antihistamine

Butibel:
belladonna extract 15 mg
butabarbital 15 mg
Uses: Anticholinergic, barbiturate

Caduet:
amlodipine 5 mg
atorvastatin 10, 20, 40, 80 mg
amlodipine 10 mg
atorvastatin 10, 20, 40, 80 mg
Uses: Antihyperlipidemic/antihypertension

Cafatine PB:
ergotamine 1 mg
caffeine 100 mg
belladonna alkaloids 0.125 mg
pentobarbital 30 mg
Uses: Migraine agent

Cafergot:
ergotamine 1 mg
caffeine 100 mg
Uses: Adrenergic blocker

Cafergot Suppositories:
ergotamine 2 mg
caffeine 100 mg
Uses: Adrenergic blocker

Caladryl:
8% calamine, camphor
2.2% alcohol
1% pramoxine
Uses: Top antihistamine

Calcet:
calcium 152.8 mg
vitamin D 100 international units
Uses: Supplement

Caltrate 600+D:
vitamin D 200 international units
calcium 600 mg
Uses: Supplement

Cama Arthritis Pain Reliever:
aspirin 500 mg
magnesium oxide 150 mg
aluminum hydroxide 125 mg
Uses: Nonopioid analgesic, antacid

Capital w/Codeine:
Per 5 ml:
acetaminophen 120 mg
codeine 12 mg

Uses: Opioid analgesic
Capozide 25/15:
captopril 25 mg
hydrochlorothiazide 15 mg
Uses: Antihypertensive
Capozide 25/25:
captopril 25 mg
hydrochorothiazide 25 mg
Uses: Antihypertensive
Capozide 50/15:
captopril 50 mg
hydrochlorothiazide 15 mg
Uses: Antihypertensive
Capozide 50/25:
captopril 50 mg
hydrochlorothiazide 25 mg
Uses: Antihypertensive
Cardec DM Syrup:
Per 5 ml:
pseudoephedrine 60 mg
carbinoxamine 4 mg
dextromethorphan 15 mg
Uses: Adrenergic, antitussive
Cenafed Plus Tablets:
triprolidine 2.5 mg
pseudoephedrine 60 mg
Uses: Antihistamine, adrenergic
Cetapred Ophthalmic Ointment:
0.25% prednisoLONE
10% sodium sulfacetamide
Uses: Ophthalmic antiinfective,
    antiinflammatory
Cheracol D Cough Formula Syrup:
dextromethorphan 10 mg
guaifenesin 100 mg
Uses: Antitussive, expectorant
Cheracol Syrup:
Per 5 ml:
codeine 10 mg
guaifenesin 100 mg
Uses: Analgesic, expectorant
Children's Cepacol Liquid:
Per 5 ml:
acetaminophen 160 mg
pseudoephedrine 15 mg
Uses: Analgesic, adrenergic

**Chlor-Trimeton Allergy 4 Hour
    Decongestant:**
pseudoephedrine 60 mg
chlorpheniramine 4 mg
Uses: Antihistamine, adrenergic
**Chlor-Trimeton 12 Hour Relief
    Tablets:**
pseudoephedrine 120 mg
chlorpheniramine 8 mg
Uses: Antihistamine, adrenergic
Chromagen:
ferrous fumarate 66 mg
vitamin B_{12} 10 mcg
vitamin C 250 mg
intrinsic factor 100 mg
Uses: Supplement
Cipro HC Otic:
Per 1 ml:
ciprofloxacin 2 mg
hydrocortisone 10 mg
Uses: Antiinfective/antiinflammatory
Claritin-D 12 Hour:
loratidine 5 mg
pseudoephedrine 120 mg
Uses: Antihistamine, adrenergic
Claritin-D 24-Hour:
loratidine 10 mg
pseudoephedrine 240 mg
Uses: Antihistamine, adrenergic
Clindex:
chlordiazepoxide 5 mg
clidinium 2.5 mg
Uses: Antianxiety, anticholinergic
Clomycin Ointment:
bacitracin 500 units
neomycin sulfate 3.5 g
polymyxin B sulfate 500 units
lidocaine 40 mg
Uses: Antiinfective, local anesthetic
Co-Apap:
pseudoephedrine 30 mg
chlorpheniramine 2 mg
dextromethorphan 15 mg
acetaminophen 325 mg
Uses: Adrenergic, antihistamine, antitussive,
    analgesic

A Safety alert   *"Tall Man" lettering

Co-Gesic:
acetaminophen 500 mg
hydrocodone 5 mg
Uses: Analgesic
Codeprex:
Codeine:
Chlorpheniramine:
Uses: Cough, rhinitis
Codiclear DH Syrup:
Per 5 ml:
hydrocodone 5 mg
guaifenesin 100 mg
Uses: Analgesic, expectorant
Codimal:
pseudoephedrine 30 mg
chlorpheniramine 2 mg
acetaminophen 500 mg
Uses: Adrenergic, antihistamine, analgesic
Codimal DH Syrup:
Per 5 ml:
hydrocodone 1.66 mg
phenylephrine 5 mg
pyrilamine 8.33 mg
Uses: Analgesic, adrenergic
Codimal DM Syrup:
Per 5 ml:
phenylephrine 5 mg
pyrilamine 8.33 mg
dextromethorphan 10 mg
Uses: Adrenergic, antitussive
Codimal-LA:
chlorpheniramine 8 mg
pseudoephedrine 120 mg
Uses: Antihistamine, adrenergic
Codimal PH Syrup:
Per 5 ml:
codeine 10 mg
phenylephrine 5 mg
pyrilamine 8.33 mg
Uses: Analgesic, adrenergic
Col-Probenecid:
probenecid 500 mg
colchicine 0.5 mg
Uses: Antigout agent
ColBenemid:
probenecid 500 mg

colchicine 0.5 mg
Uses: Antigout agent
Coldrine:
pseudoephedrine 30 mg
acetaminophen 500 mg
Uses: Decongestant, nonopioid analgesic
Col-Probenecid:
probenecid 500 mg
colchicine 0.5 mg
Uses: Antigout
Coly-Mycin S Otic Suspension:
1% hydrocortisone
neomycin base 3.3 mg/ml
colistin 3 mg/ml
0.05% thonzonium bromide
Uses: Otic antiinfective
CombiPatch 0.05/0.14:
estradiol 0.05 mg/day
norethindrone 0.14 mg/day
Uses: Estrogen, progestin
CombiPatch 0.05/0.25:
estradiol 0.05 mg/day
norethindrone 0.25 mg/day
Uses: Estrogen, progestin
Combipres 0.1:
chlorthalidone 15 mg
clonidine 0.1 mg
Uses: Antihypertensive
Combipres 0.2:
chlorthalidone 15 mg
clonidine 0.2 mg
Uses: Antihypertensive
Combipres 0.3:
chlorthalidone 15 mg
clonidine 0.3 mg
Uses: Antihypertensive
Combisor:
mometasone 0.1%
salicylic acid 5%
Uses: Corticosteroid
Combivent:
ipratropium bromide 18 mcg
albuterol 103 mcg/actuation
Uses: Bronchodilator
Combivir:
lamivudine 150 mg

Side effects: *italics* = common; ***bold italics*** = life-threatening

zidovudine 300 mg
Uses: Antiviral
Comtrex Allergy-Sinus:
chlorpheniramine 2 mg
acetaminophen 500 mg
pseudoephedrine 30 mg
Uses: Antihistamine, analgesic, decongestant
Comtrex Liquid:
Per 5 ml:
chlorpheniramine 0.67 mg
acetaminophen 108.3 mg
dextromethorphan 3.3 mg
pseudoephedrine 10 mg
Uses: Antihistamine, analgesic, antitussive, decongestant
Comtrex Maximum Strength
Caplets:
acetaminophen 500 mg
pseudoephedrine 30 mg
chlorpheniramine 2 mg
dextromethorphan 15 mg
Uses: Analgesic, decongestant, antihistamine, antitussive
Comtrex Maximum Strength Multi-Symptoms Cold, Flu Relief:
pseudoephedrine 30 mg
dextromethorphan 15 mg
chlorpheniramine 2 mg
acetaminophen 500 mg
Uses: Analgesic, decongestant, antihistamine, antitussive
Comtrex Maximum Strength Non-Drowsy Caplets:
acetaminophen 500 mg
pseudoephedrine 30 mg
dextromethorphan 15 mg
Uses: Analagesic, decongestant, antitussive
Congess SR:
guaifenesin 250 mg
pseudoephedrine 120 mg
Uses: Expectorant, decongestant
Congestac:
guaifenesin 400 mg
pseudoephedrine 60 mg
Uses: Expectorant, decongestant

Contac Cough & Chest Cold Liquid:
Per 5 ml:
pseudoephedrine 15 mg
dextromethorphan 5 mg
guaifenesin 50 mg
acetaminophen 125 mg
Uses: Decongestant, antitussive, expectorant, analgesic
Contac Cough & Sore Throat Liquid:
Per 5 ml:
dextromethorphan 5 mg
acetaminophen 125 mg
Uses: Antitussive, analgesic
Contac Day Allergy/Sinus:
pseudoephedrine 60 mg
acetaminophen 650 mg
Uses: Decongestant, analgesic
Contac Day Cold and Flu:
pseudoephedrine 60 mg
dextromethorphan 30 mg
acetaminophen 650 mg
Uses: Decongestant, antitussive, analgesic
Contac Night Allergy Sinus:
pseudoephedrine 60 mg
diphenhydrAMINE 50 mg
acetaminophen 650 mg
Uses: Decongestant, antihistamine, analgesic
Contac Night Cold and Flu Caplets:
pseudoephedrine 60 mg
diphenhydrAMINE 50 mg
acetaminophen 650 mg
Uses: Decongestant, antihistamine, antitussive, analgesic
Contac Non-Drowsy Maximum Strength 12 Hour:
pseudoephedrine 120 mg
Uses: Adrenergic
Contac Severe Cold & Flu Nighttime Liquid:
Per 5 ml:
pseudoephedrine 10 mg
chlorpheniramine 0.67 mg
dextromethorphan 5 mg

⚠ Safety alert   *"Tall Man" lettering

acetaminophen 167 mg
18.5% alcohol
Uses: Decongestant, antihistamine,
antitussive, analgesic

Coricidin:
chlorpheniramine 2 mg
acetaminophen 325 mg
Uses: Antihistamine, analgesic

Coricidin D Tablets:
chlorpheniramine 2 mg
acetaminophen 325 mg
Uses: Antihistamine, analgesic

Coricidin D Cold, Flu & Sinus:
chlorpheniramine 2 mg
acetaminophen 325 mg
pseudoephedrine sulfate 30 mg
Uses: Antihistamine, analgesic,
decongestant

**Coricidin HBP Congestion & Cough
Softgels Capsules:**
dextromethorphan 10 mg
guaifenesin 200 mg
Uses: Antitussive, expectorant

Corcidin HBP Cough and Cold:
chlorpheniramine 4 mg
dextromethorphan 30 mg
Uses: Antihistamine, expectorant

Corcidin HBP Maximum Strength Flu:
acetaminophen 500 mg
chlorpheniramine 2 mg
dextromethorphan 15 mg
Uses: Analgesic, antihistamine, expectorant

**Cortisporin Ophthalmic/Otic
Suspension:**
0.35% neomycin polymyxin B 10,000
units/ml
1% hydrocortisone
Uses: Ophthalmic antiinfective,
antiinflammatory

Cortisporin Ophthalmic Ointment:
0.35% neomycin base
bacitracin 400 units
polymyxin B 10,000 units
1% hydrocortisone
Uses: Ophthalmic antiinfective

Cortisporin Topical Cream:
0.5% neomycin sulfate
polymyxin B 10,000 units
0.5% hydrocortisone
Uses: Topical antiinfective

Cortisporin Topical Ointment:
0.5% neomycin sulfate
bacitracin 400 units
polymyxin B 5000 units
1% hydrocortisone
Uses: Topical antiinfective

Corzide 40/5:
nadolol 40 mg
bendroflumethiazide 5 mg
Uses: Antihypertensive

Corzide 80/5:
nadolol 80 mg
bendroflumethiazide 5 mg
Uses: Antihypertensive

Cosopt:
dorzolamide 2%
timolol 0.5%
Uses: Antihypertensive

Cough-X:
dextromethorphan 5 mg
benzocaine 2 mg
Uses: Antitussive, local anesthetic

Creon:
lipase 8000 units
amylase 30,000 units
protease 13,000 units
pancreatin 300 mg
Uses: Digestive enzyme

Cyclomydril Ophthalmic Solution:
0.2% cyclopentolate
1% phenylephrine
Uses: Mydriatic

Dallergy Caplets:
chlorpheniramine 8 mg
phenylephrine 20 mg
methscopolamine 2.5 mg
Uses: Antihistamine, adrenergic

Dallergy Syrup:
Per 5 ml:
chlorpheniramine 2 mg
phenylephrine 10 mg

methscopolamine 0.625 mg
Uses: Antihistamine, adrenergic
Dallergy Tablets:
chlorpheniramine 4 mg
phenylephrine 10 mg
methscopolamine 1.25 mg
Uses: Antihistamine, adrenergic
Dallergy-D Syrup:
Per 5 ml:
phenylephrine 5 mg
chlorpheniramine 2 mg
Uses: Antihistamine, adrenergic
Damason-P:
hydrocodone 5 mg
aspirin 500 mg
Uses: Analgesic
Darvocet-N 100:
propoxyphene-N 100 mg
acetaminophen 650 mg
Uses: Analgesic
Darvon Compound-65:
propoxyphene 65 mg
aspirin 389 mg
caffeine 32.4 mg
Uses: Analgesic
♣ **Darvon-N Compound:**
aspirin 375 mg
propoxyphene 100 mg
caffeine 30 mg
Uses: Analgesic
♣ **Darvon-N w/A.S.A.:**
aspirin 325 mg
propoxyphene 100 mg
Uses: Analgesic
Deconamine:
pseudoephedrine 60 mg
chlorpheniramine 4 mg
Uses: Antihistamine, decongestant
Deconamine CX:
hydrocodone 5 mg
pseudoephedrine 30 mg
guaifenesin 300 mg
Uses: Analgesic, decongestant, expectorant
Deconamine SR:
pseudoephedrine 120 mg
chlorpheniramine 8 mg

Uses: Antihistamine, decongestant
Deconamine Syrup:
Per 5 ml:
pseudoephedrine 30 mg
chlorpheniramine 2 mg
Uses: Antihistamine, decongestant
Defen-LA:
pseudoephedrine 60 mg
guaifenesin 600 mg
Uses: Decongestant, expectorant
Demi-Regroton:
chlorthalidone 25 mg
reserpine 0.125 mg
Uses: Antihypertensive
Demulen 1/35:
ethinyl estradiol 35 mcg
ethynodiol diacetate 1 mg
Uses: Oral contraceptive
Demulen 1/50:
ethinyl estradiol 50 mcg
ethynodiol diacetate 1 mg
Uses: Oral contraceptive
Depo-Testadiol:
estradiol cypionate 2 mg
testosterone cypionate 50 mg
Uses: Menopause
Desogen:
ethinyl estradiol 30 mcg
desorgestrel 0.15 mg
Uses: Estrogen, progestin
Dexacidin Ophthalmic Ointment/
Suspension:
Per ml:
0.1% dexamethasone
0.35% neomycin
polymyxin B 10,000 units/g
Uses: Ophthalmic, antiinfective/
antiinflammatory
Dexasporin Ophthalmic Ointment:
Per gram:
0.1% dexamethasone
0.35% neomycin
polymyxin B 10,000 units
Uses: Ophthalmic, antiinfective/
antiinflammatory

⚠ Safety alert   *"Tall Man" lettering

DHC Plus:
dihydrocodeine 16 mg
acetaminophen 356.4 mg
caffeine 30 mg
Uses: Analgesic

Dialose Plus:
docusate sodium 100 mg
yellow phenolphthalein 65 mg
Uses: Laxative

Di-Gel Advanced Formula:
magnesium hydroxide 128 mg
calcium carbonate 280 mg
simethicone 20 mg
Uses: Antacid, adsorbent, antiflatulent

Di-Gel Liquid:
Per 5 ml:
aluminum hydroxide 200 mg
magnesium hydroxide 200 mg
simethicone 20 mg
Uses: Antacid, adsorbent, antiflatulent

Dihistine DH Liquid:
Per 5 ml:
pseudoephedrine 30 mg
chlorpheniramine 2 mg
codeine 10 mg
Uses: Decongestant, antihistamine,
analgesic

Dilaudid Cough Syrup:
Per 5 ml:
guaifenesin 100 mg
hydromorphone 1 mg
5% alcohol
Uses: Expectorant, analgesic

Dilor-G:
dyphylline 200 mg
guaifenesin 200 mg
Uses: Bronchodilator, expectorant

Dimetane Decongestant:
brompheniramine 4 mg
phenylephrine 10 mg
Uses: Antihistamine, adrenergic

Dimetane-DX Cough Syrup:
Per 5 ml:
brompheniramine 2 mg
pseudoephedrine 30 mg
dextromethorphan 10 mg
Uses: Antihistamine, decongestant,
antitussive

Dimetapp DM Elixir:
Per 5 ml:
pseudoephedrine 5 mg
brompheniramine 2 mg
dextromethorphan 10 mg
Uses: Antihistamine, adrenergic,
expectorant

**Dimetapp Long-acting Cough Plus
Cold Syrup:**
dextromethorphan 7.5 mg
pseudoephedrine 15 mg
Uses: Antitussive decongestant

Dimetapp Sinus:
pseudoephedrine 30 mg
ibuprofen 200 mg
Uses: Decongestant, analgesic

Diovan 80 HCT:
valsartan 80 mg
hydrochlorthiazide 12.5 mg
Uses: Antihypertensive

Diovan 160 HCT:
valsartan 160 mg
hydrochlorthiazide 12.5 mg
Uses: Antihypertensive

Diurigen w/Reserpine:
chlorothiazide 250 mg
reserpine 0.125 mg
Uses: Antihypertensive

Diutensin-R:
methylclothiazide 2.5 mg
reserpine 0.1 mg
Uses: Antihypertensive

Doan's PM Extra Strength:
magnesium salicylate 500 mg
diphenhydrAMINE 25 mg
Uses: Analgesic, antihistamine

Dolacet:
hydrocodone 5 mg
acetaminophen 500 mg
Uses: Analgesic

Donnatal:
phenobarbital 16.2 mg
hyoscyamine 0.1037 mg
atropine 0.0194 mg

✦ Canada only   Side effects: *italics* = common; ***bold italics*** = life-threatening

scopolamine 0.0065 mg
Uses: Anticholinergic, barbiturate

Donnatal Elixir:

Per 5 ml:

phenobarbital 16.2 mg

hyoscyamine 0.1037 mg

atropine 0.0194 mg

scopolamine 0.0065 mg

23% alcohol

Uses: Anticholinergic, barbiturate

Donnatal Extentabs:

phenobarbital 48.6 mg

hyoscyamine 0.3111 mg

atropine 0.0582 mg

scopolamine 0.0195 mg

Uses: Anticholinergic, barbiturate

Donnazyme:

pancreatin 500 mg

lipase 1000 units

protease 12,500 units

amylase 12,500 units

Uses: Pancreatic enzymes

Dorcol Children's Cold Formula Liquid:

Per 5 ml:

pseudoephedrine 15 mg

chlorpheniramine 1 mg

Uses: Decongestant, antihistamine

Doxidan:

docusate calcium 60 mg

phenolphthalein 65 mg

Uses: Stool softener

Dristan Cold:

pseudoephedrine 30 mg

acetaminophen 500 mg

Uses: Decongestant, analgesic

Dristan Cold Maximum Strength Caplets:

pseudoephedrine 30 mg

brompheniramine 2 mg

acetaminophen 500 mg

Uses: Decongestant, antihistamine, analgesic

Dristan Cold Multi-Symptom Formula:

acetaminophen 325 mg

phenylephrine 5 mg

chlorpheniramine 2 mg

Uses: Analgesic, adrenergic, antihistamine

Dristan Sinus:

pseudoephedrine 30 mg

ibuprofen 200 mg

Uses: Decongestant, analgesic

Drixoral Allergy Sinus:

pseudoephedrine 60 mg

dexbrompheniramine 3 mg

acetaminophen 500 mg

Uses: Decongestant, antihistamine, analgesic

Drixoral Cold & Allergy:

pseudoephedrine 120 mg

dexbrompheniramine 6 mg

Uses: Decongestant, antihistamine

Drixoral Cold & Flu:

pseudoephedrine 60 mg

dexbrompheniramine 3 mg

acetaminophen 500 mg

Uses: Decongestant, antihistamine, analgesic

Drixoral Nasal Decongestant:

pseudoephedrine 120 mg

Uses: Decongestant

DT:

Per 5 ml dose:

diphtheria toxoid 2LfU

tetanus toxoid 5LfU

Uses: Vaccine

DTP:

Per 0.5 ml dose:

diphtheria toxoid 6.5LfU

tetanus toxoid 5LfU

pertussis 4LfU

Uses: Vaccine

DuoNeb:

Per 3 ml:

albuterol 3 mg

ipratropium 0.5 mg

Uses: Bronchodilator

Dura-Vent/DA:

phenylephrine 20 mg

chlorpheniramine 8 mg

methscopolamine 2.5 mg

Uses: Adrenergic, antihistamine

A Safety alert   *"Tall Man" lettering

Dyazide:
hydrochlorothiazide 25 mg
triamterene 37.5 mg
Uses: Diuretic
Dylline-GG Tablets:
dyphylline 200 mg
guaifenesin 200 mg
Uses: Bronchodilator, expectorant
Dynafed Asthma Relief:
epHEDrine 25 mg
guaifenesin 200 mg
Uses: Adrenergic, expectorant
Dynafed Plus Maximum Strength:
pseudoephedrine 30 mg
acetaminophen 500 mg
Uses: Decongestant, analgesic
Dyphylline-GG Elixir:
Per 5 ml:
dyphylline 100 mg
guaifenesin 100 mg
Uses: Bronchodilator, expectorant
E-Lor:
acetaminophen 650 mg
propoxyphene 65 mg
Uses: Analgesic
E-Pilo-1 Ophthalmic Solution:
1% epINEPHrine
1% pilocarpine
Uses: Mydriatic, miotic
E-Pilo-2 Ophthalmic Solution:
1% epINEPHrine
2% pilocarpine
Uses: Mydriatic, miotic
E-Pilo-4 Ophthalmic Solution:
1% epINEPHrine
4% pilocarpine
Uses: Mydriatic, miotic
E-Pilo-6 Ophthalmic Solution:
1% epINEPHrine
6% pilocarpine
Uses: Mydriatic, miotic
Elase Ointment:
Per gram:
fibrinolysin 1 unit
desoxyribonuclease 666.6 units
Uses: Enzyme

Elixophyllin GG Liquid:
Per 5 ml:
theophylline 100 mg
guaifenesin 100 mg
Uses: Expectorant, bronchodilator
EMLA Cream:
lidocaine 2.5 mg
prilocaine 2.5 mg
Uses: Local anesthetic
Empirin w/Codeine #3:
aspirin 325 mg
codeine phosphate 30 mg
Uses: Analgesic
Empirin w/Codeine #4:
aspirin 325 mg
codeine phosphate 60 mg
Uses: Analgesic
♣ **Empracet-60:**
acetaminophen 300 mg
codeine 60 mg
Uses: Analgesic
Endocet:
acetaminophen 325 mg
oxycodone 5 mg
Uses: Analgesic
♣ **Endodan:**
aspirin 325 mg
oxycodone 5 mg
Uses: Analgesic
Enduronyl:
methyclothiazide 5 mg
deserpidine 0.25 mg
Uses: Antihypertensive
Enduronyl Forte:
methyclothiazide 5.0 mg
deserpidine 0.5 mg
Uses: Antihypertensive
Entex PSE:
pseudoephedrine 120 mg
guaifenesin 600 mg
Uses: Adrenergic, expectorant
Epifoam Aerosol Foam:
1% hydrocortisone
1% pramoxine
Uses: Topical corticosteroid

Epzicom:
abacavir 600 mg
lamivudine 300 mg
Uses: HIV infection

Equagesic:
meprobamate 200 mg
aspirin 325 mg
Uses: Antianxiety

Eryzole:
Per 5 ml:
erythromycin 200 mg
sulfisoxazole 600 mg
Uses: Macrolide antiinfective

Esgic-Plus:
butalbital 50 mg
acetaminophen 500 mg
caffeine 40 mg
Uses: Barbiturate, analgesic

Esimil:
guanethidine 10 mg
hydrochlorothiazide 25 mg
Uses: Antihypertensive

Estratest:
esterified estrogens 1.25 mg
methyltestosterone 2.5 mg
Uses: Menopause

Estratest HS:
esterified estrogens 1.25 mg
methyltestosterone 2.5 mg
Uses: Menopause

Etrafon:
perphenazine 2 mg
amitriptyline 25 mg
Uses: Antipsychotic, antidepressant

Etrafon 2-10:
perphenazine 2 mg
amitriptyline 10 mg
Uses: Antidepressant

Etrafon A:
perphenazine 4 mg
amitriptyline 10 mg
Uses: Antidepressant

Etrafon Forte:
perphenazine 4 mg
amitriptyline 25 mg
Uses: Antipsychotic, antidepressant

Excedrin Migraine:
aspirin 250 mg
acetaminophen 250 mg
caffeine 65 mg
Uses: Migraine agent

Excedrin P.M.:
acetaminophen 500 mg
diphenhydrAMINE citrate 38 mg
Uses: Analgesic, antihistamine

Excedrin P.M. Liquigels:
acetaminophen 500 mg
diphenhydrAMINE 25 mg
Uses: Analgesic, antihistamine

Excedrin Sinus Extra Strength:
pseudoephedrine 30 mg
acetaminophen 500 mg
Uses: Decongestant, analgesic

Fansidar:
sulfidoxine 500 mg
pyrimethamine 25 mg
Uses: Antimalarial

Fedahist:
pseudoephedrine 60 mg
chlorpheniramine 4 mg
Uses: Decongestant, antihistamine

Fedahist Expectorant Syrup:
Per 5 ml:
guaifenesin 200 mg
pseudoephedrine 20 mg
Uses: Expectorant, decongestant

Fedahist Gyrocaps:
pseudoephedrine 65 mg
chlorpheniramine 10 mg
Uses: Decongestant, antihistamine

Fedahist Timecaps:
pseudoephedrine 120 mg
chlorpheniramine 8 mg
Uses: Decongestant, antihistamine

Feen-A-Mint Pills:
docusate sodium 100 mg
phenolphthalein 65 mg
Uses: Laxative

Fem-1:
acetaminophen 500 mg
pamabrom 25 mg
Uses: Nonopioid analgesic

⚠ Safety alert   *"Tall Man" lettering

Fembrt 1/5:
norethindrone 1 mg
ethinyl estradiol 5 mcg
Uses: Menopause

Ferro-Sequels:
docusate sodium 100 mg
ferrous fumarate 150 mg
Uses: Laxative, hematinic

Fioricet:
acetaminophen 325 mg
caffeine 40 mg
butalbital 50 mg
Uses: Analgesic, barbiturate

Fioricet w/Codeine:
acetaminophen 325 mg
caffeine 40 mg
butalbital 50 mg
codeine 30 mg
Uses: Analgesic, barbiturate

Fiorinal:
aspirin 325 mg
caffeine 40 mg
butalbital 50 mg
Uses: Analgesic, barbiturate

Fiorinal w/Codeine:
aspirin 325 mg
caffeine 40 mg
butalbital 50 mg
codeine 30 mg
Uses: Analgesic, barbiturate

FML-S Ophthalmic Suspension:
0.1% flurometholone
10% sulfacetamide
Uses: Ophthalmic, antiinfective/
  antiinflammatory

Gas-Ban:
calcium carbonate 500 mg
simethicone 40 mg
Uses: Antiflatulent, antacid

Gas-Ban DS Liquid:
Per 5 ml:
aluminum hydroxide 400 mg
magnesium hydroxide 400 mg
simethicone 40 mg
Uses: Antiflatulent, antacid

Gaviscon:
magnesium trisilicate 20 mg
aluminum hydroxide 80 mg
Uses: Antacid, adsorbent, antiflatulent

Gaviscon Liquid:
Per 5 ml:
aluminum hydroxide 31.7 mg
magnesium carbonate 119.3 mg
Uses: Antacid, adsorbent, antiflatulent

Gelprin:
acetaminophen 125 mg
aspirin 240 mg
caffeine 32 mg
Uses: Analgesic

Gelusil:
aluminum hydroxide 200 mg
magnesium hydroxide 200 mg
simethicone 25 mg
Uses: Antacid, adsorbent, antiflatulent

Genac Tablets:
triprolidine 2.5 mg
pseudoephedrine 60 mg
Uses: Antihistamine

Genatuss DM Syrup:
Per 5 ml:
guaifenesin 100 mg
dextromethorphan 10 mg
Uses: Expectorant, antitussive

Glucovance 1.25:
glyBURIDE: 1.25 mg
metformin: 250 mg
Uses: Antidiabetic

Glucovance 2.50:
glyBURIDE: 2.5 mg
metformin: 500 mg
Uses: Antidiabetic

Glucovance 5:
glyBURIDE: 5 mg
metformin: 500 mg
Uses: Antidiabetic

Granulex Aerosol:
Per 0.82 ml:
trypsin 0.1 mg
balsam peru 72.5 mg
castor oil 650 mg
Uses: Top enzyme

Side effects: *italics* = common; ***bold italics*** = life-threatening

Guaifenex PSE 60:
pseudoephedrine 60 mg
guaifenesin 600 mg
Uses: Decongestant, expectorant

Guaifenex PSE 120:
pseudoephedrine 120 mg
guaifenesin 600 mg
Uses: Decongestant, expectorant

Guaituss AC:
Per 5 ml:
codeine 10 mg
guafenesin 100 mg
Uses: Analgesic, expectorant

Haley's M-O Liquid:
Per 15 ml:
magnesium hydroxide 900 mg
mineral oil 3.75 ml
Uses: Laxative

Halotussin-DM Sugar Free Liquid:
Per 5 ml:
guaifenesin 100 mg
dextromethorphan 10 mg
Uses: Expectorant, antitussive

Helidac:
In a compliance package:
bismuth subsalicylate 262.4 mg tabs
metronidazole 250 mg tabs
tetracycline 500 mg caps
Uses: Antiinfective

Hemate P:
AHF/VWF 250 units/500 units, 500 units/
1000 units, 1000 units/2000 units
Uses: Hemophilia, von Willebrand disease

Humalog Mix 50/50:
insulin lispro protamine 50%
insulin lispro (rDNA) 50%
Uses: Antidiabetic

Humalog Mix 75/25:
insulin lispro protamine 75%
insulin lispro (rDNA) 25%
Uses: Antidiabetic

Humibid DM Sprinkle Caps:
dextromethorphan 15 mg
guaifenesin 300 mg
Uses: Expectorant, antitussive

Humibid DM Tablets:
dextromethorphan 30 mg
guaifenesin 600 mg
Uses: Expectorant, antitussive

HycoClear Tuss:
Per 5 ml:
hydrocodone 5 mg
guaifenesin 100 mg
Uses: Analgesic, expectorant

Hycodan:
hydrocodone 5 mg
homatropine 1.5 mg
Uses: Analgesic, mydriatic

Hycodan Syrup:
Per 5 ml:
hydrocodone 5 mg
homatropine 1.5 mg
Uses: Analgesic, mydriatic

Hycomine Compound:
chlorpheniramine 2 mg
acetaminophen 250 mg
phenylephrine 10 mg
hydrocodone 5 mg
caffeine 30 mg
Uses: Antihistamine, analgesic, adrenergic

Hycotuss Expectorant Syrup:
Per 5 ml:
guaifenesin 100 mg
hydrocodone 5 mg
10% alcohol
Uses: Expectorant

Hydergine:
dihydroergocornine 0.167 mg
dihydroergocristine 0.167 mg
dihydroergocryptine 0.167 mg
Uses: Adrenergic blocker

Hydrocet:
hydrocodone 5 mg
acetaminophen 500 mg
Uses: Opioid analgesic

Hydrogesic:
hydrocodone 5 mg
acetaminophen 500 mg
Uses: Opioid analgesic

Hydropres-50:
hydrochlorothiazide 50 mg

⚠ Safety alert   *"Tall Man" lettering

reserpine 0.125 mg
Uses: Antihypertensive
Hydroserpine:
hydrochlorothiazide 25 mg
reserpine 0.125 mg
Uses: Antihypertensive
Hydroserpine:
hydrochlorothiazide 50 mg
reserpine 0.125 mg
Uses: Antihypertensive
Hyzaar:
losartan potassium 50 mg
hydrochlorothiazide 12.5 mg
potassium 4.24 mg
Uses: Antihypertensive
Imodium Advanced:
loperamide 2 mg
simethicone 125 mg
Uses: Antidiarrheal, antiflatulent
Inderide 40/25:
propranolol 40 mg
hydrochlorothiazide 25 mg
Uses: Antihypertensive
Inderide 80/25:
propranolol 80 mg
hydrochlorothiazide 25 mg
Uses: Antihypertensive
Inderide LA 80/50:
propranolol 80 mg
hydrochlorothiazide 50 mg
Uses: Antihypertensive
Inderide LA 120/50:
propranolol 120 mg
hydrochlorothiazide 50 mg
Uses: Antihypertensive
Inderide LA 160/50:
propranolol 160 mg
hydrochlorothiazide 50 mg
Uses: Antihypertensive
Innovar:
Per ml:
droperidol 2.5 mg
fentanyl 0.05 mg
Uses: Opioid analgesic, general anesthetic
Iofed:
brompheniramine 12 mg

pseudoephedrine 120 mg
Uses: Antihistamine, adrenergic
Iofed PD:
brompheniramine 6 mg
pseudoephedrine 60 mg
Uses: Antihistamine, adrenergic
Isopap:
isometheptene 65 mg
APAP 325 mg
dicloral-phenazone 100 mg
Uses: Migraine agent
Kaletra Capsules:
lopinavir 133.3 mg
ritonavir 33.3 mg
Uses: HIV
Kaletra Solution:
Per 1 ml:
lopinavir 80 mg
ritonavir 20 mg
Uses: HIV
Lactinex:
Mixed culture of:
Lactobacillus acidophilus and
Lactobacillus bulgaricus
Uses: Supplement
Lenoltec w/Codeine No. 1:
acetaminophen 650 mg
hydrocodone 10 mg
Uses: Analgesic
Levlite:
levonorgestrel 0.100 mg
ethinyl estradiol 20 mcg
Uses: Estrogen, progestin
Levsin PB Drops:
Per ml:
hyoscyamine 0.125 mg
phenobarbital 15 mg
5% alcohol
Uses: Anticholinergic, barbiturate
Levsin w/Phenobarbital:
hyoscyamine 0.125 mg
phenobarbital 15 mg
Uses: Anticholinergic, barbiturate
Lexxel 1:
enalapril 5 mg
felodipine 5 mg

Uses: Antihypertensive

Lexxel 2:
enalapril 5 mg
felodipine 2.5 mg
Uses: Antihypertensive

Librax:
chlordiazepoxide 5 mg
clidinium 2.5 mg
Uses: Antianxiety, anticholinergic

Lida-Mantel-HC-Cream:
0.5% hydrocortisone
3% lidocaine
Uses: Antiinflammatory, analgesic

Limbitrol DS 10-25:
chlordiazepoxide 10 mg
amitriptyline 25 mg
Uses: Antidepressant, antianxiety

Lobac:
salicylamide 200 mg
phenyltoloxamine 20 mg
acetaminophen 300 mg
Uses: Skeletal muscle relaxant, analgesic

Loestrin Fe 1/20:
norethindrone acetate 1 mg/tablet
ethinyl estradiol 20 mcg/tablet
with 7 tablets of ferrous fumarate 75 mg/
    container
Uses: Oral contraceptive

Loestrin Fe 1.5/30:
norethindrone acetate 1.5 mg
ethinyl estradiol 30 mcg
Uses: Oral contraceptive

Lomotil:
diphenoxylate 2.5 mg
atropine 0.025 mg
Uses: Antidiarrheal, anticholinergic

Lomotil Liquid:
Per 5 ml:
diphenoxylate 2.5 mg
atropine 0.025 mg
Uses: Antidiarrheal, anticholinergic

Lo Ovral:
ethinyl estradiol 30 mcg
norgestrel 0.3 mg
Uses: Oral contraceptive

Lopressor HCT 50/25:
metoprolol 50 mg
hydrochlorothiazide 25 mg
Uses: Antihypertensive

Lopressor HCT 100/25:
metoprolol 100 mg
hydrochlorothiazide 25 mg
Uses: Antihypertensive

Lopressor HCT 100/50:
metoprolol 100 mg
hydrochlorothiazide 50 mg
Uses: Antihypertensive

Lorcet 10/650:
acetaminophen 650 mg
hydrocodone 10 mg
Uses: Analgesic

Lorcet-HD:
hydrocodone 10 mg
acetaminophen 300 mg
Uses: Analgesic

Lorcet Plus:
acetaminophen 650 mg
hydrocodone 7.5 mg
Uses: Analgesic

Lortab 2.5/500:
hydrocodone 2.5 mg
acetaminophen 500 mg
Uses: Analgesic

Lortab 5/500:
hydrocodone 5 mg
acetaminophen 500 mg
Uses: Analgesic

Lortab 7.5/500:
hydrocodone 7.5 mg
acetaminophen 500 mg
Uses: Analgesic

Lortab 10/500:
hydrocodone 10 mg
acetaminophen 500 mg
Uses: Analgesic

Lortab ASA:
aspirin 500 mg
hydrocodone 5 mg
Uses: Analgesic

⚠ Safety alert   *"Tall Man" lettering

Lortab Elixir:
Per 5 ml:
hydrocodone 2.5 mg
acetaminophen 167 mg
Uses: Analgesic
Losec 1-2-3A:
omeprazole 20 mg
clarithromycin 500 mg
amoxicillin 1 g
Uses: Antiinfective
Losec 1-2-3M:
omeprazole 20 mg
clarithromycin 250 mg
medtronidazole 500 mg
Uses: Antiinfective
Lotensin HCT 5/6.25:
benazepril 5 mg
hydrochlorothiazide 6.25 mg
Uses: Antihypertensive
Lotensin HCT 10/12.5:
benazepril 10 mg
hydrochlorothiazide 12.5 mg
Uses: Antihypertensive
Lotensin HCT 20/12.5:
benazepril 20 mg
hydrochlorothiazide 12.5 mg
Uses: Antihypertensive
Lotensin HCT 20/25:
benazepril 20 mg
hydrochlorothiazide 25 mg
Uses: Antihypertensive
Lotrel 2.5/10:
amlopidine 2.5 mg
benazepril 10 mg
Uses: Antihypertensive
Lotrel 5/10:
amlodipine 5 mg
benazepril 10 mg
Uses: Antihypertensive
Lotrel 5/20:
amlodipine 5 mg
benazepril 20 mg
Uses: Antihypertensive
Lotrisone Topical:
0.05% betamethasone
1% clotrimazole

Uses: Local antiinfective, antiinflammatory
Lufyllin-EPG Elixir:
Per 5 ml:
dyphylline 150 mg
epHEDrine 24 mg
guaifenesin 300 mg
phenobarbital 24 mg
Uses: Bronchodilator, expectorant
Lufyllin-GG:
dyphylline 200 mg
guaifenesin 200 mg
Uses: Bronchodilator, expectorant
Lunelle Monthly Contraceptive Injection:
25 mg medroxyprogesterone
5 mg estradiol/0.5 ml
Uses: Contraceptive
M-M-R-II:
measles
mumps
rubella
Uses: Vaccine, toxoid
Maalox:
aluminum hydroxide 200 mg
magnesium hydroxide 200 mg
Uses: Antacid, adsorbent, antiflatulent
Maalox Plus:
aluminum hydroxide 200 mg
magnesium hydroxide 200 mg
simethicone 25 mg
Uses: Antacid, adsorbent, antiflatulent
Maalox Plus Extra Strength Suspension:
Per 5 ml:
aluminum hydroxide 500 mg
magnesium hydroxide 450 mg
simethicone 40 mg
Uses: Antacid, adsorbent, antiflatulent
Maalox Suspension:
Per 5 ml:
aluminum hydroxide 225 mg
magnesium hydroxide 200 mg
Uses: Antacid, adsorbent, antiflatulent
Macrobid:
nitrofurantoin macrocrystals 25 mg
nitrofurantoin monohydrate 75 mg

Side effects: *italics* = common; ***bold italics*** = life-threatening

Uses: Antiinfective

Magnaprin:
aspirin 325 mg
magnesium hydroxide 50 mg
aluminum hydroxide 50 mg
calcium carbonate 50 mg
Uses: Nonopioid analgesic

Magnaprin Arthritis Strength:
aspirin 325 mg
magnesium hydroxide 75 mg
aluminum hydroxide 75 mg
calcium carbonate 75 mg
Uses: Nonopioid analgesic

Malarone:
250 mg atovaquone
100 mg proguanil
Uses: Malaria

Malarone Pediatric:
62.5 mg atovaquone
25 mg proguanil
Uses: Malaria

Mapap Cold Formula:
acetaminophen 325 mg
chlorpheniramine 2 mg
pseudoephedrine 30 mg
dextromethorphan 15 mg
Uses: Bronchodilator, expectorant

Marax:
epHEDrine 25 mg
theophylline 130 mg
hydrOXYzine 10 mg
Uses: Bronchodilator, sedative/hypnotic

Maxitrol Ophthalmic Suspension/ Ointment:
Per ml:
0.35% neomycin
0.1% dexamethasone
polymyxin B 10,000 units
Uses: Ophthalmic antiinfective, antiinflammatory

Maxzide:
hydrochlorothiazide 50 mg
triamterene 75 mg
Uses: Antihypertensive, diuretic

Maxzide-25 MG:
hydrochlorothiazide 25 mg
triamterene 37.5 mg
Uses: Diuretic

Medi-Flu Liquid:
Per 5 ml:
pseudoephedrine 10 mg
chlorpheniramine 0.67 mg
dextromethorphan 5 mg
acetaminophen 167 mg
18.5% alcohol
Uses: Decongestant, antihistamine, antitussive, analgesic

Medigesic:
acetaminophen 325 mg
caffeine 40 mg
butalbital 50 mg
Uses: Nonopioid analgesic

Mepergan Fortis:
meperidine 50 mg
promethazine 25 mg
Uses: Analgesic, antihistamine

Mepergan Injection:
meperidine 25 mg
promethazine 25 mg
Uses: Analgesic

Metaglip:
glipizide/metformin 2.5 mg/250 mg, 2.5 mg/500 mg, 5 mg/500 mg
Uses: Diabetes mellitus

Metimyd Ophthalmic Suspension/ Ointment:
0.5% prednisoLONE
10% sodium sulfacetamide
Uses: Ophthalmic antiinfective, antiinflammatory

Micardis HCT 40:
telmesartan 40 mg
hydrochlorthiazide 12.5 mg
Uses: Antihypertensive

Micardis HCT 80:
telmesartan 80 mg
hydrochlorthiazide 12.5 mg
Uses: Antihypertensive

Microgestin Fe 1/20:
norethindrone 1 mg
ethinyl estradiol 20 mcg
ferrous fumarate 75 mg in container

Uses: Estrogen, progestin
Microgestin Fe 1.5/30:
norethindrone 1.5 mg
ethinyl estradiol 30 mcg
ferrous fumarate 75 mg in container
Uses: Estrogen, progestin
Midol Maximum Strength Multi-Symptom Menstrual Gelcaps:
acetaminophen 500 mg
pyrilamine 15 mg
caffeine 60 mg
Uses: Analgesic
Midol PM:
acetaminophen 500 mg
diphenhydrAMINE 25 mg
Uses: Analgesic, antihistamine
Midol PMS Maximum Strength Caplets:
acetaminophen 500 mg
pyrilamine 15 mg
pamabrom 25 mg
Uses: Analgesic
Midol, Teen:
acetaminophen 400 mg
pamabrom 25 mg
Uses: Analgesic
Midrin:
isometheptene 65 mg
acetaminophen 325 mg
dichloralphenazone 100 mg
Uses: Analgesic
Minizide 1:
prazosin 1 mg
polythiazide 0.5 mg
Uses: Antihypertensive
Minizide 2:
prazosin 2 mg
polythiazide 0.5 mg
Uses: Antihypertensive
Minizide 5:
prazosin 5 mg
polythiazide 0.5 mg
Uses: Antihypertensive
Moduretic:
hydrochlorothiazide 50 mg
amiloride 5 mg
Uses: Diuretic

Monopril-HCT 10:
fosinopril 10 mg
hydrochlorthiazide 12.5 mg
Uses: Antihypertensive
Monopril-HCT 20:
fosinopril 20 mg
hydrochlorthiazide 12.5 mg
Uses: Antihypertensive
Motrin Children's Cold Suspension:
Per 5 ml:
ibuprofen 100 mg
pseudoephedrine 15 mg
Uses: Nonopioid analgesic, decongestant
Motrin IB Sinus:
pseudoephedrine 30 mg
ibuprofen 200 mg
Uses: Adrenergic, analgesic
Mucinex:
guaifenesin 600 mg or 1200 mg
Uses: Cough suppressant, expectorant
Mucinex D:
guaifenesin/pseudoephedrine 1200 mg/120 mg, 600 mg/60 mg
Uses: Expectorant, decongestant
Mucinex DM:
dextromethorphan 30 mg
guaifenesin 600 mg
Uses: Antitussive, expectorant
Murocoll-2 Ophthalmic Drops:
0.3% scopolamine
10% phenylephrine
Uses: Ophthalmic anticholinergic, mydriatic
Mycolog II Topical:
Per gram:
0.1% triamcinolone acetonide
nystatin 100,000 units
Uses: Local antiinfective, antiinflammatory
Mylanta:
aluminum hydroxide 200 mg
magnesium hydroxide 200 mg
simethicone 20 mg
Uses: Antacid, adsorbent, antiflatulent
Mylanta Double Strength Liquid:
Per 5 ml:
aluminum hydroxide 400 mg

APPENDIX

magnesium hydroxide 400 mg
simethicone 40 mg
Uses: Antacid, adsorbent, antiflatulent
Mylanta Gelcaps:
calcium carbonate 311 mg
magnesium carbonate 232 mg
Uses: Antacid, adsorbent, antiflatulent
Naldecon Senior DX Liquid:
Per 5 ml:
dextromethorphan 10 mg
guaifenesin 200 mg
Uses: Expectorant, antitussive
Naphcon-A Ophthalmic Solution:
0.25% naphazoline
0.3% pheniramine
Uses: Ophthalmic vasoconstrictor
Nasatab LA:
guaifenesin 500 mg
pseudoephedrine 120 mg
Uses: Expectorant, decongestant
NeoDecadron Ophthalmic Ointment:
0.35% neomycin
0.05% dexamethasone
Uses: Ophthalmic antiinfective, antiinflammatory
NeoDecadron Ophthalmic Solution:
0.35% neomycin
0.1% dexamethasone
Uses: Ophthalmic antiinfective, antiinflammatory
Neosporin Cream:
Per gram:
polymyxin B 10,000 units
neomycin 3.5 mg
Uses: Top antiinfective
Neosporin G.U. Irrigant:
Per ml:
neomycin 40 mg
polymyxin B 200,000 units
Uses: Antiinfective
Neosporin Ointment:
Per gram:
polymyxin B 5000 units
bacitracin zinc 400 units
neomycin 3.5 mg

Uses: Top antiinfective
Neosporin Ophthalmic Solution:
Per ml:
neomycin 1.75 mg
polymyxin B 10,000 units
gramicidin 0.025 mg
Uses: Ophthalmic antiinfective
Neosporin Ophthalmic Ointment:
Per gram:
neomycin 3.5 mg
polymyxin B 10,000 units
bacitracin zinc 400 units
Uses: Ophthalmic antiinfective
Neosporin Plus Cream:
polymyxin B 10,000 units
neomycin 3.5 mg
lidocaine 40 mg
Uses: Top antiinfective
Niferex-150 Forte:
ferrous sulfate 150 mg
vitamin B_{12} 25 mcg
folic acid 1 mg
Uses: Supplement
Norco 5/325:
hydrocodone 5 mg
acetaminophen 325 mg
Uses: Analgesic, opioid, nonopioid
Norco:
hydrocodone 10 mg
acetaminophen 325 mg
Uses: Analgesic, opioid, nonopioid
Norgesic:
orphenadrine 25 mg
aspirin 385 mg
caffeine 30 mg
Uses: Skeletal muscle relaxant, analgesic
Norgesic Forte:
orphenadrine 50 mg
aspirin 770 mg
caffeine 60 mg
Uses: Skeletal muscle relaxant, analgesic
Novacet Lotion:
sodium sulfacetamine 10%
sulfur 5%
Uses: Acne agent

A Safety alert   *"Tall Man" lettering

Novafed A:
pseudoephedrine 120 mg
chlorpheniramine 8 mg
Uses: Adrenergic, antihistamine

Novahistone Elixir:
Per 5 ml:
phenylephrine 5 mg
chlorpheniramine 2 mg
5% alcohol
Uses: Antihistamine

Novo-Gesic ✤C8:
acetaminophen 300 mg
codeine 8 mg
caffeine 15 mg
Uses: Analgesic

NuLytely:
PEG 3350/420 g
sodium bicarbonate 5.72 g
sodium chloride 11.2 g
potassium chloride 1.48 g
Uses: Laxative

NyQuil Hot Therapy:
Per packet:
acetaminophen 1000 mg
pseudoephedrine 60 mg
dextromethorphan 30 mg
doxylamine 12.5 mg
Uses: Analgesic, adrenergic, antitussive

**NyQuil Nighttime Cold/Flu Medicine
   Liquid:**
Per 5 ml:
pseudoephedrine 10 mg
doxylamine 1.25 mg
dextromethorphan 5 mg
acetaminophen 167 mg
25% alcohol
Uses: Adrenergic, antitussive, analgesic

Octicair Otic Suspension:
1% hydrocortisone
neomycin 5 mg/ml
polymyxin B 10,000 units/ml
Uses: Otic antiinflammatory, antiinfective

Opcon-A Ophthalmic Solution:
0.027% naphazoline
0.315% pheniramine
Uses: Ophthalmic vasoconstrictor

Ornade Spansules:
phenylpropanolamine 75 mg
chlorpheniramine 12 mg
Uses: Antihistamine, decongestant

Ornex:
pseudoephedrine 30 mg
acetaminophen 500 mg
Uses: Adrenergic, analgesic

Ornex No Drowsiness Caplets:
acetaminophen 325 mg
pseudoephedrine 30 mg
Uses: Adrenergic, analgesic

Orphengesic:
orphenadrine 25 mg
aspirin 385 mg
caffeine 30 mg
Uses: Analgesic

Orphengesic Forte:
orphenadrine 50 mg
aspirin 770 mg
caffeine 60 mg
Uses: Analgesic

Ortho-cept:
ethinyl estradiol 30 mcg
desogestrel 0.15 mg
Uses: Oral contraceptive

Ortho-cyclen:
ethinyl estradiol 35 mcg
norgestimate 0.25 mg
Uses: Oral contraceptive

Ortho-Novum 7/7/7:
Phase I:
0.5 mg norethindrone
35 mcg ethinyl estradiol
Phase II:
0.75 mg norethindrone
35 mcg ethinyl estradiol
Phase III:
1 mg norethinidrone
35 mcg estradiol
Uses: Oral contraceptive

Ortho-Prefest:
estradiol 1 mg (15)
norgestimate 0.09 mg (15)
Uses: Menopause

✤ Canada only   Side effects: *italics* = common; ***bold italics*** = life-threatening

Ovcon-50:
ethinyl estradiol 50 mcg
norethindrone 1 mg
Uses: Oral contraceptive

♣ **Oxycocet:**
acetaminophen 325 mg
oxycodone 5 mg
Uses: Analgesic

P-A-C Analgesic:
aspirin 400 mg
caffeine 32 mg
Uses: Nonopioid analgesic

Pain-X Topical:
0.05% capsaicin
5% menthol
4% camphor
Uses: Top analgesic

Pamprin Maximum Pain Relief:
acetaminophen 250 mg
pamabrom 25 mg
magnesium salicylate 250 mg
Uses: Analgesic

Pamprin Multi-Symptom:
acetaminophen 500 mg
pamabrom 25 mg
pyrilamine 15 mg
Uses: Analgesic

Panacet 5/500:
hydrocodone 5 mg
acetaminophen 500 mg
Uses: Analgesic

Panasal 5/500:
hydrocodone 5 mg
aspirin 500 mg
Uses: Analgesic

Pancrease Capsules:
amylase 20,000 units
protease 25,000 units
lipase 4500 units (microspheres)
Uses: Digestive enzyme

Parcopa:
carbidopa/levodopa 10 mg/100 mg, 25 mg/
100 mg/25 mg/250 mg
Uses: Parkinson's disease

Pedia Care Cold-Allergy Chewable:
pseudoephedrine 15 mg

chlorpheniramine 1 mg
Uses: Adrenergic, antihistamine

Pedia Care Cough-Cold Liquid:
Per 5 ml:
pseudoephedrine 15 mg
chlorpheniramine 1 mg
dextromethorphan 5 mg
Uses: Adrenergic, antihistamine, antitussive

**Pedia Care NightRest Cough-Cold
   Liquid:**
Per 5 ml:
pseudoephedrine 15 mg
chlorpheniramine 1 mg
dextromethorphan 7.5 mg
Uses: Adrenergic, antihistamine, antitussive

Pediacof Syrup:
Per 5 ml:
codeine 5 mg
phenylephrine 2.5 mg
chlorpheniramine 0.75 mg
potassium iodide 75 mg
5% alcohol
Uses: Opioid, narcotic analgesic,
   antihistamine

Pediazole Suspension:
Per 5 ml:
erythromycin 200 mg
sulfiSOXAZOLE 600 mg
Uses: Antiinfective

Pepcid Complete:
calcium carbonate 800 mg
magnesium hydroxide 165 mg
famotidine 10 mg
Uses: Antiulcer agent

Percocet 2.5/325:
oxycodone 2.5 mg
acetaminophen 325 mg
Uses: Analgesic

Percocet 5/325:
oxycodone 5 mg
acetaminophen 325 mg
Uses: Analgesic

Percocet 7.5/500:
oxycodone 7.5 mg
acetaminophen 500 mg
Uses: Analgesic

Percocet 10/650:
oxycodone 10 mg
acetaminophen 650 mg
Uses: Analgesic
Percodan:
oxycodone 4.88 mg
aspirin 325 mg
Uses: Analgesic
Percodan-Demi:
aspirin 325 mg
oxycodone HCl 2.25 mg
oxycodone terephthalate 0.19 mg
Uses: Analgesic
Percodan-Demi:
aspirin 325 mg
oxycodone 2.5 mg
Uses: Analgesic
Percogesic:
phenyltoloxamine 30 mg
acetaminophen 325 mg
Uses: Analgesic
Perdiem Granules:
Per teaspoon:
senna 0.74 g
psyllium 3.25 g
sodium 1.8 mg
potassium 35.5 mg
Uses: Laxative
Peri-Colace:
docusate sodium 100 mg
casanthranol 30 mg
Uses: Laxative
Peri-Colace Syrup:
Per 15 ml:
docusate sodium 60 mg
casanthranol 30 mg
Uses: Laxative
Phenaphen w/Codeine No. 3:
aspirin 325 mg
codeine 30 mg
Uses: Analgesic
Phenaphen w/Codeine No. 4:
aspirin 325 mg
codeine 60 mg
Uses: Analgesic

Phenerbel-S:
ergotamine tartrate 0.6 mg
belladonna alkaloids 0.2 mg
phenobarbital 40 mg
Uses: α-Adrenergic blocker, anticholinergic
Phenergan VC Syrup:
Per 5 ml:
phenylephrine 5 mg
promethazine 6.25 mg
Uses: Adrenergic, antihistamine
Phenergan VC w/Codeine Syrup:
Per 5 ml:
phenylephrine 5 mg
promethazine 6.25 mg
codeine 10 mg
Uses: Adrenergic, antihistamine, opioid
    analgesic
Phenergan w/Codeine Syrup:
Per 5 ml:
promethazine 6.25 mg
codeine 10 mg
Uses: Antihistamine, analgesic
Pherazine DM Syrup:
Per 5 ml:
dextromethorphan 15 mg
promethazine 6.25 mg
7% alcohol
Uses: Antitussive, antihistamine
Phillips' Laxative Gelcaps:
docusate sodium 83 mg
phenolphthalein 90 mg
Uses: Laxative
PMB-400:
conjugated estrogens 0.45 mg
meprobamate 400 mg
Uses: Oral contraceptive
Polaramine Expectorant Liquid:
Per 5 ml:
guaifenesin 100 mg
dexchlorpheniramine 2 mg
pseudoephedrine 20 mg
7.5% alcohol
Uses: Expectorant
Polycillin-PRB Oral Suspension:
Per single dose:
ampicillin 3.5 g

✦ Canada only   Side effects: *italics* = common; ***bold italics*** = life-threatening

probenecid 1 g
Uses: Antiinfective
Polycitra Syrup:
Per 5 ml:
potassium citrate 550 mg
sodium citrate 500 mg
citric acid 334 mg
Uses: Laxative
Poly-Histine Elixir:
Per 5 ml:
pheniramine 4 mg
pyrilamine 4 mg
phenyltoloxamine 4 mg
4% alcohol
Uses: Antihistamine
Polysporin Ophthalmic Ointment:
Per gram:
polymyxin B 10,000 units
bacitracin zinc 500 units
Uses: Ophthalmic antiinfective
Polysporin Topical Ointment:
Per gram:
polymyxin B 10,000 units
bacitracin zinc 500 units
Uses: Top antiinfective
Polytrim Ophthalmic Solution:
Per ml:
trimethoprim 1 mg
polymyxin B 10,000 units
Uses: Ophthalmic antiinfective
Pravigard PAC:
aspirin 81 mg
pravastin 20, 40, 80 mg
aspirin 325 mg
pravastin 20, 40, 80 mg
Uses: Antihyperlipidemic, antithrombotic
Premphase:
In a compliance package:
conjugated estrogens 0.625 mg
medroxyPROGESTERone 5 mg
Uses: Menopause
Prempro:
In a compliance package:
conjugated estrogens 0.625 mg
medroxyPROGESTERone 2.5 mg
Uses: Menopause

Premsyn PMS:
acetaminophen 500 mg
pamabrom 25 mg
pyrilamine 15 mg
Uses: Analgesic
Prevpac:
In a compliance package:
amoxicillin 500 mg caps
clarithromycin 500 mg tabs
lansoprazole 30 mg caps
Uses: Antiinfective
Primatene:
theophylline 130 mg
epHEDrine 24 mg
phenobarbital 7.5 mg
Uses: Bronchodilator, barbiturate
Primaxin 250 mg IV for Injection:
imipenem 250 mg
cilastatin sodium 250 mg
Uses: Antiinfective
Primaxin 500 mg IV for Injection:
imipenem 500 mg
cilastatin sodium 500 mg
Uses: Antiinfective
Prinzide 10-12.5:
lisinopril 10 mg
hydrochlorothiazide 12.5 mg
Uses: Antihypertensive
Prinzide 20-12.5:
lisinopril 20 mg
hydrochlorothiazide 12.5 mg
Uses: Antihypertensive
Prinzide 20-25:
lisinopril 20 mg
hydrochlorothiazide 25 mg
Uses: Antihypertensive
Probampacin Oral Suspension:
Per single dose:
ampicillin 3.5 g
probenecid 1 g
Uses: Antiinfective
Proben-C:
colchicine 0.5 mg
probenecid 500 mg
Uses: Antigout agent

⚠ Safety alert   *"Tall Man" lettering

Proctofoam-HC Aerosol Foam:
1% hydrocortisone
1% pramoxine
Uses: Topical corticosteroid

Prometh w/Codeine Syrup:
codeine 10 mg
promethazine 6.25 mg/5 ml
Uses: Antitussive, antihistamine

Prometh VCW/Codeine Syrup:
codeine 10 mg
promethazine 6.25 mg
phenylephrine 5 mg/5 ml
Uses: Antitussive, antihistamine, decongestant

Propacet 100:
propoxyphene-N 100 mg
acetaminophen 650 mg
Uses: Analgesic

Pseudo-Chlor:
pseudoephedrine 120 mg
chlorpheniramine 8 mg
Uses: Antihistamine

Pseudo-Gest Plus:
pseudoephedrine 60 mg
chlorpheniramine 4 mg
Uses: Antihistamine

P-V-Tussin:
phenindamine 25 mg
guaifenesin 200 mg
hydrocodone 5 mg
Uses: Antihistamine, analgesic

P-V-Tussin Syrup:
Per 5 ml:
chlorpheniramine 2 mg
phenindamine 5 mg
phenylephrine 5 mg
pyrilamine 6 mg
Uses: Antihistamine, decongestant

Quadrinal:
epHEDrine 24 mg
theophylline 65 mg
potassium iodide 320 mg
phenobarbital 24 mg
Uses: Adrenergic, bronchodilator,
barbiturate

Quelidrine Cough Syrup:
Per 5 ml:
dextromethorphan 10 mg
phenylephrine 5 mg
epHEDrine 5 mg
chlorpheniramine 2 mg
ammonium chloride 40 mg
ipecac 0.005 ml
Uses: Expectorant, adrenergic,
antihistamine

Quibron-300:
theophylline 300 mg
guaifenesin 180 mg
Uses: Bronchodilator, expectorant

Quibron:
theophylline 150 mg
guaifenesin 90 mg
Uses: Bronchodilator, expectorant

Quinaretic:
quinapril/hydrochlorothiazide 10 mg/
12.5 mg or 20 mg/12.5 mg
Uses: Hypertension

R&C Shampoo:
0.3% pyrethrins
3% piperonyl butoxide
Uses: Scabicide, pediculicide

Rauzide:
bendroflumethiazide 4 mg
powdered *Rauwolfia serpentina* 50 mg
Uses: Diuretic, antihypertensive

Rebetron:
interferon alfa-2b 3 million units/0.5 ml
ribavirin, PO 200 mg
Uses: Biologic response modifier, antiviral

Regroton:
chlorthalidone 50 mg
reserpine 0.25 mg
Uses: Diuretic, antihypertensive

Regulace:
docusate sodium 100 mg
casanthranol 30 mg
Uses: Laxative

Renese-R:
polythiazide 2 mg
reserpine 0.25 mg
Uses: Diuretic, antihypertensive

Repan:
acetaminophen 325 mg
caffeine 40 mg
butalbital 50 mg
Uses: Nonopioid analgesic

Respahist:
pseudoephedrine 60 mg
brompheniramine 6 mg
Uses: Adrenergic, antihistamine

Respaire-60:
guaifenesin 200 mg
pseudoephedrine 60 mg
Uses: Expectorant, adrenergic

RID Mousse:
pyrethrins 0.33%
piperonyl butoxide 4%
Uses: Scabicide, pediculicide

RID Shampoo:
0.3% pyrethrins
3% piperonyl butoxide
Uses: Scabicide, pediculicide

Rifamate:
isoniazid 150 mg
rifampin 300 mg
Uses: Antitubercular, antileprotic

Rifater:
rifampin 120 mg
isoniazid 50 mg
pyrazinamide 300 mg
Uses: Antitubercular

Rimactane/INH Dual Pack:
isoniazid 300 mg (30 tabs)
rifampin 300 mg (60 caps)
Uses: Antitubercular

Riopan Plus Suspension:
Per 5 ml:
magaldrate 540 mg
simethicone 40 mg
Uses: Antacid, adsorbent, antiflatulent

Robaxisal:
methocarbamol 400 mg
aspirin 325 mg
Uses: Skeletal muscle relaxant, analgesic

Robitussin Allergy & Cough Liquid:
dextromethorphan 10 mg
brompheniramine 2 mg
pseudoephedrine 30 mg
Uses: Antitussive, antihistamine, decongestant

Robitussin Cold & Cough Softgels:
pseudoephedrine 30 mg
guaifenesin 200 mg
dextromethorphan 10 mg
Uses: Antitussive, expectorant, decongestant

Robitussin Cold, Multi-Symptom Cold & Flu Tablets:
dextromethorphan 10 mg
guaifenesin 200 mg
pseudoephedrine 30 mg
acetaminophen 325 mg
Uses: Antitussive, expectorant, decongestant, analgesic

Robitussin Cough & Cold Infant Drops:
pseudoephedrine 6 mg/ml
dextromethorphan 2 mg/ml
guaifenesin 40 mg/ml
Uses: Decongestant, antitussive, expectorant

Robitussin Cough & Congestion Formula:
dextromethorphan 10 mg
guaifenesin 200 mg
Uses: Antitussive, expectorant

Robitussin-DM Infant Drops:
dextromethorphan 2 mg/ml
guaifenesin 40 mg/ml
Uses: Antitussive, expectorant

Robitussin-DM Liquid:
Per 5 ml:
guaifenesin 100 mg
dextromethorphan 10 mg
Uses: Expectorant, antitussive

Robitussin Flu Liquid:
dextromethorphan 5 mg
chlorpheniramine 1 mg
pseudoephedrine 15 mg
acetaminophen 160 mg
Uses: Antitussive, antihistamine, decongestant, analgesic

Robitussin Honey Cough & Cold Liquid:
dextromethorphan 10 mg

🛆 Safety alert   *"Tall Man" lettering

pseudoephedrine 15 mg
Uses: Antitussive, decongestant
Robitussin Honey Flu Multi-Symptom Liquid:
dextromethorphan 6.6 mg
pseudoephedrine 20 mg
acetaminophen 166.7
Uses: Antitussive, decongestant, analgesic
Robitussin Honey Flu Night-Time Syrup:
dextromethorphan 20 mg
chlorpheniramine 4 mg
pseudoephedrine 60 mg
acetaminophen 500 mg
Uses: Antitussive, antihistamine, decongestant, analgesic
Robitussin Honey Flu Non-Drowsy Syrup:
dextromethorphan 20 mg
pseudoephedrine 60 mg
acetaminophen 500 mg
Uses: Antitussive, decongestant, analgesic
Robitussin Maximum Strength Cough and Cold Syrup:
dextromethorphan 15 mg
pseudoephedrine 30 mg
Uses: Antitussive, adrenergic
Robitussin Night Relief Liquid:
dextromethorphan 5 mg
pyrilamine 8.3 mg
pseudoephedrine 10 mg
acetaminophen 108.3 mg
Uses: Antitussive, adrenergic
Robitussin Pediatric Cough & Cold Liquid:
Per 5 ml:
pseudoephedrine 15 mg
dextromethorphan 7.5 mg
Uses: Antitussive, adrenergic
Robitussin Pediatric Night Relief Cough & Cold Liquid:
pseudoephedrine 15 mg
chlorpheniramine 1 mg
dextromethorphan 7.5 mg
Uses: Decongestant, antihistamine, antitussive

Robitussin PM Cough & Cold Liquid:
dextromethorphan 7.5 mg
chlorpheniramine 1 mg
pseudoephedrine 15 mg
Uses: Antitussive, antihistamine, decongestant
Robitussin Sugar Free Cough Liquid:
dextromethorphan 10 mg
guaifensin 100 mg
Uses: Antitussive, expectorant
Rolaids Calcium Rich:
magnesium hydroxide 80 mg
calcium carbonate 412 mg
Uses: Antacid, adsorbent, antiflatulent
Rondec:
pseudoephedrine 60 mg
carbinoxamine 4 mg
Uses: Adrenergic
Rondec DM Drops:
Per ml.
pseudoephedrine 25 mg
carbinoxamine 2 mg
dextromethorphan 4 mg
Uses: Adrenergic, antitussive
Rondec DM Syrup:
Per 5 ml:
pseudoephedrine 60 mg
carbinoxamine 4 mg
dextromethorphan 15 mg
Uses: Adrenergic, antitussive
Rondec Oral Drops:
Per 5 ml:
pseudoephedrine 25 mg
carbinoxamine 2 mg
Uses: Adrenergic
Roxicet:
Per 5 ml:
acetaminophen 325 mg
oxycodone 5 mg
Uses: Opioid analgesic
Roxicet 5/500:
oxycodone 5 mg
acetaminophen 500 mg
Uses: Opioid analgesic

Roxicet Oral Solution:
Per 5 ml:
acetaminophen 325 mg
oxycodone 5 mg
Uses: Analgesic

Roxiprin:
aspirin 325 mg
oxycodone HCl 4.5 mg
oxycodone terephthalate 0.38 mg
Uses: Analgesic

Ru-Tuss DE:
pseudoephedrine 120 mg
guaifenesin 600 mg
Uses: Adrenergic, expectorant

Ru-Tuss Expectorant Liquid:
Per 5 ml:
guaifenesin 100 mg
pseudoephedrine 30 mg
dextromethorphan 10 mg
10% alcohol
Uses: Adrenergic, expectorant, antitussive

Ru-Tuss with Hydrocodone Liquid:
Per 5 ml:
hydrocodone: 1.7 mg
phenylephrine 5 mg
pyrilamine 3.3 mg
pheniramine 3.3 mg
phenylpropanolamine 3.3 mg
5% alcohol
Uses: Antihistamine, analgesic,
  decongestant

Ryna-C Liquid:
Per 5 ml:
pseudoephedrine 30 mg
chlorpheniramine 2 mg
codeine 10 mg
Uses: Adrenergic, antihistamine, analgesic

Ryna Liquid:
Per 5 ml:
pseudoephedrine 30 mg
chlorpheniramine 2 mg
Uses: Adrenergic, antihistamine

Rynatan:
phenylephrine 25 mg
chlorpheniramine 8 mg
pyrilamine 25 mg

Uses: Adrenergic, antihistamine

Rynatan Pediatric Suspension:
Per 5 ml:
phenylephrine 5 mg
chlorpheniramine 2 mg
pyrilamine 12.5 mg
Uses: Adrenergic, antihistamine

Rynatuss:
epHEDrine 10 mg
carbetapentane 60 mg
chlorpheniramine 5 mg
phenylephrine 10 mg
Uses: Adrenergic, antihistamine

Saleto Tablets:
115 mg acetaminophen
210 mg aspirin
65 mg salicylamide
16 mg caffeine
Uses: Nonopioid analgesic

Salutensin:
hydroflumethiazide 50 mg
reserpine 0.125 mg
Uses: Antihypertensive

Salutensin Demi:
hydroflumethiazide 25 mg
reserpine 0.125 mg
Uses: Antihypertensive

Scot-Tussin DM Liquid:
Per 5 ml:
chlorpheniramine 2 mg
dextromethorphan 15 mg
Uses: Antihistamine, antitussive

**Scot-Tussin Original 5-Action
  Liquid:**
phenylephrine 4.2 mg
pheniramine 13.3 mg
sodium citrate 83.3 mg
sodium salicylate 83.3 mg
caffeine citrate 25 mg
Uses: Adrenergic, analgesic

Scot-Tussin Senior Clear Liquid:
Per 5 ml:
guaifenesin 200 mg
dextromethorphan 15 mg
Uses: Antitussive, expectorant

A Safety alert   *"Tall Man" lettering

Sedapap-10:
acetaminophen 650 mg
butalbital 50 mg
Uses: Analgesic, barbiturate

Semprex-D:
acrivastine 8 mg
pseudoephedrine 60 mg
Uses: Adrenergic, bronchodilator

Senokot-S:
docusate 50 mg
senna concentrate 187 mg
Uses: Laxative

Septra:
sulfamethoxazole 400 mg
trimethroprim 80 mg
Uses: Antiinfective

Septra DS:
sulfamethoxazole 800 mg
trimethroprim 160 mg
Uses: Antiinfective

Septra I.V. for Injection:
Per 5 ml:
trimethoprim 80 mg
sulfamethoxazole 400 mg
Uses: Antiinfective

Septra Suspension:
Per 5 ml:
trimethoprim 40 mg
sulfamethoxazole 200 mg
Uses: Antiinfective

Ser-A-Gen:
hydrochlorothiazide 15 mg
hydrALAZINE 25 mg
reserpine 0.1 mg
Uses: Antihypertensive

Ser-Ap-Es:
hydrochlorothiazide 15 mg
reserpine 0.1 mg
hydrALAZINE 25 mg
Uses: Diuretic, antihypertensive

Silafed Syrup:
Per 5 ml:
pseudoephedrine 30 mg
triprolidine 1.25 mg
Uses: Adrenergic, antihistamine

Silaminic Cold Syrup:
Per 5 ml:
phenylpropanolamine 12.5 mg
chlorpheniramine 2 mg
Uses: Antihistamine, decongestant

Sinarest Extra Strength:
pseudoephedrine 30 mg
chlorpheniramine 2 mg
acetaminophen 500 mg
Uses: Adrenergic, antihistamine, analgesic

Sinarest No Drowsiness:
pseudoephedrine 30 mg
acetaminophen 500 mg
Uses: Adrenergic, analgesic

Sinarest Sinus:
pseudoephedrine 30 mg
chlorpheniramine 2 mg
acetaminophen 325 mg
Uses: Adrenergic, antihistamine, analgesic

Sine-Aid IB:
pseudoephedrine 30 mg
ibuprofen 200 mg
Uses: Adrenergic, analgesic

Sine-Aid Maximum Strength:
pseudoephedrine 30 mg
acetaminophen 500 mg
Uses: Adrenergic, analgesic

Sinemet 10/100:
carbidopa 10 mg
levodopa 100 mg
Uses: Antiparkinsonian

Sinemet 25/100:
carbidopa 25 mg
levodopa 100 mg
Uses: Antiparkinsonian

Sinemet 25/250:
carbidopa 25 mg
levodopa 250 mg
Uses: Antiparkinsonian

Sinemet CR 25-100:
carbidopa 25 mg
levodopa 100 mg
Uses: Antiparkinsonian

Sinemet CR 50-200:
carbidopa 50 mg
levodopa 200 mg

Uses: Antiparkinsonian

Sine-Off Maximum Strength No Drowsiness Formula Caplets:
pseudoephedrine 30 mg
acetaminophen 500 mg
Uses: Adrenergic, analgesic

Sine-Off Sinus Medicine:
pseudoephedrine 30 mg
chlorpheniramine 2 mg
acetaminophen 500 mg
Uses: Adrenergic, antihistamine, analgesic

Sinus-Relief:
acetaminophen 325 mg
pseudoephedrine 30 mg
Uses: Nonopioid analgesic

Sinutab:
acetaminophen 325 mg
chlorpheniramine 2 mg
pseudoephedrine 30 mg
Uses: Nonopioid analgesic

Sinutab Maximum Strength Sinus Allergy:
acetaminophen 500 mg
pseudoephedrine 30 mg
chlorpheniramine 2 mg
Uses: Analgesic, adrenergic, antihistamine

Sinutab Maximum Strength Without Drowsiness:
acetaminophen 500 mg
pseudoephedrine 30 mg
Uses: Analgesic, adrenergic

Sinutab Non-Drying:
pseudoepedrine 30 mg
guaifenesin 200 mg
Uses: Adrenergic, expectorant

Slo-Phyllin GG Syrup:
theophylline 150 mg
guaifenesin 90 mg
Uses: Bronchodilator, expectorant

Slow-Salt-K:
sodium chloride 410 mg
potassium chloride 15 mg
Uses: Potassium, sodium supplement

Solage:
mequinol 2%
tretinoin 0.01%

Uses: Antineoplastic

Soma Compound w/Codeine:
carisoprodol 200 mg
aspirin 325 mg
codeine 16 mg
Uses: Skeletal muscle relaxant

Synophylate-GG Syrup:
theophylline 150 mg
guaifenesin 100 mg
15% alcohol
Uses: Bronchodilator, expectorant

Soma Compound:
carisoprodol 200 mg
aspirin 325 mg
Uses: Skeletal muscle relaxant, analgesic

Spec-T Lozenge:
dextromethorphan 10 mg
benzocaine 10 mg
Uses: Antitussive, topical anesthetic

Stalevo 50:
carbidopa 12.5 mg
levodopa 50 mg
entacapone 200 mg
Uses: Parkinsonism

Stalevo 100:
carbidopa 25 mg
levodopa 100 mg
entacapone 200 mg
Uses: Parkinsonism

Stalevo 150:
carbidopa 37.5 mg
levodopa 150 mg
entacapone 200 mg
Uses: Parkinsonism

Sudafed Cold & Allergy:
pseudoephedrine 60 mg
chlorpheniramine 4 mg
Uses: Adrenergic, antihistamine

Sudafed Cold & Cough Liquicaps:
pseudoephedrine 30 mg
dextromethorphan 10 mg
guaifenesin 100 mg
acetaminophen 250 mg
Uses: Adrenergic, antitussive, expectorant, analgesic

⚠ Safety alert   *"Tall Man" lettering

Sudafed Cold & Sinus:
pseudoephedrine 30 mg
acetaminophen 325 mg
Uses: Adrenergic, analgesic
Sudafed Plus:
pseudoephedrine 60 mg
chlorpheniramine 4 mg
Uses: Adrenergic, antihistamine
Sudafed Severe Cold:
pseudoephedrine 30 mg
dextromethorphan 15 mg
Uses: Adrenergic, antitussive
Sudafed Sinus Maximum Strength:
pseudoephedrine 30 mg
acetaminophen 500 mg
Uses: Adrenergic, analgesic
Sudal 60/500:
pseudoephedrine 60 mg
guaifenesin 500 mg
Uses: Adrenergic, expectorant
Sudal 120/600:
pseudoephedrine 120 mg
guaifenesin 600 mg
Uses: Adrenergic, expectorant
Sulfimycin Suspension:
Per 5 ml:
erythromycin 200 mg
sulfiSOXAZOLE 600 mg
Uses: Macrolide antiinfective
Sultrin Triple Sulfa Vaginal Cream:
3.42% sulfathiazole
2.86% sulfacetamine
3.7% sulfabenzamide
Uses: Antiinfective
Sultrin Triple Sulfa Vaginal Tablets:
sulfathiazole 172.5 mg
sulfacetamide 143.75
sulfabenzamide 184 mg
Uses: Antiinfective
Symbyax:
olanzapine 6 mg
fluoxetine 25 mg

olanzapine 6 mg
fluoxetine 50 mg

olanzapine 12 mg

fluoxetine 25 mg
olanzapine 12 mg
fluoxetine 50 mg
Uses: Bipolar disorder
Synalgos-DC:
aspirin 356.4 mg
caffeine 30 mg
dihydrocodeine 16 mg
Uses: Analgesic
Synercid:
quinupristin 150 mg
dalfopristin 350 mg
Uses: Antiinfective
Syntest D.S.:
esterified estrogens 1.25 mg
methylTESTOSTERone 2.5 mg
Uses: Menopause
Syntest H.S.:
esterified estrogens 0.625 mg
methylTESTOSTERone 1.25 mg
Uses: Menopause
Talacen:
acetaminophen 650 mg
pentazocine 25 mg
Uses: Analgesic
Talwin Compound:
aspirin 325 mg
pentazocine 12.5 mg
Uses: Analgesic
Talwin NX:
pentazocine 50 mg
naloxone 0.5 mg
Uses: Analgesic, opioid antagonist
Tarka 182:
trandolapril 2 mg (immed rel)
verapamil 180 mg (sus rel)
Uses: Antihypertensive, calcium channel
    blocker
Tarka 241:
trandolapril 1 mg (immed rel)
verapamil 240 mg (sus rel)
Uses: Antihypertensive, calcium channel
    blocker
Tarka 242:
trandolapril 2 mg (immed rel)
verapamil 240 mg (sus rel)

Uses: Antihypertensive, calcium channel
blocker

Tarka 244:

trandolapril 4 mg (immed rel)

verapamil 240 mg (sus rel)

Uses: Antihypertensive, calcium channel
blocker

Tavist Allergy/Sinus Headache:

clemastine 0.335 mg

pseudoephedrine 30 mg

acetaminophen 500 mg

Uses: Antihistamine, adrenergic, analgesic

Tavist Sinus:

acetaminophen 500 mg

pseudoephedrine 30 mg

Uses: Analgesic, adrenergic

♣ **Tecnal:**

aspirin 330 mg

caffeine 40 mg

butalbital 50 mg

Uses: Nonopioid analgesic

Teczem:

enalapril 5 mg (extended release)

diltiazem 180 mg (extended release)

Uses: Antihypertensive, calcium channel
blocker

Tedrigen:

epHEDrine 22.5 mg

theophylline 120 mg

phenobarbital 7.5 mg

Uses: Adrenergic, bronchodilator, barbiturate

Tegrin-LT Shampoo:

0.33% pyrethrins

3.15% piperonyl butoxide

Uses: Scabicide, pediculicide

Tenoretic 50:

atenolol 50 mg

chlorthalidone 25 mg

Uses: Antihypertensive

Tenoretic 100:

atenolol 100 mg

chlorthalidone 25 mg

Uses: Antihypertensive

Terra-Cortril Ophthalmic Suspension:

1.5% hydrocortisone acetate

0.5% oxytetracycline

Uses: Ophthalmic antiinflammatory, antiinfective

**Terramycin w/Polymycin B Sulfate
Ophthalmic Ointment:**

Per gram:

polymyxin B 10,000 units

oxytetracycline 5 mg

Uses: Ophthalmic antiinfective

T-Gesic:

hydrocodone 5 mg

acetaminophen 500 mg

Uses: Analgesic

Theodrine:

epHEDrine 22.5 mg

theophylline 120 mg

Uses: Adrenergic, bronchodilator

Thera-Flu Cold & Cough Powder:

Per packet:

pseudoephedrine 60 mg

chlorpheniramine 4 mg

dextromethorphan 20 mg

acetaminophen 650 mg

Uses: Adrenergic, antihistamine, antitussive,
analgesic

**Thera-Flu Flu & Chest Congestion
Non-Drowsy Powder:**

dextromethorphan 30 mg

guaifenesin 400 mg

pseudoephedrine 60 mg

acetaminophen 1000 mg

Uses: Antitussive, expectorant, decongestant, analgesic

**Thera-Flu Flu, Cold, Cough & Sore
Throat Maximum Strength Powder:**

dextromethorphan 30 mg

chlorpheniramine 4 mg

pseudoephedrine 60 mg

acetaminophen 1000 mg

Uses: Antitussive, antihistamine, decongestant, analgesic

🛆 Safety alert   *"Tall Man" lettering

Thera-Flu Maximum Strength Flu, Cold & Cough Powder:
dextromethorphan 30 mg
guaifenesin 400 mg
pseudoephedrine 60 mg
acetaminophen 1000 mg
Uses: Antitussive, expectorant, decongestant, analgesic

Thera-Flu Non-Drowsy Flu, Cold & Cough Maximum Strength Powder:
Per packet:
pseudoephedrine 60 mg
dextromethorphan 30 mg
acetaminophen 1000 mg
Uses: Decongestant, antitussive, analgesic

Thera-Flu Severe Cold & Congestion NightTime Maximum Strength Powder:
Per packet:
pseudoephedrine 60 mg
chlorpheniramine 4 mg
dextromethorphan 30 mg
acetaminophen 1000 mg
Uses: Decongestant, antihistamine, antitussive, analgesic

Thera-Flu Severe Cold & Congestion Non-Drowsy Maximum Strength Powder:
dextromethorphan 30 mg
pseudoephedrine 60 mg
acetaminophen 1000 mg
Uses: Antitussive, decongestant, acetaminophen

Thera-Flu Severe Cold & Cough Powder:
dextromethorphan 30 mg
chlorpheniramine 4 mg
pseudoephedrine 60 mg
acetaminophen 1000 mg
Uses: Antitussive, antihistamine, decongestant, analgesic

Thera-Flu Severe Cold Non-Drowsy Packet:
dextromethorphan 30 mg
pseudoephedrine 60 mg
acetaminophen 1000 mg
Uses: Antitussive, decongestant, acetaminophen

Thera-Flu Severe Cold Non-Drowsy Tablets:
dextromethorphan 15 mg
pseudoephedrine 30 mg
acetaminophen 500 mg
Uses: Antitussive, decongestant, analgesic

Thera-Flu Severe Cold Tablets:
dextromethorphan 15 mg
chlorpheniramine 2 mg
pseudoephedrine 30 mg
acetaminophen 500 mg
Uses: Antitussive, antihistamine, decongestant, analgesic

Timentin for Injection:
Per 3.1-g vial:
ticarcillin 3 g
clavulanic acid 0.1 g
Uses: Antiinfective

Timolide 10/25:
timolol 10 mg
hydrochlorothiazide 25 mg
Uses: Antihypertensive

Titralac Plus:
calcium carbonate 420 mg
simethicone 21 mg
Uses: Antacid, adsorbent, antiflatulent

Tobra Dex Ophthalmic Suspension/Ointment:
tobramycin 0.3%
dexamethasone 0.1%
Uses: Ophthalmic antiinfective, antiinflammatory

Triacin-C Cough Syrup:
Per 5 ml:
codeine 10 mg
pseudoephedrine 30 mg
triprolidine 1.25 mg
Uses: Analgesic, adrenergic, antihistamine

Triad:
acetaminophen 325 mg
caffeine 40 mg
butalbital 50 mg
Uses: Nonopioid analgesic

✦ Canada only   Side effects: *italics* = common; ***bold italics*** = life-threatening

Tri-Hydroserpine:
hydrALAZINE 25 mg
hydrochlorothiazide 15 mg
reserpine 0.1 mg
Uses: Antihypertensive

Tri-Levlen:
Phase I:
levonorgestrel 0.05 mg
ethinyl estradiol 30 mcg
Phase II:
levonorgestrel 0.075 mg
ethinyl estradiol 40 mcg;
Phase III:
levonorgestrel 0.125 mg
ethinyl estradiol 30 mcg
Uses: Oral contraceptive

Triaminic AM Cough & Decongestant Formula Liquid:
Per 5 ml:
pseudoephedrine 15 mg
dextromethorphan 7.5 mg
Uses: Adrenergic, antitussive

Triaminic Nite Light Liquid:
Per 5 ml:
pseudoephedrine 15 mg
chlorpheniramine 1 mg
dextromethorphan 7.5 mg
Uses: Adrenergic, antihistamine, antitussive

Triaminic Sore Throat Formula Liquid:
Per 5 ml:
pseudoephedrine 15 mg
dextromethorphan 7.5 mg
acetaminophen 160 mg
Uses: Adrenergic, antitussive

Triavil 2-10:
perphenazine 2 mg
amitriptyline 10 mg
Uses: Antipsychotic, antidepressant

Triavil 2-25:
perphenazine 2 mg
amitriptyline 25 mg
Uses: Antipsychotic, antidepressant

Triavil 4-10:
perphenazine 4 mg
amitriptyline 10 mg

Triavil 4-25:
perphenazine 4 mg
amitriptyline 25 mg
Uses: Antipsychotic, antidepressant

Triavil 4-50:
perphenazine 4 mg
amitriptyline 50 mg
Uses: Antipsychotic, antidepressant

Trinalin Repetabs:
azatadine maleate 1 mg
pseudoephedrine 120 mg
Uses: Antihistamine

Triphasil:
Phase I:
levonorgestrel 0.05 mg
ethinyl estradiol 30 mcg
Phase II:
levonorgestrel 0.075 mg
ethinyl estradiol 40 mcg
Phase III:
levonorgestrel 0.125 mg
ethinyl estradiol 30 mcg
Uses: Oral contraceptive

Triple Antibiotic Ophthalmic Ointment:
Per gram:
polymyxin B 10,000 units
neomycin 3.5 mg
bacitracin 400 units
Uses: Antiinfective

Triprolidine/Pseudoephedrine Syrup (generic):
Per 5 ml
triprolidine 1.25 mg
pseudoephedrine 50 mg
Uses: Antihistamine, decongestant

Triprolidine/Pseudoephedrine Tablets (generic):
triprolidine 2.5 mg
pseudoephedrine 60 mg
Uses: Antihistamine, decongestant

Triposed Tablets:
triprolidine 150 mg
pseudoephedrine 60 mg
Uses: Decongestant, antihistamine

Trizivir:
300 mg abacavir
150 mg lamivudine
300 mg zidovudine
Uses: HIV
Truvada:
emtricitabine 200 mg
tenofovir 300 mg
Uses: HIV
Tuinal 100 mg:
amobarbital 50 mg
secobarbital 50 mg
Uses: Sedative-hypnotic
Tuinal 200 mg:
amobarbital 100 mg
secobarbital 100 mg
Uses: Sedative-hypnotic
Tusibron-DM Syrup:
Per 5 ml:
guaifenesin 100 mg
dextromethorphan 15 mg
Uses: Expectorant, antitussive
Tussionex Pennkinetic Suspension:
Per 5 ml:
chlorpheniramine 8 mg
hydrocodone 10 mg
Uses: Antihistamine, analgesic
Tussi-Organidin NR Liquid:
Per 5 ml:
codeine 10 mg
guaifenesin 100 mg
Uses: Analgesic, expectorant
Tussi-Organidin DM NR Liquid:
Per 5 ml:
guaifenesin 100 mg
dextromethorphan 10 mg
Uses: Expectorant, antitussive
Twinrix:
hepatitis A vaccine
hepatitis B vaccine
Uses: Vaccine
Two-Dyne:
acetaminophen 325 mg
caffeine 40 mg
butalbital 50 mg
Uses: Nonopioid analgesic

Tylenol Allergy Sinus, Maximum Strength Gelcaps:
acetaminophen 500 mg
chlorpheniramine 2 mg
pseudoephedrine 30 mg
Uses: Antihistamine, adrenergic, analgesic
Tylenol Children's Cold:
acetaminophen 80 mg
chlorpheniramine 0.5 mg
pseudoephedrine 7.5 mg
Uses: Antihistamine, adrenergic, analgesic
Tylenol Children's Cold Liquid:
Per 5 ml:
acetaminophen 160 mg
chlorpheniramine 1 mg
pseudoephedrine 15 mg
Uses: Antihistamine, adrenergic, analgesic
Tylenol Children's Cold Multi-Symptom Plus Cough Liquid:
Per 5 ml:
acetaminophen 160 mg
dextromethorphan 5 mg
chlorpheniramine 1 mg
pseudoephedrine 15 mg
Uses: Antihistamine, adrenergic, analgesic
Tylenol Children's Cold Plus Cough Chewable:
acetaminophen 80 mg
pseudoephedrine 7.5 mg
dextromethorphan 2.5 mg
chlorpheniramine 0.5 mg
Uses: Antihistamine, adrenergic, analgesic
Tylenol Children's Cold Plus Cough Suspension:
pseudoephedrine 15 mg
chlorpheniramine 1 mg
dextromethorphan 5 mg
acetaminophen 160 mg
Uses: Decongestant, antihistamine, antitussive, analgesic
Tylenol Children's Flu Suspension:
pseudoephedrine 15 mg
chlorpheniramine 1 mg
dextromethorphan 7.5 mg
acetaminophen 160 mg

Uses: Decongestant, antihistamine, antitussive, analgesic

Tylenol Cold Complete Formula Tablets:

acetaminophen 325 mg
chlorpheniramine 2 mg
pseudoephedrine 30 mg
dextromethorphan 15 mg
Uses: Antihistamine, adrenergic, analgesic

Tylenol Cold & Flu Severe DayTime Liquid:

dextromethorphan 5 mg
pseudoephedrine 10 mg
acetaminophen 166.7 mg
Uses: Antitussive, decongestant, analgesic

Tylenol Cold Severe Congestion Tablets:

dextromethorphan 15 mg
guaifenesin 200 mg
pseudoephedrine 32 mg
acetaminophen 325 mg
Uses: Antitussive, expectorant, decongestant, analgesic

Tylenol Cough & Sore Throat DayTime Liquid:

dextromethorphan 5 mg
acetaminophen 166.7 mg
Uses: Antitussive, analgesic

Tylenol Flu Maximum Strength Non-Drowsy Gelcaps:

dextromethorphan 15 mg
pseudoephedrine 30 mg
acetaminophen 500 mg
Uses: Analgesic, adrenergic, antitussive

Tylenol Flu NightTime Maximum Strength Liquid:

dextromethorphan 5 mg
doxylamine 2.1 mg
pseudoephedrine 10 mg
acetaminophen 167 mg
Uses: Antitussive, antihistamine, decongestant, acetaminophen

Tylenol Headache Plus, Extra Strength:

acetaminophen 500 mg
calcium carbonate 250 mg
Uses: Analgesic, antacid

Tylenol PM, Extra Strength:

acetaminophen 500 mg
diphenhydrAMINE 25 mg
Uses: Analgesic, antihistamine

Tylenol Severe Allergy:

diphenhydrAMINE 12.5 mg
acetaminophen 500 mg
Uses: Analgesic, antihistamine

Tylenol Sinus Maximum Strength:

pseudoephedrine 30 mg
acetaminophen 500 mg
Uses: Adrenergic, analgesic

Tylenol w/Codeine Elixir:

Per 5 ml:
acetaminophen 120 mg
codeine 12 mg
Uses: Analgesic

Tylenol w/Codeine No. 1:

acetaminophen 300 mg
codeine 7.5 mg
Uses: Analgesic

Tylenol w/Codeine No. 2:

acetaminophen 300 mg
codeine 15 mg

Tylenol w/Codeine No. 3:

acetaminophen 300 mg
codeine 30 mg
Uses: Analgesic

Tylenol w/Codeine No. 4:

acetaminophen 300 mg
codeine 60 mg
Uses: Analgesic

Tylox:

oxycodone 5 mg
acetaminophen 500 mg
Uses: Analgesic

Tyrodone Liquid:

Per 5 ml:
hydrocodone 5 mg
pseudoephedrine 60 mg
5% alcohol
Uses: Analgesic, adrenergic

Ultracet:

tramadol 37.5 mg
acetaminophen 325 mg
Uses: Analgesic

🅐 Safety alert   *"Tall Man" lettering

Unasyn for Injection 3 g:
ampicillin 2 g
sulbactam 1 g
Uses: Antiinfective
Uniretic:
moexipril 7.5 mg
hydrochlorothiazide 12.5 mg
or moexipril 15 mg
hydrochlorothiazide 25 mg
Uses: Antihypertensive, diuretic
Unituss HC Syrup:
hydrocodone 2.5 mg
phenylephrine 5 mg
chlorpheniramine 2 mg
Uses: Analgesic, adrenergic, antihistamine
Urised:
methenamine 40.8 mg
phenylsalicylate 18.1 mg
atropine 0.03 mg
hyoscyamine 0.03 mg
benzoic acid 4.5 mg
methylene blue 5.4 mg
Uses: Antiinfective
Urobiotic 250:
oxytetracycline 250 mg
sulfamethizole 250 mg
phenazopyridine 50 mg
Uses: Antiinfective
Vanquish:
aspirin 227 mg
acetaminophen 194 mg
caffeine 33 mg
aluminum hydroxide 25 mg
magnesium hydroxide 50 mg
Uses: Nonopioid analgesic
Vaseretic 5-12.5:
enalapril 5 mg
hydrochlorthiazide 12.5 mg
Uses: Antihypertensive diuretic
Vaseretic 10-25:
enalapril 10 mg
hydrochlorothiazide 25 mg
Uses: Antihypertensive, diuretic
Vasocidin Ophthalmic Ointment:
sulfacetamide 10%
prednisoLONE 0.5%
Uses: Ophthalmic antiinfective,
    antiinflammatory
Vasocidin Ophthalmic Solution:
sulfacetamide 10%
prednisoLONE 0.25%
Uses: Ophthalmic antiinfective,
    antiinflammatory
Vasocon-A Ophthalmic Solution:
naphazoline 0.05%
antazoline 0.5%
Uses: Ophthalmic vasoconstrictor
**Vicks 44D Cough & Head Congestion
    Liquid:**
Per 5 ml:
dextromethorphan 10 mg
pseudoephedrine 20 mg
Uses: Antitussive, adrenergic
Vicks 44E Liquid:
Per 5 ml:
dextromethorphan 6.7 mg
guaifenesin 66.7 mg
Uses: Antitussive, expectorant
**Vicks 44M Cold, Flu, & Cough
    LiquiCaps:**
dextromethorphan 10 mg
pseudoephedrine 30 mg
chlorpheniramine 2 mg
acetaminophen 250 mg
Uses: Antitussive, adrenergic, antihistamine,
    analgesic
**Vicks 44 Non-Drowsy Cold & Cough
    LiquiCaps:**
dextromethorphan 30 mg
pseudoephedrine 60 mg
Uses: Antitussive, adrenergic
**Vicks Children's NyQuil Nighttime
    Cough/Cold Liquid:**
Per 5 ml:
pseudoephedrine 10 mg
chlorpheniramine 0.67 mg
dextromethorphan 5 mg
Uses: Adrenergic, antihistamine, antitussive
Vicks Cough Silencers:
dextromethorphan 2.5 mg
benzocaine 1 mg
Uses: Antitussive, top anesthetic

Vicks DayQuil Liquid:
Per 5 ml:
dextromethorphan 3.3 mg
pseudoephedrine 10 mg
acetaminophen 108.3 mg
guaifenesin 33.3 mg
Uses: Antitussive, adrenergic, analgesic,
    expectorant

**Vicks DayQuil Multi-Symptom Cold/
    Flu Relief Liquid:**
dextromethorphan 33 mg
pseudoephedrine 10 mg
acetaminophen 108.3 mg
Uses: Antitussive, decongestant, analgesic

**Vicks DayQuil Sinus Pressure & Pain
    Relief:**
pseudoephedrine 30 mg
acetaminophen 500 mg
Uses: Adrenergic, analgesic

Vicks NyQuil Liquicaps:
pseudoephedrine 30 mg
doxylamine 6.25 mg
dextromethorphan 10 mg
acetaminophen 250 mg
Uses: Adrenergic, antihistamine, antitussive,
    analgesic

**Vicks NyQuil Multi-Symptom Cold Flu
    Relief Liquid:**
pseudoephedrine 10 mg
doxylamine 2.1 mg
dextromethorphan 5 mg
acetaminophen 167 mg
Uses: Adrenergic, antihistamine, antitussive,
    analgesic

**Vicks Pediatric Formula 44e Cough &
    Chest Congestion Relief Liquid:**
Per 5 ml:
dextromethorphan 3.3 mg
guaifenesin 33.3 mg
Uses: Expectorant, antitussive

**Vicks Pediatric Formula 44 m Multi-
    Symptom Cough & Cold Liquid:**
pseudoephedrine 10 mg
chlorpheniramine 0.67 mg
dextromethorphan 5 mg

Uses: Adrenergic, antihistamine, antitussive

Vicodin:
acetaminophen 500 mg
hydrocodone 5 mg
Uses: Analgesic

Vicodin ES:
acetaminophen 750 mg
hydrocodone 7.5 mg
Uses: Analgesic

Vicodin HP:
hydrocodone 10 mg
acetaminophen 660 mg
Uses: Analgesic

VicodinTuss:
Per 5 ml:
hydrocodone 5 mg
guaifenesin 100 mg
Uses: Analgesic, expectorant

Vicoprofen:
hydrocodone 7.5 mg
ibuprofen 200 mg
Uses: Analgesic

Vytorin:
ezetimibe: 10, 10, 10, 10 mg
simvastatin: 10, 20, 40, 80 mg
Uses: Antihyperlipidemic

Wigraine Suppositories:
ergotamine 2 mg
caffeine 100 mg
Uses: α-Adrenergic blocker

Yasmin 28:
ethinyl estadiol 30 mcg
dropirenone 3 mg
Uses: Oral contraceptive

Zestoretic 10/12.5:
lisinopril 10 mg
hydrochlorothiazide 12.5 mg
Uses: Antihypertensive

Zestoretic 20/12.5:
lisinopril 20 mg
hydrochlorothiazide 12.5 mg
Uses: Antihypertensive

Zestoretic 20/25:
lisinopril 20 mg
hydrochlorothiazide 25 mg
Uses: Antihypertensive

Ziac 2.5:
bisoprolol 2.5 mg
hydrochlorothiazide 6.25 mg
Uses: Antihypertensive
Ziac 5:
bisoprolol 5 mg
hydrochlorothiazide 6.25 mg
Uses: Antihypertensive
Ziac 10:
bisoprolol 10 mg
hydrochlorothiazide 6.25 mg

Uses: Antihypertensive
Ziks Cream:
methyl salicylate 12%
menthol 1%
capsaicin 0.025%
Uses: Analgesic, decongestant
Zydone:
hydrocodone 5 mg
acetaminophen 500 mg
Uses: Analgesic

Appendix j

High-alert drugs

The Institute for Safe Medication Practices (ISMP) recently compiled a list of the medications with the greatest potential for patient harm if they are used in error. These high-alert medications include drugs in the 19 classes listed below, as well as the specific drugs listed below. To help nurses identify these drugs, each specific drug monograph is clearly identified in this book. While care should be taken in giving any medication, nurses are advised to exercise extra precautions when administering these high-risk drugs.

Class/Category of Medications
adrenergic agonists, IV (e.g., epINEPHrine)
adrenergic antagonists, IV (e.g., propranolol)
anesthetic agents, general, inhaled and IV (e.g., propofol)
cardioplegic solutions
chemotherapeutic agents, parenteral and oral
dextrose, hypertonic, 20% or greater
dialysis solutions, peritoneal and hemodialysis
epidural or intrathecal medications
glycoprotein IIb/IIIa inhibitors (e.g., eptifibatide)
hypoglycemics, oral
inotropic medications, IV (e.g., digoxin, milrinone)
liposomal forms of drugs (e.g., liposomal amphotericin B)
moderate sedation agents, IV (e.g., midazolam)
moderate sedation agents, oral, for children (e.g., chloral hydrate)
narcotics/opiates, IV and oral (including liquid concentrates, immediate- and sustained-release)
neuromuscular blocking agents (e.g., succinylcholine)
radiocontrast agents, IV
thrombolytics/fibrinolytics, IV (e.g., tenecteplase)
total parenteral nutrition solutions

Individual Medications

abciximab
adenosine
aldesleukin
alteplase
amiodarone
anistreplase
antihemophilic factor VIII (AHF)
antithrombin III, human
ardeparin
argatroban
arsenic trioxide
asparaginase

atropine
azacitidine
basiliximab
bevacizumab
bivalirudin
bleomycin
busulfan
carboplatin
carmustine
celecoxib
cisplatin

A Safety alert   *"Tall Man" lettering

coagulation factor VIIa,
  recombinant
cyclophosphamide
cytarabine
dacarbazine
daclizumab
dactinomycin
dalteparin
danaparoid
DAUNOrubicin
digoxin
diltiazem
DOPamine
doxacurium
DOXOrubicin
droperidol
enoxaparin
epHEDrine
epINEPHrine
epirubicin
eptifibatide
etoposide
factor IX complex (human)/factor IV
fentanyl
fluorouracil
gemtuzumab
heparin
hydromorphone
ibutilide
idarubicin
ifosfamide
inamrinone
insulin
irinotecan
lepirudin
leuprolide
lidocaine (parenteral)
magnesium sulfate
melphalan
meperidine
methadone
methotrexate

milrinone
mitomycin
mitoxantrone
mivacurium
morphine
nalbuphine
nesiritide
nitroprusside
norepinephrine
oxycodone
oxymorphone
oxytocin
pancuronium
pegaspargase
pemetrexed
pentazocine
pentobarbital
pentostatin
phenobarbital
plicamycin
poractant alfa
propofol
propoxyphene
remifentanil
rocuronium
secobarbital
streptokinase
succinylcholine
tenecteplase
thiopental
tinzaparin
tirofiban
topotecan
trastuzumab
tubocurarine
urokinase
vecuronium
vinBLAStine
vinCRIStine
vinorelbine
warfarin

1. Cohen MR, Kilo CM: High-alert medications: safeguarding against errors. In Cohen MR, editor: *Medication errors*, Washington, DC, 1999, American Pharmaceutical Association.
2. High-alert medications and patient safety, *Sentinel Event Alert* 11, Nov 1999.
3. *ISMP's list of high-alert medications*, accessed 2/1/06 at http://www.ismp.org/tools/highalertmedications.pdf.

❖ Canada only   Side effects: *italics* = common; ***bold italics*** = life-threatening

Appendix k Drugs metabolized by known P450s

1A2	2B6	2C19	2C9	2D6	3A
Clozapine	Buproprion	Amitriptyline	Celecoxib	Amitriptyline	Alprazolam
Cyclobenzaprine	Cyclophosphamide	Carisoprodol	Diclofenac	Carvedilol	Buspirone
Fluvoxamine	Efavirenz	Citalopram	Flurbiprofen	Clomipramine	Calcium
Haloperidol	Ifosfamide	Clomipramine	Ibuprofen	Codeine	Channel Blockers
Imipramine	Methadone	Diazepam	Losartan	Desipramine	Carbamazepine
Mexiletine		Imipramine	Naproxen	Dextromethorphan	CycloSPORINE
Olanzapine		Lansoprazole	Phenytoin	Fluoxetine	Efavirenz
Tacrine		Nelfinavir	Piroxicam	Metoprolol	Haloperidol
Theophylline		Omeprazole	Torsemide	Nortriptyline	HIV Protease Inhibitors
Zileuton		Phenytoin	TOLBUTamide	Ondansetron	statins
Zolmitriptan		Pantoprazole	Warfarin	Oxycodone	NOT Pravastatin
				Paroxetine	Midazolam
				Propafenone	Nevirapine
				Risperidone	Tacrolimus
				Timolol	Triazolam
					Zolpidem

INHIBITORS

Cimetidine	Thiotepa	Cimetidine	Amiodarone	Amiodarone	Amiodarone
Ciprofloxacin		Felbamate	Fluconazole	Chlorpheniramine	Diltiazem & Verapamil
Fluvoxamine		Fluoxetine	Fluoxetine	Fluoxetine	Grapefruit Juice
Levofloxacin		Fluvoxamine	Fluvastatin	Haloperidol	HIV Protease Inhibitors
		Isoniazid	Metronidazole	Indinavir	Itraconazole
		Ketoconazole	Praoxetine	Paroxetine	Ketoconazole
		Lansoprazole	Zafirlukast	Ritonavir	Macrolide Antibiotics
		Omeprazple		Terbinafine	(NOT Azithromycin)
		Ticlopidine		Ticlopidine	Nefazodone

INDUCERS

Carbamazepine	Phenobarbital	Carbamazepine	Phenobarbital		Carbamazepine
Char-grilled Meat	Phenytoin	Rifampin	Rifampin		Efavirenz & Nevirapine
Rifampin	Rifampin				Rifabutin & Rifampin
Tobacco					Ritonavir
					St. John's Wort
Absent in 15%-30% of Asians	Absent in ~1% of Caucasians			Absent in 7% of Caucasians	

Copyright 2005, David A. Flockhart, MD, PhD, Indiana University School of Medicine, http://medicine.iupui.edu/flockhart/.

Appendix I

Look-alike/sound-alike drug names

Accolate	Accupril	Adipex-P	Aciphex
Accolate	Accutane	Adriamycin	Aredia
Accupril	Accutane	Adriamycin	Idamycin
Accupril	Aciphex	Advair	Advicor
Accupril	Accolate	Advicor	Advair
Accupril	Altace	Aggrastat	Aggrenox
Accupril	Aricept	Aggrastat	argatroban
Accupril	Monopril	Aggrenox	Aggrastat
Accutane	Accolate	Akarpine	atropine
Accutane	Accupril	albuterol	acebutolol
acebutolol	albuterol	Aldara	Alora
acetaminophen and codeine	acetaminophen and hydrocodone	aldesleukin	oprelvekin
		Aldomet	Adalat CC
acetaminophen and codeine	acetaminophen and oxycodone	Alkeran	Leukeran
		Allegra	Adalat CC
acetaminophen and hydrocodone	acetaminophen and codeine	Allegra	Allegra-D
		Allegra	Asacol
acetaminophen and oxycodone	acetaminophen and codeine	Allegra	Viagra
		Allegra-D	Allegra
acetaZOLAMIDE	acetoHEXAMIDE	Allegra-D	Allerx-D
acetaZOLAMIDE	acetylcysteine	Allerx-D	Allegra-D
acetaZOLAMIDE	acyclovir	allopurinol	Apresoline
acetoHEXAMIDE	acetaZOLAMIDE	Alora	Aldara
acetylcysteine	acetaZOLAMIDE	alprazolam	clonazepam
Aciphex	Accupril	alprazolam	diazepam
Aciphex	Adipex-p	alprazolam	lorazepam
Aciphex	Aricept	Altace	Accupril
Activase	Retavase	Altace	Amaryl
Actonel	Actos	Altace	Amerge
Actos	Actonel	Altace	Artane
Acular	ocular lubricants	Altace	Norvasc
acyclovir	acetaZOLAMIDE	Alupent	Atrovent
acyclovir	famiciclovir	amantadine	amiodarone
Adalat CC	Aldomat	amantadine	ranitidine
Adalat CC	Allegra	amantadine	rimantadine
Adderall	Inderal	Amaryl	Altace
adenosine	adenosine phosphate	Amaryl	Amerge
		Amaryl	Avandia
adenosine phosphate	adenosine	Amaryl	Reminyl
		Amaryl	Symmetrel

Ambien	Amen	Anusol-HC	Anusol
Ambien	Ativan	Anzemet	Aricept
Ambien	Coumadin	Apresoline	allopurinol
Amen	Ambien	Apresoline	Priscoline
Amerge	Altace	Aredia	Adriamycin
Amerge	Amaryl	argatroban	Aggrastat
Amicar	Amikin	argatroban	Orgaran
amikacin	anakinra	Aricept	Accupril
Amikin	Amicar	Aricept	Aciphex
amiloride	amlodipine	Aricept	Anzemet
aminophylline	amitriptyline	Artane	Altace
amiodarone	trazodone	Asacol	Allegra
amiodarone	amantadine	Asacol	Ansaid
amiodarone	amlodipine	Asacol	Os-Cal
amiodarone	amrinone (former	asparaginase	pegaspargase
	nomenclature	Atacand	antacid
	for inamrinone)	Atacand	Avandia
amitriptyline	aminophylline	Atarax	amoxicillin
amitriptyline	imipramine	Atarax	Ativan
amitriptyline	nortriptyline	atenolol	metoprolol
amlodipine	amiloride	Atgam	ratgam (synonym
amlodipine	amiodarone		for Thymo-
amlodipine	felodipine		globulin)
amoxicillin	Amoxil	Ativan	Ambien
amoxicillin	ampicillin	Ativan	Atarax
amoxicillin	Atarax	atorvastatin	pravastatin
amoxicillin	Augmentin	atropine	Akarpine
Amoxil	amoxicillin	Atrovent	Alupent
amphotericin B,	amphotericin B,	Atrovent	Azmacort
lipid complex	liposomal	Atrovent	Flovent
amphotericin B,	amphotericin B,	Atrovent	Natru-Vent
liposomal	lipid complex	Atrovent	Serevent
ampicillin	amoxicillin	Attenuvax	Meruvax
ampicillin	Augmentin	Augmentin	amoxicillin
ampicillin	oxacillin	Augmentin	ampicillin
amrinone (former	amiodarone	Avandia	Amaryl
nomenclature		Avandia	Atacand
for inamrinone)		Avandia	Avelox
Anaflex	Zanaflex	Avandia	Coumadin
anakinra	amikacin	Avandia	Prandin
Anaprox	Avapro	Avapro	Anaprox
Anaspaz	Antispas	Avapro	Avelox
Anbesol	Anusol	Avelox	Avandia
Ansaid	Asacol	Avelox	Avapro
antacid	Atacand	Avelox	Cerebyx
Antispas	Anaspaz	Avinza	Invanz
Anusol	Anbesol	Avonex	Lovenox
Anusol	Anusol-HC	azithromycin	erythromycin

azithromycin	vancomycin	bupivacaine	ropivacaine
azithromycin	aztreonam	Buprenex	Bumex
Azmacort	Atrovent	buPROPion	busPIRone
Azmacort	Nasacort	BuSpar	Boost bar
aztreonam	azithromycin	busPIRone	buPROPion
Bactrim	Biaxin	butalbital,	butalbital, aspirin,
Bactrim DS	Bancap HC	acetaminophen,	and caffeine
Bancap HC	Bactrim DS	and caffeine	
Baycol	Bellergal	butalbital, aspirin,	butalbital,
Beclovent	Beconase	and caffeine	acetaminophen,
Beconase	Beclovent		and caffeine
Beconase	Beconase AQ		
Beconase AQ	Beconase	Cafergot	Carafate
Bellergal	Baycol	Calan	Calan SR
Benadryl	benazepril	Calan	Colace
Benadryl	Bentyl	Calan SR	Calan
Benadryl	Benylin	Calan SR	Cardizem CD
benazepril	Benadryl	Calan SR	Cardizem SR
benazepril	benzonatate	Calciferol	calcitriol
benazepril	donepezil	calcitriol	Calciferol
benazepril	lisinopril	calcium acetate	calcium carbonate
Bentyl	Benadryl	calcium carbonate	calcium acetate
Bentyl	Bumex	calcium carbonate	calcium gluconate
Bentyl	Proventil	calcium chloride	calcium gluconate
Benylin	Benadryl	calcium gluconate	calcium carbonate
Benylin	Ventolin	calcium gluconate	calcium chloride
benzonatate	benazepril	Capoten	Catapres
benzonatate	benztropine	captopril	carvedilol
benztropine	benzonatate	Carafate	Cafergot
bepridil	Prepidil	Carbatrol	Carbrital
Betagan	Betoptic	(carbamezapine	(pentobarbitone
Betapace	Betapace AF	in U.S.)	sodium in
Betapace AF	Betapace		Australia)
Betoptic	Betagan	carbidopa	levodopa and
Betoptic	Betoptic S		carbidopa
Betoptic S	Betoptic	carboplatin	cisplatin
Biaxin	Bactrim	Carbrital	Carbatrol
bisacodyl	bisoprolol	(pentobarbitone	(carbamezapine
bisacodyl	Visicol	sodium in	in U.S.)
bisoprolol	bisacodyl	Australia)	
bisoprolol	fosinopril	Cardene	Cardizem
Boost bar	BuSpar	Cardene	Cardura
Brevibloc	Brevital	Cardene	codeine
Brevital	Brevibloc	Cardene SR	Cardizem SR
Bumex	Bentyl	Cardiem	Cardizem
Bumex	Buprenex	Cardizem	Cardene
Bumex	Nimbex	Cardizem	Cardiem
Bumex	Permax	Cardizem	Cardizem SR
		Cardizem	clonidine

Cardizem CD	Calan SR
Cardizem CD	Cardizem SR
Cardizem SR	Calan SR
Cardizem SR	Cardene SR
Cardizem SR	Cardizem
Cardizem SR	Cardizem CD
Cardura	Cardene
Cardura	Cordarone
Cardura	Coumadin
Cardura	K-Dur
Cardura	Ridaura
carteolol	carvedilol
Cartia (aspirin in New Zealand)	Cartia XT (diltiazem in U.S.)
Cartia XT	Diltia XT
Cartia XT (diltiazem in U.S.)	Cartia (aspirin in New Zealand)
Cartia XT	Procardia XL
carvedilol	captopril
carvedilol	carteolol
Cataflam	Catapres
Catapres	Capoten
Catapres	Cataflam
Ceclor	Ceclor CD
Ceclor CD	Ceclor
cefaclor	cephalexin
cefazolin	cefepime
cefazolin	cefotaxime
cefazolin	cefotetan
cefazolin	cefoxitin
cefazolin	cefprozil
cefazolin	ceftazidime
cefazolin	ceftizoxime
cefazolin	ceftriaxone
cefazolin	cefuroxime
cefazolin	cephalexin
cefepime	cefazolin
cefepime	cefotetan
cefepime	Cefotan
cefixime	cefpodoxime
Cefobid	celecoxib
Cefobid	Levbid
Cefol	Cefzil
Cefotan	Ceftin
Cefotan	Claforan
Cefotan	cefepime
Cefotan	ceftriaxone
cefotaxime	cefazolin
cefotaxime	cefotetan
cefotaxime	cefoxitin
cefotaxime	ceftazidime
cefotaxime	ceftizoxime
cefotaxime	ceftriaxone
cefotaxime	cefuroxime
cefotetan	cefazolin
cefotetan	cefepime
cefotetan	cefotaxime
cefotetan	cefoxitin
cefotetan	ceftazidime
cefotetan	ceftizoxime
cefotetan	ceftriaxone
cefoxitin	cefazolin
cefoxitin	cefotaxime
cefoxitin	cefotetan
cefoxitin	ceftriaxone
cefoxitin	cefuroxime
cefpodoxime	cefixime
cefprozil	cefazolin
cefprozil	cefuroxime
ceftazidime	cefazolin
ceftazidime	cefotaxime
ceftazidime	cefotetan
ceftazidime	ceftizoxime
ceftazidime	ceftriaxone
ceftazidime	cefuroxime
Ceftin	Cefotan
Ceftin	Cefzil
Ceftin	Cipro
Ceftin	Rocephin
ceftizoxime	cefazolin
ceftizoxime	cefotaxime
ceftizoxime	cefotetan
ceftizoxime	ceftazidime
ceftizoxime	cefuroxime
ceftriaxone	cefazolin
ceftriaxone	cefotaxime
ceftriaxone	cefotetan
ceftriaxone	cefoxitin
ceftriaxone	ceftazidime
ceftriaxone	cefuroxime
ceftriaxone	Cefotan
cefuroxime	cefazolin
cefuroxime	cefotaxime
cefuroxime	cefprozil
cefuroxime	ceftazidime
cefuroxime	ceftizoxime

cefuroxime	ceftriaxone	Clinoril	Oruvail
cefuroxime	cephalexin	clomiPHENE	clomiPRAMINE
cefuroxime	deferoxamine	clomiPRAMINE	clomiPHENE
cefuroxime	cefoxitin	clomiPRAMINE	desipramine
Cefzil	Cefol	Clonapam	Corlopam
Cefzil	Ceftin	(clonazepam in	(fenoldopam
Cefzil	Kefzol	Canada)	in U.S.)
Celebrex	Celexa	clonazepam	alprazolam
Celebrex	Cerebra	clonazepam	clonidine
Celebrex	Cerebyx	clonazepam	clorazepate
Celebrex	Celexa	clonazepam	Klonopin
celecoxib	Cefobid	clonazepam	diazepam
Celexa	Celebrex	clonazepam	lorazepam
Celexa	Cerebra	clonidine	colchicine
Celexa	Cerebyx	clonidine	Cardizem
Celexa	Zyprexa	clonidine	clonazepam
cephalexin	cefaclor	clonidine	Klonopin
cephalexin	cefazolin	clorazepate	clonazepam
cephalexin	cefuroxime	Clozaril	Clinoril
cephalexin	ciprofloxacin	Clozaril	Colazal
Cerebra	Celebrex	codeine	Cardene
Cerebra	Celexa	codeine	iodine
Cerebyx	Avelox	codeine	Lodine
Cerebyx	Celebrex	Codiclear DH	Codimal DH
Cerebyx	Celexa	Codimal DH	Codiclear DH
cetirizine	cyclobenzaprine	Cognex	Corgard
chlordiazepoxide	chlorproMAZINE	Colace	Calan
clorhexidine	chlorproMAZINE	Colace	Peri-Colace
chlorproMAZINE	chlordiazepoxide	Colace (docusate	Colace (glycerin
chlorproMAZINE	clorhexidine	sodium)	suppository)
chlorproMAZINE	chlorproPAMIDE	Colace (glycerin	Colace (docusate
chlorproMAZINE	chlorthalidone	suppository)	sodium)
chlorproMAZINE	prochlorperazine	Colazal	Clozaril
chlorproMAZINE	thioridazine	colchicine	clonidine
chlorproPAMIDE	chlorproMAZINE	Combivir	Epivir
chlorthalidone	chlorproMAZINE	Cordarone	Cardura
Cipro	Ceftin	Cordarone	Coumadin
ciprofloxacin	cephalexin	Corgard	Cognex
ciprofloxacin	levofloxacin	Corgard	Cozaar
ciprofloxacin	ofloxacin	Corlopam	Clonapam
cisplatin	carboplatin	(fenoldopam	(clonazepam
Citracal	Citrucel	in U.S.)	in Canada)
Citrucel	Hydrocil	Cortane	Cortane-B
Citrucel	Citracal	Cortane-B	Cortane
Claforan	Cefotan	Cortef	Lortab
Claritin	Claritin-D	cortisone	hydrocortisone
Claritin-D	Claritin	Cortisporin	Cortisporin (otic)
Clinoril	Clozaril	(ophthalmic)	

Cortisporin (otic)	Cortisporin (ophthalmic)
Cosopt	Trusopt
Coumadin	Avandia
Coumadin	Cardura
Coumadin	Cordarone
Coumadin	Ambien
Covera	Provera
Cozaar	Corgard
Cozaar	Hyzaar
Cozaar	Zocor
cyclobenzaprine	cetirizine
cyclobenzaprine	cyproheptadine
cyclophosphamide	cycloSPORINE
cycloSERINE	cycloSPORINE
cycloSPORINE	cyclophosphamide
cycloSPORINE	cycloSERINE
cyproheptadine	cyclobenzaprine
cytarabine	Cytosar
cytarabine	Cytoxan
CytoGam	Gamimune N
Cytosar	cytarabine
Cytosar	Cytovene
Cytosar	Cytoxan
Cytosar-U	Neosar
Cytotec	Cytoxan
Cytovene	Cytosar
Cytoxan	cytarabine
Cytoxan	Cytosar
Cytoxan	Cytotec
danazol	Dantrium
Danocrine	Dantrium
Dantrium	danazol
Dantrium	Danocrine
Darvocet	Percocet
Darvocet-N	Darvon
Darvocet-N	Darvon-N
Darvon	Darvocet-N
Darvon	Diovan
Darvon-N	Darvocet-N
Datril	Detrol
DAUNOrubicin	DOXOrubicin
deferoxamine	cefuroxime
Demedex	Demerol
demeclocycline	dicyclomine
Demerol	Demadex
Demerol	Desyrel
Demerol	Dilaudid
Denavir	indinavir
Depokene	Depakote
Depakote	Depokene
Depakote	Senokot
Depakote	Depakote ER
Depakote ER	Depakote
Depo-Estradiol	Depo-Testadiol
Depo-Medrol	Depo-Provera
Depo-Provera	Depo-Medrol
Depo-Testadiol	Depo-Estradiol
Deseril (methysergide maleate in Australia)	Desyrel (trazodone in U.S.)
Desferal	DexFerrum
desipramine	clomiPRAMINE
desipramine	imipramine
desipramine	nortriptyline
Desyrel	Demerol
Desyrel (Trazodone in U.S.)	Deseril (methysergide maleate in Australia)
Detrol	Datril
Detrol	Dextrostat
DexFerrum	Desferal
dextroamphetamine	dextroamphetamine and amphetamine
dextroamphetamine and amphetamine	dextroamphetamine
Dextrostat	Detrol
DiaBeta	Zebeta
Diamox	Dobutrex
Diastix	Keto-Diastix
Diatex (diazepam in Mexico)	Diatx (multivitamin in U.S.)
Diatx (multivitamin in U.S.)	Diatex (diazepam in Mexico)
diazepam	alprazolam
diazepam	clonazepam
diazepam	Ditropan
diazepam	Ditropan XL
diazepam	lorazepam
diazepam	midazolam

dicloxacillin	doxycycline	DOXOrubicin	DOXOrubicin
dicyclomine	demeclocycline	liposomal	
dicyclomine	diphenhydrAMINE	doxycycline	dicloxacillin
dicyclomine	doxycycline	doxycycline	dicyclomine
Diflucan	Dilantin	doxycycline	doxepin
Diflucan	Diprivan	Duratuss	Duratuss-G
digoxin	doxepin	Duratuss-G	Duratuss
Dilantin	Diflucan	Dynabac	DynaCirc
Dilaudid	Demerol	Dynacin	DynaCirc
Diltia XT	Cartia XT	DynaCirc	Dynabac
dimenhyDRINATE	diphenhydrAMINE	DynaCirc	Dynacin
Dimetapp	Donnatal	Edecrin	Eulexin
Diovan	Darvon	efavirenz	nelfinavir
Diovan	Zyban	Effexor	Effexor XR
diphenhydrAMINE	dicyclomine	Effexor XR	Effexor
diphenhydrAMINE	dimenhyDRINATE	Efudex	Eurax
diphenhydrAMINE	dipyridamole	Elavil	Enbrel
diphtheria and	tetanus toxoid	Elavil	Oruvail
tetanus toxoid		Elavil	Plavix
Diprivan	Diflucan	Eldepryl	enalapril
Diprivan	Ditropan	Eldopaque Forte	Eldoquin Forte
dipyridamole	diphenhydrAMINE	Eldoquin Forte	Eldopaque Forte
Ditropan	diazepam	Elidel	Eligard
Ditropan	Diprivan	Eligard	Elidel
Ditropan XL	diazepam	Elmiron	Imuran
DOBUTamine	DOPamine	enalapril	Eldepryl
Dobutrex	Diamox	enalapril	lisinopril
Dobutrex	DOPamine	Enbrel	Elavil
docetaxel	paclitaxel	enoxacin	enoxaparin
docusate calcium	docusate sodium	enoxaparin	enoxacin
docusate sodium	docusate calcium	Entex LA	Eulexin
Dolobid	Slo-bid	Entuss	Entuss-D
donepezil	benazepril	Entuss-D	Entuss
donepezil	doxazosin	epHEDrine	epINEPHrine
Donnatal	Dimetapp	epINEPHrine	epHEDrine
Donnatal	Donnatal Extentabs	epINEPHrine	Neo-Synephrine
Donnatal	Donnatal	epINEPHrine	norepinephrine
Extentabs		Epivir	Combivir
DOPamine	Dobutrex	Epogen	Neupogen
DOPamine	DOBUTamine	Equagesic	EquiGesic
doxazosin	terazosin	EquiGesic	Equagesic
doxazosin	donepezil	Erex	Urex
doxepin	digoxin	Erythrocin	Ethmozine
doxepin	doxycycline	erythromycin	azithromycin
DOXOrubicin	DAUNOrubicin	Eskalith	Estratest
DOXOrubicin	DOXOrubicin	esmolol	Osmitrol
	liposomal	esomeprazole	omeprazole
DOXOrubicin	idarubicin	Estrance	Evista

Estraderm	Testoderm
estradiol	ethinyl estradiol
estradiol	Risperdal
estramustine	exemestane
Estratab	Estratest
Estratest	Eskalith
Estratest	Estratab
Estratest	Estratest HS
Estratest HS	Estratest
ethinyl estradiol	estradiol
ethinyl estradiol and levonorgestrel	ethinyl estradiol and norgestrel
ethinyl estradiol and norgestrel	ethinyl estradiol and levonorgestrel
Ethmozine	Erythrocin
etidronate	etomidate
etomidate	etidronate
Eulexin	Edecrin
Eulexin	Entex LA
Eurax	Efudex
Evista	Estrace
Evista	E-Vista
E-Vista	Evista
exemestane	estramustine
famciclovir	acyclovir
famotidine	fluoxetine
famotidine	furosemide
felodipine	amlodipine
felodipine	NIFEdipine
felodipine	ranitidine
fentanyl citrate	sufentanil citrate
Fer-In-Sol	Poly-Vi-Sol
Fioricet	Fiorinal
Fioricet	Florinef
Fiorinal	Fioricet
Fleet Enema	Fleet Phospho-Soda
Fleet Phospho-Soda	Fleet Enema
Flomax	Flonase
Flomax	Flovent
Flomax	Fosamax
Flomax	Volmax
Flonase	Flomax
Flonase	Flovent
Florinef	Fioricet
Florinef	fluoride
Flovent	Atrovent
Flovent	Flomax
Flovent	Flonase
flucytosine	fluorouracil
Fludara	FUDR
fludarabine	Flumadine
Flumadine	fludarabine
fluocinolone	fluocinonide
fluocinonide	fluocinolone
fluocinonide	fluorouracil
fluoride	Florinef
fluorouracil	flucytosine
fluorouracil	fluocinonide
fluoxetine	fluphenazine
fluoxetine	fluvoxamine
fluoxetine	famotidine
fluoxetine	fluvastatin
fluoxetine	furosemide
fluoxetine	paroxetine
fluphenazine	fluoxetine
fluphenazine	perphenazine
fluphenazine	trifluoperazine
flurazepam	temazepam
fluvastatin	fluoxetine
fluvoxamine	fluoxetine
FML Forte	FML S.O.P.
FML S.O.P.	FML Forte
folic acid	folinic acid
folinic acid	folic acid
Foltex PFS	FOLTX
FOLTX	Foltex PFS
Foradil	Toradol
Fortovase	Invirase
Fosamax	Flomax
fosinopril	bisoprolol
fosinopril	furosemide
fosinopril	lisinopril
fosinopril	minoxidil
fosphenytoin	phenytoin
FUDR	Fludara
furosemide	famotidine
furosemide	fluoxetine
furosemide	fosinopril
furosemide	torsemide
Gamimune N	CytoGam
Gemzar	Zinecard
Gengraf	Prograf
gentamicin	tobramycin

gentamicin	vancomycin
glipiZIDE	glyBURIDE
Glucophage	Glucophage XR
Glucophage	Glucotrol
Glucophage	Glutofac
Glucophage XR	Glucotrol XL
Glucophage XR	Glucophage
Glucophage XR	Glucotrol
Glucotrol	Glucophage XR
Glucotrol	Glucophage
Glucotrol	Glucotrol XL
Glucotrol	glyBURIDE
Glucotrol XL	Glucophage XR
Glucotrol XL	Glucotrol
Glutofac	Glucophage
glyBURIDE	glipiZIDE
glyBURIDE	Glucotrol
glycerin	nitroglycerin
Granulex	Regranex
guaifenesin	guanfacine
guanfacine	guaifenesin
Halcion	Haldol
Haldol	Halcion
Haldol	Haldol Decanoate
Haldol	Inderal
Haldol	Stadol
Haldol Decanoate	Haldol
haloperidol	Halotestin
Halotestin	haloperidol
Hemoccult	Seracult
heparin	Levaquin
heparin	Hespan
Herceptin	Perceptin
Hespan	heparin
Humalog	Humalog Mix
Humalog Mix	Humalog
Humalog, Insulin Human	Humulin, Insulin Human
Humulin 70/30	Humulin N
Humulin 70/30	Humulin R
Humulin L	Humulin N
Humulin L (Lente)	Humulin U (Ultralente)
Humulin N	Humulin 70/30
Humulin N	Humulin R
Humulin N	Humulin U
Humulin N	Novolin N
Humulin N	Humulin L
Humulin R	Humulin 70/30
Humulin R	Humulin N
Humulin R	Humulin U
Humulin R	Novolin R
Humulin U	Humulin N
Humulin U	Humulin R
Humulin U (Ultralente)	Humulin L (Lente)
Humulin, Insulin Human	Humalog, Insulin Human
hydrALAZINE	hydrochlorothiazide
hydrALAZINE	hydrocortisone
hydrALAZINE	hydrOXYzine
hydrochlorothiazide	hydrALAZINE
hydrochlorothiazide	hydroxychloroquine
Hydrocil	Citrucel
hydrocodone	hydrocortisone
hydrocodone and acetaminophen	oxycodone and acetaminophen
hydrocodone and acetaminophen	hydromorphone
hydrocortisone	cortisone
hydrocortisone	hydrALAZINE
hydrocortisone	hydrocodone
hydromorphone	hydrocodone and acetaminophen
hydromorphone	morphine
hydroxychloroquine	hydrochlorothiazide
hydroxyurea	hydrOXYzine
hydrOXYzine	hydrALAZINE
hydrOXYzine	hydroxyurea
Hypergel	MPM GelPad Hydrogel Saturated Dressing
Hyzaar	Cozaar
Idamycin	Adriamycin
idarubicin	DOXOrubicin
IMDUR	Imuran
IMDUR	Inderal LA
IMDUR	K-Dur
imipenem	meropenem
imipenem	Omnipen
imipramine	amitriptyline
imipramine	desipramine
Imodium	Indocin
Imovax	Imovax I.D.
Imovax I.D.	Imovax

Imuran	Elmiron	Keto-Diastix	Diastix
Imuran	IMDUR	ketorolac	ketotifen
Imuran	Tenormin	ketotifen	ketorolac
Inapsine	Lanoxin	Klonopin	clonazepam
Inderal	Adderall	Klonopin	clonidine
Inderal	Haldol	K-Lor	K-Dur
Inderal	Isordil	K-Lor	K-Lyte
Inderal	Toradol	K-Lyte	K-Lor
Inderal LA	IMDUR	K Lyte	K-Lyte Cl
indinavir	Denavir	K Lyte Cl	K-Lyte
Indocin	Imodium	Kogenate	Kogenate-2
infliximab	rituximab	Kogenate-2	Kogenate
insulin	Integrilin	K-Phos Neutral	Neutra-Phos-K
insulin human	lispro, insulin human	labetolol	Lamictal
		Lacrilube	Surgilube
insulin human	isophane, insulin human	Lamicel	Lamisil
		Lamictal	labetolol
Integrilin	insulin	Lamictal	Lamisil
Invanz	Avinza	Lamictal	Lomotil
Invirase	Fortovase	Lamictal	Ludiomil
iodine	codeine	Lamisil	Lamicel
iodine	Lodine	Lamisil	Lamictal
Ismo	Isordil	Lamisil	Lomotil
isophane, insulin human	insulin human	lamivudine	lamotrigine
		lamivudine	zidovudine
Isopto Carpine	Propine	lamotrigine	lamivudine
Isordil	Inderal	Lanoxin	levothyroxine
Isordil	Ismo	Lanoxin	Inapsine
isosorbide dinitrate	isosorbide mononitrate	Lanoxin	Lasix
		Lanoxin	Levoxyl
isosorbide mononitrate	isosorbide dinitrate	Lanoxin	Lomotil
		Lanoxin	Levsin
Kaletra	Keppra	Lanoxin	Lonox
Kaopectate	Kayexalate	Lanoxin	Lovenox
Kayexalate	Kaopectate	Lanoxin	Xanax
Kayexalate	potassium acetate	Lantus, Insulin Human	Lente, Insulin Human
K-Dur	Cardura	Lasix	Lanoxin
K-Dur	IMDUR	Lasix	Lomotil
K-Dur	K-Lor	Lasix	Luvox
Keflex	Kefzol	L-Dopa	levodopa
Keflex	Norflex	L-Dopa	methyldopa
Kefurox	Kefzol	Lente, Insulin Human	lipro, insulin human
Kefzol	Cefzil		
Kefzol	Keflex	Lente, Insulin Human	Lantus, Insulin Human
Kefzol	Kefurox		
Kenalog	Ketalar	leucovorin	Leukeran
Keppra	Kaletra	leucovorin	Leukine
Ketalar	Kenalog		

leucovorin	levothyroxine
Leukeran	Alkeran
Leukeran	leucovorin
Leukeran	Leukine
Leukine	leucovorin
Leukine	Leukeran
Levaquin	heparin
Levaquin	Lovenox
Levaquin	Tequin
Levbid	Cefobid
Levbid	Lithobid
Levbid	Lopid
Levbid	Lorabid
Levlen	Tri-Levlen
levobunolol	levocabastine
levocabastine	levobunolol
levocarnitine	levofloxacin
levodopa	L-Dopa
levodopa	methyldopa
levodopa and carbidopa	carbidopa
levofloxacin	ciprofloxacin
levofloxacin	levocarnitine
levothyroxine	Lanoxin
levothyroxine	leucovorin
levothyroxine	liothyronine
Levoxyl	Lanoxin
Levoxyl	Luvox
Levsin	Lanoxin
Lexapro	loxapine
Librax	Librium
Librium	Librax
Lioresal	Lotensin
liothyronine	levothyroxine
Lipitor	Zocor
lisinopril	benazepril
lisinopril	enalapril
lisinopril	fosinopril
lisinopril	quinapril
lisinopril	Risperdal
lispro, insulin human	insulin human
lispro, insulin human	Lente, Insulin Human
Lithobid	Levbid
Lithobid	Lithostat
Lithostat	Lithobid
Lodine	codeine
Lodine	iodine
Lomotil	Lamictal
Lomotil	Lamisil
Lomotil	Lanoxin
Lomotil	Lasix
Loniten	Lotensin
Lonox	Lanoxin
loperamide	lorazepam
Lopid	Levbid
Lopid	Lorabid
Lopid	Slo-bid
Lorabid	Levbid
Lorabid	Lopid
Lorabid	Lortab
Lorabid	Slo-bid
loratadine	losartan
lorazepam	alprazolam
lorazepam	clonazepam
lorazepam	diazepam
lorazepam	loperamide
lorazepam	midazolam
lorazepam	temazepam
Lorcet	Lortab
Lortab	Cortef
Lortab	Lorabid
Lortab	Lorcet
Lortab	Luride
losartan	loratadine
losartan	valsartan
Lotensin	Lioresal
Lotensin	Loniten
Lotensin	lovastatin
Lotrimin	Lotrisone
Lotrisone	Lotrimin
Lotronex	Lovenox
Lotronex	Protonix
lovastatin	Lotensin
Lovenox	Avonex
Lovenox	Lanoxin
Lovenox	Levaquin
Lovenox	Lotronex
Lovenox	Luvox
loxapine	Lexapro
Loxitane	Soriatane
Ludiomil	Lamictal
Luride	Lortab
Luvox	Lasix
Luvox	Levoxyl

Luvox	Lovenox	methylPRED-	predniSONE
magnesium citrate	magnesium sulfate	NISolone	
magnesium sulfate	magnesium citrate	methylTESTOS-	methylPRED-
Maxipime	Moxapen	TERone	NISolone
(cefepime	(amoxacillin	metoclopramide	metolazone
hydrochloride	trihydrate in	metoclopramide	metoprolol
in U.S.)	Thailand)	metoclopramide	metronidazole
meclofenamate	mycophenolate	metolazone	medroxyPRO-
Medigesic	Medi-Gesic		GESTERone
Medi-Gesic	Medigesic	metolazone	metaxalone
medroxyPRO-	methylPRED-	metolazone	methotrexate
GESTERone	NISolone	metolazone	metoclopramide
medroxyPRO-	metolazone	metolazone	metoprolol
GESTERone		metoprolol	atenolol
mefloquine	meloxicam	metoprolol	metoclopramide
Megace	Reglan	metoprolol	metolazone
Mellaril	melphalan	metoprolol	metronidazole
meloxicam	mefloquine	metoprolol	misoprostol
melphalan	Mellaril	metoprolol	metoprolol
melphalan	Myleran	succinate	tartrate
meperidine	methadone	metoprolol	metoprolol
meperidine	morphine	tartrate	succinate
Mepron	Mepron	MetroGel	MetroGel-Vaginal
(atovaquone	(meprobamate	MetroGel-Vaginal	MetroGel
in U.S.)	in Australia)	metronidazole	metformin
meropenem	imipenem	metronidazole	methazolamide
Meruvax	Attenuvax	metronidazole	metoclopramide
mesalamine	sulfasalazine	metronidazole	metoprolol
Metadate CD	Metadate ER	metronidazole	miconazole
Metadate ER	Metadate CD	Miacalcin	Micatin
metaxalone	metolazone	Micatin	Miacalcin
metformin	metronidazole	miconazole	metronidazole
methadone	meperidine	Micro-K	Micronase
methadone	methylphenidate	Micronase	Micro-K
methazolamide	methimazole	Micronase	Microzide
methazolamide	metronidazole	Microzide	Micronase
methimazole	methazolamide	midazolam	diazepam
methohexital	methotrexate	midazolam	lorazepam
methotrexate	methohexital	midodrin	Midrin
methotrexate	metolazone	midodrine	molindone
methyldopa	L-Dopa	Midrin	midodrin
methyldopa	levodopa	mifepristone	misoprostol
methylphenidate	methadone	minoxidil	fosinopril
methylPRED-	medroxyPRO-	minoxidil	Monopril
NISolone	GESTERone	MiraLax	Mirapex
methylPRED-	methylTESTOS-	Mirapex	MiraLax
NISolone	TERone	misoprostol	metoprolol
		misoprostol	mifepristone

mitomycin	mitoxantrone
mitoxantrone	mitomycin
Moban	Mobic
Mobic	Moban
molindone	midodrine
Monoket	Monopril
Monopril	Accupril
Monopril	minoxidil
Monopril	Monoket
morphine	hydromorphone
morphine	meperidine
Moxapen	Maxipime
(amoxicillin	(cefepime
trihydrate in	hydrochloride
Thailand)	in U.S.)
MPM GelPad	Hypergel
Hydrogel	
Saturated	
Dressing	
MS Contin	OxyContin
Murocel	Murocoll-2
Murocoll-2	Murocel
Mycelex	Mycolog
Mycolog	Mycelex
mycophenolate	meclofenamate
Mylanta	Mylicon
Myleran	melphalan
Mylicon	Mylanta
Naprelan	Naprosyn
Naprosyn	Naprelan
Naprosyn	Niaspan
Narcan	Norcuron
Narcan	Nubain
Nasacort	Azmacort
Nasalcrom	Nasalide
Nasalide	Nasalcrom
Nasarel	Nizoral
Natru-Vent	Atrovent
Navane	Norvasc
Nebcin	Nubain
nefazodone	nelfinavir
nelfinavir	efavirenz
nelfinavir	nefazodone
nelfinavir	nevirapine
Neoral	Neurontin
Neoral	Nizoral
Neosar	Cytosar-U
Neo-Synephrine	epINEPHrine

Neo-Synephrine	Neo-Synephrine 12 Hour
Neo-Synephrine	norepinephrine
Neo-Synephrine 12 Hour	Neo-Synephrine
Nephrox	Niferex
Neumega	Neupogen
Neupogen	Epogen
Neupogen	Neumega
Neurontin	Neoral
Neurontin	Noroxin
Neutra-Phos	Neutra-Phos-K
Neutra-Phos-K	K-Phos Neutral
Neutra-Phos-K	Neutra-Phos
nevirapine	nelfinavir
niacin	Niaspan
Niaspan	Naprosyn
Niaspan	niacin
niCARdipine	NIFEdipine
niCARdipine	nimodipine
Nicoderm	Nitroderm
NicoDerm CQ	Nitro-Dur
NIFEdipine	felodipine
NIFEdipine	niCARdipine
NIFEdipine	nimodipine
Niferex	Nephrox
Nimbex	Bumex
Nimbex	Revex
nimodipine	niCARdipine
nimodipine	NIFEdipine
Nitro-Bid	Nitro-Dur
Nitroderm	Nicoderm
Nitro-Dur	NicoDerm CQ
Nitro-Dur	Nitro-Bid
Nitro-Dur	NitroQuick
nitroglycerin	glycerin
NitroQuick	Nitro-Dur
nizatidine	tizanidine
Nizoral	Nasarel
Nizoral	Neoral
Nolvadex	Norvasc
Norcuron	Narcan
norepinephrine	epINEPHrine
norepinephrine	Neo-Synephrine
norepinephrine	phenylephrine
Norflex	Keflex
Norflex	norfloxacin
Norflex	Noroxin

Norflex	Norvasc
norfloxacin	Norflex
norfloxacin	Noroxin
Noroxin	Neurontin
Noroxin	Norflex
Noroxin	norfloxacin
Norpramin	nortriptyline
nortriptyline	amitriptyline
nortriptyline	desipramine
nortriptyline	Norpramin
Norvasc	Altace
Norvasc	Navane
Norvasc	Nolvadex
Norvasc	Norflex
Norvasc	Vasotec
Norvir	Retrovir
Novolin 70/30	Novolin N
Novolin L	Novolin N
Novolin N	Humulin N
Novolin N	Novolin 70/30
Novolin N	Novolin L
Novolin N	Novolin R
Novolin R	Humulin R
Novolin R	Novolin N
Nubain	Narcan
Nubain	Nebcin
Nutropin	Nutropin AQ
Nutropin AQ	Nutropin
Ocufen	Ocuflox
Ocufen	Ocupress
Ocuflox	Ocufen
ocular lubricants	Acular
Ocumycin	Ocu-Mycin
Ocu-Mycin	Ocumycin
Ocupress	Ocufen
ofloxacin	ciprofloxacin
olanzapine	oxcarbazepine
omeprazole	esomeprazole
Omnipen	imipenem
opium tincture, deodorized	opium, camphorated
opium, camphorated	opium tincture, deodorized
oprelvekin	aldesleukin
Orgaran	argatroban
Ortho Tri-Cyclen	Ortho-Cyclen
Ortho Tri-Cyclen	Tri-Levlen
Ortho-Cept	Ortho-Cyclen
Ortho-Cept	Ortho-Est
Ortho-Cyclen	Ortho-Cept
Ortho-Cyclen	Ortho Tri-Cyclen
Ortho-Est	Ortho-Cept
Oruvail	Clinoril
Oruvail	Elavil
Os-Cal	Asacol
Osmitrol	esmolol
oxacillin	ampicillin
oxazepam	oxycodone
oxazepam	temazepam
oxcarbazepine	olanzapine
oxybutynin	OxyContin
oxycodone	oxazepam
oxycodone	OxyContin
oxycodone and acetaminophen	hydrocodone and acetaminophen
oxycodone and acetaminophen	oxycodone and aspirin
oxycodone and aspirin	oxycodone and acetaminophen
OxyContin	MS Contin
OxyContin	oxybutynin
OxyContin	oxycodone
paclitaxel	docetaxel
paclitaxel	paroxetine
paclitaxel	Paxil
Pamelor	Panlor SS
Panlor SS	Pamelor
papaverine	propafenone
Parafon Forte DSC	Profen Forte
Paraplatin	Platinol
Parlodel	pindolol
Parlodel	Provera
paroxetine	fluoxetine
paroxetine	paclitaxel
paroxetine	pyridoxine
Paxil	paclitaxel
Paxil	Plavix
Paxil	Taxol
Pediapred	Pediazole
Pediapred	Risperdal
Pediazole	Pediapred
pegaspargase	asparaginase
penicillamine	penicillin
penicillin	penicillamine
penicillin G potassium	penicillin G procaine

penicillin G procaine	penicillin G potassium	pneumococcal vaccine, 7-valent	pneumococcal vaccine, 23-valent (polyvalent)
pentobarbital	phenobarbital		
Pepcid	Prevacid		
Perative	Periactin	Polocaine	Pilocar
Perceptin	Herceptin	Poly-Vi-Sol	Fer-In-Sol
Percocet	Darvocet	potassium	predniSONE
Percocet	Percodan	potassium acetate	Kayexalate
Percocet	Procet	potassium acetate	potassium chloride
Percodan	Percocet	potassium	potassium
Percodan	Peri-Colace	bicarbonate	bicarbonate
Percodan	Vicodin	and potassium	and potassium
Periactin	Perative	chloride	citrate
Peri-Colace	Colace	potassium	potassium
Peri-Colace	Percodan	bicarbonate	bicarbonate
Peri-Colace	Procardia	and potassium	and potassium
Permax	Bumex	citrate	chloride
permethrin	pyrethrins, piperonyl butoxide	potassium chloride	potassium acetate
		potassium chloride	potassium citrate
		potassium chloride	sodium chloride
perphenazine	fluphenazine	potassium citrate	potassium chloride
phenazopyridine	promethazine	potassium phosphates	potassium sodium phosphates
phenobarbital	pentobarbital		
phenylephrine	norepinephrine	Prandin	Avandia
phenylephrine	phenytoin	Pravachol	Prevacid
phenytoin	fosphenytoin	Pravachol	Prinivil
phenytoin	phenylephrine	Pravachol	propranolol
physostigmine	pyridostigmine	pravastatin	atorvastatin
Pilocar	Polocaine	prazosin	terazosin
pilocarpine	proparacaine	Precare	Precose
pindolol	Parlodel	Precose	Precare
pindolol	Plendil	prednisoLONE	predniSONE
pioglitazone	rosiglitazone	predniSONE	methylPRED-NISolone
Pitocin	Pitressin		
Pitressin	Pitocin	predniSONE	potassium
Platinol	Paraplatin	predniSONE	prednisoLONE
Plavix	Elavil	predniSONE	Prilosec
Plavix	Paxil	predniSONE	primidone
Plendil	pindolol	predniSONE	pseudoephedrine
Plendil	Pletal	Premarin	Prempro
Plendil	Prilosec	Premarin	Prevacid
Plendil	Prinivil	Premarin	Primaxin
Pletal	Plendil	Premarin	Provera
pneumococcal vaccine, 23-valent (polyvalent)	pneumococcal vaccine, 7-valent	Premphase	Prempro
		Premphase	Vancenase
		Prempro	Premarin
		Prempro	Premphase
		Prepidil	bepridil

Prevacid	Prinivil
Prevacid	Pepcid
Prevacid	Pravachol
Prevacid	Premarin
Prevacid	Prilosec
Preven	Preveon
Preveon	Preven
Prilosec	Plendil
Prilosec	predniSONE
Prilosec	Prevacid
Prilosec	Prinivil
Prilosec	Prozac
Primacor	Primaxin
Primatene	ProAmantine
Primaxin	Premarin
Primaxin	Primacor
primidone	predniSONE
Prinivil	Plendil
Prinivil	Pravachol
Prinivil	Prevacid
Prinivil	Prilosec
Prinivil	Prinzide
Prinivil	Proventil
Prinzide	Prinivil
Priscoline	Apresoline
ProAmantine	Primatene
probenecid	Procanbid
procainamide	prochlorperazine
Procan SR	Proscar
Procanbid	probenecid
Procardia	Peri-Colace
Procardia	Provera
Procardia XL	Cartia XT
Procet	Percocet
prochlorperazine	chlorproMAZINE
prochlorperazine	procainamide
prochlorperazine	promethazine
Proctocort	Proctocream HC
Proctocream HC	Proctocort
Profen	Profen II
Profen	Profen LA
Profen Forte	Parafon Forte DSC
Profen II	Profen
Profen II	Profen LA
Profen LA	Profen
Profen LA	Profen II
Prograf	Gengraf
promethazine	phenazopyridine

promethazine	prochlorperazine
promethazine VC	promethazine w/codeine
promethazine VC w/codeine	promethazine w/codeine
promethazine w/codeine	promethazine VC w/codeine
promethazine w/codeine	promethazine VC
propafenone	papaverine
proparacaine	pilocarpine
Propine	Isopto Carpine
propranolol	Pravachol
propranolol	Propulsid
Propulsid	propranolol
propythiouracil	Purinethol
Proscar	Procan SR
Proscar	ProSom
Proscar	Prozac
Proscar	Provera
ProSom	Proscar
ProSom	Prozac
Protonix	Lotronex
Proventil	Bentyl
Proventil	Prinivil
Provera	Covera
Provera	Parlodel
Provera	Premarin
Provera	Procardia
Provera	Proscar
Prozac	Prilosec
Prozac	Proscar
Prozac	ProSom
pseudoephedrine	predniSONE
Pulmicort	Pulmozyme
Pulmozyme	Pulmicort
Purinethol	propythiouracil
pyrazinamide	pyridostigmine
pyrethrins, piperonyl butoxide	permethrin
Pyridium	pyridoxine
pyridostigmine	physostigmine
pyridostigmine	pyrazinamide
pyridostigmine	pyridoxine
pyridoxine	paroxetine
pyridoxine	Pyridium
pyridoxine	pyridostigmine

pyridoxine	pyrimethamine	Retavase	Activase
pyrimethamine	pyridoxine	Retrovir	Norvir
Quibron	Quibron-T	Retrovir	ritonavir
Quibron	Quibron-T/SR	Revex	Nimbex
Quibron-T	Quibron	Revex	ReVia
Quibron-T	Quibron-T/SR	ReVia	Revex
Quibron-T/SR	Quibron	Rezulin	Relafen
Quibron-T/SR	Quibron-T	Rheomacrodex	Reopro
quinocrine	quinidine	Ridaura	Cardura
quinapril	lisinopril	rifabutin	rifampin
quinidine	quinacrine	Rifadin	Rifater
quinidine	quinine	rifampin	ramipril
quinine	quinidine	rifampin	rifabutin
raloxifene	ropinirole	Rifater	Rifadin
ramipril	rifampin	rimantadine	amantadine
ranitidine	amantadine	rimantadine	ranitidine
ranitidine	rimantadine	risedronate	risperidone
ranitidine	felodipine	Risperdal	estradiol
ratgam (synonym for thymoglo-bulin)	Atgam	Risperdal	lisinopril
		Risperdal	Pediapred
		Risperdal	Requip
ReFresh (breath drops)	Refresh (lubricant eye drops)	Risperdal	reserpine
		Risperdal	risperidone
Refresh (lubricant eye drops)	ReFresh (breath drops)	Risperdal	Restoril
		risperidone	reserpine
Reglan	Megace	risperidone	Risperdal
Reglan	Renagel	risperidone	risedronate
Reglan	Robitussin	risperidone	ropinirole
Reglan	Zofran	Ritalin	Ritalin SR
Regranex	Granulex	Ritalin SR	Ritalin
Relafen	Rezulin	ritonavir	Retrovir
Remegel	Renagel	rituximab	infliximab
Remeron	Restoril	Robinul	Reminyl
Remeron	Zemuron	Robitussin	Reglan
Reminyl	Amaryl	Robitussin	Robitussin DM
Reminyl	Robinul	Robitussin AC	Robitussin DAC
Renagel	Reglan	Robitussin AC	Robitussin DM
Renagel	Remegel	Robitussin DAC	Robitussin AC
Reno-60	Renografin-60	Robitussin DM	Robitussin
Renografin-60	Reno-60	Robitussin DM	Robitussin AC
Reopro	Rheomacrodex	Robitussin DM	Rondec DM
repaglinide	rosiglitazone	Rocephin	Ceftin
Requip	Risperdal	Rondec DM	Robitussin DM
reserpine	Risperdal	ropinirole	raloxifene
reserpine	risperidone	ropinirole	risperidone
Restoril	Remeron	ropivacaine	bupivacaine
Restoril	Risperdal	rosiglitazone	pioglitazone
Restoril	Vistaril	rosiglitazone	repaglinide

Roxanol	Roxicet
Roxanol	Roxicodone
Roxanol	Roxicodone Intensol
Roxicet	Roxanol
Roxicet	Roxicodone
Roxicodone	Roxanol
Roxicodone	Roxicet
Roxicodone	Roxicodone Intensol
Roxicodone Intensol	Roxanol
Roxicodone Intensol	Roxicodone
Rynatan	Rynatuss
Rynatuss	Rynatan
Salagen	selegiline
Salbutamol (albuterol in other countries)	salmeterol
salmeterol	Salbutamol (albuterol in other countries)
salsalate	sulfasalazine
Sarafem	Serophene
selegiline	Salagen
selegiline	Serentil
selegiline	sertraline
selegiline	Serzone
Senna	Soma
Senokot	Depakote
Senokot	Sinemet
Seracult	Hemoccult
Serentil	selegiline
Serentil	Seroquel
Serentil	sertraline
Serentil	Serzone
Serentil	Sinequan
Serevent	Atrovent
Serevent	Serevent Diskus
Serevent Diskus	Serevent
Serophene	Sarafem
Seroquel	Serentil
Seroquel	Serzone
Seroquel	Sinequan
Seroquel	Symmetrel

Seroquel	sertraline
sertraline	selegiline
sertraline	Serentil
sertraline	Serzone
sertraline	Seroquel
Serzone	selegiline
Serzone	Serentil
Serzone	Seroquel
Serzone	sertraline
Serzone	Sinequan
Sinemet	Senokot
Sinemet	Sinemet CR
Sinemet CR	Sinemet
Sinequan	Serentil
Sinequan	Seroquel
Sinequan	Serzone
Sinequan	Singulair
Singulair	Sinequan
Slo-bid	Dolobid
Slo-bid	Lopid
Slo-bid	Lorabid
Slow Fe	Slow-K
Slow-K	Slow Fe
sodium bicarbonate	sodium chloride
sodium chloride	potassium chloride
sodium chloride	sodium bicarbonate
sodium phosphates	potassium phosphates
Solu-Cortef	Solu-Medrol
Solu-Medrol	Depo-Medrol
Solu-Medrol	Solu-Cortef
Soma	Senna
Soma	Soma Compound
Soma Compound	Soma
Soriatane	Loxitane
sotalol	Subdue
Stadol	Haldol
Stadol	Toradol
Subdue	sotalol
sufentanil citrate	fentanyl citrate
sulfADIAZINE	sulfasalazine
sulfADIAZINE	sulfiSOXAZOLE
sulfasalazine	mesalamine
sulfasalazine	salsalate
sulfasalazine	sulfADIAZINE

sulfasalazine	sulfiSOXAZOLE	thioridazine	Thorazine
sulfiSOXAZOLE	sulfADIAZINE	tiagabine	tizanidine
SulfiSOXAZOLE	sulfasalazine	Tiazac	Tigan
sumatriptan	zolmitriptan	Tiazac	Ziac
Suprax	Surfak	Ticlid	Tequin
Surfak	Suprax	Tigan	Tiazac
Surgilube	Lacrilube	Timoptic	Timoptic-XE
Symmetrel	Amaryl	Timoptic-XE	Timoptic
Symmetrel	Seroquel	tizanidine	nizatidine
Symmetrel	Synthroid	tizanidine	tiagabine
Synagis	Synvisc	TNKase	t-PA (synonym for
Synthroid	Symmetrel		alteplase,
Synvisc	Synagis		recombinant)
Tambocor	Temodar		
Tamiflu	tamoxifen	Tobradex	Tobrex
Tamiflu	Theraflu	tobramycin	gentamicin
tamoxifen	Tamiflu	Tobrex	Tobradex
tamoxifen	tamsulosin	TOLAZamide	TOLBUTamide
tamsulosin	tamoxifen	TOLBUTamide	TOLAZamide
Taxol	Paxil	tolcapone	tolterodine
Taxol	Taxotere	tolterodine	tolcapone
Taxotere	Taxol	Topamax	Toprol-XL
Tegretol	Toradol	topiramate	torsemide
Tegretol	Trental	Toprol-XL	Tegretol-XR
Tegretol	Trileptal	Toprol-XL	Topamax
Tegretol-XR	Toprol-XR	Toradol	Foradil
temazepam	flurazepam	Toradol	Inderal
temazepam	lorazepam	Toradol	Stadol
temazepam	oxazepam	Toradol	Tegretol
Temodar	Tambocor	Toradol	Torecan
Tenormin	Imuran	Toradol	tramadol
Tenormin	thiamine	Torecan	Toradol
Tenormin	Trovan	torsemide	furosemide
Tequin	Levaquin	torsemide	topiramate
Tequin	Ticlid	t-PA (synonym	TNKase
terazosin	prazosin	for alteplase,	
terazosin	doxazosin	recombinant)	
Testoderm	Estraderm	tramadol	Toradol
tetanus toxoid	diphtheria and	tramadol	trandolapril
	tetanus toxoid	tramadol	trazodone
tetracycline	tetradecyl sulfate	tramadol	Voltaren
tetradecyl sulfate	tetracycline	Trandate	Trental
Thalitone	Thalomid	Trandate	Tridrate
Thalomid	Thalitone	trandolapril	tramadol
Theraflu	Tamiflu	trazodone	amiodarone
thiamine	Tenormin	trazodone	tramadol
thioridazine	chlorproMAZINE	Trental	Tegretol
Thorazine	thioridazine	Trental	Trandate

Triad (butalbital, acetaminophen, caffeine)	Triad (topical)
Triad (topical)	Triad (butalbital, acetaminophen, caffeine)
triamterene	trimethoprim
Tridrate	Trandate
trifluoperazine	fluphenazine
trifluoperazine	trihexyphenidyl
trihexyphenidyl	trifluoperazine
Trileptal	Tegretol
Tri-Levlen	Levlen
Tri-Levlen	Ortho Tri-Cyclen
trimethoprim	triamterene
Tri-Nasal	Triphasil
Tri-Norinyl	Triphasil
Triphasil	Tri-Nasal
Triphasil	Tri-Norinyl
Trovan	Tenormin
Trusopt	Cosopt
Tylenol	Tylenol w/codeine
Tylenol Children's	Tylenol w/codeine
Tylenol w/codeine	Tylenol
Tylenol w/codeine	Tylenol Children's
Ultane	Ultram
Ultracef (cefadroxil in other countries)	Ultracet (acetaminophen/ tramadol hydrochloride in U.S.)
Ultracet (acetaminophen/ tramadol hydrochloride in U.S.)	Ultracef (cefadroxil in other countries)
Ultram	Ultane
Ultram	Voltaren
Unasyn	Zosyn
Uniretic	Univasc
Univasc	Uniretic
Univasc	Urispas
Urex	Erex
Uridon	Vicodin
Urised	Uricit-K
Urispas	Univasc
Urispas	Uro-Mag
valacyclovir	valgancyclovir
Valcyte	Valtrex
valganciclovir	valacyclovir
Valium	Versed
Valium	Vicodin
valsartan	losartan
Valtrex	Valcyte
Vancenase	Premphase
Vancenase	Vanceril
Vancenase AQ	Vanceril DS
Vanceril	Vancenase
Vanceril DS	Vancenase AQ
vancomycin	azithromycin
vancomycin	gentamicin
vancomycin	vecuronium
vancomycin	Vibramycin
Vantin	Ventolin
Vasocon	Vasocon A
Vasocon A	Vasocon
Vasotec	Norvasc
vecuronium	vancomycin
Ventolin	Benylin
Ventolin	Vantin
Vepesid	Versed
verapamil	Verelan
Verelan	verapamil
Verelan	Virilon
Versed	Valium
Versed	Vepesid
Versed	Vistaril
Vexol	VoSol
Viagra	Allegra
Vibramycin	vancomycin
Vicodin	Percodan
Vicodin	Uridon
Vicodin	Valium
Vicodin	Vicodin ES
Vicodin ES	Vicodin
vinBLAStine	vinCRIStine
vinCRIStine	vinBLAStine
Viracept	Viramune
Viramune	Viracept
Virilon	Verelan
Visicol	bisacodyl
Vistaril	Restoril
Vistaril	Versed
Vistaril	Zestril
Vitamin C	Vitamin E
Vitamin D	Vitamin E

Vitamin E	Vitamin C
Vitamin E	Vitamin D
Volmax	Flomax
Voltaren	tramadol
Voltaren	Ultram
VoSol	Vexol
Wellbutrin	Wellbutrin SR
Wellbutrin SR	Wellbutrin
Xalatan	Xalcom (latanoprost, timolol in other countries)
Xalcom (latanoprost, timolol in other countries)	Xalatan
Xanax	Lanoxin
Xanax	Zanaflex
Xanax	Zantac
Xanax	Zyrtec
Xigris	zydis (dosage form trademark)
Yocon	Zocor
Zagam	Zyban
zaleplon	zolpidem
Zanaflex	Anaflex
Zanaflex	Xanax
Zantac	Xanax
Zantac	Zofran
Zantac	Zyrtec
Zaroxolyn	Zyprexa
Zebeta	DiaBeta
Zemuron	Remeron
Zerit	Zestril
Zestril	Vistaril
Zestril	Zerit
Zestril	Zocor
Zestril	Zyrtec
Ziac	Tiazac
Ziac	Zocor
zidovudine	lamivudine
zidovudine	zidovudine and lamivudine
zidovudine	ziprasidone
zidovudine and lamivudine	zidovudine
Zinacef	Zithromax
Zinecard	Gemzar
ziprasidone	zidovudine
Zithromax	Zinacef
Zocor	Cozaar
Zocor	Lipitor
Zocor	Yocon
Zocor	Zestril
Zocor	Ziac
Zocor	Zoloft
Zofran	Reglan
Zofran	Zantac
Zofran	Zosyn
zolmitriptan	sumatriptan
Zoloft	Zocor
Zoloft	Zyloprim
zolpidem	zaleplon
Zonalon	Zone A Forte
Zone A Forte	Zonalon
Zosyn	Unasyn
Zosyn	Zofran
Zovirax	Zyvox
Zyban	Zagam
zydis (dosage from trademark)	Xigris
Zyloprim	Zoloft
Zyprexa	Celexa
Zyprexa	Zaroxolyn
Zyprexa	Zyprexa Zydis
Zyprexa	Zyrtec
Zyprexa Zydis	Zyprexa
Zyrtec	Xanax
Zyrtec	Zantac
Zyrtec	Zestril
Zyrtec	Zyprexa
Zyvox	Zovirax

Appendix m

FDA pregnancy categories

A   No risk demonstrated to the fetus in any trimester

B   No adverse effects in animals, no human studies available

C   Only given after risks to the fetus are considered; animal studies have shown adverse reactions, no human studies available

D   Definite fetal risks, may be given in spite of risks if needed in life-threatening conditions

X   Absolute fetal abnormalities; not to be used anytime during pregnancy

Note: **UK** = Unknown fetal risk (used in this text but not an official FDA pregnancy category).

Appendix n

Controlled substance chart

Drugs	United States*
Heroin, LSD, peyote, marijuana, mescaline	Schedule I • High abuse potential • No currently accepted medical use
Opium (morphine), meperidine, amphetamines, cocaine, short-acting barbiturates (secobarbital)	Schedule II • High abuse potential; potentially severe psychologic or physical dependence • Currently accepted medical use but may be severely restricted • Telephone orders only in emergencies if written Rx follows promptly • No refills
Glutethimide, paregoric, phendimetrazine	Schedule III • Abuse potential less than the drugs/substances in Schedules I and II; potentially moderate or low physical dependence or high psychologic dependence • Currently accepted medical use • Telephone orders permitted • Prescriber may authorize limited refills
Chloral hydrate, chlordiazepoxide, diazepam, mazindol, meprobamate, phenobarbital	Schedule IV • Low abuse potential relative to drugs/substances in Schedule III; potentially limited physical or psychologic dependence • Currently accepted medical use • Telephone orders permitted • Prescriber may authorize limited refills
Antidiarrheals with opium, antitussives	Schedule V • Lowest abuse potential; potentially very limited physical or psychologic dependence • Currently accepted medical use • Prescriber determines refills • Some products containing limited amounts of Schedule V substances (e.g., cough suppressants) available OTC to patients >18 yr

*See appendix q for Canadian controlled substance chart

Appendix o

Abbreviations

AAS argininosuccinic acid synthetase
abd abdomen
ABG arterial blood gas
ac before meals
ACE angiotensin-converting enzyme
ADA American Diabetes Association
ADH antidiuretic hormone
ALT alanine aminotransferase
ANA antinuclear antibody
AP anteroposterior
APTT activated partial thromboplastin time
ASA acetylsalicylic acid, aspirin
ASHD arteriosclerotic heart disease
AST aspartate aminotransferase (SGOT)
AV atrioventricular
bid twice a day
BM bowel movement
BMR basal metabolic rate
B/P blood pressure
BPH benign prostatic hypertrophy
BPM beats per minute
BS blood sugar
BUN blood urea nitrogen
C Celsius (centigrade)
Ca cancer
CAD coronary artery disease
cap capsule
Cath catheterization or catheterize
CBC complete blood cell count
CC chief complaint
cc cubic centimeter
CCr creatinine clearance
CHF congestive heart failure
cm centimeter
CNS central nervous system
CO₂ carbon dioxide
CONT continuous
COPD chronic obstructive pulmonary disease
CPAP continuous positive airway pressure

CPK creatine phosphokinase
CPR cardiopulmonary resuscitation
CPS carbamoyl phosphate synthetase
C&S culture and sensitivity
C sect cesarean section
CSF cerebrospinal fluid
CV cardiovascular
CVA cerebrovascular accident
CVP central venous pressure
D&C dilatation and curettage
DIC diffuse intravascular coagulation
DIR INF direct infusion
dr dram
D₅W 5% glucose in distilled water
ECG electrocardiogram (EKG)
EDTA ethylenediamine tetraacetic acid
EEG electroencephalogram
EENT ear, eye, nose, and throat
EPS extrapyramidal symptom
ESR erythrocyte sedimentation rate
EXT-
REL extended release
EXTRA-
STREN-
SUSP extra strength suspension
FBS fasting blood sugar
FHT fetal heart tones
FSH follicle-stimulating hormone
g gram
GABA γ-aminobutyric acid
GI gastrointestinal
gr grain
GT glucose tolerance test
gtt drops
GU genitourinary
H₂ histamine₂
HCG human chorionic gonadotropin
Hct hematocrit
HDCV human diploid cell rabies vaccine
Hgb hemoglobin

H & H	hematocrit and hemoglobin	**NOS**	not otherwise specified
5-HIAA	5-hydroxyindoleacetic acid	**NPO**	nothing by mouth (Lat. *nulla per os*)
HIV	human immunodeficiency virus (AIDS)	**NS**	normal saline
H₂O	water	**O₂**	oxygen
HOB	head of bed	**OBS**	organic brain syndrome
HR	heart rate	**od**	right eye
hr	hour	**OR**	operating room
IgG	immunolobulin G	**os**	left eye
IM	intramuscular	**OTC**	over-the-counter
INF	infusion	**OU**	each eye
INH	inhalation	**oz**	ounce
inj	injection	**p̄**	after
I&O	intake and output	**P56**	plasma-lyte 56
INT	intermittent	**PaCO₂**	arterial carbon dioxide tension (pressure)
IPPB	intermittent positive-pressure breathing	**PaO₂**	arterial oxygen tension (pressure)
ITP	idiopathic thrombocytopenic purpura	**PAT**	paroxysmal atrial tachycardia
IUD	intrauterine device	**PBI**	protein-bound iodine
IV	intravenous	**pc**	after meals
IVP	intravenous pyelogram	**PCWP**	pulmonary capillary wedge pressure
K	potassium	**PEEP**	positive end-expiratory pressure
kg	kilogram	**PERRLA**	pupils equal, round, react to light and accommodation
L	liter	**pH**	hydrogen ion concentration
lb	pound	**PO**	by mouth
LDH	lactic dehydrogenase	**postop**	postoperative
LE	lupus erythematosus	**PP**	postprandial
LFT	liver function test	**preop**	preoperative
LH	luteinizing hormone	**prn**	as required
LLQ	left lower quadrant	**PT**	prothrombin time
LMP	last menstrual period	**PTT**	partial thromboplastin time
LOC	level of consciousness	**PVC**	premature ventricular contraction
LR	lactated Ringer's solution	**pwd**	powder
LT	leukotriene	**qAM**	every morning
LUQ	left upper quadrant	**qh**	every hour
M	meter	**q2h**	every 2 hours
m	minim	**q3h**	every 3 hours
m²	square meter	**q4h**	every 4 hours
MAC	monitored anesthesia care	**q6h**	every 6 hours
MAOI	monoamine oxidase inhibitor	**q12h**	every 12 hours
mEq	milliequivalent	**qid**	four times daily
mg	milligram	**qPM**	every night
MI	myocardial infarction	**qs**	sufficient quantity
min	minute	**qt**	quart
ml	milliliter	**R**	right
mm	millimeter	**RAIU**	radioactive iodine uptake
mo	month	**RBC**	red blood cell count or red blood cell
Na	sodium	**RECT**	rectal
neg	negative	**RLQ**	right lower quadrant
ng	nanogram	**ROM**	range of motion

RUQ	right upper quadrant	**tsp**	teaspoon
SIMV	synchronous intermittent mandatory ventilation	**TT**	thrombin time
		UA	urinalysis
SL	sublingual	**UTI**	urinary tract infection
SLE	systemic lupus erythematosus	**UV**	ultraviolet
SOB	shortness of breath	**vag**	vaginal
sol	solution	**VMA**	vanillylmandelic acid
ss	one half	**vol**	volume
SUBCUT	subcutaneous	**VS**	vital sign
suppos	suppository	**WBC**	white blood cell count
SUS REL	sustained release	**wk**	week
syr	syrup	**wt**	weight
T&A	tonsillectomy and adenoidectomy	**yr**	year
tab	tablet	**>**	greater than
tbsp	tablespoon	**<**	less than
temp	temperature	**=**	equal
tid	three times daily	**°**	degree
tinc	tincture	**%**	percent
TPN	total parenteral nutrition	**α**	alpha
top	topical	**β**	beta
TRANS	transdermal	**γ**	gamma
TSH	thyroid-stimulating hormone		

- For a list of the Institute for Safe Medicine Practices (ISMP) error-prone abbreviations, symbols and dose designations, please see http://www.ismp.org/tools/errorproneabbreviations.pdf.
- For frequently asked questions regarding the 2006 National Patient Safety Goals, please visit the Joint Commission on Accreditation of Healthcare Organizations (JCAHO) website at http://www.jcaho.org/accredited+organizations/patient+safety/.

Appendix p

Weights and equivalents

METRIC SYSTEM
Weight

kilogram	= kg	=	1000 grams
gram	= g	=	1 gram
milligram	= mg	=	0.001 gram
microgram	= mcg	=	0.001 milligram

Volume

liter	= L	=	1 L
milliliter	= ml	=	0.001 L

AVOIRDUPOIS WEIGHT

1 ounce (oz)	= 437.5 grains
1 pound (lb)	= 16 ounces = 7000 grains

METRIC AND APOTHECARY EQUIVALENTS
Exact weight equivalents

Metric	*Apothecary*
1 mg	1/64.8 grain
64.8 mg	1 grain
324 mg	5 grains
1 g	15.432 grains
31.103 g	1 ounce = 480 grains

Exact volume equivalents

Metric	*Apothecary*		
1.00 ml	16.23 minims		
3.69 ml	1 fluidram	=	60 minims
29.57 ml	1 fluid ounce	=	480 minims
473.16 ml	1 pint	=	7680 minims
946.33 ml	1 quart	=	15,360 minims

Appendix q
High-alert Canadian medications

High-alert medications are medications that have a narrow margin of safety and when misused have the greatest potential to cause significant client harm. The Institute for Safe Medication Practices Canada (ISMP Canada) is a national nonprofit organization that independently reviews voluntary reports of medication errors and develops recommendations for safe medication practices throughout Canada to reduce the harm to clients. In 2003, the ISMP compiled a list of high-alert medications that includes medications in the 19 classes listed below, as well as the specific medications listed below. When these drugs appear in this book, each specific drug monograph is highlighted with a light color screen to help nurses identify them. While care should be taken in giving any medication, nurses are advised to exercise extra precautions when administering these high-risk drugs.

Class/Category of Medications
adrenergic agonists, IV (e.g., epINEPHrine)
adrenergic antagonists, IV (e.g., propranolol)
anesthetic agents, general, inhaled and IV (e.g., propofol)
cardioplegic solutions
chemotherapeutic agents, parenteral and oral
dextrose, hypertonic, 20% or greater
dialysis solutions, peritoneal and hemodialysis
epidural or intrathecal medications
glycoprotein IIb/IIIa inhibitors (e.g., eptifibatide)
hypoglycemics, oral
inotropic medications, IV (e.g., digoxin, milrinone)
liposomal forms of drugs (e.g., liposomal amphotericin B)
moderate sedation agents, IV (e.g., midazolam)
moderate sedation agents, oral, for children (e.g., chloral hydrate)
narcotics/opiates, IV and oral (including liquid concentrates, immediate- and
    sustained-release)
neuromuscular blocking agents (e.g., succinylcholine)
radiocontrast agents, IV
thrombolytics/fibrinolytics, IV (e.g., tenecteplase)
total parenteral nutrition solutions

Individual Medications
amiodarone, IV
colchicine injection
heparin, low molecular weight, injection
heparin, unfractionated, IV
insulin, subcutaneous and IV
lidocaine, IV

magnesium sulfate, injection
methotrexate, oral, nononcologic use
nesiritide
nitroprusside, sodium, for injection
potassium chloride, concentrate, for injection
potassium phosphates, injection
sodium chloride, hypertonic, more than 0.9% concentration, injection
warfarin

1. Cohen MR, Kilo CM: High-alert medications: safeguarding against errors. In Cohen MR, editor: *Medication errors,* Washington, DC, 1999, American Pharmaceutical Association.
2. High-alert medications and patient safety, *Sentinel Event Alert* 11, Nov 1999.
3. ISMP's list of high-alert medications, accessed 12/28/04 at http://www.ismp.org/MSAarticles/highalert.htm.
4. ISMP Canada accessed 12/28/04 at http://www.ismp-canada.org/index.htm.

Appendix r

Canadian controlled substance chart

Drugs	Canada
LSD, mescaline (peyote), harmaline, psilocin & psilocybin (magic mushrooms)	**Part J of the Food and Drug Regulation (FDR)** • Considered "restricted drugs" • High misuse potential • No recognized medical use • Marihuana exemption from FDR if produced for medical reasons
Sedatives such as barbiturates and derivatives (secobarbital), thiobarbiturates (pentothal sodium); anabolic steroids (androstanolone), weight reduction drugs (anorexiants)	**Part G of the FDR** • Controlled drugs • Misuse potential • Verbal and written prescriptions under certain conditions • Only prescribed if required for medical condition • Specified number of refills (conditions apply) • Records must be kept • May be administered under emergency situations (conditions apply)
Amphetamines; benzaphetamine; methamphetamine; phenmetrazine; phendimetrazine	**Part G of the FDR** • Designated controlled drug • May be used for designated medical conditions outlined in FDR
Benzodiazepine tranquilizers such as diazepam, lorazepam, flunitrazepam, zolpidem	**Benzodiazepines and Other Targeted Substances Regulations** • Misuse potential • Verbal and written prescriptions under certain conditions • Only prescribed if required for medical condition • Specified number of refills (conditions apply) • Records must be kept • May be administered under emergency situations (conditions apply)
Opiates: heroin, morphine, codeine >8 mg, amidones (methadone), coca and derivatives (cocaine), phencyclidine (PCP), benzazocines (analgesics such as pentazocine), fentanyls	**Narcotic Control Regulation** • High misuse potential • Written prescriptions for specific medical conditions* • Records of opiate prescription file must be kept • No refills (limited amounts in a prescription) • Heroin and methadone are subject to specific controls
Chloral hydrate, chlordiazepoxide	**Schedule F of the FDR** • Low misuse potential

*Verbal prescriptions are permitted for certain opioid preparations (such as Tylenol No. 2 and No. 3), but not for opiate alone, or opiates with 1 other active non-opioid ingredient.

Explanation of Controlled Drugs and Substances Chart for Canada

The *Canadian Controlled Drugs and Substances Act (CDSA)* is a "legislative framework for the control of substances that can alter mental processes and that may produce harm to the health of an individual and to society when diverted or misused" (*Canada Gazette*, 2003, paragraph 5) that is under the jurisdiction of Health Canada. A "controlled substance" means a substance included in Schedules I to VI. Schedules VII and VIII specify amounts of substances in Schedule II (e.g., cannabis and cannabis resin) associated of the FDR or the *Benzodiazepines and Other Targeted Substances Regulations* (Targeted Substances Regulations). Different levels of control measures are found within the various regulations that apply to licensed dealers, pharmacists, practitioners, and hospitals. Part J of the FDR regulates the use of controlled substances with no recognized medical use; substances listed in the schedule to Part J of the FDR are defined as "restricted drugs" and include such substances as LSD and mescaline. Controlled substances included in CDSA Schedules III and IV that have some therapeutic use are regulated under either Part G of the FDR or the Targeted Substances Regulations with the former having more stringent controls over distribution.

Canada Gazette. (2003). Order amending schedule III to the controlled drugs and substances act. Retrieved January 3, 2005 from http://canadagazette.gc.ca/partII/2003/20031231/html/sor412-e.html.

Department of Justice Canada. (2004). *Narcotic Control Regulations*. Retrieved January 6, 2005 from http://laws.justice.gc.ca/en/C-38.8/C.R.C.-c.1041/76122.html.

Department of Justice Canada. (2004). *Controlled Drugs and Substances Act*. Retrieved December 31, 2004 from http://laws.justice.gc.ca/en/C-38.8/.

Health Canada. (2004). *Food and Drugs Act*. Part G–Controlled Drugs. Part J–Restricted Drugs. Schedule F. Retrieved January 6, 2005 from http://www.hc-sc.gc.ca/food-aliment/friia-raaii/food_drugs-aliments_drogues/act-loi/e_index.html.

National Association of Pharmacy Regulatory Authorities (NAPRA). *Controlled Drugs and Substances Act and Regulations*. Retrieved January 6, 2005 from http://www.napra.org/docs/0/93/143.asp.

NAPRA. (2003). *Marihuana Exception (Food and Drugs Act) Regulations*. Retrieved January 6, 2005 from http://www.napra.ca/pdfs/fedleg/0307marihuana exemption.pdf.

NAPRA. *Benzodiazepines and Other Targeted Substances Regulations*. Retrieved January 6, 2005 from http://www.napra.ca/pdfs/fedleg/benzodiaz.pdf.

Appendix s
Canadian Recommended Immunization Schedules for Infants and Children

| VACCINE | MONTHS | | | | | | YEARS | | |
	2	4	6	12	18	4 TO 6	9 TO 13	14 TO 16
Hepatitis B*	3 doses	3 doses	3 doses	3 doses	3 doses	3 doses	3 doses	
Diphtheria, Pertussis, and Tetanus (DPT)	DPT	DPT	DPT		DPT	DPT		Td
								**
Haemophilus influenzae type b *** (Hib)	Hib	Hib	Hib		Hib			
Polio (inactivated polio vaccine/oral polio vaccine)	Polio	Polio	Polio		Polio	Polio		Polio
			****					****
Measles, Mumps, and Rubella ***** (MMR)				MMR	MMR	MMr		
					*****	*****		

* Adolescents who have not received hepatitis B vaccine in infancy should receive it through school programs according to the provincial and territorial policies.

** Td (tetanus and diphtheria toxoids, adult formulation).

*** Recommended schedule for both Hib-TITER® and ActHIB®.

**** If oral polio vaccine is used exclusively, boosters at 6 months and 14 to 16 years of age may be omitted.

***** The second dose of MMR is routinely recommended at either 18 months or at 4 to 6 years of age. It should be given any time before school entry provided that there is at least a 1-month interval between receipt of the first and second doses.

🍁 Canada only

Side effects: *italics* = common; ***bold italics*** = life-threatening

Index

Entries can be identified as follows: *Combination Products,* DISEASES/DISORDERS,
DRUG CATEGORIES, generic names, Trade Names.

Entries can be identified as follows: *Combination Products,* DISEASES/DISORDERS,
DRUG CATEGORIES, generic names, Trade Names.

Entries can be identified as follows: *Combination Products,* DISEASES/DISORDERS,
DRUG CATEGORIES, generic names, Trade Names.

Entries can be identified as follows: *Combination Products*, DISEASES/DISORDERS, *DRUG CATEGORIES*, generic names, Trade Names.

Entries can be identified as follows: *Combination Products*, DISEASES/DISORDERS, *DRUG CATEGORIES*, generic names, Trade Names.

Entries can be identified as follows: *Combination Products*, DISEASES/DISORDERS, *DRUG CATEGORIES*, generic names, Trade Names.

Entries can be identified as follows: *Combination Products,* DISEASES/DISORDERS, *DRUG CATEGORIES,* generic names, Trade Names.

Entries can be identified as follows: *Combination Products*, DISEASES/DISORDERS, *DRUG CATEGORIES*, generic names, Trade Names.

Entries can be identified as follows: *Combination Products*, DISEASES/DISORDERS, *DRUG CATEGORIES*, generic names, Trade Names.

Entries can be identified as follows: *Combination Products,* DISEASES/DISORDERS,
DRUG CATEGORIES, generic names, Trade Names.

Entries can be identified as follows: *Combination Products,* DISEASES/DISORDERS, *DRUG CATEGORIES,* generic names, Trade Names.

Entries can be identified as follows: *Combination Products,* DISEASES/DISORDERS,
DRUG CATEGORIES, generic names, Trade Names.

Entries can be identified as follows: *Combination Products,* DISEASES/DISORDERS,
DRUG CATEGORIES, generic names, Trade Names.

Entries can be identified as follows: *Combination Products*, DISEASES/DISORDERS, *DRUG CATEGORIES*, generic names, Trade Names.

Entries can be identified as follows: *Combination Products,* DISEASES/DISORDERS,
DRUG CATEGORIES, generic names, Trade Names.

Entries can be identified as follows: *Combination Products*, DISEASES/DISORDERS, *DRUG CATEGORIES*, generic names, Trade Names.

Entries can be identified as follows: *Combination Products,* DISEASES/DISORDERS,
DRUG CATEGORIES, generic names, Trade Names.

Entries can be identified as follows: *Combination Products,* DISEASES/DISORDERS, *DRUG CATEGORIES,* generic names, Trade Names.

Entries can be identified as follows: *Combination Products,* DISEASES/DISORDERS, *DRUG CATEGORIES,* generic names, Trade Names.

Entries can be identified as follows: *Combination Products,* DISEASES/DISORDERS, *DRUG CATEGORIES,* generic names, Trade Names.

Entries can be identified as follows: *Combination Products,* DISEASES/DISORDERS,
DRUG CATEGORIES, generic names, Trade Names.

Entries can be identified as follows: *Combination Products,* DISEASES/DISORDERS,
DRUG CATEGORIES, generic names, Trade Names.

Entries can be identified as follows: *Combination Products*, DISEASES/DISORDERS,
DRUG CATEGORIES, generic names, Trade Names.

Entries can be identified as follows: *Combination Products*, DISEASES/DISORDERS, *DRUG CATEGORIES*, generic names, Trade Names.

Entries can be identified as follows: *Combination Products,* DISEASES/DISORDERS, *DRUG CATEGORIES,* generic names, Trade Names.

Entries can be identified as follows: *Combination Products,* DISEASES/DISORDERS,
DRUG CATEGORIES, generic names, Trade Names.

Entries can be identified as follows: *Combination Products,* DISEASES/DISORDERS, *DRUG CATEGORIES,* generic names, Trade Names.

Entries can be identified as follows: *Combination Products*, DISEASES/DISORDERS,
DRUG CATEGORIES, generic names, Trade Names.

Entries can be identified as follows: *Combination Products,* DISEASES/DISORDERS, *DRUG CATEGORIES,* generic names, Trade Names.

Entries can be identified as follows: *Combination Products*, DISEASES/DISORDERS, *DRUG CATEGORIES*, generic names, Trade Names.

Entries can be identified as follows: *Combination Products,* DISEASES/DISORDERS,
DRUG CATEGORIES, generic names, Trade Names.

Entries can be identified as follows: *Combination Products*, DISEASES/DISORDERS, *DRUG CATEGORIES*, generic names, Trade Names.

Entries can be identified as follows: *Combination Products*, DISEASES/DISORDERS,
DRUG CATEGORIES, generic names, Trade Names.

Entries can be identified as follows: *Combination Products,* DISEASES/DISORDERS, *DRUG CATEGORIES,* generic names, Trade Names.

Entries can be identified as follows: *Combination Products,* DISEASES/DISORDERS,
DRUG CATEGORIES, generic names, Trade Names.

Entries can be identified as follows: *Combination Products,* DISEASES/DISORDERS, *DRUG CATEGORIES,* generic names, Trade Names.

Entries can be identified as follows: *Combination Products,* DISEASES/DISORDERS, *DRUG CATEGORIES,* generic names, Trade Names.

Mosby's 2007 Nursing Drug Reference Companion CD-ROM

Use *Mosby's 2007 Nursing Drug Reference Companion CD-ROM* to find drug information fast! This five-in-one CD-ROM provides you with the top 28 prescribed drugs in the United States, a drug interactions tool, patient teaching guides, herbal monographs, and calculators.

This Companion CD-ROM includes:

- **Top 28 Drugs**
  Complete, printable information on the 28 most commonly prescribed drugs in the United States.

- **Drug Interactions Tool**
  Use this powerful drug interactions tool for instant access to drug-drug, drug-diet, and drug-lab test interactions.

- **Patient Teaching Guides**
  Select up-to-date English and Spanish patient teaching handouts for hundreds of the most commonly used drugs.

- Over 25 **Clinical Calculators** and the most commonly used **Herbs and Natural Supplements**.

Contact Us
For further information, visit us at http://www.us.elsevierhealth.com or call us at (800) 545-2522.

Mini CD-ROM
This mini CD-ROM will work in your CD-ROM drive. Place it on the inner ring of the tray, as shown, and follow the on-screen installation instructions.

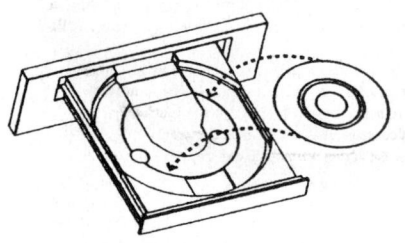

This mini-CD does not work in:
  Floppy Drives
  Slot Drives
  Zip Drives
  Stereos
Insert this mini-CD into your CD-ROM drive as shown at left.

Important
No credit or refund will be issued on this book if the CD envelope has been opened, torn, or otherwise tampered with.

Companion CD-ROM to accompany *Mosby's 2007 Nursing Drug Reference*

MINIMUM SYSTEM REQUIREMENTS

Windows®
98SE, 2000, NT, ME, or XP operating system
200 MHz Intel Pentium® II processor or faster
64 MB or more of installed RAM
30 MB free hard disk space
2× or faster CD-ROM drive
800 × 600 monitor or larger
256 Colors

Software Requirement
Adobe Acrobat Reader®
This product was designed to work with Internet Explorer 5.5 or higher; or Netscape 6.1 or higher. Other browsers may work; however, if problems occur, your first step should be to make sure the product is running Internet Explorer 6.0.

INSTALLATION INSTRUCTIONS

If the autorun feature is on, the program will automatically start after the CD is inserted into the CD-ROM drive. If the program does not launch automatically, follow these steps.
1. Start Microsoft Windows® and insert the CD-ROM.
2. Click the *Start* button from the Taskbar and select the *Run* option.
3. Type d:\sctup.cxc (where "d:\" is your CD-ROM drive) and press *Enter*.
4. Follow the on-screen instructions for installation.

TECHNICAL SUPPORT

Technical support for this product is available between 7:30 AM and 7 PM CST, Monday through Friday. Before calling, make sure that your computer meets the minimum system requirements to run this software. Inside the United States, call (800) 692-9010. Outside the United States, call (314) 872-8370. You may also fax your questions to (314) 523-4932.

You may also contact Technical Support via e-mail at:
technical.support@elsevier.com

For access to a list of *Frequently Asked Questions (FAQ),* as well as troubleshooting tips, please visit our website at **http://www.us.elsevierhealth.com/TechSupport**

Produced in the United States of America.

Part number: 9996025705

Pentium, Windows, and Adobe Acrobat Reader are registered trademarks.

Formulas for drug calculations

Surface area rule:

$$\text{Child dose} = \frac{\text{Surface area (m}^2)}{1.73 \text{ m}^2} \times \text{Adult dose}$$

Calculating strength of a solution:

$$\textit{Solution Strength:} \quad \textit{Desired Solution:}$$
$$\frac{x}{100} = \frac{\text{Amount of drug desired}}{\text{Amount of finished solution}}$$

Calculating flow rate for IV:

$$\text{Rate of flow} = \frac{\text{Amount of fluid} \times \text{Administration set calibration}}{\text{Running time}}$$

$$\frac{x}{1} = \frac{\text{(ml) (gtt/min)}}{\text{min}}$$

Calculation of medication dosages:

Formula method:

$$\frac{\text{Amount ordered}}{\text{Amount on hand}} \times \text{Vehicle} = \text{Number of tablets, capsules, or amount of liquid}$$

Vehicle is the drug form or amount of liquid containing the dosage. Amounts used in calculation by formula must be in same system.

Ratio—proportion method:

1 tablet:tablet in mg on hand: :x tablet order in mg

Know or have: :Want to know or order

Multiply means and extremes, divide both sides by known amount to get x. Amounts used in equation must be in same system.

Dimensional analysis method:

$$\text{Order in mg} \times \frac{1 \text{ tablet or capsule}}{\text{What 1 tablet or capsule is in mg}}$$

$$= \text{Tablets or capsules to be given}$$

If amounts are in different systems:

$$\text{Order in mg} \times \frac{1 \text{ tablet or capsule}}{\text{What 1 tablet or capsule is in g}} \times \frac{1}{1000 \text{ mg}}$$

$$= \text{Tablets or capsules to be given}$$

Nomogram for calculation of body surface area

Place a straight edge from the patient's height in the left column to the patient's weight in the right column. The point of intersection on the body surface area column indicates the body surface area (BSA). (Reproduced in Behrman RE, Kliegman RM, Jenson HB: *Nelson textbook of pediatrics*, ed 17, Philadelphia, 2004, WB Saunders; Nomogram modified from data of E. Boyd by CD West.)

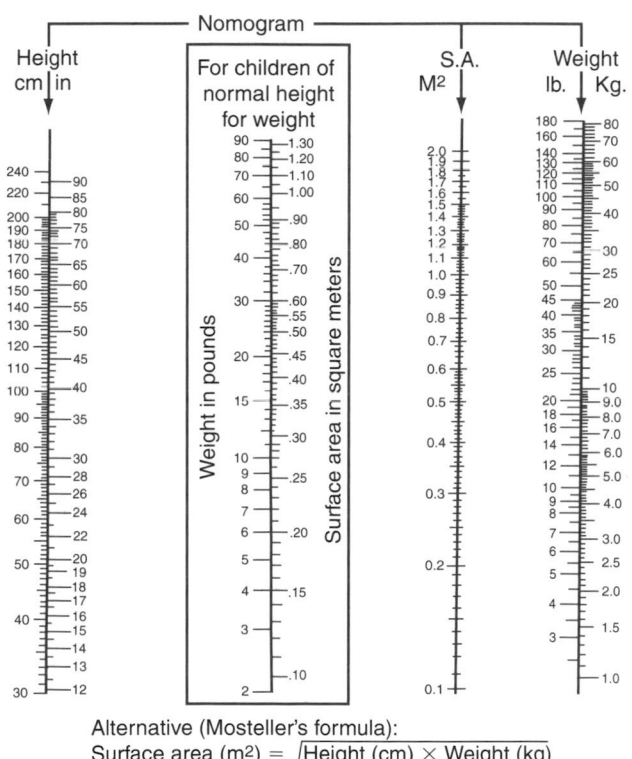

Alternative (Mosteller's formula):

$$\text{Surface area (m}^2) = \sqrt{\frac{\text{Height (cm)} \times \text{Weight (kg)}}{3600}}$$

alprazolam (℞)

(al-pray'zoe-lam)
Apo-Alpraz ✦, Novo-Alprazol ✦,
Nu-Alpraz ✦, Xanax, Xanax XR
Func. class.: Antianxiety
Chem. class.: Benzodiazepine

Controlled Substance Schedule IV
Do not confuse:
alprazolam/lorazepam

> **Controlled substances clearly identified**

...ortical levels of
CNS, including limbic system, reticular
formation

Uses: Anxiety, panic disorders, anxiety
with depressive symptoms

Investigational uses: Depression,
social phobia, premenstrual dysphoric
disorders

DOSAGE AND ROUTES

Anxiety disorder
• *Adult:* **PO** 0.25-0.5 mg tid, not to
exceed 4 mg/day in divided doses
• *Geriatric:* **PO** 0.125-0.25 mg bid;
increase by 0.125 as needed

Panic disorder

> **Geriatric, pediatric and other special doses included throughout**

...tid may increase,
...el tabs (Xanax XR)
...mg initially, mainte-

...phoric disorders
...ng bid-qid, starting on
day 16-18 of menses, taper over 2-3 days
when menses occurs

Social phobia
• *Adult:* **PO** 2-8 mg/day

Hepatic dose
• Reduce dose by 50%

Available forms: Tabs 0.25, 0.5, 1, 2
mg; oral sol 1 mg/ml; tabs, ext rel (Xanax
XR) 0.5, 1, 2, 3 mg

SIDE EFFECTS

CNS: Dizziness, drowsiness, confusion,
headache, anxiety, tremors, stimulation,
fatigue, depression, insomnia, hallucinations

*CV: Orthostatic hypotension, **ECG
changes, tachycardia,*** hypotension

EENT: Blurred vision, tinnitus, mydriasis

GI: Constipation, dry mouth, nausea,
vomiting, anorexia, diarrhea

INTEG: Rash, dermatitis, itching

Contraindications: Pregnancy (D),
hypersensitivity to benzodiazepines,
narrow-angle glaucoma, psychosis, addiction, addiction

Precautions: Elderly, debilitated, hepatic disease

> **Pregnancy considerations appear under contraindications (D or X) or precautions (A, B, or C)**

PHARMACOKINETICS

PO: Onset 30 min, peak 1-2 hr, duration 4-6 hr, therapeutic response 2-3
days; metabolized by liver, excreted by
kidneys; crosses placenta, breast milk,
half-life 12-15 hr

> **Pharmacokinetic information presented in a new boxed format**

INTERACTIONS

A substrate of CYP3A4
Increase: alprazolam action—
cimetidine, disulfiram, erythromycin,
fluoxetine, isoniazid, ketoconazole,
metoprolol, propoxyphene, oral contraceptives,
valproic acid

Increase: CNS depression—
anticonvulsants, alcohol, antihistamines,
sedative/hypnotics

Decrease: sedation—xanthines

Decrease: alprazolam action—
barbiturates, rifampin

Decrease: action of levodopa

Drug/Herb
Increase: CNS depression: cat's claw,
chamomile, cowslip, echinacea, goldenseal, hops, kava, licorice, Queen Anne's
lace, skullcap, St. John's wort, valerian,
wild cherry

Drug/Food
Increase: drug level; grapefruit juice

Drug/Lab Test
Increase: AST/ALT, alk phosphatase

> **Interactions are written out and reorganized**